Clinics in Developmental Medicine Nos 173/174
ORTHOPAEDIC MANAGEMENT IN
CEREBRAL PALSY, 2ND EDITION

© 2007 Mac Keith Press
30 Furnival Street, London EC4A 1JQ

Editor: Hilary M. Hart
Managing Editor: Michael Pountney
Project Manager: Edward Fenton

First published in this edition 2007

British Library Cataloguing-in-Publication data
A catalogue record for this book is available from the British Library

ISBN: 9781898683520

Typeset by Keystroke, 28 High Street, Tettenhall, Wolverhampton
Printed by The Lavenham Press Ltd, Water Street, Lavenham, Suffolk
Mac Keith Press is supported by Scope

Clinics in Developmental Medicine Nos 173/174

Orthopaedic Management in Cerebral Palsy, 2nd edn

HELEN M. HORSTMANN AND EUGENE E. BLECK

2007
Mac Keith Press
Distributed by Blackwell Publishing

A.M.D.G.

To our loving and patient spouses, Anne and John

To the Bleck offspring: John, Mary, Daniel, Patrick and Jayne

To the Horstmann daughters: Helen, Caroline, Anne, Mary, Sara and Jane

and

To the children and adults with cerebral palsy and their valiant families
whom we have had the privilege of serving

AUTHORS' APPOINTMENTS

Helen Meeks Horstmann, M.D.
Hospital of the University of Pennsylvania

Children's Hospital of Philadelphia
Philadelphia, Pennsylvania

Eugene E. Bleck, M.D.
Stanford University
Palo Alto, California

CONTENTS

PREFACE TO THE FIRST MAC KEITH PRESS EDITION

When the first edition of this book* went out of print, many of my orthopaedic colleagues around the world asked me if there would be a new edition. The result is this new monograph on the same subject. Many colleagues told me that they liked the first edition because it was concise and well illustrated. In this new volume I have again tried to be as concise as possible without omitting important details, particularly in surgical procedures. I have drawn attention to the pitfalls of surgery, in the hope that the unintended results of instant and dramatic change in form and function due to the intervention will not be disappointing too often.

This is not a comprehensive work on all aspects of cerebral palsy. The associated defects and developmental problems (e.g. convulsive disorders, communication and education) are touched on, to give orthopaedic surgeons a perspective on the complexity of the condition and enable them to be conversant about it with their colleagues in pediatrics, general practice, neurology, and physical medicine and rehabilitation. In case more information on a particular defect in function is wanted, I have included a list of suggestions for further reading.

When indicated, I have added new sections and new information. In descriptions of operative procedures I have attempted to reference new procedures reported in the literature. The procedures I recommend have been tested with my own experience, although I am sure that other surgeons have their own preferences.

The format remains essentially the same, because of my opinion that the patient should be treated comprehensively rather than as isolated anatomical parts. Accordingly, the major sections are on spastic hemiplegia, spastic diplegia and total body involvement, with the operative procedures most commonly needed to correct the structural deformity in each of these three categories of geographical involvement. However, procedures described in one section will apply in another section when a particular deformity occurs. For example, the management of spastic equinus is in the chapter on hemiplegia, but would equally apply to equinus in diplegia.

The surgical treatment of paralytic scoliosis has changed so dramatically in the past six years that an entire chapter is devoted to it. I have updated the chapter dealing with neurobiology and its importance in the use of physical therapy. A separate chapter is devoted to physical therapy because physicians are usually asked to approve of a particular therapy program, or to certify it (in the United States a prescription is required). Consequently, a critique of current methods seems important if the physician's advice or authority to approve is requested. It would be most unwise for the physician to take responsibility for recommending the management of a child with cerebral palsy, and be detached from the physical and occupational therapists and their methods.

Some chapters such as those on the family and counseling might seem to have more to do with philosophy than science. So be it. No apology needs to be made for an apparent lack of science. Medicine, after all, fulfils a social need: it is an applied science and an art. To rise above the mere technocrat, the physician needs a philosophical base from which to work in this difficult, often frustrating, and sometimes depressing field.

I would like to acknowledge here the painstaking task of translating the entire first edition of my book into Chinese by Dr Cheng Chao-peng, Fourth Municipal Hospital, Zhengzhou, Henan, People's Republic of China. Despite my fairly intense efforts to find a publisher, I have failed to find any (including international agencies) to undertake the publication in Chinese. Perhaps with the growing awareness of China's importance in the world, this might be accomplished eventually.

Dr Sue Jenkins, Dr Martin Bax and Mr Edward Fenton of the Mac Keith Press deserve my thanks for all of their careful editing and many useful suggestions.

As in the first edition, I must thank the people of France: specifically Mme John Pila of Lyon who allowed us to use her villa in the 'presqu'Île Giens', Dr and Mrs Eric Bérard and their children who were our constant source of guidance in the ways of French living, and the people of the village of Giens-Hyères, for allowing us to live so well while writing. To them I say: 'Je vous prie de croire dans mes sentiments très amicaux.'

Eugene E. Bleck, 1987

*Published by W.B. Saunders Company, 1979.

PREFACE TO THE NEW EDITION

Twenty years have elapsed since the publication of the first Mac Keith edition of this book. The senior author finally succumbed to the invitation for a revision. The consent of Dr Helen Meeks Horstmann, pediatric orthopaedic surgeon of Philadelphia, to be coauthor was most gratifying. She lends her contemporary experience that give the revision a reality of present practice rather than too much of the past by the senior author.

While the clinical characteristics of cerebral palsy have remained unchanged since the previous edition, newer approaches to relieving spasticity of the muscles have evolved rapidly. A review of selective posterior rootlet rhizotomy, botulinum toxin intramuscular injections, and intrathecal baclofen are included in the text. Although these new modalities are not strictly in the context of orthopaedic management, they can impact on management. The contemporary orthopaedic surgeon should have a reasonably detailed knowledge of the indications, the results and the limitations of these methods. It is apparent that orthopaedic surgery for cerebral palsy still lives. Current orthopaedic surgery is a distillation of a half-century of clinical practice. In the process it has been streamlined; older surgical procedures have been either abandoned or modified. Gait analysis laboratories are now commonplace. They allow more objective analysis of preoperative gait abnormalities and efficacy of surgical treatment. Gait analysis is confined to those who walk—primarily spastic hemiplegia and diplegia.

As a result of more critical analyses of the results of physical therapy methods such as the Gross Motor Function Measure, many 'systems' of physical therapy have been modified or abandoned. In their place muscle strengthening and attainment of functional goals have been emphasized. The impetus for restoration of muscle strength has been dramatic reduction of the spasticity after selective posterior root rhizotomy and the concomitant weakness of muscles. The postoperative weakness created the need for muscle strengthening with active exercise and functional activities particularly in spastic diplegia.

The success of intrathecal baclofen in reducing the severe spasticity of muscles in the patient with total body involvement is replacing attempts to reduce muscle tone and abnormal reflexes through physical therapy alone. Instead the focus has shifted to assistive technology to compensate for mobility and communication deficits.

We have included a chapter with basics and highlights of neurobiology as they apply to neural development, prognosis and management with neuropharmacologic agents. We hope that detailing some of the reality of the biology and chemistry of the central nervous system will allow the clinician and his or her patients to avoid untested and unproven treatments.

We thank all the authors of papers and books who have provide much of the new knowledge in the clinical and basic science areas pertaining to cerebral palsy. Particularly we thank our colleagues and friends who have inspired and encouraged us along the way, especially Drs James Gage, Jacqueline Perry, Leon Root, Martin Bax, Dean MacEwen and David Sutherland. We thank the many authors who gave us permission to reproduce or redraw their illustrations to illuminate the subject. Thank you to Michael Pountney, managing editor at Mac Keith Press and Dr Hilary Hart, book editor at Mac Keith. Finally, we are grateful for the editorial expertise and patience of our senior Mac Keith Press editor, Ed Fenton. Thank you especially to our spouses, Anne Bleck and John Horstmann, for their support and encouragement for this book and our demanding careers.

EUGENE E. BLECK, M.D.

1

CLASSIFICATION, EPIDEMIOLOGY AND ETIOLOGY

HISTORY

It was a London physician, William John Little (1810–94), who published the first clinical report of cerebral palsy in 1843 (Fig. 1.1). Twenty years later he read an influential paper to the Obstetrical Society of London entitled 'On the influence of abnormal parturition, difficult labors, premature birth, and asphyxia neonatorum on the mental and physical condition of the child, especially in relation to deformities' (Little 1862). Little's description of the syndrome was so complete and accurate that by the end of the 19th century the syndrome was widely known as Little's Disease (Wilkins and Brody 1969, Accardo 1982, Schifrin and Longo 2000). Little had an equinovarus deformity of his left foot due to the paralysis of poliomyelitis contracted at age 4 years. After medical school he sought treatment for his foot deformity and found Frederick Louis Stroymeyer in Hanover, Germany. In 1836 Stroymeyer did a successful correction of Little's left foot equinus with a simple stab-wound subcutaneous tenotomy of the Achilles tendon. When Little returned to London he performed the first subcutaneous tenotomy of the Achilles to correct a talipes equinovarus (club foot) in London on August 10, 1837—the same year that Victoria became Queen. After licensure by the Royal College of Physicians, he began his practice of orthopaedic surgery. In 1840 he raised sufficient funds to open the Orthopaedic Infirmary in London's Bloomsbury Square. The demand for his services was so great that he moved to a large mansion in Hanover Square that subsequently became the Royal Orthopaedic Hospital in 1845 (Jones 1949).

Sir William Osler (1849–1919) coined the durable term 'cerebral palsy' in his clinical study of children at the Infirmary for Nervous Diseases in Philadelphia, Pennsylvania, in his 1889 book *The Cerebral Palsies of Children* (Osler 1987).

In Vienna, Sigmund Freud (1856–1939) expanded the clinical description of cerebral palsy, leaving no doubt that the condition was not a single disease but a collection of motor disorders related to lesions of the brain originating during infancy or at birth (Freud 1968). Freud's description of spastic diplegia

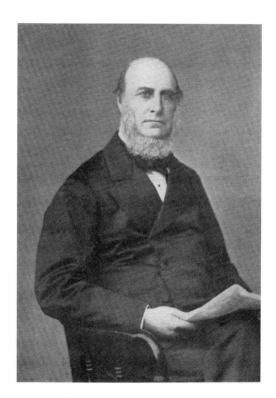

Fig. 1.1. William John Little.

is so complete that it remains as relevant in 2005 as it was at the end of the 19th century. Freud could not find any neuropathological lesions that correlated with the clinical findings. As Freud became more interested in neuroses, he abandoned cerebral palsy. In letters to William Fliess on the origins of psychoanalysis (1887–1902) he wrote: 'I am fully occupied with children's paralysis, in which I am not the least interested' (quoted in Accardo 1982). He went on to create a new medical discipline: psychiatry.

Of particular relevance to this text is Winthrop M. Phelps (1894–1971), an orthopaedic surgeon. His paper 'Cerebral birth injuries: their orthopaedic classification and subsequent treatment' is considered to be the first major classic on the subject after Little's publication in 1862 (Bick 1976, Phelps 1990)[1]. Phelps proposed that children with cerebral palsy should be helped to achieve their full potential as individuals. Toward this end he established the Children's Rehabilitation Institute in Baltimore, Maryland, where he emphasized a holistic approach rather than focusing on only the mechanical or neurological aspects of cerebral palsy (Slominski 1984).[2] Phelps was the first president of the American Academy for Cerebral Palsy founded in 1947.

DEFINITIONS

CEREBRAL PALSY

Despite attempts to label the syndrome differently (e.g. static encephalopathy, permanent brain damage, or the French 'infirme moteur cérébrale'), the term 'cerebral palsy' has been adopted and understood worldwide (Stanley and Alberman 1984, Stanley et al. 2000).

Perhaps the most relevant description is Ingram's (Haslam et al. 1955): 'Cerebral palsy is used as an inclusive term to describe a group of non-progressive disorders occurring in young children in which disease of the brain causes impairment of motor function. The impairment of motor function may be the result of paresis, involuntary movement or incoordination, but motor disorders which are transient or are the result of progressive disease of the brain or attributable to abnormalities of the spinal cord are excluded.'

Other clinicians have offered more succinct definitions. According to Rang (1990), 'Cerebral palsy is the result of an insult to the developing brain that produces a disorder of movement and posture that is permanent but not unchanging.' Bax (2001) defined it as a disorder of movement and posture resulting from a condition of non-progressive brain damage that occurred in infancy or childhood. Although the brain lesion is static, the musculoskeletal manifestations change over time, and secondary complications arise as the child ages (Fennell and Dikel 2001).

The consensus is that cerebral palsy is not a single disease entity but a group of conditions in which different factors acting at different times in fetal development produce varying degrees of damage to the developing brain (Pharoah et al. 1996).

The scope implied by the term 'cerebral palsy' assumes importance in epidemiological studies. At an international meeting in Brioni, Yugoslavia, in 1990, epidemiologists agreed that cerebral palsy was 'an umbrella term covering a group of non-progressive, but often changing, motor impairment syndromes secondary to lesions or anomalies of the brain arising in the early stages of its development' (Mutch et al. 1992). Despite years of debate and discussion, the name 'cerebral palsy' remains firmly entrenched in the lexicon of clinical terms.

---

1 Read before the section of Orthopaedic Surgery, New York Academy of Sciences, January 15, 1932.
2 'The treatments should constitute a regular part of the daily routine and the average length of time is an hour a day. The rest of the day the condition should be forgotten. Patients become "stale" as in too prolonged or constant training for any reason.' (Bick 1976, Phelps 1990.)

To further address issues raised by improved understanding of brain disorders with refined technological advances, a panel of internationally recognized experts on 'cerebral palsy' convened in 2004 to generate a report on the definition and classification of cerebral palsy (Rosenbaum et al. 2006). Their final wording of the definition of cerebral palsy came up as follows:

> 'Cerebral palsy (CP) describes a group of permanent disorders of the development of movement and posture, causing activity limitation, that are attributed to non-progressive disturbances that occurred in the developing fetal or infant brain. The motor disorders of cerebral palsy are often accompanied by disturbances of sensation, perception, cognition, communication, and behavior, by epilepsy, and by secondary musculoskeletal problems.'

TONE

We read and hear this term often; physical therapists in particular seem to have fondness for 'tone'. They speak of 'hypertonicity', and 'tone'-inhibiting plasters, rather than using expressions which emphasise terms such as 'spasticity' or 'spastic paralysis'. Muscle tone has two characteristics: (1) slight resting tension, and (2) involuntary resistance to mechanical stretch (Gamble 1988). The tension and resistance to stretch are due to viscoelastic properties and nerve impulses (McMahon 1984). 'Tone' can be thought of as the set point from which the muscle can contract to enable us to move against gravity: to enable us to shift between reciprocal inhibition and co-contraction (Helsel et al. 2001). The brain and spinal cord ultimately control the level of tension we call 'muscle tone'. This control is exerted through the stretch reflex in which stretching the intrafusal muscle fiber in the muscle spindle activates the 1a afferent neuron that synapses with the α motor neuron in the spinal cord. The resultant efferent action potentials cause the extrafusal muscle to contract that relaxes the stretch on the spindle (Truex and Carpenter 1969). Hypotonia, extremely low tone, can be noted transiently with some frequency in cerebral palsy but may also persist. It is usually accompanied by motor weakness. It can also be noted underlying hypertonia. Quantitating tone is subjective at best (Fig. 1.2).

REFLEXES

A reflex is a simple motor action, stereotyped and repeatable; it is elicited by a sensory stimulus, the strength of the motor action being graded with the intensity of the stimulus. Konrad Lorenz, who studied animal behavior in the field in 1950, suggested that many of the individual motor actions and motor responses of

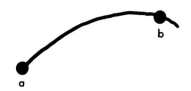

Fig. 1.2. Graphic representation of hypotonia (or flaccid paralysis). Motor control permits going from points *a* to *b*, but weakness causes the limb to 'fall off' the terminal point. (Redrawn from Gesell and Amatruda 1947.)

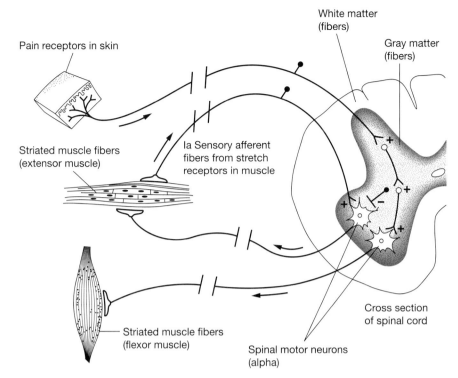

Pain receptors in skin

White matter
(fibers)

Gray matter
(fibers)

Striated muscle fibers
(extensor muscle)

Ia Sensory afferent
fibers from stretch
receptors in muscle

Cross section
of spinal cord

Striated muscle fibers
(flexor muscle)

Spinal motor neurons
(alpha)

Fig. 1.3. Muscle reaction to sensory information. Stretch of extensor muscle causes activation of 1a fibers in the spindle organ of the extensor muscle, which then activates the alpha spinal motor neurons causing muscle contraction (stretch reflex). Pinching the skin over the extensor muscle, however, excites motor neurons to the flexor muscles, creating a flexion reflex, which the extensor motor neurons are inhibited through inhibitory interneurons. (Redrawn from Thompson *et al.* 2000, by permission.)

animals could be described as fixed action patterns: 'instinctual, stereotyped and characteristic of a given species' (Shepherd 1994). The characteristics of these are a complex motor act, involving a specific temporal sequence of component acts; it is generated internally, or elicited by a sensory stimulus. The stimulus acts as trigger, and should cause release of the motor act (Shepherd 1994). A *myostatic reflex* occurs when the muscle that was stretched contracts and the reflex feeds back to the stretched muscle via the neural circuit through the spinal cord. It is also called a stretch reflex because it is elicited by stretch (Fig. 1.3) (Thompson *et al.* 1993, Shepherd 1994).

SPASTICITY

Spasticity is usually described as a condition of increased sensitivity of the muscle to stretch, resulting in contraction from the recruitment of all the fibers within the muscle. The continuous contraction of a spastic muscle when it responds to passive or active stretch (e.g. during walking) can be called a myostatic reflex, i.e. contraction of the muscle feeds back to cause more contraction. Spasticity can be defined as velocity-dependent resistance to movement associated with exaggerated deep-tendon reflexes (Young 1994) (Fig. 1.4).

DYSKINESIA

Dyskinesia connotes involuntary movements of the limbs that may be of several different types: dystonia, athetosis, chorea, ballismus or tremor. *Dystonia* is posturing of the limb, neck or spine due to abnormal continuous muscle tone. The posture disappears when the patient is relaxed or sleeping and does not result in muscle shortening, i.e. contracture (Fig. 1.5). *Athetosis*

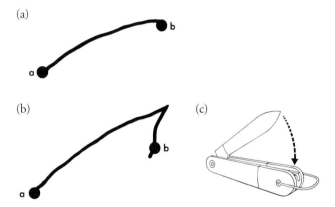

Fig. 1.4. (*a*) Graphic representation of normal motor control from points *a* to *b*. (*b*) Graphic representation of spastic motor control: the patient reaches the mark but then overshoots it. (*c*) Symbolic representation of a spastic muscle which on stretch responds like a clasp knife. (Redrawn from Gesell and Amatruda 1947.)

is continuous writhing movements of the limbs, head and neck (Fig. 1.6). Subsumed under athetosis is *ballismus* characterized by violent jerking movements of primarily the proximal joints and *chorea* characterized by random disorganized muscle contractions primarily of the distal joints[3] (Fig. 1.7), while a tremor results in an almost vibratory type of involuntary movement, usually of the hands (Fig. 1.8). Rigidity has persistent elevated tone throughout a motion rather than extraneous movement. The persistent tone can be felt while passively extending a limb with continuous resistance similar to the feeling of bending a lead pipe (Fig. 1.9*a*)

---

3 Chorea: the abnormal movement characteristics should be easy to remember from its Latin and Greek roots (*chorea*, dance; χορεια, choral dance).

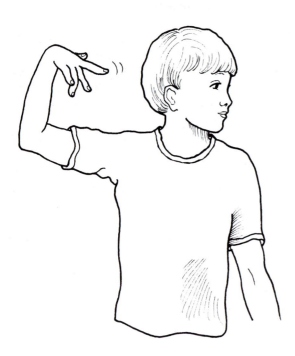

Fig. 1.5. Typical dystonic posture of upper limb in hemidystonia.

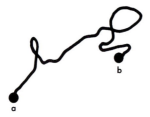

Fig. 1.6. Graphic representation of motor control in athetosis: getting to the mark with convoluted motions. (Redrawn from Gesell and Amatruda 1947.)

or with periodic and patterned resistance as movement in a cogwheel (see Fig. 1.9b). Another common expression of rigidity is in Parkinsonism where there is degeneration of the substantia nigra in the midbrain. Patients who have dyskinesias sometimes develop structural changes such as scoliosis and degenerative arthritis of the spine or hips. Their orthopaedic problems can be

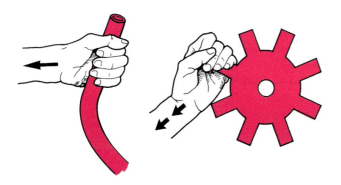

Fig. 1.9. Rigidity. *Left*: lead-pipe type. *Right*: cogwheel type.

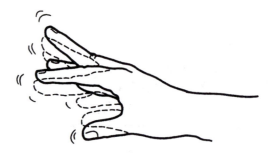

Fig. 1.7. Chorea: involuntary movement of the digits.

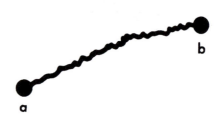

Fig. 1.8. Graphic representation of tremor. (Redrawn from Gesell and Amatruda 1947.)

surgically treated as in patients who have no paralysis. Muscle contractures are uncommon.

Dystonia is frequently confused with spasticity. Dystonic postures are not amenable to orthopaedic surgery. *Tension athetosis* described by Phelps does seem different from spasticity. These patients are usually total body involved, and overzealous release of presumed spastic muscles can result in the opposite deformity, e.g. total hip-flexor 'release' can become a postoperative extension contracture of the hip. To differentiate spasticity from tension athetosis, as defined by Phelps, rapid flexion and extension of the involved limb joints results in the relaxation of the muscles, whereas in spasticity increased muscle spasticity is observed (Fig. 1.10).

When examined using electromyography, muscle in athetosis (in contrast to spasticity) demonstrates tonic patterns of electrical activity on both voluntary and involuntary movements. Hallett (1983) found excessive firing of muscle action potentials in both agonist and antagonist muscle groups. Classification based upon electromyographic analysis has been tried, but it has not succeeded in defining what we can observe by clinical examination.

Ataxia involves uncoordinated voluntary movements due to disordered cerebellar function and results in gait disturbances and uncoordinated volitional muscle use. Simple and predominant ataxia in cerebral palsy is less common than ataxia layered on a more predominant motor dysfunction such as spasticity. An ataxic gait is uncoordinated and wide-based (Fig. 1.11). Falls are frequent due to difficulty with standing balance. Control of the upper extremities is marked by dysmetria where spatial relationships are misjudged, and/or by intention tremor. With dysmetria, past-pointing or overreaching are hallmarks.

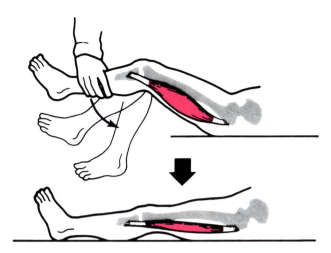

Fig. 1.10. In contrast to spasticity, in tension athetosis the resistance and response of the muscle to repetitive and fast stretch relaxes ('flails').

(a)

(b)

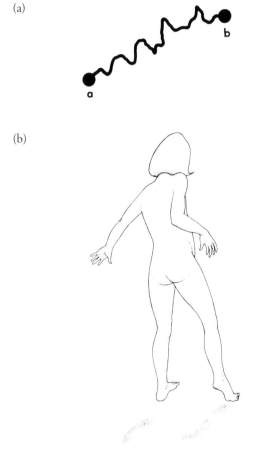

Fig. 1.11. (*a*) Graphic representation of ataxic motor performance (redrawn from Gesell and Amatruda 1947). (*b*) Typical ataxic wide-based gait. (Redrawn from Ducroquet 1968.)

INFANTILE REFLEXES AND AUTOMATISMS

Infantile reflexes and automatisms can be considered as 'fixed action patterns'. They are a complex motor act elicited by a sensory stimulus. Examples are the Babinski sign, the Moro reflex, and the tonic neck reflexes (Baird and Gordon 1983).

CLASSIFICATION

To be valid, a classification has 'to be repeatable in relation to the same subject, both by the same and different observers'. It also needs to be sensitive, i.e. efficient in labeling cases which may or may not fall into a class according to an established reference. This ability to classify correctly cases which are not 'genuine' is called 'specificity' (Alberman 1984a).

Table 1.I shows the classification that many of us have used. It lists the physiological classification as the type of movement disorder with the common risk factors and the topographical classification according to the limb and trunk involvement. Ideally we would have a classification based on etiology, but it would be dependent on new technological advances in the study of the brain (Mutch *et al.* 1992). Most properly it is difficult to assign a single factor to etiology; more often there may be multiple risk factors (Uvebrant 1988, Aicardi 1998, Ebebol-Tysk *et al.* 1998).

The Swedish classification was adopted by epidemiologists at an international conference at Brioni, Yugoslavia, in 1990 (Table 1.II). The classification has the merit of simplicity and takes account of the fact that most studies group together spastic and ataxic diplegia, and chorea-athetosis and dystonia as forms of dyskinesia (Mutch *et al.* 1992).

Some Australian epidemiologists have pointed out that 'cerebral palsy is a term of convenience applied to a group of motor disorders of central origin defined by clinical description' (Badawi *et al.* 1998). They warn that it is not a diagnosis and does not imply anything about the pathology, etiology or prognosis. There must be motor impairment that arises from malfunction of the brain. It must be non-progressive and be manifested early in life.

Because this monograph is concerned mainly with the orthopaedic management of the spastic type of cerebral palsy, the classification submitted attempts to be precise in describing the characteristics and the topographic involvement of spastic paralysis.

SPASTIC DIPLEGIA

The term spastic diplegia is now universally preferred over paraplegia. Osler called it 'bilateral spastic hemiplegia'. The mental picture we have of a child with spastic diplegia is one who has obvious spasticity in the lower limbs, and none in the upper limbs except for fine-motor coordination defects. Most were born preterm with a birthweight less than 2500 g, and their prognosis for life function is generally good (Fig. 1.12).

SPASTIC HEMIPLEGIA

In spastic hemiplegia, the major and obvious involvement is in the upper and lower limbs on the same side (Fig. 1.13).

SPASTIC PARAPLEGIA

Paraplegia means that there is absolutely no involvement in the upper limbs, and no associated defects. The importance of precision in describing a patient as paraplegic is that if the child

TABLE 1.IA
Classification of movement disorders: physiologic (according to the movement disorder)

Type	Major clinical findings	Etiology: common risk factors
1. Spasticity (pyramidal)	Increased stretch reflex in muscles, i.e. hypertonicity of 'clasp knife' (Fig. 1.4) Hyperreflexia (deep tendon reflexes) Clonus Positive Babinski sign	Preterm birth Perinatal hypoxia Cerebral trauma Rubella (maternal), Familial
2. Dyskinesia (athetoid or extrapyramidal cerebral palsy)		
a. Tension type	Tension can be 'shaken out' of limb by examiner (Fig. 1.10) Extensor pattern (usually) Normal or depressed reflexes Paralysis of upward gaze Deafness (frequently)	Kernicterus due to Rh incompatibility

b. Dystonia	Intermittent distorted posturing of limbs, neck, trunk (Fig. 1.5)
	No contractures
	Full range of joint motion when relaxed
		Neonatal jaundice
		Hyperbilirubinemia
		Cerebral hypoxia
		    Perinatal 67%*
		    Prenatal 21%

c. Chorea	Spontaneous jerking of distal joints (fingers and toes) (Fig. 1.7)	Same as above
d. Ballismus (rotary, flailing)	Uncontrolled involuntary motions of proximal joints (shoulders, elbows, hips and knees) (Fig. 1.6)	Same as above
e. Rigidity	Rigid limbs Lead-pipe type—continuous resistance to passive motion (Fig. 1.9) Cogwheel type—discontinuous resistance to passive motion (Fig. 1.9)	Same as above
3. Ataxia	Lack of balance (Fig. 1.11a, b) Uncoordinated movement Dysmetria Dysarthia Wide-based gait—sways while walking Flexible pes valgus (common)	Prenatal 25%* Unknown 41%
4. Tremor	Rare Intentional or non-intentional (Fig. 1.8) Rhythmic or non-rhythmic	
5. Atonia	Rare Hypotonia of limbs and trunk (Fig. 1.2) Seen shortly after birth, usually evolves to athetosis	Cerebral hypoxia
6. mixed	Spasticity and dystonia Usually total body involved	Encephalitis Cerebral hypoxia Birth trauma

*% incidence from Aicardi (1998).

TABLE 1.IB
Classification of movement disorders: topographical

Type	Major clinical findings	Etiology: common risk factors
Monoplegia	Rare, usually a lower limb Probably hemiplegia Ask the child to run to unmask hemiplegia with elbow flexion on the same side	Same as hemiplegia
Hemiplegia	Spastic upper and lower limbs on the same side	Prenatal 42% Perinatal 16% Pre- and perinatal 9% Unknown in 34% (Uvebrant 1988)
Paraplegia	Lower limb spasticity spasticity only Completely normal upper limb function	Familial, hereditary Rule out spinal cord lesion
Diplegia	Major spasticity of lower limbs (1.11) Minor involvement of upper limbs Slight motor inco-ordination of finger movement	Preterm birth Low birthweight < 2500 g
Triplegia Three limb dominated bilateral spastic	Three limbs with gross spasticity Usually all four limbs, but one limb less involved and more functional	Perinatal 47% Very preterm infants
Total body involved	Spastic and/or athetosis all four limbs	Prenatal 50%–55% Quadriplegia Brain malformations Perinatal 30% Cerebral anoxia Postnatal 15%–20% (Edebol-Tysk et al. 1989)

TABLE 1.II
Swedish classification of cerebral palsy (Mutch *et al.* 1992)

Ataxic	Diplegic*
	Congenital (simple)
Dyskinetic	Mainly choreoathetotic*
	Mainly dystonic*
Spastic	Hemiplegic
	Tetraplegic
	Diplegic*

*Grouped together in epidemiologic studies. Almost all who have spastic diplegia have deficient postural equilibrium reactions in varying degrees with deficient posterior equilibrium reactions at a minimum (see Chapter 2).

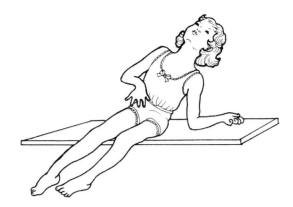

Fig. 1.14. Total body involvement: spastic, athetoid or mixed quadriplegia with abnormal control (disequilibrium) of the trunk, head and neck. Usually an extensor pattern predominates.

without involvement of the trunk must be rare. Lack of postural balance reactions of the trunk is usual (Fig. 1.14).

ASSESSMENT OF SEVERITY

It is difficult to precisely quantify the severity of the spasticity, athetosis, dysequilibrium or ataxia. Clinicians most frequently use the terms 'mild, moderate or severe' which depend on the perceptions and experience of the examiner.

ASHWORTH SCORES FOR SEVERITY OF SPASTICITY (TABLE 1.III)

With the advent of direct methods of treatment to relieve spastic paralysis using selective posterior rootlet rhizotomy and intrathecal baclofen, the Ashworth scoring method has been used by clinicians who report their results. The method of assessment is clinical, i.e. 'hands-on' (Ashworth 1964, Albright 1995). Its accuracy obviously depends on the perception of the one who does the testing. At various symposia on the results of rhizotomy, the problem of discerning score 3 from score 4 has often been raised.

One study attempted to show the reliability between raters in the assessment of elbow-flexor spasticity (Bohannan and Smith 1987). Using a statistical method of correlation they found that the raters' judgement and reliability were good (p<0.001). It is possible that the relatively light weight of the upper limbs in contrast to the lower limbs, and the ease of doing the test while sitting, affect the interrater reliability.

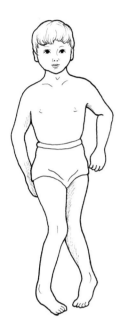
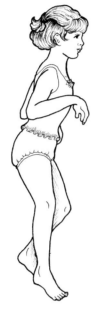

Fig. 1.12. Spastic diplegic posture: upper limbs grossly normal; hips flexed, adducted and internally rotated; knees flexed; ankle and foot in equinus.

Fig. 1.13. Hemiplegic posture: flexed elbow, wrist and fingers; equinus of the ankle and foot.

has genuine paraplegia, the diagnosis may not be cerebral, and a spinal-cord lesion (tethered cord or tumor), or hereditary spastic paraplegia should be considered.

TRIPLEGIA

Triplegia exists if we are describing definite and gross spastic paralysis in three limbs. An alternative term has been coined: 'three-limb-dominated bilateral spastic cerebral palsy' (Aicardi 1998). In this text the surgical treatment applicable would be that done in hemiplegia (upper limb) and diplegia.

TOTAL BODY INVOLVEMENT

The term 'total body involvement' has replaced quadriplegia or tetraplegia as more descriptive and has been generally accepted as a term appropriate for those who have obvious involvement of all four limbs, together with abnormal posturing and movement of the trunk, head and neck. Spastic paralysis of four limbs

TABLE 1.III
Ashworth scores in assessment of severity of spasticity

Ashworth score	Muscle tone (resistance to movement of limb in flexion or extension)
1	No increase in tone
2	Slight increase in tone, giving a 'catch' when limb moved
3	More marked increase in tone; passive movements difficult
4	Considerable increase in tone; passive movements difficult
5	Affected part rigid in flexion or extension

Skøld and associates (1998) attempted to correlate the Ashworth scale (modified) with electromyographic measurements in 15 men who had spastic quadriplegia due to a spinal cord injury. They recorded muscle action potentials simultaneously while flexing and extending the knee joints. They concluded that the electrical activity of the muscles showed a positive correlation with the Ashworth scores ($p<0.05$), and considered these results a validation of the accuracy of the Ashworth method.

DYNAMOMETRY
The assessment of severity with dynamometers to measure muscle force is a technique that has been developed to quantify severity of spasticity that would provide a more objective evaluation of outcomes of surgery or physical therapy. However, no reports of the use of dynamometry in measuring the outcome of orthopaedic surgery, rhizotomy or physical therapy methods can be found. These instruments use a strain-gauge torque sensor to measure passive resistance to stretch primarily of the calf muscles. Similar instruments have been reported by Otis *et al.* (1983), Price *et al.* (1991), Boiteau *et al.* (1995) and Engsberg *et al.* (1996). Engsberg and colleagues used the hamstrings. Despite these measurement tools, the Ashworth scales continue to be used in the assessment of outcomes of posterior rootlet rhizotomy.

ELECTROMYOGRAPHY
Electromyography seems limited in quantifying the degree of spasticity in the muscles tested. One should be cautious in placing too much emphasis on the peaks and volume of electrical discharges recorded graphically. As pointed out by M.P. Murray (personal communication), the volume and strength of the electrical discharges is dependent upon the density of motor endplates in the muscle. For example, the orbicularis oris muscles are packed with motor endplates and will have stronger and denser muscle-firing, while the peroneus longus (with more sparsely distributed motor units) will have less proportionate firing, especially when recorded with fine-wire or needle electrodes. Electromyography, however, is very useful when combined with kinematic studies of walking to ascertain the timing of the muscle contraction and relaxation. Perry (1992) made the case that electromyographic signals can be quantified using a computer for digital sampling, rectification and integration of the data.

INSTRUMENTED MOTION ANALYSIS
The optical recording of movement of the lower limbs and trunk in ambulatory patients appears to be the best way to measure abnormal movement compared to normal standards. The cadence, velocity, step length and the range of motion of the principal joints in gait are easy to measure (Chapter 3 provides more detail on these methods).

ENERGY REQUIREMENTS
Energy expenditure for walking or for wheelchair mobility can be measured to rate efficiency. Heart rate during the activity, compared with the resting state, is a simple way of assessing energy requirements for the individual patient. Measurements of oxygen consumption at rest and with activity are a more complex, but also more accurate method of analysis (see Chapter 3).

BALANCE MEASUREMENTS
In the patient who can stand unassisted, the objective measurement of balance should be relatively easy, with either piezoelectric force-plates or strain-gauge platforms linked to a computer program. We developed this kind of instrumentation and computer analysis in the study of postural mechanisms in idiopathic scoliosis (Adler *et al.* 1986). A more detailed description of methods of measurement of postural equilibrium and results can be found in Chapter 3.

PHOTOGRAPHY AND CINEMATOGRAPHY
Multiple sequential still photographs of walking have been used for over a century, ever since Eadweard Muybridge responded to a request from Senator Leland Stanford (founder of Leland Stanford Junior University) and proved that his racehorse had all four feet off the ground at one time (Muybridge 1887). Cinematography, used for many years, has been replaced with videotape recording. Photographic methods do allow a gross perception of the appearance of the subject when walking as observational gait analysis, but here too the assessment of severity of the spastic paralysis or another motion disorder is dependent on the perception of the viewer.

ASSESSMENT OF FUNCTION
In recent years analysis of function rather than measurement of severity has been increasingly emphasized as most important in the assessments of results of physical therapy, surgery and rehabilitation methods. Terver and colleagues (1981) devised a numerical score of functional abilities in both independence and efficiency in a prospective study of goal-setting for 71 children with total body involvement.

The Gross Motor Function Measure (Russell *et al.* 1989) is being increasingly used in the assessment of results of physical therapy and other types of specific treatment. The details of this particular assessment of function are presented in Chapter 6.

DISABILITY: IMPAIRMENT, ACTIVITY LIMITATION AND PARTICIPATION RESTRICTION
The World Health Organization has proposed a definition of terminology of impairment, activity limitation and participation (World Health Organization 2001). All of the following definitions are used 'in the context of health experience'. *Impairments* are problems in body function or structure such as a significant deviation or loss. *Activity limitation* is the umbrella term for impairments, activity limitations and participation restrictions. It refers to difficulties that an individual may have in executing activities. *Participation restrictions* are problems that an individual may experience in involvement in life situations.

All of our patients with cerebral palsy are impaired, and have some activity limitation and participation restriction in varying degrees depending on social, cultural and environmental barriers. Our role is to help these individuals cope with their disability so that they can lead as normal a life as possible.

EPIDEMIOLOGY AND ETIOLOGY

PREVALENCE

Epidemiological information is needed by public health administrators and clinicians when planning for services and special programs. *Prevalence* is a term used by epidemiologists. In school-age children, for example, it can be used in a particular geographic area. The word 'prevalence' is chosen rather than the commonly used 'incidence' because of Alberman's (1984a) recommendations: 'Prevalence is the number of cases of the disease present during a certain time-period.' Because cerebral palsy is by definition a permanent condition, birth prevalence is expressed as the number of cerebral palsy cases per 1000 neonatal survivors. The very early diagnosis of cerebral palsy is hazardous because some infants who have an early neurological abnormality may have none by the age of 7 years. Therefore overinterpretation of birth prevalence data needs to be tempered (Nelson and Ellenberg 1982).

In 1984, birth-prevalence rates were remarkably similar in all Western countries: close to 2 per 1000 (Paneth and Kiely 1984). Despite the advance in prevention of hemolytic anemia of the newborn, and improved obstetric and neonatal care, the prevalence of cerebral palsy in the 1990s has remained the same in most developed countries at 2–2.5/1000 children born (Stanley and Blair 1991, Rosen and Dickinson 1992, Stanley and Watson 1992, Yeargin-Allsopp *et al.* 1992, Thompson *et al.* 1993, Hagberg *et al.* 1996, Pharoah *et al.* 1998, Stanley *et al.* 2000).

ETIOLOGY: CAUSAL PATHWAYS

Although clinicians who deal with patients who already have cerebral palsy can contribute little to prevention (this task belongs to pediatricians, obstetricians, family physicians and neonatologists), the orthopaedic surgeon, other clinicians and therapists should be aware of past and current studies of epidemiology and etiology. Parents often ask the physician's opinion on the cause of their child's cerebral palsy. As doctors of medicine, they are expected to be professionals who can read and interpret the medical scientific literature. Some mothers feel guilty about the unexpected impairment of their child. Other parents may assume the unexpected outcome is the physician's fault.

'Brain damage, birth trauma and lack of oxygen' do not pass the test of scientific scrutiny as major causes in the 21st century. Litigation against obstetricians and gynecologists accounts for the highest indemnity payments of any specialty. Almost one-third of the awards in Australia were for brain-damaged babies (Stanley *et al.* 2000). The 2001 California Large Loss Trend Study confirms that in California birth-injury cases were again the most frequent and costly of all categories. The major claims for indemnity were delays in recognizing fetal distress, delays in performing caesarian-sections, and failure to perform prenatal diagnostic tests. From a total of 24 indemnity awards, totalling

$69,482,951, nine were claimed as birth injuries, accounting for $37,482,922 (Medical Underwriters of California 2001). This continuing trend stems from 'the popular belief that cerebral palsy was caused mostly in the intrapartum period and was therefore avoidable by modern obstetrics fuelled the increase in litigation against obstetricians' (Freeman and Freeman 1992, Stanley *et al.* 2000).

Physicians and the public need to be informed that prenatal factors and events are responsible for the majority of outcomes of birth of a child with cerebral palsy. Among the many etiological prenatal factors, one can cite the very large study of the possible causes of bilateral spastic cerebral palsy in Germany and Sweden, in which no etiology was found in 44% of the cases (Krägeloh-Mann *et al.* 1995). We need to prevent time, energy and money being wasted in unjustified and excessive liability claims and divert it from the courts to biomedical research on epidemiology and etiology. From these we derive what always should be preeminent: prevention.

The search for risk factors and prevention goes on apace throughout the developed world and with more interest in the less developed world. We have cited only a few of these reports for the interest of the clinician. While causation of most of cerebral palsy remains elusive, some risk factors are known and preventative measures, although limited in the majority of cases, can be implemented. In the past we succumbed to the easy way of trying to identify a single causative event for the child with cerebral palsy. The most notable was birth asphyxia in an apparent stillbirth who had heroic resuscitation and was kept alive in an intensive care unit (Stanley *et al.* 2000). Because many cases often have antecedents that combine to causation, Stanley and colleagues (2000) proposed 'causal pathways' as risk factors. These pathways have been divided into prenatal, very preterm birth (before 32 weeks of gestation) and extreme preterm birth (before 28 weeks of gestation), intrauterine growth restriction, signs of birth asphyxia, multiple pregnancy, and postnatally acquired cerebral palsy. The reason for this etiological approach is to discern possible preventative measures.

PRENATAL PATHWAYS (Fig. 1.15)

> *'The humane foetus tho no bigger than a Green Pea, yet is furnished with all its parts.'*
>
> (Antonj van Leeuwenhoek, 1683)[4]

Brain development although complex is orderly on a time table from conception to birth. By 20 weeks the glia form and neurons migrate to form the various structures of the brain; circuits and connections develop after 20 weeks and by about 36 weeks the cortex, cerebellum and basal ganglia are formed but immature. Motor development continues up to puberty. Normal neuron development and neuronal migration can be interrupted by a

---

4 Quoted by England, M.A. (1983) *Color Atlas of Life before Birth.* Chicago: Yearbook Medical Publishers and special arrangement with Wolfe Medical Publications.

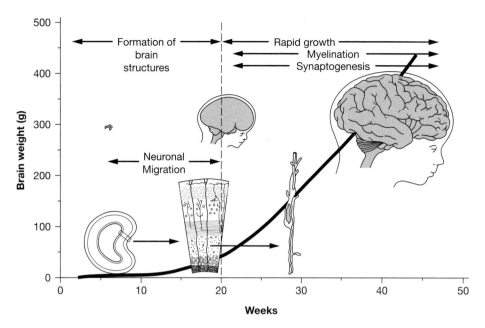

Fig. 1.15. Progression of brain development from gestation to early postnatal life. Reproduced by permission from *Stanley et al.* 2000; illustration by courtesy of M. Squires.

number of agents or events with a resultant motor disorder. The effect of such noxious influences depends on when it occurs during gestation. Table 1.IV is a list of prenatal causes of the cerebral palsy syndrome.

The TORCH group of infections (Toxoplasma gondii, rubella, cytomegalovirus and herpes), transmitted from mother to fetus, tend to cause congenital brain malformations during the first and second trimesters; while in the third trimester, when the brain is already formed, these agents tend to cause destructive lesions (Barkovich and Girard 2003). In their study of fetal brains using magnetic resonance imaging (MRI) in 178 patients with known prenatal infections, 23% had cerebral abnormalities. The most prevalent and virulent were found to be toxoplasmosis (97 cases, with 15% abnormal MRI), cytomegalovirus (37 cases, with 39% abnormal MRI), varicella (17 cases, with 18% abnormal MRI).

Toxoplasma gondii is a parasite that infects millions all over the world. It may be dismaying to cat-lovers to learn that the domestic cat is a major carrier of the parasite. Its source is raw or poorly cooked meat of hogs or pigs that have ingested soil infected with the parasite from cat feces (the US Public Health Service advises that cooked meat should have an internal temperature of 155°F for safe eating). The infection is rare in the United States, accounting for only 37 cases per year between 1982 and 1986 (Schantz and McAuley 1991).

Still toxoplasma gondii causes neurologic impairment and chorioretinitis with inflammation of the retina and uveal tract which causes blindness. The reported prevalence of toxoplasmosis in various countries includes the following. In Turkey, 694 of 1149 (60.4%) pregnant women were IgG-positive, indicating previous infection, and 35 (3%) were IgM-positive, i.e. recently

TABLE 1.IV
Causes of, and risk factors for, cerebral palsy (from Reddihough and Collins 2003)

Preconception	Prenatal	Perinatal	Postnatal
Irregular menses	Brain malformation	Intrapartum hypoxia	Infection, e.g. meningitis, septicemia
Maternal intellectual disability	Vascular events	Sarnat grade III encephalopathy	Traumatic brain injury
Maternal seizures	Maternal infection	Hypoglycemia	Near-drowning
Maternal thyroid disease	Metabolic disorders	Infection	Stroke
Advanced paternal age	Toxins	Preterm birth	Neonatal seizures
	Genetic syndromes	Low birthweight	Sepsis
	Pre-eclampsia in term infants	Low placental weight	Respiratory disease
	Antepartum hemorrhage	Low Apgar scores	In preterm infants: patent ductus
	Multiple-birth pregnancy	Prolapsed cord	arteriosus, complicated neonatal course
	In utero death of co-twin	Hemorrhage	
		Traumatic delivery	
		Cephalopelvic disproportion	
		Abnormal fetal presentation	
		Maternal shock	
		Chorioamniotis	
		Prolonged second stage of labor	
		Emergency cesarean section	

infected (Harma *et al.* 2004); from Saudi Arabia, of 1400 sampled in a cross-section of people, the incidence of inactive toxoplasmosis (positive IgG) was 26% and 25% in two different towns, while active toxoplasmosis (positive IgM) was 4.9% and 3.8% (Al-Qurashi 2004); from Brazil, 195 of 364,130 or 0.05% neonates tested positive for toxoplasma gondii-specific IgM (Neto *et al.* 2004); in southern Italy, 2.9% of infants 0 to 15 months had antibodies (Leogrande 1992).

The *rubella* virus damages the embryo with resultant deafness, blindness, microcephaly, cerebral palsy, mental retardation and heart defects. If the infection occurs a month before conception the risk to the fetus is 42%, and if it occurs between conception and the 12th week, the risk is 52%. Rubella vaccine developed in 1969 has made the rubella syndrome rare. Immunization between the ages of 1 and 2 years confers lifelong immunity (Batshaw and Perret 1992).

Cytomegalovirus infection is more common than supposed, with an intrauterine infection rate varying between 2 and 20 per livebirths. However, not all children who have the infection have neurological manifestations. It is thought to account for 5%–10% of the cases of cerebral palsy with the major disability of deafness and microcephaly (Stanley *et al.* 2000). Based on a retrospective review of MRI and computerized tomography (CT) scans in 15 patients who had a cytomegalic infection of the brain, Barkovich and Lindan (1994) concluded that the damage by the virus occurs between 16 and 24 weeks of gestation. Among the abnormalties was lissencephaly (smooth brain-agyria), focal dysplasia of the cortex, small cerebella, and delayed myelination.

Herpes virus transmission in utero is extremely low, despite the stubborn persistence of the virus in the mother. In one study using enzyme immunoassay to detect type-specific antibodies, the annualized rate of herpes simplex infection, type 2, was only 0.58% of pregnant women. None of the infants born had any defects (Boucher *et al.* 1990). Death of the infant due to encephalitis can occur, but with acyclovir therapy the mortality decreased to 20%; 40% of the survivors were normal after a year of treatment.

The most dramatic prevention of athetosis was derived from the knowledge of *Rh factor incompatibility* as the cause of the hemolytic anemia of the newborn (erthryoblastosis fetalis), kernicterus, and deafness. As a result of Rh immunization of Rh negative mothers, intrauterine diagnosis and transfusion of the fetus, and early diagnosis of neonatal jaundice with treatment by intravascular transfusions (92.1% with no residual disability; Doyle *et al.* 1993) and phototherapy, athetosis with deafness has practically disappeared in Western countries. Anti-D immunization of the mother when done routinely has dramatically dropped this severe and generally untreatable chorioathetosis (Stanley and Alberman 1984) These good results continue.

Iodine deficiency as a cause of spastic diplegia, mental retardation[5] and deafness was first discovered in the Jimi Valley of New Guinea (Pharoah *et al.* 1971). Since then it is the most common cause of preventable brain damage in the world. The World Health Organization estimated in 1993 that 1.6 billion people were at risk for iodine deficiency (Stanley *et al.* 2000). Iodized salt is the obvious answer.

Methyl mercury toxicity responsible for structural malformation of the brain has apparently disappeared since the first report from Minamata Bay, Japan, of an epidemic of neurological symptoms and signs.[6] The causative agent was contamination of the fish with methyl mercury from the discharge of vinyl chloride and acetaldehyde into the sea (Stanley 1984). A similar outbreak occurred in Iraq in 1972 due to consumption of bread made from wheat treated with a mercury fungicide (Amin-Zaki 1974).

Alcohol is the commonest teratogen accounting for fetal growth failure. Its prohibition in pregnancy goes back at least as far as Biblical times.[7] Bertrand and colleagues (2004) described the characteristics of the syndrome as facial abnormailites that include smooth philtrum (groove under the nose); thin vermilion border (upper lip); small palpebral fissures; growth deficits with size below the 10th centile in height or weight; CNS deficits including microcephaly under the 10th centile; brain abnormalities; cognitive and/or motor delays; and social-skill problems. In the United States the prevalence is approximately 2 per 1000 livebirths; alarmingly 73% of 12- to 34-year-old women had consumed alcohol at some time during their pregnancies (Hansen and Ulrey 1993). Although the syndrome occurs mainly with very high levels of maternal consumption, pregnancy outcome studies show that low-birthweight babies are born to mothers imbibing more modest amounts, 140 g of absolute alcohol per week, or about two drinks per day (Larroque 1992).

Smoking during pregnancy has long been recognized as a factor in low birthweight, as has been recently documented (Kyrklund-Blomerg and Cnattingius 1998). Cotinine accumulates in the fetal fluid compartments as early as 7 weeks of gestation in active and passive smokers (Jauniaux *et al.* 1999).[8]

Drug abuse has progressed from marijuana in the 1960s, to heroin in the 1970s and cocaine in the 1990s (Peters and Thorell 1991). None of these recreational drugs is known as a teratogenic agent. Studies of cocaine use during pregnancy do not indicate obstetric, perinatal or neonatal complications. Preterm birth has been suggested as associated with cocaine use (Koren and Graham 1992, Martin *et al.* 1992). The lifestyle of the mother as it affects

---

6 Minamata is in the Kumamoto Prefecture of Kyushu, the southernmost major island of Japan. Mercury poisoning (Minamata disease) was first diagnosed in 1956 following the pumping of waste from the Chisso Company. Approximately 2000 people died and a further 13,000 were affected. The Japanese government has now declared the waters mercury-free.

7 And the angel of the Lord appeared unto the wife of Manoah and said unto her: "Behold now thou art barren, but thou shalt conceive, and bear a son. Now therefore beware, I pray thee, and drink no wine nor strong drink." . . . And the woman bore a son and called his name Samson; and the child grew.' (Judges 13:3–4; 13:24; quoted by Goldberg 1987.)

8 Cotinine: 1-methyl-5(3-pyridyl)-2-pyrrolidinone, anagram of nicotine. One of the major detoxification products of nicotine; eliminated rapidly and completely by the kidneys.

---

5 'Learning disability' in UK usage.

child development is thought to be a possible important environmental factor (Singer *et al.* 1991).

Glucose-6-phosphate dehydrogenase deficiency (G6PD) is the commonest enzyme deficiency in humans and the cause of jaundice, kernicterus, death or spastic cerebral palsy. It has been observed primarily in Middle Eastern and Mediterranean populations. The hemolytic crises responsible for these effects is due to interactions with specific drugs or ingestion of *fava beans*. The WHO Working Group was successful in prevention by community-wide screening for the G6PD deficiency, education and successful treatment of jaundice with phototherapy (Meloni *et al.* 1992). Fava beans may not be the whole story; a study of Thais and south-east Asians with G6PD deficiency and who ate fava beans found no evidence of hemolytic anemia (Kitayaporn 1991).

Familial cerebral palsy is rare. A study in Sweden showed that only 1.5% of all cerebral palsy cases were autosomal recessive inherited conditions. Even rarer were sex-linked and dominant inheritance (Stanley 1984). Familial spastic paraplegia has little or no involvement of the upper limbs and no associated defects of cognition or speech. The symptoms usually appear later in childhood with no abnormal birth or gestation history. Dominant inheritance is usual although recessive types do occur. The types of familial spastic paraplegia and congenital ataxias with autosomal dominant and recessive inheritance have been extensively reviewed by Aicardi (1998).

PATHWAYS INVOLVING VERY PRETERM BIRTH

Very preterm birth is defined as birth before 32 weeks of gestation; extreme preterm birth occurs prior to 28 weeks of gestation. Birthweight was formerly used as a proxy for gestational age (preterm birthweight less than 2500 g). Very preterm birth is the strongest predictor of cerebral palsy. The rate of cerebral palsy among survivors born at less than 33 weeks of gestation is 30 times higher than those born at term (Stanley *et al.* 2000). The relationship between preterm birth and cerebral palsy has been confirmed with studies in the 1990s (al-Rajeh *et al.* 1991, Escobar *et al.* 1991, Rosen and Dickinson 1992, Bhushan *et al.* 1993, Meberg and Broch 1995).

PREVALENCE

The problem with reporting prevalence is that outcome studies cannot be claimed to be accurate in discerning cerebral palsy in neonates until probably at least 4–7 years after birth; so the investigator has to wait for the child to grow up to make sure of the diagnosis and the neurological impairment (Nelson and Ellenberg 1982). Astbury *et al.* (1990) made the same point in their prospective study of 53 extremely low-birthweight (<1000 g) babies who were survivors at ages 1, 2 and 5 years. Thirteen had impairments at 5 years, but only seven were identified at 1 year and 17 at 2 years. This data on underestimation at 1 year and overestimation at 2 years suggest the most reliable estimation of adverse sequelae of extremely low-birthweight infants might not be possible until school age, i.e. 5–6 years.

In Western Australia, spastic diplegia in over 40% was the most common outcome of preterm birth. Spastic hemiplegia evolved in 25.2%, 15.6% with spastic quadriplegia and 4.8% with other types. The reports in the medical literature cited strongly suggest that preterm babies had prenatal factors to cause cerebral palsy rather than events solely in the perinatal period. Those who wish more details on the subject should consult the text of Stanley *et al.* (2000).

INTRAUTERINE INFECTION

Intrauterine infection is an additional pathway to cerebral palsy not only in preterm but in term infants. Group B hemolytic streptococci are among the most common bacteria causing neonatal meningitis (Haslam *et al.* 1977). Gram-negative bacterial meningitis due to Eschericha coli and Listeria monocytogenes are considered the next most common. Nosocomial infections, usually Streptococcus group B arising from the nursery are occasional (Aicardi 1998).

Among the adverse risk factors in very preterm babies was chorioamnionitis and maternal infection in a study from Oxford (Murphy and MacKenzie 1995). Maternal infection in normal-birthweight infants indicated that 22% of the children had cerebral palsy versus 2.9% of the control children in a four-county study in northern California (Grether and Nelson 1997).

In an extensive review, McCormick (1985) concluded that 'despite increased access to antenatal services, only moderate declines in the proportion of low birth weight infants has been observed, and almost no change has occurred in the proportion of those with very low birth weight at birth'. Since 1985 survival rates of very low-birthweight infants has been improved, but the rate of cerebral palsy appears the same (Stanley and Watson 1992).

INTRAUTERINE GROWTH RESTRICTION

Intrauterine growth restriction, leading to babies being born too small for gestational age (SGA), is another pathway to cerebral palsy suggested by Stanley and colleagues (2000). However, the underlying mechanisms are not clear. Is growth restriction an epiphenomenon of early pregnancy factors such as malformations or viral infections? Antepartum rather than intrapartum stress may be an event that causes a neurological disability to emerge.

NEONATAL ASPHYXIA

According to Stanley and Colleagues (2000), 'The "traditional" pathways of fetal heart rate abnormalities, as measured by electronic monitoring in labour followed by a "suboptimal" obstetric response (not expediting delivery), birth asphyxia, neonatal encephalopathy and cerebral palsy does not occur for most cases of cerebral palsy. Even where clinical signs are suggestive it is impossible to prove. . . . The major effects of electronic monitoring of the fetal heart in labour are in increase in cesarean section rate and a reduced rate of neonatal seizures; it has no impact on the rates of cerebral palsy.'

Prolonged and difficult labor, breech birth, prolapsed umbilical cord, meconium staining and birth trauma have all been thought to be associated with cerebral palsy. Prenatal problems complicate the analysis of the etiology as well, so the examining physician should be cautious in assigning an etiology to a single event or entity occurring at birth.

Birth asphyxia has long been recognized as causative of brain damage. Half a century ago Ranck and Windle (1959) studied experimental neonatal asphyxia in monkeys. Asphyxia in those newborn monkeys that survived beyond 25–30 minutes indicated brain damage. Neonatal asphyxia appears to be overdrawn as a cause of cerebral palsy. It is may be an important etiology in non-western countries as reflected in a report from Medan, Sumatra, Indonesia, in which 27.5% of 40 cases of cerebral palsy were judged due to neonatal asphyxia (Lubis *et al.* 1990).

Nelson and Ellenberg (1981) studied the Apgar scores of 49,000 infants followed to the age of 7 years. Apgar scores were recorded at 1, 5, 10 and 20 minutes. 55% of the children with cerebral palsy had Apgar scores of 7 at 10 minutes; 53% of those with cerebral palsy had a score of 7 at 5 minutes. Of the 99 children who had scores of 0–3 at 10, 15 and 20 minutes, 12% had cerebral palsy, and 11% were mentally retarded. However, three-quarters of the survivors of severe asphyxia had intact neurological functions when examined at the age of 7 years. This study refuted the old assumption that most cases of cerebral palsy were due to lack of oxygen or birth trauma. Freeman and Nelson (1988) found few cases of cerebral palsy which met the criteria of a substantial hypoxic episode, with subsequent effects to prove the impact of the hypoxic event. Further, although hypoxic events are not uncommon around the birth process, they found no single event to be a predictor of subsequent cerebral palsy with a reasonable degree of medical certainty.

Nelson and Grether (1998) revisited asphyxia. Of 46 children born with unexplained cerebral palsy in four California counties (1983–85), eight who had quadriplegia were associated with tight nuchal cords compared with 15 of 378 controls born with tight nuchal cords. No asphyxiating conditions were found with spastic diplegia or hemiplegia. Intrapartum abnormalities were common in both groups. The role of umbilical cord prolapse in asphyxia remains in doubt, if not absolutely refuted by the Oxford study of 56,283 births which found cord prolapse in 2.3 per 1000 births and one death from asphyxia (Murphy and MacKenzie 1995).

Nelson and Grether (1999), on the basis of a detailed study of children who had a history of birth asphyxia, concluded that most of the depressed infants had conditions other than asphyxia that may have caused the cerebral palsy. This study included 366 full-term singleton surviving infants born in four northern California counties (1983–85). Of these, 84 had moderate to severe cerebral palsy. From this group they found 18 who had a 5-minute Apgar score of less than 6, 20 who needed intubation in the delivery room, and five who had a blood pH of 7.0 or less. Only 19 of the children with cerebral palsy had at least two criteria of asphyxia (when three criteria were used, the prevalence of cerebral palsy was only 0.019 per 1000). In seven of the 19 there was evidence of maternal or infant infection,

and in eight an abnormal coagulation factor, thrombosis or thrombocytopenia. In nine, there were other complications predating birth.

A meta-analysis of 42 published studies was derived from 1312 studies and 81 articles between 1966 and 1997 on the relationship of the Apgar score, umbilical blood pH, or the Sarnat grading of encephalopathy (van de Riet *et al.* 1999).[9] The strongest predictors of neonatal death were an umbilical artery pH less than 7 and Sarnat grade III encephalopathy. The strongest associations for predicting cerebral palsy were a Sarnat grade III encephalopathy (versus grade II) and a 20-minute Apgar score of 0–3 (versus 4–6).

From Norway comes an analysis of the possible etiology of 129 cases of dyskinetic and dystonic forms of cerebral palsy (Foley 1992). No relationship to clinical severity was found among those who had kernicterus, abnormal birth or asphyxia. This led to the conclusion that abnormal birth and asphyxia are not the cause of cerebral damage, but only manifestations of a pre-existing condition that made the infant more susceptible to stress at birth.

In Western Australia, *multiple birth* has been recognized as an increased risk-factor for cerebral palsy, ranging from a prevalence of 28/1000 survivors in triplets (47 times more often than singleton births) to 7.3 for twins. However, these risks were similar for singletons who had low birthweights and for children who were of low birthweight and were survivors of multiple births (Petterson *et al.* 1993).

In California, twin pregnancies produced a child with cerebral palsy 12 times more often than singleton pregnancies (Grether *et al.* 1993). In Osaka, Japan, the prevalence of cerebral palsy in multiple births was 1.5% for twins, 8% for triplets, and 42.9% for quadruplets born after 1977 (Yokoyama *et al.* 1995). In the 1990s, paradoxically, multiple births (especially triplets and quadruplets) have increased while the birth rate in most Western countries has remained stable, low or falling. This increase in multiple births appears to be due partly to older women having delayed pregnancy, but is primarily due to the prominent use of fertility-enhancing drugs and interventions (in vitro fertilization) in developed countries (Stanley *et al.* 2000). These multiple births often result in very preterm low-birthweight infants who are at greater risk for a neurological impairment. Papiernik (1991) opined that most supermultiple pregnancies are the result of ovulation-inducing drugs.

The survival of very preterm infants has been improved by the advances in neonatology. The survival rates of infants with birthweights of 501–800 g increased from 20% in the period 1979–84, to 59% in 1989–94. Cerebral palsy in these survivors has not resulted in an increased rate of major developmental

---

9 Sarnat grades entail three levels of encephalopathy in term infants arising from a hypoxic–ischaemic event (Aicardi 1998). I: first 24 hours, then diminish. Jitteriness, irritability, facile Moro response. II: lethargy and obtundation for more than 24 hours. Hypertonus on simulation, weakness in upper limbs, diminished spontaneous movements. May improve in 48–72 hours. If it persists, it evolves to grade III: stupor, coma, convulsions first 24 hours; profound hypotonia; reflexes abolished.

problems at 1 year; the decline was from 13%–20% to 7% in the same time-frames (Grögaard *et al.* 1990, O'Shea *et al.* 1997).

In contrast to the foregoing optimistic report, a paper in 1998 reviewed the literature of 42 studies on mortality rates and prevalence of major neurodevelopmental disabilities over time of extremely preterm infants suggests that more of the small and/or early born babies survived, but resulted in a steadily increasing prevalence of children with disabilities (Ericson and Kallen 1998, Lorenz *et al.* 1998).

POSTNATAL ACQUIRED CEREBRAL PALSY

When the acute phase of a cerebral insult in a previously normal child has evolved into a non-progressive motor disorder, the child is then labeled as having cerebral palsy, though neurologists prefer the term 'static encephalopathy'. However, more studies have shown that prenatal metabolic conditions or clotting disorders that cause brain damage and become progressive after birth can be responsible for the signs of cerebral palsy (Stanley *et al.* 2000).

Infection is the leading cause of postnatal encephalopathy (60%), followed by head injury (20%). Postnatal central nervous system infections, either bacterial or viral, accounted for the etiology of postnatal cerebral palsy in 47%–63% of the cases in New York, Chicago and Western Australia (Stanley and Blair 1984). *Haemophilus influenzae* was the most common cause of meningitis in Western Australia followed by *Streptococcus pneumoniae* and *Neisseria meningitidis* (Hanna and Wild 1991). The Swedish Register reported that during the period of the lowest rate of postnatally acquired cerebral palsy (1987–90), when there was a rate of 1.09/10,000 livebirths, there were no cases of central nervous system infection as a cause (Stanley *et al.* 2000).

Cerebral anoxia due to near drowning, suffocation and postoperative or intraoperative cardiac arrest accounts for 2%–13% of the cases reported. Cerebral vascular accidents vary with the location of the report from about 5% to 12%. The residual brain damage from tumors in childhood was found to be a cause of a motor disorder in 8% of cases from New York (Stanley 1984).

Lead encephalopathy accounted for 2.4% of 624 postnatal cases studied in Chicago (Stanley 1984). Campaigns to reduce lead exposure in paint (dust from old paint), gasoline and old lead pipes in houses, which have resulted in a decline the prevalence of childhood lead poisoning, is a public health success story in the United States (Markowitz 2000; see also Javier *et al.* 1999, Ellis and Kane 2001).

Cow urine encephalopathy is an exotic cause of cerebral palsy in Nigeria, attributed to application to the skin and ingestion of the cow's urine mixed with mixed with tobacco leaves, citrus medica and ocinium vera leaves for the general health of children. When used in larger amounts, status epilepticus and a vegetative state occurred and evolved into cerebral palsy and non-motor brain damage (Nottidge and Okogbo 1991).

BRAIN PATHOLOGY AND IMAGING IN CEREBRAL PALSY

In 1897, Freud declared: 'I should like to make two statements prior to embarking on a detailed presentation of the subject: (1) hemiplegic and diplegic forms present the same anatomical findings so cannot be distinguished as far as the pathological anatomy is concerned; (2) from the very start one must abandon any expectation that infantile cerebral palsy can be characterized by a topical factor, such as localization of the affection.' In Freud's time, pathologists assiduously pursued postmortem studies. Porencephaly, hydrocephalus, intracerebral bleeding, cortical agenesis, atrophy, lobar sclerosis and chronic meningitis were among the pathological anatomical findings reported. In our time, pathological studies have indicated that ischemic damage to the brain was present in 44% of the stillborns after 27 weeks of gestation. Of the 165 brains studied at the Radcliffe Infirmary, Oxford, 90 liveborn infants who survived less than 3 days had evidence of ischaemic damage of prenatal origin (Squier and Keeling 1991).

Due to the advance of brain-imaging technology we seem to be a bit closer to a classification of cerebral palsy based on the pathological lesion in the brain and the etiology (Okumura *et al.* 1997a, b). Some examples might be 'periventricular leukomalacia palsy' (spastic diplegia); 'cystic basal ganglia (putamen) motion disorder', i.e. athetosis (Rutherford *et al.* 1992). Ultrasonography, CT and MRI have advanced our knowledge of the pathological changes in the brain, many of which appear to be antenatal in origin. Single proton emission computed tomography (SPECT), positron emission tomography (PET) and proton spectroscopy (MRS) are used for research (Aicardi 1998).

Computerized tomography has given way to the superior definition of the brain by MRI. CT scans of the brains of hemiplegic children have demonstrated that 57% of the lesions studied were of prenatal origin. Periventricular atrophy suggested periventricular leukomalacia associated with preterm birth (Wiklund *et al.* 1991, Wiklund and Uvebrant 1991). Cranial CT was reported to be a good predictor of an adverse neurological outcome in newborns who had a symptomatic congenital cytomegalovirus infection. In these newborns, CT depicted abnormalities in 70% with intracerebral calcifications as the most frequent finding (Boppana *et al.* 1997).

Cranial ultrasonography has been extensively used to discern leukomalacia and other brain pathologies shortly after birth (Govaert and de Vries 1997). As a predictor of cerebral palsy, cerebral ultrasonography has often been used to test the efficacy of treatment regimens (e.g. indomethacin for intraventricular hemorrhage) in the low-birthweight newborns as a predictor of cerebral palsy (Allan *et al.* 1997). Ultrasonography was deemed the most powerful predictor of cerebral palsy in low-birthweight babies (Rogers *et al.* 1994, Pinto-Martin *et al.* 1995). Ultrasonography in children at the age of 6 years revealed that no child with a normal ultrasound scan developed cerebral palsy, while almost all of those who had major lesions did develop it (Johgmans *et al.* 1997). Minor lesions, however, did not predict later outcomes. The correlation with perceptual–motor problems in these children born preterm was low. Ultrasonography through the posterolateral fontanelle revealed cerebellar hemorrhage in preterm infants that was clinically silent; long-term follow-up of the neurodevelopmental outcome is not yet known (Merrill et al. 1998).

Magnetic resonance imaging is more accurate in depicting pathological changes in the brain, but clinical correlations with the specific motor disorder are yet to be determined. Okumura and colleagues (1997a, b) used MRI images of the brain in 152 patients who had spastic cerebral palsy. They related the MRI findings to gestational age and type of cerebral palsy. They found that 90% of the patients who had periventricular leukomalacia (the commonest finding in spastic diplegia) had been born between 25 and 32 weeks of gestation.

Among those born at full term, an MRI study showed three major pathological findings: (1) gyral anomalies (polymicrogyria); (2) periventricular leukomalacia indicative of late second to early third trimester injury; and (3) watershed cortical or deep gray nuclear damage consistent with later-trimester, perinatal, or postnatal injury (Truitt et al. 1992).[10] In a retrospective study of cerebral palsy in term infants, MRI studies indicative of defective neuronal migration and cerebral infarctions suggested that the brain pathology was frequently due to prenatal factors (Sugimoto et al. 1995). MRI studies in children who had extrapyramidal cerebral palsy displayed hyperintense signals in the putamen and thalamus that were considered to be indicators of a hypoxic–ischaemic encephalopathy (Hoon et al. 1997). Other signal abnormalities in the basal ganglia were thought to represent genetic and metabolic diseases, as well as mitochondrial and organic acid metabolism disorders.

Proton MR spectroscopy was used to detect ratios of choline, creatine, and N-acetylaspartate in preterm and term neonates (Vigneron et al. 2001). Barkovich and colleagues (1999) applied the technique in 31 asphyxiated term neonates. Many had ratios of these metabolites that correlated significantly with the neurodevelopmental outcome. However, three with watershed injuries had normal clinical outcomes, i.e. false positives. Quantitative analysis of brain MRI studies and neurodevelopmental outcomes at age 12 months of 53 asphyxiated neonates by Coskun et al. (2001) revealed a strong correlation with an anterior watershed injury of the brain.

Brain imaging continues to unravel the mystery of cerebral palsy of prenatal and perinatal origin and its clinical effects. Martin Bax (personal communication) believes that all children diagnosed with cerebral palsy should have an MRI study of the brain, and he is currently conducting a study with a European consortium. No parent has refused to see 'a picture' of their child's brain. Currently most infants and young children need sedation or general anesthesia during MRI, although more up-to-date MRI facilities are eliminating the need for this.

Fast MRI has made in utero diagnoses of suspected brain lesions depicted by ultrasonography (Simon et al. 2000). Lesions such as heterotopia (displacement of cerebral gray matter into the deep white matter), callosal anomalies and posterior malformtions were discovered prenatally. In all cases the referring physician thought that in utero brain imaging was valuable and facilitated parent counseling.

PREVENTION

'Never have a meeting on cerebral palsy without including prevention.'

(Ronnie Mac Keith)

From the epidemiological data and a heavy dose of proposed preventative measures, it appears that we have used a pound of prevention for an ounce of cure. The progress continues to be slow despite intensive efforts by obstetricians and neonatologists.

ANTENATAL PREVENTION
Magnesium sulfate in utero and antenatal corticosteroids have been tried as prophylaxis against preterm birth and cerebral palsy. The results are mixed with positives and negatives. A study in Finland claimed that after 1990 antenatal dexamethasone reduced the incidence of parenchymal hemorrhage and cerebral palsy in neonates that had an average weight of 1291 g (Salokorpi et al. 1997). Cooke (1999), using cranial ultrasonography in newborn infants whose mothers had prophylactic corticosteroids, reported improved survival rates and a decrease in cerebral hemorrhage and cerebral palsy after 1990.

In utero exposure to magnesium sulfate as a 'tocolytic' (an agent to reduce uterine contractions) was suggested as a protective effect from cerebral palsy in very low-birthweight (<1500 g) infants (Nelson and Grether 1995, Schendel et al. 1996, Grether et al. 1998). However, to assess the results an estimated 1,000,000 pregnancies would be required to generate the number of eligible gravid women—a formidable undertaking as a multicenter trial (Rouse et al. 1996).

A detailed investigation of perinatal predictors in singleton very low-birthweight children compared 50 who developed cerebral palsy and 22 with other neurological impairments with 72 neurologically normal very low-birthweight children. No significant differences in neurological outcomes in the children whose mothers had pregnancy-induced hypertension, tocolytic agents (magnesium sulfate), or corticosteroids (Wilson-Costello et al. 1998). Another study entailing sonography of the brain to determine the effect of magnesium sulfate exposure, and periventricular leukomalcia and intraventricular hemorrhage in preterm babies, found that maternal magnesium sulfate was not associated with a reduction in abnormal sonograms and obviously had no protective effect (Canterino et al. 1999).

Prenatal care programs for women 'at risk' for preterm birth have been instituted in various US and European venues (Buescher et al. 1988, Covington et al. 1988, Ernest et al. 1988, Freda et al. 1988, Mueller-Heuback et al. 1989, Kindt et al. 1991, Ruckhaberle et al. 1992). Lequien et al. (1990) reported a study over two periods, 1980–1982 and 1983–1985, in which they

---

10 'Watershed': an area of marginal blood flow at the extreme periphery of a vascular bed.

noted a dramatic increase in preterm infants born after the induction of labor for reasons of fetal distress. They found a statistically significant lower gestational age and birthweight compared to spontaneously born infants, and concluded that these trends would counter the presumed efficacy of prevention policies.

Smoking during pregnancy increases the risk of low birthweight. Smoking appeared to overlap predictors of low birthweight that included race, no previous livebirths, and body weight under 100 pounds (Micheliutte *et al.* 1992). The yields of tar, nicotine and carbon monoxide seemed to be important in one study in which mothers who smoked low-toxin yield cigarettes had babies of similar birthweights as non-smoking mothers (Peacock *et al.* 1991).

SOCIAL, CULTURAL AND BEHAVIORAL FACTORS
One study emphasized the effect of maternal age, social and demographic status, prenatal health and behavior on neonatal outcomes. Of four primiparous age groups (13–15, 16–18, 19–21, 22–30 years old), the youngest mothers had the least weight gain, and gave birth to babies of lower birthweights with shorter gestation periods. A major conclusion was that interventions should emphasize the prevention of pregnancy in young adolescents and betterment of social and economic conditions (Ketterlinus *et al.* 1990).

ETHICAL ISSUES
Steinberg (1993) attempted to offer a perspective on the dispute of whether the intensive neonatal care programs should be continued in very low-birthweight infants. The argument in the 1980s was whether to save infants weighing below 2500 g. In the 1990s no one disputes the policy of treating babies below 1500 g. The debate centers on saving extremely low-weight infants, below 1000 g, 'micronates'. Outcome studies of these micronates indicate that the mortality rate approached 90% at below 26 weeks' gestational age. At follow-up 23% of the survivors had a physical impairment. By 1987 the survival rates had improved to 50%. In another study 71% of the deaths occurred in the first 48 hours of life. Survival rates of infants weighing 500–799 g have varied from 5% to 61% with increasing survivorship as birthweights increased. The incidence of severe neurological sequelae varies considerably among reports. Because there are few prognostic factors for mortality or morbidity in the individual baby and that the resultant disability may be mild or moderate and successfully managed, Steinberg (1993) came down on the side of the preservation of life.

PERINATAL
Fetal electronic monitoring of preterm infants with the aim of reducing the incidence of cerebral palsy is controversial and mostly negative (Freeman 1990). A study by Shy and colleagues (1990) showed there was no benefit from it. Furthermore the incidence of cerebral palsy was higher in the monitored babies than in the non-monitored. Nevertheless, routine fetal monitoring has become the standard of care in delivery facilities. As

reported in 10 relevant studies, cesarean delivery resulted in no significant difference in the rates of cerebral palsy (Scheller and Nelson 1994). Fetal monitoring has been used to determine fetal distress and if found, an indication for cesarean section occurs.

Nelson and associates (1996) did a study of fetal monitoring of 155,636 children born between 1983 and 1985 in four California counties. They identified 95 singleton infants whose birthweight was at least 2500 g and survived until the age of 3 years with moderate or severe cerebral palsy. Of these 78 had fetal monitoring and were compared with 300 of 378 controls. Their results showed that specific abnormal findings of the fetal heart rate were associated with the risk of cerebral palsy, but the false-positive rate was extremely high. Because of the high false-positive rate, the authors expressed concern that if these indications for cesarean section were widely used, many cesarean sections would be of no benefit and would risk potential harm to the mother.

Phototherapy for *hyperbilirubinemia* was found as effective as management with only exchange transfusions in a follow-up study at 1 and 6 years of 1339 newborns from six neonatal care centers. The incidence of cerebral palsy in the phototherapy group and the control exchange transfusion group was the same, at 5.8% and 5.9% (Scheidt *et al.* 1990). The neurological effect of bilirubin serum levels on the rate of cerebral palsy was determined in a 6-year follow-up study of 224 control children with birthweights less than 2000 g treated with exchange transfusions (Scheidt *et al.* 1991). The rates of cerebral palsy were not significantly higher in children whose bilirubin levels were at the maximum or in those whose levels remained low. No association was found between the IQ and the bilirubin level or its time of exposure.

In this chapter we have examined the basics of our study of cerebral palsy and its care. This includes an early history of modern medical care, definitions, classifications, our tools for assessing the severity of the problems, predictive tools and preventative measures. Continued refinement of these areas will help sort out effective care and early counseling for families of affected children. Subsequent chapters will further deepen the discussion of the definitions and assessment tools, and show some of the outcomes of the medical, therapeutic and orthopaedic management of cerebral palsy.

REFERENCES

Accardo, P.J. (1982) 'Freud on diplegia—commentary and translation.' *American Journal of Diseases of Children*, **138**, 452–456.

Adler, N., Bleck, E.E., Rinsky, L.A., Young, W. (1986) 'Balance reactions and eye–hand coordination in idiopathic scoliosis.' *Journal of Orthopaedic Research*, **4**, 102–107.

Aicardi, J. (1998) *Diseases of the Nervous System in Childhood, 2nd edn.* London: Mac Keith Press with Cambridge University Press; Philadelphia, J.B. Lippincott, pp. 348–355.

Alberman, E. (1984a) 'Describing the cerebral palsies: methods of classifying and counting.' *In* Stanley, F., Alberman, E. (Eds) *The Epidemiology of the Cerebral Palsies. Clinics in Developmental Medicine, No. 87.* London: Spastics International Medical Publications with Heinemann Medical; Philadelphia: J.B. Lippincott, pp. 27–31.

—— (1984b) 'World health initiatives.' *In* Stanley, F., Alberman, E. (Eds) *The Epidemiology of the Cerebral Palsies. Clinics in Developmental Medicine, No.*

87. London: Spastics International Medical Publications with Heinemann Medical; Philadelphia: J.B. Lippincott, pp. 32–34.

Albright, L. (1995) 'Spastic cerebral palsy. Approaches to drug treatment.' *CNS Drugs*, **4**, 17–27.

Allan, W.C., Vohr, B., Makuch, R.W., Katz, K.H., Ment, L.R. (1997) 'Antecedents of cerebral palsy in a multicenter trial of indomethacin for intraventricular hemorrhage.' *Archives of Pediatric and Adolescent Medicine*, **151**, 580–585.

Al-Qurashi, A.R. (2004) 'Newborn screening for congenital infectious diseases.' *Journal of the Egyptian Society of Parasitology*, **34**, 23–34.

al-Rajeh, S., Bademosi, O., Awada, A., Ismail, H., Al-Shammasi, S., Dawodu, A. (1991) 'Cerebral palsy in Saudi Arabia: a case-control study of risk factors.' *Developmental Medicine and Child Neurology*, **33**, 1048–1052.

Amin-Zaki, L., Elhassani, S., Majeed, M.A., Clarkson, T.W. (1974) 'Intrauterine methyl-mercury poisoning in Iraq.' *Pediatrics*, **54**, 587–579.

Ashworth, B. (1964) 'Preliminary trial of carisoprodol in multiple sclerosis.' *Practitioner*, **192**, 540–542.

Astbury, J., Orgill, A.A., Bajuk, B., Yu, V.Y. (1990) 'Neurodevelopmental outcome, growth and health of extremely low birthweight survivors: how soon can we tell?' *Developmental Medicine and Child Neurology*, **32**, 582–589.

Badawi, N., Watson, L., Petterson, B., Blair, E., Slee, J., Haan, E., Stanley, F. (1998) 'What constitutes cerebral palsy?' *Developmental Medicine and Child Neurology*, **40**, 520–527.

Baird, H.W., Gordon, E.C. (1983) *Neurological Evaluation of Infants and Children. Clinics in Developmental Medicine, Nos 84/85*. London: Spastics International Medical Publications with Heinemann Medical; Philadelphia: J.B. Lippincott.

Barkovich, A.J., Lindan, C.E. (1994) 'Congenital cytomegalovirus infection of the brain: imaging analysis and embryologic considerations.' *American Journal of Neuroradiology*, **15**, 703–715.

—— Baranski, K., Vigneron, D., Partridge, J.S., Hallam, D.K, Hajnai, B.L., Ferriero, D.M. (1999) 'Proton MR spectroscopy for the evaluation of brain injury in asphyxiated, term neonates.' *American Journal of Neuroradiology*, **20**, 1399–1405.

—— Girard, N. (2003) 'Fetal brain infections.' *Child's Nervous System*, **19**, 501–517.

Batshaw, M.L., Perret, Y.M. (1992) *Children with Disabilities*. Baltimore: Paul H. Brookes, pp. 45–46.

Bax, M. (2001) 'What's in a name?' *Developmental Medicine and Child Neurology*, **43**, 75.

Bertrand, J., Floyd, R.L., Weber, M.K. (2004) *Fetal Alcohol Syndrome: Guidelines for Referral and Diagnosis*. Atlanta, GA: US Department of Health and Human Services, CDC.

Bhushan, V., Paneth, N., Kiely, J.L. (1993) 'Impact of improved survival of very low birth weight infants on recent secular trends in the prevalence of cerebral palsy.' *Pediatrics*, **91**, 1094–1100.

Bick, E.M. (1976) *Classics of Orthopaedics*. Philadelphia: J.B. Lippincott, pp. 140–148.

Blair, E., Stanley, F.J. (1988) 'Intrapartum asphyxia: a rare cause of cerebral palsy.' *Journal of Pediatrics*, **112**, 515–519.

Bleck, E.E., Nagel, D.A. (1982) *Physically Handicapped Children: A Medical Atlas for Teachers, 2nd edn*. Orlando, FL: Grune & Stratton.

Bohannon, R.W., Smith, M.B. (1987) 'Interrater reliability of a modified Ashworth scale of muscle spasticity.' *Physical Therapy*, **67**, 206–207.

Boiteau, M., Malouin, F., Richards, D.L. (1995) 'Use of a hand-held dynamometer and a Kin-Com dynamometer for evaluating spastic hypertonia in children: a reliability study.' *Physical Therapy*, **75**, 796–802.

Boppana, S.B., Fowler, K.B., Vaid, Y., Hedlund, G., Stagno, S., Britt, W.J., Pass, R.F. (1997) 'Neuroradiographic findings in the new born period and long term outcome in children with symptomatic cytomegalovirus infection.' *Pediatrics*, **99**, 109–414.

Boucher, F.D., Yasukawa, L.L., Bronzan, R.N., Hensliegh, P.A., Arvin, A.M., Prober, C.G. (1990) 'A prospective evaluation of primary genital herpes simplex virus type 2 infections acquired during pregnancy.' *Pediatric Infectious Disease Journal*, **9**, 499–504.

Buescher, P.A., Meis, P.T., Ernest, J.M., Moore, M.L., Michielutte, R., Sharp, P. (1988) 'A comparison of women in and out of a prematurity prevention project in North Carolina prenatal care region.' *American Journal of Public Health*, **78**, 264–267.

Canterino, J.S., Verma, U.L., Visintainer, P.F., Figueroa, R., Klein, S.A., Tejani, N.A. (1999) 'Maternal magnesium sulfate and the development of neonatal periventricular leukomalacia and intraventricular hemorrhage.' *Obstetrics and Gynecology*, **93**, 396–402.

Cooke, R.W. (1999) 'Trends in incidence of cranial ultrasound lesions and cerebral palsy in very low birthweight infants 1982–1993.' *Archives of Disease in Childhood. Fetal and Neonatal Edition*, **80**, F115–117.

Coskun, A., Lenquin, M., Segal, M., Vigneron, D.B., Ferriero, D.M., Barkovich, A.J. (2001) 'Quantitative analysis of MR images in asphyxiated neonates: correlation with neurodevelopmental outcomes.' *American Journal of Neuroradiology*, **22**, 400–405.

Covington, D.L., Carl, J., Daley, J.G., Cushing, D., Churchill, M.P. (1988) 'Effects of the North Carolina Prematurity Prevention Program among public patients delivering at the New Hanover Memorial Hospital.' *American Journal of Public Health*, **78**, 1493–1495.

Critchley, M. (Ed.) (1978) *Butterworths Medical Dictionary, 2nd edn*. London: Butterworths.

Doyle, L.W., Kelly, E.A., Rickards, A.L., Ford, G.W., Callanan, C. (1993) 'Sensorineural outcome at 2 years for survivors of erythroblastosis treated with fetal intravascular transfusions.' *Obstetrics and Gynecology*, **81**, 931–935.

Ducroquet, P. (1968) *Walking and Limping*. Philadelphia: J.B. Lippincott.

Edebol-Tysk, K., Hagberg, B., Hagberg, G. (1989) 'Epidemiology of spastic tetraplegic cerebral palsy in Sweden. II. Prevalence, birth data and origin.' *Neuropediatrics*, **20**, 46–52.

Ellenberg, J.H., Nelson, K.B. (1979) 'Birthweight and gestational age in children with cerebral palsy or seizure disorders.' *American Journal of Diseases of Children*, **133**, 1044–1048.

Ellis, M.R., Kane, K.Y. (2001) 'Lightening the lead load in children.' *American Family Physician*, **62**, 545–554, 559–560.

Engsberg, J.R., Olree, K.S., Ross, S.A., Park, T.S. (1996) 'Quantitative clinical measure of spasticity in children with cerebral palsy.' *Archives of Physical Medicine and Rehabilitation*, **77**, 594–599.

—— (1998) 'Spasticity and strength changes as a function of selective dorsal rhizotomy.' *Journal of Neurosurgery*, **88**, 1020–1026.

Ericson, A., Kallen, B. (1998) 'Very low birth weight boys at age of 19.' *Archives of Disease in Childhood. Fetal and Neonatal Edition*, **78**, F171–174.

Ernest, J.M., Michielutte, R., Meis, P.J., Moore, M.L., Sharp, P. (1988) 'Identification of women at high risk for pre-term-low-birthweight births.' *Preventative Medicine*, **17**, 60–72.

Escobar, G.J., Littenberg, B., Petitti, D.B. (1991) 'Outcome among surviving very low birthweight infants: a meta-analysis.' *Archives of Disease in Childhood*, **66**, 204–211.

Fennell, E.B., Dikel, T.N. (2001) 'Cognitive and neurophyschological functioning in children with cerebral palsy.' *Journal of Child Neurology*, **16**, 58–63.

Foley, J. (1992) 'Dyskinetic and dystonic cerebral palsy and birth.' *Acta Paediatrica (Norway)*, **81**, 57–60.

Freda, M.C., Damus, K., Merkatz, I.R. (1988) 'The urban community as the client in preterm birth prevention: evaluation of a program component.' *Social Science and Medicine*, **27**, 1439–1446.

Freeman, J.M., Nelson, K.B. (1988) 'Intrapartum asphyxia and cerebral palsy.' *Pediatrics*, **82**, 240–249.

—— Freeman, A.D. (1992) 'Cerebral palsy and the 'bad baby' malpractice crisis: New York State sheds light toward the end of the tunnel.' *American Journal of Diseases of Children*, **146**, 725–727.

Freeman, R. (1990) 'Intrapartum fetal monitoring—a disappointing story.' *New England Journal of Medicine*, **322**, 624–626.

Freud, S. (1968) *Infantile Cerebral Paralysis*. (Trans. by Russin, L.A.) Coral Gables, FL: University of Miami Press, p.158.

Gamble, J.G. (1988) *The Musculoskeletal System—Physiological Basics*. New York: Raven Press, p. 123.

Gesell, A., Amatruda, C.S. (1947) *Developmental Diagnosis, 2nd edn*. New York: Harper & Row.

Goldberg, M.J. (1987) *The Dysmorphic Child*. New York: Raven Press, pp. 358–364.

Govaert, P., de Vries, L.S. (1997) *An Atlas of Brain Sonography. Clinics in Developmental Medicine, Nos 141/142*. London: Mac Keith Press with Cambridge University Press; Philadelphia: J.B. Lippincott.

Grether, J.K., Nelson, K.B., Cummins, S.K. (1993) 'Twinning and cerebral palsy: experience in four northern California counties, birth 1983 through 1985.' *Pediatrics*, **92**, 845–858.

—— Nelson, K.B., Emery, E.S. 3rd, Cummins, S.K. (1996) 'Prenatal and perinatal factors and cerebral palsy in very low birth weight infants.' *Journal of Pediatrics*, **128**, 407–414.

—— —— (1997) 'Maternal infection and cerebral palsy in infants of normal birth weight.' *Journal of American Medical Association*, **278**, 207–211. (Erratum, 1998, *Journal of the American Medical Association*, 14, 279.)

—— Hoogstrate, J., Selvin, S., Nelson, K.B. (1998) 'Magnesium sulfate tocolysis and risk of neonatal death.' *American Journal of Obstetrics and Gynecology*, **178**, 1–6.

Grögaard, J.B., Lindstrom, D.P., Parker, R.A., Culley, B., Stahlman, M.T. (1990) 'Increased survival rate in very low birth weight infants (1500 grams or less): no association with increased incidence of handicaps.' *Journal of Pediatrics*, **117**, 139–146.

Hagberg, B., Hagberg, G., Olow, I., Van Wendt, L. (1996) 'The changing panorama of cerebral palsy in Sweden. VII: Prevalence and origin in birth year period 1987–1990.' *Acta Pediatrica*, **85**, 954–960.

Hallett, M. (1983) 'Analysis of abnormal voluntary and involuntary movements with surface electromyography.' *Advances in Neurology*, **39**, 907–917.

Hanna, J., Wild, B.E. (1991) 'Bacterial meningitis in children under the age of five years in Western Australia.' *Medical Journal of Australia*, **155**, 160–164.

Hansen, R.L., Ulrey, G.L. (1993) 'Knowns and unknowns in the outcomes of drug-dependent women.' *In* Anastasiow, N.J., Harel, S. (Eds) *At-Risk Infants.* Baltimore: Paul H. Brookes, p.136.

Harma, M., Harma, M., Gungen, N., Demir, N. (2004) 'Toxoplasmosis in prgnatn women in Sanliurfa, Southeastern Anatolia City, Turkey.' *Journal of the Egyptian Society of Parasitology*, **34**, 519–525.

Haslam, R.H.A., Allen, J. R., Dorsen, M.M., Kanofsky, D.L., Ingram, T.T.S. (1955) 'A study of cerebral palsy in the childhood population of Edinburgh.' *Archives of Disease in Childhood*, **30**, 85–98.

—— Allen, J.R., Dorsen, M.M., Kanofsky, D.L., Mellito, E.D., Norris, D.A. (1977) 'The sequelae of group B-hemolytic streptococcal meningitis in early infancy.' *American Journal of Diseases of Children*, **131**, 845–849.

—— (1984) 'A historical review of the definition and classification of the cerebral palsies.' *In* Stanley, F., Alberman, E. (Eds) *The Epidemiology of the Cerebral Palsies. Clinics in Developmental Medicine, No. 87.* London: Spastics International Medical Publications with Blackwell Scientific; Philadelphia: J.B. Lippincott, pp. 1–11.

Helsel, P., McGee, J., Graveline, C. (2001) 'Physical management of spasticity.' *Journal of Child Neurology*, **16**, 24–30.

Hoon, A.H. Jr, Reinhardt, E.M., Kelley, R.I., Brieter, S.N., Morton, D.H., Naidu, S.G., Johnston, M.V. (1997) 'Brain magnetic resonance imaging in suspected extrapyramidal cerebral palsy: observations in distinguishing genetic-metabolic from acquired causes.' *Pediatrics*, **131**, 240–245.

Jauniaux, E., Gulbis, B., Acharya, G., Thiry, P., Rodeck, C. (1999) 'Maternal tobacco exposure and cotinine levels in fetal fluids in the first half of pregnancy.' *Obstetrics and Gynecology*, **93**, 25–29.

Javier, F.C. 3rd, McCormick, D.P., Alcock. W. (1999) 'Lead screening among low-income children in Galveston, Texas.' *Clinical Pediatrics*, **38**, 655–660.

Johgmans, M., Meercuri, E., de Vries, L., Dubowitz, L., Henderson, S.E. (1997) 'Minor neurological signs and perceptual-motor difficulties in prematurely born children.' *Archives of Disease in Childhood. Fetal and Neonatal Edition*, **76**, F9–14.

Jones, A.R. (1949) 'William John Little.' *Journal of Bone and Joint Surgery*, **31B**, 123–126.

Ketterlinus, R.D., Henderson, S.H., Lamb, M.E. (1990) 'Maternal age, sociodemographics, prenatal health and behavior: influence on neonatal risk factors.' *Journal of Adolescent Health Care*, **11**, 423–431.

Kindt, J., Retzke, U., Ketscher, K.D., Gabler, G. (1991) 'Decreases in premature birth rate through consequent application of diagnostic and therapeutic standards in pregnancy monitoring.' *Zentralblatt für Gynakologie*, **113**, 431–437.

Kitayaporn, D., Charoenlarp, P., Pattaraarechachai, J., Phlopoti, T. (1991) 'G6pd deficiency and fava bean consumption do not produce hemolysis in Thailand.' *Southeast Asian Journal of Tropical Medicine and Public Health (Thailand)*, **22**, 176–182.

Koren, G., Graham, K. (1992) 'Cocaine in pregnancy: analysis of fetal risk.' *Veterinary and Human Toxicology*, **34**, 263–264.

Krägeloh-Mann, I., Hagberg, B., Meisner, C., Haas, G., Eeg-Olofsson, K.E., Selbmann, H.K., Hagberg, B., Michaelis, R. (1995) 'Bilateral spastic cerebral palsy—a collaborative study between South-West Germany and West Sweden. III. Etiology.' *Developmental Medicine and Child Neurology*, **37**, 191–203.

Kyrklund-Blomberg, N.B., Cnattingius, S. (1998) 'Preterm birth and maternal smoking: risks related to gestational age and onset of delivery.' *American Journal of Obstetrics and Gynecology*, **179**, 1051–1055.

Larroque, B. (1992) 'Alcohol and the fetus.' *International Journal of Epidemiology*, **21** (Suppl. 1), 8–16.

Leogrande, G. (1992) 'Studies on the epidemiology of child infections in the Bari area (south Italy).V. Epidemiology of Toxoplasma gondii infections.' *Microbiologica*, **15**, 237–241.

Lequien, P., Delecour, M., Puech, F., Lecoutour, X., Dubos, J. P., Valat, A. S., Kacet, N., Moriso, C., Germillet, C., Pierrat, V. (1990) 'Evolution of the prematurity before the 32nd week from 1980 to 1985 in a tertiary perinatal center in Lille, France.' *European Journal of Obstetrics, Gynecology and Reproductive Biology*, **34**, 59–65.

Little, W.J. (1862) 'On the influence of abnormal parturition, difficult labor, premature birth and asphyxia neonatorum, on the mental and physical condition of the child, especially in relation to deformities.' *Transactions of the Obstetrical Society of London*, **3**, 293.

Lorenz, J.M., Wooliver, D.E., Jetton, J.R., Paneth, N.A. (1998) 'Quantitative review of mortality and developmental disability in extremely premature infants.' *Archives of Pediatrics and Adolescent Medicine*, **152**, 425–435.

Lubis, M.U., Tjipta, G.D., Marbun, M.D., Saing, B. (1990) 'Cerebral palsy.' *Paediatrica Indonesia*, **30**, 65–70.

Markowitz, M. (2000) 'Lead poisoning: a disease for the next millennium.' *Current Problems in Pediatrics*, **30**, 62–70.

Martin, M.L., Khoury, M.J., Cordero, J.F., Waters, G.D. (1992) 'Trends in rates of multiple vascular disruption defects, Atlanta, 1968–1989: is there evidence of a cocaine teratogenic epidemic?' *Teratology*, **45**, 674–653.

McCormick, M.C. (1985) 'The contribution of low birth weight to infant mortality and childhood morbidity.' *New England Journal of Medicine*, **312**, 82–90.

McMahon, T.A. (1984) *Muscles, Reflexes, and Locomotion.* Princeton: Princeton University Press.

Meberg, A., Broch, H. (1995) 'A changing pattern of cerebral palsy. Declining trend for incidence of cerebral palsy in the 20-year period 1970–89.' *Journal of Perinatal Medicine*, **23**, 395–402.

Medical Underwriters of California (2001) *California Large Loss Trend Study.* 6250 Claremont Ave., Oakland, CA 94618–1324; www.miec.com

Merrill, J.D., Piecuch, R.E., Fell, S.C., Barkovich, A.J., Goldstein, R.B. (1998) 'A new pattern of cerebellar hemorrhage in preterm infants.' *Pediatrics*, **102**, E62.

Meloni, T., Forteleoni, G., Meloni, G.F. (1992) 'Marked decline of favism after neonatal glucose-6-phosphate dehydrogenase screening and health education.' *Acta Haematologica (Switzerland)*, **87**, 29–31.

Michielutte, R., Ernest, J.M., Moore, M.L., Meis, P.J., Sharp, P.C., Wells, H.B., Buescher, P.A. (1992) 'A comparison of risk assessment models for term and preterm low birthweight.' *Preventative Medicine*, **21**, 98–109.

Mueller-Heuback, E., Reddick, D., Barnett, B., Bente, R. (1989) 'Preterm birth prevention: evaluation of a prospective controlled randomized trial.' *American Journal of Obstetrics and Gynecology*, **160**, 1172–1178.

Murphy, D.J., MacKenzie, I.A. (1995) 'The mortality and morbidity associated with umbilical cord prolapse.' *British Journal of Obstetrics and Gynaecology*, **102**, 826–830.

Mutch, L., Alberman, E., Hagberg, B., Kodama, K., Perat, M.V. (1992) 'Cerebral palsy epidemiology: where are we now and where are we going?' *Developmental Medicine and Child Neurology*, **34**, 547–555.

Muybridge, E . (1887) *Animals in Motion.* (Reprinted 1957.) New York: Dover.

Nelson, K.B., Ellenberg, J.H. (1981) 'Apgar scores as a predictor of chronic neurologic disability.' *Pediatrics*, **68**, 36–44.

—— —— (1982) 'Children who outgrew cerebral palsy.' *Pediatrics*, **69**, 529–536.

—— Grether, J.K. (1995) 'Can magnesium sulfate reduce the risk of cerebral palsy in very low birthweight infants?' *Developmental Medicine and Child Neurology*, **95**, 263–269.

—— Dambrosia, J.M., Ting, T.Y., Grether, J.K. (1996) 'Uncertain value of electronic fetal monitoring in predicting cerebral palsy.' *New England Journal of Medicine*, **334**, 613–618.

—— Grether, J.K. (1998) 'Potentially asphyxiating conditions and spastic cerebral palsy in infants of normal birth weight.' *American Journal of Obstetrics and Gynecology*, **179**, 507–513.

18

—— —— (1999) 'Selection of neonates for neuroprotective therapies: one set of criteria applied to a population.' *Archives of Pediatrics and Adolescent Medicine*, **153**, 393–398.

Neto, E.C., Rubin, R., Schulte, J., Giugliani, R. (2004) 'Newborn screening for congenital infectious diseases.' *Emerging Infectious Diseases*, **10**, 1053–1068.

Nottidge, V.A., Okogbo, M.E. (1991) 'Cerebral palsy in Ibadan, Nigeria.' *Developmental Medicine and Child Neurology*, **33**, 241–245.

Okumura, A., Kato, T., Kuno, K., Hayakawa, F., Watanabe, K. (1997a) 'MRI findings in patient with spastic cerebral palsy. I: Correlation with gestational age at birth.' *Developmental Medicine and Child Neurology*, **39**, 363–368.

—— —— —— —— —— (1997b) 'MRI findings in patient with spastic cerebral palsy. II: Correlation with type of cerebral palsy.' *Developmental Medicine and Child Neurology*, **39**, 369–372.

O'Shea, T.M., Klinepeter, K.L., Goldstein, D.J., Jackson, B.W., Dillard, R.G. (1997) 'Survival and developmental disability to infants with birth weights of 501–800 grams, born between 1979 and 1994.' *Pediatrics*, **100**, 982–986.

Osler, W. (1987) *The Cerebral Palsies of Children, Classics in Developmental Medicine, No.1.* London: Mac Keith Press with Blackwell Scientific; Philadelphia: J.B. Lippincott.

Otis, J.C., Root, L., Pamilla, J.R., Kroll, M.A. (1983) 'Biomechanical measurement of spastic plantarflexors.' *Developmental Medicine and Child Neurology*, **25**, 60–66.

Paneth, N., Kiely, J. (1984) 'The frequency of cerebral palsy: a review of population studies in industrialized nations since 1950.' *In* Stanley, F., Alberman, E. (Eds) *The Epidemiology of the Cerebral Palsies. Clinics in Developmental Medicine, No. 87.* London: Spastics International Medical Publications with Heinemann Medical; Philadelphia: J.B. Lippincott, pp. 46–56.

Papiernik, E. (1991) 'The very tiny baby, multiple births, and other questions about preterm deliveries.' *Current Opinion in Obstetrics and Gynecology*, **4**, 4–7.

Peacock, J.L., Bland, J.M., Anderson, H.R., Brooke, O.G. (1991) 'Cigarette smoking and birthweight: type of cigarette smoked and a possible threshold effect.' *International Journal of Epidemiology*, **20**, 405–412.

Perry, J. (1992) *Gait Analysis. Normal and Pathological Function.* Thorofare, NJ: Slack, pp. 386–395.

Peters, H., Thorell, D.J. (1991) 'Fetal and neonatal effects of maternal cocaine use.' *Journal of Obstetric, Gynecologic, and Neonatal Nursing*, **20**, 121–126.

Petterson, B., Nelson, K.B., Watson, L., Stanley, F. (1993) 'Twins, triplets, and cerebral palsy in births in Western Australia in the 1980s.' *British Medical Journal*, **307**, 1239–1243.

Pharoah, P.O., Butterfield, I.H., Hetzel, B.S. (1971) 'Neurological damage to the fetus resulting from severe iodine deficiency during pregnancy.' *Lancet*, **i**, 308–301.

—— Platt, M. J., Cooke, T. (1996) The changing epidemiology of cerebral palsy.' *Archives of Disease in Childhood. Fetal Neonatal Edition*, **75**, F169–173.

—— Cooke, T., Johnson, M.A., King, R., Mutch, L. (1998) 'Epidemiology of cerebral palsy in England and Scotland.' *Archives of Disease in Childhood. Fetal and Neonatal Edition*, **79**, F21–25.

Phelps, W.M. (1990) 'Cerebral birth injuries: their orthopaedic classification and subsequent treatment, 1932.' *Clinical Orthopedics and Related Research*, **253**, 4–11.

Pinto-Martin, J.A., Riolo, S., Cnaan, A., Holzman, C., Susser, M.W., Paneth, N. (1995) 'Cranial ultrasound prediction of disabling and non-disabling cerebral palsy at age two in a low birth weight population.' *Pediatrics*, **95**, 249–254.

Price, R., Bjornson, K.F., Lehman, J.F., McLaughlin, J.F., Hayes, R.M. (1991) 'Quantitative measurement of spasticity in children with cerebral palsy.' *Developmental Medicine and Child Neurology*, **33**, 585–595.

Ranck, J.B., Windle, W.F. (1959) 'Brain damage in the monkey Macacca mulatta by asphyxia neonatorum.' *Experimental Neurology*, **1**, 130–154.

Rang, M. (1990) 'Cerebral palsy.' *In* Morrissy, R.T. (Ed.) *Lovell and Winter's Pediatric Orthopaedics, 3rd edn.* Philadelphia: J.B. Lippincott.

Reddihough, D.S., Collins, K.J. (2003) 'The epidemiology and causes of cerebral palsy.' *Australian Journal of Physiotherapy*, **49**, 7–12.

Rogers, B., Msall, M., Owens, T., Guernsey, K. Brody, A., Buck, G., Hudak, M. (1994) 'Cystic periventricular leukomalacia and type of cerebral palsy in preterm infants.' *Journal of Pediatrics*, **125**, S1–8.

Rosen, M.G., Dickinson, J.C. (1992) 'The incidence of cerebral palsy.' *American Journal of Obstetrics and Gynecology*, **167**, 417–423.

Rosenbaum, P., Paneth, N., Leviton, A., Goldstein, M., Bax, M., Damiano, D., Dan, B., Jacobsson, B. (2007) 'Definition and classification of cerebral palsy.' *Developmental Medicine and Child Neurology*, **49**, suppl. 109.

Rouse, D.J., Hauth, J.C., Nelson, K.G., Goldenberg, R.L. (1996) 'The feasibility of a randomized clinical perinatal trial: maternal magnesium sulfate for the prevention of cerebral palsy.' *American Journal of Obstetrics and Gynecology*, **175**, 701–705.

Ruckhaberle, K.E., Viehweg, B., Reichel, S., Schninagl, A. (1992) 'Evaluation of efforts in prenatal care for the prevention of prematurity.' *Zentralblatt für Gynakologie*, **114**, 231–237.

Russell, D.J., Rosenbaum, P.L., Cadman D.T., Gowland, C., Hardy, S., Jarvis, S. (1989) 'The gross motor function measure: a means to evaluate the effects of physical therapy.' *Developmental Medicine and Child Neurology*, **31**, 341–352.

Rutherford, M.A., Pennock, J.M., Murdoch-Eaton, D.M., Cowan, F.M., Dubowitz, L.M. (1992) 'Athetoid cerebral palsy with cysts in the putamen after hypoxic–ischaemic encephalopathy.' *Archives of Disease of Children*, **67**, 846–850.

Salokorpi, T., Sajaniemi, N., Hallback, H., Kari, A., Rita, H., Von Wendt, L. (1997) 'Randomized study of the effect of antenatal dexamethasone on growth and development of premature children at the corrected age of 2 years.' *Acta Pediatrica*, **86**, 294–298.

Schantz, P.M., McAuley, J. (1991) 'Current status of food-borne parasitic zoonoses in the United States.' *Southeast Asian Journal of Tropical Medicine and Public Health*, **22** (Suppl.), 65–71.

Scheidt, P.C., Bryla, D.A., Nelson, K.B., Hirtz, D.G., Hoffman, H.J. (1990) 'Phototherapy for neonatal hyperbilirubinemia: six-year follow-up of the National Institute of Child Health and Human Development clinical trial.' *Pediatrics*, **85**, 455–463.

—— Graubard, D.I., Nelson, K.B., Hirtz, D.B., Hoffman, H.J., Gartner, L.M., Bryla, D.A. (1991) 'Intelligence at six years in relation to neonatal bilirubin levels: follow-up of the National Institute of Child Health and Human Development Clinical Trial of Phototherapy.' *Pediatrics*, **87**, 797–805.

Scheller, J.M., Nelson, K.B. (1994) 'Does cesarean delivery prevent cerebral palsy or other neurologic problems of childhood?' *Obstetrics and Gynecology*, **83**, 624–630.

Schendel, D.E., Berg, C.J., Yeargin-Allsopp, M., Boyle, C.A., Decoufle, F. (1996) 'Prenatal magnesium sulfate exposure and the risk for cerebral palsy or mental retardation among very low-birth-weight children aged 3–5 years.' *Journal of the American Medical Association*, **276**, 1805–1810.

Schiffrin, B.S., Longo, L.D. (2000) 'William John Little and cerebral palsy. A reappraisal.' *European Journal of Obstetrics, Gynecology, and Reproductive Biology*, **90**, 139–144.

Shepherd, G. M. (1994) *Neurobiology, 3rd edn.* New York and Oxford: Oxford University Press.

Shy, K.K., Luthy, D.A., Bennett, F.C., Whitfield, M., Larson, E.B., van Belle, G., Hughes, J.P., Wilson, J.A., Stenchever, M.A. (1990) 'Effects of fetal heart-rate monitoring, as compared with periodic auscultation, on the neurologic development of pre-term infants.' *New England Journal of Medicine*, **322**, 588–593.

Simon, E.M., Goldstein, R.B., Coakley, F.V., Filly, R.A., Broderick, K.C., Musci, T.J., Barkovich, A.J. (2000) 'Fast MR imaging of fetal CNS anomalies in utero.' *American Journal of Neuroradiology*, **21**, 1688–1698.

Singer, L.T., Garber, R., Kliegman, R. (1991) 'Neurobehavioral sequelae of fetal cocaine exposure.' *Journal of Pediatrics*, **119**, 667–672.

Sköld, C., Harms-Ringdahl, K., Hultling, C., Levi, R., Seiger, A. (1998) 'Simultaneous Ashworth measurements and electromyographic recordings in tetraplegic patients.' *Archives of Physical Medicine and Rehabilitation*, **79**, 959–965.

Slominski, A.H. (1984) 'Winthrop Phelps and the Children's Rehabilitation Institute.' *In* Scrutton, D. (Ed.) *Management of Motor Disorders of Children with Cerebral Palsy. Clinics in Developmental Medicine, No. 90.* London: Spastics International Medical Publications with Blackwell Scientific; Philadelphia: J.B. Lippincott, pp. 59–74.

Squier, M., Keeling, J.W. (1991) 'The incidence of prenatal brain injury.' *Neuropathology and Applied Neurobiology*, **17**, 29–38.

Stanley, F. (1984) 'Prenatal risk factors in the study of the cerebral palsies.' *In* Stanley, F., Alberman (Eds) *Epidemiology of the Cerebral Palsies. Clinics in Developmental Medicine, No. 87.* London: Spastics International Medical

Publications with Blackwell Scientific; Philadelphia: J.B. Lippincott, pp. 87–97.

—— Alberman, E. (1984) 'Birthweight, gestational age and the cerebral palsies.' *In* Stanley, F., Alberman, E. (Eds) *The Epidemiology of the Cerebral Palsies. Clinics in Developmental Medicine, No. 87.* London: Spastics International Medical Publications with Blackwell Scientific; Philadelphia: J.B. Lippincott, pp. 57–68.

—— Blair, E. (1984) 'Postnatal risk factors in the cerebral palsies.' *In* Stanley, F., Alberman, E. (Eds) *The Epidemiology of the Cerebral Palsies. Clinics in Developmental Medicine, No. 87.* London: Spastics International Medical Publications with Blackwell Scientific; Philadelphia: J.B. Lippincott, pp. 135–149.

—— Blair, E. (1991) 'Why have we failed to reduce the frequency of cerebral palsy?' *Medical Journal of Australia*, **154**, 623–626.

—— Watson, L. (1992) 'Trends in perinatal mortality and cerebral palsy in Western Australia 1967–1985.' *British Medical Journal*, **304**, 1658–1663.

—— Blair, E., Alberman, E. (2000) *Cerebral Palsies: Epidemiology and Causal Pathways. Clinics in Developmental Medicine, No. 151.* London: Mac Keith Press with Cambridge University Press; Philadelphia: J.B. Lippincott.

Steinberg, A. (1993) 'Ethical issues in early intervention.' *In* Anastasiow, N.J., Harel, S. (Eds) *At-Risk Infants.* Baltimore: Paul H. Brookes.

Sugimoto, T., Woo, M., Nishida, N., Araki, A., Hara, T., Yasuhara, A., Kobayashi, Y., Yamanouchi, Y. (1995) 'When do brain abnormalities in cerebral palsy occur? An MRI study.' *Developmental Medicine and Child Neurology*, **37**, 285–292.

Terver, S., Levai, J.P., Bleck, E.E. (1981) 'Les buts raisonnables que l'on peut fixer à un infirme moteur cérébrale gravement handicapé.' *Motricité Cérébrale*, **2**, 55–68.

Thompson, C.M., Buccimazza, S.S., Webster, J., Malan, A.F., Molteno, C.D. (1993) 'Infants of less than 1250 grams birth weight at Groote Schuur Hospital: outcome at 1 and 2 years of age.' *Pediatrics*, **91**, 961–968.

Thompson, R.F. (2000) *The Brain: A Neuroscience Primer.* New York: Worth.

Truex, R.C., Carpenter, M.D. (1969) *Human Neuroanatomy.* Baltimore: Williams & Wilkins.

Truitt, C.L., Barkovich, A.J., Koch, T.K., Ferriero, D.M. (1992) 'Cerebral palsy: MR findings in 40 patients.' *American Journal of Neuroradiology*, **13**, 67–78.

Uvebrant, P. (1988) 'Hemiplegic cerebral palsy. Aetiology and outcome.' *Acta Paediatrica Scandinavica*, Suppl. **354**, 1–100.

van de Riet, J.E., Vandenbussche, F.P., Le Cessie, S., Keirse, M.J. (1999) 'Newborn assessment and long-term adverse outcome: a systematic review.' *American Journal of Obstetrics and Gynecology*, **180**, 1024–1029.

Vigneron, D.B., Barkovich, A.J., Noworolski, S.M., von dem Bussche, M., Henry, R.G., Lu, Y., Patridge, J.C., Gregory, G., Ferriero, D.M. (2001) 'Three-dimensional proton MR spectroscopic imaging of premature and term neonates.' *American Journal of Neuroradiology*, **22**, 1424–1433.

Wilkins, R.H., Brody, L.A. (1969) 'Little's Disease.' *Archives of Neurology*, **20**, 217–224.

Wiklund, L.M., Uvebrant, P., Flodmark, O. (1991) 'Computed tomography as an adjunct in the etiological analysis of hemiplegic cerebral palsy: II. Children born at term.' *Neuropediatrics (Germany)*, **22**, 121–128.

—— Uvebrant, P. (1991) 'Hemiplegic cerebral palsy: correlation between CT morphology and clinical findings.' *Developmental Medicine and Child Neurology*, **33**, 512–513.

Wilson-Costello, D., Borawski, E., Friedman, H., Redline, R., Fanaroff, A.A., Hack, M. (1998) 'Perinatal correlates of cerebral palsy and other neurologic impairment among very low birth weight children.' *Pediatrics*, **102**, 315–322.

World Health Organization (2001) *International Classification of Functioning, Disability and Health. Short version.* Geneva: World Health Organization, p. 12.

Yeargin-Allsopp, M., Murphy, C.C., Oakley, G.P., Sikes, R.K. (1992) 'A multiple-source method for studying the prevalence of developmental disabilities in children: the Metropolitan Atlanta Developmental Disability Study.' *Pediatrics*, **89**, 624–630.

Yokoyama, Y., Shimizu, T., Hayakawa, K. (1995) 'Prevalence of cerebral palsy in twins, triplets and quadruplets.' *International Journal of Epidemiology*, **24**, 943–948.

Young, R.R. (1994) 'Spasticity: a review.' *Neurology*, **44**, S12–20.

2

PHYSICIAN'S NEUROLOGICAL AND ORTHOPAEDIC ASSESSMENT

'We have no routines in our clinic. When you have routines, everyone stops thinking.'

(Douglas Buchanan, MD)

ROLE OF THE ORTHOPAEDIST: DOCTOR OR TECHNICIAN?

The orthopaedist usually acts as a consultant upon referral of a pediatrician, family practitioner, neurologist or physiatrist, and consequently does not need to concentrate on the detailed examination of associated defects common to cerebral palsy. However, the surgeon does need to have at least a working knowledge of medical problems beyond the malfunction of the locomotor system. The surgeon is supposed to be a doctor of medicine first and an orthopaedic surgeon second. There are many excellent texts and chapters devoted to behavioral, intellectual, visual, communication, gastrointestinal, gynecological, urinary and pulmonary problems in developmental disabilities, of which cerebral palsy is one (Paine and Oppé 1966, Beadle 1982, Baird and Gordon 1983, Goble 1984, Rubin and Crocker 1989, Bratshaw and Perret 1992, Aicardi 1998). In addition, papers on a wide variety of associated defects in cerebral palsy can be accessed in the journal *Developmental Medicine and Child Neurology*. In some clinics the orthopaedic surgeon assumes the role of the primary physician to whom the child and parents can relate and obtain information. The important thing is that the parents should have access to one doctor who has a comprehensive view of the child and a perspective on a reasonable achievement of goals for ultimate functioning as an optimally independent person.

Occasionally the etiology of an orthopaedic or neuro-muscular condition will not have been diagnosed (for example, a unilateral valgus deformity of the foot with peroneal spasticity). In these instances the orthopaedic surgeon will have to use all the diagnostic skills he or she can muster: being aware of the refinements of certain parts of the neurological examination, and as with all patients, doing a complete physical examination to collect the data necessary to form an opinion. Although recent practice styles under the rubric of efficiency and cost-containment seem to favor paramedical personnel (e.g. nurse practitioners and physician's assistants) to obtain the clinical data of the history and physical examination for the physician, it seems wise for the doctor to personally take a good part of the history face-to-face and do the actual examination of the patient. For the physician not to do this time-consuming task misses the *Gestalt* of the patient–physician encounter. Furthermore, as Aicardi (1998) reminds us, 'the diagnosis of cerebral palsy is essentially clinical. Neuroimaging can have confirmatory value in some cases. Electromyography that may shed some light on the mechanisms has no place in practical diagnosis except for the exclusion of other conditions that share with CP some weakness or hypotonia.'

HISTORY OF THE PRESENT PROBLEM

MEDICAL RECORDS

Where available, medical records should be scanned for pertinent information on the prenatal, perinatal and postnatal events, and the child's development. Records may contain useful information on past treatment, especially if surgery has been performed. In view of the common complaint by patients that not enough time has been spent with them, rather than read the record in isolation, we prefer to bring the past record into the examining room, and scan the record with the parents. In this way we can ask them questions to clarify certain parts of the history.

Basic one-time historical data should be included in the consultant's record. A nurse or physician's assistant can obtain this information from the parents, and record it on a standard form. Birthdate, sex and ethnic background are obviously required. The details of the prenatal, perinatal and postnatal histories are often clues to the etiology. The family history will indicate possible genetic factors. A knowledge of convulsive disorders, medications, immunizations and allergies is necessary for preoperative planning and postoperative care. For the basic one-time data acquisition, Bleck (1987) published the form designed for use in our clinic. It assured, more or less, that important past historical data were included. But we found that physicians, in particular, hate forms and questionnaires. Nevertheless a checklist form or template designed by the physician and staff of the clinic or office still seems a good idea and helps with chart organization. The readers can construct their own forms. Figure 2.1 suggests items that might be included as a one-time background data-form. A companion form (Fig. 2.2) can record on each visit the important growth data of height and weight, as well as leg-length measurements in following a discrepancy, and radiographic measurements of a scoliosis.

It is essential for the physician to listen to the history (beyond the details from the past record and the one-time database). After the usual introductions, which include talking directly to the child, the physician should ask what the problems are. The clinician can delve into the history in more detail and gain insight into the parent's perception of their child's behavior: what their expectations might be, what fears they have and what hostilities are harbored. Some of this conversation might best take place without the child being present. This process will not only establish an all-important rapport, but may also reveal the diagnosis.

Serial Orthopaedic Measurements								
Name				**Record No**				
Visit No. Date	1	2	3	4	5	6	7	8
Height cm								
Weight kg								
Leg length Right cm								
Left cm								
Scoliosis:								
T__ to T__ Rt__ Lt__								
T__ to L__ Rt__ Lt__								
L__ to L__ Rt__ Lt__								
Risser 0-5								
Menarche								
Orthosis Surgery								

Code for Orthosis=O in box; Surgery=S in box with date.
Etiology of scoliosis_____
Non-ambulatory patient?_____
Independent walker?_____
Dependent walker?_____

Fig. 2.2. Example of format for recording growth measurement data serially, particularly useful in leg-length discrepancy and scoliosis follow-up to determine progression. Three curve patterns: thoracic, thoracolumbar, lumbar. If a double major curve, record the thoracic and lumbar segments separately, indicating curve to the right (Rt) or left (Lt).

Patient Identification:
1. Date:_____
2. Name:_____
3. Birth Date:_____
4. Record #_____
5. Sex:__Male=1 Female=2
6. Ethnic background(codes)___
7. Age problem first noted:____
8. Problem first noted by(codes)_
  1-Patient 2-Parent 3-Relative
  4-Friends 5-GP 6-Paediatrician
  7-Orthopaedist 8-Teacher
9. Other physicians consulted:
Name:_____
Address:_____
Name:_____
Address:_____
10. Chief Problem:✓
  1.Cerebral Palsy__2. Limps__
  3.Falls easily__4.Clumsy__
  5.Toes-in__6.Tips toes__
  7.Not walking__8.Other_____
11. Prior treatments(codes)
  None-1 Physical therapy-2
  Braces-3 Special Shoes-4
  Plaster casts-5 Surgery-6
12. Past Surgery and dates:
_____
_____
_____
13. Name of surgeon/institution:
_____
Address:_____
_____
14. Childhood diseases/illnesses:
_____
_____
15. Recent exposure to and date:
  Rubella?__ __ __
  Measles?__ __ __
  Chickenpox?__ __ __
  Tuberculosis?__ __ __
16. Family History:

Mother_____ Father_____
Siblings-No.___Ages:__,__,__,
17. Familial-Genetic disease:
  Bleeding disorder?_____
Diabetes?_____
  Other?_____
18. **Allergies?**_____
19. Current Medications:_____
20. Prenatal and Perinatal History
  Pregnancy Normal?_____
  Bleeding?____Eclampsia?____
21. Gestation(weeks)____
22. Birth Weight(kg/ lbs)_____
23. Labor-hours?____Induced?___
24. Breech?____C-Section?____
25. Heart-Respiratory Problem?___
26. Isolette?___
27. Rh mother?___Rh immuniz.?__
28. Blood transfusion?___
29. Jaundice?____Phototherapy?__
30. Hypoglycemia?___
31. Convulsions-1st week?___
32. Abnormal blood chemistry?____
Early Childhood Development
33. Fussy baby?_____Colic?____
34. Convulsions?_____
35. Sat alone(months)_____
36. Walked(months)_____
37. Talked(months)_____
38. Dominant hand?R___L___0___
Later Childhood Development
39. Grade in School_____
40. Special School or Classes?___
41. Academic Status(codes)_____
  Average=1 Below average=2
  Above average=3
42. Sports(code)_____
  None=0 Minimal=1
  Average=2 Above Average=3

Fig. 2.1. Format for 'one-time' background information. Numbers on left-hand side of column are for computer data input as desired.

ORTHOPAEDIC NEUROLOGICAL EXAMINATION

TOOLS

The tools required are simple: toys, some small wooden blocks, round beads or pebbles, various objects of readily identifiable shape (triangles, circles and squares), a few coins, objects with differing textures, a tape measure, a goniometer, a small reflex hammer, a pocket flashlight, a wax pencil, a right-angled triangle, and a rule 5–8 cm long. The wax pencil and right-angled triangle are useful for drawing on radiographs when explaining the findings to parents; the metric ruler can be used to measure discrepancies of anatomy (particularly the hip) visualized by radiography. One instrument not needed in the examination of children with cerebral palsy is a sharp pin or needle! Loss of pain sensation in these children must be very rare.

SPACE

If space is limited, it is more important to have a large corridor or waiting-room than a large examination room. Because cerebral palsy is defined primarily as a disorder of motion, the child must have adequate space in which to demonstrate movement. A corridor 2.5 m wide and at least 9 m long is necessary for observational gait analysis. This corridor should be well lit, carpeted with a compact firm surface, warm and well ventilated. The examination room should be large enough to contain a padded table, 75 cm wide, 75 cm high and 185 cm long. A step stool is important, to enable us to observe the child's climbing ability. There should be room for three chairs, for members of the family and observers (such as a social worker).

The physical-therapy gym—a room crowded with physical therapists cooing, singing and using rattles and bells (presumably for 'stimulation')—is not conducive to a thorough examination and a thoughtful discussion with the parents. The environment should be quiet and calm.

CLOTHING

To be adequately examined, children should be undressed to their underwear, and socks and shoes removed. Gowns ought to be abolished! For many years we have used shorts for boys and girls, and a triangular halter for girls who want their modesty protected. If keeping cloth garments on hand is a problem, we have found disposable paper shorts and halters practical and cost-effective.

SEQUENCE OF EXAMINATION

The sequence of the examination described here has evolved over the years. Others will have their own style of proceeding. The objective of the sequences, and the blend of the neurological with the orthopaedic examination, is to avoid shifting the child too often from one position to another as will occur when the orthopaedic examination is totally separate from the neurological. The purpose of the examination is to collect accurate data, effectively and efficiently, for the best possible analysis of the problem. It is the means by which the ends are achieved: a rationale for the recommended management, and a record that will permit subsequent evaluations.

The following sequences of the examination depend upon the age of the child and the status of his or her locomotor system.

For infants and young children (under the age of 6 years), start with the assessment of the upper limbs while the child is in the security of the mother's lap.

For older children who can stand and walk (with or without external supports), begin with assessment of the standing posture, then the observational gait analysis, then (with the child sitting) the upper limbs are examined and tested for function and sensation, and finally the lower limbs are assessed.

The child should be seated, with knees flexed over the edge of the table; then (1) check deep-tendon reflexes and the Babinski sign and its modifications (Chaddock's sign); and (2) obtain the position and the range of motion of the foot and its degree of axial rotation and tibial–fibular torsion.

The lower limbs can be assessed with the child lying first supine and then prone on the table.

For children who cannot walk or stand, obviously the spine and sitting posture need to be examined in this position. The spine and pelvis alignments are most effectively observed with the child sitting (assisted by the parents) with legs over the edge of the table.

INDIRECT EXAMINATION

We observe the child's behavior, verbal ability, facial configuration and expression, eye contact, head control, drooling, general build, nutrition and mood (see Baird and Gordon 1983). One can sense supportive, depressed or hostile parents. If the child is not sitting but moving about on the floor, movement disorders, postures, and hand preference can be ascertained. Appropriate toys should be available. During this time it should be possible to see how the child communicates.

INFANTILE AUTOMATISMS AND POSTURAL RESPONSES

'Posture accompanies movement like a shadow; movement begins in posture and ends in posture.'
(Sherrington, quoted by Rushworth 1964)

The supine posture of the infant and young child (less than 7 years old) who cannot stand or walk, or the child older than 7 years who has never walked, is best examined *after* the upper-limb and sitting-posture assessments. Retraction and abduction of the shoulders, elbow flexion, and an extension of the trunk and lower limbs is called the *tonic labyrinthine reflex*. It is common in infants who have central nervous system lesions. When such infants are placed prone, the upper and lower limbs assume a flexed position. These postural abnormalities of a delayed development of the central nervous system were described by Magnus, and were thought to originate in the brainstem mediated through the upper cervical nerve roots (Bobath 1954) (Fig. 2.3).

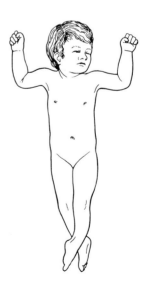

Fig. 2.3. Tonic labyrinthine reflex. When the baby is supine, the shoulders are abducted and elbows flexed, the spine is extended, and the lower limbs extended and abducted.

Infantile automatisms and postural responses can be tested while the infant or child is supine. Seven tests are considered valid for prognosis of walking, but only after the age of 12 months (Bleck 1975). The tests are performed in the following sequence. (See Chapter 5 for the interpretation of these responses for the purpose of a locomotor prognosis.)

1. *Asymmetric tonic neck reflex.* With the child supine, turn the head to one side and then the other. A positive response is flexion of the upper and lower limbs on the skull side, and extension on the face side—the 'fencing' position. The reflex may be found to a minor degree in normal infants up to the age of 7 months, but it is never normal if it can always be imposed and the child cannot move his or her limbs out of their position while the head is held turned to the side (Paine and Oppé 1966) (Fig. 2.4). In some children with cerebral palsy, only the upper limb may manifest the obvious reflex concomitant with lesser degrees of postural change in the lower limb; and the reflex may be positive with head turning to one side only.

2. *Neck-righting reflex.* This is positive if the shoulder girdle and trunk turn simultaneously when the head is turned. It is never normal if the child can be rolled over and over like a log (Fig. 2.5). In its transient but imposable form it disappears in all unaffected infants by 10 months of age (Paine and Oppé 1966).

3. *Moro reflex.* This is precisely defined and should not be confused with the startle response, which is normal in infants and throughout childhood. A startle is a mass myoclonic movement which can occur during sleep, with a sudden noise or anything that evokes fear. It is thought to be a cortical release phenomenon that decreases with maturation (Baird and Gordon 1983). The Moro reflex is a sudden abduction and extension of the upper limbs with spreading of the fingers followed by an embrace. The best way to elicit the response is by lifting, gently with the right hand under the upper thoracic spine and the left hand under the

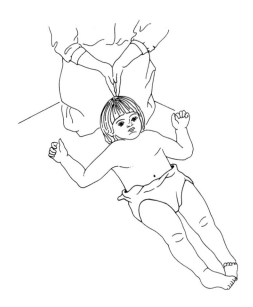

Fig. 2.6. Moro reflex elicited by a loud noise, jar of the table, or sudden extension of neck. The complete response is abduction of the upper limbs followed by the embrace.

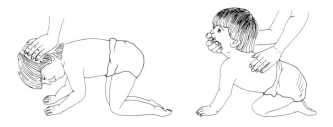

Fig. 2.7. Symmetrical tonic neck reflex. (*a*) Flexion of head causes flexion of forelimbs and extension of hindlimbs. Hindlimb extension is often suppressed due to predominant flexor pattern of spasticity. (*b*) Extension of head causes extension of forelimbs and flexion of hindlimbs.

head, and then dropping the left hand to allow neck extension (Baird and Gordon 1983). Suddenly jarring the examining table or making a loud noise is a more startling way to obtain the Moro reflex. In unaffected infants it disappears by age 6 months (Fig. 2.6).

4. *Symmetric tonic neck reflex.* The child is placed in the quadruped (crawling) position. When the head is flexed ventrally, flexion of the forelimbs and extension of the hindlimbs results (Fig. 2.7); extension of the head and neck causes extension of the forelimbs and flexion of the hindlimbs (Fig. 2.7). A positive reflex is normal up to the age of 6 months.

5. *Parachute reaction.* The child is prone and lifted horizontally from the table and then quickly lowered to the tabletop (not dropped!) With this movement, protective extension of the upper limbs and hands is automatic and is developed in all children by age 12 months (Paine and Oppé 1966) (Fig. 2.8). If the child has severe involvement of one upper limb, the protective placement of the upper limbs may be unilateral; if so, the test is still valid and positive.

6. *Foot-placement reaction.* With the child held by the chest and axillae, the dorsal surface of the feet is brought upward

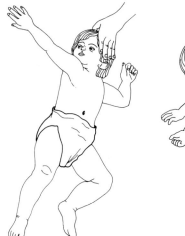

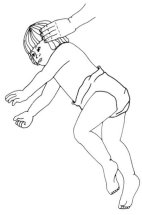

Fig. 2.4. Asymmetrical tonic neck reflex. When the head is turned, the limbs flex on the skull side (occipital) and extend on the face side.

Fig. 2.5. Neck-righting reflex. When the head is turned, the trunk and limbs turn to the same side.

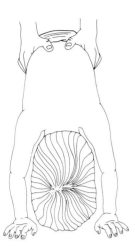

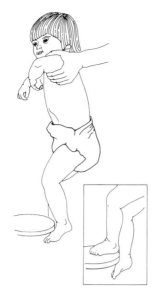

The *Landau reflex* is useful in documenting hypotonia. When the hypotonic infant (in cerebral palsy hypotonia often precedes athetosis) is raised in the horizontal prone position from the table, a collapse into the shape of an upside-down 'U' is classic. The true Landau reaction in unaffected infants is extension of the head and neck beyond the shoulder level, and extension of the spine. Spinal extension to form a concavity is not present in all infants until the age of 12 months (Baird and Gordon 1983). When the normal child is in this position, passive flexion of the head and neck causes loss of extensor tone. It has been used to assess the motor development of infants (Cupps *et al.* 1976).

THE HEAD

The head circumference should always be measured and compared with normal measurements (Fig. 2.11). Measurement is easier if done when the child is supine and before s/he gets too tired and irritable. In babies, the fontanelles should be palpated for evidence of closure. Bleck always auscultates the skull for a bruit. Rarely, one may find a vascular anomaly of the brain to explain the etiology of spastic hemiplegia.

Fig. 2.8. Parachute reaction. Child is lifted from table in prone position and suddenly lowered or tipped onto the tabletop. Normal response (after age 11 months) is automatic extension of the upper limbs and placement of hands on table's surface. With noticeable involvement of one upper limb, positive response can be unilateral.

Fig. 2.9. Foot-placement reaction. Child is lifted by axilla and torso so that the dorsa of the feet come up against underside of the table or chair. Automatic symmetrical or asymmetrical placement of feet on surface is normal response.

against the edge of the tabletop or chair (usually the edge of a plain unpadded chair or table-top is best). Automatic foot placement on the tabletop or chair surface occurs either symmetrically or asymmetrically. This response is normal in all infants. Suppression of it occurs with voluntary control, usually by the age of 3 or 4 years (Fig. 2.9).

7. *Extensor thrust.* When the child is lifted by the axilla and suspended, and then lowered so that the feet touch the floor or tabletop, it is always abnormal if there is definite and progressive extension of the lower limbs progressing upward into the trunk (Gesell and Amatruda 1947) (Fig. 2.10). Normal infants will flex their legs with this maneuver.

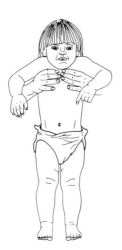

Fig. 2.10. Extensor thrust. When the child is suspended vertically in space and then lowered so that the feet touch the tabletop, progressive extension of the lower limbs progressing superiorly from the feet to the trunk is abnormal.

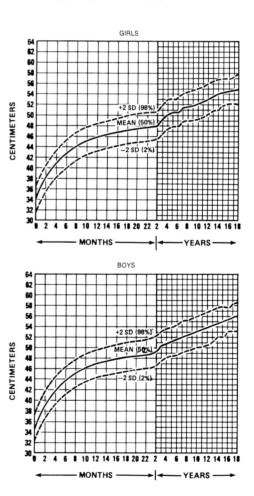

Fig. 2.11. Head circumference for girls (*top*) and boys (*bottom*). Head circumference below –2SD almost always indicates mental retardation. If head circumference approaches –4 SD, serious mental retardation is likely. Children with growth failure, but normal intelligence, have normal head circumferences. (From O'Connell *et al.* 1965.)

STANDING POSTURE

The standing posture should be observed from three views: lateral, posterior and anterior.

The *lateral* view permits observation of the head and neck position, thoracic kyphosis, lumbar lordosis, pelvic inclination and the position of the hip, knee, and ankle joints, and the feet (Figs 2.12, 2.13).

The extent of thoracic kyphosis and lumbar lordosis can be estimated by placing a meter rule against the mid-thoracic spine and sacrum. When significant thoracic kyphosis is suspected, the ruler deviates posteriorly from the perpendicular (Fig. 2.14). Additionally, the distance between the edge of the ruler and the mid-lumbar spine is a clinical measurement of lordosis. In normal children, this distance is no more than 4 cm (Fig. 2.14).

The *posterior* view will discern scoliosis which has been noted for many years as more common in children with total body involvement than in children without cerebral palsy (Robson 1968, Balmer and MacEwen 1970, Samilson and Bechard 1973, Madigan and Wallace 1981). Currently scoliosis is estimated to occur in 25% of patients with cerebral palsy and very frequently in non-ambulatory total body involved children in approximately 60%–75% (Thomson and Banta 2001). Scoliosis is indicated by inequality in the height of shoulders or pelvis, and a shift of the trunk that creates unilateral loin fullness. A retractable tape-measure in a spool serves nicely as a plumb-line which can be dropped from the tip of the first thoracic spinous process to delineate spinal alignment and balance. When the spine is perfectly balanced ('compensated'), the plumb-line from the first thoracic vertebra will cross the mid-sacrum and the gluteal fold.

An essential test for structural scoliosis is to ask the child to flex the trunk forward 90º at the hips with the upper limbs extended downward and forward, and to avoid trunk rotation as much as possible, with palms together (as if at prayer.) With the

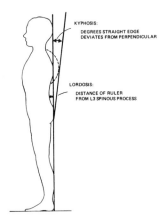
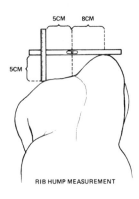

Fig. 2.14. Assessment of standing posture with a ruler or yardstick placed against sacrum and thoracic spinous processes. With kyphosis, straight edge deviates posteriorly from perpendicular. The distance from straight edge to mid-lumbar spine is gross estimate of lordosis (normal 3–4 cm).

Fig. 2.15. Posterior view of chest and thoracic spine with patient flexed forward 90º.

examiner's vision directed level with the spine, asymmetry of the posterior thorax can be seen. A rib hump denotes rotation of the thoracic vertebra to the convex side of a structural scoliosis. The rib hump can be measured as indicated in Figure 2.15.

These findings of rib hump, unilateral loin fullness, shoulder height inequality and pelvic obliquity are indications for a radiographic examination. These same indications exist if the child can be examined only when seated.

A good way of measuring the range of spine flexion is with a tape-measure that spans the spinous processes from the first thoracic vertebra to a prominent spine of the sacrum. This distance is first measured with the patient standing erect, and then with the trunk flexed 90º at the hips. Normally the difference between the standing and the flexed distances is 10–13 cm: a difference in measurement of 7 cm or less indicates limited flexion of the spine.

Heel positions. From the posterior view the position of the heels should be recorded: neutral, varus (inverted) or valgus (everted) alignment.

In the *anterior* view of the posture the examiner can observe: (1) asymmetry of the chest (usually secondary to structural thoracic scoliosis with chest depression on the convex side of the curve); (2) asymmetry of the limbs; (3) the position of the femur whether internally, externally or neutrally rotated, adducted or abducted; (4) the femoral–tibial alignment in varus (bowed knees) or valgus (knock knees); (5) medial or lateral rotation of the foot; (6) varus (inverted) or valgus (everted) position of the foot; and (7) hallux valgus, flexion or clawing of the toes.

EQUILIBRIUM REACTIONS

If the child can stand without support, this is the time to test for the all-important standing equilibrium reactions (see Chapter

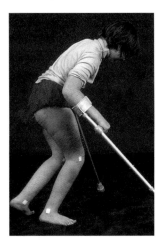
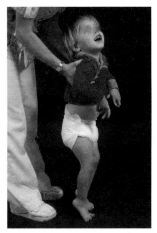

Fig. 2.12. Lateral view of teenager with uncorrected hip and knee-flexion contractures balanced by crutches.

Fig. 2.13. Lateral view of standing posture supported. Spastic diplegia, severe flexion of hips and knees, no lumbar lordosis.

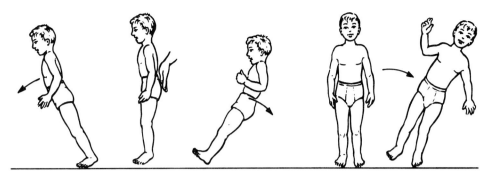

Fig. 2.16. Standing equilibrium reactions. The child is gently pushed forward, backward and from side to side. Lack of normal equilibrium reactions is easily demonstrated—the child topples over without normal stepping response.

5 for their prognostic significance). The child is pushed gently from side to side, anteriorly and posteriorly (Fig. 2.16). Normal children will maintain their balance with ease, and with a prompt righting response to regain stability, but children who have deficient equilibrium reactions will topple over like 'felled pine trees' (Hagberg *et al.* 1972) (Fig. 2.17).

In children who have normal equilibrium reactions, but who seem to be clumsy or ataxic, the familiar Romberg sign (performed with feet together and eyes closed) will document cerebellar ataxia (Baird and Gordon 1983).

Instrumented measurement of postural balance in children has been reported by Rose *et al.* (2002). A summary of this method is contained in Chapter 3. Another study of measuring balance in children with cerebral palsy using instrumentation confirmed that one-leg standing and walking on a line were reliable clinical indicators of balance (Liao *et al.* 2001).

A quick check on balance. The status of balance mechanisms can be further ascertained in those children who have good equilibrium reactions and negative Romberg signs if they can hop on one foot. If they can do this by the age of about 6 years, proceed no further. If not, a child should be able to stand on one foot and then the other for at least 10 seconds; inability to do this by the age of 5 years is evidence of impaired motor function. Children with spastic diplegia or hemiplegia who can walk independently often fail the unilateral standing balance test, either on one side or both.

Effect of equilibrium reactions on gait. During the gait cycle, ability to maintain posture while standing on one limb alone is

necessary. If unable to maintain balance on one limb, the patient leans to the side of the single stance limb to counteract the tendency to fall to the opposite side. This is often mistaken for a positive Trendelenberg sign which indicates weak hip-abductor muscles when the trunk bends to the opposite side of the stance limb. In spastic paralysis the excessive firing of muscles during level gait appears to be enhanced by the muscle contraction to counter the tendency to fall while attempting to regain balance on the stance limb. Crutches and walkers compensate for loss of balance and smooth the gait. This is why postoperative results appear better after surgery of the lower limbs in patients who use external supports to compensate for balance. In the examination of patients who walk without external supports and have an ungainly gait pattern, I have found the following test useful to indicate the effect of loss of balance reactions: stand behind the patient while grasping the sides of the head with both hands while walking behind the child. Stabilization of the head with the examiner's hands seems to transmit the examiner's normal equilibrium reactions to the patient. We know of no exercises or treatments that can overcome defective central balance mechanisms. However, in recent years attempts have been made to improve declining balance in older men and women by special training programs. The hope is to prevent frequent falling and fractured hips. Lack of good postural balance reactions, particularly on single-limb stance, explains why people begin to make shorter steps as they age.

WALKING

'It is distinctly human; it permits us to view the world in an upright manner, though not always acting in an upright way.'
(Vernon Inman MD[1])

OBSERVATIONAL GAIT ANALYSIS
The observation of the child's walking pattern is one of the most important parts of the examination, especially for the surgeon. The process is called 'gait analysis', with gait being defined as 'bipedal plantigrade progression'. The clinical examination of walking can be called 'observational gait analysis', which means describing what the examiner *sees*, as opposed to analysis by

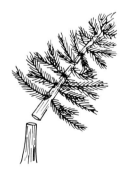

Fig. 2.17. The fall of the child who has abnormal equilibrium reactions has been likened to a 'felled pine tree'. When the standing posture is perturbed, the child does not have the righting response and topples over (From Hagberg *et al.* 1972.)

---

1 Professor of Orthopaedic Surgery, lectures on gait, 1960–70, University of California, San Francisco.

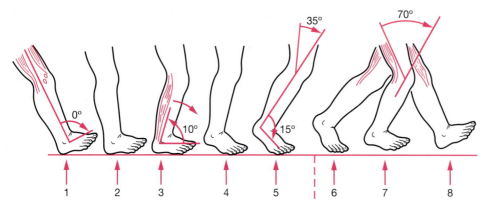

Fig. 2.18. Terminology of the events in the gait cycle (adapted from Perry 1967). (1) Initial contact. Ankle is flexed 0º; knee extended; hip flexed 30º; synchronous activity of hamstrings and quadriceps. (2) Loading response. Ant. tibialis, quadriceps muscles. Double limb support and deceleration and absorption of impact. (3) Mid-stance. Foot flat on floor; ankle dorsiflexed 10º; gastrocnemius-soleus contracts to prevent forward acceleration of the tibia. (4) Terminal stance. The gastroc-soleus inhibits dorsiflexion and creates propulsion by active plantarflexion at the ankle. Weightbearing is shifted to the forefoot. (5) Pre-swing, 35º–40º of knee flexion. Double limb support. (6) Initial swing ('pickup'). Knee flexion an additional 35º to prevent toe-drag; here hip flexion need be only 30º–35º. After pick-up, the knee-flexors relax. Ankle progressively dorsiflexes, and the ankle plantarflexes again (15º–20º) when the limb passes the opposite supporting limb. Toe clearance is minimal and may be only 1 cm. Rectus femoris active. (7) Mid-swing. Muscles not active as they switch from active quadriceps to active hamstring. (8) Terminal swing ('reach'). Knee extends for maximum stride-length, hip flexes about 30º and ankle remains flexed. Knee extends primarily by passive swinging with the hamstrings decelerating.

instruments and measurements. The *terminology* of the gait cycle can be used in clinical narrative descriptions of the position of the head, upper limbs, trunk, pelvis, femora, knees, ankles and feet while walking.

Stance phase begins with heel contact and ends with toe-off. Stance is 60% and *swing* is 40% of the gait cycle. To further improve observations, the gait cycle has been divided into eight phases when describing joint and muscle function (Perry 1967, 1975) (Fig. 2.18).

Perry (1992) has pointed out that during stance phase there are three changes of the fulcrum of motion, the so-called three foot-rockers (Fig 2.19). The first rocker occurs at loading response when the heel contacts the ground and serves as the axis of the forces of gait. This shifts to the ankle during mid-stance and later to the forefoot during terminal stance. During the first rocker the

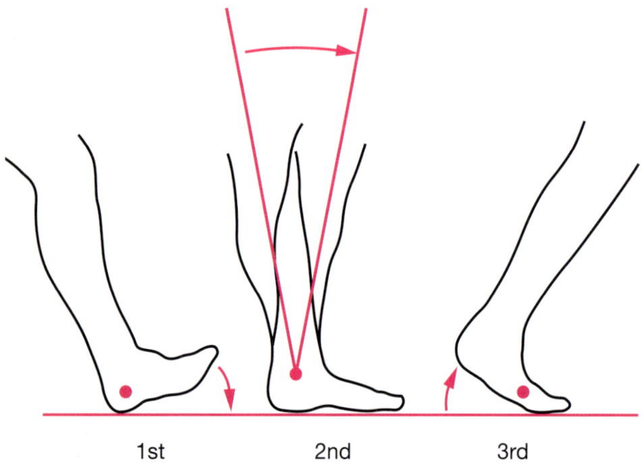

pretibial muscles are lengthening (eccentric contraction) to control and decelerate dorsiflexion of the foot and control flexion at the knee. There is shock absorption as the heel hits the ground. As the stance phase progresses ground reaction forces shift and pass anterior to the ankle and the ankle becomes the fulcrum (second rocker). The posterior capsule of the knee stabilizes the extended knee. Mid-stance is a period of energy conservation. At the beginning of mid-stance there is eccentric (lengthening) contraction of the soleus soon joined by the gastrocnemius to control the forward progression of the tibia. The other limb is in mid-swing.

During terminal stance, the gastroc-soleus contracts (shortens), creating concentric motion and producing forward propulsion and active plantarflexion. The fulcrum of motion progresses to the forefoot creating the third rocker of stance phase. In terminal stance heel rise occurs with ankle dorsiflexion. Perry feels this involves a shift to the forefoot rocker in a 'roll-off' mechanism rather than a 'push-off'. Gage (2004), on the other hand, notes the concentric contraction of the gatroc-soleus in terminal stance creating acceleration. This, together with other posterior calf muscles, generates about 50% of the propulsive forces in normal walking. Hence he uses the term push-off. The other propulsive forces come from the hip-extensors during loading response and hip-flexors during initial and terminal swing (Winter 1991). The knee creates little propulsive power during normal gait but it does in running and some pathologic gait conditions.

Step length is the distance between the same point on each foot (right to left or left to right) during double-limb support; *stride length* is the distance traversed by the same point of the same foot during two successive steps (right to left, or left to right). Stride length can be estimated. Perry (1975) has pointed out that stride length is dependent on the stance rather than the swing

Fig. 2.19. Three foot rockers. 1st: heel rocker; 2nd: ankle rocker; 3rd: forefoot rocker.

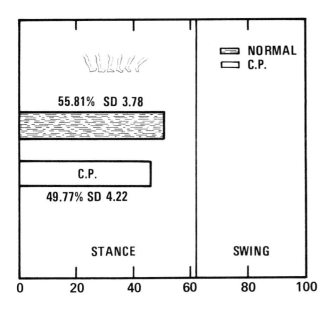

Fig. 2.20. Comparison of percent of gait cycle in normal children and in cerebral palsy (spastic diplegia). Stance phase is shorter in spastic gait patterns. (From Csongradi *et al.* 1979.)

limb during level walking. In spastic paralysis of the lower limbs, stride length can be limited by restrictions in the range of motion of the hip, knee and ankle; such limitations would account for the short swing of the opposite limb when the weightbearing limb is in mid-stance. Our studies have confirmed that the majority of children with spastic diplegia had shorter stance phases and faster cadences than normal children (Bleck 1975, Csongradi *et al.* 1979) (Fig. 2.20).

Cadence is the number of steps per minute, and *velocity* is meters traveled per minute. In studies of the gait in normal children it is apparent that as the child matures, the stride length and cadence increase and the base of the gait narrows (Burnett and Johnson 1971, Statham and Murray 1971). Stride length is related to the height of the child varying from approximately 30% of the height at 2 weeks after independent gait is achieved to 63%–72% at 61–70 weeks (Burnett and Johnson 1971).

The base of the gait, as measured from heel to heel, can be estimated. In a normal person, the base of the gait as measured from heel to heel is 5–10 cm (though in some individuals it can be as narrow as 1 cm, which accounts for scuffing of the medial aspect of the heel counter of the shoes, or the wearing out of the inside cuffs of trousers). Other parameters of the normal gait cycle can be helpful. For example, when assessing the gait of the patient with a view to surgery or orthotics, it is useful to know that normally the knee flexes 35º at pre-swing and must flex 70º for the foot to clear the ground (Fig. 2.18).

CORONAL-, TRANSVERSE- AND SAGITTAL-PLANE OBSERVATIONS

The patient should be viewed from the coronal plane, each segment at a time—head, trunk, upper limbs, pelvis, hips, knees, feet and ankles. It can be helpful to narrow the field of vision for each joint by partially closing your hand to form a sort of

telescope or by using a rolled-up magazine or newspaper as a scope. Transverse-plane motions particularly of the femora can be seen with excessive internal rotation of the femur during stance, and of course the internal or external rotation of the foot in the stance phase. The sagittal-plane joint motions of the hip, knee, ankle and foot can be estimated from the lateral view while walking. It is possible to estimate with fair accuracy, for example, the initial range of knee flexion in the swing phase and in terminal swing. Equinus on terminal stance and dorsiflexion of the ankle on swing can be easily observed. Excessive vertical oscillations of the head might be noted as evidence of lower-limb malfunction to keep the center of gravity of the body on a low sinusoidal curve during forward progression.

The type of motion disorder can often be diagnosed by observation of the gait, and applying the descriptive terminology delineated in Chapter 1. Spastic gait patterns are distinct from athetoid types of either the rotatory (ballismus) or dystonic forms. A purely ataxic gait is characteristic. A relatively new and erudite term, 'titubation', describes the shaking of the trunk and head with the staggering, reeling and stumbling gait of ataxia (Baird and Gordon 1983, p. 100).

Although accurate measurements cannot be made with careful observation alone, we need to remember that all laboratory findings must be correlated with clinical examinations. Indeed, most gait laboratories use videotape recordings of the patient's walking pattern as a check on the analog and digital data generated.

GAIT MECHANICS

Conducive to astute observational gait analysis is an understanding of the accepted mechanical theories of walking based upon experimental evidence and the principles of physics.

The ballistic walking model is comparable to a projectile moving through space, because once the swing phase begins, forward movement occurs entirely by the action of gravity (McMahon 1984). *The center of gravity* is a fixed point in a body through which the force of gravitational attraction acts (Kelley 1971) (Fig. 2.21). In the human body the center of gravity is located just anterior to the first and second sacral segments (Braune and Fischer 1898, cited by Brunnstrom 1962). If the lower limbs are not considered, the center of gravity of the trunk only is just anterior to the 11th thoracic vertebra (Hellebrant 1938, cited by Brunnstrom 1962). In children, the center of gravity of the whole body is at first located at about the level of the 11th thoracic vertebra, just anterior to the vertebral column where the vena cava enters the abdomen through the diaphragm; with maturation of the child, the center of gravity descends to its adult level anterior to the sacrum. The location of the center of gravity can be estimated as 55% of the total height, measured from the soles of the feet.

Many of the postural abnormalities of patients with cerebral palsy seen during walking appear to be adjustments of the trunk and limbs to maintain the center of gravity when equilibrium reactions are deficient or when there are structural abnormalities of the trunk. Because the head, upper limbs and trunk represent

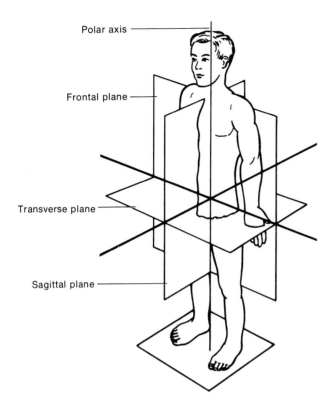

Polar axis

Frontal plane

Transverse plane

Sagittal plane

Fig. 2.21. The center of gravity of the body is the point where all planes (coronal, sagittal and transverse) converge, just anterior to the second sacral segment. (Redrawn from Kelley 1971.)

70% of the bodyweight, this mass (known as HAT, i.e. head, arms and trunk) has to be balanced and supported by the lower limbs. With anatomical shifts of the trunk, as might occur in scoliosis, balance is shifted and off-center. The lower limbs usually accommodate these changes by moving the feet wider apart (Perry 1975).

The *vertical displacement of the center of gravity* is at the core of the mechanics of walking. The most efficient instrument of motion on earth's surface is the wheel because its center of gravity remains perfectly level, horizontal to the ground and without oscillation in its path of motion (Fig. 2.22). In human gait the vertical displacement of the center of gravity attempts to approximate the action of the wheel by minimizing the displacement and tracing a trajectory as a low sinusoidal curve. This saves energy. If the lower limbs in humans were unarticulated sticks, a 'compass gait' with high-amplitude oscillations of the center of gravity would result, with consequent increased energy expenditure (Fig. 2.22).

The five major determinants of gait in the ballistic model of walking are responsible for maintaining the lowest possible sinusoidal path of the center of gravity (Saunders *et al.* 1953, McMahon 1984).

1. *Pelvic rotation.* At normal walking speed, the amplitude of motion of the pelvis in rotation is ±3°. Rotation increases at greater speeds. Pelvic rotation effects lengthening of the lower limb, and thus allows a longer step length and a greater radius for rotation of the hip. Walking racers exaggerate their pelvic rotation, which allows continued walking at high speeds rather than progression to running (McMahon 1984).

2. *Pelvic tilt.* Tilt of the pelvis in the coronal plane causes an angular displacement of 5° or more. The hip on the swing side falls lower than the hip on the stance limb. The lowering of the swing limb occurs just before toe-off, and accordingly the trajectory of the center of gravity is further lowered. As the pelvis dips, knee flexion of the swing limb must occur so that the advancing foot does not strike the ground on forward movement.

3. *Knee flexion.* Knee flexion in the stance phase further lowers the sinusoidal path of the center of gravity.

4. *Plantarflexion of the stance ankle.* At heel strike, the ankle plantarflexes and the knee flexes to shorten the limb. As the trunk passes over the stance limb, the knee then extends and the heel rises to effect lengthening of the limb.

5. *Lateral displacement of the pelvis.* The shift of the trunk is normally no more than 4–5 cm during gait. Excessive displacement would occur if the lower limbs were parallel to each other. The normal anatomy of adduction of the femora and the resultant valgus angle between the femur and tibia prevents excessive displacement.

While the ballistic model of walking explains how gravity alone determines the dynamics of gait, the model assumes no muscular torques at the joints of the swing limb; hence it cannot represent running, or walking at very low or high speeds (McMahon 1984). Extrinsic joint torque is defined as that produced by the forces of gravity and inertia. It tends to flex or extend the joint depending on the line of application of the force from the ground or floor either behind the joint or in front of it. The intrinsic joint torque is defined as due to muscle forces that flex the joint (Sutherland 1984).

A moon-walk might demonstrate the low oscillations of displacement of the body's center of gravity. On the moon, the time of swing phase must be increased 2½ times; so the walking speed for a given step length can be only about 40% of what it is on earth. This explains why the Apollo astronauts on the moon preferred to move about in a series of jumps rather than restrict their walking speed. The maximal jump height on the moon is said to be 4 metres (McMahon 1984).

Gait laboratory studies have shown that normally the pelvis and lower limb segments rotate internally throughout swing, and at mid-stance abrupt external rotation of these segments occurs. The function of the subtalar joint is to absorb the torques generated by the foot–floor reaction when these changes in rotation take place.

In spastic paralysis of the lower limbs, motion is often restricted in the joints that affect the major determinants of gait. If external rotation at the hip joint is limited, then pelvic rotation (the first determinant) will be restricted; the degree of pelvic rotation internally (i.e. anteriorly) is permitted by the degree of hip external rotation. With this kind of restriction, the path of the center of gravity would have higher peaks and valleys, and the gait would be less efficient. If knee flexion were limited (e.g. by a spastic quadriceps muscle), then the gait would be compass-like,

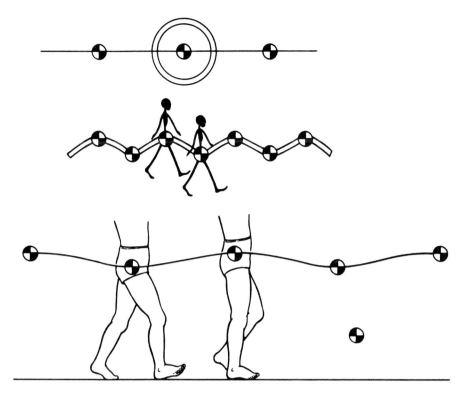

Fig. 2.22. Pathways of the center of gravity in lateral projection. *Top*: in the wheel, the center of gravity (the axis) remains horizontal, making it the most efficient instrument of forward motion. *Center*: in human walking, if the knee joint is eliminated, the center of gravity rises and falls precipitously. This increases energy expenditure. *Bottom*: in normal gait the oscillations of the center of gravity result in a low sinusoidal curve. The major determinants of gait (pelvis, hip, knee, foot and ankle) serve to keep the center of gravity as close as possible to that of the wheel, thus conserving energy.

the arc of the center of gravity would rise, and energy expenditure would increase. Compensation for restricted ankle motion can be accomplished by exaggerated movements of the hip and knee. Because central nervous system integration may be deficient in cerebral palsy, these compensatory mechanisms are not often adequate.

The lower-limb movement patterns and ranges of joint motion during walking have been measured and standards are known; these standards of measurement are described in Chapter 3. The role of the muscles during gait has been determined by electromyography. The normative data derived from electromyography, and its possible applications in cerebral palsy, are also covered in the next chapter.

RUNNING

Running is different from walking. In walking there are two periods of double support: initial heel contact with the advancing limb and toe-off with the opposite limb. The two events are replaced by a 'double float' when neither foot is on the ground. In running stance is always less than swing to accommodate this period of 'double float' (Gage 1991). A study of both walking and running in children with spastic diplegia found that they increased their velocity by increasing their cadence, and distinctly different from normal healthy children (David *et al.* 1993). The ankle kinematics (ranges of motion) and kinetics (ground reaction forces, joint moments and powers) when the children with spastic

diplegia ran were more similar to the gait patterns of normal children and transferred the energy between adjacent joints comparable to normal children. The authors suggested that running should be part of the assessment in children with spastic diplegia. Running is very useful in observing the spasticity of the elbow-flexor muscles that is not noticed in level walking in some who have spastic hemiplegia. This particularly true when you examine a child who has what appears to be a monoplegia with a spastic equinus with varus or valgus of the foot.

SITTING POSTURE

The sitting posture will be either supportive ('propped') or unsupportive. Children who are hypotonic, or who have cerebral damage, usually do not have the normal lumbar lordotic curve, so the spine is rounded posteriorly. The lower limbs of the child who has total body involvement are frequently extended. When the manual supports of the seated child are removed, automatic protective placement of the extended upper limb and hand usually denotes good function of the hand and limb. Scoliosis, a posterior rib hump, and the levels of the pelvic brim can be discerned.

DEEP-TENDON AND PLANTAR REFLEXES

Deep-tendon reflexes and the plantar responses can be checked when the infant or young child is seated on the mother's lap, or when the older child sits with his knees flexed over the table edge. The biceps, triceps, and the periosteal–radial reflexes in the upper limb, and the quadriceps and Achilles reflexes in the lower limb, are hyperactive in spasticity and normal or absent in ataxia. While these responses are classic, variations occur according to age and severity of the spastic paralysis. In infants under 1 month of age, the predominant flexor pattern suppresses the triceps reflex, and the Achilles reflex may be weak or absent. Severe spasticity, rigidity, or a long-standing severe contracture of the triceps surae muscles may eliminate the ankle jerk response. The crossed adductor response, in which tapping of the patellar tendon results in adduction of the opposite hip, indicates severe spasticity. This crossed spread of the quadriceps reflex can be normal in infants up to the age of 8 months, and in 2% of infants at the age of 12 months (Paine and Oppé 1966, Baird and Gordon 1983).

The *Babinski sign* is best induced by gently stroking the lateral plantar aspect of the foot with a blunt instrument (e.g. a key or the handle of a reflex hammer). Joseph Babinski in 1896 noticed that the response was best obtained when the limb was slightly flexed and the muscles were well relaxed. Ordinarily, this state of the limb is achieved with the patient seated and the legs hanging over the table edge. The positive response consists of extension and spreading of the toes—usually strongest in the great and second toes (Baird and Gordon 1983). Many other ways of eliciting the Babinski sign have been described. I have found *Chaddock's sign* one of the better alternatives. The lateral aspect of the dorsum of the foot is gently stroked from the heel to the forefoot with the end of a key or the tip of the reflex hammer handle. Fanning and extension of the toes will occur if the sign is positive (Mayo Clinic, Department of Neurology 1991).

ASSOCIATED DEFECTS: CRANIAL NERVES

Because the major associated defects (convulsive, learning and behavioral disorders excepted) are related to dysfunction of the cranial nerves, the examination of these nerves is presented. The sitting posture is the most practical for these observations.

III, IV and VI. Eye mobility is frequently affected in cerebral palsy. Esotropia or exotropia is easy to see. While esotropia is more common in the general population than exotropia, in low-birthweight children children both esotropia and exotropia can be seen in the same frequency (O'Connor *et al.* 2002). Pupil inequality is uncommon, and most often seen in patients with hemiplegia due to cerebrovascular conditions, brain tumors, or after head injuries. Paralysis of the upper gaze is common in tension athetosis due to kernicterus. Nystagmus is sometimes seen in ataxia. The eye-righting reflex means that when the neck is flexed, extended and rotated, the eyes should follow the movement of the head. Absence of this reflex indicates brainstem injury. The absence of eye movements with rotation of the head, or turning of the eyes to the side opposite of head rotation, has been called 'doll's eyes' (oculocephalic reflex, 'doll's head', Mayo Clinic, Department of Neurology 1991). The normal eye-reflex response may be delayed a few weeks in normal infants (Baird and Gordon 1983). Visual acuity testing and funduscopic examinations are best left to the ophthalmologist.

VII and XII. On inspection of the mouth and face, inequality of facial muscle function is sometimes seen in upper motor-neuron lesions. The corner of the child's mouth on the affected side may not move when crying or smiling, or he may not be able to wrinkle the forehead. In less severe unilateral lesions, the only finding may be a wide palpebral fissure on the affected side (Baird and Gordon 1983).

Athetoid movements of the orbicularis oris muscle, and muscles of mastication, are fairly common. They indicate a general motor disorder, rather than cranial nerve paralysis.

IX. If the child can open his mouth, paralysis of the pharyngeal muscles may be seen. The only manifestation of paralysis may be a slight dropping of the palatal arch. Despite paralysis, both sides of the arch may elevate when saying 'aah'. In his lectures on cerebral palsy, Meyer Perlstein (1960–66) gave some useful clinical tips: if swallowing is more difficult with fluids, spasm of the pharyngeal muscles should be suspected; if difficulty in swallowing is greater with solids, paralysis of these muscles may be present.

VIII. Gross hearing defects can be ascertained by asking the parents whether they think the child hears, and by watching the child's reaction to sounds out of his visual field, *e.g.* by shaking a few grains of sand in a cardboard cylinder. In suspicious cases, referral for audiometry and otolaryngeal consultation is indicated.

UPPER-LIMB ASSESSMENT

Where to position the infant or child for a good assessment of upper-limb and hand function depends on the age of the child, the status of his postural development, and the motor disorder. For the infant or toddler, the mother's lap is usually best; for the older child with hemiplegia, a desk and chair should be used; for the child who cannot sit unsupported and has gross involvement of one or both upper limbs, use a wheelchair with a seat insert and a lap-tray. The child with no gross involvement of the upper limbs can be examined sitting with the knees flexed over the edge of the table; most often this is a child who has spastic hemiplegia or diplegia. For a more refined assessment of fine-motor hand function, a chair and desk will be required.

Assessment of the upper limbs should include measurement of the passive and active ranges of motion of the shoulder and elbow; in this process spasticity, athetosis, dystonia or ataxia can be recognized. Chorea will be demonstrated when the child is asked to hold his arms and hands extended forward; the sign of chorea is involuntary 'wormlike' movements of the fingers (Fig. 1.4).

One good way to begin the assessment is to give the child an object that requires the use of both hands; wooden or plastic eggs within eggs or barrels within barrels are ideal. When the child grasps the object, one can see lateralization of hand function, the quality of grasp and release, and the ability of the hands to cross the midline. Gross grasp and release can be tested by handing the child a cylindrical stick or similar object (Fig. 2.23). To test fine motion of the fingers and pinch, small wooden beads or hard-coated sweets are useful (Fig. 2.24).

Gross spasticity of the wrist and digit muscles requires a more detailed examination, which must be precise if surgery is planned. Palpation of the spastic wrist flexors, as the wrist is extended, identifies which of these tendons is spastic and contracted (Fig. 2.25). If the thumb is indwelling in the palm, measurement of the web space while pulling the thumb into abduction will define the spastic abductor hallucis. Limited extension of the interphalangeal joint of the thumb, with the wrist held in the neutral position and the metacarpal–phalangeal joint in extension,

indicates a spastic flexor pollicis longus muscle. If the fingers are consistently flexed in the palm, two maneuvers are necessary to determine if one or the other or both finger-flexor muscles are spastic and contracted: (1) extend and hold the wrist in the neutral position, and extend and hold the metacarpal–phalangeal joints in neutral extension; the resistance to extension of the proximal interphalangeal joints while extending the distal joint will indicate the extent of spasticity and contracture of the flexor digitorum superficialis (Fig. 2.26); (2) with the wrist and metacarpal–phalangeal joints in the same position, stabilize the proximal interphalangeal joint in extension; flexion and resistance to extension of the distal interphalangeal joint implies a spastic and contracted flexor digitorum profundus muscle (Fig. 2.26).

In patients who have wrist- and finger-flexion postures, the ability to extend the fingers voluntarily is tested by holding the wrist in extension; if active extension of the fingers occurs at the metacarpal–phalangeal joints, then the extensor digitorum muscles of the fingers have a good chance of functioning if the wrist- and finger-flexion contractures are relieved with surgery. If the fingers will extend only by dropping the wrist into flexion to open the grasp, then anything done to correct wrist flexion will seriously compromise function due to a permanent fist position. If there is doubt about voluntary control of wrist and finger extension, the median nerve can be blocked at the elbow with a local anesthetic to eliminate most of the flexor muscle function, and the quality of active wrist and finger extension will be evident. Currently, botulinium A toxin injection of the flexor muscle mass might be used instead of a local anesthetic block. But its effects may last from a few weeks to a few months. Chapter 6 covers the current status of botulinium A toxin in cerebral palsy. For precision in terms of describing active and passive motion of the thumb and digits, see Figure 2.27. Additional assessment techniques are described in the section on hand surgery in spastic hemiplegia (Chapter 7).

Fine motor incoordination of the hand is often seen in the child with spastic diplegia, ataxia, localized chorea, and the rare case of tremor. It can be discerned with the following simple tests:

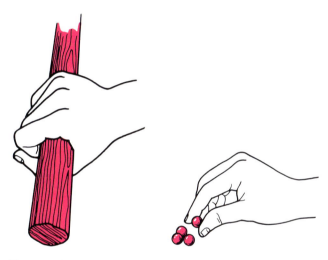

Fig. 2.23. Grasp testing.　　**Fig. 2.24.** Pinch testing.

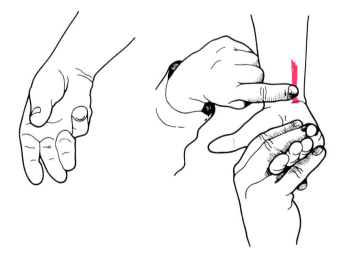

Fig. 2.25. To test for spastic wrist-flexor: flex wrist then gradually extend; palpate contracted and spastic tendon (flexor carpi ulnaris or radialis).

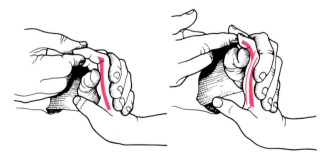

Fig. 2.26. To test for spastic and contracted flexor digitor superficialis: extend wrist and metacarpal–phalangeal joint and stabilize both. With distal interphalangeal joint stabilized, attempt to extend proximal interphalangeal joint. *Above right*: test for spastic and contracted flexor digitorum profundis: extend and stabilize wrist, metacarpal–phalangeal joint and proximal interphalangeal joint. Then attempt to extend distal interphalangeal joint.

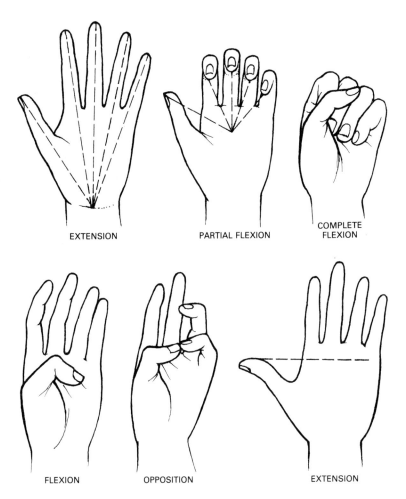

EXTENSION · PARTIAL FLEXION · COMPLETE FLEXION

FLEXION · OPPOSITION · EXTENSION

Fig. 2.27. Terminology to describe motion of the digits, and linear measurements to record ranges of motion. *Top*: for *opening capacity* of each finger, measure the distance from the extended finger to the distal flexion crease of the wrist. For *closing capacity* of the fingers, measure distance from tips of the fingers to the mid-palmar crease at the third metacarpal. *Bottom*: to measure *opposing capacity of the thumb* to the fingers, measure distance in centimeters between the tip of the thumb and the tip of each finger. (Note: this is 'pulp' pinch; 'key' pinch is just as useful and may be better—see Moberg 1976 and Chapter 7 in this volume.) To measure the *opening and closing of the thumb* in extension/abduction or flexion/adduction, measure distance from the tip of the thumb to the head of the fifth metacarpal in both extension and flexion.

(1) ask the child to touch each fingertip to the thumb in as rapid a succession as possible; (2) rapidly pronate and supinate the forearm to discover dysdiadochokinesis; (3) with both hands resting, palms down on the desk or tabletop, ask the child to mimic your own hand movements (e.g. tapping the fingers as if typing or playing the piano, or rapidly pronating and supinating one hand). With these latter movement tests, mirror movements in the opposite resting hand may be discovered. However, mirror motions can be normal in some children up to the age of 6 or 7 years. Mirror movements are fairly frequent in children who have hemiplegia on attempted voluntary manipulations with the hemiplegic hand.

Other tests for visual–motor coordination that can be useful are drawing tests. The simplest to use for a developmental estimate is the Slosson Drawing Co-ordination test (Alcorn and Nicholson 1972). A 3-year-old should be able to copy a circle and a vertical line, a 4½-year-old a square, a 5-year-old an x, a 5½-year-old a triangle, and a 6-year-old a diamond. With children 6 years of age or more, start by asking them to copy a diamond. If they can, proceed no further. More elaborate tests of hand function and visuomotor coordination are usually the province of the occupational therapist and psychologist, to whom the physician can refer the child when indicated (Baird and Gordon 1984).

The *Elliott and Connolly classification of hand movements* (1984) is an assessment based upon intrinsic movements of the digits in the hand. The descriptive terminology is appealing, e.g. 'pinch', 'dynamic tripod' (holding a pencil), 'squeeze' (compressing the barrel of a syringe), 'twiddle' (rolling a nut on a threaded bolt), 'rock' (holding a thin disc in the palm and rotating it, 'radial roll' (as in snapping the thumb), 'index roll' (rolling a pea-sized object between the pulp of the thumb and index finger), plus combinations of manipulative movements termed 'steps' and 'slides'. For a complete detailed description of these tests, the original paper in *Developmental Medicine and Child Neurology* should be studied. Despite what appears to be a superior method of analysis of hand function, the paucity of references to these tests in the literature suggests that hand surgeons and occupational therapists have not adopted this method assessment of function.

In children who have to use wheelchairs, hand use should be part of the assessment. We can observe whether or not the child can move a manual wheelchair independently and efficiently, and if so, whether with both hands or only one, and in what positions the hands and fingers are placed to propel the chair.

Sensory examination is frequently neglected in cerebral palsy, possibly because of a failure to appreciate the all-important role of sensation in intellectual development, but more likely because sensory assessment is tedious.

In the hierarchy of the external senses touch was considered the most important in the philosophical discourses of Thomas Aquinas (1224–74) (McInerny 1984). Thomas Aquinas believed that touch was wedded to a physical change. For example, when the hand feels a cold object and keeps it there for a time, the temperature of the body (37.5°C) gradually warms the cold object until the temperatures become equal. We hear such terms as 'deficient sensory perception', 'sensory retraining' and 'sensory integration' applied to the child with cerebral palsy, without knowing exactly what is meant or their implications for the child and attempts at remediation. Recognizing a deficiency in the sense of touch is important, to understand the possible limitations of hand function in the child.

One recent study on kinesthetic performance of children with spastic and athetoid cerebral palsy, when compared with age-matched normal children, demonstrated that those with spasticity had the greatest number of errors on kinesthetic tests (children with athetosis were less prone to error) when analyzed against the normal control's performance. The authors suggested that attempts to apply 'reafference theory' with methods using feedback of movement should not be done using the sense of touch in patients with cerebral palsy, but rather should use intact sensory systems, i.e. vision and hearing (Opila-Lehman *et al.* 1984).

Stereognosis is the most common defect. Generally, aster-ognosis in spastic hemiplegia seems to accompany the degree of atrophy of the upper limb. Testing for shape recognition with the hands is even more important if surgery is planned (Tachdjian and Minear 1958, Ferlic 1966). The child has to be old enough to verbalize shape and texture (or if non-verbal, communicate with symbols or drawings). The child is asked to identify objects while blindfolded, or vision occluded with the examiner's hand. For shape identification we use pieces of wood cut into a triangle, square, and circle (or perhaps coins, for more sophisticated children); for texture recognition, use two ping-pong balls: one smooth and one rough (Goldner 1974) (Fig. 2.28).

Another way to test for stereognosis is with dermographics. Again the child is blindfolded. The examiner traces an Arabic numeral (1–9) on the palm of the hand, and the child is asked to identify it. As in the tests for shape and texture identification, in hemiplegic hands the opposite (presumed neurologically intact) hand can serve as a control.

The most sensitive test for adequate sensation is the two-point discrimination test as modified by Moberg (1976). It was

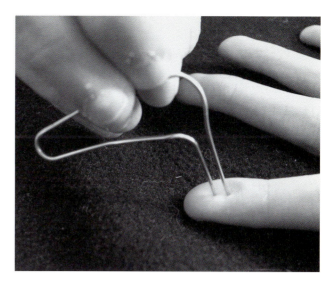

Fig. 2.29. Moberg's test instrument for the two-point discrimination test: a wire paper-clip reconfigured and bent. Tips can be spread apart to a measured distance (5 mm). To do the two-point discrimination test on the pulp of the fingers and thumb, both patient and examiner must be seated. The examiner uses free hand to stabilize the digit on the tabletop (Moberg 1976). A measured 10 g of pressure by the examiner is more accurate.

used almost exclusively in the assessment of paralysis of the hands in spinal cord and peripheral nerve injuries, and often to discern the sensory impairment due to nerve entrapments at the wrist (carpal tunnel syndrome). We have used Moberg's two-point paper-clip discrimination test in 51 patients with cerebral palsy and aged 6–20 years. We found it to have significantly higher sensitivity and slightly lower specificity testing tactile sensation compared with shape recognition (Belanos *et al.* 1989). The advantages of using two-point discrimination testing rather than shape recognition is that the subject has only to answer 'one' or 'two'. Depending on the intellectual level of the patient, articulation of the shape may be difficult, if not impossible. Furthermore, the ordinary paper clip is readily available every-where. Lesny *et al.* (1993) also found deficient two-point discrimination on eight points in the upper extremities in all children who had cerebral palsy. Moberg's 'microsurgical' two-point discrimination test on the digits of cerebral palsied children should be conducted according to his instructions (Moberg 1976). The examiner and patient are both comfortably seated so that the examiner's and the patient's hands can rest securely on the table or desk. The finger to be tested is held firmly against the tabletop with the examiner's free hand. The test instrument is an ordinary paper-clip, unfolded so that the two free ends are at the same level, and then bent 90° in the middle of the reconfigured clip (Fig. 2.29). The ends of the clip are spread 5 mm for testing; the patient just has to say 'one' or 'two'.

LOWER-LIMB ASSESSMENT

'I fancy that the American, quite apart from any love of money, has a great love of measurement. He will mention the exact size or weight of things, in a way which appears to us as irrelevant.

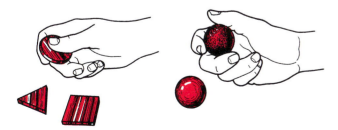

Fig. 2.28. Stereognosis test objects: 5 mm plywood triangle, square and disc for shape recognition; smooth and rough (covered with flock paint) ping-pong balls for texture recognition.

It is as if we were to say that a man came to see us carrying three feet of walking stick and four inches of cigar.'

(G.K. Chesterton, *What I Saw in America*)

RANGES OF MOTION

Despite Chesterton's acerbic comment, some scientific description of the abnormalities in the limbs that include a range of motion and other measurements seems essential. To be certain, measurements ought to be made with the goniometer. It is accepted that in clinical practice an experienced examiner can reliably estimate the range of motion of joints visually. However, as much as a 30% difference in the range of motion with the single observational method has been reported (Lea and Gerhardt 1995). Interobserver variability has been such that only less or more than 5° is acceptable as a true decrease or increase in joint motion (Greene and Heckman 1994). Lea and Gerhardt (1995) advised that all measurements of the range of motion should be made three times. If the total range is less than 50°, a 5° variation is judged to be valid; if the range is over 50°, a 10° variation among measurements is deemed acceptable.

The goniometer should be an improvement over the observational method. The problem with the two-limb goniometer is locating the axis of rotation of the joint, the long axes of the limb, and that the true vertical and horizontal positions can only be estimated. All joint measurements should start from the 'neutral zero position' which is extension for most joints rather than 180° to avoid confusion (Greene and Heckman 1994). It is tedious and time-consuming for the physician to accurately measure important passive and active motions of the major joints. Perhaps this task can be done by the physical therapist, who is generally more patient and likely to take the time.

The accuracy of goniometric measurements in cerebral palsy has been questioned. McDowell and colleagues (2000) recorded three consecutive measurements of six joint ranges in 12 children with cerebral palsy, and measurement was repeated 1 week later. A randomized blinded study with masked goniometers showed same-day and different-day errors of ± 10 to 14°in the foot/thigh angle, abduction and internal rotation of the hip. Ankle dorsiflexion and popliteal angles on the same day had similar errors in the range of ± 18 to 28° that increased on different days. The watchword as expected was 'caution' in using ranges of motion for clinical decisions.

To add more doubt on the value of passive joint ranges of motion in cerebral palsy, McMulkin *et al.* (2000) correlated kinematic data from gait analysis in 80 adolescents with cerebral palsy and 30 unaffected controls. They were unequivocal with their findings: there was no correlation between the static physical examination measurements and the dynamic ranges of motion recorded with instrumented gait analysis.

But another word of caution seems indicated before abandoning estimation of the range of joint motion measured passively. Motion analysis data will not necessarily confirm whether or not a joint contracture is present, e.g. knee-flexion contracture or fixed equinus. As with all laboratory investigations, instrumented gait analysis requires clinical correlations.

Mechanical or electronic inclinometers have been proposed and are available for more accurate measurements (Lea and Gerhardt 1995). The mechanical inclinometers are less expensive and offer limited advantages over the electrical ones. Whether these instruments would be simple enough for use with children who have cerebral palsy compared to the goniometric method and useful in clinical decisions is questionable.

Normal standards for passive ranges of motion, angular and torsional measurements, radiographic parameters, growth of bones etc. can be extracted from the veritable mine in Hensinger's text (1986). Staheli *et al.* (1985) have published normal rotations of the lower-limb anatomy. Time-oriented serial examination forms are very useful when evaluating a patient over a period of years.

Measurement of the active range of motion of joints and spine depends on the willingness of the patient, their maximal effort, and the muscle strength. In cerebral palsy, active motion also depends on voluntary control that the child may not have.

MUSCLE STRENGTH

Muscle testing, using the standards and grading originally developed for poliomyelitis, is too well known to be worth repeating here. While it is true that in cerebral palsy, muscle-strength testing will be altered due to lack of voluntary control, or limited due to spasticity and/or contracture, at least some idea of the muscle function can be gained. Recently, muscle strengthening exercises have been shown to be important in improving function in spastic diplegia.

Leg length should always be measured with the patient supine. We emphasize this because it is often overlooked. The proper way to measure leg length is with a tape measure (preferably a metal one) from the anterior superior iliac spine to the medial malleolus. If the patient has a flexion contracture of the knee joint, obviously this measurement will be affected. In such instances, the measurement can be from the anterior superior iliac spine to the medial knee joint space, and from the medial joint space to the medial malleolus. The addition of the two gives a reasonable estimate of the limb length. Asymmetrical adduction contractures of the hip result in the illusion of a short limb. Therefore measurement of the *actual* (rather than the apparent) limb length is important. Because we don't walk on our medial malleoli, measurement to the plantar surface of the heel might be more accurate particularly if there is a foot deformity and a small foot on one side.

Another method of estimating leg-length discrepancy, if the patient can stand unsupported and has no contractures in the knees or ankles, is to level the pelvis with wood blocks in increments of 5 mm–4 cm in height. The patient should not be fat. If so, the crests of the ilium will be difficult to see and palpate.

Hip, supine measurements. The range of *abduction* of each hip is measured with the hips flexed 90° and extended (normally 45°–60°). The range of *flexion* varies in children (110°–125°). *Hip-flexion contracture* is common and is measured in two ways. In the classic *Thomas test*, the hip is flexed on the abdomen to flatten the lumbar spine, and the opposite hip is gently pushed to its maximum extension. The angle that the femur subtends with the tabletop is a measure of the degree of hip-flexion deformity (Fig. 2.30). This test is unreliable. Varying degrees of hip-flexion deformity can be produced in the same patient, depending on how far the hip is pushed onto the abdomen and how much pelvic femoral fixation is present due to spastic and contracted hamstrings (Fig. 2.30). Lee *et al.* (1997) used gait analysis of patients who had hip-flexion contractures, and reported a weak correlation between the degree of hip-flexion contracture measured by the Thomas test and peak hip extension during gait and was a poor predictor of anterior pelvic tilting. The Thomas test can confirm spasticity and contracture of the iliopsoas by grasping the femoral condyles on the side which is to be measured, and attempting to rotate the femur externally. External rotation will be blocked when the iliopsoas is spastic. In contrast to spastic paralysis of the iliopsoas, if the hip-flexion contracture is due to the iliotibial band, the hip can be easily externally rotated. Contracture of the iliotibial band is most often seen in flaccid paralysis due to poliomyelitis or in muscle diseases, e.g. muscular dystrophy.

Hip, prone measurements. A second, more accurate, and preferred method of measuring the contracture is *prone hip-extension test* (Staheli 1977). The patient is prone with the pelvis over the table's edge and the lower limbs hanging free in flexion. The examiner places one hand on the posterior superior iliac spines, while the other hand brings one lower limb gradually and slowly into extension. The point at which the pelvis begins to move anteriorly is the point of the hip-flexion deformity; the angle subtended by the femur and the horizontal plane is measured (Fig. 2.31). Bartlett *et al.* (1985) compared four different measuring techniques for a hip-flexion contracture in patients with spastic diplegia and myelomeningocele. They found that the least reliable measurements were with the Thomas test in cerebral palsy. The conclusion was that considering the ease of measurement, the reliability and reproducibility, the prone extension test of Staheli was best in cerebral palsy and the Thomas test better in myelomeningocele.

The normal range of hip extension (i.e. no flexion contracture) is at least zero, and may be as much as 20º in some children. All newborn infants have a flexion contracture of the hip with a mean value of 28º (Haas *et al.* 1973). At 6 weeks of age, the contracture decreases to a mean of 19º, and at 3–6 months to 7º (Coon *et al.* 1975).

With the patient still prone, internal (medial) and external (lateral) rotation are measured. The measurements are made with the knees flexed 90º and the pelvis stabilized by the examiner (or by a parent, nurse, or student) to avoid overestimation of hip rotation due to lateral rolling of the pelvis (Fig. 2.32). Staheli *et al.* (1985) delineated normal ranges of medial and lateral hip rotation in children and adults. Medial rotation was greatest in infants less than 1 year old and gradually decreased from the age of 7 or 8 years to a mean value at skeletal maturity to a mean

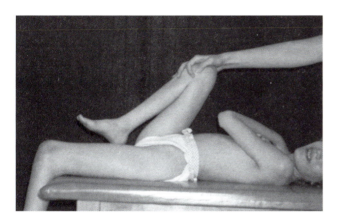
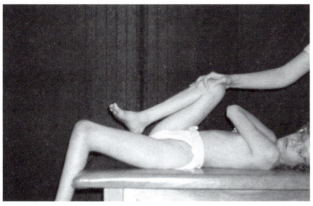
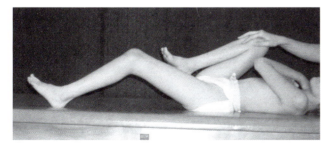

Fig. 2.30. *Above*: Thomas test for hip-flexion contracture. *Center and below*: the variability of the Thomas test in the same patient. Which one is the correct degree of contracture? When the hamstrings are contracted, the pelvis will rock posteriorly in varying degrees, thereby giving varying degrees of apparent flexion contracture.

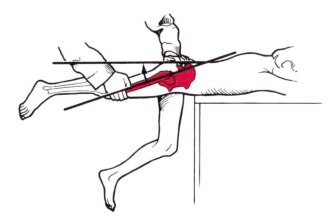

Fig. 2.31. Prone hip-flexion contracture test (Staheli 1977). Patient lies prone with pelvis off the examining table. Put one hand on the posterior superior iliac spines. As the hip to be tested is brought into extension, the point of contracture is when the pelvis begins to move anteriorly.

(a)

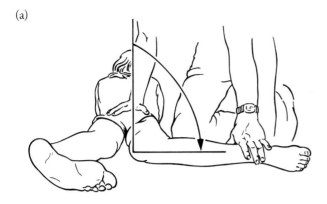

(b)

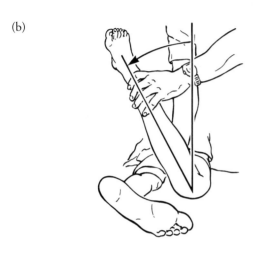

Fig. 2.32. (*a*) Measurement of internal rotation of the hip in extension. Patient prone; one hand should always be firmly placed on the pelvis to stabilize it and minimize pelvic rotation. (*b*) Measurement of external rotation of the hip.

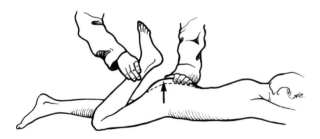

Fig. 2.33. Rectus femoris stretch test (Ely test). With patient prone, quick flexion of the knee causes buttock to rise if there is spasticity of the rectus femoris. Resistance to the flexion can be felt and represents quadriceps spasticity. This test also causes action potentials in the iliopsoas (From Perry *et al.* 1976.)

of 50º in males (range 25º–65º) and a mean of 40º in females (range 16º–60º). Lateral rotation in infants less than 1 year old had a mean value of almost 70º and medial rotation declined at about the same age a mean of 45º (range 25º–65º). In contrast

2 Phelps gracilis test. With the patient prone, knees flexed and hip abducted, extend one knee. If the hip adducts on progressive extension of the knee, gracilis spasm and contracture are confirmed (Keats 1965).

to the data on medial rotation where females had a greater degree of passive motion (mean 7º more than males), no sex difference was found in the measurements of lateral rotation.

With the patient still prone, spasticity of the quadriceps muscle can be estimated with the prone rectus femoris test, in which the knee is rapidly flexed and its resistance to flexion is felt. Buttock elevation is supposed to be indicative of the complete positive test (Fig. 2.33). This is not a pure rectus femoris test. Stretch electromyograms have shown that in this test the iliopsoas muscle has the same number of action potentials as the rectus femoris (Perry *et al.* 1976).

Stretch tests about the hips are limited in specificity (Perry *et al.* 1976). The adductors are sensitive to the hip-adductor stretch texts (i.e. abducting the hips quickly) with the hips and knees flexed, or to Phelps gracilis,[2] and also to the Thomas test. Electromyographic data show that both the straight leg-raising and the gracilis tests induce the same amount of electrical activity of the medial hamstrings. The Thomas test produces similar amounts of electrical activity in both the iliopsoas and the rectus femoris. The adductors are sensitive to the hip adductor stretch tests (i.e. abducting the hips quickly) with the hips and knees flexed, or to the Phelps gracilis test, and also to the Thomas test.

Knee. Spasticity and contracture of the hamstrings are reliably measured with the straight leg-raising or the popliteal angle measurement. The hamstrings are almost exclusively active on electromyograms with straight leg-raising (Perry *et al.* 1976). To palpate the hamstrings and obtain a better estimate of contracture, flex the hip 90º and then extend the knee to the limit permitted by the contracture. The degree of contracture is measured as the angle which the tibia subtends with the neutral and normal extension expected at the knee joint (0º); this angle is the popliteal angle (Fig. 2.34). The mean popliteal angle in newborns was reported to be 27º (SD 6.3º) with a range of 20º–40º that decreased to zero by age 1 year (Reade *et al.* 1984). In children, Tardieu (1984) considered a 20º popliteal angle to be normal.

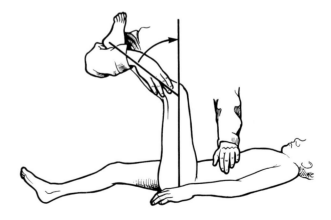

Fig. 2.34. Test for hamstring spasm and contracture. Patient supine; hip flexed 90º and knee extended to point of resistance. The angle between the neutral extended position of the knee and the tibia is the 'popliteal angle'.

'Tight hamstrings' are quite usual in the normal population. A study of 369 children selected from the non-orthopaedic clinics at the Prince of Wales Children's Hospital in Randwick, Australia determined that under the age of 2 years the maximum angle was 180º (0) in all children. After the age of 2 years the angle decreased rapidly to plateau at 155º (25º) at age 6 years. An angle greater than 125º (55º) suggested significant hamstring tightness (Kuo *et al.* 1997).

In Denmark a study of 769 children and adolescents from seven schools and 10 kindergartens measured the popliteal angles (Reimers *et al.* 1993). They found that 75% of the boys and 40% of the girls over age 10 years had tight hamstrings with popliteal angles greater than 40º; 10% of the boys over age 10 years had angles greater than 60º. The data from these two studies and others that reported similar results ought to temper any zeal to lengthen the hamstring muscles in children who have cerebral palsy based solely on the static tests for hamstring contracture. Observational and/or instrumented gait analysis will discern whether the decreased popliteal angle is functionally significant. To demonstrate the point to students and residents in the clinic, Bleck often did the popliteal angle measurement on students and residents. Many had angles greater than 20º, usually were athletic, and had no functional impairment.

The position of the patella is noted; whether it is riding above its normal location in the patellar–femoral groove. (In orthopaedic sports medicine circles the cryptic code words are, 'patella alta' for high, and the opposite: 'patella baja' for low.) To discover the amount of flexion contracture of the knee joint, the limb is extended so it lies flat on the table. If firm pressure on the anterior aspect of the knee joint fails to extend the knee to the zero position, a flexion contracture of knee joint (posterior capsule) in addition to the hamstring contracture is likely.

Voluntary control of the quadriceps and its strength within the range allowed by a knee flexion contracture can be estimated with the child lying supine and with legs flexed over the table's edge (Evans 1975). Simultaneous extension of both knees seems easier for most patients. Those who have unilateral voluntary control of knee extension seem to have better walking patterns.

With the patient in this sitting position, quadriceps spasticity might be elicited by quickly pushing the knees into flexion. Those patients who have severe quadriceps spasticity will not be able to have their knees passively flexed to 90º, and the increased stretch reflex can be seen easily.

Pendulum test. With the patient seated and the legs hung over the table edge, the leg is allowed to fall with the force of gravity and oscillate as a pendulum easily provides visualization of quadriceps and hamstring spasticity. Fowler and colleagues (2000) used electrogoniometers on the thigh to measure the degree of motion, and surface electrodes on the muscles for electromyography to confirm relaxation (Fig. 2.35). They measured the number of oscillations, their duration, the excursion of the first backward swing, and the first swing excursion between the starting and resting angles. The first swing was the best predictor of the degree of spasticity in cerebral palsy and had a good correlation with the Ashworth scales of severity. But whether the data from the pendulum test can be related to walking or other functions is not known (Graham 2000).

Tibial–fibular torsion and foot rotation. For language purists, the normal degree of tibial–fibular rotation should be called 'version' and the abnormal 'torsion' (2 standard deviations from the mean, Staheli 1990). This fixed rotation of the tibia is measured as the expression of the angle between an imaginary line through the tips of the medial and lateral malleoli of the ankle and the polar axis of the proximal articular surface of the tibia (Fig. 2.36). Since Le Damany's treatise on torsion of the tibia (1909), many methods of measurement have been described together with anatomical and clinical studies (Hutter and Scott 1949, Dupuis 1951, Khermosh *et al.* 1971, McSweeny 1971, Staheli and Engel 1972, Engel and Staheli 1974, Ritter *et al.* 1976, Kobyliansky *et al.* 1979, Malekafzali and Wood 1979, Staheli *et al.* 1985). The results of all the different types of measurement show variations of a few degrees of normal tibial rotation, but all are generally in agreement on mean values (Fig. 2.37).

Unless a formal and reportable study is planned by the examiner, elaborate instrumentation and calculations to measure

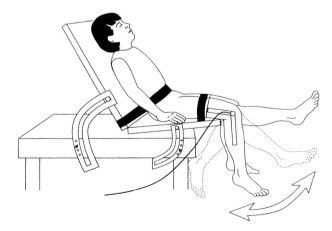

Fig. 2.35. Pendulum test. Patient seated, electrogoniometer in place, right lower-limb movement observed after leg is dropped. (From Fowler *et al.* 2000; reproduced by permission of Mac Keith Press.)

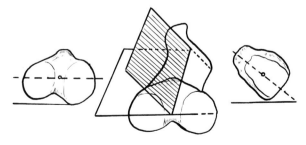

Fig. 2.36. Tibial torsion is the angle formed by the intersection of the two planes constructed between the proximal and distal ends of the tibia (*center*). The coronal plane is through the proximal articular surface of the polar axis (*left*). The other plane is through the distal articular surface of the tibia in a line which bisects the medial malleolus and the articular facet for the fibula (*right*).

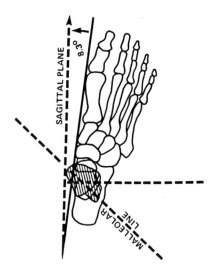

Fig. 2.37. Axial deviation of the foot from the line of progression in the mid-sagittal plane. (Adapted from Elftman 1969.)

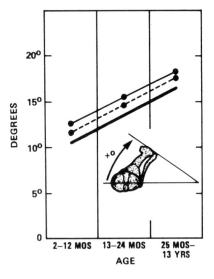

Fig. 2.38. Mean external tibial–fibular torsion in normal children. Three series of measurements: Bleck and Minaire 1983 (top line, normal children), Bleck and Minaire 1983 (dashed line, in-toed children with no external tibial–fibular torsion as measured), Staheli and Engel 1972 (bottom line, normal).

tibial–fibular torsion are too time-consuming to be worthwhile. But, it is necessary to do some estimate of tibial–fibular torsion to avoid the unintended consequences of femoral derotation osteotomy when the patient has a compensatory external tibial–fibular torsion creating a duck walk, or after a subtalar or triple arthrodesis correction of a pes valgus that results in pigeon toeing.

The bottom line is the direction of the foot along the line of progression during the stance phase of gait. Normally the toe-out, the axial rotation of the foot, is a mean of +8.3° (SD 3.5°) (Elftman 1945, 1969)[3] (Fig. 2.38). Variations from the mean and

3   These data on foot rotation were used in the mass production of artificial limbs for military personnel who lost lower limbs during World War II— all foot pieces were set externally rotated from the leg at 7° at the Naval Amputation Center, Mare Island, California.

standard deviations are due to femoral rotation, tibial–fibular torsion, and persistent fetal medial deviation of the neck of the talus (Attenborough 1966, Bleck and Minaire 1983

Visual goniometric measurement. The patient sits with knees flexed over the table edge and with the hip in neutral rotation. An imaginary line through the femoral condyles is visualized; this line would be roughly parallel to the one through the polar axis of the proximal tibial surface. The second line is between the tips of the malleoli. One arm of the goniometer is placed parallel to the table edge and the other arm is placed in line with the oblique line constructed through the tips of the malleoli, the transmalleolar axis (Fig. 2.39).

With this method of measurement, the normal mean angles with this method according to age were approximately as follows: 0–12 months, 7° (SD 4. l°); 13–24 months, 10° (SD 2°); 25 months–13 years, 13° (SD 3°); and in the older children and adults the mean value was 22°.

In the study by Staheli *et al.* (1985), in which a photographic method was used, the infant under age 1 year had a mean transmalleolar axis of about 0° (SD 20°) and by age 8 years had increased to 20° (range 0° to about 35°; and in the skeletally mature, the mean remained at 20° with a range of 0°–45°. In a personal communication, J.L. Goldner (1999) maintained that a part of the tibial torsion is rotation in the knee joint. With the knee flexed to 90° it is possible to rotate the tibia when assessing tibial torsion. Therefore no attempt should be made to manually hold the tibia in rotation, medial or lateral, when estimating the degree of tibial torsion.

The *thigh–foot angle* is a measurement of the rotation of the foot at the ankle with reference to the midline of the thigh

(a)   (b)

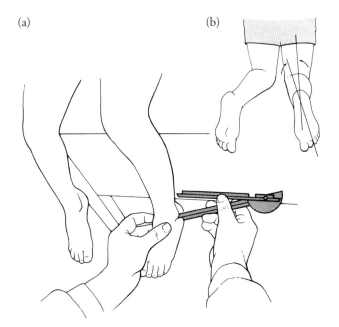

Fig. 2.39. (*a*) clinical measurement of tibial–fibular torsion: knee flexed 90° over the table edge; hip in neutral rotation. One limb of the goniometer is parallel to the table edge, and the other limb of the goniometer is placed in a line through the tips of the medial and lateral malleoli. (*b*) measurement of thigh–foot angle. Patient is prone, with knee flexed 90°.

(Staheli and Engel 1972, Bleck 1982, Staheli *et al.* 1985). The patient lies prone, and the knee is flexed to 90º; the foot is dorsiflexed to neutral (the measurement is limited to those children who do not have equinus deformities of the ankle). In dorsiflexing the ankle, one has to avoid everting or inverting the foot. One arm of the goniometer is placed on a line that bisects the heel, and the other arm of the goniometer is placed directly over the visualized mid-line of the thigh.[4] The medial or lateral deviation of the foot from the line on the mid-thigh is the thigh–foot angle. It is a lower angle than that for tibial torsion, but it does roughly parallel the angle of the transmalleolar axis with a mean of +10º and a range from –3º to +20º. It remains practically the same in children and adults. The foot-progression angle refers to the angle made by the long axis of the foot and the line of progression of walking (Staheli 1985, 1990, 1993).

Foot and ankle range of motion. The range of dorsiflexion of the ankle is measured with the heel held in inversion in order to get a true estimate of the dorsiflexion; holding the foot in varus locks the mid-tarsal joints and prevents a false measurement of dorsiflexion of the ankle; simply dorsiflexing the entire foot as a unit can add dorsiflexion at the talonavicular joint (Fig. 2.40). The classic test to differentiate gastrocnemius muscle contracture from that of the soleus muscle was described by Silfverskiöld (1923). In this test, if dorsiflexion of the foot with the knee flexed is greater than that with the knee extended, then the gastrocnemius is implicated as the main site of the contracture (Fig. 2.41). If there is no change in dorsiflexion of the ankle with this maneuver, then contracture of both muscles is present. Electromyographic studies of these muscles in performance of the Silfverskiöld test demonstrated that both muscles show increased action potentials, regardless of the position of the knee joint (Perry *et al.* 1974). No clear-cut differences in gastrocnemius and soleus spasticity were found in three of Perry's eight cases, in spite of positive Silfverskiöld tests in all. The only case in which I would

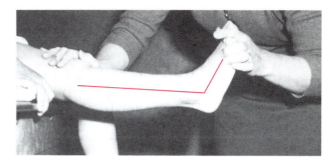

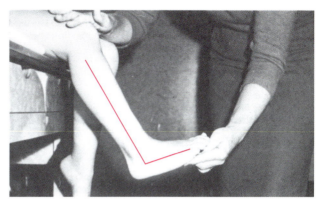

Fig. 2.41. Silfverskiöld test for gastrocnemius versus soleus contracture. *Top*: with knee extended and foot in varus, passively dorsiflex the ankle and note the limited range of ankle dorsiflexion. The same maneuver is repeated with the knee flexed 90º. If the ankle dorsiflexes easily when the knee is flexed, gastrocnemius contracture alone is presumed.

implicate the gastrocnemius alone as the source of the equinus (and contracture), is when the foot (with hind-foot held in inversion) can be passively dorsiflexed with great ease when the knee if flexed 90º. If any force is required to dorsiflex the foot in this position, I consider the test negative (EEB).

Voluntary dorsiflexion of the foot is frequently absent. It is worth noting if the patient can dorsiflex the foot. Frequently active dorsiflexion can be obtained only with the flexor withdrawal ('confusion reflex'). This phenomenon is observed by flexing the knee 90º over the table's edge, and asking the patient to flex the hip actively while the examiner resists flexion of the thigh by manual pressure on the anterior portion of the mid-thigh (Fig. 2.42). To test whether or not the confusion test is useful in predicting active swing-phase contraction of the tibialis anterior muscle, a gait analysis was done on 23 patients who had cerebral palsy (David *et al.* 1993). The result was that 33% showed abnormal swing-phase dorsiflexion and 61% had abnormal swing-phase plantarflexion. Conclusion: the confusion test is a patterned response, but does not predict swing-phase action of the tibialis anterior during gait.

Varus of the foot can be due to a spastic posterior tibial muscle which inverts the hind-foot, or an overactive anterior tibial muscle which inverts the mid-foot, or both. If the varus position of the foot can be corrected passively, the deformity is 'dynamic' versus 'fixed'. Quick eversion of the heel may demonstrate an increased stretch reflex in the posterior tibial muscle; in this case, its tendon can be palpated and seen more prominently posterior to the medial malleolus.

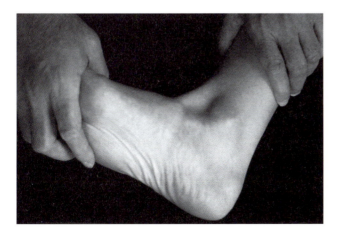

Fig. 2.40. For an accurate measurement of the range of passive dorsiflexion of the ankle, the foot must be held in varus (inversion) to stabilize the talonavicular joint and prevent dorsiflexion at the mid-tarsal joints.

4 The line that bisects the heel rest is visualized as the major axis of an ellipse formed by the heel on weightbearing.

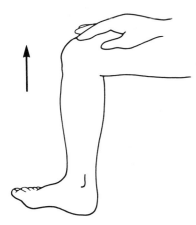

Fig. 2.42. Flexor withdrawal reflex. Patient seated with hips and knees flexed 90º. Examiner's hand is on the anterior surface of the thigh. The patient is instructed to flex the hip against the resistance of the examiner's hand. Automatic dorsiflexion of the ankle occurs in a positive response.

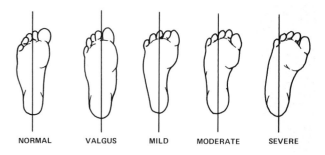

NORMAL   VALGUS   MILD   MODERATE   SEVERE

Fig. 2.43. Assessment of forefoot adduction based upon the heel bisector method in which the plantar aspect of the heel is visualized as an ellipse. The heel bisector is the major axis of the ellipse (Bleck 1971, 1982, 1983). Normal: bisects toes 2 and 3; metatarsus adductus: mild, toe 3; moderate, 3 and 4; severe, 4 and 5.

Valgus of the foot appears to be due primarily to spastic peroneal muscles which overpower the inverters of the foot. A quick inversion of the foot may elicit the stretch reflex in the peroneal muscles which will offer resistance to this motion. The degree of 'fixed' valgus deformity should be ascertained by manipulating the foot into the corrected position. Usually equinus is a component of the valgus of the hind- and mid-foot, and therefore to correct the deformity passively, the foot must be kept in equinus (see Chapter 8 for more details about preoperative assessment of equinovalgus deformities of the foot). Luckily for those who hate measuring inversion or eversion of the foot (subtalar joint), there is no good technique to measure the range of motion.

Forefoot adduction deformity (spastic metatarsus adductus) is found by inspection of the plantar aspect of the foot while the examiner holds the heel in one hand and the head of the first metatarsal medially is cupped by the palm and web space of the thumb; the forefoot is then abducted against the fixed heel. Limited or no passive abduction of the forefoot indicates a fixed forefoot adduction deformity. One way to assess the metatarsal adduction deformity is to visualize the plantar weightbearing surface of the heel as an ellipse; the major axis of this ellipse defines the center line of the foot (Bleck 1971, 1983, Bleck and Minaire 1983). In the normal foot, this line ('heel bisector') passes through the second and third toes; in moderate metatarsus adductus it passes between the third and fourth toes, and between the fourth and fifth toes in severe adductus (Fig. 2.43). If dynamic metatarsus adductus has been noted during the gait examination, passive abduction of the forefoot is possible and the tendon of the spastic abductor hallucis can be palpated on the medial aspect of the head of the first metatarsal.

Deformities of the toes to be looked for are hallux valgus and toe-flexion contractures. Hallux valgus rarely occurs in isolation, but rather is secondary to a valgus deformity of the foot.

A cavus deformity is excessive forefoot equinus and a fixed deformity. In ordinary terms it is a 'high arch'. The forefoot equinus can be compounded by a calcaneus deformity of the hind-foot (an excessive dorsiflexed position of the calcaneus) (Fig. 2.44). The diagnosis is usually made by a perception of what constitutes a 'high arch'—how high is high, and how low is low? To overcome subjectivity in this evaluation, the angle between the horizontal weightbearing surface of the head and the shaft of the first metatarsal can be measured (Fig. 2.45). This angle should be measured on maximum passive dorsiflexion of the foot, or on photographs of the medial side of the foot when the patient is standing. In normal feet, this angle is between 15º and 30º, an angle of 40º or more denotes a cavus deformity.

TYPE OF MOTION DISORDER

By the time this detailed orthopaedic and neurological examination has been completed, the examiner should have no difficulty in deciding whether the motion disorder can be classified as spastic, athetoid, dystonic, tension athetoid, ataxic, tremor or mixed. Even though there are patients who have mixed athetosis and spasticity, we try to avoid taking this easy route, and prefer as much diagnostic precision as possible. Also based upon observations during the examination, one should have little difficulty in formulating an opinion on the geographic involvement hemiplegia, diplegia, triplegia (or three-limb-dominated bilateral spastic cerebral palsy: Aicardi 1998), quadriplegia (we prefer total body involved). The standard format for recording the diagnosis is, for example: 'cerebral palsy, spastic diplegia, etiology preterm birth and low birthweight', or 'cerebral palsy, athetosis, total body involved, etiology, perinatal hypoxia', etc.

In the course of examining the joints for ranges of motion assessment of *severity of spasticity* can be estimated according to the Ashworth scale as delineated in Chapter 1 and added to your diagnostic impression. Also you might use the pendulum test described in this chapter, but more studies are needed to determine whether the values obtained are reproducible and sensitive. Caution in interpretation is advisable. Furthermore, the pendulum test is applicable only to the lower limb and not the upper limbs.

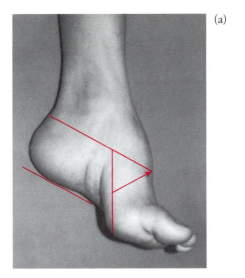

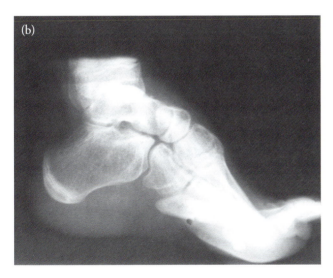

Fig. 2.44. (*a*) Cavus deformity of the foot. The primary deformity is excessive forefoot equinus which can be measured as indicated in Figure 2.42 with the foot dorsiflexed to its maximum amount, or with the patient standing. (*b*) Radiograph, lateral projection of the foot and ankle, depicts marked forefoot plantarflexion (equinus).

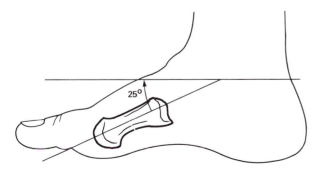

Fig. 2.45. Measurement of forefoot equinus. Horizontal line is parallel to the weight-bearing surface of the heel; the second line is along the shaft of the first metatarsal. The normal angles range from 10º–20º; 30º–40º moderate cavus ('high arch'); <40º represents severe cavus.

The classification according to the child's motor function in the age range of 6–12 years in five levels can be added to the diagnosis using the Gross Motor Performance Measure and Classification (Palisano *et al.* 1997), usually done by the physical therapist as summarized in Chapter 3.

SUMMARY

The sequence of the examination will be according to one's own style and thought process in data collection. We have resisted the temptation to be 'au courant' by constructing an algorithm. These diagrams or little boxes with arrows pointing downward, sideways and obliquely, as a guide on what to do next in the diagnosis and treatment of cerebral palsy, seem too complex to be useful. The diagnosis and management of cerebral palsy cannot be reduced to a simple road map with occasional detours: it is more like the maze at Hampton Court, and only repetition of the experience of examining children makes the process easier. '*Repetitio mater est studiorum*' (repetition is the mother of studies).

However, for those who have read the preceding pages and would like some guidance based upon my own style (EEB), I suggest the following order of the examination.

Infants and children aged 5 years (± 2 years). Begin with child sitting on mother's lap, then assess the upper limbs, followed by the head and associated defects, deep tendon reflexes and plantar responses, sitting posture, supine posture, and lower limbs.

Older children (aged 7 years, ± 2 years) who cannot walk. Begin with child seated in the wheelchair, then assess the upper limbs, the head and associated defects, sitting posture, deep tendon reflexes and plantar responses, supine posture, and lower limbs.

For children who can stand and walk (with or without aids). First assess standing posture, then equilibrium reactions, walking, sitting posture, deep tendon reflexes and plantar responses head and associated defects, upper limbs, supine posture (if walking is functional, no need to test locomotor prognostic signs), and lower limbs.

TIME

Physicians can only give their time, and no computer program has yet been devised to produce 'artificial intelligence' that will decrease the time needed for examination and data collection (Winograd 1985). The time for a complete assessment, recording all the data in a record, making necessary referrals, and above all talking with the parents will be at least 60 minutes. If the child has not been previously diagnosed, or if the condition is complex (e.g. total body involved, or spastic diplegia versus hemiplegia), 90 minutes will not be too long. If skeletal radiographs are necessary (excluding computerized axial tomography and magnetic resonance imaging etc.), another 30–45 minutes will be required, depending on the efficiency of the radiographic services. In the growing child, reevaluations are almost always necessary every 6 months and will take at least 30 minutes. Parents usually have many questions and anxieties, which must be answered patiently.

In the United States there is a growing trend to make the physician 'more productive', by insisting that the time spent with patients must be restricted so that the volume of patients per physician can be increased. The proposed practice of medicine by 'Megacorporate Health Care' promises to exclude such luxuries as 'personal consultation-time with the practitioner'. Based upon what is known of these corporate practices, it is predicted that proper assessments of conditions such as cerebral palsy will be done only for 'relatively affluent individual consumers' (Freedman 1985). In the two decades since the last edition of this book (Bleck 1987), more 'managed' care has captured many more people for health care insurance in the USA[5]. We hope that physicians will reject and dispel the illusion that a rapid screening process and quick examinations under the rubric of efficiency can replace proper medical diagnosis and advice.

Ironically, when things go wrong in patient care (usually due to errors in judgement), much more time is spent with attorneys and courts (or in societies less litigious than the United States, in explanations and filing reports) than was spent on the initial and subsequent assessments of the patient. Furthermore the fees paid, the money spent and the awards granted are considerably more than what was deemed to be the just fee on the first visit (Sanderson 1981).

The *team approach* arose after World War II, probably because of the greater interest by physicians in children with long-term orthopaedic impairments, and the growth of medical science and practice which permitted more effective management of complex conditions such as cerebral palsy and spina bifida. Many medical and paramedical specialists were educated to deal with the specific problems presented by such children. The public was not niggardly in providing funds to service the multiple needs of disabled children and their parents. The team approach meant that every child with cerebral palsy was seen by a member of the team: pediatrician, neurologist, ophthamologist, orthopaedic surgeon, physiatrist, audiologist, physical and occupational therapists, speech therapist, psychologist and social worker (and in clinics within special schools, the teacher) regardless of the needs of the particular child. After some 25 years of this kind of team approach, it has been seriously questioned as a viable model. McCollough (1984) reported that such teams are inordinately expensive, and recommended a more rational and modified approach. The physician who assumes responsibility for the overall patient management should refer only to those specialists who are required to assess a particular problem in a particular child. The medical and paramedical specialists should be available for consultation, but each child does not have to run through a mill with every member of the team taking a little piece of the child.

Up to the 1990s the orthopaedic surgeon most often assumed the role of the primary treating physician. Surgery has a powerful effect in forging a strong relationship with the orthopaedic surgeon and to whom parents turn for advice and referral. But with the advent of botulinum toxin, selective posterior rootlet rhizotomy and intrathecal baclofen this leadership might devolve to the neurosurgeon, physiatrist, or neurologist. As pediatricians have become more interested and active in the diagnosis and management of cerebral palsy and other chronic disabilities in children they can be the primary treating physician who refers to other specialists for advice and treatment options.

REFERENCES

Aicardi, J. (1998) *Diseases of the Nervous System in Childhood.* London: Mac Keith Press with Cambridge University Press; Philadelphia: J.B. Lippincott, pp. 226–227.

Alcorn, C.L., Nicholson, C.L. (1972) 'Validity of the Slosson Drawing Coordination Test with adolescents of below-average ability.' *Perceptual Motor Skills,* **34**, 261–262.

Attenborough, D.G. (1966) 'Severe congenital talipes equinovarus.' *Journal of Bone and Joint Surgery,* **48B**, 31–39.

Baird, H.W., Gordon, E.C. (1983) *Neurological Evaluation of Infants and Children. Clinics in Developmental Medicine, Nos 84/85.* London: Spastics International Medical Publications with Heinemann Medical; Philadelphia: J.B. Lippincott.

Balmer, G.A., MacEwen, G.D. (1970) 'The incidence of scoliosis in cerebral palsy.' *Journal of Bone and Joint Surgery,* **52B**, 134–136.

Bartlett, M.D., Wolf, L.S., Shurtleff, D.B., Staheli, L.T. (1985) 'Hip flexion contractures: a comparison of measurement methods.' *Archives of Physical Medicine and Rehabilitation,* **66**, 620–625.

Beadle, K. (1982) 'Communication disorders.' *In* Bleck, E.E., Nagel, D.A. (Eds) *Physically Handicapped Children: A Medical Atlas for Teachers.* Orlando, Florida: Grune & Stratton.

Belanos, A.A., Bleck, E.E., Firestone, P., Young, B.A (1989) 'Comparison of sterognosis and two-point discrimination testing of the hands in children with cerebral palsy.' *Developmental Medicine and Child Neurology,* **31**, 371–376.

Bleck, E.E. (1971) 'The shoeing of children: sham or science.' *Developmental Medicine and Child Neurology,* **13**, 188–195.

—— (1975) 'Locomotor prognosis in cerebral palsy.' *Developmental Medicine and Child Neurology,* **17**, 18–25.

—— (1982) 'Developmental orthopaedics. III: Toddlers.' *Developmental Medicine and Child Neurology,* **24**, 533–555.

—— (1983) 'Metatarsus adductus: classification and relationship to outcomes of treatment.' *Journal of Pediatric Orthopaedics,* **3**, 2–9.

—— Minaire, P. (1983) 'Persistent medial deviation of the neck of the talus: a common cause of in-toeing in children.' *Journal of Pediatric Orthopaedics,* **3**, 149–159.

—— (1987) *Orthopaedic Management in Cerebral Palsy. Clinics in Developmental Medicine, No. 99/100.* London: Mac Keith Press with Blackwell Scientific; Philadelphia: J.B. Lippincott.

Bobath, B. (1954) 'A study of abnormal reflex activity in patients with lesions of the central nervous system.' *Physiotherapy,* **40**, 259–289.

Bratshaw, M.L., Perret, Y.M. (1992) *Children with Disabilities.* Baltimore: Paul H. Brooks.

Brunnstrom, S. (1962) *Clinical Kinesiology.* Philadelphia: F.A. Davies.

Burnett, C.N., Johnson, E.W. (1971) 'Development of gait in childhood. Part I. Method.' *Developmental Medicine and Child Neurology,* **13**, 196–206.

Coon, V., Donato, G., Houser, C., Bleck, E.E. (1975) 'Normal ranges of motion of the hip in infants, six weeks, three months and six months of age.' *Clinical Orthopaedics and Related Research,* **110**, 256–260.

Csongradi, J., Bleck, E.E., Ford, W.F. (1979) 'Gait electromyography in normal and spastic children.' *Developmental Medicine and Child Neurology,* **21**, 738–748.

Cupps, C., Plescia, M.G., Houser, C. (1976) 'The Landau reaction: a clinical and electromyographic analysis.' *Developmental Medicine and Child Neurology,* **18**, 43–53.

David, J.R., Holland, W.C., Sutherland, D.H. (1993) 'Significance of the confusion test in cerebral palsy.' *Journal of Pediatric Orthopaedics,* **13**, 717–721.

Dupuis, P.V. (1951) *La Torsion Tibiale.* Paris: Masson.

---

5 A search of the Medline/PubMed database for 'managed care' from 1987 to December 2002 resulted in 30,083 publications, of which 1505 were initially displayed for retrieval.

Elftman, H. (1945) 'Torsion of the lower extremity.' *American Journal of Physical Anthropology*, **3**, 255–256.

—— (1969) 'Dynamic structure of the human foot.' *Artificial Limbs*, **13**, 49–58.

Elliott, J.M., Connolly, K.J. (1984) 'A classification of manipulative hand movements.' *Developmental Medicine and Child Neurology*, **26**, 283–296.

Engel, G.M., Staheli, L.T. (1974) 'The natural history of torsion and other factors influencing gait in childhood. A study of the angle of gait, tibial torsion, knee angle, hip rotation, and development of the arch in normal children.' *Clinical Orthopaedics and Related Research*, **99**, 12–17.

Evans, E.B. (1975) 'The knee in cerebral palsy.' *In* Samilson, R.L. (Ed.) *Orthopaedic Aspects of Cerebral Palsy. Clinics in Developmental Medicine, Nos 52/53.* London: Spastics International Medical Publications with Heinemann Medical; Philadelphia: J.B. Lippincott.

Ferlic, D.C. (1966) 'Sensory status of the hand as related to reconstructive surgery of the upper extremity in cerebral palsy.' *Clinical Orthopaedics and Related Research*, **46**, 87–92.

Fowler, E.G., Nwigwe, A.I., Ho, T.W. (2000) 'Sensitivity of the pendulum test for assessing spasticity in persons with cerebral palsy.' *Developmental Medicine and Child Neurology*, **42**, 182–189.

Freedman, S.A. (1985) 'Megacorporate health care.' *New England Journal of Medicine*, **312**, 579–582.

Ford, F., Stevik, A.C., Csongradi, J. (1975) 'EMG telemetry study of spastic gait patterns in cerebral palsied children.' *Developmental Medicine and Child Neurology*, **17**, 307. (Abstract.)

Gage, J.R. (1991) *Gait Analysis in Cerebral Palsy. Clinics in Developmental Medicine, No. 121.* London: Mac Keith Press with Cambridge University Press; Philadelphia: J.B. Lippincott.

Gesell, A., Amatruda, C.S. (1947) *Developmental Diagnosis, 2nd edn.* New York: Hoeber.

Goble, J. (1984) *Visual Disorders in the Handicapped Child.* New York: Marcel Dekker.

Goldner, J.L. (1974) 'Upper extremity tendon transfers in cerebral palsy.' *Orthopedic Clinics of North America*, **5**, 389–414.

Graham, H.K. (2000) 'Pendulum test in cerebral palsy.' *Lancet*, **355**, 2184.

Greene, W.B., Heckman, J.D. (1994) *The Clinical Measurement of Joint Motion.* Rosemont, IL: American Academy of Orthopaedic Surgeons.

Haas, S.S., Epps, C.H. Jr, Adams, J.P. (1973) 'Normal ranges of hip motion in the newborn hip.' *Clinical Orthopaedics and Related Research*, **91**, 114–118.

Hagberg, B., Sanner, G., Steen, M. (1972) 'The dysequilibrium syndrome in cerebral palsy.' *Acta Paediatrica Scandinavica*, **226** (Suppl.), 1–63.

Hensinger, R.N. (1986) *Standards in Pediatric Orthopedics: Tables, Charts and Graphs Illustrating Growth.* New York: Raven Press.

Hutter, C.G., Scott, W. (1949) 'Tibial torsion.' *Journal of Bone and Joint Surgery*, **31A**, 511–518.

Ingram, T.T.S. (1984) 'A historical review of the definition and classification of the cerebral palsies.' *In* Stanley, F., Alberman, E. (Eds) *The Epidemiology of the Cerebral Palsies. Clinics in Developmental Medicine, No. 87.* London: Spastics International Medical Publications with Heinemann Medical; Philadelphia: J.B. Lippincott.

Keats, S. (1965) *Cerebral Palsy.* Springfield, IL: C.C. Thomas.

Kelley, D.L. (1971) *Kinesiology, Fundamentals of Motion Description.* Englewood Cliffs, NJ: Prentice-Hall.

Khermosh, O., Lior, G., Weissman, S.L. (1971) 'Tibial torsion in children.' *Clinical Orthopaedics and Related Research*, **79**, 25–31.

Kobyliansky, E., Weissman, S.L., Nathan, H. (1979) 'Femoral and fibial torsion. A correlation study in dry bones.' *International Orthopaedics*, **3**, 145–147.

Kuo, L., Chung, W., Bates, E., Stephen, J. (1997) 'The hamstring index.' *Journal of Pediatric Orthopaedics*, **17**, 78–88.

Lea, R.D., Gerhardt, J.J. (1995) 'Current concept review: range of motion measurements.' *Journal of Bone and Joint Surgery*, **77A**, 784–798.

Le Damany, P. (1909) 'La torsion du tibia. Normal, pathologique, expérimentale.' *Journal d'Anatomie et Physiologie*, **45**, 589–615.

Lee, L.W., Kerrigan, D.C., Della Croce, U. (1997) 'Dynamic implications of hip flexion contractures.' *Archives of Physical Medicine and Rehabilitation*, **76**, 502–508.

Lesny, I., Stehlik, A., Tomasek, J., Tomankova, A., Havlicek, I. (1993) 'Sensory disorders in cerebral palsy.' *Developmental Medicine and Child Neurology*, **35**, 402–405.

Liao, H.F., Mao, P.J., Hwang, A.W. (2001) 'Test–retest reliability of balance test in children with cerebral palsy.' *Developmental Medicine and Child Neurology*, **43**, 180–186.

Madigan, R.R., Wallace, S.L. (1981) 'Scoliosis in the institutionalized cerebral palsy population.' *Spine*, **6**, 583–590.

Malekafzali, S., Wood, M.B. (1979) 'Tibial torsion—a simple clinical apparatus for its measurement and its application to a normal adult population.' *Clinical Orthopaedics and Related Research*, **145**, 154–157.

Mayo Clinic, Members of the Department of Neurology (1991) *Clinical Examinations in Neurology.* St Louis: Mosby Year Book.

McCollough, N.C. III (Chairman) (1984) *Proceedings of the Conference on The Critical Needs of the Child with Long Term Orthopedic Impairment.* Washington, DC.

McDowell, B.C., Hewitt, V., Nurse, A., Weston, T., Baker, R. (2000) 'The variability of goniometric measurements in ambulatory children with spastic paralysis.' *Gait and Posture*, **12**, 114–121.

McInerny, R. (1984) *St Thomas Aquinas. Six Lectures on the Saint and His Thought.* Notre Dame, IN: University of Notre Dame Press.

McMahon, T.A. (1984) *Muscles, Reflexes, and Locomotion.* Princeton, NJ: Princeton University Press.

McMulkin, M.L., Guilliford, J.J., Williamson, R.V., Ferguson, R.L. (2000) 'Correlation of static to dynamic measures of lower extremity range of motion in cerebral palsy and control populations.' *Journal of Pediatric Orthopaedics*, **20**, 366–369.

McSweeny, A. (1971) 'A study of femoral torsion in children.' *Journal of Bone and Joint Surgery*, **53B**, 90–95.

Moberg, E. (1976) 'Reconstructive hand surgery in tetraplegia, stroke, and cerebral palsy: some basic concepts in physiology and neurology.' *Journal of Hand Surgery*, **1A**, 29–34.

O'Connell, E.J. Feldt, R.H., Stickler, G.B. (1965) 'Head circumference, mental retardation and growth failure.' *Pediatrics*, **36**, 62–66.

O'Connor, A.R., Stephenson, T.J., Johnson, A., Tobin, M.J., Ratib, S., Fielder, A.R. (2002) 'Strabismus in children of birth weight less than 1701 g.' *Archives of Ophthalmology*, **120**, 767–773.

Opila-Lehman, J., Short, M.S., Trombly, C.A. (1984) 'Kinesthetic performance of athetoid and spastic cerebral palsied and non-handicapped children.' *Orthopaedic Transactions*, **8**, 104. *Developmental Medicine and Child Neurology*, **26**, 241. (Abstract.)

Paine, R.S., Oppé, T.E. (1966) *Neurological Examination of Children. Clinics in Developmental Medicine, Nos 20/21.* London: Spastics International Medical Publications with Heinemann Medical; Philadelphia: J.B. Lippincott.

Palisano, R.J., Rosenbaum, P.I., Walters, S.D., Russell, D., Wood, E., Galuppi, B. (1997) 'Development and reliability of a system to classify gross motor function in children with cerebral palsy.' *Developmental Medicine and Child Neurology*, **39**, 214–213.

Perry, J. (1967) 'The mechanics of walking.' *Physical Therapy*, **47**, 778–801.

—— (1975) 'Cerebral palsy gait.' *In* Samilson, R.L. (Ed.) *Orthopaedic Aspects of Cerebral Palsy. Clinics in Developmental Medicine, Nos 52/53.* London: Spastics International Medical Publications with Heinemann Medical; Philadelphia: J.B. Lippincott.

—— (1992) *Gait Analysis: Normal and Pathological Function.* Thorofare, NJ: Slack.

—— Hoffer, M.M., Giovan, P., Antonelli, D., Greenberg, R. (1974) 'Gait analysis of the triceps surae in cerebral palsy.' *Journal of Bone and Joint Surgery*, **56A**, 511–520.

—— Antonelli, D., Plut, J., Lewis, G., Greenberg, R. (1976) 'Electromyography before and after surgery for hip deformity in children with cerebral palsy.' *Journal of Bone and Joint Surgery*, **58A**, 201–208.

Reade, E., Horn, L., Hallurn, A., Lopopolo, R. (1984) 'Changes in popliteal angle measurement in infants up to one year of age.' *Developmental Medicine and Child Neurology*, **26**, 774–780.

Reimers, J., Brodersten, A., Pedersen, M.D. (1993) 'The incidence of hamstring shortness in Danish Children 3–17 years old.' *Journal of Pediatric Orthopaedics*, **2**, 173–175.

Ritter, M.A., DeRosa, G.P., Babcock, J.L. (1976) 'Tibial torsion.' *Clinical Orthopaedics and Related Research*, **120**, 159–163.

Robson, P. (1968) 'The prevalence of scoliosis in adolescents and young adults with cerebral palsy.' *Developmental Medicine and Child Neurology*, **10**, 447–452.

Rose, J., Wolff, D.R., Jones, V.K., Bloch, D.A., Ochlert, J.W., Gamble, J.G. (2002) 'Postural balance in children with cerebral palsy.' *Developmental Medicine and Child Neurology*, **44**, 58–63.

Rubin, I.L., Crocker, A.C. (1989) *Developmental Disabilities: Delivery of Medical Care for Children and Adults.* Philadelphia: Lea & Febiger.

Rushworth, G. (1964) *The Role of the Gamma System in Movement and Posture.* New York: Association for the Aid of Crippled Children.

Samilson, R.L., Bechard, R. (1973) 'Scoliosis in cerebral palsy.' *In* Ahstrom, J.P. (Ed.) *Current Practice in Orthopaedic Surgery, Vol. 5.* St Louis: C.V. Mosby.

Sanderson, R.R. (1981) 'Medical practice and malpractice.' *Legal Aspects of Medical Practice*, **9**, 1–7.

Saunders, J.B., Inman, V.T., Eberhart, H.D. (1953) 'The major determinants in normal and pathological gait.' *Journal of Bone and Joint Surgery*, **35A**, 543–558.

Si1fverskiöld, N. (1923) 'Reduction of the uncrossed two joint muscles of the one-to-one muscle in spastic conditions.' *Acta Chirurgica Scandinavica*, **56**, 315–330.

Staheli, L.T. (1977) 'The prone hip extension test.' *Clinical Orthopaedics and Related Research*, **123**, 12–15.

—— (1990) 'Lower positional deformity in infants and children: a review.' *Journal of Pediatric Orthopaedics*, **11**, 559–563.

—— Engel, G.M. (1972) 'Tibial torsion. A method of assessment and a survey of normal children.' *Clinical Orthopaedics and Related Research*, **86**, 183–186.

—— Corbett, B.S., Wyss, C., King, H. (1985) 'Lower-extremity rotational problems in children.' *Journal of Bone and Joint Surgery*, **67A**, 39–47.

Statham, L., Murray, M.P. (1971) 'Early walking patterns of normal children.' *Clinical Orthopedics and Related Research*, **79**, 11–24.

Sutherland, D.H. (1984) *Gait Disorders in Childhood and Adolescence.* Baltimore: Williams and Wilkins.

Tachdjian, M.O., Minear, W.L. (1958) 'Sensory disturbances in the hands of children with cerebral palsy.' *Journal of Bone and Joint Surgery*, **40A**, 85–90.

Tardieu, G. (1984) *Le Dossier Clinique de L'Infirmité Motrice Cérébrale, 3rd edn.* Paris: Masson.

Thomson, J.D., Banta, J.V. (2001) 'Scoliosis in cerebral palsy: an overview and recent results.' *Journal of Pediatric Orthopaedics, Part B*, **10**, 6–9.

Winograd, T. (1985) 'Artifical intelligence may be over-sold.' *Campus Report, Stanford University, California*, Feb. 27, pp. 1, 10.

Winter, D.A. (1991) *The Biomechanics and Motor Control of Human Gait: Normal, Elderly and Pathological, 2nd edn.* Waterloo, Ontario: University of Waterloo Press.

3
SPECIAL ASSESSMENTS AND INVESTIGATIONS

This chapter includes only those special assessment tools that should be of interest to the orthopaedic surgeon and other clinicians who deal with cerebral palsy. These include the physical and occupational therapist's assessments with developmental tests, the Gross Motor Function Measure and Classification, radiology, photography, instrumented gait analysis, myoneural blocks and psychological testing. Not included are special laboratory examinations such as blood, urine and cerebrospinal fluid for metabolic defects, chromosomal analysis, electroencephalography, or details of neurometric examinations. There is ample literature about these specialized subjects (Baird and Gordon 1983, Aicardi 1998, pp. 32–154).

PHYSICAL AND OCCUPATIONAL THERAPIST'S ASSESSMENTS

A complete motor assessment includes the following examinations with the data recorded on special forms so that the status of the motor system can be followed as the child matures: (1) assessment of the severity of the spasticity; (2) passive ranges of motion of the limb joints; (3) active ranges of motion to delineate selective motor control; (4) manual muscle strength tests; (5) developmental and motor maturity evaluations.

CLINICAL SEVERITY ASSESSMENT

> '*There is not a clear "best test" or comprehensive quantitative measure of spasticity.*'
>
> (Skinner 1992)

The advent of selective posterior rootlet rhizotomy in spastic paralysis created a need for assessment of the severity of the spasticity. Although attempts have been made to use instrumentation to determine resistance to stretch of a single muscle group (e.g. calf or knee), these methods are limited to only the one muscle (Tripp and Harris 1991). Electromyographs made in response to stretch are not quantitative. The electrical response of muscle-action potentials either in motion analysis or in stretch tests cannot be used for assessment of the degree of spastic paralysis. Consequently, the clinical observational tests of Ashworth have come into use in almost all outcome studies of selective posterior rootlet rhizotomy and intrathecal baclofen (Ashworth 1964, Albright 1995). Table 1.I details the Ashworth scoring of spasticity. Chutorian and Root (1994) modified the scoring system in the assessment of effects of botulinum A intramuscular injections (grading from 0, 1, 1+, 2, 3, 4). It seems obvious that the Ashworth scores are dependent on the perceptions of the examiner. In the original Ashworth scoring the difference between score 3 and 4 may be difficult to discern and between 2 and 3 in the modification by Chutorian and Root. In an interobserver manual testing of elbow-flexor muscles the ratings between therapists of a modified Ashworth test was 86.7% (Bohannon & Smith 1987).

QUANTIFYING SPASTICITY

ELECTROMYOGRAPHY
Skinner (1992) emphasized that there is no accepted technique for relating the electromyographic (EMG) signal to the muscle force in spastic paralysis. The H-wave response is thought to reflect the excitability of the alpha motor neuron at the spinal cord level. It is evoked in able-bodied individuals by stimulation of the posterior tibial nerve and recording the response of the plantar muscles. The H-wave response bypasses the muscle spindle. The values in spastic paralysis overlap the normals and can be changed by local and environmental factors.

MEASUREMENT OF RESISTANCE TO PASSIVE MOTION
The *pendulum drop test*, in which the knee is dropped from full extension over the edge of a table with the patient lying supine, has been used to observe oscillations of the knee in flexion due to spasticity of the quadriceps. The amplitude and frequency of oscillations have been measured and reduced by a formula to a number which is used to assess the severity of the spasticity (Fowler *et al.* 2000). The details of this test have been discussed in Chapter 2.

Dynanometers have been tested in measuring the torque resistance of the ankle when put through a range of motion from dorsiflexion to plantarflexion manually in both unaffected individuals and in patients with spasticity. The latter showed greater torque resistance in response to stretch velocity than in unaffected persons. The results were repeatable (Otis *et al.* 1983).

Motorized foot plates were used in a Spasticity Measurement System (Lehman *et al.* 1989). The system measures the torque in response to a 5° arc of motion near the patient's maximum dorsiflexion. The torque response consisted of an elastic component that was dependent on displacement and not velocity, and a viscous component that was dependent on velocity. The oscillations ranged in frequency from 3 to 12 Hz. The children with spastic paralysis were compared with able-bodied children. Those with spasticity showed a response that depended on a viscoelastic response as seen in adults.

As noted by Skinner (1992), the tests for resistance to passive motion appear suitable for children and are repeatable and reliable. Nevertheless, they do not seem to be used very much in the assessment of outcomes in rhizotomy or intrathecal baclofen. Rather, a review of the results of these direct assaults on the spastic muscles shows a reliance on only the Ashworth clinical scores.

DEEP-TENDON REFLEX MEASUREMENT
Because the deep-tendon reflexes are hyperactive in spastic paralysis, several laboratories have made quantitative measurements of the deep-tendon reflex. In a prospective study of posterior rootlet rhizotomy, Skinner (1992) used an electromechanical hammer that recorded the force used with a transducer when tapping the patellar tendon with the knee flexed. An angular accelerometer strapped to the shin recorded the angular acceleration in response to the tendon tap. Surface electrodes recorded an electromyogram of the quadriceps to identify the data. When he studied the children with rhizotomy, Skinner (1992) found significant reduction of the angular acceleration of the shin in response to the hammer blow 6 months and 12 months postoperative selective posterior rootlet rhizotomy.

Although the foregoing laboratory investigations to quantify spasticity have their limitations, they may be useful when studying the efficacy of various interventions: physical therapeutic, pharmacologic, surgical, and those using nerve blocks. The results will either refute, confirm or modify the clinical impressions of the effectiveness of the particular agent or method. For example, given the current enthusiasm by some therapists for electrical stimulation in cerebral palsy, the work of Robinson and associates (1988a, b) seems important. They found that electrical stimulation of spastic muscles in spinal-cord injuries caused fatigue of the muscles that reduced spasticity, but had little effect in the long term. In children, instrumented tests can be time-consuming and anxiety-producing, as well as adding to the expense of treatment.

PASSIVE AND ACTIVE RANGE OF MOTION OF LIMBS
The measurement of the passive range of joint motion in the limbs was described in Chapter 2. Muscle-strength testing requires active voluntary control of the limb which is either present, or absent, or limited in range of joint motion due to muscle and joint contractures or spasicity. To assess voluntary control and strength in the lower limbs of the child with spastic diplegia in a making a decision for selective posterior rootlet rhizotomy, one neurosurgeon (W. Peacock, personal communication) told me that he asks the child to squat and rise. While not measurable, it seems to be a quick and easy method of assessment of not only strength and voluntary control, but also of the integrity of balance reactions (equilibrium). Those who can do it would seem to have a better prognosis for a good outcome of surgery including rhizotomy.

INFANT AND CHILD DEVELOPMENT ASSESSMENT

'All too often, children are examined but not looked at.'
(Aicardi 1998)

Why should orthopaedic surgeons and other specialists be bothered with developmental assessment? Doctors who deal with children with cerebral palsy and their parents need to have at least some basic knowledge of child development and to be conversant with the variety of assessment tests that have been developed. Growth and development are important in the practice of pediatric orthopaedics if these physicians go beyond being mere surgical technicians.

Aicardi (1998) urged the physician not only to look at the test results, but also to observe the quality of the activity observed as well as such unquantifiable behaviors as 'intensity of gaze' and 'directed attention' as described by Brazelton and Nugent (1995). The qualitative approach takes experience and practice that comes only with time.

NEONATAL AND INFANT SCREENING
Due to the enormous interest in outcomes of infants born 'at risk' (e.g. due to preterm birth, low birthweight, perinatal hypoxia), numerous developmental screening tests have been devised. These tests have been used in many clinical investigations of infants to determine the natural history of development of infants born 'at risk', and to judge the efficacy of 'early intervention' for such infants. During the last quarter of the 20th century, with growing awareness of child development and hopes for effective 'early intervention', many other tests were formulated for their predictive value of future neurological and psychological problems (Brazelton 1973, Touwen 1976, Prechtl 1977, Dubovitz and Dubovitz 1981, Nelson and Ellenberg 1982, Amiel-Tison and Grenier 1983, Stanley and Alberman 1984, Harel and Anastasiow 1985, Egan 1990, Brazelton and Nugent 1995). Infant screening tests have contributed to our knowledge of the epidemiology of cerebral palsy and its natural history of infants deemed 'at risk' (Nelson and Ellenberg 1978, 1982).

Most of these tests can be administered by therapists, especially the *Denver Developmental Screening test*. The Denver test is by far the most popular initial screening test for identifying suspected development delay (Frankenburg and Dodds 1967, Frankenburg *et al.* 1971, Baird and Gordon 1983). This test has been standardized for infants born in other cultures and societies (Federal Republic of Germany: Flehmig *et al.* 1973; UK: Bryant *et al.* 1974; USA: Barnes and Stark 1975, Frankenburg *et al.* 1975; South Africa: Super 1976; Netherlands: Cools and Hermanns 1977; Japan: Ueda 1978; Israel: Shapira and Harel 1983). A plethora of other developmental tests for the infant and child up to the age of 3 years to identify children who are predicted to have or have cerebral palsy have been published (Paine and Oppé 1966, Bayley 1969, Brazelton 1973, 1984, Sheridan 1975, 1978, Prechtl 1977, Saint-Anne Dargassies 1977, Touwen 1979, Amiel-Tison and Grenier 1983, Harris 1989).

One would think that no more tests would be needed. Yet reports of tests continued into the 1990s. The *Early Motor Pattern Profile* consists of 15 items of variations in muscle tone, reflexes and movement in a standardized format using a 3-point scale: 2 if the abnormality is severe and present all of the time; 0 if none present, 1 if inconsistent or partial (Morgan and Alag 1996). These authors tested 1247 high-risk infants who were followed to a minimum of 36 months of age. The predictive value was 89.4, sensitivity was 87.1, and specificity was 97.8 at 6 months and a bit lower at 12 months. The authors stated that the test takes only a few minutes and can be incorporated into the routine pediatric office visit.

Six motor milestones to screen preterm infants for cerebral palsy were found to be more effective in serial screening than any individual milestone alone (Allen and Alexander 1997). The six milestones were: roll prone to supine, roll supine to prone, sit with support, sit without support, crawl and cruise. When the 173 high-risk infants were re-examined at 18–24 months, 18% who had delays in more than four milestones had cerebral palsy.

The ultimate simplicity for early identification of cerebral palsy is the *popliteal angle* (Johnson and Ashurst 1989). The test was described in response to a letter to the editor as testing one leg at a time with the baby supine. The hip was flexed on the abdomen and the knee extended. The health visitor measured the angle 'by eye'. The angle used was between the thigh and the leg with a 'passing angle' of 140º; a failed test occurred when this angle was less than 100º. The specificity was 92% but the sensitivity was only 51%. It was more sensitive but less specific for infants of less than 30 weeks gestational age. Only 12% of infants who failed the test were diagnosed as cerebral palsy. Of major importance to clinicians is that the health visitors 'were remarkably accurate' in their increased concern about the infant based on their impressions that exceeded the popliteal angle predictions at 92.7% sensitivity and 80.4% specificity.

PRESCHOOL DEVELOPMENT ASSESSMENT
Watch the child standing, walking, moving, looking, talking and playing. A good simple developmental test for preschool children (ages 2–5 years) was published originally by Paine and Oppé (1966) and reintroduced by Baird and Gordon (1983). The motor age of the child is determined by the observations of postural and functional activities related to what is considered

normal for age. For example, at 7 months the infant assumes the quadruped position, at 9 months pulls self to standing, at 13 months walks alone. Cumulative percentiles for achievement of sitting, walking, and talking were developed by Neligan and Prudham (1969) (Table 3.I). Of pertinence to the orthopaedist, walking occurred in the 97th centile at 18 months. The physician, even the orthopaedist, should have some working knowledge of developmental milestones. Parents and teachers want to discuss the problems of their child's lack of development. For what is expected of a child's abilities at a certain age, the list by Aicardi (1998) should be appealing to the therapist and physician (Table 3.II).

Developmental screening tests for the child over 3 years of age can be used to identify children who may have neurologically based problems so that special care and attention can be given to them during their education. These tests are additions to the neurological examinations for gros- and fine-motor skills (Baird and Gordon 1983). Recommended and commonly used tests are: the Peabody Picture Vocabulary test (Coop *et al.* 1975), the Slosson Oral Reading test (Erford and Luce 2005), the Draw-a-Person test (Dykens 1996), the Slosson Drawing Co-Ordination test (Alcorn and Nicholson 2002) and the Bender-Gestalt test (Patel and Bharucha 1972). This last test has given consistent results and has been judged to be dependable (Baird and Gordon 1983).

Bax and Whitmore (1973, 1987) used a battery of tests and the traditional physician's examination and observations of 5-year-old children about to enter school. They then followed up the educational and behavioural outcomes at the ages of 7 and 10 years. They found that the neurodevelopmental score alone did not give as good a prediction of future difficulties as the school doctor's clinical judgement. Three cheers for the traditional physician–observer who takes the time do it!

TABLE 3.I
Cumulative percentiles for four standard developmental milestones (Neligan and Prudham 1969)

Milestone	Percentile	Age (mths)
Sitting	3rd	5
	50th	6
	97th	10
Walking	3rd	8–9
	50th	13–14
	97th	18
Single words	3rd	9
	50th	12
	97th	21
Sentences: boys	3rd	17.5
	50th	24
	97th	>36
Sentences: girls	3rd	16
	50th	23
	97th	36

Girls tend to be slightly more advanced than boys in communication skills.

TABLE 3. II
Selected developmental milestones (Aicardi 1998, pp. 817–21)

Developmental milestone	Approximate age first noted
Gaze contact	1–2 hours
Smile	0–6 weeks
Vocalizing other than crying	2–8 weeks
Social smile	2–3 months
Begins to lift head in prone position	2–4 months
Laughs aloud	2–4 months
Bimanual (visually guided) coordination in reaching objects	4–6 months
Pulls to stand holding onto furniture	5–10 months
Sits steadily unsupported	7–10 months
Responds to own name	7–10 months
Sits upright on floor	8–10 months
Pincer grip	9–12 months
Waves goodbye	9–12 months
Holds out object to adult but will not release it	9–12 months
One word with meaning	9–14 months
Simple pretend play (e.g. 'peek-a-boo')	10–14 months
Walks unsupported	10–16 months
Holds out object to adult and will release it	11–14 months
Shakes head for 'No'	12–16 months
Complex pretend play	18–24 months
Goes up and down stairs alone, both feet on each step	20–26 months
Uses 'I', 'Me', 'You'	2–2½ years
Mutual play with other children	2–2½ years
Five-word sentences comprehensible to strangers	2–3 years
Mainly dry by day	2–5 years
Mainly dry by night	2½–6 years
Speech generally intelligible to strangers	2½–5 years
(Imaginary companion—not universal)	(3–4 years)
Skips on one foot	3½–4½ years
Tells stories	3½–4½ years
Draws a person	3½–4½ years
Emerging time concepts: distinguishes morning/evening	4½–6 years

BEYOND TRADITIONAL MILESTONES TO THE CHILD'S 'INNER WORLD'

Aicardi (1998, pp. 817–21) provided a summary of new insights into the child's 'inner world' of development beyond the traditional milestones: shared attention (wanting to share other people's attention to points of reference, e.g. a light on the ceiling), social referencing (your perception of other person's interpretation of an event), the 'eye-direction detector' construct (see what others see), executive functions (planning, sequentially arrange events, and delayed gratification), central coherence (seek meaning, pattern and coherence from details presented), and more complex forms of social interactions (social competence, empathy, mentalizing ability, a theory of the mind). For more discussion of these fascinating new ideas of child development, Aicardi (1998, pp. 817–21) can provide a springboard for further study.

ASSESSMENT OF FUNCTION

'*Bald numbers rarely tell a full story and clinical sensitivity in the interpretation of results is vital.*'

(Rosenbaum 1992)

Although motor age determinations can be used in special studies and prognosis (Beals 1966), we must remember that normal children do not perform and develop on an exact timetable, and allowances must be made for considerable individual variations (Table 3.I). Another problem is that a motor age does not always tell us how a child functions, or what adaptations to function independently have occurred. Testing for functional abilities is probably more important in evaluating and following children. Functions in eating, daily hygiene, toileting, dressing, mobility, and communication skills, when scored for independence and completion in a practical time, or performed with equipment and adaptations, are most informative. Many physical and occupational therapists in the past developed their own forms, and some have been published (Coley 1978, Bleck and Nagel 1982, Tardieu 1984). These proposed measures of function were not universally adopted and were not subjected to reliability and reproducibility analysis, and were not quantitative. The need for better testing of function of the child with cerebral palsy seems to have been stimulated by the many years of physical therapy systems that promised improvement (unfortunately in some instances perceived as a 'cure'), but without a systematic method of assessing their efficacy.

Palisano *et al.* (1997) used the *Peabody Developmental Gross Motor Scale* to evaluate infants who received physical therapy, but found the scale not responsive to change in infants with cerebral palsy over a 6-month period. As a result of their study the authors could not recommend this method to evaluate the direct effects of physical therapy; however, it could be recommended for a global assessment as part of other evaluation systems.

The *Gross Motor Function Measure* (GMFM)[1] was developed to quantitate changes in motor function of children with cerebral palsy (Russell *et al.* 1989). The need was to overcome assessment of children who have cerebral palsy measured by using tests developed for normal child populations. The test is termed 'criterion-referenced' in which the person is reassessed on a set of activities previously evaluated, i.e. before and after an intervention. A companion to the GMFM is the Gross Motor Performance Measure (GMPM). It attempts to quantitate quality of function (Boyce *et al.* 1991), i.e. how well a child performs a subset of the same gross motor functions. The GMFM defines how much the child can do (Russell *et al.* 1993, 2003).

The Gross Motor Function Measure quantitates changes in function of children with cerebral palsy. It defines how much the child can do.

The GMFM consists of five dimensions that a normal 5-year-old can accomplish. The five dimensions are: (A) lying and rolling; (B) sitting; (C) crawling and kneeling; (D) standing; and (E) walking, running and jumping. The original test consisted of 88 items to be scored. The authors use a 4-point Likert scale. Values of 0–3 are assigned to the four categories: 0 = does not initiate;

---

1 As much as I abhor the proliferation of abbreviations in medical articles, I use them for these two tests. EEB

1 = initiates (less than 10% of the task); 2 = partially completes (10 to less than 100% of the task); 3 = completes. Explicit definitions for partial and complete achievement in each item are essential for proper administration and scoring (Russell *et al.* 1993). A percentage score is calculated for each dimension and a total score is derived from the mean of the five dimension scores. Those who wish to use this measure should consult the *Gross Motor Function Measure (GMFM-66 and GMFM-88) User's Manual* (Russell *et al.* 2003).

The measure has been found to have an acceptable level of reliability in reproducibility and intrarater and interrater testing. Boyce and colleagues (1995) pursued further studies to validate the measure of gross motor performance in detecting changes in the quality of movement in children with cerebral palsy from birth to 12 years. They reported validity across the diagnoses, severity and age groups, but the relationships of parent's and therapist's ratings were not evident.

The *Gross Motor Function Classification System* is divided into five levels. Each level is divided into segments according to the age range: before the 2nd birthday, from age 2 to the 4th birthday, from age 4 to the 6th birthday, from age 6 to 12 years (Palisano *et al.* 1997) (Table 3.III). For details of the level at the various ages, the entire publication should be consulted. Palisano and associates (1997), with 48 experts in the field, used a nominal group process and Delphi survey consensus methods to achieve a consensus on the validity and revisions of the classification system. The interrater reliability was 0.55 for children less than two years old and 0.75 for children from 2 to 12 years. Scandinavian experts confirmed its reliability in children with cerebral palsy or brain damage (Nordmark *et al.* 1997). They found that its interrater and intrarater reliabilities were good; the interrater reliability was 0.77 and 0.88 at the first and second assessments respectively.

Since its introduction, the GMFM has been revised and simplified to 66 items (GMFM-66) (Russell *et al.* 2000). Applying

TABLE 3.III
Gross Motor Function Classification System (Palisano *et al.* 1997)

Level I: walks without restrictions; limitations in more advanced gross motor skills.

Level II: walks without assistive devices; limitation walking outdoors and in the community.

Level III: walks with assistive mobility devices; limitations walking outdoors and in the community.

Level IV: self-mobility with limitations; children are transported or use power mobility outdoors and in the community.

Level V: self-mobility is severely limited even with the use of assistive technology. These children have no means of independent mobility and are transported. Some achieve self-mobility using a power wheelchair with extensive adaptations.

In a former classification of mobility the descriptive terms that seem to conform to the Gross Motor Function Classification System levels were:

Level I = independent walker in household, neighborhood and community
Level II = neighborhood walker
Level III= household walker
Level IV= physiological walker (in physical therapy room)
Level V = non-walker

this measure to 537 children with varying degrees of cerebral palsy showed high test–retest reliability and the 66-item test to be a better assessment tool for motor development than the 88-item GMFM. A subset of 228 children were tested a 12 months. Although the GMFM has been shown to be responsive in infants under the age of 24 months with cerebral palsy or motor delay (Kolobe *et al.* 1998), Russell and colleagues (2000) found that the 66-item measure detected less change in children older than age 5 years regardless of the severity of the cerebral palsy. Accordingly, they thought that a disability inventory such as the *Pediatric Evaluation of Disability Inventory* (PEDI), from the New England Medical Center Hospitals, might be a better assessment tool (Feldman *et al.* 1990, Ketelaar *et al.* 1998). The PEDI was designed to assess function of disabled children, from age 6 months to 7 years. The three dimensions developed to identify functional status and change were: (1) functional skill level; (2) caregiver assistance; and (3) modifications or adaptive equipment used (Feldman *et al.* 1990).

Nordmark *et al.* (2000) used the GMFM and the PEDI at 6 and 12 months postoperative selective dorsal rhizotomy in 18 children who had spastic diplegia. They found that both measures were sensitive to changes in function, but the PEDI detected significant changes earlier in cases of mild impairment. But in a group with more severe impairment the changes in function were noted only with the PEDI. They recommended that both instruments be used as they are complementary.

The GMFM has been increasingly used in outcome assessments of various treatments of cerebral palsy: physical therapy (Russell *et al.* 1989, Bower *et al.* 1996), muscle performance and physical fitness in cerebral palsy (Parker *et al.* 1993), electrical stimulation following rhizotomy (Steinbok *et al.* 1997), selective posterior rootlet rhizotomy (Steinbok *et al.* 1997, McLaughlin *et al.* 1998, Wright *et al.* 1998), intrathecal baclofen in a single case report (Almeida *et al.* 1997), and correlation with gait analysis (Damiano and Abel 1996, Drouin *et al.* 1996).

Because the GMFM-66 consists of 22 fewer items, the authors believe it should take less time to administer (Russell *et al.* 2000). A limitation is the need for a computer program to score the test. The software program calculates the score based on the 66 items with a standard error (Burrows 1999). One major difference in this new program is that no zero scores are recorded if the item was not administered or that the child did not perform. In this case the new format includes the response as 'not tested'.

Rosenbaum (1992) made the valid point that 'surrogate' measures such as Ashworth scale, gait analysis, and range of motion measurements do not necessarily translate into improved motor function after selective posterior rootlet rhizotomy and cannot be claimed as success in improving gross motor function. Conversely, rhizotomy might improve motor function without altering the range of motion or the spasticity. Hence the need to use a measure of function such as the GMFM and the PEDI in the assessment of outcomes.

Therapists and other clinicians have also recognized a need for a classification for fine motor activity of the upper limbs for children with cerebral palsy. Accordingly the Manual Ability

TABLE 3.IV
Manual Ability Classification System (MACS) (Eliasson *et al.* 2006)

I: handles objects easily and successfully.

II: handles most ojects but with somewhat reduced quality and/or speed of achievement.

III: handles objects with difficulty; needs help to prepare and/or modify activities.

IV: handles a limited selection of easily managed objects in adapted situations.

V: does not handle objects and has severely limited ability to perform even simple actions.

Classification (MACS) was devised in Sweden (Eliasson *et al.* 2006, Table 3.IV). The reliability and validity of the test has been confirmed in a study out of Britain (Morris *et al.* 2006). MACS assesses how the hands work together to handle objects and accomplish tasks. As with GMFCS, there are five levels with Level 1 categorizing the most functional hand usage. This will be discussed in more detail in Chapter 5 under prognosis for upper-limb function.

OTHER ROLES OF PHYSICAL THERAPISTS IN ASSESSMENT

Special investigations that can be performed by the therapist include photography, videotape recording, assessment of balance, energy requirements and instrumented gait analysis to help the physician in clinical decisions and outcome studies. The therapist must recognize structural changes in the musculoskeletal system that would impair function (e.g. subluxation of the hip, flexion contracture of the knee and scoliosis). Early discernment of such potential problems, and alerting the physician to them, enables the physician to appropriate radiographic investigations.

Special perceptual and visual–motor tests for the evaluation of learning disabilities including dyslexia have been popular in the United States, parallel with the great interest and concomitant funds allocated to improve the education of children. The most widely applied tests (usually by occupational therapists) were those of Frostig (Frostig 1963, Frostig and Horne 1964) and Ayres (1972, 1978); they were often requested by the teachers. When these tests were positive, therapists initiated special remediation programs with the intent of improving academic performance. In follow-up studies most of these tests and remedial program were discounted (Feagans 1983). The ultimate outcome of the hoped-for help by teachers in shifting some of the educational role to physical and occupational therapists for remedial exercises for perceptual disorders seems to have allowed the reversion to the traditional role of teachers, i.e. to teach.

RADIOLOGY

Plain radiographs are essential for the diagnosis and for surgical treatment of structural changes in the skeleton. Infants and children who have adduction and/or flexion spasticity of the hip musculature should have an anterior–posterior radiograph of

the hips (with the hips held in the neutral abduction/adduction and rotation) at approximately 6-monthly intervals, in order to make the early diagnosis of subluxation. Scrutton and Baird (1997) recommended surveillance measures of hips based on a study of 166 children who had bilateral cerebral palsy (spastic diplegia and total body involved). They recommended anterior–posterior projections of the pelvis and hips with the child lying supine, with the limbs parallel and the hips in neutral rotation. If there was a flexion posture of the hips, they placed padding under the legs to flex the hips and flatten the lumbar spine. The measurements used were the migration percentage and the acetabular index (Reimers 1980, Eklof *et al.* 1988) to ascertain subluxation (normal migration index chosen was equal to or less than 33%) (Fig. 3.1). In Eklof's study the 98th percentile of migration increased up to 4 years of age, to 16%, and at age 12 or more years it was 24%; higher percentages represented subluxation.

The study of Scrutton and Baird (1997) indicated that the acetabular index did not correlate well with the migration percentage at 4–5 years. However, an acetabular index of 30° or more at 30 months indicated a hip problem by 5 years.[2] The migration percentage is the simplest way to monitor the hip for the purpose of preventing with surgery subluxation and dislocation in bilateral cerebral palsy. While Scrutton and Baird recommended radiological surveillance at 30 months, the study group of a hip surveillance clinic at the Royal Children's Hospital in Melbourne, Australia, recommended that *all* children with bilateral cerebral palsy should have a radiograph of the pelvis with the lower limbs in the correct position before the age of 18 months (Dobson *et al.* 2002).

Children who have bilateral spastic cerebral palsy and whose pelvic radiograph shows a migration percentage of the hip greater than 15% should have radiographic surveillance every 6 months.[3] In particular, children with total body involved cerebral palsy (spastic quadriplegia) and a poor prognosis for walking, and those who have spastic diplegia with delayed walking or are dependent on external supports (crutches or walkers), are at risk for hip subluxation. Opinions as to the time for surgical inter-vention vary from a 40% to a 60% migration percentage. Dobson and colleagues (2002) settled on 40%. The question as to the age and type of surgery is addressed in Chapter 8. Earlier is clearly better than later—before the age of 4 years. These guidelines are summarized in Table 3.V. They must of course be individualized for each child.

If there are clinical signs of scoliosis, a single anterior–posterior radiograph of the spine and pelvis (made with the patient standing or sitting) should be made. More projections will be necessary if orthotic or surgical treatment is planned. If a leg-length discrepancy of significance (more than 1 cm) is found,

---

2 Pelvic rotation distorts the acetabular angle. To be assured that the pelvis is in neutral rotation, the width of the obturator foramina should be approximately 1:1.
3 Reimers' study of able-bodied children's hips showed that the 90th centile of children by age 4 years had a migration percentage of 10% and migration of less than 1% per year (Reimers 1980).

PERCENT OF SUBLUXATION

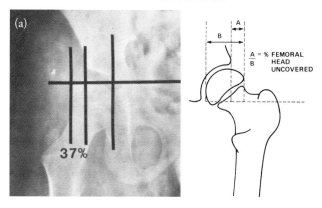

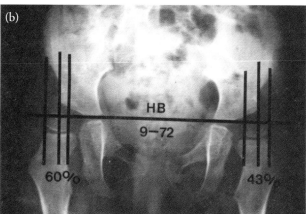

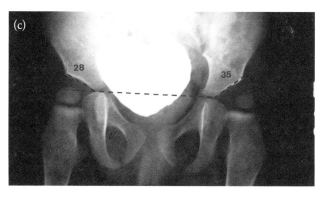

Fig. 3.1. (*a*) Measurement of the migration percentage of a hip from the anterior–posterior radiograph. The upper limit of migration is 15%. (*b*) Anterior–posterior radiograph of the pelvis and both hips with measurement of the migration index showing bilateral subluxation. (*c*) Anterior–posterior radiograph of a 3-year-old with spasticity in both lower limbs. The right hip shows and acetabular index of 35º and the left 28º. The right hip is at definite risk for progressive subluxation; surgery required. Note that the widths of the obturator foramina are equal in a ratio of 1:1; this ensures that the acetabular angle measurement has not been distorted by rotation of the pelvis.

special leg-length films are the only accurate way to document and then follow the shortening of the limb in the growing child most often in spastic hemiplegia and rarely more than 2 cm at skeletal maturity (< 2 cm is not clinically significant). Radiographs of the other bones and joints are usually made when the history and clinical examination indicate they are necessary.

Parents today are rightly concerned about overexposure to radiation. Despite the promise of magnetic resonance imaging (MRI) to reduce the need for radiation, skeletal structures do not visualize as well as in radiographs. MRI is considerably more expensive. Furthermore, imaging artifacts are noted in the presence of metallic implants near the anatomy of interest. Non-ferromagnetic metallic implants are now used (Guermazi *et al.* 2003). Therefore, although prudence in ordering radiographs in children is required, there is no other way for a correct diagnosis and treatment to be accomplished. Parents need to be more informed with objective information on radiographic dosages and risks of cancer. With special filters and modern radiographic equipment, the dosages per projection to various anatomical parts can be determined and related to what is deemed to be safe. Since radiographic equipment differs, each radiographic unit would be advised to prepare its own data for publication. This kind of data has helped us give parents a perspective, and has reduced anxiety.

Computerized tomography (CT) has been available since the 1970s.[4] It virtually eliminated invasive procedures such as pneumoencephalography in the diagnosis of suspected lesions of the brain (e.g. hydrocephalus, porencephalic cysts). Cranial CT has been shown to predict an adverse neurodevelopmental outcome in a long-term follow-up study of 56 children who had symptomatic congenital cytomagalovirus infections in the newborn period. 90% of the newborns who had an abnormal scan developed at least one sequela of the disease (Boppana *et al.* 1997).

MRI of the brain has largely supplanted cranial CT: but, for skeletal structures, CT is superior to MRI. It is especially useful in the analysis of abnormalities in the hip joint. It is faster than MRI and allows a better visualization of the femoral head in relation to the acetabulum and the configuration of the acetabulum than plain radiographs so that surgical reconstruction can be more accurately designed and performed (Lasda *et al.* 1978, Weiner *et al.* 1978, Terver *et al.* 1982, Mahboubi *et al.* 1986, Horstmann *et al.* 1987) (Fig. 3.2).

Three-dimensional (3D) CT that defines the pathological skeletal anatomy of established subluxation and dislocation of the hips in cerebral palsy have been increasingly used to plan

4 Dr Geoffrey Hounsfield, an engineer at the EMI Laboratories in Middlesex, England, had worked as a sound engineer for the Beatles, who later financed the research laboratory. The first paper on CT scanning was published in 1973. In 1979 Dr Hounsfield shared the Nobel Prize for Medicine with Alan M. Cormack (Webb 1990).

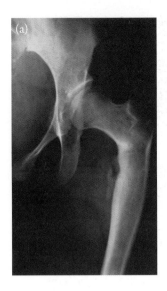
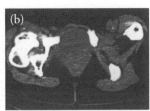

Fig. 3.2. (*a*) Anterior–posterior radiograph of 19-year-old female with spastic diplegia, totally disabled because of hip pain. Was referred after femoral osteotomy and subsequent removal of the internal fixation device. (*b*) CT scan of patient's hip shows severe femoral torsion, erosion on the anterior femoral head, and an irregular acetabulum

the appropriate surgical reconstruction (Abel *el al.* 1994). Measurements of the femoral neck-shaft angles were more than 99% accurate, and acetabular anteversion measurements had more than 96% accuracy. In complex distorted hip anatomy, 3D imaging is impressive in defining exactly the problems to be addressed with surgery (Fig. 3.3).

BRAIN IMAGING

MRI has become the standard investigation in the diagnosis of lesions of the spinal cord and brain (Mumenthaler 1990, Aicardi 1998). This tremendous technical advance has practically eliminated invasive myelography and pneumoencephalography in adults and children. It is painless and, except in infants and young children, does not usually require sedation or general anesthesia. The latter are necessary to keep the child immobile during the scanning.

We have not reached the stage of classifying cerebral palsy according to the precise cerebral pathology. Some progress has been reported. MRI studies of six patients who had extrapyramidal cerebral palsy with a history of intrapartum asphyxia showed lesions in the putamen and thalamus (Menkes and Curran 1994). Byrne *et al.* (1990) studied brain MRIs in 15 term infants who had hypoxic–ischemic encephalopathy during the neonatal period, and at 4 and 8 months of age. Cerebral palsy developed in nine infants, and two had an abnormality of 'tone' and delayed motor milestones. Brain abnormalities and/or delayed myelination were observed at age 8 months in all nine infants who developed cerebral palsy. Hayakawa *et al.* (1997) studied the brains of 34 children with spastic quadriplegia using the axial proton density, T2- and T1-weighted images. All had abnormal findings. Term infants who had no adverse perinatal events had 62.5% prevalence of congenital anomalies, and those who did have adverse events had a variety of brain lesions. 75% of preterm infants had periventricular leukomalacia.

Spasticity of the lower limbs is not always cerebral in origin. Upper spinal-cord lesions and anomalies are known to cause spastic paraplegia. The alert physician who finds no birth or developmental history compatible with cerebral palsy and no upper-limb paralysis or associated defects common to cerebral palsy, must think of the spinal cord. Such lesions are rare, but for the particular child who has a spinal-cord lesion causing spastic paraplegia that might be resolved with surgery, rarity is a non-issue.

Neurosonography has also identified brain pathology in cerebral palsy. Cystic periventricular leukomalacia was diagnosed in 31 preterm infants manifested primarily by cysts in the middle-posterior or posterior periventricular regions. Clinically, all had cerebral palsy: 54% quadriplegia, 42% diplegia and 4% hemiplegia. In quadriplegia there were larger and more extensive cysts (Rogers *et al.* 1994). Hoon and colleagues (1997) have found the brain MRI a useful diagnostic tool in children who 'appear' to have cerebral palsy. They have found characteristic signals in hypoxic–ischemic encepathalopathies, genetic–metabolic, mitochondrial and organic acid metabolic disorders. Another study using cranial ultrasound in 33 preterm infants was compared with an MRI at 44 weeks' postmenstrual age. The neurodevelopmental outcome was assessed at age 3 years in 31 of these children.

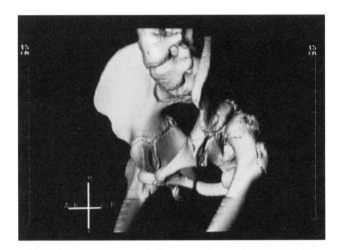

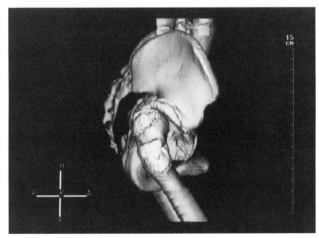

Fig. 3.3. Three-dimensional CT scan of the hip of a 14 year old boy, total body involved cerebral palsy, non-ambulatory. Note the posterior and lateral subluxation of the hip with mainly a shallow acetabulum posteriorly. (Reproduced by courtesy of Hank Chambers MD, San Diego, California.)

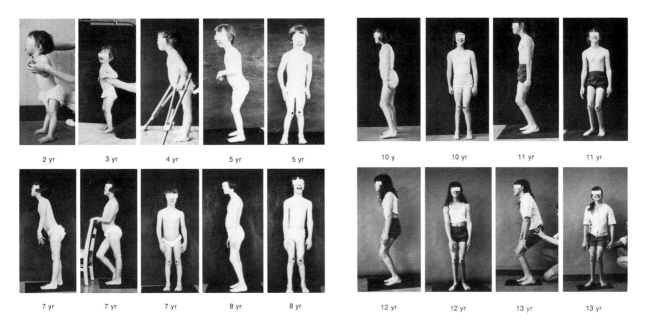

Fig. 3.4. A physical therapist's serial photographs of a child with spastic diplegia from age 2 years to 13 years. Hip-flexion contracture and internal rotation of the hips evident at age 5 years. At age 10 years a bilateral derotation subtrochanteric femoral osteotomy and the result 1 year postoperatively shows a flexed knee posture as a compensation for the increased hip-flexion contracture.

The finding of periventricular leukomalacia with ultrasound was the best predictor for the clinical outcome. MRI was not recommended at 44 weeks' postmenstrual age for predicting neurodevelopmental outcome.

What do these brain-imaging studies tell us? For all those who care for children with cerebral palsy, they confirm that we are dealing with a real brain lesion, while most of our interventions are outside the brain in the periphery of the limbs, trunk and sense organs. The studies also confirm that there is defined brain neuronal pathology which we have to accept and deal with as best we can with our limited therapeutic methods.

CLINICAL PHOTOGRAPHY

Monochrome or color photographs continue to be useful for recording changes in posture as the child develops, in cases of scoliosis and fixed foot deformities (Fig. 3.4). We have found Polaroids or digital pictures useful in our clinics; they can be seen immediately, retaken if the views are not satisfactory, and mounted in the record. Instant Polaroid photos or those made with the new digital cameras and printers linked to the computer avoid the tedious cataloguing of negatives, printing, sorting and finally mounting in the record.

SIMPLE AND PRIMITIVE METHODS OF GAIT ANALYSIS

VIDEOTAPE RECORDING

To record gait patterns, mobility and upper-limb functions, videotape recordings have replaced cinematography. As with photographic films, the major disadvantage is the need to splice serial tapes of one patient into a sequence. Special computerized video systems, which can search for and retrieve specific tapes, allow us to overcome this difficulty. Although the recording of walking and function can be of value in following a patient's progress (or lack of it), viewing films takes time (which always seems limited) over and beyond that required for a re-examinations of the patient. Videotape recordings with slow-motion playback have been used for clinical studies (Rodda and Graham 2001). Although instrumented gait analysis permits more objective data, video recordings are usually done at the time of gait analysis to serve as a reference and check on the graphic and numerical data generated by instrumented gait analysis.

PEDOGRAPHY

Measuring footprints made by walking is a simple and inexpensive way to record some elements of the gait cycle; but in the 21st century it is likely to become increasingly distrusted, and to be seen as barely worth the effort and time for the limited information obtained. In fact, no reports in the medical literature using pedography can be found since our own laboratory at Stanford reported on the results of oral Dantrolene sodium in cerebral palsy many years ago (Ford *et al.* 1976).

INSTRUMENTED MOTION ANALYSIS

'*Before computer-based gait analysis was available, surgeons would start with a spastic child who walked abnormally and ended with a spastic child who walked differently, but it was very difficult to tell exactly what surgery had accomplished.*'

(Gage 1992)

'*Is it all that it's cracked up to be?*'

(Watts 1994)

'Measure twice, cut once.'

(Old principle of carpentry)

PERSPECTIVES ON THE STATE OF
THE QUESTION

One of the first attempts at more objective gait analysis began with the horse at the farm of Senator Leland Stanford of California. At the Senator's farm (which subsequently became the site of Stanford University), Muybridge using timed-phase photography proved that the Senator's racehorse had all four feet off the ground at times when running. The measurement and analysis of human walking began in the latter part of the 19th century when Marey (1873) made records of running and walking. The development of photography permitted Muybridge (1901) to record with multiple exposure the gait of horses, humans and other animals.

The advance of electronic technology launched more sophisticated instrumented gait analysis by the late Vernon Inman MD and colleagues at the University of California, Berkeley (Inman *et al.* 1981). Part of the stimulus to study gait came during the 1950s to fulfil the need for better design of artificial limbs necessitated by the Korean War casualties, and the availability of electronic instruments, primarily the oscilloscope, video cameras and computers.

Further development and definition of the gait cycle was pioneered by Jacqueline Perry (1975, 1992) and its application in defining walking patterns and muscle contractions timed with the events in the gait cycle in persons who had cerebral palsy at the Rancho Los Amigos Hospital, Downey, California. David Sutherland (1984) at the San Francisco Shriners Hospital established a gait analysis laboratory and subsequently established a very sophisticated gait analysis system in San Diego in 1970. His efforts stimulated James R. Gage (2004), first at the Newington Children's Hospital and then at the Gillette Children's Hospital in St Paul, Minnesota, to apply and develop further advances in instrumented gait analysis in cerebral palsy.

Since the early 1990s the principles of the instrumentation used for gait analysis have not changed appreciably. The basic terminology has remained essentially the same in dividing the walking cycle into the swing and stance phases. Subdivision of each phase of the cycle was refined by Perry (1992), who divided the cycle into three tasks (A, B and C) and added the duration of the phase as a percentage of the gait cycle (Adams and Perry 1994). Task A, weight acceptance, has two phases: phase 1, initial contact when the foot touches the floor (instantaneous); and phase 2: loading response, when both feet are in contact with floor (initial double stance 0–10 %). Task B, single-limb support, also has two phases: phase 3: mid-stance, which begins when the other foot is lifted and continues until the weight is over the forefoot (10%–30%); and phase 4, terminal stance, which begins with heel rise and continues until the other foot strikes the ground (30%–50%). Task C, limb advancement, has four phases: phase 5, pre-swing, beginning with initial contact of the other limb and ends with toe-off on the same side (50%–60%); phase 6, initial swing, when the foot clears the floor (60%–73%);

phase 7, mid-swing, when the swinging limb is opposite the stance limb (73%–87%); and phase 8, terminal swing, which ends when the foot strikes the floor (87%–100%).

A further refinement of the basic functions of walking was made again by Perry (1974) and also adopted by Gage (2004) to describe how momentum throughout the stance phase is implemented by the concept of *three foot rockers*: (1) *heel rocker*—the initial contact of the heel with the ground until the foot is flat with controlled lowering of the foot by lengthening of the ankle dorsiflexors (eccentric contraction); heel strike is often prevented by spastic plantar flexors of the ankle or weakness of the dorsiflexors as in peroneal nerve palsy (foot drop); (2) *ankle rocker*—the foot is flat on the ground while the tibia advances forward controlled by the lengthening of the ankle plantarflexors (eccentric contraction); spasticity of the plantarflexors prevents the forward acceleration of the tibia with a resultant hyperextension of the knee as compensation; and (3) *forefoot rocker*—push-off due to shortening of the gastrocnemius–soleus muscles (concentric contracture). Push-off assists the firing of the psoas muscle and helps to drive the ipsilateral knee into flexion. Weakness of the calf muscles prevents push-off and accounts for the crouched gait in cerebral palsy (usually as the result of overlengthening of the Achilles tendon).

Rather than cope with all of the phases of gait and their measurements, the gait analysis laboratory at the Gillette Children's Hospital of St Paul, Minnesota, devised and tested a single number to represent the deviation of a gait pattern from normal (Schutte *et al.* 2000). They combined 16 independent variables from 16 selected variables derived from instrumented gait analysis. This number that is interpreted as a deviation from the normal gait is the sum of square of these variables. This single number method to define a gait as abnormal and to what degree according to an increasing index score seems to be a rather quick way to summarize all events in the gait cycle. However, it would not give the data on any particular joint–muscle complex of the lower limb as responsible for the abnormal pattern.

OBSERVATIONAL GAIT ANALYSIS

Watts' question may seem unduly pejorative, but it is maybe right to question whether every patient with cerebral palsy and who is able to walk (i.e. those with spastic diplegia and hemiplegia), and has surgery proposed, needs an instrumented computer-based gait analysis rather than mere observation. Not every physician in the world who wishes to treat with either orthopaedic surgery, posterior rootlet rhizotomy, or myoneural blocks with botulinum toxin, has access to a conveniently located gait laboratory, and the patients may not be able to afford the expensive technology and personnel needed. Furthermore, the prevalence of cerebral palsy is relatively low compared with other diseases that are of greater personal and public concern, e.g. heart disease, cancer and AIDS. Therefore public or private insurance schemes in less developed countries may tend to constrain this additional expenditure when healthcare budgets must be allocated to more pressing needs such as control of infectious diseases, care of motorcycle accident trauma, provision of adequate nutrition, maternal and child care and care of the aging population.

However, instrumented gait analysis and the publication of results of muscles responsible for abnormal gait patterns in cerebral palsy has unquestionably greatly enhanced the decision process for orthopaedic surgery in spastic diplegia and hemiplegia. A study of 38 patients with static encephalopathy at the Children's Hospital of Los Angeles concluded that postoperative gait analysis caused a change in patient care in 84%, either to surgery, bracing or specific physical therapy (Kay *et al.* 2000).

Instrumented gait analysis and the publication of results of muscles responsible for abnormal gait patterns in cerebral palsy has greatly enhanced the decision process for orthopaedic surgery in spastic diplegia and hemiplegia.

Instrumented gait analysis studies have eliminated the rationale for some common orthopaedic procedures in spastic diplegia and have also added new and more effective operations. Instrumented gait analysis has been used to demonstrate the efficacy of selective posterior rootlet rhizotomy in spastic diplegia and the effectiveness of botulinum toxin in relieving spasticity of the muscle injected. The recent medical literature confirms the increasing use of instrumented gait analysis in clinical research studies. Without instrumented gait analysis, no refereed journal is likely to publish a report on outcomes of walking after surgical procedures, orthotics, myoneural blocks, or intrathecal baclofen in cerebral palsy. These reports are referenced and detailed in Chapter 6 under the particular treatment method discussed.

Some doubt on the efficacy of gait analysis and its clinical application was expressed in a review of the literature by Hailey and Tomie (2000) of Edmonton, Canada. These authors thought it was a potentially useful technology, but that more systematic study and assessment of clinical outcomes should be done. They raised the question as to whether the costs (averaging C$2000 per examination) would be offset by the decrease in follow-up surgical procedures and hospital costs, as claimed by proponents of instrumented gait analysis. In this study the literature did not provide convincing data to support the proposition, although it may be correct.

Observational gait analysis depends on the physician's and/or therapist's knowledge of the basic elements of the gait cycle and joint motions in the sagittal, transverse and coronal planes. Instrumented gait analysis and its terminology have enhanced the power of observation only. A 'Full Body Observational Gait Analysis Form' was developed by clinicians at the Pathokinesiology and Physical Therapy Departments of the Rancho Los Amigos Medical Center, Downey, California (Adams and Perry 1994). The form is used to identify 33 commonly observed gait deviations and their occurrence during the phases of the gait cycle.

In observing gait it is useful to focus on one joint linkage at a time in the three planes. Cupping the hand over one eye or using a rolled-up magazine as a sort of telescope facilitates concentration on the particular joint and its movement. The surgeon needs to know the generic terminology used to describe the events observed during level walking, i.e. stance, swing, toe-off, initial contact, etc. Stance phase includes initial contact, loading response mid-stance, terminal stance and pre-swing; swing phase includes initial swing, mid-swing and terminal swing. Adams and Perry (1994) advocated videotaping of the gait to enable the clinician to do multiple viewing for analysis and to prevent patient fatigue. Rodda and Graham (2001) used observational gait analysis in the sagittal plane and video recording with slow-motion replay to classify postural/gait patterns in spastic hemiplegia and diplegia.

Observations have been coupled with the data on joint range of motion and the clinical evidence of spasticity of the muscles. However, when static measurements of hip, knee and ankle ranges of motion were compared with kinematic data derived from gait analysis in 80 adolescents with cerebral palsy and 30 unaffected controls, McMulkin *et al.* (2000) of the Shriner's Hospital in Spokane, Washington, did not find a good correlation. Although this report throws cold water on the correlation of the static physical examination (e.g. popliteal angle, hip-flexion contracture etc.), with patience and practice observational gait analysis combined with the examination of the lower-limb joints can be surprisingly close to the measurements of the kinematic data from instrumented gait analysis. The value of observing the gait is confirmed by the fact that all gait laboratories videotape the individuals to check on the match of the graphic data derived from the instrumented gait analysis.

The surgeon learns from the gait laboratory to be a 'trained observer'. Unfortunately most graduate orthopaedic education pays insufficient attention to the question of how to describe the gait of a patient using universally accepted terms derived from gait analysis.[5]

'Observational evaluation of gait is fundamental to any examination of the child with spastic diplegia; therefore, all orthopaedic surgeons should be better trained to do this.'

(Sussman 1992)

Observational gait analysis reliability was first studied in children who wore knee–ankle–foot orthoses viewed on videotape by three 'expert' observers (Krebs *et al.* 1985). Total agreement between and within observers occurred in two-thirds. The authors concluded in this limited study that observational gait analysis was convenient but only moderately reliable. A limitation of 'naked eye' viewing is that the eye can see only about 16 frames a second. If the events in the gait cycle do not last as long as 1/16th of a second, the action will be missed. Because many activities occur simultaneously at the various joints, you can

5 Terms such as walking 'with the knees bent' and 'toeing-in' represent crude observations and not analysis. Instead use gait cycle terms. For example, on initial contact the knee extends to zero and on swing the knee flexes initially an estimated 20° and only 30° on completion of swing. The femora internally rotate during mid-stance approximately 30° so that on forward progression the feet are medially rotated 10° from the line of progression. The base of the gait is approximately 10 cm.

view only one event at a time (Gage 2004). Viewing one joint at a time implies that you are able to combine the various segments into a whole.

Numerous other studies have evaluated gait analysis reliability. Maathius and coworkers (2005) from the Netherlands noted good intraobserver but not interobserver reliability in interpreting gait studies done on nine spastic hemiplegic and 15 spastic diplegic children at a 6-week interval. Mackey *et al.* (2003) from New Zealand evaluated the repeatabity of kinematic measurements in children with spastic hemiplegia and noted high levels of reliability on sagittal gait data, a slightly less coeffecient of multiple correlations for transverse and frontal plane measurements and good to moderate repeatability of kinematic studies of tasks through the upper limbs.

Using the Observational Gait Scale, inter- and intra-observer reliability was noted for knee and foot position in midstance, initial foot contact and heel rise but not for heel position or base of support. Lest we be complacent, Kerr Graham's group from Australia (Dobson *et al.* 2006) have recently reviewed existing classifications of gait and found that many classifications evaluated sagittal gait data only, and no single classification addressed all of the variations of patterns noted in gait in cerebral palsy. This area will no doubt continue to evolve so that gait studies can be more objectively interpreted especially by different reviewers.

As Gage *et al.* (1987) pointed out, it was the EMG evidence of rectus femoris firing during the swing phase that convinced him of the need to release and transfer the spastic rectus femoris tendon. Now that we all know this, is gait laboratory analysis necessary in every case? If you are not sure, the answer is yes. The kinematic and EMG data might convince you to do a distal rectus femoris transfer at the time of fractional hamstring lengthening. Most major gait laboratories are directed by a physician, often with the assistance of a physical therapist; together they perform the traditional examination of the muscles and joints and correlate these findings with the data derived from the instrumented gait analysis. A principle in medicine remains true: all laboratory investigation results must be correlated with the clinical examination. If your clinical impression is grossly different from that shown in the gait analysis data, you might look again at either or both. In the decision process for surgery, repeat examinations are crucial. When specific surgical procedures are scheduled in advance, the findings and surgical recommendations should be committed to writing. Then when the patient returns for the preoperative visit, reexamine the child without first reading the original notes. If you come to the same conclusion the second time, you are more likely to be right than wrong.

All results of laboratory investigations must be correlated with the clinical findings.

Watts (1994) contended that when preoperative gait analysis is done, postoperative gait analysis is not often reported following orthopaedic surgical procedures. His reason at the time was that some third-party insurers (private and public) refused to pay for postoperative assessments. This is no longer true. Most major gait laboratories do routine postoperative analysis. When surgical decision-making is optimal and enhanced with gait studies, it should ensure fewer trips to the operating room. The texts of Sutherland (1984) and Gage (2004) displayed impressive pre- and postoperative results of orthopaedic surgery in spastic diplegia. Since 1994 many more studies on pre- and postoperative outcomes of orthopaedic surgery in spastic diplegia have appeared in the literature (Gage 1995, Scott *et al.* 1996, Yngve and Chambers 1996, Miller *et al.* 1997, O'Byrne *et al.* 1997, Sutherland *et al.* 1997, Chambers *et al.* 1998, Deluca *et al.* 1998, Stefko *et al.* 1998, Fabry *et al.* 1999, Rethlefsen *et al.* 1999, Granata *et al.* 2000, Steinwender *et al.* 2000). Kay *et al.* (2000) reported on the value of postoperative gait analysis in defining appropriate further treatment which may cause a change in the perceptions of the public and private insurers. In this report of 38 patients who had postoperative gait analyses, this caused recommendations for a change in care in 84% (surgery in 42%, bracing in 53%, and specific physical therapy in 21%).

Laboratory gait (or motion) analysis does entail costs and charges have to be made. The costs are in equipment, space, and personnel including the physician time. The costs need to be borne either by the patient, or by the insurer, or by a research grant, or by the institution. What should be evident is that a large amount of time is required to synthesize the massive amount of data generated in instrumented gait analysis with the clinical findings and then make a thoughtful decision for surgery. As Reimers (1992) reminded us, 'It is important to expend the energy required to make the best possible decision.' And in the words of Rang (1990): 'The decision is more important than the incision.'

CLINICAL OBSERVATIONS AND EXAMINATION VERSUS INSTRUMENTED GAIT ANALYSIS DATA IN ORTHOPAEDIC SURGICAL OUTCOMES

Two studies have compared the surgical outcome based on the clinical examination alone or with gait analysis data. Lee *et al.* (1992) compared the surgical outcome of 23 ambulatory children with cerebral palsy based on clinical examination alone or with gait analysis data. They did postoperative gait assessments 1 year postoperatively. Sixteen were improved and seven were not. They found that those who had not improved had had operations that differed from those recommended by gait analysis. EMG recordings postoperatively did not differ from those done preoperatively.

DeLuca *et al.* (1997) compared surgical recommendations by clinicians who made surgical decisions based on the clinical examination and observational videotape gait analysis with those made using kinematic, kinetic and EMG data. Gait analysis data changed the surgical recommendations in 52% of the patients. Cook *et al.* (2003) noted how gait analysis altered the type of surgical procedure recommended in 106 of 267 operations. Gait analysis was particularly important in decisions regarding soft-tissue surgery for tone-related problems while decisions regarding bone surgery were more frequently not altered based on the gait studies.

Damiano and Abel (1996) studied the correlation between the GMFM and gait analysis parameters of 32 children with spastic cerebral palsy, and noted strong correlation of cadence and normalized velocity with the GMFM. Gait analysis and the GMFM scoring system were complimentary measures because gait is representative of the general motor status in cerebral palsy.

Selective posterior rootlet rhizotomy and botulinum toxin have generated a flood of papers on results with gait analysis before and after in ambulatory patients (see Chapter 6).

In comparison, instrumented gait analysis has not been reported to document improved gait patterns in cerebral palsy with and without a specific physical therapy regimen or with oral medications proposed as 'muscle relaxants'.

The natural history of spastic diplegia was suggested with gait analysis in one longitudinal study of 32 months of 18 children with spastic diplegia (Johnson et al. 1997). That gait stability deteriorated was evidenced by increasing double support and decreasing single support time. Popliteal angles also decreased, together with losses of excursions of the knee, ankle and pelvis. This study on the natural progression of gait function in spastic diplegia should be valuable when evaluating changes in gross motor function over a period of time.

ARE GAIT ANALYSIS DATA REPRODUCIBLE?
To have validity, investigations should be reproducible within a short time-frame on the same day and a few succeeding days. Kirkpatrick et al. (1994) recorded walking velocity and vertical ground reaction forces from 15 normal children and 11 with spastic cerebral palsy. Both parameters had low individual variations during over consecutive days. Watts (1994) asked whether children with cerebral palsy may walk differently inside the laboratory confines, but it is hard to imagine how such a question could be resolved. White and colleagues at the University of Aberdeen (1999) also found that the most reproducible force parameter data derived from a force platform was the vertical ground reaction force. Other force parameters had high variability and were not considered reliable measures of gait.

Another variable to remember is that walking speed probably affects the electromyogram Detrembleur et al. (1997) studied the EMG patterns of ankle muscles of normal children aged between 4 and 12 years when walking at different speeds. They found that the pattern of muscle firing changed significantly with the speed of progression, and was independent of growth. This observation may be important in assessing abnormal or prolonged muscle firing in ambulatory children when planning tendon lengthening or transfers. Fast walking progressing to running by children who have spastic diplegia appears to stress the central nervous system so that the effects of the spastic muscles become more evident. Children who have been trained to walk in physical therapy gyms usually walk with a controlled gait pattern—'the clinic walk'. But when they are outdoors on the playground their abnormal patterns of locomotion become evident—a sobering observation.

A study from Karl Franzens University of Gräz, Austria (Steinwender et al. 2000), found that the repeatability of kinetic and kinematic data derived from the gait analysis was lower in 20 children who had spastic diplegia than in 20 normal controls. They surmised that this lower repeatability in children with spastic diplegia was due to restricted joint motion and errors due to inadvertent marker placement used in all gait analysis systems.

DOES EVERY PATIENT NEED GAIT ANALYSIS?
Instrumented gait analysis assists in better decision-making for surgery. Gait analysis adds objectivity in prospective studies of walking to determine out comes of surgery, and the efficacy of orthotics, physical therapy and drug therapy.

The debate about the value of gait analysis in cerebral palsy might be settled if we surgeons acknowledge the contributions of our colleagues who have published their gait analysis data of the effects of specific orthopaedic surgical procedures. Surgeons who do not have access to gait analysis laboratories can apply the published knowledge derived from the laboratories to select the proper operative procedure with reasonable assurance. But they must examine and re-examine the child, do a thorough observational gait analysis, and then perform the specific procedures. Unsatisfactory outcomes can be minimized but, due to the many variables in the human condition, not completely eliminated. As orthopaedic surgery in spastic hemiplegic and diplegic cerebral palsy has evolved, it has become more selective and simplified. It is not the surgical technique itself that counts, but the selection of the proper procedure for the particular patient.

In surgery for cerebral palsy it is not the surgical technique that counts, but the selection of the proper procedure.

COMPONENTS OF GAIT ANALYSIS
(GAGE 1992, 1995)
The following are standard components of gait analysis.

1. Dynamic EMG to record muscle firing in the lower limbs while walking and coordinated with the phases of the gait.

2. Kinematics—the recording of the ranges of motion between the links in the lower limbs, velocity and acceleration without measurement of forces that caused the forward progression. Data are generated from all three body planes: coronal, sagittal and transverse.

3. Kinetics—the measurement of forces that cause forward progression: the mechanisms of ground reaction forces (GRF), joint moments and joint powers. These are measured simultaneously with the joint range of motion and force-plate data.

4. Energy expenditure by steady-state oxygen requirements and/or carbon dioxide production after 6 minutes of walking or by measurement of heart rate and walking speed. Another way to measure energy costs during walking is with inverse dynamics using kinetic and kinematic data.

5. Videotape recording and clinical observation.

6. Clinical assessment of balance (equilibrium reactions). Assessment of posterior, anterior and lateral equilibrium reactions

should be included in the gait analysis report. Objective measurement is feasible using the force plate, but normative standards need to be developed for the particular laboratory. Measurement while standing in one place is probably not going to be as informative as a mechanism to perturb the subject with a standard degree of tilt of the electronic force-plate platform (an instrumented Romberg sign).

LIMITATIONS OF INSTRUMENTED GAIT ANALYSIS

Tylkowski (1992) delineated some limitations of the technology available. When asked to walk for gait analysis, the child does so 'on command' and thus reacts differently from when walking spontaneously outside a laboratory. The child will be burdened with devices such as the electrodes, reflective markers and adhesive tapes. The reflective devices or light-emitting diodes taped to the lower limbs used to obtain the kinematic data can have considerable motion as the skin glides over the subcutaneous fat or from the underlying muscle contraction. Patients also have limited tolerance for fine wire insertions. Trailing cables impede walking and wireless telemetry systems add noise and interfere with the signals so that filtering is necessary. In one study that compared walking with and without electrodes, the data showed that surface electrodes caused a large decrease in cadence; wire electrodes caused significant decreases in step length and walking velocity (Young *et al.* 1989). For EMG data, do you get the best information from individual walks or a summation of many walks? Can the level of electrical activity be related to the work output of the muscle and the clinical grade of muscle strength?

Force-plate data may be impossible or irregular in patients who use crutches or walkers unless they can cross the plate without the crutch or walker touching it. In these patients who use external supports the ground reaction forces may be distributed between the upper and lower limbs.

Ways of locating true joint center are still in development, and true joint motion calculations are not well established. Kinematic data generation assumes the linked segment model in many systems and we have to acknowledge that anatomic motions are not recorded. Despite the imperfections in modern instrumented gait analysis, we have well standardized norms for EMG and kinematic data that can be clinically useful and reasonably accurate to judge a significant abnormality of muscle action and joint motion. The linear data of step length, stride length, cadence and velocity appear to be on sound and reliable footing with the technology used. Instrumented gait analysis has limited application in those patients who can barely walk, need walkers, and classified as level III GMFM classification ('physiological walkers'—walking only in therapy spaces) or level II GMFM ('household walkers'). Usually a child with this degree of involvement will have surgery recommended for an isolated deformity such as a contracture of the knee joint beyond the 15° functional range, subluxation of the hip, or a hip-adduction contracture.

GAIT LABORATORY EQUIPMENT

ELECTROMYOGRAPHY

Like most other laboratories, we have used EMG biotelemetry systems, to avoid the 'spaghetti effect' with wires from the patient to the recording instruments, and to allow freedom of movement. The action potentials of the muscles chosen for study (up to eight) are recorded from surface miniature electrodes or indwelling fine-gauge teflon-coated stainless steel wire (0.0045 inches in diameter). Intramuscular wire electrodes are used when recording from an isolated muscle (e.g. posterior tibial). Surface electrodes are satisfactory for large muscle groups (e.g. hip adductors, hamstrings). The original investigative studies used wire electrodes for greater accuracy. However, for clinical use whenever possible, especially in children, surface electrodes are preferred. Wire electrodes are now used in muscles too far from the surface to record the electrical activity accurately. In the lower limb the iliacus

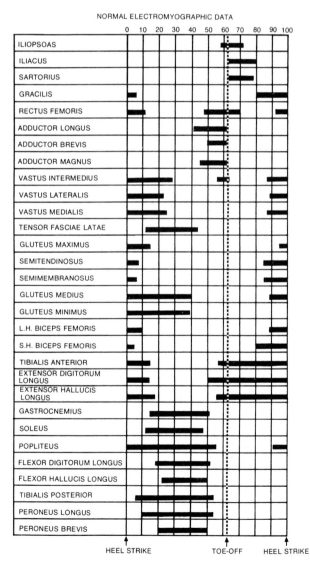

Fig. 3.5. Normal EMG recordings of muscles of the lower limb. (By courtesy of R. Mann and J. Hagy, Shriner's Hospital for Crippled Children, San Francisco, California.)

Varus

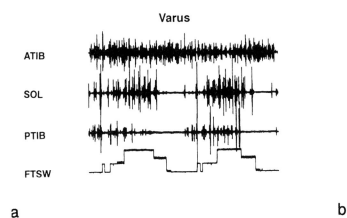

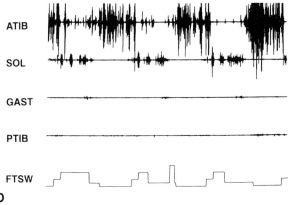

a

b

Fig. 3.6. Raw record recording of abnormal muscle action potentials in level walking: (*a*) continuous anterior tibial (ATIB) firing; premature soleus (SOL) onset in terminal swing rather than in mid-stance; (*b*) posterior tibial (PTIB) action missing in terminal stance. Foot switch (FTSW) recording to differentiate stance from swing phase. (*c*) Prolonged anterior tibial (ATIB) action, premature soleus (SOL) action, and no significant activity in the gastrocnemius (GAST) and posterior tibial (PTIB). (Reproduced by permission from Perry 1992, Fig. 18.15, p. 397.)

(iliopsoas), and the tibialis posterior muscles are usually studied with fine wire electrodes. Action potentials from the muscles can be processed in several ways for easy-to-see graphic displays, but a raw record is usually necessary to be sure of the quality of the processed signals.

During the swing and stance phase of gait 3D ranges of joint motion are simultaneously recorded using optoelectronic systems. EMG is recorded from surface electrodes or the fine wires, and the foot-switch lead wires are connected to a radio transmitter. In our system each EMG electrode has its own miniature battery-operated transmitter (Fig 3.5). The patient walks at least 10m on a walkway. Two photocells at each end of the walkway are used as a timing device. Data are transmitted via

RF into a bank of receivers. The amplified signals from the receivers were fed into an oscilloscope for visual assessment. A light beam oscillograph was used in the past for permanent recording on light sensative paper. Modern systems record data directly to a computer. Data analysis by the computer detects the onset and termination of the EMG signals and the phases of gait through the ground reaction force or by foot-switches. A graphic printout of muscle activity timed with the stance and swing phases of gait completes the process. In this way a comprehensive report can be produced. The physician compares the patient's EMG with the normal data on muscle activity during gait (Figs 3.6, 3.7). The EMG data can be presented in a variety of forms (Fig. 3.8).

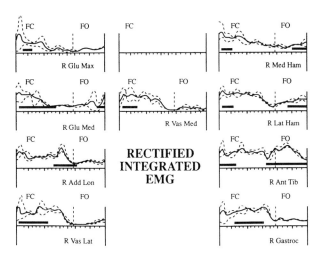

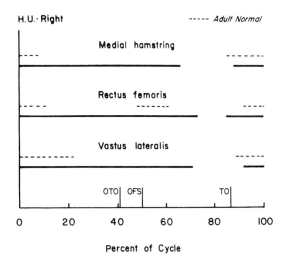

Fig. 3.7. Rectified integrated EMG action potentials of lower-limb muscles during level walking of a patient with cerebral palsy. The signals are integrated and then rectified with a machine-directed averaging to separate 'noise' from the muscle signal according to preset parameters of the operator. The wavy darker lines are the rectified integrated signals. The horizontal dark lines at the bottom of each graphic display are the expected normal muscle contractions during gait. FC, foot contact (stance phase); FO, foot off (swing phase). (Reproduced by permission from Gage 1991, Fig. 2.7, p. 25.)

Fig. 3.8. A simplified way of graphically depicting muscle firing during gait. A 9-year-old girl who had severe lower-limb spasticity and used a walker. The solid horizontal lines represent the recorded muscle action potentials during gait; the dotted line above represents normal adult muscle contractions. The upper recording shows prolonged contraction of both the quadriceps and hamstrings during stance and swing phases. OTO, opposite toe-off; OFS, opposite foot strike; TO, toe-off. (Reproduced by permission from Sutherland 1984, Fig. 9.3, p. 145.)

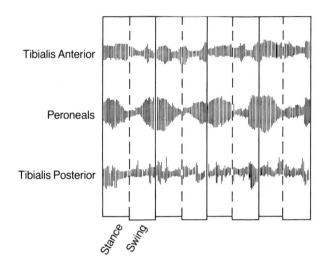

Tibialis Anterior

Peroneals

Tibialis Posterior

Stance Swing

Fig. 3.9. Gait electromyograms redrawn from 'raw' recording by the optical method on photosensitive paper. Eight-year-old patient with spastic diplegia; postoperative subtalar extra-articular arthrodesis (Grice). *Top*: right foot; shows extent of muscle-action potentials coordinated with stance and swing phases of gait. Foot in balanced neutral position despite almost continuous low-level activity of the anterior and posterior tibial muscles. (Reproduced by permission from Bleck 1987, Fig. 3.11, p. 80.)

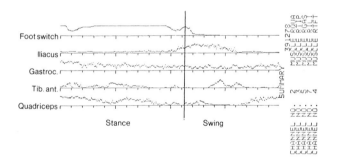

Foot switch
Iliacus
Gastroc.
Tib. ant.
Quadriceps

Stance Swing

Fig. 3.10. Automated EMG record of on-and-off signals during gait of a 12-year-old boy with spastic diplegia and postoperative iliopsoas recession. The iliacus fires normally shortly before and in the initial swing phase. The gastrocnemius is contracting continuously; anterior tibial fairly normal; quadriceps contraction is prolonged in stance. (Reproduced by permission from Bleck 1987, Fig. 3.8, p. 77.)

Publications and reports on the clinical usefulness in preoperative and postoperative studies of dynamic EMG and joint ranges of motion have appeared in the past 25 years (Perry *et al.* 1976, Griffin *et al.* 1977, Perry and Hoffer 1977, Simon *et al.* 1978, Baumann 1980, 1984, Sutherland and Baumann 1981, Frazier *et al.* 1982, Hoffer and Perry 1983, Knutsson 1983, Bose and Goh 1984, Fabian *et al.* 1984, Gage *et al.* 1984, Mederios 1984, Skinner and Lester 1984, Sutherland 1984, Adler *et al.* 1989, Gage 1992, 1994, 1995, 2004, Perry 1992). Clinical applications of gait electromyograms of selected muscles in patients with cerebral palsy are displayed in Figures 3.9 to 3.12. In cerebral palsy, the use of EMG alone to demonstrate changes in muscle firing before and after surgery appeared to be of limited value in two good studies (Waters *et al.* 1982, Gage *et al.* 1984). However, when planning specific muscle surgery, electromyography (e.g. posterior tibial, anterior tibial, rectus femoris) is

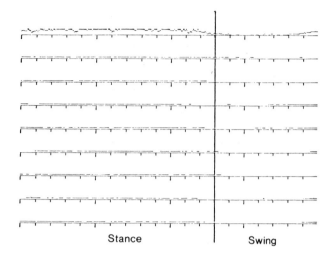

Stance Swing

Fig. 3.11. Automated EMG record of on-and-off recording of signals from the rectus femoris. On top summary plot of several gait cycles showing continuous stance-phase activity.

STANCE % ACTIVITY							
	RF	34.70	−3.80	1.66	0.00	0.00	−19.02
	VM	38.65	−4.05	3.56	0.00	0.00	−10.64
	MH	50.76	0.00	0.00	0.00	0.00	0.00

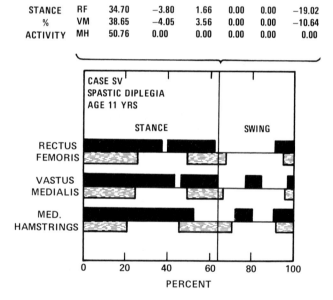

CASE SV
SPASTIC DIPLEGIA
AGE 11 YRS

STANCE SWING

RECTUS FEMORIS

VASTUS MEDIALIS

MED. HAMSTRINGS

0 20 40 60 80 100
PERCENT

Fig. 3.12. Conversion of gait EMG of the rectus femoris (RF), vastus medialis (VM), and medial hamstrings (MH) a patient with spastic diplegia into digital form (top) as a percentage of action in the stance and swing phases of gait. The bottom part are the electromyograms of the muscles redrawn for clarification. This was our first documentation of a co-contraction of the hamstrings and the quadriceps during gait in spastic diplegia.

helpful in making decisions on transfer or lengthening of the muscle–tendon unit.

When planning specific muscle surgery (e.g. posterior tibial, anterior tibial, rectus femoris) electromyography is helpful in making decisions on transfer or lengthening of the muscle-tendon unit.

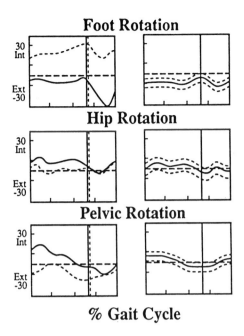

Foot Rotation

Hip Rotation

Pelvic Rotation

% Gait Cycle

Fig. 3.14. Transverse-plane kinematics of the lower limbs for the same child with diplegia shown in Figure 3.14. Left column, abnormal, preoperative cerebral palsy; normal kinematics right side. Patient data represented by a solid line for the right lower limb and a dotted line for the left. Stance phase to the left separated from the swing phase by the vertical line. Horizontal dotted line (abscissa) is the zero joint position. Ordinate to the far left represents the degrees of motion. (Reproduced by permission from Gage 1991, Fig. 8.5, p. 161.)

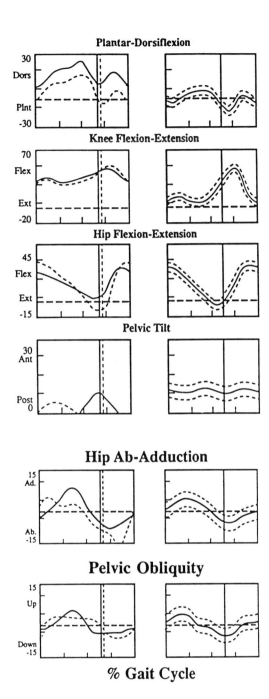

Plantar-Dorsiflexion

Knee Flexion-Extension

Hip Flexion-Extension

Pelvic Tilt

Hip Ab-Adduction

Pelvic Obliquity

% Gait Cycle

Fig. 3.13. Lower-limb kinematics of a child with diplegia, with intoeing and crouch gait. Abnormal (left column) and normal (right column) of lower-limb kinematics. Solid lines represent the mean values of normal; the dotted lines = 2 ± standard deviations. Top four are sagittal-plane kinematics; bottom two are coronal-plane. Stance phase to the left of the vertical line, swing to the right. Horizontal dotted line (abscissa) is the zero position. Ordinate at far left represents degrees of motion. The patient's data is represented by a solid line for the right lower limb and the dotted line for the left lower limb. (Reproduced by permission from Gage 1991, Figs 8.3 and 8.4, p. 161.)

KINEMATICS

Most laboratories use an optical tracking system that use either illuminated markers (diodes) on the patient's limbs and trunk (Selspot—Sweden) or reflective markers taped to the skin with the light source from the camera (e.g. Vicon—Oxford Metrics, UK, CODA-3). Target locations can be on the shoulder girdles to identify the trunk, pelvis, thighs, knees, legs and feet. Three targets are required on each body segment to give 3D localization. The elimination of the upper limbs simplifies the tracking. All data are programmed for processing and display via a micro-processor and printer. Motion analysis seems more useful than electromyography in the overall assessment of a gait problem in a child with cerebral palsy (Figs 3.14, 3.15).

KINEMATIC GAIT ANALYSIS FOR CLASSIFICATION OF GAIT PATTERNS

Kinematics has been used for the classification of gait patterns in cerebral palsy in three studies and one used kinetics only. All studies were done in the sagittal plane of the lower limbs. The sagittal view is how we usually visualize the gait and simplifies the attempts at classification. Winters *et al.* (1987) at the Newington Children's Hospital classified gait patterns in hemiplegia into four groups, and recommended either an orthosis or specific surgery in a particular group.

From the Central Remedial Clinic in Dublin are two reports of gait pattern recognition using kinematic data. Kelly *et al.* (1997) differentiated idiopathic toe-walkers from mild spastic diplegia. Able-bodied children, when asked to toe-walk, had the same pattern as those with the idiopathic type. O'Byrne *et al.* (1998) described eight gait patterns in cerebral palsy in 55

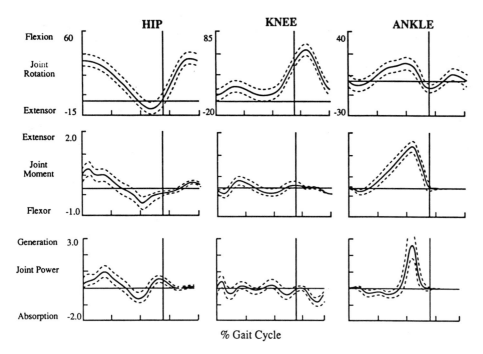

Fig. 3.15. Normal sagittal-plane kinetics of the hip, knee, and ankle based on an average field of 31 children. Top-row graphs display measurements in degrees. *Middle row:* the three joints (Nm/kg). Powers in the same three joints in the bottom row expressed as units of watts/kg. Positive power means the muscle is contracting concentrically (accelerating); if negative, the contraction is eccentric (decelerating). (Reproduced by permission from Gage 1991, Fig. 8.6, p. 162.)

hemiplegic and 91 diplegic patients. They used the predominant clinical features as typical of each group, such as a mobile crouch with the hips flexed, a stiff crouch with toe-walking, a severe crouch, a mild and severe knee recurvatum, and three foot and ankle abnormal patterns. No treatment suggestions were given. The point made was that these patterns could be recognized 'automatically' using the instrumented gait analysis with the CODA-3 optico-electronic scanner system.

Winters *et al.* (1987), using kinematic data in the sagittal plane and EMG data, defined four gait patterns in 46 patients with spastic hemiplegia. Davids *et al.* (1999) used computer-based gait analysis to differentiate the gait pattern of 17 children with spastic cerebral palsy and 23 with the dyskinetic type. Those who had dyskinesia had a significantly wider base of support, a small step profile (step length divided by step width), and a more variable maximal lateral acceleration than those who were either unaffected or had spasticity.

Davids *et al.* (1998) using gait analysis studied running in children who had spastic diplegia compared with able-bodied controls. Kinematic and kinetic data from the sagittal plane revealed that the walking gait pattern of children with cerebral palsy was similar to the running pattern of unaffected children. Kinetic data confirmed that children with cerebral palsy depend more on their hip muscles for power generation when they increase the velocity of their gait compared to unaffected children. But they increased their velocity by increasing their cadence that is different and less energy-efficient than that used by unaffected children.

KINETICS

Kinetics describes the causes of motion: ground reaction forces, joint moments and powers. A *moment* is a force acting at a distance about an axis of rotation to cause angular acceleration about the axis, e.g. the joint, expressed as Newton meters (Nm—the force times the distance from the center of rotation). To compare moments among individuals, the moments (Nm) are divided by the subject's bodyweight (Nm/kg). When walking, the ground reaction forces produce the external movement of the joints and are balanced by the internal moments generated by muscle action. *Joint power* is net joint moment × joint angular velocity (watts/kg). *Of the total energy in walking, 54% is from the hip, 10% from the knee, and 36% from the ankle (Gage 1992).*

To gather kinetic data one needs a force plate, which is a rigid platform suspended on force transducers of either piezoelectric crystals or stiff springs with strain gauges. This sensitive electronic scale measures vertical, horizontal and lateral forces, moments about the joints, their trajectories and the potential and kinetic energies of each limb segment when the patient's foot hits the ground or floor. Calculations of changes in mechanical energy of the center of mass of the body during walking, running, and other activities can be made (McMahon 1984, Winter 1987, Gage 2004). Gait analysis incorporating kinetics in cerebral palsy patients resulted in the realization that both muscle and ground reaction forces work on bony lever arms to produce a moment about a joint (Gage 1994). What was formerly thought to be just muscle weakness became 'lever arm dysfunction'—the force was acting on an inadequate or maldirected lever arm. Orthopaedics 'can do much more to correct the skeletal levers than correct inadequate muscle forces' (Gage 1994). Force-plate data during the gait of young children with cerebral palsy may be limited because the children frequently step off or miss the plate; it is more reliable in older children and adolescents (Gage *et al.* 1984, Gage 2004). Obviously force-plate data are not reliable if the patient depends on external supports during walking.

Hullin *et al.* (1996), at the Princess Margaret Rose Orthopaedic Hospital, Edinburgh, studied the gait in spastic hemiplegia with kinetic data. They discerned five gait patterns, though they did not relate these to any particular treatment: (I) minimal gait problem, a drop foot and normal kinetics with weak anterior tibial muscles; (II) flexed knee with normal hip extension and a functionally 'tight' gastrocnemius; (III) flexed hip and flexed knee with functionally tight gastrocnemius and hip-flexors; (IV) knee hyperextension and tibial 'arrest' with a functionally tight soleus; and (V) knee hyperextension and persistent ankle dorsiflexion in which the patient had abnormally high anterior–posterior shear forces, but the gastrocnemius and soleus were not 'tight'.

NORMATIVE DATA

Normative data for muscle activity, and the range of motion of the pelvis and lower limb joints during level walking, have been available for a long time (Murray 1967, Sutherland and Hagy 1972, Sutherland *et al.* 1980, Chao *et al.* 1983).

LINEAR MEASUREMENTS: CADENCE, VELOCITY, STRIDE LENGTH AND STEP LENGTH

An individual's basic walking capability consists of their stride characteristics: walking speed (velocity), stride length and step rate. The velocity is the time required to cover a designated distance expressed as meters/second (m/s) or meters/minute (m/min). Cadence is steps per minute. Stride length is the distance or interval between the first and second contact of the same foot with the ground (i.e. right foot–right foot). Step length is the interval between one foot and the other (i.e. left foot–right foot). Normative data of linear measurements during gait for both adults and children have been published (see Tables 3.VI and 3.VII).

BALANCE (POSTURAL EQUILIBRIUM) ANALYSIS

The importance of postural balance mechanisms (equilibrium reactions) in cerebral palsy has been one of my 'hobby horses' (Bleck 1994). Defective equilibrium reactions seem as important as the spasticity of the muscles or the athetosis for the disabling gait of patients and the lack of sitting balance in the total body

TABLE 3.VI
Linear measurements of the walking cycle for normal adults

Parameter	Right	Left
Opposite toe-off (%)	15.62	15.38
Opposite heel strike	51.56	49.23
Single stance	35.94	33.85
Toe-off (%)	65.62	64.62
Step length (cm)	60.30	60.70
Stride length (cm)	120.10	121.00
Cycle time (sec)	1.08	1.10
Cadence (steps/min)	109.85	109.84
Walking velocity (cm/sec)	110.43	110.43

% refers to percentage of the gait cycle. From Gage *et al.* (1984).

TABLE 3.VII
Average linear measurements of walking in children*

Age (years)	1	2	3	7
Duration single-limb stance (per cent of gait cycle)	32.1	33.5	34.8	36.7
Toe-off (per cent of gait cycle)	67.1	67.1	65.5	62.4
Walking velocity (cm/sec)	63.7	71.8	85.8	114.3
Step length (cm)t	21.6	27.5	32.9	47.9
Stride length (cm)	43	54.9	67.7	96.5
Ratio of pelvic span to ankle ('base of gait')		1-1.5	2	2.5

*From Sutherland (1984). All measurements show a gradual increase with maturation except cadence which decreases. Most changes occur between the ages of one and four years. Step length has a linear relationship with leg length.

Note: Lower limb-joint motions in children are only slightly different from adults. The same is true for gait electromyograms (Sutherland *et al.* 1980). For adult measurements of joint ranges of motion and electromyographic data, see Figures 3.5 and 3.15. For accurate graphs of lower-limb-joint ranges of motion in children, see Sutherland (1984).

involved patients. During walking one must be able to support the trunk over only one limb as single stance shifts from limb to limb in forward progression. This means that lateral balance is essential as the body shifts about 2 cm to the supporting limb (Perry 1975). If the patient lacks unilateral standing balance, due to the brain lesion, then the patient will fall to the swing limb when standing on other limb. This falling to one side is often confused with the Trendelenberg sign, which is due to insufficient hip-abductor muscle function. It is not known if there is a relationship between the degree of defective equilibrium reactions and the abnormal and prolonged muscle contractions during the gait of a patient with cerebral palsy. In patients who can stand alone, balancing ability should be measured to show the integrity of the postural mechanisms (Figs. 3.16, 3.17). This kind of

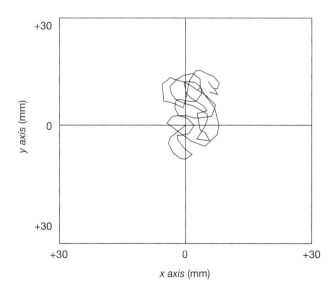

Fig. 3.16. Graphic display of the extent of postural sway in a child with spastic diplegia. Data obtained from standing on a force plate and calculation of deviations from the center of pressure over time (see Table 3.VI). (By courtesy of Dr J. Rose; see Wolff *et al.* 1998.)

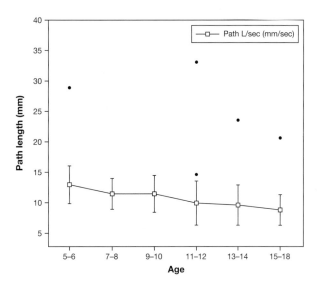

Fig. 3.17. Path length values ±1 S.D. for 92 non-disabled children and adolescents and for five children with spastic diplegic cerebral palsy with eyes open. Path length in mm/second is a measure of deviations from the center of pressure while standing on the force place. ● spastic diplegia, ❑ non-disabled. (From Wolff et al. 1998, by permission.)

objective analysis allows a more accurate opinion on the status of a patient with ataxia due to a variety of causes.

BALANCE STUDIES IN ADULTS
Murray et al. (1975) used force-plate analysis to measure postural stability in men and found that it began to deteriorate around the age of 50 years—hardly surprising to those of us plummeting to, or already in, the *troisième age*. Yet a study using dynamic posturography in healthy persons suggested that in 234 elderly subjects compared with 34 young controls, there were only small declines in balance between the ages of 70 and 85 years. Significant balance impairment appeared due to age-related disease rather than the consequence of aging (Wolfson et al. 1992). However, Ciamicioli et al. (1997) using dynamic posturography found that functionally evident quantitative changes in balance occurred with aging independent of typical geriatric pathologic conditions. Balance assessment that included dynamic posturography in 700 adults were correlated with brain MRI. The changes in the brain were significantly correlated with the poorer balance measures found (Tell et al. 1998).

Since the 1990s the medical literature has reflected a proliferation of reports of instrumented balance measurements ('posturography') mainly in aging adults, after stroke and traumatic brain injury. In the aging population the objective was to prevent falls by balance training and exercise (Judge et al. 1993, Di Fabio and Seay 1997, Fishman et al. 1997). Because of the growing interest in Chinese culture, a report on the effects of *Tai Chi Quan* in improving balance showed that it had no effect when postural stability was measured by instrumented platforms (Wolf et al. 1997). This ancient Chinese form of exercise delayed the onset between the first or multiple falls in older individuals without any associated measures of improved postural stability. The authors thought that *tai chi* appeared

successful because it promoted confidence rather than improving body sway measurements.

There have been a few reports on the effects of drugs on measured postural sway. Triazolam (Halcion®) was found to increase postural sway in six healthy male volunteers (Robin et al. 1991). Perhaps standing balance ought to be tested, before and after prescribing 'muscle relaxants' for patients who have cerebral palsy,

BALANCE STUDIES IN CHILDREN
Kowalski and Di Fabio (1995) studied balance reactions and motor proficiency in 21 children and adolescents. The authors suggested that such tests might reveal hidden deficits in motor performance, assist the evaluation of anticonvulsant side-effects, and be useful in a rehabilitation program. Sitting balance in 17 patients who had spastic cerebral palsy was measured 3 months after selective posterior rhizotomy (Yang et al. 1996). Using the Chattecx Balance System (Chattanooga Group, Hixson, TN, USA) the authors reported improvement in sitting balance postoperatively except for the non-visual testing condition.

Hadders-Algra et al. (1999) used ultrasound to study 13 preterm children with abnormal brain scans, 13 preterm children with normal brain scans, and 13 children born at term, using multiple EMG of the neck, trunk and leg muscles and kinematics while sitting on a movable platform. The 13 preterm children who had ultrasonographic evidence of lesions of the periventricular white matter were compared with a control group of 13 who had normal neonatal brain scans. Preterm children had a higher sensitivity to platform velocity than full-term children, and also lacked the ability to modulate the EMG amplitudes as recorded in the initial sitting position. The inability to modulate the postural responses was not related to the periventricular lesions, but to preterm birth itself. The correlation of the clinical findings with the ultrasonographic evidence of pathology was not absolute, inasmuch as only three of the preterm infants who had periventricular leukomalacia had cerebral palsy (nine had minor neurological signs and one was normal).

MEASUREMENT OF BALANCE IN CHILDREN AND ADOLESCENTS WITH CEREBRAL PALSY
The postural equilibrium measuring system we used originally was devised for a study of postural mechanisms in scoliosis (Adler et al. 1986). The system consisted of two foot-plates, with two strain gauges in each plate, interfaced to a minicomputer and printer plotter. The computer was programmed to display the center of foot pressure on the plates while the patient stood. An additional test was an 'instrumented Romberg sign' in which the platform was tilted sinusoidally 4° posteriorly eight times per minute. The tests were done with eyes open and closed.

The computer program draws an X–Y axis and graphically displays the center of foot pressure and its change over time. The computer also calculates (as a function of body weight) the average center of foot pressure, and draws five concentric circles corresponding to 5%, 10%, 20%, 40% and 60% of the

TABLE 3.VIII
Average balance values (SD) for children with cerebral palsy and children without disability (from Rose *et al.* 1999)

	N	Eyes	Age (years)	Path mm/sec	ARD Mm	Frequency Hz	Ds mm2/sec	HI
CP	23	Open	11.2–4.7 (5–18)	15.0–7.6 (5.7–32.2)*	8.4–5.1 (2.9–24.5)**	0.31–0.08 (0.21–0.49)**	50.30–61.40 (4.7–255.7)*	0.22–0.08 (0.03–0.37)*
Normal	92	Open	10.9–3.7 (5–18)	10.8–3.3 (4.2–20.0)	4.9–1.5 (2.2–12.4)	0.37–0.08 (0.23–0.67)	16.40–12.90 (1.3–88.6)	0.25–0.09 (0.08–0.68)
CP	23	Closed	11.2–4.7 (5–18)	18.3–8.7 (7.4–43.7)*	9.2–5.1 (2.7–24.0)**	0.35–0.10 (0.14–0.52)**	73.97–85.20 (8.3–399.4)*	0.17–0.08 (0.07–0.35)
Normal	92	Closed	10.9–3.7 (5–18)	14.0–4.6 (6.4–34.1)	5.4–1.9 (2.4–13.2)	0.43–0.08 (0.27–0.72)	28.91–28.03 (6.8–244.5)	0.18–0.05 (0.06–31)

*p<0.05 **p 0.005

Center of pressure calculations: Path, path length per second; ARD, average radial displacement;
Freq, mean frequency of sway; Ds, Brownian random motion measures of short-term diffusion coefficient; HI, long-term scaling exponent as calculated in a previous report (Wolff *et al.* 1998).

bodyweight around the average center. The printer provides a graphic display of postural sway (Fig. 3.16).

Rose *et al.* (1999, 2002) analyzed postural control using a force plate in 23 ambulatory children and adolescents with spastic diplegia, ages 5–18 years. They stood on a force plate for 30 seconds with eyes open and closed. The data were compared with those previously obtained from 92 age-matched children without a disability (Wolff *et al.* 1998). From the center-of-pressure plots generated by the computer program, average balance values were determined for those who had spastic diplegia and the matched normal controls (Table 3.VIII). Abnormal balance was defined as being present where values were greater than 2 standard deviations compared with the controls. Eight of the 23 children with spastic diplegia had abnormal balance values.

The relatively high percentage of children with cerebral palsy (65%) who had normal balance when standing indicated that postural control for simply standing alone was not a major problem in the majority. Average values for path length, average radial displacement and diffusion coefficient as center-of-pressure measures were significantly higher for those with cerebral palsy compared to controls (p<0.05). Abnormal values were highest in the youngest children and in those who had hamstring lengthening (60%). Data obtained with eyes open and closed revealed no difference in the values, and implied that those with cerebral palsy had normal dependence on visual feedback to maintain balance.

In Taiwan, Liao and colleagues (2001) tested the reliability of balance tests in children with cerebral palsy compared with children who had no disabilities. They used the Smart Balance Master System and the Bruininks–Oseretsky Test of Motor Proficiency (BOTMP) as a subtest. The Smart Balance Master System that measured postural sway had good to moderate reliability; the subtest (BOTMP) had 100% agreement in one-legged standing and walking on a line.

These studies indicate that patients who have abnormal postural control may be partially documented with objective measurements. The data should be important in the pre- and postoperative assessments as well as in outcome studies of physical therapy or orthoses. Further study to measure the effects of an instrumented perturbation of the standing posture (comparable to the Romberg sign) may show more correlation with the clinical observations and tests of postural balance observed in so many patients with spastic diplegia: with the slightest push backward they are apt to stumble or fall. It remains to be reported whether balance is improved by physical therapeutic treatments such as exercise, orthopaedic surgery, rhizotomy, baclofen or as-yet undiscovered pharmaceuticals.

ENERGETICS

The measurement of energy expenditure while walking can be useful in the evaluation of the efficacy of walking aids, wheelchairs, orthotics, physical therapy and surgery in cerebral palsy. Oxygen-consumption measurements reflect the energy cost of activity. Oxygen consumption indicates aerobic energy-production by the muscles, in contrast to the anaerobic type in which glucose and phosphorus are metabolized without oxygen to convert adenosine diphosphate to adenosine triphosphate, with its high-energy phosphate bonds. In anaerobic metabolism, lactic acid is the end product. Anaerobic metabolism is limited in energy production; almost 19 times more energy will be produced by the aerobic method (Waters *et al.* 1978).

Duffy *et al.* (1996) studied the rate of oxygen consumption in children who had cerebral palsy or spina bifida. They found that it was significantly higher in children with spastic diplegia than in those who had hemiplegia or spina bifida. They surmised that children with diplegia may have consumed more oxygen when walking due to their abnormal equilibrium reactions and their inability to control their walking speed.

Csongradi *et al.* (1979) reported that the cadence of children who had spastic diplegia was faster than in normal controls. These children could not slow down. The opposite conclusion on walking speeds in spastic diplegia was reached by Campbell and Ball (1978) who studied the energetics of walking in children with spastic diplegia and in normal children. In their study of 6- to 13-year-old children, those with spastic diplegia had slower walking speeds than the normal controls, and their heart rates and energy costs were greater.

Although oxygen-consumption studies are important in clinical research, the methods have been found to be especially cumbersome for children (Shephard 1975, Sutherland 1978, Ghosh *et al.* 1980). It is simpler to measure heart rate, and its relationship to oxygen consumption is linear from the resting state to the submaximal exercise levels in normal and disabled persons with the slope of the linear relationship differing in the two groups (Poulsen and Asmussen 1962, Ganguli and Datta 1978, Rose *et al.* 1989) (Fig. 3.18).

Rose *et al.* (1989, 1991) used an energy-expenditure index (Physiological Cost Index, PCI) derived from the average number of heartbeats per unit distance walked (heartbeats per minute divided by meters per minute). Each participant in this study was used as his or her own control by measuring the heartbeat in the resting state. Rose found that, in children with cerebral palsy, the energy cost was lower when wheeled walking aids were used rather than 'quad canes'. Wolfe (1978) measured the effects of floor surface on energy costs in wheelchair propulsion, and found that oxygen uptake per minute was higher on carpets; but it made no difference whether pneumatic or hard rubber tires were used.

Heart rate can be conveniently monitored by an electro-cardiographic telemetry system, to allow walking to be as natural as possible. The heart rate is measured by asking the child to walk a standard distance, and monitoring the heart rate for the last 2 minutes of a 5-minute period of walking (Medeiros 1984). This simple instrumentation is within the capabilities of almost any facility. Since Rose's introduction of measuring energy consumption by heart rate, there are reports that favor oxygen-consumption studies as more accurate and reliable.

The newer technology of measurement from Cosmed of Rome, Italy, appears to have made oxygen-consumption measurement in children easier and with reasonable repeatable results. The lightweight portable telemetric system for oxygen consumption, Cosmed K2, was compared with the stationary breath-by-breath system using a treadmill (Corry *et al.* 1996). The equipment did not affect the gait pattern, and repeatability was stated to be satisfactory. But it was unreliable in detecting differences of less than 10% in a single individual.

The group at the Alfred I. duPont Institute, Delaware, used the Cosmed K2 instrumentation to measure oxygen consumption in five children who had cerebral palsy with five unaffected children (Bowen *et al.* 1998). They found no significant differences in the percentage of variability of the oxygen cost and consumption or the PCI between the children with cerebral palsy and the normal children. The oxygen cost was the most reliable measurement with an average variability of 13.2% for the cerebral palsy group and 13.9% for the normal group. The heart-rate method (PCI) was found to be the least reliable with variability of 20.3%–20.5% in the two groups studied.

Bowen and coworkers (1999) compared oxygen consumption in eight children with cerebral palsy, and eight who had muscular dystrophy. Oxygen cost and consumption were higher in the children with cerebral palsy. Despite their muscle weakness the children who had muscular dystrophy had normal oxygen cost and consumption. Because of these observations the authors concluded that energy measurements should not be used as the only outcome measure for patient with cerebral palsy who might have changes in muscle strength. This observation may be important in assessment of outcomes of tendon/muscle unit lengthenings, rhizotomy, botulinum toxin or intrathecal baclofen.

From the Royal Children's Hospital in Melbourne, Australia, is a report that further questioned the validity of the heart-rate method (Boyd *et al.* 1999). In this study they compared the repeatability of the low-technology method of the PCI, using the heart rate, with high-technology oxygen-consumption methods (Cosmed K4) in five children and four adults without a disability. The repeatability for the oxygen-cost method was 13%, but the standard deviation in adults was 6%–72%, and even higher in children, at the 91% and 95% ranges. Accordingly, they questioned the validity of the heart-rate method as an outcome measure.

One might think that energy requirements would ideally be included in every gait analysis. In practice, however, even in large series of patients with postoperative orthopaedic surgery,

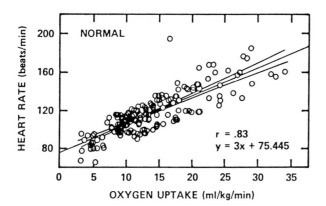

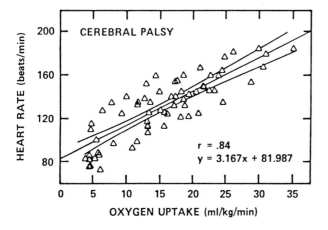

Fig. 3.18. Scatterplots and linear regression line with 95% confidence limits around the means for heart rate vs oxygen uptake. (*a*) 18 normal children walking on a treadmill in a range of speeds from 22 to 131 m/min. (*b*) 13 children with cerebral palsy walking on a treadmill at the same range of speeds. The slope of the relationship between the two was no groups was not significantly different (0.30 normals; 0.32 cerebral palsy). (Reproduced by permission from Rose *et al.* 1989.)

selective posterior rootlet rhizotomy or myoneural blocks we do not find records of oxygen-cost data or PCI in the reports, probably due to cost and time constraints.

When dealing with the individual child or adolescent with cerebral palsy, the simple radial pulse rate can be effective in showing how to redirect the efforts of walking to more efficient mobility. In some patients who have severe spastic paralysis and poor equilibrium reactions (GMFM levels III, IV, V), the drive to keep them walking—often instigated by parents and therapists—can deplete them of the energy required for learning and engaging in social exchange. The direction needs to be changed to mobility. It is simple to count the radial pulse per minute while resting and after walking 5 minutes. The difference between the two pulse rates can provide an effective demonstration of the extraordinary energy the child is expending. The result can provide parents with a powerful demonstration of why a wheelchair would allow the child or adolescent to use his energy more profitably, by using his brain, rather than by struggling to walk a few steps.

MYONEURAL BLOCKS

Botulinum-A toxin has replaced alcohol for myoneural blockade of the motor end plates of spastic muscles muscle in the lower limb (O'Brien 1995). Instead of using the myoneural block as a temporary diagnostic measure to test the effects of elimination of the spastic muscle force prior to orthopaedic surgery in equivocal cases, e.g. adductor myotomy or gastrocnemius–soleus lengthening, the toxin has become part of the treatment. The evidence is the plethora of reports attesting to its efficacy as a proposed treatment in the 1990s.

The objective of myoneural blocks with alcohol, local anesthetics or phenol was to eliminate the stretch reflex of the spastic muscle temporarily by altering the sensitivity of the muscle-spindle receptors; the muscle is 'paralyzed'. Alcohol, except in the upper limbs because of long duration damage to the peripheral nerves, might be used in lieu of botulinum toxin where costs are a major consideration, but the duration of its effect is short (1–6 weeks).

The only virtue of alcohol is that it is inexpensive compared with botulinum toxin. But with alcohol a general anesthetic was usually necessary because the pain with an alcohol block is considerable and may cause muscle soreness for a day or two. In contrast, botulinum toxin is practically painless when injected so that anesthesia is not usually necessary and the duration of its effect is usually 3–6 months.

Phenol can be destructive to the muscle, nerves, skin and subcutaneous tissue and can cause extreme pain if injected into or in proximity to a sensory nerve. Phenol can cause destruction of the nerve, muscle atrophy and necrosis. Skin sloughs can occur. Phenol is not recommended for myoneural blockade.

Preceding the myoneural blocks, it is important to record the gait on film or videotape. If motion-analysis laboratory facilities are available, gait EMG and kinematics are the ideal objective methods for recording lower-limb motion.

A contraindication to the use of myoneural blocks is an obvious fixed deformity due to a definite contracture of the muscle. A deformity that is mainly dynamic can often be determined by clinical examination, if the child is relaxed and a slow stretch of the muscle is applied. When in doubt, complete relaxation under general anesthesia can differentiate contracture from spasticity alone.

Botulinum, alcohol and lidocaine blocks are given into the muscle bellies that can be identified by knowledge of gross anatomy, and into the motor endplates for muscles close to the surface of the skin such as the gastrocnemius, adductor longus, the hamstrings and selected upper-limb muscles (Fig. 3.19). Deeper muscles such as the iliopsoas or the posterior tibialis require a Teflon-coated hollow needle for electomyographic confirmation and then injection of the agent. A hollow needle electrode can be used so that with electric stimuli the action of the muscle can be observed, the agent injected, and the 'muscle put to sleep' (A. Campos da Paz Jr, personal communication).

BOTULINUM-A TOXIN
Judging from the plethora of reports in the literature it seems evident that botulinum toxin has evolved into a method of treatment rather than for diagnostic myoneural blocks (Russell *et al.* 1997); Dysport is the trade name of the European

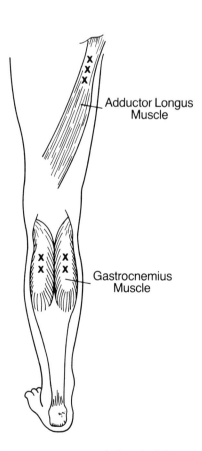

Fig. 3.19. Common injection sites in the lower limb for a myoneural block with botulinum toxin or alcohol. *Caution: take care to map the course of the lateral popliteal nerve as is crosses the lateral head of the gastrocnemius to the neck of the fibula.*

formulation of botulinum-A toxin (Watanabc *et al.* 1998). Chapter 6 discusses its use as treatment of spasticity and dystonia. Dosage is usually 5 units/kg (ranging from 1 to 2 units/kg for the gastrocnemius heads for a total of 100–320 units). Koman *et al.* (1996) stated that the maximum dose is 6 units/kg; toxicity is dose related. When injecting the toxin, respiratory support and antitoxin should be available.[6] The paralytic effect on the particular muscle injected lasts from 3 to 6 months. If the purpose of the block is to decide on surgery, its longer duration than either alcohol or lidocaine might be a disadvantage for the surgeon and the patient who expect a more timely decision. But alcohol injections are probably not advisable in the upper limbs, or in deep muscles such as the posterior tibial in the lower limbs.

ALCOHOL

The pioneers in alcohol injection of muscles originally intended the method as a therapeutic modality (Hariga *et al.* 1964, Tardieu *et al.* 1964, 1971, 1975, Hariga 1966, Tardieu and Hariga 1972). It was hoped that the results of eliminating the stretch reflex in a specific muscle, primarily the gastrocnemius, would allow neurological restructuring so that correction of the deformity would be permanent. These intentions have been modified now that more follow-up experience has been gained. As initiated by Carpenter and Mikhail (1972), the method is not useful so much for therapy as for diagnosis and evaluation.

Diluted alcohol of 45%–50% concentration is recommended in a dose of 5 ml per kg bodyweight (Carpenter and Mikhail 1972, Carpenter 1983). Injection of 3–4 ml of diluted alcohol into several areas of the muscle bellies is a simple procedure. The most common and accessible muscles which have been injected are the gastrocnemius and the adductor longus (Fig. 3.19). Alcohol injection into the hamstrings was less reliable (Carlson *et al.* 1984). Commonly alcohol injections were done under brief general anesthesia; hospitalization was not usually required.

The effect of the alcohol block lasts 2–6 weeks, giving all observers ample time to determine if surgical treatment of the equinus or hip-adduction deformity might improve gait function (Carpenter and Mikhail 1972, Carpenter and Seitz 1980, Carpenter 1983, Carlson *et al.* 1984). We did 45% alcohol myoneural blocks of the gastrocnemius in children (usually under age 5 years) who had a dynamic equinus and could not tolerate an ankle–foot orthosis because of severe spasticity. In this way direct surgical intervention might be avoided and sufficient time can elapse to allow further development of the child's equilibrium reactions as the nervous system matures (to the age of 3–4 years). The same principles of delaying surgical lengthening of the spastic calf muscles in young children appears to be obtained with intramuscular botulinum toxin injections.

Another use of the gastrocnemius blocks has been in the rare case of disabling equinus in a child with hemidystonia. In this condition there is no contracture of the muscle, and a decision might be made after the block on whether or not a gastrocnemius neurectomy would partially relieve the disabling equinus, which is usually controlled with a plastic ankle–foot orthosis after the neurectomy. The myoneural block can demonstrate if an undesirable 'athetoid shift' of the dystonia to the ankle dorsiflexors might occur following the permanent gastrocnemius neurectomy. Botulinum-A toxin myoneural blocks currently appear to be the treatment of choice for dystonia.

The only complication with myoneural 45% alcohol blocks is the injection into a peripheral nerve such as the lateral popliteal nerve as it crosses over the lateral head of the gastrocnemius. Alcohol destroys nerve fibers. If peroneal nerve paralysis occurs, an intractable dynamic varus deformity of the foot is the result; but complete recovery can be expected in 3 months. This complication may be avoided by mapping on the skin the course of the lateral popliteal nerve as it emerges from the popliteal fossa to become the peroneal at the fibula neck and using a surface nerve stimulator before injection.

LOCAL ANESTHETICS

Lidocaine is useful for a temporary (1- to 2-hour) myoneural block of muscles in adolescents and adults who will tolerate needle injections. The dose of lidocaine should not exceed the toxic limits of about 1 mg/kg of body weight. Excessive dosages can result in convulsions and cardiac arrest. If larger volumes of lidocaine are needed to infiltrate an entire muscle, a 0.5% solution is safer.

Lidocaine (0.5%) infiltrated into spastic upper-limb muscles such as the finger- and wrist-flexors can help determine if the patient has active extension of the wrist and/or fingers preliminary to the decision to lengthen the affected muscle–tendon unit. The problem with lidocaine is its relatively short duration of action, so effects must be observed at once. Lidocaine can also cause light-headedness and anxiety in children, which will preclude accurate observations and analysis of its effect on gait.

Bupivacaine (Sensorcaine®) when injected has a rapid onset and longer duration of anesthesia than Lidocaine. It is not recommended for children under age 12 years because of its toxicity. At all ages, the risks include acute emergencies of the cardiovascular system—even cardiac arrest. When bupivacaine is used, oxygen and cardiopulmonary resuscitative equipment and personnel should be on hand (AstraZeneca product information 2000)[7]. Because of the increased toxicity, it is probably not used for myoneural blocks in patients who have cerebral palsy.

PHENOL

Aqueous phenol has been used as a temporary but long-acting neurolytic agent in spastic paralysis.

Its use in cerebral palsy is discussed for historical interest only. There seems to be no indication for intramuscular phenol injections or direct application to an isolated nerve to the muscle. It has a short-term anesthetic effect, and a long-term destructive

---

6 Botulinum antitoxin from Center for Disease Control and Prevention, Atlanta, GA, USA.

7 *Physicians' Desk Reference, 2000,* Montvale, NJ: Medical Economics Co.

effect. Nerve fibers of all diameters are destroyed. Phenol blocks can last for 6 months to over a year. We have not used phenol because it is difficult to control the degree of tissue destruction. Direct injection into perineural tissue by open surgical exposure may result in undesirable and long-term overactivity of antagonistic spastic muscles. For example, a phenol injection of a motor point in the posterior tibial muscle could 'uncover' underlying spasticity of the peroneal muscles, with the result that a dynamic varus deformity of the foot would become a valgus deformity (Herman 1976). If phenol is inadvertently injected subcutaneously, skin necrosis and slough can occur (R.L. Samilson, personal communication).

PSYCHOLOGICAL TESTS

Even though the surgeon or physician is not trained or equipped to perform psychological testing, he or she will have to consider the intellectual functioning of the child when advising treatment or management in achieving functional goals. Consequently, some familiarity with the interpretation of psychological tests is advisable. Even though a high incidence of mental retardation was reported in cerebral palsy (Hohman 1953), the changing etiology of cerebral palsy should make us wary of overgeneralizing. Non-verbal ability is not necessarily an indication of mental retardation: witness the success of non-verbal communication techniques, from sign language to advanced computer technology and artificial voice devices. Mental retardation is not predictive of the ability to walk (Shapiro *et al.* 1979). Certainly no child should be rejected for surgical treatment solely on the grounds of presumed intellectual status. We all know of examples of normal or superior intelligence in some very severely impaired persons with cerebral palsy. The case of Christy Brown (documented in his book *My Left Foot*, and the subsequent film) is one notable example.

Table 3.IX is a guide for labeling the degree of mental retardation. Most persons with athetosis have normal intellects and some are of above-average intelligence; children who have spastic diplegia usually succeed in regular school although they may have some specific learning problems; those who have total body involved spastic paralysis (quadriplegia) seem to have a higher incidence of retardation; those with less motor involvement such as ataxia or spastic hemiplegia due to cerebral maldevelopment appear to have more mental retardation.

TABLE 3.IX
Level of mental retardation according to IQ

Level	IQ scale	
	Stanford–Binet	*Wechsler*
(Borderline*)	(69–84)	(70–84)
Mild	52–68	55–69
Moderate	36–51	40–54
Severe	20–35	25–39
Profound	#19	#24

*Since the American Association on Mental Deficiency adopted its 1973 definition, persons who score in the borderline range are not considered mentally retarded. (From Baird and Gordon 1983, p. 121.)

As pointed out by Baird and Gordon (1983), definitions of retardation can be based upon function. Children with cerebral palsy whose test scores show them to be ineducable— approximately 50% according to Illingworth (1958) and Nelson and Ellenberg (1978)—can nevertheless learn a sufficient number of skills without formal 'schooling' to achieve reasonable independence for adult living. The increasing use of rehabilitation engineering technology and adaptive devices in recent years greatly enhances this prospect.

As any psychologist knows, referral of babies and toddlers for 'psychological testing' may be inappropriate because the estimate of intellectual performance is based mainly upon motor development and developmental tests, and may be inaccurate in terms of prognosis. As the intellectually impaired baby and toddler matures, the gap from the expected mental development of the normal child grows wider (Fig. 3.20).

At least two IQ tests 3 months apart that show an IQ level of less than 70 are necessary before a diagnosis of mental retardation can be accepted. At the ages of 7–8 years the standardized tests such as the WISC-8 have shown high reliability (Aicardi 1998, p. 826). That the IQ is stable over long periods of time from the ages of 7–13 years was impressively shown in a study of 800 children followed in Dunedin (Moffitt *et al.* 1993).

Good psychological testing at the appropriate age does have validity, even though there is lack of standardization for children with cerebral palsy. For groups of children the test–retest reliability was thought to be 98%, and 90% for an individual child (Baird and Gordon 1983).

Fennell and Dikel (2001) concluded that children with cerebral palsy should have 'neuropsychological' assessment rather than rely solely on the global IQ or vocational outcomes. Among the neuropsychological measures were semantic comprehension, expressive language function, short-term memory, non-verbal reasoning and academic skills. These authors expressed the hope that future studies would delineate the relationship between

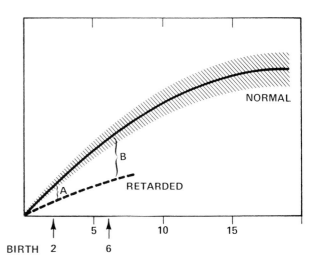

Fig. 3.20. As the child who is mentally retarded matures the discrepancy in intelligence between this child and the normal becomes wider. (Redrawn from Bray 1969, and Bleck and Nagel 1982.)

brain lesions depicted in the MRI studies and their effects on neuropsychological functions.

Learning disorders are discovered when the child enters school. In cerebral palsy these usually take the form of specific problems in reading, for instance, or mathematics. Behavior problems do occur, and have been estimated as being five or six times more prevalent in cerebral palsy than in the normal healthy child. It is also accepted that in families who have psychopathology, and have understandable stress coping with their disabled child, psychodynamics may influence behavioral problems (Aicardi 1998, p. 833).

The past decade and a half has seen a tremendous enhancement of tools to evaluate the child with cerebral palsy. Technological improvements bring these studies within the reach of far more clinicians than previously. These allow us to be more objective and critical in our recommendations, and to better assess the outcomes of our therapies. Only by utilizing these tools will we continue to refine our treatment plans.

REFERENCES

Abel, M.F., Wenger, D.R., Murbarak, S.J., Sutherland, D.H. (1994) 'Quantitative analysis of hip dysplasia in cerebral palsy: a study of radiographs and 3-D reformatted images.' *Journal of Pediatric Orthopaedics*, 14, 283–289.

Adams, J.M., Perry, J. (1994) 'Gait analysis: clinical application.' *In* Rose, J., Gamble, J.G. (Eds) *Human Walking*. Baltimore: Williams and Wilkins, p. 143.

Adler, N.T., Bleck, E.E., Rinsky, L.A., Young, W. (1986) 'Balance reactions and eye–hand coordination in idiopathic scoliosis.' *Journal of Orthopaedic Research*, 4, 102–107.

—— Bleck, E.E., Rinsky, L.A. (1989) 'Gait electromyograms and surgical decisions for paralytic deformities of the foot.' *Developmental Medicine and Child Neurology*, 31, 287–292.

Aicardi, J. (1998) *Diseases of the Nervous System in Childhood, 2nd edn.* London: Mac Keith Press with Cambridge University Press; Philadelphia: J.B. Lippincott.

Albright, L. (1995) 'Spastic cerebral palsy, approaches to drug treatment.' *Practical Therapeutics*, 4, 17–27.

Alcorn C.L., Nicholson, C.L. (1972) 'Validity of the Slosson Drawing Coordination Test with adolescents of below-average ability.' *Perceptual Motor Skills*, 34, 261–262.

Allen, M.C., Alexander, G.R. (1997) 'Using motor milestones as a multistep process to screen preterm infants for cerebral palsy.' *Developmental Medicine and Child Neurology*, 39, 12–16.

Almeida, G.L., Campbell, S.K., Girolami, G.L., Penn, R.D., Corcos, D.M. (1997) 'Multidimensional assessment of motor function n a child with cerebral palsy following intrathecal administration of baclofen.' *Physical Therapy*, 77, 751–764.

Amiel-Tison, C., Grenier, A. (1983) *Neurological Evaluation of the Newborn and the Infant.* New York: Masson USA.

Ashworth, B. (1964) 'Preliminary trial of carisoprodol in multiple sclerosis.' *Practitioner*, 192, 540–542.

Ayres, A.J. (1972) 'Characteristics of types of sensory integrative dysfunction.' *Journal of Learning Disabilities*, 5, 336–343.

—— (1978) 'Learning disabilities and the vestibular system.' *Journal of Learning Disabilities*, 11, 18–29.

Baird, H.W., Gordon, E.C. (1983) *Neurological Evaluation of Infants and Children. Clinics in Developmental Medicine, Nos 84/85.* London: Spastics International Medical Publications with Heinemann Medical; Philadelphia: J.B. Lippincott.

Barnes, K.E., Stark, A. (1975) 'Denver Developmental Screening Test: a normative study.' *American Journal of Public Health*, 65, 363–369.

Baumann, J.U. (1980) 'Gait analysis and its benefit to the patient.' *Progress in Orthopaedic Surgery*, 4, 103–107.

—— (1984) 'Clinical experience of gait analysis in the management of cerebral palsy.' *Prosthetics and Orthotics International*, 8, 29–32.

Bax, M.C.O., Whitmore, I. (1973) 'Neurodevelopmental screening in the school entrant medical examination.' *Lancet*, ii, 368–370.

—— (1987) 'The medical examination of children on entry to school. The results and use of neurodevelopmental assessment.' *Developmental Medicine and Child Neurology*, 29, 40–55.

Bayley, N. (1969) *Bayley Scales of Infant Development.* New York: Psychological Corporation.

Beals, R.K. (1966) 'Spastic paraplegia and diplegia: an evaluation of non-surgical and surgical factors influencing the prognosis for ambulation.' *Journal of Bone and Joint Surgery*, 48A, 827–846.

Bleck, E.E., Nagel, D.A. (Eds) (1982) *Physically Handicapped Children: A Medical Atlas for Teachers, 2nd Edn.* Orlando, FL: Grune & Stratton.

—— (1994) 'A sense of balance.' *Developmental Medicine and Child Neurology*, 36, 377–378.

Bohannon, R.W., Smith, M.B. (1987) 'Interrater reliability of a modified Ashworth scale of muscle spasticity.' *Physical Therapy*, 67, 206–207

Boppana, S.B., Fowler, K.B., Vaid, Y., Hedlund, G., Stagno, S., Britt, W.J., Pass, R.F. (1997) 'Neuroradiographic findings in the newborn period and long-term outcome in children with symptomatic congenital cytomagalovirus infection.' *Pediatrics*, 99, 409–414.

Bose, K., Goh, J.C. (1984) 'Gait analysis in clinical practice.' *Journal of Western Pacific Orthopaedic Association*, 21, 57–62.

Bowen, T.R., Lennon, N. Castagno, P., Miller, F., Richards, J. (1998) 'Variability of energy-consumption measures in children with cerebral palsy.' *Journal of Pediatric Orthopaedics*, 18, 738–742.

—— Miller, F., Mackenzie, W. (1999) 'Comparison of oxygen consumption measurements in children with cerebral palsy to children with muscular dystrophy.' *Journal of Pediatric Orthopaedics*, 19, 133–136.

Bower, E., McLellan, D.L., Arney, J., Campbell, M.J. (1996) 'A randomized controlled trial of different intensities of physiotherapy and different goal-setting procedures in 44 children with cerebral palsy.' *Developmental Medicine and Child Neurology*, 38, 226–237.

Boyce, W., Gowland, C., Hardy, S., Rosenbaum, P., Lane, M., Plews, N., Goldsmith, C., Russell, D.J. (1991) 'Development of a quality-of-movement measure for children with cerebral palsy.' *Physical Therapy*, 71, 820–832.

—— Gowland, C., Rosenbaum, P.L., Lane, M., Plews, N., Goldsmith, C.H., Russell, D.J., Wright, V., Potter, S., Harding, D. (1995) 'Gross Motor Performance Measure: validity and responsiveness of a measure of quality of movement.' *Physical Therapy*, 75, 603–613.

Boyd, R., Fatone, S., Roda, J., Olesch, C., Starr, R., Cullis, E., Gallagher, E., Carlin, J.B., Nattrass, G.R., Graham, K. (1999) 'High- or low-technology measurements of energy expenditure in clinical gait analysis?' *Developmental Medicine and Child Neurology*, 41, 676–682.

Brazelton, T.B. (1973) *Neonatal Behavioral Assessment Scale. Clinics in Developmental Medicine, No. 50.* London: Spastics International Medical Publications with Heinemann Medical.

—— (1984) *Neonatal Behavioral Assessment Scale. Clinics in Developmental Medicine, No. 88.* London: Spastics International Medical Publications with Blackwell Scientific; Philadelphia: J.B. Lippincott.

—— Nugent, J.K. (Eds) (1995) *Neonatal Behaviour Assessment Scale, 3rd Edn. Clinics in Developmental Medicine, No. 137.* London: Mac Keith Press.

Bryant, G.M., Davies, K.J., Newcombe, R.G. (1974) 'The Denver Developmental Screening Test. Achievement of test items in the first year of life by Denver and Cardiff infants.' *Developmental Medicine and Child Neurology*, 16, 474–484.

Burrows, L. (1999) *Gross Motor Ability Estimator* [software]. Hamilton, Ontario, Canada: *CanChild* Centre for Childhood Disability Research, McMaster University. (Software available from http://www.fhs.mcmaster.ca/canchild.)

Byrne, P., Welch, R., Johnson, M.S., Darrah, J., Piper, M. (1990) 'Serial magnetic resonance imaging in neonatal hypoxic–ischemic encephalopathy.' *Journal of Pediatrics*, 117, 694–700.

Camp, B.W., Van Natta, P.A. (1971) 'The validity of the DDST.' *Child Development*, 42, 474–485.

Campbell, J., Ball, J. (1978) 'Energetics of walking in cerebral palsy.' *Orthopaedic Clinics of North America*, 9, 374–377.

Carlson, W., Carpenter, B., Wenger, D. (1984) 'Myoneural blocks for preoperative planning in cerebral palsy surgery.' *Developmental Medicine and Child Neurology*, 26, 252–253. (Abstract.)

Carpenter, E.B. (1983) 'Role of nerve blocks in the foot and ankle in cerebral palsy: therapeutic and diagnostic.' *Foot and Ankle*, **4**, 164–166.

—— Mikhail, M. (1972) 'The use of intramuscular alcohol as a diagnostic and therapeutic aid in cerebral palsy.' *Developmental Medicine and Child Neurology*, **14**, 113–114. (Abstract.)

—— Seitz, D.G. (1980) 'Intramuscular alcohol as an aid in management of spastic cerebral palsy.' *Developmental Medicine and Child Neurology*, **22**, 497–501.

Chambers, H., Lauer, A., Kaufman, K. Cardelia, J.M., Sutherland, D. (1998) 'Prediction of outcome after rectus femoris surgery in cerebral palsy: the role of cocontraction of the rectus femoris and vastus lateralis.' *Journal of Pediatric Orthopaedics*, **18**, 703–711.

Chao, E.Y., Laughmann, R.K., Schneider, E., Stauffer, R.N. (1983) 'Normative data of knee joint motion and ground reaction forces in adult level walking.' *Journal of Biomechanics*, **16**, 219–233.

Chutorian, A.B., Root, L. (1994) 'Management of spasticity in children with Botulinum-A toxin.' *International Pediatrics*, **9** (Suppl. 1), 35–43.

Ciamicioli, R., Panzer, V.P., Kaye, J. (1997) 'Balance in the healthy elderly: posturography and clinical assessments.' *Archives of Neurology*, **54**, 976–981.

Coley, I. (1978) *Pediatric Assessment of Self-Care Activities*. St Louis: C.V. Mosby

Cook, R.E., Schneider, I., Hazlewood, M.E., Hillman, S.J., Robb, J.E. (2003) 'Gait analysis alters decision-making in cerebral palsy.' *Journal of Pediatric Orthopaedics*, **23**, 292–295.

Cools, A.T.M., Hermanns, J.M.A. (1977) *Denver Developmental Screening Test*. Amsterdam: Swets & Zeitlinger.

Coop, R.H., Eckel, E., Stuck, G.B. (1975) 'An assessment of the Pictorial Test of Intelligence for use with young cerebral-palsied children.' *Developmental Medicine and Child Neurology*, **17**, 287–292.

Corry, I.S., Duffy, C.M, Cosgrave, A.P., Graham, H.K. (1996) 'Measurement of oxygen consumption in disabled children by the Cosmed K2 portable telemetry system.' *Developmental Medicine and Child Neurology*, **38**, 585–593.

Csongradi, J, Bleck, E., Ford, W.F. (1979) 'Gait electromyography in normal and spastic children, with special reference to the quadriceps femoris and hamstring muscles.' *Developmental Medicine and Child Neurology*, **21**, 738–748.

Damiano, D.L., Abel, M.F. (1996) 'Relation of gait analysis to gross motor function in cerebral palsy.' *Developmental Medicine and Child Neurology*, **38**, 389–396.

Davids, J.R., Bagley, A.M., Bryan, M. (1998) 'Kinematic and kinetic analysis of running in children with cerebral palsy.' *Developmental Medicine and Child Neurology*, **40**, 528–535.

—— Foti, T., Dabelstein, J., Blackhurst, D.W., Bagley, A. (1999) 'Objective assessment of dyskinesia in children with cerebral palsy.' *Journal of Pediatric Orthopaedics*, **19**, 211–214

—— —— Bagley, A. (1999) 'Voluntary (normal) versus obligatory (cerebral palsy) toe-walking in children: a kinematic, kinetic, and electromyographic study.' *Journal of Pediatric Orthopaedics*, **19**, 461–469.

DeLuca, P.A., Davis, R.B. 3rd, Õunpuu, S., Rose, S., Sirkin, R. (1997) 'Alterations in surgical decision making in patients with cerebral palsy based on three-dimensional gait analysis.' *Journal of Pediatric Orthopaedics*, **17**, 608–614.

—— Õunpuu, S., Davis, R.B., Walsh, J.H. (1998) 'Effect of hamstring and psoas lengthening on pelvic tilt in patients with spastic diplegic cerebral palsy.' *Journal of Pediatric Orthopaedics*, **18**, 712–718.

Detrembleur, D., Willems, P., Plaghki, L., (1997) 'Does walking speed influence the time pattern of muscle activation in normal children?' *Developmental Medicine and Child Neurology*, **39**, 803–807.

Di Fabio, R.P., Seay, R. (1997) 'Use of the "fast evaluation of mobility, balance, and fear" in elderly community dwellers: validity and reliability.' *Physical Therapy*, **77**, 904–917.

Dick, N.P., Cariand, J. (1975) 'Development of preschool-aged children of different social and ethnic groups: implications for developmental screening.' *Journal of Pediatrics*, **87**, 125–132.

Dobson, F., Boyd, R.N., Parrott, J., Nattrass, G.R., Graham, H.K. (2002) 'Hip surveillance in children with cerebral palsy impact on the surgical management of spastic hip disease.' *Journal of Bone and Joint Surgery*, **84B**, 720–726.

—— Morris, M.E., Baker, R., Graham, H.K. (2006) 'Gait classification in cerebral palsy: a systematic review.' *Gait and Posture*, Feb. 18.

Drouin, L.M., Malouin, F., Richards, C.L., Marcoux, S. (1996) 'Correlation between the gross motor function measure scores and gait spatiotemporal measures in children with neurological impairments.' *Developmental Medicine and Child Neurology*, **38**, 1007–1019.

Dubovitz, L., Dubovitz, V. (1981) *The Neurological Assessment of the Preterm and Full Term Infant, Clinics in Developmental Medicine, No. 79*. London: Spastics International Medical Publications with Heinemann Medical; Philadelphia: J.B. Lippincott.

Duffy, C.M., Hill, A.E., Cosgrove, A.P., Corry, I.S., Graham, H.K. (1996) 'Energy consumption in children with spina bifida and cerebral palsy: a comparative study.' *Developmental Medicine and Child Neurology*, **38**, 238–243.

Dykens, E. (1996) 'The Draw-a-Person task in persons with mental retardation: what does it measure?' *Research in Developmental Disability*, **17**, 1–13.

Egan, D.F. (1990) *Developmental Examination of Infants and Preschool Children. Clinics in Developmental Medicine, No.112*. London: Mac Keith Press with Blackwell Scientific; Philadelphia: J.B. Lippincott.

Eklof, O., Ringertz, H., Samuelsson, L. (1988) 'The percentage of migration as indicator of femoral head position.' *Acta Radiologica*, **29**, 363–366.

Eliasson, A.C., Krumlinde-Sundholm, L., Rosblad, B., Beckung, E., Arner, M., Ohrvall, A.M., Rosenbaum, P. (2006) 'The Manual Ability Classification System (MACS) for children with cerebral palsy: scale development and evidence of validity and reliability.' *Developmental Medicine and Child Neurology*, **48**, 549–554.

Erford, B.T., Luce, C.L. (2005) Reliability and validity of scores of the Slosson Auditory Perception Skills Screener.' *Perceptual Motor Skills*, **101**, 891–897.

Fabian, D., Hicks, R., Tashmarm, S. (1984) 'Pre- and postoperative gait analysis in patients with spastic diplegia: a preliminary *report.'Journal of Pediatric Orthopaedics*, **4**, 715–725.

Fabry, G., Liu, X.C., Molenaers, G. (1999) 'Gait pattern in patients with spastic diplegic cerebral palsy who underwent staged operations.' *Journal of Pediatric Orthopaedics B*, **8**, 33–38.

Feagans, L. (1983) 'A current view of learning disabilities.' *Journal of Pediatrics*, **102**, 487–493.

Feldman, A.B., Haley, S.M., Coryell, J. (1990) 'Concurrent and construct validity of the Pediatric Evaluation of Disability Inventory.' *Physical Therapy*, **70**, 602–610.

Fennell, E.B., Dikel, T.N. (2001) 'Cognitive and neuropsychological functioning in children with cerebral palsy.' *Journal of Child Neurology*, **16**, 58–63.

Fishman, M.N., Colby, L.A., Sachs, L.A., Nichols, D.S. (1997) 'Comparison of upper extremity balance tasks and force platform testing in persons with hemiparesis.' *Physical Therapy*, **77**, 1052–1062.

Flehmig, I., Schimm, M., Uhde, J., Van Bernuth, H. (1973) *Denver-Entwicklungsskalen (Denver Development Scales)*. Stuttgart: Thieme.

Ford, F., Bleck, E.E., Aptekar, R.G., Collins, F.J., Stevik, D. (1976) 'Efficacy of dantrolene sodium in the treatment of spastic cerebral palsy.' *Developmental Medicine and Child Neurology*, **18**, 770–783.

Fowler, E.G., Nwigwe, A.I., Ho, T.W. (2000) 'Sensitivity of the pendulum test for assessing spasticity in persons with cerebral palsy.' *Developmental Medicine and Child Neurology*, **42**, 182–189

Frankenburg, W.K., Dodds, J.B. (1967) 'Denver developmental screening test.' *Journal of Pediatrics*, **71**, 181–491.

—— Camp, B.W., Van Natta, P.A. (1971) 'The validity of the DDST.' *Child Development*, **42**, 474–485.

—— Dick, N.P., Carland, J. (1975) 'Development of preschool-aged children of different social and ethnic groups: implications for developmental screening.' *Journal of Pediatrics*, **87**, 125–132.

Frazier, J., Garland, D.F., Jordan, C., Perry, J. (1982) 'Electromyographic gait analysis before and after operative treatment for hemiplegic equinus and equinovarus deformity.' *Journal of Bone and Joint Surgery*, **64A**, 284–288.

Frostig, M. (1963) 'Visual perceptual development and school adjustment *programs.'American Journal of Orthopsychiatry*, **33**, 367–368.

—— Horne, D. (1964) *The Frostig Program for Development of Visual Perception*. Chicago: Follett.

Gage, J.R. (1992) 'Computer based decision making.' *In* Sussman, M.D. (Ed.) *The Diplegic Child*. Rosemont, IL: American Academy of Orthopaedic Surgeons, pp. 187–199. (1994) 'The role of gait analysis in the treatment of cerebral palsy.' *Journal of Pediatric Orthopaedics*, **14**, 701–702.

—— (2004) *The Treatment of Gait Problems in Cerebral Palsy. Clinics in Developmental Medicine Nos 164/5* . London: Mac Keith Press with Cambridge university Press; New York: Cambridge University Press.

—— Fabian, D., Hicks, R., Tasman, S. (1984) 'Pre- and postoperative gait analysis in patients with spastic diplegia: a preliminary report.' *Journal of Pediatric Orthopaedics*, **4**, 715–725.

—— Perry, J.H., Peicks, R.R., Koop, S., Werntz, J.R. (1987) 'Rectus femoris transfer to improve knee function of children with cerebral palsy.' *Developmental Medicine and Child Neurology*, **29**, 159–166.

—— DeLuca P., Renshaw, T. (1995) Gait analysis: principles and applications. Emphasis on its use in cerebral palsy.' *Journal of Bone and Joint Surgery*, 77**A**, 1607–1623.

Ganguli, S., Datta, S.R. (1978) 'A new method for prediction of energy expenditure from heart rate.' *Journal of the Institution of Engineers (India)*, **58**, 57–61.

Ghosh, A.K., Tibarewala, B., Chakaraborty, S., Ganguh, S., Bose, K. (1980) 'An improved approach for performance evaluation in lower extremity involvement.' *Journal of Biomedical Engineering*, **2**, 121–125.

Granata, K.P., Abel, M.F., Damiano, D.L. (2000) 'Joint angular velocity in spastic gait and the influence of muscle tendon lengthening.' *Journal of Bone and Joint Surgery*, **82A**, 174–186.

Griffin, P.P., Wheelhouse, W.W., Shiavi, R. (1977) 'Adductor transfer for adductor spasticity: clinical and electromyographic gait analysis.' *Developmental Medicine and Child Neurology*, **19**, 783–789.

Guermazi, A., Miaux, Y., Zaim, S., Peterfy, C.G., White, D., Genant, H.K. (2003) 'Metallic artifacts in MR imaging: effects of main field orientation and strength.' *Clinical Radiology*, **58**, 322–328.

Hadders-Algra, M., Brogren, E., Katz-Salamon, M., Forssberg, H. (1999) 'Periventricular leukomalacia and preterm birth have difference detrimental effects on postural adjustments.' *Brain*, **122**, 727–740.

Hailey, D., Tomie, J.A. (2000) 'An assessment of gait analysis in the rehabilitation of children with walking difficulties.' *Disability Rehabilitation*, **22**, 275–280.

Harel, S., Anastasiow, N.J. (Eds) (1985) *The At-Risk Infant:Psycho/Socio/Medical Aspects*. Baltimore and London: Paul H. Brooks.

Hariga, J. (1966) 'Influences sur la motricité de la suppression des effecteurs gamma par alcoolisation des nerfs périphériques.' *Acta Neurologica Belgica*, **66**, 607–611.

—— Tardieu, G., Gagnard, L. (1964) 'Effets de l'application d'alcool dilué sur le nerf. Confrontation de l'étude dynamographique de l'étude histologique chez le chat décérébré.' *Revue Neurologique*, **111**, 472–474.

Harris, S.R. (1989) 'Early diagnosis of spastic diplegia, spastic hemiplegia, and quadriplegia.' *American Journal of Diseases of Children*, **144**, 958–959.

Hayakawa, K., Kanda, T., Hasimoto, K., Okuno, Y., Yamori, Y. (1997) 'MR of spastic tertraplegia.' *American Journal of Neuroradiology*, **18**, 247–253.

Herman, R. (1976) 'Postural control and therapeutic implications.' *In* Murdoch, G. (Ed.) *The Advance in Orthotics*. London: Edward Arnold.

Hoffer, M.M., Perry, J. (1983) 'Pathodynamics of gait alterations in cerebral palsy and the significance of kinetic electromyography in evaluating foot and ankle problems.' *Foot and Ankle*, 4, 128–134.

Hohman, L.B. (1953) 'Intelligence levels in cerebral palsied children.' *American Journal of Physical Medicine*, **32**, 282–290.

Hoon, A.H. Jr, Reinhardt, E.M., Kelley, R.I., Breiter, S.N., Morton, D.H., Naidu, S.B., Johnston, M.V. (1997) 'Brain magnetic resonance imaging in suspected extrapyramidal cerebral palsy: observations in distinguishing genetic–metabolic from acquired causes.' *Journal of Pediatrics*, **131**, 240–245.

Horne, D. (1964) *The Frostig Program for Development of Visual Perception*. Chicago: Follett.

Horstmann, H.M., Mahboubi, S. (1987) 'The use of computed tomography scan in unstable hip reconstruction.' *Journal of Computed Tomography*, **11**, 364–369.

Hullin, M.G., Robb, J.E., Loudon, I.R. (1996) 'Gait patterns in children with hemiplegic spastic cerebral palsy.' *Journal of Pediatric Orthopaedics B*, **5**, 247–251,

Illingworth, R.S. (1958) 'The early diagnosis of cerebral palsy.' *Cerebral Palsy Bulletin*, 2, 6–8.

Knutsson, E. (1983) 'Analysis of gait and isokinetic movements for evaluation of antispastic drugs or physical therapies.' *Advances in Neurology*, **39**, 1013–1034.

Inman, V.T., Ralston, H.J., Todd, F. (1981) *Human Walking*. Baltimore: Williams and Wilkins.

—— Rose, J., Gamble, J.G. (Eds) (1994) *Human Walking, 2nd Edn*. Baltimore: Williams and Wilkins.

Johnson, A., Ashurst, H. (1989) 'Is the popliteal angle measurement useful in early identification of cerebral palsy?' *Developmental Medicine and Child Neurology*, **31**, 457–465.

Johnson, D.C., Damiano, D.L., Abel, M.F. (1997) 'The evolution of gait in childhood and adolescent cerebral palsy.' *Journal of Pediatric Orthopaedics*, **17**, 392–396.

Judge, J.L., Lindsey, C., Underwood, M., Winsemius, D. (1993) 'Balance improvements in older women: effects of exercise training.' *Physical Therapy*, **73**, 254–262.

Kay, R.M., Dennis S., Rethlefsen, S., Skaggs, D.L., Tolo, V.T. (2000) 'Impact of postoperative gait analysis on orthopaedic care.' *Clinical Orthopedics and Related Research*, **374**, 259–264,

Kelly, I.P., Jenkinson, A., Stephens, M., O'Brien, T. (1997) 'The kinematic patterns of toe walkers.' *Journal of Pediatric Orthopaedics*, **17**, 478–480.

Ketelaar, M., Vermeer, A., Helders, P.J. (1998) 'Functional motor abilities of children with cerebral palsy: a systematic literature review of assessment measures.' *Clinical Rehabilitation*, **12**, 369–380.

Kirkpatrick, M., Wytch, R., Cole, F., Helms, P. (1994) 'Is the objective assessment of cerebral palsy gait reproducible?' *Journal of Pediatric Orthopaedics*, **14**, 705–708.

Kolobe, T.H., Palisano, R.J., Stratford, P.W. (1998) 'Comparison of two outcome measures for infants with cerebral palsy and infants with motor delay.' *Physical Therapy*, **78**, 1062–1072.

Koman, L.A., Mooney, J.F. III, Smith, B.P. (1996) 'Neuromuscular blockade in the management of cerebral palsy.' *Neurology*, **11**, Supplement 1, S23–28.

Kowalski, K., Di Fabio, R.P. (1995) 'Gross motor and balance impairments in children and adolescents with epilepsy.' *Developmental Medicine and Child Neurology*, **37**, 604–619.

Krebs, D.E., Edelstein, J.E., Fishman, S. (1985) 'Reliability of observational kinematic gait analysis.' *Physical Therapy*, **65**, 1027–1033.

Lasda, N.A., Levinsohn, E.M., Yuan, H.A., Bunnell, W.P. (1978) 'Computerized tomography in disorders of the hip.' *Journal of Bone and Joint Surgery*, **60A**, 1099–1102.

Lee, E.H., Goh, J.C., Bose, K. (1992) 'Value of gait analysis in the assessment of surgery in cerebral palsy.' *Archives of Physical Medicine and Rehabilitation*, **73**, 642–646.

Lehman, J.F., Price, R., DeLateur, B.J., Hinderer, S., Traynor, C. (1989) 'Spasticity: quantitative measurements as a basis for assessing the effectiveness of therapeutic intervention.' *Archives of Physical Medicine and Rehabilitation*, **70**, 6–15.

Liao, H.F., Mao, P.J., Hwang, A.W. (2001) 'Test–retest reliability of balance tests in children with cerebral palsy.' *Developmental Medicine and Child Neurology*, **43**, 180–186.

Maathuis, K.G., van der Schans, C.P., van Iperen, A., Rietman, H.S., Geertzen, J.H. (2005) 'Gait in children with cerebral palsy: observer reliability of Physician Rating Scale and Edinburgh Visual Gait Analysis Inteval Testing scale.' *Journal of Pediatric Orthopedics*, **25**, 268–272.

Mackey, A.H., Lobb, G.L., Walt, S.E., Stott, N.S. (2003) 'Reliability and validity of the Observational Gait Scale in children with spastic diplegia.' *Developmental Medicine and Child Neurology*, **45**, 4–11.

Mahboubi, S., Horstmann, H.M. (1986) 'Femoral torsion: CT measurement.' *Radiology*, **160**, 843–844.

Marey, E.J. (1873) *La Machine Animale. Locomotion Terrestre (Bipèdes) et Aérienne*. Paris: Baillière.

McLaughlin, J.F., Bjornson, K.F., Astley, S.J., Graubert, C., Hays, R.M. Roberts, T.S., Price, R., Temkin, N. (1998) 'Selective dorsal rhizotomy: efficacy and safety in an investigator-masked randomized clinical trial.' *Developmental Medicine and Child Neurology*, **40**, 220–232.

McMahon, T.A. (1984) *Muscles, Reflexes, and Locomotion*. Princeton, NJ: Princeton University Press.

McMulkin, M.L., Guilliford, J.J., Williamson, R.V., Ferguson, R.L. (2000) 'Correlation of static to dynamic measures of lower extremity range of motion in cerebral palsy and control population.' *Journal of Pediatric Orthopaedics*, **20**, 366–369.

Medeiros, J.M. (1984) 'Clinical application of gait analysis.' *Paper presented at symposium on the Pathokinesiology of Cerebral Palsy, Advances in Applied and Clinical Research, Division of Physical Therapy, School of Medicine, University of North Carolina, Chapel Hill; and at the Olympic Scientific Congress, University of Oregon, Eugene, OR.*

Menkes, J.H., Curran, J. (1994) 'Clinical and MR correlates in children with extrapyramidal cerebral palsy.' *American Journal of Neuroradiology*, **15**, 451–457.

Miller, F., Cardoso Dias, R., Lipton, G.E., Albarracin, J.P., Dabney, K.W., Castagno, P. (1997) 'The effect of rectus EMG patterns on the outcome of rectus femoris transfers.' *Journal of Pediatric Orthopaedics*, 17, 603–607.

Moffitt, T.E., Caspi, A., Harkness, A.R., Silva, P.A. (1993) 'The natural history of change in intellectual performance: who changes? How much? Is it meaningful?' *Journal of Child Psychology and Psychiatry*, 34, 455–506.

Morgan, A.M., Aldag, J.C. (1996) 'Early identification for cerebral palsy using a profile of abnormal motor patterns.' *Pediatrics*, 98, 692–697.

Morris, C., Kurinczuk, J.J., Fitzpatrick, R., Rosenbaum, P.L. (2006) 'Reliability of the manual ability classification system for children with cerebral palsy.' *Developmental Medicine and Child Neurology*, 48, 950–953.

Mumenthaler, M. (1990) *Neurology*. New York: Thieme Medical, p. 32.

Murray, M.P. (1967) 'Gait as a total pattern of movement.' *American Journal of Physical Medicine*, 46, 290–322.

—— Seireg, A.A., Sepic, S.B. (1975) 'Normal postural stability and steadiness: quantitative assessment.' *Journal of Bone and Joint Surgery*, 57A, 510–516.

Muybridge, E. (1901) *The Human Figure in Motion, An Electrophotographic Investigation of Consecutive Phases of Muscular Action*. London: Chapman and Hall.

Neligan, G., Prudham, D. (1969) 'Norms for four standard developmental milestones by sex, social class and place in family.' *Developmental Medicine and Child Neurology*, 11, 413–422.

Nelson, K.B., Ellenberg, J.H. (1978) 'Epidemiology in cerebral palsy.' *Advances in Neurology*, 25, 21–435.

—— —— (1982) 'Children who "outgrew" cerebral palsy.' *Pediatrics*, 69, 529–536.

Nordmark, E., Hagglund, G., Jarnlo, G.B. (1997) 'Reliability of the gross motor function measure in cerebral palsy.' *Scandinavian Journal of Rehabilitation Medicine*, 29, 25–8.

—— Jarnlo G.B., Hagglund, G. (2000) 'Comparison of the Gross Motor Function Measure and Pediatric Evaluation of Disability Inventory in assessing motor function in children undergoing selective dorsal rhizotomy.' *Developmental Medicine and Child Neurology*, 42, 245–252.

O'Brien, C. (1995) 'Clinical issues in the management of spasticity with botulinum toxin.' *In* O'Brien, C., Yablon, S. (Eds) *Management of Spasticity with Botulinum Toxin. Proceedings of the 12th World Congress of International Federation of Physical Medicine and Rehabilitation, March 27–31, 1995, Sydney, Australia*. Littleton, CO: Postgraduate Institute for Medicine, pp. 17–23.

O'Byrne, J.M., Kennedy, A., Jenkinson, A., O'Brien, T.M. (1997) 'Split tibialis posterior tendon transfer in the treatment of spastic equinus foot.' *Journal of Pediatric Orthopaedics*, 17, 481–485.

—— Jenkinson, A., O'Brien, T.M. (1998) 'Quantitative analysis and classification of gait patterns in cerebral palsy using a three-dimensional motion analyzer.' *Journal of Child Neurology*, 13, 101–108.

Otis, J.C., Root, L., Pamilla, J.R., Kroll, M.A. (1983) 'Biomechanical measurement of spastic plantarflexors.' *Developmental Medicine and Child Neurology*, 25, 60–66.

Paine, R.S., Oppé, T.E. (1966) *Neurological Examination of Children. Clinics in Developmental Medicine, Nos 20/21*. London: Spastics International Medical Publications with Heinemann Medical.

Palisano, R., Kolobe, T.H., Haley, S.M., Lowes, L.P., Jones, S.L. (1997) 'Validity of the Peabody Developmental Gross Motor Scale as an evaluative measure of infants receiving physical therapy.' *Physical Therapy*, 75, 939–948.

—— Rosenbaum, P., Walter, S., Russell, D., Wood, E., Galuppi, B. (1997) 'Development and reliability of a system to classify gross motor function in children with cerebral palsy.' *Developmental Medicine and Child Neurology*, 39, 214–223.

Parker, D.F., Carriere, L. Hebestreit, H., Salsberg, A., Bar-Or, O. (1993) 'Muscle performance and gross motor function of children with spastic cerebral palsy.' *Developmental Medicine and Child Neurology*, 35, 17–23.

Patel, S., Bharucha, E.P. (1967) 'The Bender Gestalt test as a measure of perceptual and visuo-motor defects in cerebral palsied children.' *Developmental Medicine and Child Neurology*, 14, 156–160.

Perry, J. (1974) 'Kinesiology of lower extremity bracing.' *Clinical Orthopaedics and Related Research*, 102, 20–31.

—— (1975) 'Cerebral palsy gait.' *In* Samilson, R.L. (Ed.) *Orthopaedic Aspects of Cerebral Palsy. Clinics in Developmental Medicine, Nos 52/53*. London: Spastics International Medical Publications with Heinemann Medical; Philadelphia: Lippincott.

—— (1992) *Gait Analysis: Normal and Pathological Function*. Thorofare, NJ: Slack.

—— Hoffer, M.M., Antonelli, D., Plut, J., Lewis, G., Greenberg, R. (1976) 'Electromyography before and after surgery for hip deformity in cerebral palsy.' *Journal of Bone and Joint Surgery*, 58A, 201–208.

—— —— (1977) 'Preoperative and postoperative dynamic electromyography as an aid in planning tendon transfers in children with cerebral palsy.' *Journal of Bone and Joint Surgery*, 59A, 531–537.

Poulsen, E., Asmussen, E. (1962) 'Energy requirements of practical jobs from pulse increase and ergometer test.' *Ergonomics*, 5, 33–36.

Prechtl, H.F.R. (1977) *The Neurological Examination of the Full Term Newborn Infant. Clinics in Developmental Medicine, No. 63*. London: Spastics International Medical Publications with Heinemann Medical; Philadelphia: J.B. Lippincott.

Rang, M. (1990) 'Cerebral palsy.' *In* Morrissy, R.E. (Ed.) *Lovell and Winter's Pediatric Orthopaedics, 3rd Edn*. Philadelphia: J.B. Lippincott, pp. 465–506.

Reimers, J. (1980) 'The stability of the hip in children: a radiological study of the results of muscle surgery in cerebral palsy.' *Acta Orthopaedica Scandinavica* (Suppl. 184), pp. 1–100.

—— (1992) 'Clinically based decision making for surgery.' In Sussman, M.D. (Ed.) *The Diplegic Child*. Rosemont, IL: American Academy of Orthopaedic Surgeons.

Rethlefsen, S., Tolo, V.T., Reynolds, R.A., Kay, R. (1999) 'Outcome of hamstring lengthening and distal rectus femoris transfer surgery.' *Journal of Pediatric Orthopaedics*, B, 8, 75–79.

Robin, D.W., Hasan, S.S., Lichtenstein, M.J., Shiavi, R.G., Wood, A.J. (1991) 'Dose-related effect of triazolam on postural sway.' *Clinical Pharmacology and Therapeutics*, 49, 581–588.

Robinson, C.J., Kett, N.A., Bolam, J.M. (1988a) 'Spasticity in spinal cord injured patients: I. Short-term effects of surface electrical stimulation.' *Archives of Physical Medicine and Rehabilitation*, 69, 598–604.

—— —— —— (1988b) 'Spasticity in spinal cord injured patients: 2. Initial measures and long-term effects of surface electrical stimulation.' *Archives of Physical Medicine and Rehabilitation*, 69, 862–868.

Rodda, J., Graham, H.K. (2001) 'Classification of gait patterns in spastic hemiplegia and spastic diplegia: a basis for a management algorithm.' *European Journal of Neurology* (Suppl. 5), 98–108.

Rogers, B., Msall, M., Owens, T., Guernsey, K., Brody, A., Buck, G., Hudak, M. (1994) 'Cystic periventricular leukomalacia and type of cerebral palsy in preterm infants.' *Journal of Pediatrics*, 125, S1–8.

Rose, J., Gamble, J.G., Medeiros, J., Burgos, A., Haskell, W.J. (1989) 'Energy cost of walking in normal children and in those with cerebral palsy: comparison of heart rate and oxygen uptake.' *Journal of Pediatric Orthopaedics*, 9, 276–279.

—— Gamble, J.G., Lee, J., Lee, R., Haskell, W.L. (1991) 'The energy expenditure index: a method to quantitate and compare walking energy expenditure for children and adolescents.' *Journal of Pediatric Orthopaedics*, 11, 571–578.

—— Wolff, D.R., Jones, V.K., Bloch, D.A., Gamble, J.G. (1999) 'Postural control analysis in patients with cerebral palsy.' *Paper presented at the North American Gait Conference, Dallas, TX*.

—— —— —— Ochlert, J.W., Gamble, J.G. (2002) 'Postural balance in children with cerebral palsy.' *Developmental Medicine and Child Neurology*, 44, 58–63.

Rosenbaum, P.L. (1992) 'Clinically based outcomes for children with cerebral palsy: Issues in the measurement of function.' *In* Sussman, M.D. (Ed.) *The Diplegic Child*. Rosemont, IL: American Academy of Orthopaedic Surgeons, pp. 125–132.

Russell, B.S., Tilton, A., Gormley, M.E. Jr (1997) 'Cerebral palsy: a rational approach to a treatment protocol, and the role of botulinum toxin in treatment.' *Muscle and Nerve*, Suppl., 6, S181–193.

Russell, D.J., Rosenbaum, P.L., Cadman, D.T., Gowland, C., Hardy, S., Jarvis, S. (1989) 'The gross motor function measure: a means to evaluate the effects of physical therapy.' *Developmental Medicine and Child Neurology*, 31, 341–352.

—— —— —— (1991) 'The gross motor function measure: a means to evaluate the effects of physical therapy.' *Developmental Medicine and Child Neurology*, 31, 341–352.

—— —— Gowland, C., Hardy, S., Lane, M., Plews, N., McGavin, H., Cadman, D., Jarvis, S. (1993) *Gross Motor Function Measure Manual*, Hamilton, ON, Canada: *CanChild* Centre for Childhood Disability Research, McMaster University.

—— Avery, L.M., Rosenbaum, P.L., Raina, P.S., Walter, S.D., Palisano, R.J. (2000) 'Improved scaling of the Gross Motor Function Measure for children with cerebral palsy: evidence of reliability and validity.' *Physical Therapy*, **80**, 873–884.

—— —— Lane, M., Rosenbaum, P. (2003) *Gross Motor Function Measure (GMFM-66 and GMFM-88), User's Manual. Clinics in Developmental Medicine, No. 159.* London: Mac Keith Press with Cambridge University Press.

Saint-Anne Dargassies, S. (1977) *Neurological Development in Full Term and Premature Neonates.* Amsterdam: Excerpta Medica; New York: Elsevier North-Holland.

Schutte, L.M., Narayanan, U., Stout, J.L., Selber, P., Gage, J.R., Schwartz, M.H. (2000) 'An index for quantifying deviations from normal gait.' *Gait and Posture*, **11**, 25–31.

Scott, A.C., Chambers, D., Caine, T.E. (1996) 'Adductor transfer in cerebral palsy: long-term results studied by gait analysis.' *Journal of Pediatric Orthopaedics*, **16**, 741–746.

Scrutton, D., Baird, G. (1997) 'Surveillance measures of the hips of children with bilateral cerebral palsy.' *Archives of Disease in Childhood*, **56**, 381–384.

Shapira, Y., Harel, S. (1983) 'Standardization of the Denver Developmental Screening Test for Israeli children.' *Israeli Journal of Medical Science*, **19**, 246–251.

Shapiro, B.K., Accardo, P.J., Capute, A.J. (1979) 'Factors affecting walking in a profoundly retarded population.' *Developmental Medicine and Child Neurology*, **21**, 369–373.

Shephard, R. (1975) 'Efficiency of muscular work.' *Physical Therapy*, **55**, 476–481.

Sheridan, M.D. (1975) *Children's Developmental Progress from Birth to Five Years. The STYCAR Sequences, 3rd Edn.* Windsor: NFER.

—— (1978) *Sheridan Stycar Developmental Sequences.* Windsor: NFER.

Simon, S.R., Deutsch, S.D., Nuzzo, R.M., Mansour, J.M., Jackson, J.L.F., Koskinen, M., Rosenthal, R.K. (1978) 'Genu recurvatum in spastic cerebral palsy.' *Journal of Bone and Joint Surgery*, **60A**, 822–894.

Skinner, S.R. (1992) 'Direct measurement of spasticity.' *In* Sussman, M.D. (Ed.) *The Diplegic Child.* Rosemont, IL: America Academy of Orthopaedic Surgeons, pp. 31–34.

—— Lester, D.K. (1984) 'Dynamic EMG findings in valgus hindmost deformity in spastic cerebral palsy.' *Paper read at Annual Meeting of American Academy for Cerebral Palsy and Developmental Medicine, Washington, DC.*

Stanley, F., Alberman, E. (1984) *The Epidemiology of the Cerebral Palsies. Clinics in Developmental Medicine, No. 87.* London: Spastics International Medical Publications with Blackwell Scientific; Philadelphia: Lippincott.

Stefko, R.M., de Swart, R.J., Dodgin, D.A., Wyatt, M.P., Kaufman, K.R., Sutherland, D.H., Chambers, H.G. (1998) 'Kinematic and kinetic analysis of distal derotational osteotomy of the leg in children with cerebral palsy.' *Journal of Pediatric Orthopaedics*, **18**, 81–87.

Steinbok, P., Reiner, A.M., Beauchamp, R., Armstrong, R.W., Cochrane, D.D., Kestle, J. (1997) 'A randomized clinical trial to compare selective posterior rhizotomy plus physiotherapy with physiotherapy alone in children with spastic diplegic cerebral palsy.' *Developmental Medicine and Child Neurology*, **39**, 178–184.

—— Kestle, J.R. (1997) 'Therapeutic electrical stimulation following selective posterior rhizotomy in children with spastic diplegic cerebral palsy: a randomized clinical trial.' *Developmental Medicine and Child Neurology*, **39**, 515–520.

Steinwender, G., Saraph, V., Scheiber, S., Zwick, E.B., Uitz, C., Hackl, K. (2000) 'Intrasubject repeatability of gait analysis data in normal and spastic children.' *Clinical Biomechanics*, **15**, 134–139.

—— —— —— —— Linhart, W. (2000) 'Assessment of hip rotation after gait improvement surgery in cerebral palsy.' *Acta Orthopaedica Belgica*, **66**, 259–264.

Super, C.M. (1976) 'Environmental effects on motor development. The case of African infant precocity.' *Developmental Medicine and Child Neurology*, **18**, 561–567.

Sussman, M.D. (Ed.) (1992) *The Diplegic Child-Evaluation and Management.* Rosemont, IL: American Academy of Orthopaedic Surgeons, p. 205.

Sutherland, D.H. (1978) 'Gait analysis in cerebral palsy.' *Developmental Medicine and Child Neurology*, **20**, 807–813.

—— (1984) *Gait Disorders in Childhood and Adolescence.* Baltimore and London: Williams and Wilkins.

—— Hagy, J.L. (1972) 'Measurement of gait movements from motion picture films.' *Journal of Bone and Joint Surgery*, **54A**, 787–797.

—— Olshen, R., Cooper, L., Woo, S.K. (1980) 'The development of mature gait.' *Journal of Bone and Joint Surgery*, **64A**, 336–353.

—— Baumann, J.U. (1981) 'Correction of paralytic foot drop by external orthoses.' *In* Black, J., Doubleton, J.H. (Eds) *Clinical Biomechanics.* Edinburgh: Churchill Livingstone.

—— Olshen, R., Cooper, L., Wyatt, M., Leach, J., Mubarak, S., Schultz, P. (1981) 'The pathomechanics of gait in Duchenne muscular dystrophy.' *Developmental Medicine and Child Neurology*, **23**, 3–22.

—— Zilberfaarb, J.J., Kaufman, K.R., Wyat, M.P., Chambers, H.G. (1997) 'Psoas release at the pelvic brim in ambulatory patients with cerebral palsy: operative technique and functional outcome.' *Journal of Pediatric Orthopaedics*, **17**, 563–570.

Tardieu, C., Tardieu, G., Hariga, J., Gagnard, L., Velin, J. (1964) 'Fondement expérimental d'une thérapeutique des raideurs d'origine cérébrale. Effect de l'alcoolisation ménagée du nerf moteur sur le réflexe d'étirement de l'animal décérébré.' *Archives françaises de Pédiatrie*, **21**, 5–23.

Tardieu, G. (1984) *Le Dossier Clinique de l'Infirmité Motrice Cérébralé, 3ème Edn.* Paris: Masson.

—— Tardieu, C., Hariga, J. (1971) 'Infiltrations par l'alcool à 45° des points moteurs, des racines par voie épidurale on du nerf tibial postérieur. Leurs indications et contre indications dans les divers modes de spasticité (expérience de dix ans).' *Revue Neurologique*, **125**, 63–68.

—— Hariga, J. (1972) 'Selective partial denervation by alcohol injections and their results in spasticity.' *Reconstructive Surgery and Traumatology*, **13**, 18–36.

—— Got, C., Lespargot, A. (1975) 'Indications d'un nouveau type d'infiltration au point moteur (alcool à 96°). Applications cliniques d'une étude expérimentale.' *Annales de Medicine Physique*, **18**, 539–557.

Tell, G.S., Lefkowitz, D.C., Diehr, P., Elster, A.D. (1998) 'Relationship between balance and abnormalities in cerebral magnetic resonance imagine in older adults.' *Neurology*, **55**, 73–79.

Terver, S., Dillingham, M., Parker, B., Bjorke, A., Bleck, E.E., Levai, J.P., Teinturier, P., Viallet, J. F. (1982) 'Étude de l'orientation réelle du cotyle grâce au tomodensitomètre axial on scanner.' *Journal de Radiologie*, **63**, 167–173.

Touwen, B.C.L. (1976) *Neurological Development in Infancy. Clinics in Developmental Medicine, No. 58.* London: Spastics International Medical Publications with Heinemann Medical; Philadelphia: J.B. Lippincott.

—— (1979) *The Examination of the Child with Minor Neurological Dysfunction, 2nd edn. Clinics in Developmental Medicine, No. 71.* London: Spastics International Medical Publications with Heinemann Medical; Philadelphia: J.B. Lippincott.

Tripp, E.J., Harris, S.R. (1991) 'Test–retest reliability of isokinetic knee extension and flexion torque measurements in persons with spastic hemiparesis.' *Physical Therapy*, **71**, 390–396.

Tylkowski, C.H. (1992) 'Limitations of Technologic Assessment.' *In* Sussman, M.D. (Ed.) *The Diplegic Child.* Rosemont, IL: American Academy of Orthopaedic Surgeons, pp. 163–171.

Ueda, R. (1978) 'Standardization of the Denver Developmental Screening Test on Japanese children.' *Developmental Medicine and Child Neurology*, **20**, 647–656.

Watanabe, Y., Bakheit, A.M., McLellan, D.L. (1998) 'A study of the effectiveness of botulinum toxin type As (Dysport) in the management of muscle spasticity.' *Disability and Rehabilitation*, **20**, 62–65.

Waters, R.L., Hislop, H.J., Perry, J., Antonelli, D. (1978) 'Energetics: application to the study and management of locomotor disabilities.' *Orthopaedic Clinics of North America*, **9**, 351–356.

—— Frazier, J., Garland, D.E., Jordan, C., Perry, J. (1982) 'Electromyographic gait analysis before and after operative treatment for hemiplegic equinus and equinovarus deformity.' *Journal of Bone and Joint Surgery*, **64A**, 284–288.

Watts, H.G. (1994) 'Gait laboratory analysis for preoperative decision making in spastic cerebral palsy: is it all it's cracked up to be?' *Journal of Pediatric Orthopaedics*, **14**, 701–702.

Webb, S. (1990) *The Watching of Shadows. The Origins of Radiological Tomography.* Bristol: Adam Hilger.

Weiner, D.S., Cook, A.J., Hoyt, W.A., Oravec, C.E. (1978) 'Computed tomography in the measurement of femoral anteversion.' *Orthopedics*, **1**, 299–306.

White, R., Agouris, E., Selbie, R.D., Kirkpatrick, M. (1999) 'The variability of force platform data in normal and cerebral palsy gait.' *Clinical Biomechanics (Bristol, Avon)*, **14**, 185–192.

Winter, D.A. (1987) *The Biomechnanics and Motor Control of Human Gait.* Waterloo, Ontario: University of Waterloo Press.

Winters, T.F. Jr, Gage, J.R., Hicks, R. (1987) 'Gait patterns in spastic hemiplegia in children and young adults.' *Journal of Bone and Joint Surgery*, **69A**, 437–441.

Wolf, S.L., Barnhart, H.X., Ellison, G.L., Coogler, C.E. (1997) 'The effect of Tai Chi Quan and computerized balance training in postural stability in older subjects. Atlanta FICSIT Group. Frailty and injuries: cooperative studies on intervention techniques.' *Physical Therapy*, 77, 371–381.

Wolfe, G. (1978) 'Influence of floor surface with energy cost of wheelchair propulsion.' *Orthopaedic Clinics of North America*, **9**, 367–370.

Wolff, D.R., Rose, J., Jones, V.K., Bloch, D.A., Oehlert, J.W., Gamble, J.G. (1998) 'Postural balance measurements for children and adolescents.' *Journal of Orthopaedic Research*, **16**, 271–275.

Wolfson, L., Whipple, R., Derby, C.A., Amerman, P., Murphy, T., Tobin, J.N., Nasher, L. (1992) 'A dynamic posturography study of balance in healthy subjects.' *Neurology*, **42**, 2069–2075.

Wright, F.V., Sheil, E.M., Drake, J.M., Wedge, J.H., Naumann, S. (1998) 'Evaluation of selective dorsal rhizotomy for the reduction of spasticity in cerebral palsy: a randomized controlled trial.' *Developmental Medicine and Child Neurology*, **40**, 239–247.

Yang, T.F., Chan, R.C., Wong, T.T., Bair, W.N., Kao, C.C., Chuang, T.Y., Hsu, R.C. (1996) 'Quantitative measurement of improvement in sitting balance in children with spastic cerebral palsy after selective posterior rhizotomy.' *Archives of Physical Medicine and Rehabilitation*, **75**, 348–352.

Yngve, D.A., Chambers, C. (1996) 'Vulpius and Z-lengthening.' *Journal of Pediatric Orthopaedics*, **16**, 759–764.

Young, C.C., Rose, S.E., Biden, E.N., Wyatt, M.P., Sutherland, D.H. (1989) 'The effect of surface and internal electrodes on the gait of children with cerebral palsy, spastic diplegic type.' *Journal of Orthopaedic Research*, **7**, 732–737.

4
NEUROBIOLOGY

'Everything should be made as simple as possible, but not simpler.'

(Albert Einstein)

Despite Einstein's advice and admonition, it is impossible to describe, compress and simplify all the known anatomical, histological, neurophysiological and chemical details that comprise the human brain—in which the cerebral cortex area is 2.5 square feet, and contains 25 billion neurons interconnected with more than 100,000 kilometers of axons that have 3×10^{14} synapses (Nolte 2002). A search of the Medline database between 1990 and 2007, on the specific topic of neurobiology, will not garner as many references as there are neurons and axons in the human brain, but something in the region of 3700 citations: much more than can be summarized in this chapter. Consequently we can only present a drastically brief review of some selected and possibly relevant neurobiological studies. We can highlight those aspects that seem particularly applicable to cerebral palsy. Those who wish more in-depth knowledge should consult the two textbooks on neurobiology referenced at the end of the chapter (Shepherd 1994, Thompson 2000) and the contemporary reviews of Rakic cited in the references (Fig. 4.1).

The pioneering silver nitrate staining of the brain cells and their dendrites by Camillo Golgi, of Pavia, Italy, led in 1885 to the monumental work by Santiago Ramón y Cajal of Barcelona, Spain. His publications between 1888 and 1891 described the staining of the central nervous system and proved that each nerve cell was a separate entity with dendrites and axons. Wilhelm Waldeyer of Berlin in 1891 consolidated this new knowledge that cells comprised the nervous system and named the nerve cell a 'neuron' (Shepherd 1994). Such was the state of our understanding of the brain and its function during the first half of the 20th century.

In the 1950s our appreciation and knowledge of the complexity of brain function leapt forward beyond the anatomical and the concept of the brain as a 'black box' of electrical circuits. The great leap was initiated by the application of the electron microscope to cell biology in the 1950s, by the ability to make

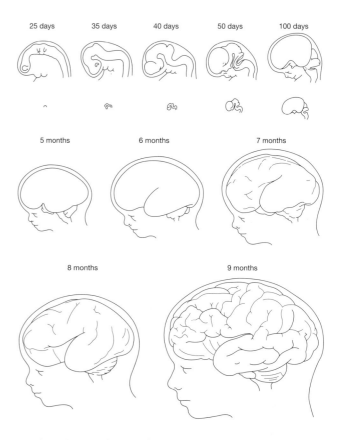

Fig. 4.1. Schematic diagram of human brain development, ages 25 days to 9 months of gestation. (Redrawn from Thompson 2000, p.318, by permission.)

precise recordings of electrical signals from the neuron and axon with microelectrodes, and primarily by the advance of the molecular biology that explains how neuron to neuron connections (synapses) are made by chemical neurotransmitters secreted to receptors on the cell membrane. Only half a century has elapsed since we appreciated that the function of the neuron is dependent on its protein composition and synthesis which is encoded in the desoxyribonucleic acid (DNA) of the cell—the double helix of two strands of loosely bonded aminoacids. From the DNA, a single strain of ribonucleic acid (RNA) becomes the template for the sequences of the amino acids to form the proteins and their replication. Due to the work of neuroscientists we now know that synaptic transmission of some 10 trillion synapses of an estimated 100 billion neurons are almost all chemical (25 billion are in the cerebral cortex).

'*We are what we are because our brains are basically chemical machines.*'

(R.F. Thompson, 2000)

NEUROGENESIS

It is well known now that the entire process of central nervous system development is under genetic control (also called 'innate'). In other words, humans, animals and insects have inherited the processes of development. Of the estimated 100,000 genes in the chromosome (DNA) of mammalian cells, the brain uses an estimated 30,000 to 50,000 unique to the brain (Thompson 2000). It is now accepted that genes regulate and control brain development and how pathological processes can stop or alter it (Rubenstein and Rakic 1999).

'*I now recognize that the development of the nervous system is not only more complicated than we had imagined, but it may be more complicated than we can imagine.*'

(Pasko Rakic 1999a)

Cell birth occurs from the precursor cells (neuroblasts) of the embryonic neural tube and crest. From the cells of the neural tube are derived the neurons, astrocytes, oligodendroglial and ependymal cells. Those that arise from the neural crest are the dorsal and autonomic ganglia, the bipolar auditory cells and the chromaffin cells of the adrenal medulla. Cells which share their origin from both the tube and the crest are the pia mater, arachnoid, microglial and Schwann cells (Shepherd 1994).

NEURONS

The neurons are all generated in 60 days in the monkey (gestation 165 days) and in 100 days in the human. Two classes of neurons exist: excitatory principal cells and inhibitory interneurons. Principal neurons are those that are acted on by other neurons and send their messages through myelinated axons (Fig. 4.2). The two types of principal neurons are the motor neurons and the sensory neurons. The sensory neurons are located adjacent to the spinal cord in groups, termed 'ganglia'. Interneurons send their axons to nearby neurons; some have no long axon or no axon. The larger axons are sheathed in a kind of membrane insulator, a fatty sort of substance, myelin. The smaller axons have no myelin such as the slow-conducting pain fibers. The myelinated axons conduct information faster (Fig. 4.3)

The neuron has only one axon, but many extensions or branches (dendrites) that connect with other neurons. On the spine are multiple spines that are the locus of the synapse (from the Ancient Greek word for a connection or junction). In the

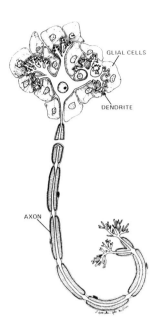

Fig. 4.2. Neuron: the main cell of the brain and spinal cord. It is surrounded and supported by glial cells, as an immobile 'Buddha in a cage with a long tail, the axon', as Dr Douglas Buchanan used to describe it. The cross-hatched areas surrounding the axon in nodal fashion is the myelin sheath. (Reproduced by permission from Bleck and Nagel 1982.)

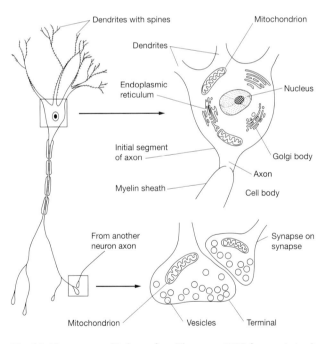

Fig. 4.3. Neuron parts. (Redrawn from Thompson 2000, by permission.)

cerebral cortex the dendritic spines are few in the fetal brain and increase in number with maturation (Fig. 4.4). The spines are affected in some cerebral neurological diseases such as Down syndrome where they are tiny and thin. Conversely, those in the cerebral cortex are affected by environmental influences. Animals raised in mazes and with toys had thicker cortices than those

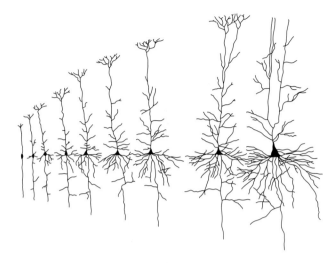

Fig. 4.4. Pyramidal cell growth and differentiation of dendritic trees and axon collaterals from fetus to adult. (Redrawn from Shepherd 1994, Fig.30.4, p.659, by permission.)

raised in barren cages. Raising an animal in the dark results in a reduction of synapses in the visual cortical areas (Shepherd 1994) (Fig. 4.5). Domesticated animals have long been known to have smaller brains that those reared in the wild. These observations appear to have lent credence to the recent past and current drive to encourage 'enriched' environments for infants and children (e.g. 'infant stimulation', the Federal funding for Head Start preschool programs in the United States). Within the neurons are chemical engines, the major one being in the mitochondria that manufacture from glucose and oxygen adenosine triphosphate (ATP) that has high-energy phosphate bonds. Other chemical manufacturing of transmitter substances occurs in the clumps of endoplastic reticulum, Nissl bodies, and in small vesicles of the Golgi apparatus. The axon is filled with microtubules that

transport chemical substances such as the neurotransmitters to and from the synaptic transmitters.

GLIAL CELLS AND ASTROCYTES

'Nobody ever thinks that glia are interesting.'
(Barbara Barres 1997/1998)

Glial cells of two types, oligodendrocytes and astrocytes, comprise a network in the brain. It used to be thought they were merely supporting cells that kept the neurons like a Buddha in a cage. Observations of glial cells in vitro show that some move around. They do multiply and clear out cellular debris. Another function is to form the myelin for the axon sheaths (Thompson 2000). Glial cells make the neurotransmitter messengers, the receptors that translate the messengers, and the channel that carry out the instructions (Barres 1997/1998, Barres and Raff 1999, Ullian *et al.* 1999). Glial cells wrap around the synapses between neurons as they release the chemical transmitters (Meyer-Franke and Barres 1999) (Fig. 4.6).

The astrocyte is special because it forms the blood–brain barrier. The brain has a very rich blood supply, taking a full 16% of the total blood supply in the body while occupying only 2% of the body's space. A barrier is necessary to keep out toxic substances from the brain. The astrocyte has many pods that hook onto the wall of the blood vessels forming a continuous fatty barrier (Fig. 4.7). The barrier prevents substances not soluble in fat from entering the blood supply of the brain. The blood–brain barrier has pertinence in the use of oral baclofen in cerebral palsy. It is limited in crossing the blood–brain barrier so that its effect on reducing spasticity is minimal. Hence, the intrathecal route of administration of baclofen is much more effective and clinically useful.

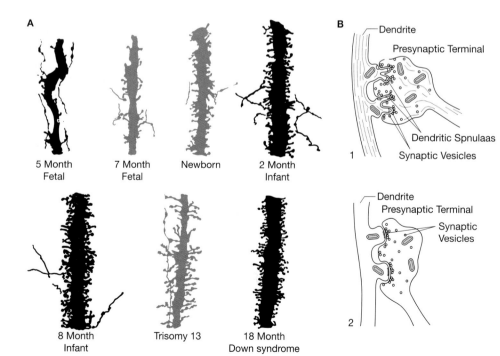

Fig. 4.5. (*a*) Apical dendrites in human cortical pyramidal neurons with increased quantity of spines with maturation compared with the thin and tiny spines in Down syndrome. (*b*) Effects of deprivation on dendritic spines in lateral geniculate nucleus of dogs: 1, normal; 2, raised in the dark. (Redrawn from Shepherd 1994, Fig. 30.6, p.663, by permission.)

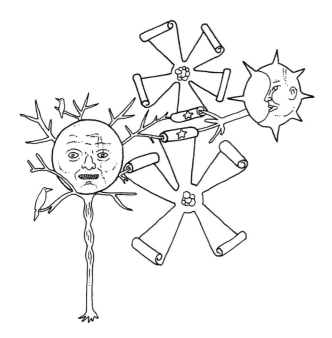

Fig. 4.6. Glial cells wrap around synapses. Neurons communicate by sending chemicals across the synapses. (Redrawn from Wells, W. 'Filled with glia.' *Stanford Medicine,* Winter 97/98.)

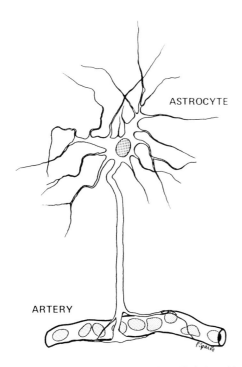

Fig. 4.7. Astrocyte. Its extensions hook onto the wall of a brain blood vessel to form a fatty blood–brain barrier. (Reproduced by permission from Bleck and Nagel 1982.)

NEURON MIGRATION FROM BIRTHPLACE TO CORTEX

The developmental period of neurons and their migration in mammals including humans ranges between 10 and 25 weeks of gestation (Sidman and Rakic 1973, Letinic *et al.* 2002).

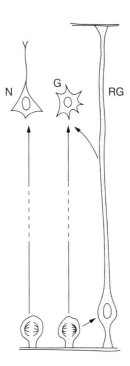

Fig. 4.8. Neuron and glial origins including dual-cell-line theory of glia through transient radial glia. (Redrawn from Shepherd 1994, Fig. 9.5, p.201, by permission.)

Disruptions of neuronal migration have been found in developmental and movement disorders, e.g. lissencephaly.[1]

Glia assume great importance by providing transient radial glia as a scaffold upon which the neurons at birth placed close to the cerebral ventricle climb to their permanent resting place to the surface of the cerebral cortex where they form the six layers (Rakic and Lombroso 1998; Rakic 1999a) (Fig. 4.8). Axons travel a long way to their target synapses by growth cones that have amoeboid movements that push away obstacles in their path (Fig. 4.9). The neurons are guided along the glial highway to their final location by molecular cues specified by the genetic code. Ion channels, neurotransmitter receptors and intracellular Ca^{2+} orchestrate the neuronal migration to final destination (Komuro and Rakic 1998). Another chemical, discovered in 1951, is the nerve growth factor (NGF)—a peptide of the large family of cytokines that include the neurotransmitters, acetylcholine, serotonin, and catecholamine.

Interruptions of neuron migration on a specific day of gestation prevent the neurons from arriving at the right place at the right time. Neurons in the wrong place do not form the right synaptic connections. Examples of such neurological disasters have been the effect of cocaine use by the mother during pregnancy (other disruptions occur with alcohol, ionizing radiation, and viruses (Rakic 1999b). Such effects of cocaine as noted in monkey models are permanent and cannot be restored to a normal neuron position.

---

1 Lissencephaly (from the Greek λισσος, smooth, and ᾽εγκεφαλος, brain): absence of gyri.

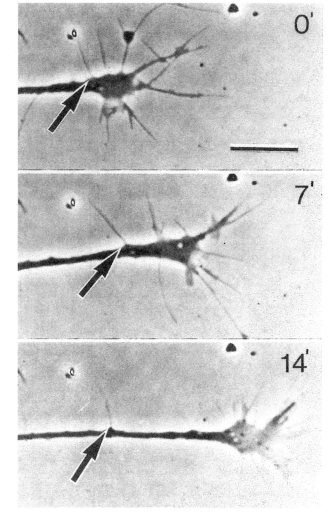

Fig. 4.9. Growth-cone (club-like with protruding filaments) movement in tissue culture at 7-second intervals. (From Thompson 2000, by permission.)

'*No amount of training will entice misrouted cells to move into the proper position. . . . A brain damaged by cocaine during intrauterine life cannot be fully rehabilitated.*'

(Rakic 1999b, p. 99)

According to Rakic (2000), the majority of 'postmitotic neurons have their traveling itinerary, final address, as well as a hint of their phenotypic determination at the time of their birth in the proliferative zone well before arriving at their place of residence'. Most neurons respect their interdivisional borders, but there are 'newborn neurons that do not obey the law and trespass into foreign territories'. Rakic (2000) made these comments on the report of the origin of the precerebellar system by Rodriguez and Dymecki (2000). During phylogenesis, major anatomical brain structures and their functional links evolve in a coordinated way independently of evolutionary change in other structures (Barton and Harvey 2000). Migrating neurons that cross into foreign territories are 'like ancestors who come from the same homeland and then drift apart, only to reconnect later in life; neurons born in the same region may ultimately become

permanent residents in different brain subdivisions and eventually develop specific synaptic contacts with one another' (Rakic 2000).

CORTICAL CELL DIFFERENTIATION

Cell differentiation is the next step in development; however, in some cells this begins before migration. It overlaps considerably with other stages of development. Initial mapping of cortical neurons occurs because of well defined patterns of gene expression of molecules that are regulated by programs intrinsic to the cortical cells before there are afferent inputs from the thalamus (Donoghue and Rakic 1999). As well as inputs from the thalamus, chemical factors, particularly Ca^{2+}, in the cell environment determine the differentiation. The thalamus does not influence the initial regional mapping of the cortex but is essential for its maturation (Rakic 2002a).

CORTEX DEVELOPMENT

The sequence is the same in all regions (sensory, motor, association or limbic) (Shepherd 1994). Research has indicated that the cortex developed as a whole rather by than by regions in sequence, and suggests a basic cortical plan under common genetic control. As we all might recall from our initial studies of neuroanatomy the brain was parceled into areas of specific function by a German neurologist, Kobinian Brodmann (1909), now known as 'cytoarchitectonic areas' (Rakic 1999a), as the locus of vision, language, motor and sensory systems, emotion etc. Due to the advance of neuroscientific tools we now know that these cortical areas are interconnected.

'*The cells of our brain are organized as functional units—as maps of our bodies on which are superimposed maps of the outside world as perceived through our senses, and then maps of our experience over time, our memories. These interconnecting cortical maps hold our secrets not only for success but also to the limits of our species.*'

(Rakic 1999a, p. 90)

CELL MATURATION

The time for maturation varies in different regions of the central nervous system, and in humans continues for some time after birth. Ramifications of the neuronal dendrites commence just after birth. By 6 months of age the rate of growth of dendritic processes is striking. The dendrites increase in size and length but not in number up to the age of 15 months. By the age of 2 years, neuronal differentiation is essentially complete. After 2 years the growth continues, but at a reduced rate (Schade and Von Groenigen 1961) (Fig. 4.10).

The brain regions do not develop synchronously. Cell multiplication is most rapid in the forebrain and is complete at 18 weeks of gestation. Cell growth is rapid in the first 3 months of gestation but myelination continues until about the age of 3 years (Fig. 4.11). Cerebellar growth starts about half way through gestation and is complete by about 18 months (Dobbing and Sands 1973, Rakic 1999a). The acceleration of change in the

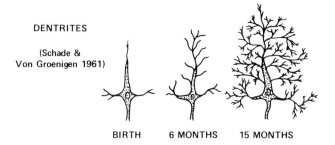

DENTRITES

(Schade &
Von Groenigen 1961)

BIRTH   6 MONTHS   15 MONTHS

Fig. 4.10. Schematic drawing of dendritic arborization from birth to 15 months. (Reproduced from Schade and Von Groenigen 1961, by permission.)

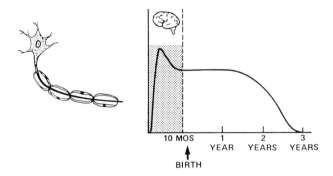

10 MOS   1 YEAR   2 YEARS   3 YEARS

BIRTH

Fig. 4.11. Schematic drawing of central nervous system cell-growth velocity from fertilization of the ovum to the age of 3 years (Reproduced from Dobbing and Sands 1973, by permission.)

developing brain has been compared to driving an automobile on a highway: the greater the rate of acceleration, the greater the stress on the controlling mechanism, and the greater chance for disaster when the mechanisms are blocked or sidetracked (Neligan 1974).

SYNAPTIC TRANSMISSION

'Such a special connection of one nerve cell with another might be called a synapse.'

(Charles Sherrington 1897, quoted by Shepherd 1994)

The neurons connect with other neurons through the dendrites via gap junctions. The two types of synapses are electrical and chemical. The gap junctions vary between 0.1 and 10 μm. They carry either electric current or low-molecular-weight substances (chemical neurotransmitters). The electric synapses have low resistance and act quickly. They are rigid and cannot be altered except through major structural change.

Cortical synapses rapidly increase in density during fetal life, reach their peak in early childhood (age 2–4 years), and then decline during sexual maturation to a density that remains the same at the adult level until another decline at senility (Fig. 4.12). The monumental effort by Rakic (1985) identified over 500,000 synapses in 25,000 electron micrographs from 22 monkeys. In humans the number of synpases is estimated in

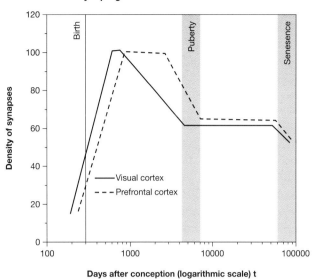

Synaptogenesis in human cerebral cortex

Fig. 4.12. The relative density of synapses in the human cerebral cortex according to days of function after conception to senescence (100,000 days). (Adapted by permission from Rakic 1999a, based on the data of Huttenlocher and Dabholkar and reproduced from Bourgeois *et al.* in Gazzaniga, M.S., Ed., *Cognitive Neuroscience, 2nd edn.* Boston: MIT Press.)

trillions; 100,000 per second are lost in humans during puberty.[2] The position of the cells and their connections with other brain cells are critical to function. As surmised by Rakic (1999a), the 'importance of being well placed and having the right connections' explains why a loss of 0.001% of neurons in a particular brain location can result in 100% loss of function.

Chemical synapses are predominant through the nervous system. They function through the release of a neurotransmitter. In contrast to the electrical synapses, the chemical ones can be altered by chemicals, and so are plastic. In the first half of the 20th century, neuroscientists persevered in the research that gave neurochemicals predominance in synaptic transmission (Valenstein 2002). Among these pioneers were Otto Loewi, an Austrian pharmacologist, who in 1921 discovered the best-known neurotransmitter, acetylcholine, now in the forefront of spastic muscle management with botulinum toxin, and further elaborated by Henry Dale and colleagues in England in 1935 (Shepherd 1994).

' "The war of the sparks and the soups"—electrical versus chemical synaptic transmission waged between electrophysiologists and pharmacologists extended over two world wars—stimulated the research that gave pharmacologists their victory.'

(Valenstein 2002)

---

2 Loss of synapses extrapolated from the macaque in which 20,000 synapses in the neocortex are lost per second (in the human the time for sexual maturation is longer and the cortex is 10 times larger).

ACETYLCHOLINE

The neuromuscular junction is of particular interest to us working in the field of cerebral palsy. The junction is between the motor neuron's axon (presynatic terminal) and the muscle (postsynaptic terminal). When we move a muscle the nerve impulse from the neuron through its axon causes a release of the chemical, acetylcholine (ACh) contained in small vesicles at the terminal end. The impulse opens calcium ion (Ca^{2+}) channels in the membrane so that the ACh containing vesicles cross the junction cleft, release the acetylcholine and act on the nicotinic acetylcholine receptor (nAChR), so called because its action is mimicked by nicotine. The receptor is a five-chain polypetide protein with a molecular weight of approximately 270,000. When the acetylcholine reaches the muscle membrane, sodium ion (Na^+) channels open and sodium ions rush in. The muscle membrane potential become slightly less negative. The action potential spreads through the sarcolemmal membrane of the muscle and releases calcium ions to cause interaction of the muscle proteins, actin and myosin. Muscle contraction occurs (Fig. 4.14). As a bit of seemingly good news to smokers, the nicotinic receptors for acetylcholine are particular for skeletal muscle, but not for cardiac muscle. The bad news for smokers is that there are many nicotine-acetylcholine receptors in the brain, perhaps accounting for addiction to nicotine (Thompson 2000).

The acetylcholine released at the junction is broken down to acetate and choline by acetylcholineterase. The products return to the terminal and are reused. The source of choline is food. At the risk of starting a dietary fad opposed to the current low cholesterol diets, it should be stated that egg yolk is rich in choline.

The acetylcholine transmitter has become relevant with the current use of botulinum myoneural injections to reduce the spasticity of muscles in cerebral palsy. The neurotoxin blocks the release of acetylcholine.

GAMMA AMINO BUTYRIC ACID (GABA)

Gamma amino butyric acid (GABA) is a fast inhibitory neurotransmitter distributed in the gray matter of the brain and in local interneurons presumed to be inhibitory. It is derived from the amino acid, glutamine, which is converted to glutamate. As with choline, the source of glutamine is food. Similar to acetylcholine it is stored in vesicles in the terminus of the axon. When it is released the chloride ion (Cl^-) channels open so that the inside of the membrane is negatively charged. The postsynaptic potential is inhibitory, i.e. it decreases the excitability of the neuron. GABA has its receptors: GABA$_A$ that binds to such compounds (called *ligands*) such as benzodiazepines (e.g. diazepam), barbiturates, picrotoxin, and steroids (Shepherd 1994). GABA$_B$ receptors bind to baclofen and open channels selective for potassium ions (K^+) (Fig. 4.15). Baclofen, now used intrathecally to reduce muscle spasticity, is an analog of GABA and is thought to effect blocking of the GABA$_B$ receptors in the superficial layers of the spinal cord as well as in the brain.

Other chemical transmitters are glycine (confined mainly to the spinal cord and brainstem), and two catecholamines:

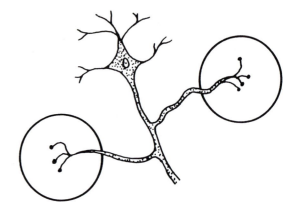

Fig. 4.13. Schematic representation of axonal sprouting (Edds 1953, Liu and Chambers 1958).

norepinephrine, the main transmitter of ganglion cells of the sympathetic nervous system, and dopamine, three-quarters of which is in the basal ganglia. Serotonin is widely distributed in the brain. It is manufactured from the amino acid tryptophan in food. Among foods, bananas are loaded with tryptophan (Thompson 1993).

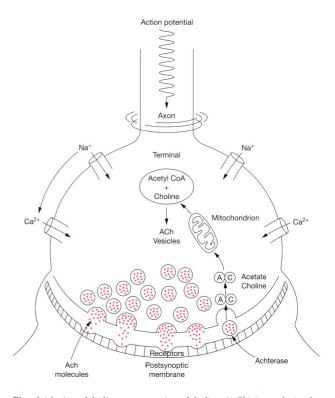

Fig. 4.14. Acetylcholine synapse. Acetylcholine (ACh) is made in the axon terminal by the mitochondrion from acetyl coenzyme A and choline and stored in vesicles. When the action potential arrives at the terminal calcium changes are opened and Ca^{2+} (calcium ions) enter the terminal, trigger the vesicles to fuse with the membrane and release acetylcholine molecules into the synaptic cleft. The ACh molecules attach to the receptors on the opposite membrane (postsynaptic) and trigger opening of sodium ion (Na^+) channels. The ACh is immediately separated into choline and acetate by the enzyme acetylcholineterase. Choline and acetate return to the terminal and reused. (Redrawn from Thompson 2000.)

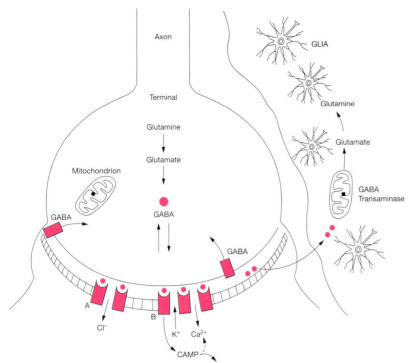

Fig. 4.15. GABAergic synapse. Gamma amino butyric acid (GABA) is synthesized from glutamine and from glutamate. It is stored in the axon terminal and released by exocytosis into the synaptic cleft where it binds with either $GABA_A$ or $GABA_B$ receptors on the postsynaptic membrane. $GABA_A$ receptors are coupled to a chloride ion (Cl^-) channel. It is a binding site for benzodiazepines, e.g. Valium. The $GABA_B$ receptors are linked through a G protein and/or another chemical, $_cAMP$, to potassium ion (K^+) and calcium ion (Ca^{2+}) channels. These are blocked by baclofen. GABA binds to presynaptic receptors and return to the terminal. It also enters the glial where it is restored in the mitochondria to glutamate and glutamine that re-enters the terminal to start the process of synthesis of GABA all over again. (From Shepherd 1994.)

NEW NEURONS?

'People seem to have difficulty accepting that a 75-year-old individual has 75-year-old neurons.'

(Pasko Rakic)

Of particular importance in dealing with children and adults who have the clinical manifestations of neuronal damage and death is the 'general rule, in both invertebrates and vertebrates, that once the processes of development are complete there is little or no further generation of new nerve cells' (Shepherd 1994). À propos of growing older and smelling the roses, an exception is the development of new receptor neurons in the olfactory bulb. As the receptor neuron dies it sends out an unknown signal to its precursor cells so that mitosis begins anew. The neurons send out axons to the right synaptic target in the olfactory bulb. The remodeling goes on throughout adult life (Shepherd 1994, Kornack and Rakic 2001a, b).

The limits of neurogenesis in primates were been shown by Rakic (1985). In an extremely detailed and tedious method of measuring DNA replication with radioactive [3H] thymidine, no evidence was found in 12 Rhesus monkey brains of any neuronal replication (regeneration). With the exception of the granule neurons in the dentate gyrus of the hippocampus, the olfactory bulb and the cerebellum, the neurons generated during early development are not replaced (Kornack and Rakic 1999). Only in those neurons in the dentate gyrus does neurogenesis continue beyond sexual maturity. This limitation of new neurons to the hippocampus and olfactory bulb was reinforced by the scientific studies of Kornack and Rakic (2001a, b). In the adult monkey (5.5–16.5 years of age), one new granule cell in the dentate gyrus is generated each day per 24,000 existing cells (Rakic 2002b).

The stability of the original neurons of the brain is in striking contrast to neuron and axon regeneration in fish, amphibians and birds that have provided hypotheses for various passive manipulations aimed at influencing the development of brain-damaged infants (infants-at-risk).

'One can speculate that a prolonged period of interaction with the environment, as pronounced as it is in all primates, especially humans, requires a stable set of neurons to retain acquired experience in the pattern of their synapses.'

(Rakic 1985)

Gould and co-authors (1999) burst upon the news media that in the adult macaque monkey prefrontal, parietal, and temporal lobes of the neocortex acquired new neurons throughout adulthood.

This startling news was preceded by Shankle *et al.* (1998) who published their findings of large additions of neurons that alternated with comparable losses in the human neocortex during the early years of postnatal life. This revolution in neurobiology on the stability of neurons was questioned and refuted by the studies of Rakic (2002c). The basis of the refutation was that the methods which used incorporation of BrdU as a sign of cell division and proof of new neurons was that these were old neurons that synthesized the DNA as part of the apoptotic process.[3] These presumed new neurons had BrdU-labelled nuclei that were endothelial cells which were misinterpreted as

---

3 BrdU: 5-Bromodeoxyuridine: a thymidine analogue that is incorporated into replicating DNA of dividing cells and thus can be detected in these cells or their subsequent progeny by using immunochemistry (Kornack and Rakic 2001a, b).

a migrating stream of cortical neurons. The conclusions of the pioneer Ramón y Cajal (1928), who found rare mitosis in the nerve cells in his histological preparations, and who stated that our birth neurons are irreplaceable (with the exception of those in the dentate gyrus and olfactory bulb), remain intact (Rakic 2002c).

Programmed cell death and apoptosis is an established phenomenon in the development of the central nervous system as well as in non-neural tissues.[4] Apparently death of up to 75% of the cells occurs in some regions of the brain in a gene-programmed and regulated system. Two classes of cysteine proteases, proteolytic enzymes (caspases), are involved in the execution of neurons by degradation before the formation of synaptic connections (Oppenheim *et al.* 2001). Some neurons have to die to allow normal brain development. The accepted view is that cell death occurs to match the size of each neuronal population to the size of its target fields and to eliminate neurons with erroneous or inadequate projections. An important finding in brain development (morphogenesis) was severe malformations of the brain in mutant mice which were deficient in the pro-apoptotic genes for specific caspases responsible for normal programmed cell death (Kuan *et al.* 2000). Billions of neurons compete to innervate their targets, and some of them lose out (Shepherd 1994). In the embryo several motor neurons send axons to a muscle fiber. But in the end, only one neuron and axon dominates a muscle fiber. Overlap of innervation ceases after the competition is over.

NEUROPLASTICITY

The theoretical aspects of neuroplasticity continue as hope and promise to reverse the devastating injuries of the brain and spinal cord (Trojan and Pokorny 1999). Research using advanced technology continues to enhance knowledge of the morphological or functional plasticity of the nervous system (Cohen *et al.* 1998, Thompson *et al.* 2005).

Brain. Some indication that the brain may be resilient to extensive damage is from the clinical results of hemispherectomy for intractable epilepsy (Villablanca and Hovda 1999). Studies show remarkable recovery in experimental hemispherectomy in cats that were postnatal up to 60 days, but not when done in late fetal or adult life. The long-term effect at all ages was a loss of neurons remote from the operative site.

We do know that some humans make a partial recovery from brain injury despite the strong evidence that the neurons degenerate irreversibly after a specific injury (Ramón y Cajal 1928, Windle 1956, Clemente 1964). Adults have sometimes recovered remarkably from cerebral vascular accidents (Rosner 1974). The mechanism of recovery is not regeneration of a dead neuron, but is due almost entirely to the capability of synapses to modify their function, be replaced, and to increase or decrease

in number when necessary. After brain damage the restoration of cortical function is a recognized process of two factors: (1) activation of silent synapses probably mediated by the neurotransmitter GABA which exerts trophic actions on the principal neurons (Wolff *et al.* 1993, Swann *et al.* 1999); (2) sprouting of axons of neighboring undamaged axons over a period of weeks and months. Many molecules among which are neurotrophins, nitric oxide, integrins are active in this process. The molecular basis of neuronal plasticity was identified in the past as an extremely complicated chemical process and remains so (Black *et al.* 1985, Nirenberg *et al.* 1985). Nerve growth factors, neuropeptides, gangliosides and many other substances such as serotonin (Azmitia 1999) and phospholipids are active in the process.

Some molecules block regeneration; among these are the chondroitin sulphate proteoglycans that form perineuronal nets surrounding the neurons (Fox and Caterson 2002, Pizzorusso *et al.* 2002). Pizzorusso and colleagues used an enzyme, chondroitinase ABC, to blow away the net surrounding the neurons and allow them to form synapses with one another more freely and promise to restore function in the visual cortex.

Another protein, Nogo, in the membrane of nerve fibers inhibits regeneration of axons gives hope that this discovery will lead to promotion of recovery after strokes and spinal cord injuries. (Goldberg and Barres 2000). Hormones can influence greater axonal sprouting in the nucleus retroambiguus of the caudal medulla oblongata as reported in ovariectomized female Rhesus monkeys treated with estrogen compared with the control monkeys (Vanderhorst *et al.* 2002).

A rare report pertaining to brain reorganization in cerebral palsy was described by neuroscientists from Melbourne, Australia (Briellmann *et al.* 2002). They studied a 15-year-old girl with a perinatal left sided subcortical lesion depicted by functional magnetic resonance imaging (MRI) at 3 Telsa. She had a hemiparesis, mirror limb movements and normal language. Hand movements induced asymmetric bilateral activation of the motor cortex with predominant activation one the opposite right side of the lesion. Language activated the uninvolved right cerebral hemisphere. These findings suggest alternative cortical organization with a subcortical lesion, i.e. plasticity.

Apparent recovery of damaged neurons seems to occur not so much by regeneration as by development of behavioral maneuvers which mask the less specific motor functions. The masking of neurological deficits can be spectacular. Reports abound in clinical and laboratory reports (Geschwind 1974). Recovery of near-normal behavior after hemispherectomy is well known, and recovery of normal speech after ablation of cortical areas for speech has been observed. Despite these examples of dramatic recovery, there are patients who do not recover from brain lesions. Small lesions have produced large functional deficits.

Recovery in immature nervous systems has been presumed to be superior to that in adults. Most of this presumption has been based upon the greater regenerative ability of lower vertebrates such as amphibia and reptiles (Kerr 1975). Past research indicated that the immature nervous system may be less plastic than

---

4 Apoptosis (from the Greek ’απο, off, and πτωσις, a falling): single deletion of scattered cells by fragmentation into membrane-bound particles which are phagocytosed by other cells.

originally envisaged (Goldman 1972, 1974, Lawrence and Hopkins 1972, Berman and Berman 1973). The experimental data indicated that damage to the central nervous system during its period of rapid growth may result in more destruction of ultimate function than injury during the more stable phases of brain development (Teuber 1971, Goldman 1972, 1974, Brunner and Altman 1974, Goldberger 1974, Neligan 1974, Schneider and Jhaveri 1974). But contemporary neuroscience indicates that plasticity in adults is restricted compared to newborns.

'Fasting is good for your neurons and enhances synaptic plasticity.'
(Mattson *et al.* 2003)

In the current climate of concern about obesity in adults and children in the United States, the research by Mattson, Duan, and Guo of the Gerontology Research Center, National Institute of Aging (2003), provides impressive data that intermittent fasting or reduction in caloric intake protects neurons from degeneration in animal models, enhances synaptic plasticity and stimulates the production of new neurons from stem cells. These effects seem to be the result of cell stress that induces the production of proteins such as the brain-derived neurotrophic factor that enhance neuronal plasticity.

In keeping with the contemporary fascination with food's effect on health, pharmacologists from Mahidol University, Bangkok, suggested that long-term garlic consumption may be good for you. It would be good too for the economy of Gilroy, California—the 'Garlic Capital of the World'. They reported that male rats, 7–8 months old, improved their physical performance and learning behavior from ingestion of garlic (*Allium sativum)* at a low dose as well as with pentoxifylline, a blood rheological and antiplatelet agent[5] (Sookvanichsilp *et al.* 2002). The rationale for consumption of pentoxifylline was not stated except perhaps as control substance along with water. Of course this experiment with garlic would need confirmation. One wonders if 25–50 children in a classroom all exhaling garlic breath would outweigh the presumed benefits of a daily diet laced with garlic, but then again if they lived in Sicily it would probably not be noticed.

SPINAL CORD
Liu and Chambers (1959) were the first to prove that neurons have an innate ability to form new connections when other cells are lost (Edds 1953) (Fig. 4.13). They demonstrated axonal sprouting in the cat spinal cord after experimental transaction of the spinal cord pyramidal tract and found that several years later the field of termination was larger on the side of the tract lesion. This observation suggested that dorsal root fibers give off collateral sprouts to fill the vacated synaptic spaces.

Many contemporary references have to do with experimental neuroplasticity of the spinal cord after injury. With the use of

functional MRI somatosensory cortical representations in the brain were found after a 5-year absence of sensorimotor function at and below the shoulders in a person who had a high-level cervical spinal-cord injury. Brain activity was observed with vibratory stimulation and voluntary movements of the body parts below and above the lesion. Cortical representations were preserved (Corbetta *et al.* 2002).

In experimental animals, hemisection of the spinal cord in adults and neonates indicated that the timing of the lesion is important. True sparing of function may have been restricted to motor patterns not directly affected by the lesion because in young animals these patterns had not yet developed at the time of the injury (Bergman and Goldenberger 1983). Although axonal sprouting in experimental animals can be demonstrated, the extent of functional recovery is unknown (Tsukahara and Murahami 1983).

In adult rats subjected to complete spinal-cord resection spinal-cord transplants with neurotrophins acted as a bridge that reestablished projections from the central nervous system supraspinal centers; neurotrophin treatment was essential for axonal growth. A 2-week delay in the delivery of the spinal-cord transplant yielded increased axonal growth and increased function recovery (Bregman *et al.* 2002).

RHIZOTOMY
Studies of posterior root rhizotomies in experimental deafferentation suggested that function may be recoverable but is inhibited by the remaining intact system. When a single upper limb of a monkey was deafferented by cutting of the dorsal spinal roots, permanent impairment of all spontaneous limb movement resulted (Mott and Sherrington 1895, Lassek 1953, Twitchell 1954). In addition, reflex activity unrelated to the dorsal-root sensory nerves was impaired, e.g. the static labyrinthine reflexes (Denny-Brown 1966). If both limbs were deafferented (as in patients with selective posterior rootlet rhizotomy), functional recovery occurred spontaneously (Knapp *et al.* 1963, Taub and Berman 1968). In a monkey in which the posterior root rhizotomy was done in only one limb and the opposite limb restricted in movement, recovery of the deafferented limb was enhanced (Fig. 4.16). With this evidence we might conclude that forced use of the deafferented limb discouraged recovery, and that the intact sensory system in the normal limb selectively

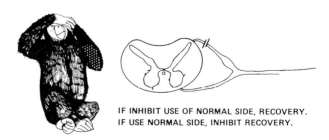

IF INHIBIT USE OF NORMAL SIDE, RECOVERY.
IF USE NORMAL SIDE, INHIBIT RECOVERY.

Fig. 4.16. Deafferentation of one limb with posterior root rhizotomy in a monkey; the motor system is intact.

---

5 Pentoxifylline (Trental,® Adventis Pharmaceuticals), used primarily for chronic occlusive arterial disease.

inhibited recovery of the normal intact limb (Taub *et al.* 1973). As in the deafferentation experiments in animals, children with spastic diplegia who have a bilateral selective posterior rootlet rhizotomy have partially deafferented lower limbs and marked muscular weakness immediately postoperatively, and then slowly recover.

Similar phenomena have been observed in pyramidal-tract lesions in which recovery was enhanced by secondary lesions of the contralateral cerebral hemisphere (Bard 1938, Semmes and Chow 1955) and also of the ventrolateral funiculus of the spinal cord (Goldberger 1969). These findings implied an inhibitory process in the contralateral hemisphere. Amphetamines were thought to improve recovery by suppression of some of the inhibitory cortical areas (Beck and Chambers 1970). Amphetamines act on catecholamine receptors and at the synapses for norepinephrine and dopamine (Thompson 2000).

Classic operant conditioning methods have achieved near-normal function in deafferented limbs (Bossom and Ommaya 1968). Liu and Chambers (1971) reported that monkeys could be trained to perform accurate and complicated maneuvers with their deafferented limbs without visual guidance. These maneuvers were performed with little or no feedback from the limb. Thus it was concluded that training methods 'unmasked' latent abilities in the central nervous system.

Leonard *et al.* (1984) performed cortical ablations in neonatal and adult cats. They analyzed the function of the cats with neurological tests and motion analysis. They found that the neonatal cats had a more prolonged emergence of reflexes and had fewer deficits than the adult cats. Motion analysis (kinematics) of the neonates showed that abnormalities of their locomotion were compensated for during a later phase of development, and the deficit was masked. These results indicated two possible mechanisms: (1) behavioral plasticity, which means masking of the deficits by movements different from the normal; and (2) neurological plasticity, e.g. axonal sprouting.

The vestibular system appears most adaptable. The vestibulo-ocular system and its reflex can be easily altered by visual training with inverted prisms. In human experiments, when people wore spectacles that inverted their visual field (Fig. 4.17), they were initially helpless: but with time they recovered and could move about normally. The synaptic circuits in the vestibular reflexes seem to be easily rearranged (Miles and Fuller 1974, Gonshor and

Melvill-Jones 1976a, b). We have known for a long time that lesions of the vestibular system due to unilateral labyrinthectomies or neuronitis do not produce long-lasting symptoms, and compensation readily occurs. As with conditioned motor behaviour, these brainstem systems are almost independent of cortical control and are influenced primarily by lesions of the cerebellum and its nuclei (Llinas *et al.* 1975)

As an example of central nervous system plasticity the effects of weightlessness on the vestibular system is the experience of astronauts during and after space flight. After returning to earth they were unable to stand on a narrow rail with eyes open on the first day, but recovered later. Standing was almost impossible with eyes closed, and this deficit in balance lasted longer before returning to normal. The data clearly show that postural mechanisms are affected by weightlessness. The hypothesis is that a 'pattern center' of the brain adapts during space flight, and then reverses upon return to earth. This distributed system is used for the maintenance of thee standing posture. It receives information from the vestibular organ, the muscle and tendon receptors, and tactile receptors from the skin and deeper tissues (e.g. joints) (Shepherd 1994).

PERIPHERAL NERVOUS SYSTEM

Repair and regrowth of axons through severed and repaired peripheral nerves has long been known (Freed *et al.* 1985). The best example of functional recovery due to axonal growth is in the resuturing of severed peripheral nerves. Experiments have shown that axonal growth can be enhanced by refinements in suturing the cut ends to minimize scar formation that obstructs axon growth across the sutured nerve. Trophic and growth substances that promote neuronal growth (e.g. nerve growth factor, ganglioside, glycoproteins, heart-conditioned medium, neuronotrophic factors induced by the lesion) have been investigated and found to promote peripheral nerve regeneration. Reorganization of the brain in response to peripheral nerve injuries or amputation appears evident in human and animal studies. Following such peripheral injuries expansion of sensory and motor system representations occur at several levels in the spinal cord, brainstem, thalamus and cortex. Motor function after stroke may be due to the adjacent cortical areas taking over function or the use of alternative pathways. After peripheral injury the significance of motor reorganization for function is uncertain (Chen *et al.* 2002).

In a review of postnatal histogenesis in various sites of the peripheral nervous system, Geuna *et al.* (2002) of Torino, Italy, focused on the autonomic nervous system's myenteric system in a search for postnatal neuron additions.[6] Based on their review of experimental and clinical studies, they suggested that residual neural crest cells could be multipotent stem cells as a peripheral reserve pool that could be a 'powerful therapeutic tool' for clinicians to treat degenerative diseases of the peripheral nervous system. Schematically this theory implies that under different

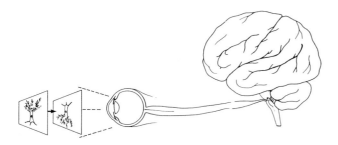

Fig. 4.17. Representation of brainstem adaptation of reversal of the visual image with inverted prism spectacles demonstrating the great adaptability of the vestibulo-ocular system.

6 Myenteric: pertaining to the muscular coat of the intestines.

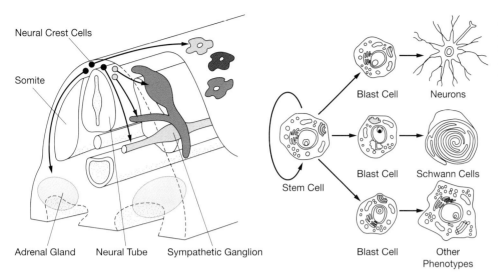

Fig. 4.18. (*a*) Migration pathways of neural-crest cells. (*b*) Neural-crest stem cells in vitro differentiate into various phenotypes such as neurons and Schwann cells. These can then self-replicate. (Redrawn from Shepherd 1994, by permission.)

Neural Crest Cells

Somite

Adrenal Gland   Neural Tube   Sympathetic Ganglion

Blast Cell   Neurons

Stem Cell

Blast Cell   Schwann Cells

Blast Cell   Other Phenotypes

conditions as the neural crest cells migrate they differentiate into different final phenotypes (Fig. 4.18).

STEM CELLS

Implantation of stem cells to restore lost or damaged neurons has generated much excitement by scientists and the press in recent years. Embryonic stem cells in particular have been proposed as pluripotential to replace damaged components of the central nervous system in neurodegenerative and neurodevelopmental diseases (Gokhan and Mehler 2001). Adult bone marrow stromal cells have been converted to neurons, according to Woodbury and colleagues (2002), suggesting that these marrow cells are multidifferentiated and the neural differentiation is due to a quantitative modulation of gene expression. Thus far, experiments with stem cells have been confined to laboratory animals. Current reports indicate that a great deal of laboratory research will be needed before giving hope to children with cerebral palsy that on the near horizon their neurons can be replaced and restore lost functions of the brain.

Riess *et al.* (2002) of the Head Injury Center, University of Pennsylvania School of Medicine, evaluated mice that had a cortical impact brain injury and transplanted neural stem cells. They observed improved motor function in the animals, but cognitive dysfunction was not affected. Histological studies showed that the transplanted neurons differentiated into neurons or glia.

Rats that had middle cerebral artery occlusions to simulate stroke had MHP36 stem cells implanted into the parenchyma or infused into the right ventricle. Spatial learning did not improve with parenchymal implants, but those that had stem cells infused into the right ventricle improved spatial learning. Implanted cells occupied both sides of the rat brains (Modo *et al.* 2002).

NEUROCHEMICAL TRANSMITTERS AND THE BRAIN IN CEREBRAL PALSY

A search for neurochemical transmitter abnormalities in the cerebral palsy and the administration of a magic bullet was reported by two neuroscientists from Moscow, Russia (Mashilov

and Kogan 1992), and subsequently by Brin and colleagues also from Russia (Brin *et al.* 1994, Brin and Mashilov 1996). They investigated plasma cortisol, plasma somatotrophic hormones, plasma prolactin, and dopamine-β-hyroxylase levels in 102 children who had cerebral palsy. Fifteen who had either post-traumatic, infectious or 'allergic' encephalopathy were used as controls. They found increases in levels of cortisol in spastic diplegia, of somatotrophic hormones in hyperkenetic forms and spinal cord injury, of prolactin in spastic diplegia and hemiplegia, and hyperkinesia. Dopamine-β-hydroylase activity was lower in spastic diplegia ($p<0.001$), hyperkinesia ($p<0.01$) and spastic hemiplegia ($p<0.05$). It was also lower in those who had spinal cord diseases than in spinal cord injury patients ($p<0.001$). Armed with this biochemical information they treated dopamine deficient patients with carbidopa-levodopa. Their report seemed to indicate 'improvement' in some children, but not all, leading them to classify their patients as 'dopamine correctable' and 'uncorrectable'.

Brin and colleagues (1994) described the investigation of plasma catecholamine and serum dopamine-β-hydroylase levels in 21 children with spastic diplegia. These children were defined as having 'clinical signs of central catecholaminergic neuro-mediation deficiency and were administered a single daily dose of 60 mg of carbidopa-levodopa. The result was stated as having 'a good clinical effect'. In 1996 these same Russian scientists reported the effect of carbidopa-levodopa with a daily dose of 62.5 mg in 110 patients with cerebral palsy. The levels of adrenocorticotropic hormones (ACTH), hydrocortisone, soma-totropic hormone, and prolactin were elevated in those with cerebral palsy. With *Nakom* administration the 'dopamine dependent' children had 'normalization' of the biochemical and clinical indices.

Lest the reader becomes enthusiastic for dopamine replace-ment treatment of cerebral palsy, the studies reported would need repeating and confirmation.[7] Altering brain chemistry with

7 In a literature search from 1996 to February 2003 no subsequent reports of replacement therapy with dopamine in cerebral palsy have been found.

drugs can be tricky and dangerous. The unintended effect of irreversible tardive dyskinesia with the use of antipsychotic drugs (haloperidol—a dopamine blocker) should be a warning flag that brain chemistry can be altered for the worse with drugs.[8]

The administration of interferon alpha-2a in the treatment of hemangiomas in infants induced spastic diplegia in five that persisted in three and recovery in two (Barlow *et al.* 1998). The known side-effects of interferon alpha treatment in adults includes central nervous system symptoms of depression, cognitive and behavioral changes, anorexia, somnolence and seizures. The authors suggested that in very young infants interferon gamma may cause disruption of normal myelination, damage to the glia and induce coagulation defects. However, MRI studies of the brains and spinal cords in these infants were normal.

These observations appear to have led Grether and colleagues (1999) to search for clues of elevated neonatal interferons[9] in 31 children with spastic diplegia and hemiplegia. They found that in 14 of 31 children with spastic diplegia and hemiplegia compared with 65 in a control group had concentrations of alpha, beta, and gamma interferons exceeding the control group. In addition levels of cytokines such as interleukins, 1,6,8, tumor necrosis factor-alpha, transforming growth factor-beta, chemokines, certain neuropeptides and thyroid hormones differed from the controls. These inflammatory markers were increased in those who had spastic diplegia, but near normal in those with hemiplegia. Because viruses and bacteria are the most efficient natural inducers of interferons alpha-2a and beta, Barlow and colleagues (1998) wondered if elevated interferon levels were a manifestation of subclinical infections in the mothers.

PHYSICAL THERAPEUTIC APPLICATIONS OF 'NEUROPLASTICITY?

In some ways the term 'neuroplasticity' is unfortunate because it can be used as a canard to justify all sorts of experimental treatments and educational programs in children who have impairments of cerebral function. Therapists have been encouraged to use an 'an eclectic approach' based on 'physiologic evidence' to 'utilize all weapons to combat lesion changes' using 'neuroplastic phenomena' to guide the new pathways of axonal and dendritic development. The hypothesis is that 'reorganization of the CNS is ongoing, and long-term physiotherapy (over many years) can continue to enhance recovery' (Stephenson 1993).

The hope that neuroplasticity will respond to improved passive 'therapies' for central nervous system injury remains a paradigm for rehabilitation by 'enhancement' of neurologic recovery with 'manipulating the brain and spinal cord' (Dobkin 1993). These concepts of neuroplasticity continue to be attractive

in keeping the difficult process of rehabilitation of neurological injury and disease going and giving hope. But thus far the results in cerebral palsy after years of dedicated attempts to improve sensory and motor development or alleviating the spasticity or athetosis or dysequilibrium with *passive* movements and stimuli do not indicate a significant change in either motor or sensory behavior.

THE MOTOR UNIT

Comprising the motor unit is a single motor neuron, the neuromuscular junction, and the muscle fibers innervated (Fig. 4.19). The number of muscle fibers varies with the size and function of the muscle. The number of muscle fibers supplied by a single motor neuron depends on the function of the muscle. Small muscles for fine movement have between one and three muscle fibers per nerve fiber. A large muscle will have over 150 fibers per nerve and some such as the gastrocnemius will have a ratio of 2000:1 (Rose and McGill 1998, Thompson 2000).

The motor neurons corresponding to the muscle are set inside a motor centre, a 'motor neuron pool'. In this pool is a mix of small and large neurons. The small ones have slow rates of contraction, small contraction force and moderate resistance to fatigue, while the large ones have the largest and fastest conducting axons and fatigue rapidly. As might be expected, there are intermediate motor neurons whose properties fall in between the two other types (Shepherd 1994). The variation of the motor neurons and synapses account for the ability to change from the low activity of standing still to running and jumping by increasing the recruitment of motor units as the need for specific muscle activity arises.

> '*Motoneuron properties are exquisitely matched to the properties of the motor units supplying the muscle and the properties of the muscles themselves.*'
>
> (Shepherd 1994, p. 450)

The skeletal muscle fibers are cells that are organized in smaller units, myofibrils. These fibrils are broken down into

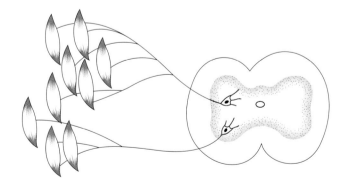

Fig. 4.19. The motor unit comprised of a single motor neuron and its axon and all the muscle fibers it innervates. The single motor axon can go to only two muscle fibers or as many as 100 depending on the size of the muscle. (From Thompson 2000, by permission.)

---

8 A persistent extrapyramidal syndrome of dystonia and rigidity was reported in a 58-year-old woman with cerebral palsy while being treated for vomiting with dopamine antagonists: metoclopramide combined with prochlorperazine (Factor and Matthews 1991).

9 Interferons are small (molecular weight 26,000–38,000 daltons) glycoproteins that are antiviral in homologous cells through a cellular metabolic process involving synthesis of a double-stranded RNA which is an intermediate in the replication of RNA viruses.

myofibrils whose ultratructure is comprised of the two inter-locking muscle proteins filaments, actin and myosin. The microscopic contracting unit of these proteins is called a sar-comere. The thicker myosin filaments have protruding heads that are at right angles to the thinner actin filaments. The myosin heads bind to the actin filaments. When acetylcholine releases at the neuromuscular junction, calcium ions are released by depolarization of the muscle membrane. This causes the adjacent enveloping chains of another protein, tropomysin bound to troponin, the calcium binding site, to move aside to expose the myosin heads. The heads then bind so that the sliding action occurs to cause muscle contraction (Thompson 2000).

Dantrolene sodium used to relax spastic muscles exerts its effects beyond the myoneural junction. It acts probably by inter-fering with the release of calcium ions (Ca^{2+}) from the sarcoplasmic reticulum. But it also has a central nervous system effect causing drowsiness and dizziness in some subjects.[10] Cyclobenzaprine is stated to relieve skeletal muscle spasm not by acting on the muscle, but at the level of the brainstem through suggested reduction in tonic somatic motor activity by the influences of both the alpha and gamma motor systems.[11]

SPINAL REFLEXES

Because some physical therapy systems in the past (and perhaps still in the present) were attempts to diminish, alter or use spinal reflexes, the known neurophysiology of the reflexes is briefly reviewed. The reflex arc consists of the alpha motor neuron in the spinal cord and its axon to the muscle and the sensory input via afferent 1a fibers back to the motor neuron. The stretch reflex is a monosynaptic one—only one set of synapses is between the sensory fibers and the motor neuron. When the muscle is stretched the sensation travels back to the motor neuron and the muscle contracts: the *stretch reflex* with which we are very familiar in cerebral palsy of the spastic type.

The *flexion reflex* is the other familiar one in cerebral palsy. It is a defensive action against bodily injury and a polysynaptic reflex because more than one synapse is involved. An example is a needle stick in your finger; you jerk away. The fast pain receptors in the skin connect to the interneurons in the spinal cord to stimulate the motor neurons for flexor muscles.

Within the muscle fibers is another sensory system, the gamma motor system, with its own neuron in the spinal cord. Sensors to stretch are in a muscle spindle that contains small muscle fibers (intrafusal) innervated by the gamma motor neuron. The spindle lies within and is parallel to the large contractile fibers (extrafusal). When stretch of the muscle occurs activation of the muscle spindle results in activation of the alpha motor neuron and the muscle contracts (Fig. 4.20). With respect to other than slow and gradual manual stretching of the tight muscle, it would seem that you get more contraction in return.

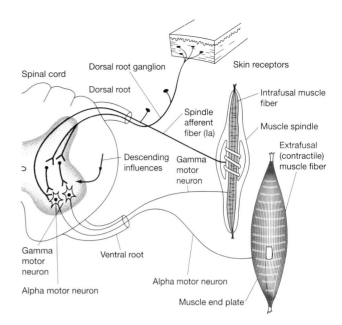

Fig. 4.20. The α motor neuron in the spinal cord and its axon innervating the muscle (extrafusal). Feedback from the muscle (intrafusal) sensory stretch organ innervated by its own neuron in the cord, the γ motor neuron. The stretch receptor in the muscle spindle sends it information back to the α motor neuron causing contraction of the extrafusal muscle. The intrafusal muscle fibers in the spindle organ are in parallel to the extrafusal fibers. The more stretch you do, the more contraction you get. (From Thompson 2000, by permission.)

The Golgi tendon organ is an afferent nerve fiber that lies within the tendon insertions to bone. Like the muscle spindle it provides stretch or relaxation signals to the motor neuron, but is activated with fairly rapid change in muscle tension. It has a slower discharge rate than the muscle spindle organ.

The higher motor centers in the brain all act on the motor neurons to affect the reflex activity of the spinal cord via descending pathways from the brain to the spinal cord. This higher central control is the basic principle in posterior rootlet rhizotomy in the patient who has cerebral palsy with spastic paralysis of the limbs.

The *neurophysiologic basis of muscle spasticity* in cerebral palsy remains unresolved. Based on experimental observations in human participants who had spastic hemiplegia, Rymer (1992) proposed two possible explanations for the increased stretch reflexes: (1) increased motor neuron excitability due to sustained or tonic descending depolarizing input to the spinal motor neurons; (2) and increase in the synaptic responses elicited by muscle stretch. His observations led him to conclude that 'in all likelihood' the spasticity is due to a reduction in effective motor neuron thresholds resulting from sustained depolarization of the motor neurons. It is still uncertain whether this depolarization is caused by increased excitatory descending impulses from the higher centers or reduced stimuli from the descending or regional inhibitory systems. Whatever the origin, the problem resides in the supraspinal center's white matter.

---

10 Proctor & Gamble, Cincinnati, OH, Product information, *Physicians' Desk Reference 1997*. Montvale, NJ: Medical Economics, p. 2131.
11 Merck & Co., West Point, PA, Product information, *Physicians' Desk Reference 1997*. Montvale, NJ: Medical Economics, pp. 1701–1702.

MOTOR BEHAVIOR

More and more research clearly indicates that we have genetically inherited 'innate' movement patterns (Grillner 1985). These patterns are coordinated neural circuits in the brain and spinal cord; despite being innate, they can be modified by experience and by sensory inputs in order to adapt to the immediate environment.

Wilson (1968) first suggested that there might be built-in circuits for motor behavior. To study the flight-control system of the locust, he cut the sensory nerves to the wings and then stimulated the central nervous system with a noise pattern. With the noise he was able to obtain replicas of the flight pattern from the motor neurons of the locust. Flight for the locust is thus a 'motor score' written in the brain, so there is no need for direct stimulation and sensory input from its wings. Shik *et al.* (1966) provided additional evidence of an innate central program for gait in the cat. These Soviet scientists prepared a mesencephalic cat by surgical decerebration and then applied gradations of electrical current to the remaining brain. With varying degrees of electrical stimulation (10–20 mA) the cat walked, trotted and ran (Fig. 4.21). Corresponding brainstem areas for locomotion have been found in primates, reptiles and fish. Those of us from farms know that the chicken can run after its head has been chopped off—central program generators at work.

Experimental data indicate that even when movement-related afferent inputs from the limb or body has been abolished, the locomotor circuits can be activated. The current view is that locomotor output is produced by the central nervous system and spinal cord which house central program generators (cpGs). Sensory feedback from muscle and joint receptors in the limbs is important; without this the system breaks down.

The decision to take a step is sufficient to begin walking. Signals are channeled through the basal ganglia to the spinal-cord central program generators. While the loss of equilibrium sensation severely compromises walking, this loss can be com-pensated for by a treadmill which prevents the animal from falling; experimental animals adapt the speed of locomotion to that of the treadmill.

The brainstem centers control the spinal rhythm generators by spontaneous and modulating discharges which facilitate the phases of the gait cycle. Although the cerebellum is very important for the perfection of the movement patterns, it has no direct connections with the spinal cord. In the hierarchy of the central nervous system it is in the middle between the spinal cord and the cortex. It controls muscle tone, balance and sensorimotor coordination, and modulates sensory feedback from the limbs.

Grillner's (1985) experiments with the lamprey formed the hypothesis that individual central program generators exist to be used alone or in combination. If we wish to walk, we call on an ensemble of central program generators. But if we only want to move the big toe, we just call on one. Other evidence of 'hard-wired' motor synergies was suggested by Ghez *et al.* (1983). The onset of contraction of different muscle groups reflected the property of the total system. Further evidence of an innate central system of locomotion was provided by Forssberg and Svartengren (1983), who found retention of the extensor pattern in the cat gastrocnemius after it had been surgically transposed to a dorsiflexor action. They concluded that the spinal motor network had little plasticity.

The 19th-century concept of the cerebral cortex as the supreme commander is no longer tenable. Rather it is one part of a 'distributive system'—a combination of cortical and subcortical centers. It is often the middle of signal processing. Any cortical region can be significant for its synaptic connections and its connections to other cortical and subcortical regions. These synaptic circuits generate the special functions. The human attributes we have are in the organization of the synaptic circuits of the cortex (Shepherd 1994).

ENVIRONMENT

'The old debate of nature vs nurture has been rendered obsolete.'
(Shepherd 1994)

All now recognize that both the genetic program and environmental factors are operative in function of the neuron. The cortical synapses are sensitive to environmental influences. For example, the removal of a rodent's eye reduces the number of spines (which make synapses) on apical dendrites in the visual cortex; in these newborn rodents, either the spines are lost or the dendrites fail to mature. When animals are raised in enriched environments, with toys to play with and mazes to run in, their cortices are thicker and synapses larger than those raised in barren cages. Cortices of wild animals can be 30% thicker than domesticated ones. Dendritic spines are reduced in some types of human mental retardation. In monkeys when one eye is closed at birth, there is expansion of the ocular-dominance columns of the cortex of the normal eye. This expansion depends upon noradrenaline (norepinephrine) in the cells of the cortex and midbrain. The relatively few noradrenaline neurons clustered in

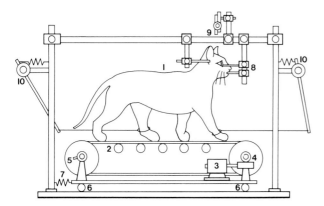

Fig. 4.21. Mesencephalic cat preparation. (1) Cat with cerebral cortex removed; (2) treadmill to record gait; (3) electric motor; (4) brake; (5) belt-speed marker; (6) rollers; (7) dynamometer; (8) stereotaxic instrumentation; (9) stimulating electrodes to the mesencephalon; (10) pick-up to measure displacement of the limbs. (Adapted from Shik *et al.* 1966.)

the locus ceruleus in the midbrain send multiple branching axons to almost every region of the central nervous system where multiple synapses occur (Shepherd 1994).

Held and Hein (1963), in a unique experiment using kittens where one was active and the other was pulled in a gondola in a room painted with striped walls, showed loss of normal behaviors in the passively stimulated kitten. The kitten that walked and pulled the gondola had normal responses to visually guided tasks. The obvious conclusion is that active movement is necessary to integrate visual motor control mechanisms and has bearing on attempts by passive therapies to change motor behavior in cerebral palsy.

Self-controlled movement remains essential for the development of the central nervous system (Connolly 1969). Contemporary reports from different countries reinforce the need for active use ('dynamic therapy') in central nervous system motor behavior in humans and experimental animals (the Netherlands, Hadders-Algra 2001; Finland, Schalow 2001; New York, USA, Schieber 2002).

> '*Learning is an adaptive change in behaviour caused by experience.*'
>
> (Neurobiologist's definition; Shepherd 1994)

Learning is an adaptive change in behavior caused by experience. 'Adaptive' means that a change in behavior has some meaning for survival of the animal and species. 'Change' implies a difference between behavior before and after the event. The change must be specific in the nervous system and independent of ongoing maturation (Shepherd 1994). Learning is intimately linked to memory which is the storage and recall of experiences. It is essential for learning. It can involve almost any neuronal or cellular process.

Synapses are responsible for acquisition and storage of memories in which neurotransmitters are operative: N–Methyl-D-Aspartate (NMDA) activation and GABAergic inhibition. The recent studies by Donchin *et al.* (2002) indicate that these neurotransmitters are involved in the acquisition, but not in the recall of new motor memories in humans.

Goldberger (1969) pointed out that monkeys, who had cerebral cortical lesions and then passive manipulations to assist recovery, performed well under test conditions. When conditioned stimuli were applied, however, monkeys exhibited little improvement in spontaneous behavior. For example, a monkey in which only the pyramidal tract cortex has been preserved may be trained to feed itself or to grasp an object if the conditioned stimulus is applied, but is unable to perform the task voluntarily. Conditioned motor behavior is patterned, and therefore inaccessible to cortical volition when the cortex is damaged. Hepp-Reymond *et al.* (1970) reported that conditioned behavior remained unchanged despite extensive cortical and pyramidal tract lesions.

Memory is important for retention of motor skills that are developed by practice as anyone who has learned to play the piano, a musical instrument, or to use a typewriter/computer keyboard. A fascinating report from Lübeck, Germany (Fischer *et al.* 2002), confirms that practice makes perfect in learning finger skills and is enhanced by 33.5% following sleep. Walker and colleagues (2002) at Harvard University conducted experiments that found a 20% increase in motor speed without the loss of accuracy in motor skill performance after a night's sleep. That sleep is essential for storing and optimizing motor skills is hardly surprising, but it is good to know that experimental data support this common perception. 'At eight years, to bed at eight' was favorite child-rearing advice to parents by a wise pediatrician friend.

The idea of 'environmental enrichment' of infants 'at-risk', or diagnosed as having cerebral palsy, has led some therapists to try and stimulate such infants with bells, rattles, tambourines and by singing songs. In the 1980s, the pediatric neurologist P.C. Ferry (1981, 1986) had the temerity to question the neurobiological basis of infant stimulation programs (see also Chapter 6). Yet in my (EEB) frequent visits to developing countries in Asia and South America over the same time period I found that these western therapy programs continued to be used. One wonders if this 'technology transfer' absorbs time and money that could be used more effectively in prevention of cerebral palsy as well as eradication of infectious diseases (e.g. tuberculosis, malaria, AIDS). Experimental brain trauma in rats subjected to enriched environments improved spatial memory only in male rats and not females. Motor recovery was unaffected (Wagner *et al.* 2002).[12]

In contrast to the foregoing study, adult mice (age 10–20 months) exposed to an enriched environment had a fivefold increase in neurogenesis in the hippocampus. Significant improvements in learning and motor behavior occurred. This led to the conclusion that old mice as well as old humans benefit from leading an active and challenging life: another strike for activity's effect on brain plasticity (Kempermann *et al.* 2002). It would be important not to overdraw the significance of this data. We know and accept that new neurons develop postnatally in the hippocampal gyrus as well as the olfactory bulb, but new cortical neurons are not replaceable (Rakic 2001).

CEREBRAL CORTEX, HUMAN BEHAVIOR, LEARNING AND MEMORY

A complete exposition of this complex subject is beyond the intended readership of this text. However, some general remarks seem pertinent, because from the 1950s to the 1990s there was an explosion of manipulative educational and infant treatment programs for cerebral palsy. Many of these programs were based on presumptions that the brain was a 'black box' and could be programmed as a computer by passive inputs.

Contemporary evidence dispels our old concepts that all intelligence, cognitive abilities, affective behavior and tem-

---

12 Spatial memory: memory of a particular place, e.g. in a maze, located in a 'place recognition neuron' in the hippocampus. Learning 'where' for rats is like learning 'what' for humans (Thompson 2000).

perament reside solely within the billions of cells of the cerebral cortex. Instead the new idea is that these functions are mediated by a system of cortical and subcortical centers. The cerebellum has been recognized as important not only in motor function but sensory as well. Its functions are mainly inhibitory. In contrast to the cerebral cortex its 'wiring diagram' is the same throughout and its cytoarchitectonic organization is the same in all mammals from mouse to human (Thompson 1993).

We used to accept the evolutionary idea that the size of the forebrain and cortical development was linear. We were taught that the neocortex first appeared in amphibians; in reptiles and birds sensory systems were projected through the thalamus from the cortex; and finally, in mammals, the cortex grew larger with the inputs from the thalamus and basal ganglia. Thalamic input was shown to be unnecessary by the research using developing mouse embryos by Fukuchi-Shimigori and Grove (2001).In their study they showed that by genetic manipulation and site of production of Growth Factor 8 (fibroblasts) the map of the cerebral cortex could be amazingly altered.

It is conceded that the forebrain and cortex have not undergone gradual and linear evolutionary change, but that species have developed their forebrains independently. We also know that the functions of neuritic tracts are mediated differently among species. Various animal species have neither a typical tract nor a center for a given function. These independently evolving structures are termed 'homoplastic'[13] (Shepherd 1994). Genetic markers have identified behavioral phenotypes such as those that comprise a number of mental retardation syndromes, e.g. Lesch-Nyhan syndrome, 9p deletion syndrome and others listed by the Society for the Study of Behavioral Phenotypes (their website, www.ssbp.co.uk, lists condensed information on 38 syndromes primarily of mental retardation).

' The detailed analysis of behaviour and its infrastructures, such as the analysis of the biochemical pathway between gene and behaviour, opens our understanding of the mechanisms of behavior.'

(Bax 2002)

Psychological development in infants appears to be 'canalized' (Kagan 1982)—a term describing the common behavioral changes and developmental milestones in infants between the ages of 17 and 24 months. These include the sense of right and wrong, emergence of speech, self-awareness in actions and in recognition, memory for the past and maintenance of an active memory. These behavioral events occur in parallel as the central nervous system matures. In the rat, a sevenfold increase in the number of synapses was found in the parietal cortex between the 12th and 26th days after birth. Similar increases in synaptic connections occur in the primate and human after birth. Programmed cell death and synaptic remodeling occur at the same time. All of these events take place under genetic regulation. The neuron reaches maturity under the influences of its own environment.

The old belief that developmental milestones in cognition, emotion and behavior were determined almost solely by the social interactions of parents and children, meant that differences of behavior had to be due to differing family experiences. Although we cannot deny the importance of family experiences in human development, we also need to recognize the effects of innate characteristics that appear on a biologically determined timetable. Even Freud eventually recognized that innate maturational forces in infants would have common developmental profiles (Kagan 1982). Thus parents are not the sole and only sculptors of their children. Anyone who has raised more than one child or has observed children in other families and cultures can acknowledge the common developmental profiles of infants and children as well as their inherited behavioral traits. Two longitudinal studies of 200 pairs of twins, aged 14–20 months, in the areas of temperament, emotion, cognition and language, confirmed the genetic factors were operative at 14 and 20 months primarily in cognition and memory (Emde *et al.* 1992, Plomin *et al.* 1993). Perhaps in individual and family relationships, the adage that 'blood is thicker than water' has biological validity.

Kagan (1982) gave numerous examples of canalization of infant development. One is the anxiety of infants between the ages of 8 and 12 months when separated from the mother. This is true in infants worldwide including blind infants, and infants in kibbutzim in Israel, in villages in Guatemala, in Indian villages in Central America, in day-care centers and in nuclear families. All have maximum distress at about 15 months, but by the third birthday they no longer fuss or cry on separation. Eight-month-old infants show no fear of infants the same age. However, by the middle of the second year they become inhibited, circumspect and timid, and cling to the mother. Again this characteristic mood disappears in the third year. This fearfulness has been observed in all social classes, races and groups. This fear seems to be neurobiologically based due to the new cognitive functions resulting from the growth of the central nervous system among which are the maturation of the frontal and rhinal cortices, hippocampus, and integration of the limbic system.

As further evidence of neurobiological development the studies by Liston and Kagan (2002) show that long-term memory in infants improves through the second year and indicate that at 9 months the hippocampus and regions of the frontal cortex are not fully mature. Therefore early assumptions that memory enhancement is entirely due to experience has been modified. However, Kagan (2001) noted that the biological constraints are weakest in semantic (meaning and development of words) networks as these are influenced by history, economy, religion, geography and social structures.

Cerebral cortical functions are not compartmentalized in local regional centers. The cortical area is one part of a larger interconnecting system. For example, seeing an object requires connections from the occipital lobe to the motor outputs in the parietal and frontal lobes; grasping it requires additional connections to the eye fields in the frontal cortex to coordinate eye movements with our fingers. Neurochemicals are also important for the function of cortical systems. When dopamine was

13 Homoplastic: similar in form and structure, but not in origin.

selectively suppressed in the frontal cortex of monkeys by injections of 6-hydroxydopamine, the monkeys could not remember the location of a test object; these results were comparable to those obtained by prefrontal lobotomy. The effects of dopamine depletion were reversed by dopamine agonists.

Maps of the somatosensory cortical systems in humans have become increasingly detailed and have shown to be plastic (Shepherd 1994). Punctate electrical stimulation of the cortex by Penfield and colleagues in Montreal between the 1930s and the 1950s gave us a map of the body surface on the postcentral gyrus of the cerebral cortex ('the homunculus') (Penfield and Rasmussen 1952). The cortex receives information from the several subdivisions of the thalamus. The plasticity of the cortical representations is exemplified by experiments in which a digit of the animal is amputated and its area in the map disappears only to be filled in by expansion of area by the skin of the adjacent digit.

CLINICAL IMPLICATIONS FOR CEREBRAL PALSY

Given the complexity and distribution of central nervous system functions that make us human, it seems clear that a highly localized cerebral lesion does not usually explain the motor, sensory and cognitive defects commonly observed in cerebral palsy. Not only is the brain a chemical machine: it is also very complicated. This review of neurobiology is only to provide a framework to understand that we who are engaged in the diagnosis and management of cerebral palsy are dealing with a biological reality.

The biological evidence that neurons are irreplaceable should assist our understanding of the prognosis in cerebral palsy. The existence of innate central motor programs within the spinal cord and brain ought to make us wary of passive manipulative treatments presumed to restore locomotor ability in infants and children. The data on maturation of the neurons, and their connections during the first 3 years of life, might temper our zeal in ascribing developmental progress solely to early special educational schemes or treatment methods.

Doing and perfecting the task by active self-controlled activity has a firm neurobiological basis. 'Enriched environments' for developing children at the appropriate time, consistent with maturation of the nervous system, seems logical. The once-fashionable habit of playing Mozart to infants, to enhance their eventual academic ability, does not seem to be supported by the neurobiological evidence.

While the administration of brain-altering drugs, electrical stimulation and neuron transplants are fascinating experiments in animals, their direct clinical application to solve the problem of the brain disorder cerebral palsy seems limited thus far in the third millennium. Meanwhile, we will have to be content to manage the child with cerebral palsy based upon its effects on the peripheral anatomy such as muscle-strengthening exercises and skill learning (e.g. typing, playing the piano, participating in sports), orthopaedic surgery, neurosurgery for rhizotomy, myoneural blockades with neurotoxins, and blocks of

neurochemical synapses. We know now that the brain is not a computer but a chemical machine.

REFERENCES

Azmitia, E.C. (1999) 'Serotonin neurons, neuroplasticity, and homeostasis of neural tissue.' *Neurophamarcology*, 21 (2 Suppl.), 33S–45S.

Bard, P. (1938) 'Studies on the cortical representation of somatic sensibility.' *Harvey Lectures*, 33, 143–169.

Barlow, C.F., Priebe, C.J., Mulliken, J.B., Barnes, P.D., MacDonald, D., Folkman, J., Ezekowitz, A.B. (1998) 'Spastic diplegia as a complication of interferon alpha-2a treatment of hemangiomas in infancy.' *Journal of Pediatrics*, 132, 527–530.

Barres, B. (1997/1998) In Wells, W. (Ed.) *Stanford Medicine*, Winter 97/98.

—— Raff, M.C. (1999) 'Axonal control of oligodendrocyte development.' *Journal of Cell Biology*, 147, 1123–1128.

Barton, R.A., Harvey, P.H. (2000) 'Mosaic evolution of brain structures in mammals.' *Nature*, 405, 1055–1058.

Bax, M.C.O. (2002) 'Re-thinking the brain: a frog leaps'. *Developmental Medicine and Child Neurology*, 44, 723.

Beck, C.H., Chambers, W.W. (1970) 'Speed, accuracy and strength of forelimb movement after unilateral pyramidotomy in rhesus monkeys.' *Journal of Comparative and Physiological Psychology*, 70, 1–22.

Bergman, B.S., Goldenberger, M.E. (1983) 'Infant lesion effect: II. Sparing and recovery of function after spinal cord damage in newborn and adult cats.' *Brain Research*, 285, 119–135.

Berman, A.J., Berman, D. (1973) 'Fetal deafferentation: the ontogenesis of movement in the absence of peripheral sensory feedback.' *Experimental Neurology*, 38, 170–176.

Black, I.R., Adler, J.E., Dreyfus, C.F., Jonakait, G.M., Katz, D.M., LaGamma, E.F., Markey, K.M. (1985) 'Neurotransmitter plasticity at the molecular level.' *In* Abelson, P.H., Butz, E., Snyder, S.H. (Eds) *Neuroscience.* Washington, DC: American Association for the Advancement of Science, pp. 30–39.

Bleck E.E., Nagel, D.A. (1982) *Physically Handicapped Children. A Medical Atlas for Teachers.* New York: Grune and Stratton.

Bossom, J., Ommaya, A.K. (1968) 'Visuo-motor adaptation in prismatic transformation of the retinal image in monkeys with bilateral dorsal rhizotomy.' *Brain*, 91, 161–172.

Bregman, B.S., Coumans, J.V., Dai, H.N., Kuhn, P.L., Lynskey, J., McAtee, M., Sandhu, F. (2002) 'Transplants and neurotrophic factors increase regeneration and recovery after spinal cord injury.' *Progress in Brain Research*, 137, 257–273.

Briellmann, R. S., Abbott, D., F., Caflisch, U., Archer, J.S., Jackson, G.D. (2002) 'Brain reorganization in cerebral palsy: a high-field functional MRI study.' *Neuropediatrics*, 33, 162–165.

Brin, I.L., Drozdov, A.Z., Kovaleva, I.A., Filatova, T.S., Kogan, B.M. (1994) 'Catecholamines and the dopamine-beta-hydroxylase activity of the blood plasma in motor pathology in children: the role of central and peripheral mechanisms.' *Zhurnal Nevropatologii i Psikhiatrii Imeni S.S. Korsakova*, 94, 7–12. (Russian.)

—— Mashilov, K.V. (1996) 'The effect of low doses of nakom on the hormonal secretion of hypothalamo–hypophyseal–adrenal system in patients with infantile cerebral palsy.' *Zhurnal Nevropatologii i Psikhiatrii Imeni S.S. Korsakova*, 96, 51–54. (Russian.)

Brodmann, K. (1909) *Vergleichende Localisationsationslehre der Grosshir-hinde.* Leipzig: Barth.

Brunner, R.L., Altman, J. (1974) 'The effects of interference with the maturation of the cerebellum and hippocampus on the development of adult behavior.' *In* Stein, P.G., Rosen, J.J., Butters, N. (Eds) *Plasticity and Recovery of Function in the Central Nervous System.* New York: Academic Press.

Chen, R., Cohen, L.G., Halett, M. (2002) 'Nervous reorganization following injury.' *Neuroscience*, 111, 761–763.

Clemente, C.D. (1964) 'Regeneration in the vertebrate central nervous system.' *International Review of Neurobiology*, 6, 257–301.

Cohen, L.G., Ziemann, U., Chen, R., Classen, J., Hallett, M., Gerloff, C., Butefisch, C. (1998) 'Studies of neuroplasticity with transcanial magnetic stimulation.' *Journal of Clinical Neurophysiology*, 15, 305–324.

Connolly, K. (1969) 'Sensory motor coordination: mechanism and plans.' *In* Wolff, P.H., Mac Keith, R. (Eds) *Planning for Better Learning. Clinics in Developmental Medicine, No. 33.* London: Spastics International

Medical Publications with Heinemann Medical; Philadelphia: J.B. Lippincott.

Corbetta, M., Burton, H., Sinlciar, R.J., Conturo, T.E., Akbudak, E., McDonald, J.W. (2002) 'Functional reorganization and stability of somatosensory-motor cortical topography in a tetraplegic subject with late recovery.' *Proceedings of the National Academy of Sciences of the USA*, **99**, 17066–17071.

Denny-Brown, D. (1966) *The Cerebral Control of Movement.* Liverpool: University of Liverpool Press.

Dobbing, J., Sands, J. (1973) 'Quantitative growth and development of the human brain.' *Archives of Disease in Childhood*, **48**, 757–767.

Dobkin, B.H. (1993) 'Neuroplasticity. Key to recovery after central nervous system injury.' *Western Journal of Medicine*, **159**, 56–60.

Donchin, O., Sawaki, L., Madupu, G., Cohen, L.G., Shadmehr, R. (2002) 'Mechanisms influencing acquisition and recall of motor memories.' *Journal of Neurophysiology*, **88**, 2114–2123.

Donoghue, M.J., Rakic, P. (1999) 'Molecular evidence for the early specification of presumptive functional domains in the embryonic primate cerebral cortex.' *Journal of Neuroscience*, **19**, 5967–5979.

Edds, M.V. (1953) 'Collateral nerve degeneration.' *Quarterly Review of Biology*, **28**, 260–275.

Emde, R.N., Plomin, R., Robinson, J.A., Corley, R., DeFries, J., Fulker, D.W., Reznick, J.S., Campos, J., Kagan, J., Zahn-Wacler, C. (1992) 'Temperament, emotion, and cognition at fourteen months: the MacArthur Longitudinal Twin Study.' *Child Development*, **63**, 1437–1455.

Factor, S.A., Matthews, M.K. (1991) 'Persistent extrapyramidal syndrome with dystonia and rigidity caused by combined metoclopramide and prochlorperazine therapy.' *Southern Medical Journal*, **84**, 526–528.

Ferry, P.C. (1981) 'On growing new neurons: are early intervention programs effective?' *Pediatrics*, **67**, 38–41.

—— (1986) 'Infant stimulation programs. A neurologic shell game?' *Archives of Neurology*, **43**, 281–182.

Fischer, S., Hallschmid, M., Elsner, A.L., Born, J. (2002) 'Sleep forms memory for finger skills.' *Proceedings of the National Academy of Sciences of the USA*, **99**, 11987–11991.

Forssberg, H., Svartengren, G. (1983) 'Hardwired locomotor network in cat revealed by a retained motor pattern to gastrocnemius after muscle transposition.' *Neuroscience Letters*, **41**, 283–288.

Fox, K., Caterson, B. (2002) 'Neuroscience: enhanced: freeing the brain from the perineuronal net.' *Science*, **298**, 1187–1189.

Freed, W.J., Medinaceli, L. de, Wyatt, R.J. (1985) 'Promoting functional plasticity in the damaged nervous system.' *Science*, **227**, 1544–1552.

Fukuchi-Shimogori T, Grove E.A. (2001) 'Neocortex patterning by the secreted signaling molecule FGF8.' *Science*, **294**, 1071–1074.

Geschwind, N. (1974) 'Late changes in the nervous system: an overview.' In Stein, P.G., Rosen, J.J., Butters, N. (Eds) *Plasticity and Recovery of Function in the Central Nervous System.* New York: Academic Press.

Geuna, St., Barrione, P., Filogamo, G. (2002) 'Postnatal histogenesis in the peripheral nervous system.' *International Journal of Developmental Neuroscience*, **20**, 475–479.

Ghez, C., Vicario, D., Martin, J.H., Yumiga, H. (1983) 'Sensory motor processing of target central control motor programs.' *Advances in Neurology*, **39**, 61–92.

Gokhan, S., Mehler, M.F. (2001) 'Basic and clinical neuroscience applications of embryonic stem cells.' *Anatomical Record*, **15**, 142–156.

Goldberg, J.L., Barres, B.A. (2000) 'Nogo in nerve regeneration.' *Nature*, **403/6768**, 369–370.

Goldberger, M.E. (1969) 'The extrapyramidal systems of the spinal cord. II: Results of combined pyramidal and extrapyramidal lesions in the macaque.' *Journal of Comparative Neurology*, **135**, 1–26.

—— (1974) 'Recovery of movement after central nervous system lesions in monkeys.' In Stein, P.G., Rosen, J.J., Butters, N. (Eds) *Plasticity and Recovery of Function in the Central Nervous System.* New York: Academic Press.

Goldman, P.S. (1972) 'Developmental determinants of cortical plasticity.' *Acta Neurobiologiae Experimentalis*, **32**, 495–511.

—— (1974) 'An alternative to developmental plasticity: heterology of central nervous system structures in infants and adults.' In Stein, P.G., Rosen, J.J., Butters, N. (Eds) *Plasticity and Recovery of Function in the Central Nervous System.* New York: Academic Press.

Gonshor, A., Melvill-Jones, G. (1976a) 'Short term adaptive changes in the human vestibulo-ocular reflex arc.' *Journal of Physiology*, **256**, 361–379.

—— —— (1976b) 'Extreme vestibulo-ocular adaptation induced by prolonged optical reversal of vision.' *Journal of Physiology*, **256**, 381–414.

Gould, E., Reeves, A.J., Graziano, M.S., Gross, C.G. (1999) 'Neurogenesis in the neocortex of adult primates.' *Science*, **286**, 548–552.

Grether, J.K., Nelson, K.B., Dambrosia, J.M., Phillips, T.M. (1999) 'Interferons and cerebral palsy.' *Journal of Pediatrics*, **134**, 342–332.

Grillner, S. (1985) 'Neurobiological bases of rhythmic motor acts in vertebrates.' *Science*, **228**, 143–149.

Hadders-Algra, M. (2001) 'Early brain damage and the development of motor behavior in children: clues for therapeutic intervention?' *Neural Plasticity*, **8**, 31–49.

Held, R., Hein, A. (1963) 'Movement-produced stimulation with development of visually guided behavior.' *Journal of Comparative and Physiological Psychology*, **56**, 872–876.

Hepp-Reymond, M.C., Wiesendanger, M., Brunnert, A., Mackel, A., Unger, R., Wespi, J. (1970) 'Effects of unilateral pyramidotomy on conditioned finger movement in monkeys.' *Brain Research*, **24**, 544.

Kagan, J. (1982) 'Canalization of early psychological development.' *Pediatrics*, **70**, 474–483.

—— (2001) 'Biological constraint, cultural variety, and psychological structures.' *Annals of the New York Academy of Sciences*, **49**, 973–979.

Kempermann, G., Gast, D., Gage, F.H. (2002) 'Neuroplasticity in old age: sustained fivefold induction of hippocampal neurogenesis by long-term environmental enrichment.' *Annals of Neurology*, **5**, 133–134.

Kerr, F.W.L. (1975) 'Structural and functional evidence of plasticity in the central nervous system.' *Experimental Neurology*, **48**, 16–31.

Knapp, H.D., Taub, E., Berman, A.V. (1963) 'Movements in monkeys with deafferentated limbs.' *Experimental Neurology*, **7**, 305–315.

Komuro, H., Rakic, P. (1998) 'Orchestration of neuronal migration by activity of ion channels, neurotransmitter receptors and intracellular Ca^{2+} fluctuations.' *Journal of Neurobiology*, **37**, 110–130.

Kornack, D.R., Rakic, P. (1999) 'Continuation of neurogenesis in the hippocampus of the adult macaque monkey.' *Proceedings of the National Academy of Sciences of the USA*, **96**, 5768–5773.

—— (2001a) 'The generation, migration, and differentiation of olfactory neurons in the adult primate brain. *Proceedings of the National Academy of Sciences of the USA*, **98**, 4752–4755.

—— —— (2001b) 'Cell proliferation without neurogenesis in adult primate neocortex.' *Science*, **294**, 2127–2130.

Kuan, C-Y., Roth, K.A., Flavell, R.A., Rakic, P. (2000) 'Mechanisms of programmed cell death in the developing brain.' *Trends in Neuroscience*, **23**, 291–197.

Lassek, A.M. (1953) 'Inactivation of voluntary motor function following rhizotomy.' *Journal of Neuropathology and Experimental Neurology*, **12**, 83–87.

Lawrence, D.G., Hopkins, D.A. (1972) 'Developmental aspects of pyramidal motor control in the rhesus monkey.' *Brain Research*, **40**, 117–119.

Leonard, C.T., Robinson, G.A., Goldberger, M.E. (1984) 'Development and recovery of function in brain damaged neonates of cats.' *Developmental Medicine and Child Neurology*, **26**, 243. (Abstract.)

Letinic, K., Zoncu, R., Rakic, P. (2002) 'Origin of GABAergic neurons in the human neocortex.' *Nature*, **417**, 645–649.

Liston, C., Kagan, J. (2002) 'Brain development: memory enhancement in early childhood.' *Nature*, **419**, 896.

Liu, C.N., Chambers, N.W. (1958) 'Intraspinal sprouting of dorsal root axons.' *Archives of Neurology and Psychiatry*, **79**, 46–61.

—— (1971) 'A study of cerebellar dyskinesia in bilaterally deafferentated forelimbs of the monkey (Macca mulatta and Macca speciosa).' *Acta Neurobiologiae Experimentalis*, **31**, 263–289.

Llinas, R., Walton, K., Hillman, D.E. (1975) 'Inferior olive: its role in motor learning.' *Science*, **190**, 1230–1231.

Mashilov, C.V., Kogan, B.M. (1992) 'Biologic basis of cerebral palsy.' *In* Sussman, M.D. (Ed.) *The Diplegic Child*. Rosemont, IL: American Academy of Orthopaedic Surgeons, pp. 59–64.

Mattson, M.P., Duan, W., Guo, Z. (2003) 'Meal size and frequency affect neuronal plasticity and vulnerability to disease: cellular and molecular mechanisms.' *Journal of Neurochemistry*, **84**, 417–431.

Meyer-Francke, A., Barres, B.A. (1999) 'Astrocyte-induced adhesion of axons and oligodendrocytes.' *Journal of Neuroscience*, **19**, 1049–1061.

Miles, F.A., Fuller, J.H. (1974) 'Adaptive plasticity in the vestibulo-ocular responses of the rhesus monkey.' *Brain Research*, **80**, 512–516.

Modo, M., Stroemer, R.P., Tang, E., Patel, S., Hodges, H. (2002) 'Effects of implantation of stem cells on behavioral recovery from stroke damage.' *Stroke*, **33**, 2270–2278.

Mott, F.W., Sherrington, C.S. (1895) 'Experiments on the influence of sensory nerves upon movement and nutrition of the limbs.' *Proceedings of the Royal Medical Society of London*, **57**, 81–88.

Müller, H.W., Gebicke-Härter, P.J., Hangen, D.H., Shooter, E.M. (I 985) 'A specific 37,000-Dalton protein that accumulates in regenerating but not in nonregenerating mammalian nerves.' *Science*, **228**, 499–501.

Neligan, G.A. (1974) 'The human brain growth spurt.' *Developmental Medicine and Child Neurology*, **16**, 677–678.

Nirenberg, M., Wilson, S.P., Higashida, H., Rotter, A., Krueger, K.E., Busis, N., Ray, R., Kenimer, J.G., Adler, M. (1985) 'Modulation of synapse formation by cyclic adenosine monophosphate.' *In* Abelson, P.H., Butz, E., Snyder, S.H. (Eds) *Neuroscience*. Washington, DC: American Association for the Advancement of Science, pp. 118–129.

Nolte, J. (2002) *The Human Brain, 5th edn*. St Louis: CV Mosby.

Oppenheim, R.W., Flavell, R.A., Vinsant, S., Prevette, D., Yuan, Chia-Y., Rakic, P. (2001) 'Programmed cell death of developing mammalian neurons after genetic deletion of caspases.' *Journal of Neuroscience*, **21**, 4752–4760.

Parella, P., Barro, G. (1973) 'Behavioral development after forelimb deafferention on day of birth in monkey with and without blinding.' *Science*, **181**, 959–960.

Penfield, W., Rasmussen, T. (1952) *The Cerebral Cortex of Man*. New York: Macmillan.

Pizzorusso, T., Medini, P., Berardi, N., Chierzi, S., Fawcett, J.J., Maffei, L. (2002) 'Reactivation of ocular dominance plasticity in the adult visual cortex.' *Science*, **298**, 1248–1251.

Plomin, R., Emde, R.N., Braungart, J.M., Campos, J., Corley, R., Fulker, D.W., Kagan, J., Reznick, J.S., Robinson, J., Zahn-Waxler, C. (1993) *Child Development*, **64**, 1354–1376.

Rakic, P. (1985) 'Limits of neurogenesis in primates.' *Science*, **227**, 1054–1056.

—— (1999a) 'The importance of being well placed and having the right connections.' *Annals of the New York Academy of Sciences*, **882**, 90–106.

—— (1999b) 'Discriminating migrations.' *Nature*, **400**, 315–316.

—— (2000) 'Illegal immigrations.' *Neuron*, **27**, 409–410.

—— (2001) 'Neocreationism—making new cortical maps.' *Science*, **294**, 1011–1012.

—— (2002a) 'Evolving concepts of cortical radial and areal specification.' *Progress in Brain Research*, **136**, 265–280.

—— (2002b) 'Neurogenesis in the adult primate neocortex: an evaluation of the evidence.' *Nature Reviews. Neuroscience*, **3**, 65–71.

—— (2002c) 'Adult neurogenesis in mammals: an identity crisis.' *Journal of Neurosciences*, **22**, 614–618.

—— Lombroso, P.J. (1998) 'Development of the cerebral cortex: I. Forming the cortical structure.' *Journal of the American Academy of Child and Adolescent Psychiatry*, **37**, 116–117.

Ramón y Cajal, S. (1928) *Degeneration and Regeneration of the Nervous System*. (Translation by May, R.M. from the 1913 Spanish edition.) London: Oxford University Press.

Riess, P., Zhang, E., Saatman, K.E., Laurer, H.L., Longhi, L.G., Raghupathi, R., Lenzlinger, P.M., Lifshitz, J., Boockvar, J., Neugebauer, E., Snyder, E.Y., McIntosh, Y.K. (2002) 'Transplanted neural stem cells survive, differentiate, and improved neurological motor function after experimental traumatic brain injury.' *Neurosurgery*, **51**, 1043–1052.

Rodriguez, C.I., Dymecki, S.M. (2000) 'Origin of the precerebellar system.' *Neuron*, **27**, 475–486.

Rose, J., McGill, K.C. (1998) 'The motor unit in cerebral palsy.' *Developmental Medicine and Child Neurology*, **40**, 270–277.

Rosner, B.S. (1974) 'Recovery of function and localization of function in historical perspective.' *In* Stein, D.B., Rosen, J.J., Butters, N. (Eds) *Plasticity and Recovery of Function in the Central Nervous System*. New York: Academic Press.

Rubenstein, J.L., Rakic, P. (1999) 'Genetic control of cortical development.' *Cerebral Cortex*, **9**, 521–523.

Rymer, W.Z. (1992) 'The neurophysiologic basis of spastic muscle hypertonia.' *In* Sussman, M.D. (Ed.) *The Diplegic Child*. Rosemont, IL: American Academy of Orthopaedic Surgeons, pp. 21–29.

Schade, J.P., Von Groenigen, W.B. (1961) 'Structural organization of the human cerebral cortex. 1. Maturation of the middle frontal gyrus.' *Acta Anatomica*, **47**, 74–111.

Schalow, G. (2001) 'On-line measurement of human CNS re-organization.' *Electromyography and Clinical Neurophysiology*, **41**, 225–242.

Schieber, M.H. (2002) 'Training and synchrony in the motor system.' *Journal of Neuroscience*, **22**, 5277–5281.

Schneider, G.E., Jhaveri, S.R. (1974) 'Neuroanatomical correlates of spared or altered function after brain lesion in the newborn hamster.' *In* Stein, P.G.,

Rosen, J.J., Butters, N. (Eds) *Plasticity and Recovery of Function in the Central Nervous System*. New York: Academic Press.

Semmes, J., Chow, K.L. (1955) 'Motor effects of lesions of the precentral gyrus and of lesions sparing this area in monkeys.' *Archives of Neurology and Psychiatry*, **73**, 546–566.

Shankle, W.R., Landing, B.H., Rafii, M.S., Schiano, A., Chen J.M., Hara, J. (1998) 'Evidence for a postnatal doubling of neuron number in the developing human cerebral cortex between 15 months and 6 years.' *Journal of Theoretical Biology*, **191**, 115–140.

Shepherd, G.M. (1994) *Neurobiology, 3rd edn*. New York and Oxford: Oxford University Press.

Shik, M.L., Severin, F.C., Orlovskii, G.N. (1966) 'Control of walking and running by means of stimulation of the mid-brain.' *Biofizika*, **11**, 659–666.

Sidman, R.L., Rakic, P. (1973) 'Neuronal migration, with special reference to developing human brain: a review.' *Brain Research*, **62**, 1–35.

Sookvanichsilp, N., Tiangda, D., Yuennan, P. (2002) 'Effects of raw garlic on physical performance and learning behavior in rats.' *Phytotherapy Research*, **16**, 732–736.

Stephenson, R. (1993) 'A review of neuroplasticity. Some implications for physiotherapy in the treatment of lesions of the brain.' *Physiotherapy*, **79**, 699–704.

Swann, J.W., Pierson, M.G., Smith, K.L., Lee, C.L. (1999) 'Developmental neuroplasticity roles in early life seizures and chronic epilepsy.' *Advances in Neurology*, **79**, 203–216.

Taub, E., Berman, A.J. (1968) 'Movement and learning in the absence of sensory feedback.' *In* Freedman, S.J. (Ed.) *Neuropsychology of Spatially Oriented Behavior*. Homewood, IL: Dorsey Press.

—— Parella, P., Barro, G. (1973) 'Behavioral development after forelimb deafferention on day of birth in monkey with and without blinding.' *Science*, **181**, 959–960.

Teuber, H.L. (1971) 'Mental retardation after early trauma to the brain: some issues in search of facts.' *In* Angle, C.R., Bearing, E.A. Jr (Eds) *Physical Trauma as an Etiological Agent in Mental Retardation*. Bethesda, MD: National Institutes of Health.

Thompson, R.F. (2000) *The Brain. A Neuroscience Primer, 3rd edn*. New York: Worth.

Thompson, P.M., Sowell, E.R., Gogtay, N., Giedd, J.N., Vidal, C.N., Hayashi, K.M., Leow, A., Nicolson, R., Papoport, J.L., Toga, A.W. (2005) 'Structural MRI and brain development.' *International Review of Neurobiology*, **67**, 285–323.

Trojan, S., Pokorny, J. (1999) 'Theoretical aspects of neuroplasticity.' *Physiological Research (Czech Republic)*, **48**, 87–97.

Tsukahara, N., Murahami, F. (1983) 'Axonal sprouting and recovery of function after brain damage.' *Advances in Neurology*, **39**, 1073–1084.

Twitchell, T.E. (1954) 'Sensory factors in purposive movement.' *Journal of Neurophysiology*, **17**, 239–252.

Ullian, E.M., Sapperstein, S.K., Barres, B. (1999) 'Glia enhance presynaptic maturation and function.' *Society for Neuroscience Abstracts*, **25**, 519.

Valenstein, E.S. (2002) 'The discovery of chemical neurotransmitters.' *Brain and Cognition*, **49**, 73–95.

Vanderhorst, V.G., Terasawa, E. Ralston, H.J. 3rd (2002) 'Axonal sprouting of a brainstem-spinal pathway after estrogen administration in the adult female rhesus monkey.' *Journal of Comparative Neurology*, **454**, 82–103.

Villablanca, J.R., Hovda, D.A. (1999) 'Developmental neuroplasticity in a model of cerebral hemispherectomy and stroke.' *Neuroscience*, **95**, 625–637.

Wagner, A.K., Kline, A.E., Sokoloski, J., Zafonte, R.D., Capulong, E., Dixon, C.E. (2002) 'Intervention with environmental enrichment after experimental brain trauma enhances cognitive recovery in male but not female rats.' *Neuroscience Letters*, **334**, 165–168.

Walker, M.P., Brakefield, T., Morgan, A., Hobson, J.A., Stickgold, R. (2002) 'Practice with sleep makes perfect: sleep-dependent motor skill learning.' *Neuron*, **35**, 205–211.

Wilson, D.M. (1968) 'The flight control system of the locust.' *Scientific American*, **218**, 83–90.

Woodbury, D., Reynolds, K., Black, I.B. (2002) 'Adult bone marrow stromal cells express germline, ectodermal, endodermal, and mesodermal genes prior to neurogenesis.' *Journal of Neuroscience Research*, **69**, 908–917.

Wolff, J.R., Joo, F., Kasa, P. (1993) 'Modulation by GABA of neuroplasticity in the central and peripheral nervous system.' *Neurochemistry Research*, **18**, 453–461.

Windle, W.F. (1956) 'Regeneration of axons in the vertebrate central nervous system.' *Physiological Reviews*, **36**, 427–440.

5
PROGNOSIS AND STRUCTURAL CHANGES

The prognosis for function of a child with cerebral palsy is uppermost in the minds of parents who consult the physician or therapist. Parents want to anticipate and plan. Prognosis and natural history are also extremely important in assessing the outcome of treatment: whether this involves surgery, physical or occupational therapy, or a neuropharmacological approach. For this we need to understand the structural changes that have occurred in the brain, and in the muscles, bones and joints due to the motor disorder as the child grows into adulthood. If possible, we also need to know what further changes in the musculoskeletal system will cause further disability in adult life.

MOTOR PROGNOSIS

WALKING PROGNOSIS TESTS
When a child is diagnosed as having cerebral palsy, the first question asked by the parents is always 'Will he walk?' The second is usually 'When?' and the third is 'What can we do to make him walk?' Prognostic tests for eventual walking of the infant with cerebral palsy older than 12 months have been reported as reliable. No longer can the clinician evade the question of predicting walking, and no longer can xyz special therapies be credited as effective in creating the ability to walk. Before embarking on 'treatment' it should be essential to consider the prognosis and natural history.

No longer can the clinician evade the question of predicting walking and no longer can xyz special therapies be credited as effective in creating the ability to walk.

Predictability should be within a probability, i.e. 80% or better. To try to answer the questions of parents concerned with walking ability of their child with something more than a shrug or a categorical 'Never!' Bleck (1975) did a prospective study of infants and children with cerebral palsy. The study was based upon testing for retained infantile automatisms which should not be present at age 12 months or later and postural reflexes which should be present at that time. Bleck tested 73 infants and children who were 12 months of age or older and not walking. A prognosis for walking was given, and then they were followed to the age of at least 7 years. The oldest patient followed at the time of publication in 1975 was born in 1962.

The following seven tests (Fiorentino 1963; see also Chapter 2) were done and one point assigned if the automatism was definitely and unequivocally present or the normal postural reflex was absent: (1) asymmetric tonic neck reflex, one point; (2) neck right reflex, one point; (3) Moro reflex, one point; (4) symmetric tonic neck reflex, one point; (5) extensor thrust, one point; (6) parachute reaction (should be present), one point if absent; (7) foot-placement reaction (should be present), one point if absent.

A score of two points or more gave a poor prognosis for walking, a one-point score was a guarded prognosis ('might walk'), and a zero score indicated a good prognosis.

The results were analyzed after the child's 7th birthday. To qualify as walkers, children had to walk a minimum of 15 meters without falling. Those who could walk with crutches were also considered functional walkers in the study. Children who walked only with the aid of a mobility device or only in parallel bars were not considered functional walkers. The accuracy of these predictions was 94.5%.

Of the 73 children followed, 54 became ambulatory while 19 never walked. Sixteen of these non-ambulators had been given an initial poor prognosis (2 points or more), and all had total body involvement with either spastic paralysis in all four limbs or athetosis. Three of 49 children with an initially good prognosis never walked. One was seen at age 10 months, but when he returned at 16 months the prognosis was downgraded to poor. Bleck concluded this prognostic testing was not reliable before the age of 12 months. Another child had severe seizure disorder necessitating heavy anticonvulsant medications. The third child with an initially good prognosis walked only limited distances at age 7. In subsequent follow-up of seven children who had a score of one point and a guarded prognosis, all eventually did walk with crutches; but generally by the age of 10–12 years, and most depended upon their wheelchairs for anything but short distances in the home. These patients had a strong extensor thrust, and although their lower limbs were in extension posture, the absence of flexion of the knee precluded efficient walking. Their energy consumption was too great.

In 1997, Bleck repeated these prognostic signs in children who were not walking over the age of 7 years in the United States and other countries confirming their reproducibility and predictability (unpublished observations). The three most important predictors are: (1) absent parachute reaction; (2) the persistent asymmetrical tonic neck reflex; and (3) the extensor thrust.

Sala and Grant (1995) also found that primitive reflexes and postural reactions as well as the gross motor skills and the type of cerebral palsy were the main factors in predicting walking. Badell-Ribera (1985), in a prospective study of 50 children with spastic diplegia who became independent walkers, noted that they had achieved sitting and crawling between ages 18 and 30 months.

A 22-year study by Campos da Paz *et al.* (1994) of 272 patients with the spastic type of cerebral palsy related the prognosis to the attainment of three motor milestones: head balance, sitting, and crawling. Those who walked independently or with support had achieved head balance by 9 months; those who never walked failed to achieve head balance by 20 months. All children who walked were able to sit by 24 months; the majority who were unable to sit unsupported by 36 months were unable to walk. If crawling was achieved by 30 months, walking eventually occurred; if crawling could not be done by 61 months, they failed to walk (Fig. 5.1).

Molnar and Gordon (1974) studied 233 non-walking children with cerebral palsy, and found that under the age of 2 years the ability to sit independently was not a good predictor of walking; *inability to sit alone after the age of 4 years did predict non-walking.*

AGE OF WALKING

In Bleck's study it was observed that walking ability reached a plateau by the age of 7 years. An interesting coincidence is the 'age of reason' declared by theologians in not permitting children younger than age 7 years to receive their first communion in the Church. Crothers and Paine's data on walking ability (1959) show practically the same age when no further walking occurred (Fig. 5.2). A study by Beals (1966) also showed that motor performance in children who had spastic diplegia reached a plateau at age 7 years (Fig. 5.3). The data on development of mature gait by Sutherland *et al.* (1980) confirmed that all gait electromyograms, major determinants of gait and linear measurements were of the adult type at age 7 years.

All of our children with hemiplegia walked between the ages of 18 and 21 months. Most children with spastic diplegia were walking by 48 months. In another study by Robson (quoted by Chaplais and MacFarland 1984) the mean age of walking for hemiplegic children was 15 months, and 24 months for spastic diplegia. In the study by Campos da Paz *et al.* (1994) independent walking occurred by 34 months, but for those who walked with external support the time was up to 108 months.

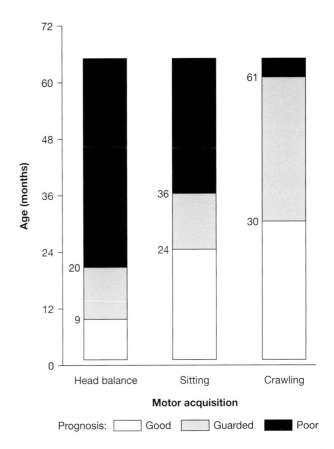

Fig. 5.1. Prognosis according to ages of attainment of milestones: head balance, sitting and crawling. Head balance before 9 months indicates a good prognosis and after 20 months, poor prognosis for motor control. Sitting by 24 months favors a good prognosis. Crawling by 30 months may indicate a good prognosis. (Reproduced from Campos da Paz *et al.* 1994, by permission.)

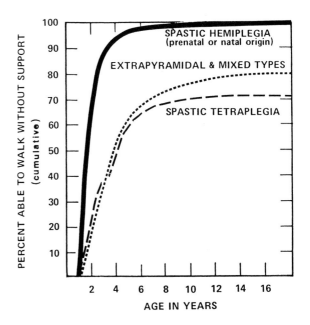

Fig. 5.2. Percentage of 289 patients with cerebral palsy able to walk according to age. Note that the ability to walk ceases for all groups about the age of 7 years. (Redrawn from Crothers and Paine 1959.)

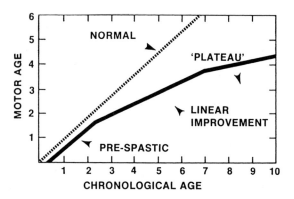

Fig. 5.3. Graphic representation of progressive improvement in motor performance of children with spastic diplegia. Note no change after age 7 years. (Redrawn from Beals 1966.)

TABLE 5.I
Walking prognosis in spastic diplegia

Severity index	Prognosis
12 or more	Free walking by 7 years
10–11	Lowest score consistent with free walking
9	Crutch walking
9–0	No walking

From Beals (1966)

Generally parents become concerned if their child is not walking by 18 months. Late walkers were defined by Johnson *et al.* (1990) as not walking by the age of 18 months in a population of 4275 infants who either weighed less than 2000 g at birth or had an admission to a special-care neonatal nursery. Using a questionnaire, home health visitors in the Oxford region of the UK identified 410 late walkers. Of these 33% had cerebral palsy diagnosed at the age of 3 years and concluded that late walking is a simple marker of morbidity in the low-birthweight infant.

In a detailed study of 242 late-walking children (Chaplais and MacFarland 1984), 5.8% were found to have some neurological abnormality (3.5% having cerebral palsy). Late walkers otherwise were called 'idiopathic'; 48% of these children had bottom shuffling as their method of locomotion. A positive family history for delayed walking was found in 50% of their first-degree relatives. The age of walking was 19.5 months in 50% and 24 months in 97%. These idiopathic and probably genetically determined late walkers had general hypotonia and increased joint laxity.

The prognosis of at-risk infants before the age of one year demands great caution. Nelson and Ellenberg (1982), who examined 32,000 children before age 1 year and again at 7 years, showed that the diagnosis of cerebral palsy was made early in 229, but at age 7 years 118 of these were free of motor disability. In this group, about 20% had early-intervention physical therapy. This study clearly demonstrates children who 'outgrew' cerebral palsy. *Motor prognosis should not be made before the age of 12 months.* This is not surprising, given what we know about central nervous system development (see Chapter 4).

OTHER PROGNOSTIC INDICATORS FOR WALKING

To predict walking in children who had spastic diplegia, Beals (1966) devised a motor quotient and a severity index. The motor quotient was derived by division of the chronological age divided by the motor age. Motor age was determined by standard tests such as those referenced in Chapter 3. The prognosis according to the motor quotient was as follows: if 30 or more, free walking

would occur; if 16 or below, no ambulation could be expected. The test results were uniform up to the age of 2 years; at later ages (to the age of 5) they had increasing variability. A major finding of this study was that motor gains reached a plateau or ceased between the ages of 6 and 7 years (Fig. 5.3).

Beals (1966) also devised a severity index based upon the motor age in months for 3-year-old children (Table 5.I). These scores were applied to the anticipated locomotor functional goals when considering orthopaedic surgery. If the severity index was 0–9, surgery was not recommended for the goal of free walking; an index of 10–11 indicated that walking was a reasonable goal to be enhanced by surgery. If the severity index was 12–18, free ambulation was thought possible, but surgery was recommended only to improve gait.

Italian neurologists found only two predictive factors for walking in 31 children with either spastic diplegia or triplegia, aged 9–18 months, and followed to a mean of 30 months (Fedrizzi *et al.* 2000). They used an 18-item functional assessment ranging from lifting the head when prone to walking without support. At the end of the follow-up, 58% walked either independently or with external support; 42% did not walk. Visual acuity was important; all who walked had normal vision. None of the children who did not walk were able to rise upright from the prone position before age 18 months. Most who became independent walkers were able to rise from the prone position by 18 months and all by 24 months.

Bose and Yeo (1975) proposed a scoring system to determine severity of gross motor function at any age. Their objective was to select children who might benefit most from treatment and to assess the results of treatment programs. Similar scoring methods were devised by Forbes and McIntyre (1968) and Reimers (1972). All of these systems used demerit points (e.g. sitting impossible, −30; standing impossible, −30; and a total score below 25 indicating that walking was possible). These methods of scoring described the extent of the disability, but had limited predictive value. In a literature search no further references to these scoring methods in predicting ambulation were found. Numerical scores have been helpful in assessing potential for functional goals and in assessing results of management to achieve goals by us. These methods and results are described in Chapter 6.

Mental retardation has little if any effect on the ability to walk (Molnar and Gordon 1974). Shapiro *et al.* (1979) studied 152 children with profound mental retardation (IQ below 25) who had neither an acquired nor a progressive degenerative disease, and found that walking began at a mean age of 30 months. The majority (95.2%) of the children who had no major neurological disability walked by age 6 years. Walking occurred in 63.6% of those who had both mental retardation and seizure disorders, and in only 10% who also had cerebral palsy. These authors concluded that 'cognition is a less important determinant of the ability to walk than is the basic neurological integrity'. It is evident that motor assessment alone cannot determine mental retardation.

PROGNOSIS FOR GROSS MOTOR FUNCTION

The Gross Motor Function Measure (GMFM), developed by the Canadians (Russell *et al.* 1989, Palisano *et al.* 1997) and now widely used to assess children who have cerebral palsy, evolved into the Gross Motor Function Classification System (GMFCS; Wood and Rosenbaum 2000, Palisano *et al.* 2000) (Table 5.II) Rosenbaum and colleagues (2002) developed from 2,632 assessments at 19 treatment facilities useable data in 657 children aged 1–13 years. All children were treated with a variety of developmental therapies. By using scores derived from the GMFM of 66 items the authors showed differences in the rates and limits of motor development according to the severity of the cerebral palsy.[1] From the scores of the GMFM they constructed five motor-development curves—one for each of the five levels in the classification system (Fig. 5.4). The rate parameters from non-linear growth models were transformed to the age in years when children are expected to reach 90% of their motor development potential. The result was a trend for faster progression to the limit of their potential as severity of the impairment increased. For example, children at level III can be expected to reach 90% of their potential by about 3.7 years. The curves reach a plateau at about the age of 7 years for all levels.

The curves of progress in motor function were developed from children with cerebral palsy who did not use assistive devices

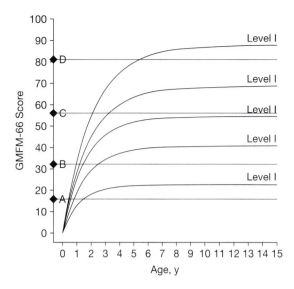

Fig. 5.4. Predicted Average Development by the Gross Motor Function Classification System Levels. The black diamonds on the vertical axis identify 4 Gross Motor Function Measure-66 (GMFM-66) that predict when children are expected to have a 50% chance of completing that item successfully. Item 21 (◆A) (GMFM-66) assesses whether a child can lift and maintain his/her head in a vertical position with trunk support by a therapist while sitting. Item 24 (◆B) assesses whether when in a sitting position on a mat, a child can maintain sitting supported by his/her arms for 3 seconds. Item 69 (◆C) measures a child's ability to walk forward 10 steps unsupported. Item 87 (◆D) assesses the task of walking down ten steps alternating feet with arms free. (Adapted from Rosenbaum *et al.* 2002 by permission of the *Journal of the American Medical Association*)

such as crutches or walkers and the scores obtained probably represent the lower limit of what children at each level can accomplish. Posterior rootlet rhizotomy, botulinum toxin injections and intrathecal baclofen do not have a major impact on function as measured by the GMFM-66 (Rosenbaum *et al.* 2002).

As cautioned by the authors, motor function levels as defined in this study do not take into account the quality and efficiency of movement, cognitive, emotional or environmental factors. However, the use of this prognostic data in developing children with cerebral palsy should be very useful in planning interventions and judging progress over time. It should help in modifying parental expectations on how much therapy is appropriate for their child.[2] As most of us know, 'the unstated goal of improving motor function at all costs (financial and otherwise) sometimes is not appropriate' (Kinsman 2002) although demanded by parents, sometimes by therapists and physicians.

'The unstated goal of improving motor function at all costs (financial and otherwise) sometimes is not appropriate.'

(Kinsman 2002)

TABLE 5. II
Gross Motor Function Classification System levels for children with cerebral palsy between the ages of 6 and 12 years (Palisano *et al.* 1997)

Level I
Walks without restrictions; limitations in more advanced gross motor skills.

Level II
Walks without assistive devices; limitations in walking outdoors and in the community.

Level III
Walks with assistive mobility devices; limitations in walking outdoors and in the community.

Level IV
Self-mobility with limitations; children are transported or use power mobility outdoors and in the community.

Level V
Self-mobility is severely limited even with the use of assistive devices
Editor note: These GMF levels were given in Chapter 3, but to spare the reader time and page flipping I have repeated them here–Repetitio Mater Est Studiorum.

---

1 The GMFM focuses on the extent of achievement of various gross motor function activities primarily in mobility and postural control, e.g. sitting, kneeling, standing on one foot, which a typical 5-year-old could accomplish. The scale is from 0 to 100; it measures change in gross-motor function and has been validated for cerebral palsy (Russell *et al.* 2002).

2 In common usage in cerebral palsy the word means physical therapy or physiotherapy that has been labeled with particular suffixes such as 'neurodevelopmental', 'Bobath', 'sensory-motor integration', Vojta, patterning, hippo, aqua.

Rosenbaum and colleagues (2002) sound a note of caution that the prognostic data should not be exaggerated by those who wish to cut costs and limit services. 'It is extremely important that parents, therapists, program managers, third-party payers, and other decision makers not assume further therapy is unhelpful or unnecessary when the curves appear to level off. Continuing efforts should be made to address ways both to increase independent activity and to promote participation of children with disabilities, as well as to address secondary impairments that may arise.' Examples of continuing efforts to improve function are usually discerned by the adolescent with cerebral palsy whose walking is inefficient and fatiguing. They tire of battling therapists' and physicians' dictates to keep struggling with exercises and take to their wheelchairs for mobility and more social experiences and educational advancement. As delineated in this chapter, structural changes in the skeleton do occur to give rise to pain and further restrictions in motor function.

EQUILIBRIUM REACTIONS

Standing equilibrium reactions, the testing for which was described in Chapter 2, are important to determine whether or not the child needs external support to walk. Children may have good prognostic signs for walking, but be unable to do so without external aids to compensate for the lack of balance. If the standing equilibrium reactions are good from side to side (lateral reactions) but deficient fore (anteriorly) and aft (posteriorly), crutches are required for support. Four-legged walkers are needed for those who have deficient equilibrium reactions in all directions. Children with spastic diplegia usually have good side-to-side and fore reactions but are poor aft. They fall backward easily with the slightest push. Despite this, they can walk independently. Table 5.III is from a study of equilibrium reactions in 116 spastic diplegic children.

Of all the motor problems in cerebral palsy, deficient equilibrium reactions interfere the most with functional walking.

Of all the motor problems in cerebral palsy, deficient equilibrium reactions interfere the most with functional walking. The need to balance on one foot and then the other in walking

stresses all of their lower-limb and trunk muscles. When external support is added, the gait immediately becomes smoother and more even. Holding the head of such children and following them while they walk is often an impressive demonstration that the major disability is not the spastic paralysis or the athetosis but the lack of balance. If we can find some way of correcting the defects in the postural mechanisms, we will have reached a milestone in therapy. Some children with spastic diplegia who needed crutches were able to do without them in the household after about the age of 10 years. Orthopaedic surgery will not necessarily alter the need for crutches or walkers—a point that needs to be emphasized to both child and parent preoperatively. Indeed crutches or walkers improve the results of lower-limb surgery, and can cover a multitude of sins.

PROGNOSIS FOR UPPER-LIMB FUNCTION

Beals (1966) used his severity index (determinations of motor age at 3 years) to predict upper-limb function. The tests included the upper limbs. The severity index scores and the prognosis for upper-limb function are shown in Table 5.IV. The most significant finding in this study was that intelligence paralleled the upper-limb severity index.

In children younger than 3 years, some generalizations appear valid. The prognosis for upper-limb function is poor when the child has no limb dominance (lateralization of hand use), or when the upper limbs are unable to cross the midline of the trunk. When stereognostic sensation in the hand is deficient, function will always be compromised. The child will have to use visual feedback exclusively to control the hands.

Is left-handedness an indicator of neurological impairment? It appears not. In a study of 114 extremely low-birthweight infants compared with 145 term infants as controls, non-right-handedness was determined at the age of 8 years (Saigal *et al.* 1992). An association between neurological impairment and non-right-handedness was found, but there was no evidence that some sort of early brain lesion resulted in subtle cognitive defects or suboptimal school performance of the non-right-handed extremely low-birthweight children.

Grip forces were found excessive in a study of 12 children with cerebral palsy compared with normal children (Eliasson *et al.* 1991). This result seemed to be due to a compensation for the lack of anticipatory control and the inefficient sensory motor integration of the hand.

Beckung and Hagberg (2002) in Göteburg, Sweden, devised a system for grading bimanual fine motor function (BFMS)

TABLE 5.III
Equilibrium reactions and need for walking aids*

Walking status	Standing equilibrium reactions			%
	Poor in all planes	Poor posterior Poor anterior Good lateral	Poor posterior Good anterior Good lateral	
Not walking	10			8.6
Walker (4-point ambulator)	5			4.3
Crutches		18		15.5
Independent			83	71.5
Totals	*15*	18	83	99.9

*Based on a 1979 study of 116 children with spastic diplegia (S. Miranda, personal communication).

TABLE 5.IV
Upper-limb function prognosis

Severity index	Prognosis
0–6	Profound disability
7–11	Moderate disability
12–17	Mild disability

From Beals (1996)

parallel with activity limitations according to the GMFCS. They found a strong correlation (0.74) between the two systems (p<0.001). Restriction in mobility was best predicted by the GMFCS, learning disability and the BFMS assessment. Restrictions in participation by the 176 children with cerebral palsy appeared to be, not surprisingly, motor function and learning disability.

Eliasson and colleagues from Sweden (2006), building on the above, described the Manual Ability Classification System (MACS). This parallels the GMFCS with broad gradations of fine motor skills. MACS evaluates the ability to handle objects, the quality and speed with which this is done, and the dependence on assistance or adaptations. There are five levels of fine motor skills (Table 3.IV). At level I, objects are handled easily, successfully but there could be some minor limitations involving dexterity or strength. There is independence in daily activities. At level II, objects are handled with reduced quality or speed. Compensatory modes can be employed to handle objects such as using a surface for support. At level III, handling objects is slow, qualitatively poor and requires supervision. Objects need to be set up in order to be handled successfully. At level IV only some parts of activities can be done. Handling objects requires assistance or adaptive equipment. At level V, the child is unable to handle objects, requires total assistance and highest activity is extremely limited to a very simple activity, e.g. pushing a button.

As the MACS instrument is used it will no doubt undergo further refinement but currently it seems to solve the issue of standardization of hand function so that children with cerebral palsy will be more readily evaluated and progress charted.

PROGNOSIS FOR FUNCTION IN ADULTS WITH CEREBRAL PALSY

While the focus of medical care in cerebral palsy is on children, the reality is that in the world life expectancy has increased to 65 years. In developed countries a long life is a statistical fact.[3] So childhood (to age 18 years) is only 25%–30% of the average life-span. Childhood is important for preparation, but most of living a life is an adult venture. For cerebral palsy, the reality is that the child with cerebral palsy becomes the adult with cerebral palsy and so it is with many chronic disabling neuromuscular or orthopaedic conditions in childhood such as spina bifida, osteogenesis imperfecta, and arthrogryposis.

Childhood is important for preparation, but most of living a life is an adult venture.

It is only in relatively recent years that the issues confronting the adult with cerebral palsy have been studied (Thomas *et al.* 1985, 1989, Bax *et al.* 1988). As children with cerebral palsy grow up they become absorbed into the adult medical-care world, where services are less focused on the specific problems of cerebral palsy. Because the prevalence of cerebral palsy is only 2.0–2.5 per 1000 livebirths, they can be hidden from view and concern as they age and live in a community.

Although cerebral palsy is a non-progressive motor disorder, musculoskeletal pain and problems occur as reflected in sporadic reports from around the world between 1993 and 2002 (Table 5.V). Functional deterioration ranged from a high of 97% in Australia (Cathels and Reddihough 1993) to a low of 25% of young adults in activities of daily living and 10%–30% for indoor and outdoor mobility in the Netherlands (van der Dussen *et al.* 2001). What clinical and environmental factors are responsible for this wide discrepancy in percentages of deteriorating function can only be assumed. One might guess that it could be Dutch pea soup (*Snert*) that made their reported experience less pessimistic than others.

The most detailed report of particular interest to orthopaedic surgeons on the fate of adults with cerebral palsy is a study by Murphy and colleagues (1995) of 101 adults in the San Francisco Bay area of the USA. The type of cerebral palsy was almost equally

TABLE 5.V
Functional deterioration in adults with cerebral palsy

Authors	Country	Per cent deterioration of function or number of cases reported
Cathels and Reddihough (1993)	Australia	97% continuing impairment/disability
Nagashima *et al.* (1993)	Japan	10 adults—cervical cord compression
Murphy *et al.* (1995)	USA, Duluth, MN	76% multiple musculoskeletal problems* 63% occurred under age 50 years
Ando and Ueda (2000)	Japan	35% primarily with involuntary head and neck movements
Andersson and Mattsson (2001)	Sweden	35% decreased walking and 9% stopped. 18% pain every day; 80% contractures 60% physically active; 54% not limited in community mobility
van der Dussen *et al.* (2001)	The Netherlands	75% independent ADL. 90% independent mobility in doors 70% outdoors
Bottos *et al.* (2001)	Italy	72 adults—function, walking distance declined

*See text and Table 5.VI for details

---

3 USA males 74.1; females 79.5; Japan 80. Sources: *World Population Prospects: The 1998 Revision* (United Nations publication Volumes I and II, Sales Nos. E.99. XIII.8 and E99.XIII.9. National Center for Health Statistics, US Department of Health and Human Services, Division of Data Services, Hyattsville, MD, 20782-2003, reviewed November 5 2002).

TABLE 5.VI
Musculoskeletal symptoms and complications, 76 adult
patients with cerebral palsy ages 19–74 years

Pain or deformity	N=76
Neck pain	46
Back pain	36
Pain in weightbearing joints	23
Hand paresthesias	10 (sensory distribution of median and ulnar nerves)
Overuse syndrome	6 (chronic repetitive and atypical use of joints or muscles)
Torticollis	3
Upper-limb contractures	22
Lower-limb contractures	64
Scoliosis	58 (> 20º–40º= 23; >40º=8)
Hip dislocation/subluxation	15
More than one problem	44

Adapted from Murphy *et al.* (1995)

divided between the spastic and dyskinetic types (athetosis, chorea or dystonia) who had ages ranging from 19 to 74 years (mean 42.6 years). Sixty-seven used wheelchairs, but 26 of them had previously been walking. 30% had a history of fractures. Fifty-seven had a total of 191 orthopaedic surgical procedures of which three were most common: Achilles tendon lengthening, adductor release, hamstring lengthening. Neck and back pain were very common complaints, along with pain in weightbearing joints, and hand paresthesias diagnosed as carpal tunnel syndrome in 20% of the dyskinetic group (Table 5.VI).

Although the 101 subjects assessed by Murphy *et al.* (1995) included only one adult with dyskinesia who had a cervical myelopathy, this late neurological complication has been reported over the years especially in Japan (Yamashita and Kuroiwa 1979, Nishihara *et al.* 1984, Fuji *et al.* 1987).[4]

The problem appears to be continuing in Japan. The experience of neurologists in Toyko might alert physicians who follow patients with cerebral palsy, particularly those who have spasticity and or athetosis affecting involuntary movements of the head and neck, might be recalled if progressive deterioration of function occurs in a patient (Nagashima *et al.* 1993). Ten patients, age 24–58 years, who had been ambulatory and independent in activities of daily living despite spasticity and/or dyskinesia, declined in function. Heralding the decline was numbness and pain in the upper limbs. This progressive dysfunction was attributed to cervical spinal canal narrowing and spinal cord shrinkage. The Japanese experience of late progressive neurological symptoms and findings in adults with athetosis or dystonia should alert clinicians to the possibility of cervical spinal cord compression.

4   Why the Japanese have more cases of cervical myelopathy in cerebral palsy than other countries might be due to a higher incidence of dyskinetic forms. Cervical myelopathy is relatively common in Japan due to ossification of the posterior longitudinal ligaments of the cervical spine without any neurological disease. When a paper on the subject was read by a Japanese orthopaedic surgeon at a Western Pacific Orthopaedic Association meeting in Bangkok, 1985, the author said 'at first we thought it might be due to soy sauce', but further investigation failed to show this association.

'The Japanese experience of late progressive neurological symptoms and findings in adults with athetosis or dystonia should alert clinicians to the possibility of cervical spinal cord compression.'
(Nagashima *et al.* 1993)

Reports concerning the deterioration of function in adults with cerebral palsy followed for 20–30 years from childhood are scarce. It is rare for a physician, therapist, or social worker to have a continuous record of functional abilities from childhood and a follow-up for years. Studies focus on the current status of the adults in a geographic area; several reports cover only young adults (17–30 years). Continuing follow-up and clinical data recording entails stability and longevity of the investigator and of the patient (in the USA 50% of the population is estimated to change residence every year) and as usual, financial support.

LIFE EXPECTANCY

Because our management of children with cerebral palsy is directed toward their adult years, it is important to have data on life expectancy. Schlesinger *et al.* (1959) and Cohen and Mustacchi (1966) did studies on longevity in cerebral palsy. The latter study reported that in 1416 persons with cerebral palsy the cumulative survival rate was 83% compared with 98% of the population at that time. Those who had the spastic type had a survival rate of 98%. As expected (Schlesinger *et al.* 1959, Cohen and Kohn 1979), those who died early were severely involved.

Based on a Medline search of English-language publications related to cerebral palsy, Rapp and Torres (2000) concluded that depending on the clinical status and the age at which survival is calculated, 65%–90% of the children survive until adulthood.

A massive study of 24,768 individuals in California derived from records of those who received services from 1980 to 1996 determined life expectancies of adults who had cerebral palsy (Strauss and Shavelle 2001). Adults who lacked skills in mobility and feeding had shortened life expectancies, as short as 11 years in those who had the worst function. Using the database from the California Department of Developmental Services, Singer and colleagues (1998) calculated the 'excess death rate' (EDR) depending on the functional level of the individual. Those with less severe cerebral palsy had an EDR of 6 per 1000 in contrast to those who had spastic quadriplegia with rate of 16 per 1000.

A survival analysis of children with cerebral palsy born between 1966 and 1989 by Hutton and Pharoah (2002) in a defined geographic area of the United Kingdom found that a severe motor disability had a 30-year survival of 42%. Reduced survival rates were in severe cognitive disability (62%) and severe visual disability (38%). The 10-year survival of low-birthweight (<2500 g) infants improved from 89% in 1989 to 97% in 1996.

In summary it appears that the life expectancy of children who have spastic hemiplegia and diplegia functioning at GMFCS level I, II or III (walk with or without assistive devices) will have a life expectancy comparable to the population with no motor disability. Those who are level IV and V (non-walkers) may have a shorter lifespan.

STRUCTURAL CHANGES

In cerebral palsy, structural changes in the musculoskeletal system due to the brain lesion are acquired after birth. Spastic paralysis accounts for the alterations in the structure and function of the muscles and secondarily in the bones and joint. Skeletal deformities occur less often in athetosis. Spinal curvature may be the result of defective postural mechanisms. Structural change, unless prevented by orthopedic surgery, occurs with the passage of time and may not cause serious disability until the child becomes 'obsolete' (i.e. an adult).[5] Therefore, as part of the prognosis we should look ahead and recognize what can happen to compromise function as the child matures, becomes an adult and goes on living.

BRAIN

Small lesions can make large impairments and large lesions small impairments.

The structural changes in the brain can arise from prenatal, perinatal and postnatal causes. The major source for the following brief description is Wigglesworth (1984). *Prenatal lesions* such as porencephaly, encephalomalacias and hydrocephalus represent the effects of intrauterine damage which might be due to cytomegalovirus, toxoplasmosis or cerebral ischemia. Wigglesworth found pathological evidence of acute anoxic damage in stillborns. The basal nuclei and brainstem showed dead neurons and reactive gliosis. In some of these cases he found histories of maternal respiratory arrest during the second trimester of pregnancy. The infants died because of damage to the respiratory center. This may be the case in infants who survive episodes of maternal hypoxia *in utero* and afterwards developed cerebral palsy, which is thought to have a genetic origin. Placental infarction due to pre-eclampsia or antepartum uterine hemorrhage may cause fetal cerebral ischemia.

Genetic and chromosomal defects or teratogenic agents do not ordinarily result in severe malformations of the brain. Genetically determined metabolic defects result in subtle changes which often are not seen at the structural level.

Perinatal causes are the familiar direct trauma at birth and resultant tearing of the tentorium or vein of Galen. With such tears the hemorrhage from the veins impairs the cerebral circulation that results in anoxic neuronal damage.

Neonatal hypoxia produces variable effects. The pattern of cerebral damage is affected by those regions of the brain that have higher metabolic activity and require greater blood flow. In the infant up to term, the areas with the greatest metabolic activity are the nuclei of the spinal cord, brainstem, midbrain, thalamus and basal ganglia. The effects of hypoxia vary from infant to infant and depend upon the status of the infant's circulatory system and cerebral perfusion.

Brain hemorrhage in the newborn is the most common phenomenon in both preterm and term infants; it has been recognized in 40%–50% of all newborns with birthweights less than 1500 g. Bleeding is from the microcirculation and arises in the subependymal cell plate near the head of the caudate nucleus. Bleeding occurs with greater frequency in the respiratory distress syndrome, which is characterized by hypercapnia and metabolic acidosis. Bleeding can break through to the ventricles. Reducing the cerebral neonatal hemorrhage is the challenge to neonatologists (Perlman *et al.* 1985). The extent of cerebral damage due to subependymal and intraventricular hemorrhage can be quite variable. There might be a small or large ventricular clot, or extensive spread of blood into the brain tissue, or CSF obstruction with secondary hydrocephalus.

It is thought that hemorrhage and ischemia often coexist. Ischemia results in periventricular leukomalacia. This structural change in the brain which occurs more frequently in preterm infants is believed to be responsible for cerebral palsy; the majority of these cases have spastic diplegia. At postmortem, the areas of affected brain show softening and early coagulation necrosis. In later stages white spots due to areas of fat-laden histiocytes are found, and still later after birth glial scars and cystic areas are found.

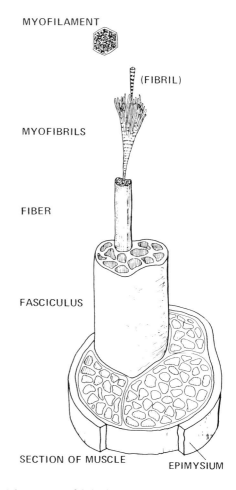

Fig. 5.5. The structure of skeletal muscle. The myofilament is comprised of the two major muscle proteins, actin and myosin. (Reproduced from Bleck & Nagel 1982.)

5 'Adults are obsolete children' (Oscar Wilde).

Bilirubin encephalopathy is due to the cellular effects of bilirubin. It alters cell function by depressing cell respiration, by affecting the mitochondrial chemistry of oxidative phosphorylation, and by inhibiting the formation of protein from the amino acids. The pathological postmortem findings are bilirubin stains of brain regions similar to those affected by cardiac arrest: thalamus, basal ganglia, midbrain and brainstem.

Wigglesworth (1984) states that after 28 weeks of gestation, the capacity of the fetal brain for remodeling is greater than that of older fetuses and infants. At this age only rudimentary connections are present. Recovery from fetal cerebral ischemia may be greater than at a later age. In general, large lesions produce significant neurological signs. However, there are reports of infants who have small brain lesions yet have major disabilities, and conversely infants with large lesions have had minor difficulties. All we can conclude from these accounts is that as cerebral imaging techniques become more and more feasible, clinicians need to be prudent in predicting the eventual severity of the neurological manifestations based solely upon presumed cerebral damage depicted in the brain images.

MUSCLE (Fig. 5.5)

MUSCLE CONTRACTION, TENSION, TONE

The basic functional unit of muscle, the motor unit, consists of a motor neuron, the neuromuscular junction and the muscle fibers innervated by the motor neuron (Fig. 5.6).

In spastic paralysis in children, there is excessive contraction of the involved muscles and with growth, some muscles become contracted. Excessive contractions of the muscles are due to increased stretch reflexes, which are a function of the spinal-cord reflex arc. In addition to the cross-sectional size of the muscle and the length, number and arrangement of its fibers in generating movement of the limb joints and the force exerted, other properties of the muscle and its tendon are operative.

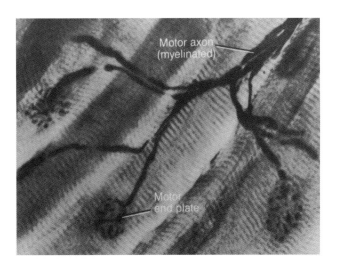

Fig. 5.6. The motor unit under electron microscopy. The myelinated motor axon terminates at the motor endplate at the neuromuscular junction and innervates the skeletal muscle fibers. (Reproduced from Carnack 1987, by permission.)

If the nerve supply to a muscle is cut experimentally, stretch of the muscle produces only a small increase in tension, due to the inherent elastic properties of the muscle and its tendon. Muscle 'tone' is frequently used to define the status of spastic muscles. But what is it? It seems as if tone is used to define resistance to movement. Noting the absence of electrical activity in resting muscle, i.e. no reflex activity, 'muscle tone' is a combination of inertia, spring stiffness, viscosity and thixotropy (Walsh 1992). Thixotropy connotes a property of a substance to change state during agitation, stirring or movement. Muscles exhibit this property when overstretched by developing stiffness. Short-range stiffness has been attributed to the formation of cross-bridges between the actin and myosin filaments in the muscle which are disrupted by excessive motion and then reform after the motion ends (Hill 1968).

Muscles can be stretched about 3% of their length before breaking down, and tendons about 6% of their length before rupturing (Alexander 1984). The stretch reflex is responsible for the greatly increased tension in muscle action. The elastic properties of the muscle and tendon probably serve as springs to store energy during walking and running as 'flexible force transmitting elements' (Alexander 1984, Walsh 1992). Very short muscle fibers can have disproportionately long tendons as in the human flexor pollicis longus. As a fascinating example of tendon function, Walsh cited the observations of Alexander (1989) on the rudimentary plantaris muscle and its tendon in the camel. This muscle consists of fibers only about 2 mm long with a tendon about 125 cm long that courses from the posterior aspect of the knee to the toe. The tendon serves as a passive spring. 'In this exceptional case, the best muscle is no muscle at all.' Australians will immediately recognize the same mechanism in the kangaroo as it bounces along, storing energy in its tendons on landing, and releasing the energy on ascending (Alexander 1988).

MUSCLE CONTRACTURE

Where is the contracture in spastic muscles? We observe that prolonged spasticity in the muscle of a growing child often leads to a shortening of the muscle ('myostatic contracture'). Histological studies with ordinary staining techniques and light microscopy fail to show fibrosis that would be expected. O'Dwyer *et al.* (1989) found no structural changes in spastic muscles except a decrease in the number of sarcomeres per fiber (Fig. 5.7). The muscle shortens.

From the work of Tardieu (1984) and colleagues (1971, 1977, 1979, 1982), it appears that in normal cats the length of the sarcomere in the muscle fiber remains constant for a given angle of ankle dorsiflexion, irrespective of the age or size of the animal, and is an adaptation to skeletal growth. When the cat's triceps surae muscle is immobilized, the tension-extension curve is more abrupt; the muscle has decreased strength, histological evidence of atrophy, and (with electron microscopy) a decrease in the number of sarcomeres. This decrease in the number of sarcomeres was also noted in the muscle biopsies of the calf muscles in children with cerebral palsy. The continued studies by these French physicians indicated that there were two different

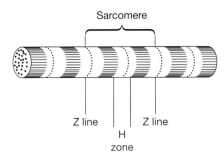

Fig. 5.7. A sarcomere; the distance between two z lines comprises the repeating sacromere of the myofibril, the contractile element, of about 1/1000 of a millimeter in diameter. The dark bands are the A bands (anisotropic, so-called because of rotation of the plane of polarized light away from the eye). The lighter bands are I bands (isotropic because of minimal influence of polarized light). Z lines (Zwischenscheibe) bisect the I bands. The A bands are bisected by Hensen's zones (H zones). (Redrawn and adapted from Gamble 1988.)

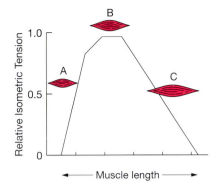

Fig. 5.8. Length-tension curve of skeletal muscle. Maximum tension at resting length (B). Either shortening (A) or lengthening (C) the muscle reduces isometric tension. (Redrawn and adapted from Gamble 1988 and Moseley 1992.)

types of spastic contracture ('hypoextensibility') in children with cerebral palsy: (I) defective 'trophic' regulation—the sarcomeres failed to increase in number during skeletal growth, and (II) normal growth regulation. In type (I), plaster-casting to stretch the muscle had no effect, but surgery did effect elongation of the muscle; in type (II) plaster-casting was more effective when tolerated. Tabary *et al.* (1971) in his study of biopsies of the spastic triceps surae muscles in 17 patients who had lengthenings of these muscles found notable increases in the length of the sarcomeres with light and electron microscopy.

In children the muscles add length in response to the elongation of the bones. Ziv *et al.* (1984) in their experimental studies in mice who have a genetic spasticity of the lower limbs suggested that muscle growth occurs at the musculotendinous junction which they termed the 'growth plate' of the muscle. New sarcomeres are added in response to the stretching of growth by the bone. When the muscle is spastic it cannot keep pace with the bone growth by adding sarcomeres. The muscle is not shortened, but merely fails to grow as rapidly at the bone. The result is a relative contracture (Moseley 1992).

Another probable cause of muscle stiffness in spasticity was described by Booth and colleagues (2001) of the Department of Zoology, Oxford University. They found convincing evidence of collagen I accumulation quantified by hydroxyproline in biopsies of the vastus lateralis muscle in 26 children with spastic diplegia or quadriplegia. This increased collagen was found in the spastic muscle's endomyesium. They also reported fibrotic regions with sparse muscle fibers. These pathological changes correlated with the severity of the spasticity according to the Ashworth Scale, ambulatory status, selective muscle control and clonus.

EFFECT OF CASTING

If the joint is immobilized in a fixed position with a plaster or fiberglass cast beyond its resting position (usually the gastrocnemius–soleus in spastic equinus), the muscle accommodates immediately to the stretch by elongation of its sarcomeres. After

a longer period of time, additional sarcomeres are added so that their normal length is restored (Moseley 1992).

EFFECT OF MUSCLE RELEASE (MYOTENOTOMY), LENGTHENING, OR TRANSFER

After release of the origin of the muscle, e.g. hip adductors, the muscle will reattach to surrounding structures and function as it did before release. If it does not find a new attachment, it will become functionless. If the tendon or muscle is cut, no new sarcomeres will be added, the muscle fails to grow, sarcomeres will be lost and the muscle fibers will shorten. Semitendinosus tenotomy has been a common procedure to relieve contracted hamstring muscles. It permanently eliminates this muscle's function. Lengthening of a muscle's tendon (e.g. Achilles) reduces muscle length as the sarcomeres decrease their lengths. Compensation occurs by reduction in the number of sarcomeres.

The effect of surgical lengthening on the muscle tension can be surmised from the well-known Blix parabolic curve of length-tension relationships (Fig. 5.8). Maximum isometric tension is present at the top of the curve at the muscle's resting length where the maximum number of cross bridges can form between the myosin and actin filaments (Gamble 1988).[6] Immediately after lengthening its maximal strength of its resting tension state will be reduced. Later on after the muscle has adjusted to its sarcomere length and restores its resting length, it will function on the down slope of the Blix curve. Its strength will be reduced. The shortened muscle will continue to function in actions that do not require 100% of its strength. Lengthening of a bipennate muscle will result in a greater loss of strength than in a unipennate muscle which has a relatively smaller number of long fibers. A greater number of the bipennate muscle-fiber excursions will be effected (Fig. 5.9). After lengthening the muscle–tendon unit will be normal in length, but the muscle will be shorter and its tendon longer (Moseley 1992).

---

6 Isometric tension: when the muscle is held at a fixed length, i.e. no work is done. Isotonic contractions: the muscle shortens under a constant load. Eccentric contractions maintain tension while the muscle is being stretched, e.g. deceleration of the leg during swing and stance phases of gait.

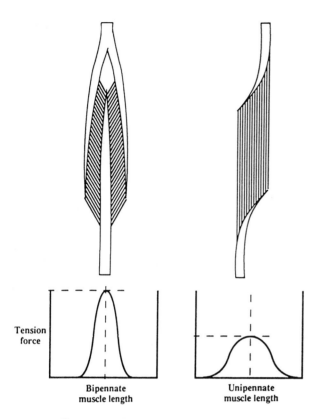

Fig. 5.9. Differences in architecture of muscles results in differing strength for the same cross-sectional area. The muscle with all short fibers has a strong but short excursion, while the muscle with long fibers has a less powerful but longer excursion. (From Moseley 1992, by permission.)

Delp and Zajac (1992) used computer modeling of simulated tendon lengthening to determine the reduction of muscle force in the commonly lengthened lower-limb muscles. The reduction in strength varies with the cross-sectional area of the muscle, its optimal fiber length,[7] pennation angle[8] and tendon length. In some muscles small changes in tendon length cause large changes in muscle force (Fig. 5.10). Pennation angles vary from 30º for the soleus, to 0º for the long head of the biceps femoris. Optimal fiber-length ratios to tendon length ranged from 0.6 for the short head of the biceps to 10 for the tibialis posterior. The computer model calculated that the maximum isometric moment[9] generated by the soleus decreased 30% with a 1 cm tendon lengthening and so theoretically argues against Achilles lengthening because it does lengthen the soleus. But lengthening of the iliopsoas tendon of 1–2 cm decreased its flexion moment by only 4% and 9% respectively and confirms the clinical impression of relative preservation of strength of this major hip-flexor when lengthened. Delp and Zajac (1992) added a caution that the data obtained did not take into account the effects of

spastic paralysis on the muscle. The calculations were based on the assumption of healthy person who was 180 cm tall.

Tendon transfer is a change in the relative position of origin to insertion, and has the same effect as lengthening. If the maximum isometric force of a muscle decreases with 1.5 cm of lengthening, the muscle force decreases the same amount if the tendon transfer decreased the distance from origin to insertion 1.5 cm. Because the muscle is sensitive to length change, the transfer should ensure that the muscle fibers are at optimal length. Generally a lower-limb tendon transfer, e.g. anterior tibial, should place the muscle under enough tension to simulate its resting length for maximum isometric tension. This becomes a matter of surgical judgement. A bit too tight is better than too loose. An old surgical rule in tendon transfers in the forearm to the hand and wrist was to pull out the muscle to its maximum length and then relax it by one-third.

MUSCLE PATHOLOGY IN CEREBRAL PALSY
In patients who had cerebral palsy and scoliosis, we found with histochemical staining of muscle biopsies neuropathic changes on both sides of the spinal curve. We found similar changes in spinal muscle biopsies in cases of idiopathic scoliosis (Bleck *et al.* 1976). These changes were alterations from the normal size and shapes as well as the distribution of fiber types.

Castle *et al.* (1979) and Romanini *et al.* (1989) used histochemical techniques in their studies of muscle biopsies of limb muscles in children with cerebral palsy and found variable atrophy and hypertrophy in type-1 and type-2 muscle fibers from normal controls. Castle and colleagues thought that the major influence on fiber-type change in cerebral palsy was due to the daily functioning of the spastic muscle.

Rose and colleagues (Rose *et al.* 1994, Rose and McGill 1998) studied the histochemistry and ultrastructure of muscle biopsies of 10 children with spastic diplegia (seven of the lateral gastrocnemius, two of the iliacus, and one of the medial hamstrings), and found significant combined coefficients of variation for type-1 and type-2 fibers. The predominance of type-1 and type-2 fibers was greater ($p \leq 0.03$) in those with cerebral palsy (67.1 %, SD 15.0%) than in controls (54.6%, SD 3.8%). The total fiber area per 100 fibers between type 1 and type 2 was significantly different from the controls ($p \leq 0.002$). In this study energy expenditure during walking was determined in eight of the subjects and electromyograms were done in six. The variations in type-1 fiber area correlated positively with the energy expenditure index ($p \leq 0.026$) as well as with the variation of type-1 and type-2 fibers ($p \leq 0.03$)[10] (Fig. 5.11). The duration of the electromyographic action potentials were 2.74 times longer during waking in the subjects with cerebral palsy.

---

7 Optimal muscle-fiber length—the length of the fiber at which active force peaks.
8 The pennation angle (from the Latin *pennatus*, feather) is the angle between the muscle fibers and its tendon.
9 Moment: a force acting at a distance about an axis of rotation to cause angular acceleration about that axis (force x distance from the center of rotation = Newton meters, Nm).

10 Type-1 fibers are slow twitch, mainly aerobic, oxidative, resistant to fatigue. Type-2 fibers are fast twitch, mainly anaerobic, store intracellular glycogen, and fatigue rapidly. Type 2a are high glycolytic and oxidative enzymes; type 2b, mainly glycolytic metabolism.

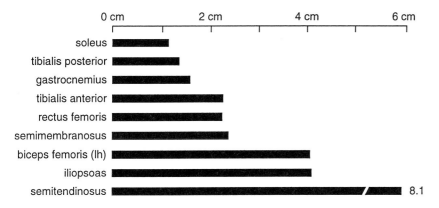

Fig. 5.10. Tendon length changes to reduce muscle spasticity by 50% in a 1.8m adult with knee flexion at 20°. (From Delp and McGill 1992.)

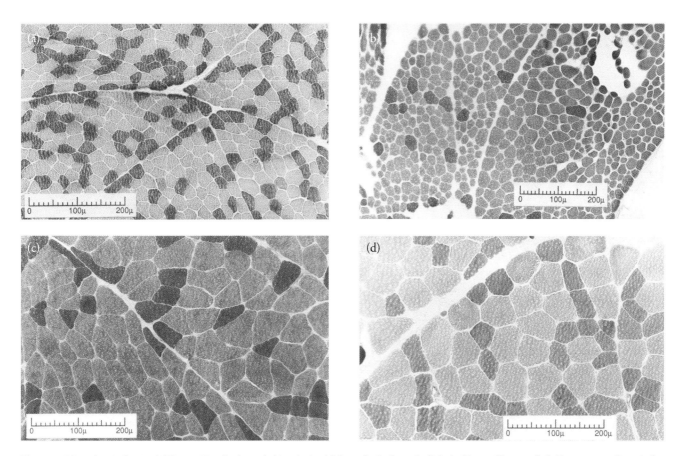

Fig. 5.11. Histochemical stains (ATPase, pH 9.4) of muscle biopsies in children who had spastic diplegia. Type-2 fibers are dark. Energy expenditure index (EEI) represents heart beats/meter) normal 0.48 ± 0.15). Electromyographic activity (EMG as % of gait cycle). Normal controls of gastrocnemius muscle 35 ± 6.3% and hamstring muscle 22 ± 5.4%. (A) Age 5 years, lateral gastrocnemius (× 50). Fairly normal distribution of type-1 and type-2 fibers. Type-1 light (63%), type-2 dark (37%). EEI 0.91. EMG 61%. (B) Age 5 years, lateral gastrocnemius (× 40), 98% type-1 fibers, 2% type 2. EEI 1.25. EMG 73%. (C) Age 10 years, medial hamstring (× 50), type 1, 73%, type 2, 27%. EEI 1.00. EMG 78%. (D) Age 14, iliacus (× 50) type 1, 63%; type 2, 37%. EEI 0.83. EMG not done. (By courtesy of Jessica Rose, PhD, PT, Motion Analysis Laboratory, Lucille Salter Packard Childrens Hospital at Stanford, Stanford, CA.)

In the study by Rose *et al.* (1994), preponderance of type-1 fibers was similar to the muscle pathology in myopathies, particularly to genetic dystrophies, and similar to the muscle biopsies in patients who have upper motor neuron lesions such as Parkinsonism and strong spasticity. Because chronic electrical stimulation of muscles at low frequency results in transformation toward type-1 fibers and increased fiber size as well as a decrease in calcium transport proteins, the increased variability in fiber size in cerebral palsy suggested the changes found in the muscles were due to prolonged stimulation that occurs in spastic paralysis. It may be that the in the muscle subjected to heightened reflex activity and spasticity, type-2 fibers respond as they do selectively to high-frequency stimulation (100 Hz) (Grimby *et al.* 1976, Jakobsson *et al.* 1988).

Based on the studies of the muscle fiber variables from the normal in the spastic muscles, Rose makes a convincing case for resistance exercises in cerebral palsy. Muscle strengthening regimens have generally been ignored in children and adults with cerebral palsy on the premise that the spastic muscle is too strong (J. Rose, unpublished observations).

EFFECTS OF IMMOBILIZATION
Because immobilization of joints and limbs is so commonly used as a method of treatment, to overcome or prevent contractures and for postoperative care, the histological effects on muscle fibers merit review. Cooper (1972) studied the effects of plaster immobilization in the adult cat soleus, gastrocnemius and flexor digitorum longus muscles. With 2 weeks of immobilization, the muscle nuclei became more prominent. In 4 weeks the nuclei were centrally located; muscle fibers were irregular in shape and size, and vacuolar degeneration of fibers was evident. After 6–22 weeks of immobilization, there was hyaline and granular degeneration but the sarcolemmic tubes were preserved. When the data were combined with those of other experiments, Cooper (1972) concluded that complete regeneration would occur in 3 months. Cooper also noted an increase in the contraction and relaxation times of muscles during immobilization. These experimental results seem clinically applicable. Should the immobilization of the limbs of patients who have had tendon lengthenings or tenotomies of spastic muscles be for only 3 weeks whenever possible? And is it probable that the good short-term results reported after plaster immobilization (inhibitive casting) for equinus deformities were due to the muscle atrophy and degeneration which occurs with immobilization?

JOINTS

HIP
The most common and serious structural change is subluxation and dislocation of the hip. This is an acquired deformity, as can be appreciated by serial radiographs of the hip beginning in the 6-month-old infant who has spasticity of the hip musculature. The configuration of the hip is normal. Due to the combination of the abnormal pull of spastic muscles, femoral torsion and the status of weightbearing subluxation is generally apparent about the age of 30–36 months with secondary acetabular dysplasia occurring after the age of 5 years. An exception would be the infant who has both a congenital dislocation of the hip and cerebral palsy; these patients' radiographs will show acetabular dysplasia very early in life. However, the incidence of congenital dislocation of the hip is only about 1 per 1000 livebirths; consequently it is not often observed in cerebral palsy. The genesis of the acquired dislocation of the hip will be discussed more fully in Chapter 9.

In patients who walk with crutches, subluxation of the hip will be 'silent' without pain for many years. Eventually, in the adolescent or young adult years, pain ensues and becomes disabling due to degenerative arthritis (Figs 5.12, 5.13). Later, subluxation of the hip results in secondary deformities of the femoral head (Fig. 5.14); the lateral aspect of the head is flattened due to the pressure of the gluteal muscles, and the ligamentum

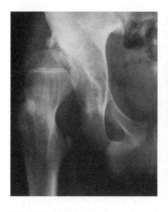 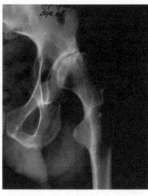

Fig. 5.12. A 'silent' subluxation of the hip which pain made evident in an 18-year-old man with spastic diplegia; walked independently with crutches.

Fig. 5.13. 61-year-old woman, spastic diplegia, used crutches. Subluxation of the hip and progressive painful degenerative joint disease.

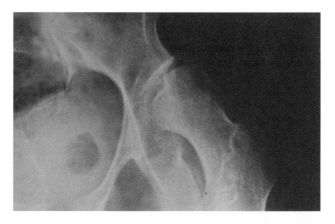

Fig. 5.14. Anterior–posterior radiograph of the hip in an 18-year-old male with spastic diplegia and independent walking with crutches. Subluxation of the hip and acetabular dysplasia. The femoral head is flattened laterally and osteoporotic. The notch in the medial central portion of the head is due to the pressure of the ligamentum teres.

teres produces a deep groove in the femoral head medially (Samilson *et al.* 1972). In dislocated hips, the femoral head articular cartilage will undergo degeneration as well as deformation (Fig. 5.15).

KNEE
Patients who walk with flexed knees develop a cephalad displacement of the patella ('patella alta') (Fig. 5.16). In older patients this can cause disabling pain due to articular cartilage degeneration (chondromalacia patellae). Deformations of the patella are common in patients who have flexed knee postures (Lottman 1976). Young patients, ranging in age from 10 to 14 years, can have knee pain with tenderness at the inferior pole of the patella. Lateral radiographs of the knee show fragmentation of the lower pole of the patella. This lesion is comparable to the sporting disability 'jumper's knee'. In cerebral palsy it is probably the constant pull of the patellar tendon on the distal pole of the patella that produces the symptoms and the radiographic findings (Cahuzac *et al.* 1979). If you live long enough and see adults you

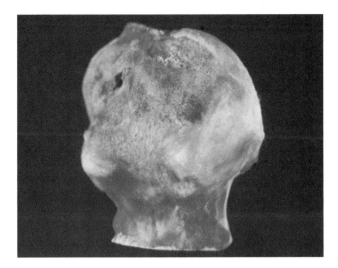

Fig. 5.15. Photograph of femoral head and neck removed in 20-year-old patient with spastic total body involvement and dislocation of the hip. Hip pain became disabling, whether in bed or wheelchair. In this anterior view of the femoral head, note extensive erosion of cartilage on the anterior and medial surfaces, and irregular contour and flattening of lateral surface. Head and neck excised because the usual surgery of subtrochanteric rotation osteotomy and pelvic osteotomy was impossible given the extensive degenerative changes.

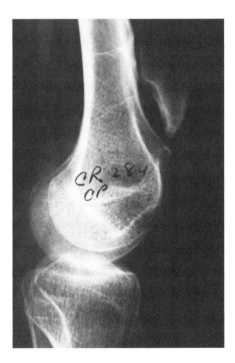

Fig. 5.16. Lateral radiograph of knee of 28-year-old man with spastic triplegia; independent walking with crutches. Had severe flexed knee gait up to the age of 12 years when he had correction with bilateral hamstring lengthening. A spastic quadriceps maintained his knee posture in extension on stance phase with ability to flex 40° on swing phase. Note cephalad displacement of patella and severe structural changes. Severe and unremitting knee pain. He has a university degree and works full time. Solution: patellectomy. The articular surface of the patella was totally covered with shredded, destroyed articular cartilage.

will encounter patients who can no longer walk due to disabling degenerative arthritis of the knee induced by long-standing flexion contractures of the knee beyond 20°. These are patients who were asymptomatic with their flexed-knee gaits until the age of 35–40 years.

ANKLE

Equinus of the ankle is the most common deformity in spastic cerebral palsy. It is not known whether the persistence of a significant ankle equinus (beyond 10°) causes disabling symptoms in adult life, because almost all patients have correction of equinus before adulthood. It seems logical and common experience that prolonged tiptoe walking would result in painful areas over the metatarsal heads. At the end of the day we all know that women in high heels kick off their shoes, and executive women in major cities walk to lunch wearing performance shoes, i.e. sneakers. These women know that walking on toes in not comfortable. Orthopaedic surgeons who care for ballerinas know that their toes wear out; taping and padding of feet of these performers is common.

Valgus deformities of the ankle joint can be a secondary change to severe pes valgus. Although we have not followed patients with valgus deformities of the distal tibial articular surface through adult life, it seems likely that these ankle joints would undergo painful degenerative arthritis. Orthopaedic surgeons who have followed adult patients with malunited fractures of the distal tibia could no doubt confirm this prediction. The abnormal tilt of the ankle joint and weightbearing will cause degenerative joint changes eventually.

FOOT

Foot varus and valgus deformities are due to subluxations at the talonavicular and calcaneocuboid joints. In the case of varus deformities, the secondary and painful condition is increased pressure with callosities on the lateral border of the foot over the base of the fifth metatarsal. In valgus deformities, the abnormal pressure is over the medial aspect of the first metatarsal head and the great toe, which is secondarily displaced into valgus. Usually adults with severe valgus deformities have to wait until past the age of 50 years before they notice disabling symptoms. These are usually due not only to the callosities on the medial border of the forefoot and great toe, but also due to degenerative arthritic changes in the talonavicular joint. Severe pes cavus does cause symptoms, usually beginning about the age of 12 years, and metatarsus adductus and hallux valgus with bunion become troublesome in adolescence. Painful flexion contractures of the toes seem to develop in the late adolescent or young adult years. The mechanisms of these foot deformities are amplified in Chapters 8 and 9.

UPPER LIMBS

The most notable skeletal change in the upper limb in patients with spasticity of the elbow flexors and the pronator teres is a posterior subluxation and (in some) a dislocation of the head of the radius. Posterior bowing of the ulna may accompany this

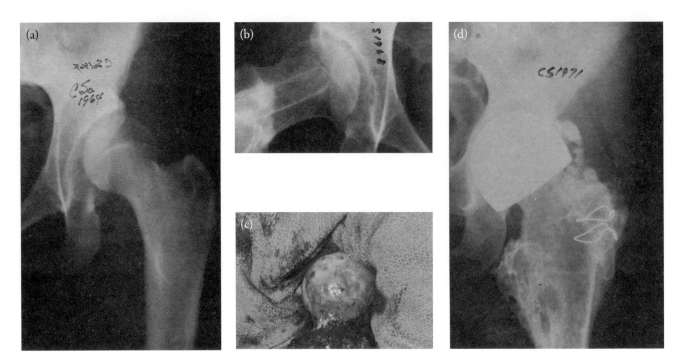

Fig. 5.17. (*a*) Anterior–posterior radiograph of the hip of a 19-year-old woman who had athetosis and spastic paralysis of the lower limbs and walked independently. Complained of severe hip pain and a crunching sound in the hip on movement. (*b*) Lateral radiograph of the same patient, after a derotation and varus subtrochanteric osteotomy had failed to relieve symptoms. (*c*) Femoral head of the same patient at time of cup arthroplasty. Large areas of the femoral head articular cartilage were eroded and not visible in the plain radiographs as shown. (*d*) Same patient, cup arthroplasty; postoperative heterotopic ossification, but motion maintained and pain-free (a more contemporary reconstruction would probably be a total hip replacement).

displacement of the radial head. This change can explain the limitation of elbow extension and the futility of gaining complete elbow extension with passive stretching or surgery.

ARTICULAR CARTILAGE

Cartilage degeneration occurs when the opposing articular surfaces are not in contact. This certainly seems to be the case in a paralytic dislocation of the hip of long duration. Complete disappearance of large segments of the articular surface of the femoral head is often seen. Similar destruction of cartilage occurs in subluxation and may be quite difficult to discern with radiographic studies until much later, when joint margin osteophytes and narrowing of the joint surface become obvious (Fig. 5.17 *a–c*). Experimental studies have demonstrated joint cartilage degeneration in non-contact opposing surfaces (Bennett and Bauer 1937, Hall 1969). In addition, cartilage needs movement of the joint for its nutrition from the synovial fluid; the nutrition of the cartilage cells is by diffusion, which occurs with movement (Ingelmark and Saaf 1948, Maroudas *et al.* 1968, Sood 1971, Freeman 1972). Articular cartilage needs movement to survive and to repair itself; Salter (Salter *et al.* 1984, Salter 1993) showed the positive effects of continuous passive motion in surgical defects of the articular cartilage of the rabbit knee joint. The clinical application of this work has been the increasing use of continuous passive motion machines in postoperative knee surgery where the integrity of the cartilage has been defective.

Compression of articular cartilage will also cause degeneration. In experimental animals, joints subjected to continuous compressive forces show gross and histological degenerative changes (Salter and Field 1960, Salter and McNeil 1965). Evidence of compression of the articular surface of the talus and degenerative changes in the ankle joint have been noted in cases of talipes equinovarus when forced manipulations of the foot with plaster casts were applied to correct the equinus deformity. It has been said that 'ligaments are hard and cartilage is soft',[11] which should subdue enthusiasm for attempts to correct a contracture by forced positioning of the joints in plaster or orthoses.

JOINT CONTRACTURE

Joint capsule contracture is superimposed on the myostatic contracture if the latter is unrelieved for several years. The major joints affected are the elbow, hip, knee and ankle. Contracture is thought to happen because of reorganization of the connective tissue that prevents the collagen fibers from gliding (Kottke 1966). Swinyard and Bleck (1985) believe that the lack of joint motion in the developing fetus causes the well-known severe joint contractures in children with arthrogryposis (multiple congenital contracture syndrome).

Experimental immobilization of rat knee joints demonstrated proliferation of subsynovial intracapsular fibers in the infrapatellar and intercondylar spaces of the knee. Connective tissue extended between joint surfaces to form adhesions and the cartilage degenerated (Evans *et al.* 1960). Parallel changes in human knee-

---

11 The late Mirhan O. Tachdjian MD (Annual International Pediatric Orthopaedic Seminars, San Francisco and Chicago).

joint immobilization for prolonged periods have been described (Enneking and Horowitz 1972).

BONES

OSTEOPOROSIS[12]

Osteoporosis of the bones does occur in cerebral palsy, but practically always in total body involved patients who are dependent on their wheelchairs and spend much of their time in bed. These patients are unable to be helped in and out of a chair. These effects are overwhelmingly due to the lack of the stress of weightbearing, and thus the effects of gravity on the bones. Since the work of Dalen and Olsson (1974), who clearly demonstrated the effects of physical activity on bone mineral content, there have been many other reports on calcium loss from the bones due to the lack of gravity. Definite loss of bone calcium has been shown in astronauts during their anti-gravity periods in flight.

Henderson *et al.* (1995) studied the incidence of osteoporosis in the proximal femora and lumbar spine in 139 children with cerebral palsy at a mean age of 9 years (range 3–15 years). They found the functional level of walking highly correlated with bone-mineral density. The earlier the child walked the better the bone density ($p<0.0005$). For years enforced standing using devices was thought to prevent osteoporosis. The authors point out that these attempts to simulate household ambulation are problematic. How much passive standing can be tolerated and for how long is not known. One study in which standing programs were discontinued resulted in no loss of bone density. Anticonvulsants were not correlated with a decrease in bone density. Those who had an intake of less than 500 mg of calcium per day had significantly lower bone-mineral densities ($p<0.05$). General good nutrition had more importance than calcium intake. Lee and Lyne (1990) reported a 42% incidence of vitamin D abnormalities in severely disabled children and young adults who had pathological fractures.

PATHOLOGICAL FRACTURES

It is not known how to prevent osteoporosis in these severely involved patients. It is well known that they are prone to fractures (McIvor and Samilson 1966, Bleck and Kleinman 1984, Brunner and Doderlein 1996). The most common fracture in Brunner and Doderlein's patients were supracondylar fractures of the femur.[13] These occur within the first year after surgery of the lower limb, due to the decreased bone mineral due to immobilization.

Most of the fractures can be treated conservatively in splints, plasters or traction. Plates and screws and intramedullary nails are not apt to hold very well in demineralized relatively soft bone. Could botulinum toxin selective myoneural blocks be used while healing of the bone occurs if muscle spasticity is causing difficulty in maintaining reasonably satisfactory alignment of the fracture fragments?

SHAFTS OF LONG BONES

The shafts of the long bones are rarely if ever deformed in spastic paralysis. Anterior bowing of the femoral shaft cannot be attributed to the spasticity of the hip-flexors. Measurements of the femoral shaft with lateral radiographs of the hip and femur in normal children, compared with 27 children who had spastic hip flexion deformities, failed to demonstrate any significant change from the normal anterior bow of the femur which had a mean of 7° and a range of 1°–20° (Bleck 1968).

TORSIONAL DEFORMATION OF BONES

Torsional deformation of the bones is their major structural change.[14] There is significant abnormal femoral anteversion for age (femoral torsion) in children with subluxation and dislocation of the hip, as well as with spastic hip-flexion internal rotation gait patterns (Lewis *et al.* 1964, Beals 1969, Bleck 1971, Baumann 1972, Fabry *et al.* 1973). In a detailed study, von Lanz and Mayet (1953) found that normal femoral anteversion is an average of 12° at the fourth embryonic month increasing to 35° at age 1–3 years with a progressive decrease to an adult man of 12° with a mean variation from 5°–20° (Hensinger 1986). The study by Fabry and colleagues (1973) reported the range of femoral anteversion as 31.3° at 1 year of age, progressively decreasing to skeletal maturity to 14°–15°. These same authors assessed femoral torsion in 91 patients with cerebral palsy. In this group the degree of torsion at age 3 years remained essentially the same throughout growth. Femoral torsion in children who have cerebral palsy at age 4 years does not improve with time (Fig. 5.18).

Bobroff *et al.* (1999) analyzed the femoral anteversion and neck-shaft angle using a trigonometric fluoroscopic method in 147 patients (267 hips) with cerebral palsy. At young ages the femoral anteversion in the cerebral palsy group was similar to that of the normal children. However, the femoral anteversion did not decrease as the child with cerebral palsy grew older in contrast to normal children in whom the degree of femoral anteversion decreased. Neck-shaft angles were greater in the children with cerebral palsy than in normal children. No significant differences in these angles were found between those who had spastic hemiplegia, diplegia or quadriplegia.

---

12 Osteoporosis is the most common type of osteopenia, a decrease in the amount of bone tissue in the skeleton; the bone that is present has a normal proportion of mineral to matrix. Because the compressive strength of bone is proportional to the square of its apparent density, decreasing the density by a factor of two decreases the compressive strength by a factor of 4 (Gamble 1988).

13 The supracondylar femoral fracture is known as the *Oops fracture*. When attempting to stretch a knee flexion contracture into extension in a patient who has osteoporotic bone, a snap may be heard above the knee. The therapist murmurs 'Oops!' Instead of the knee-joint capsule stretching, the bone gives way, and the knee-flexion deformity is suddenly corrected.

14 *Torsion* is the preferred term when the degree of twist is greater than 2 SD from the mean. *Version* is the term when the twist is within the limits of normal for the age of the individual. So *femoral anteversion* (if you wish to be precise) only means that the twist of the head, neck and trochanter of the femur is normal.

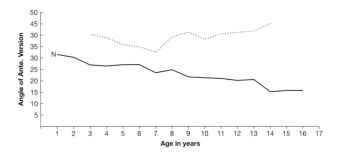

Fig. 5.18. The angle of femoral anteversion in 432 normal children from age 1 year to 16 years showing a gradual decrease (dark line) and in 91 children who had cerebral palsy (dotted line) with no change in the femoral anteversion angle from age 3 years to 14 years. (Redrawn from Fabry *et al.* 1973, Hensinger 1986.)

FEMORAL NECK-SHAFT ANGLES

The neck-shaft angles in children were not substantially different from the adult population (135º–140º) in a study by Laplaza *et al.* (1993). The neck-shaft angles are remarkably constant varying from 130º to 140º in embryonic life settling at age 4–6 years to approximately 135º (von Lanz and Mayet 1953, Shands and Steele 1958, Watanabe 1974, Hensinger 1986) (Fig. 5.19).

Neck-shaft angles greater than this are termed 'coxa valga'. With excessive femoral anteversion in cerebral palsy, anterior–posterior radiographic projections create the illusion of coxa valga—the radiograph is merely a two-dimensional shadow of the bones.[15] This radiographic illusion led to the practice of restoring the femoral neck-shaft angles with an adduction (varus) sub-trochanteric femoral osteotomy when the logical operation would have been derotation osteotomy. It is uncertain whether persistent and excessive femoral anteversion of the proximal femur (femoral torsion) in independently ambulatory patients results in late degenerative arthritis.

With excessive femoral anteversion in cerebral palsy anterior–posterior radiographic projections create the illusion of coxa valga–the radiograph is merely a two-dimensional shadow of the bones.

Ruwe *et al.* (1991) compared a clinical measurement of femoral anteversion with radiographic techniques. With the patient prone, the degree of internal rotation of the hip to the point of maximum greater trochanteric prominence varied only 4º from the radiographic measurements in 59 patients (91 hips). A quick check of internal rotation measured with the patient prone and the knees flexed 90º will indicate femoral anteversion greater than the mean for age if the range of internal rotation is greater than 70º and external rotation less than 40º–45º. The normal total rotation, both internal and external should add up to about 90º. The only trap to this estimation is in children who have excessive ligamentous laxity where the total range of motion of rotation will be greater than 100º without excessive femoral anteversion (torsion).

The percentage of hip migration can be quantified by examining a radiograph of the hip (Fig. 5.20). A transverse line is drawn through the triradiate cartilage of each hip. Perpendicular lines at the lateral edge of the femoral head, lateral edge of the acetabulum (Perkins line) and the medial edge of the femoral head. The distance from the edge of the acetabulum to the lateral edge of the femoral head is the amount of head uncovered by the acetabulum (A). Dividing this by the width of the femoral head (B) gives the migration index of Reimers (1980). Hence the migration index is the percentage of uncovering of the femoral head. In normal hips the edge of the femoral head lies within the edge of the acetabulum while problematic hips in cerebral palsy displace laterally, superiorly and usually somewhat posteriorly. Additionally, as hips in children with cerebral palsy develop dysplasia, the edge of the acetabulum erodes and broadens, giving less tightness in the joint.

External tibial–fibular torsion (beyond the mean of 23º) has often been observed in patients who have internally rotated hip walking patterns (Le Damany 1909). This external tibial–fibular torsion develops as a compensatory change to the gait associated with internal femoral torsion (excessive anteversion) (Somerville 1957) (Fig. 5.21).

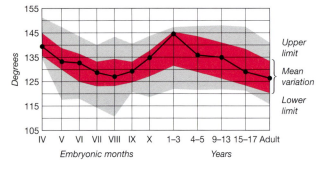

Fig. 5.19. Neck-shaft angle in embryonic life and to the adult showing little variation. (Redrawn from von Lanz and Mayet 1953 and Hensinger 1986.)

15 You can demonstrate the effect of the shadow cast by a two-dimensional object if you place your hand and wrist (or if you want, a specimen of the upper end of the femur) in front of a beam of light. As you rotate your limb it is easy to see how the shape of the shadow changes.

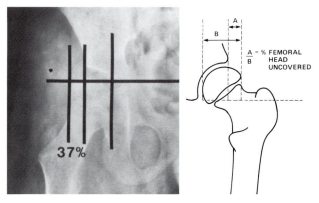

Fig. 5.20. Percentage of subluxation of the hip can be quantitated by dividing the amount of head uncovered (A) by the width of the head (B).

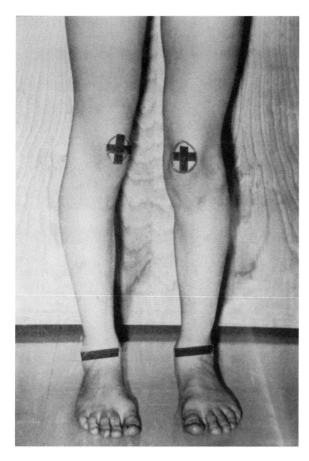

Fig. 5.21. Photograph of lower limbs of a 14-year-old boy with spastic diplegia and a hip internal rotation gait. The line of progression of the feet is almost normal in appearance due to compensatory excessive external tibial–fibular torsion of 45º.

SPINE

SCOLIOSIS, KYPHOSIS, LORDOSIS

Scoliosis is the most common and serious structural change in the spine of patients with cerebral palsy, and is more frequent and severe in non-walkers who have total body involvement. Pelvic obliquity often accompanies the scoliosis, though not necessarily due to asymmetrical adduction contractures of the hips or dislocation. The subject of scoliosis in cerebral palsy will be dealt with more fully in Chapter 9.

Kyphosis without scoliosis is seen in cerebral palsy but rarely progresses to a severe degree (> 60º). It begins as a postural defect and is flexible. If it persists throughout growth it can become a fixed structural deformity.

Lordosis is usually due to increased anterior pelvic inclination secondary to a flexion contracture of the hips in patients who stand and walk. Like kyphosis it is initially flexible, but as the child grows it becomes structural and fixed due to lack of mobility at the lumbosacral articulation. Young adult patients who have fixed flexion contractures of the hip (usually > 20º) develop an almost horizontal sacrum, and complain of low back pain when erect. Hip-flexion contractures in growing children should be treated surgically to prevent later possibly disabling low back pain.

Japanese radiologists compared the radiographs of the lumbar spine from 84 patients with spastic diplegia (mean age 20.1 years) with those from normal controls. Spondylolysis of the fifth lumbar vertebra was found in 21%. In this study it was presumed that the hip flexion contracture was the primary deformity causing the lumbar lordosis manifested by a decrease in the sacrofemoral angle and an increase in Ferguson's angle (1934).[16] Spondylolisthesis was found in three patients. In those over age 9 years low back pain increased in incidence from 38% in those aged 10–19 years to 64% of those over 30 years. Low back pain occurred in 55% of those who had a spondylolysis, but also in 41% of those who did not have spondylolysis (Harada *et al.* 1993).

A completely opposite conclusion was reached by Hennrikus *et al.* (1993) in a study of 50 ambulatory patients with cerebral palsy. Only one patient had a spondylolysis, one had spondylolisthesis (grade I, asymptomatic), and only six had low back pain. There was no correlation with the hip-flexion contracture, sacrofemoral angle, or increasing age. The practical clinical implication of this study was that periodic radiographic examinations of the lumbar spine in patients with cerebral palsy and no back pain are not necessary.

The practical clinical implication of this study was that periodic radiographic examinations of the lumbar spine in patients with cerebral palsy and no back pain are not necessary.

CERVICAL SPINE: DEGENERATIVE CHANGES

Degenerative arthritis of the cervical spine can occur in patients who have athetosis. The constant involuntary movements and dystonia of the neck muscles seem responsible for the arthritic changes in the intervertebral facet joints. These patients can have disabling symptoms due to constant neck pain, often accompanied by radicular pain in an upper limb. Because athetosis has plummeted in incidence in California over the past 30 years, only once did we (EEB) do an anterior spinal fusion at the fifth cervical interspace in the case of a 20-year-old woman who had athetosis and unremitting neck pain and unilateral upper-limb radicular pain. She became asymptomatic immediately postoperatively and had remained so for 10 years.

Angelini *et al.* (1982) reported an unusual cervical myelopathy in a 12-year-old girl who had dystonic and spastic quadriplegia. Radiographic examination revealed anterior slipping of the 4th cervical vertebra, which was eliminated with general anesthesia. These authors concluded that her signs and symptoms were due to intermittent spinal-cord compression due to the subluxation which was secondary to the torsion dystonia. Fortunately athetosis is becoming rare, at least in the USA.

16 Ferguson's angle is that angle between the superior border of the first sacral vertebra and a line parallel to the horizontal plane. The sacrofemoral angle is constructed as the angle between the superior surface of the first sacral vertebra and the long axis of the femoral shaft with the patient standing as erect as possible during the lateral projection of the sacrum and proximal femur and lower lumbar spine.

Harada *et al.* (1996) reported a 51% incidence of disc degeneration of the cervical spine in 180 patients who have athetosis. The disc degeneration was estimated at eight times the frequency seen the normal population. In this radiographic study instability at the 3rd and 4th and 5th and 6th cervical interspaces were found in 17% and 27% respectively. More ominous for spinal-cord function was a higher incidence of spinal-canal stenosis at the 4th and 5th cervical levels. Miwaka *et al.* (1997) had two patients with dystonic athetosis who were bedridden due to a cervical radiculopathy and myelopathy. Both recovered and were able to walk after an anterior and posterior decompression and fusion.

PELVIC OBLIQUITY AND 'WINDBLOWN' LOWER LIMBS

Fulford and Brown (1976) proposed that position in infancy and childhood might be responsible for deformities in cerebral palsy. They described children who had windswept lower limbs, facial asymmetry, a 'bat' ear and plagiocephaly.[17] They suspected that these deformities have a positional etiology, and suggested that somehow asymmetrical postures and positions should be prevented. Letts *et al.* (1984) studied windblown hips in cerebral palsy. They found the sequence of development was dislocation of the hip, scoliosis, and then pelvic obliquity. Their solution was early recognition of hip subluxation in the infant and 'aggressive' treatment, presumably surgery. Nwaobi and Sussman (1990) addressed the same deformity using electromyography in 13 patients who had spastic quadriplegia and a windblown deformity. They found the hip adductor muscles had electrical activity in all positions of the hip. The electromyographic activity of the abductor muscles increased when the hip was adducted from 4° abduction to 0° adduction. In the abducted hip the abductors had minimal electrical activity at 25° abduction. On the basis of the electrical activity data, the authors thought that a minimum of 25° of bilateral hip abduction would be necessary in designing special seating for this group of patients. Keeping the hips in neutral position may be insufficient in preventing the windblown deformity.

SUMMARY

Structural changes of the musculoskeletal system in cerebral palsy occur frequently, despite the efforts of physicians, surgeons, therapists and orthotists. Most of these skeletal deformities cause few symptoms in the growing child. Disabling pain develops many years later in adult life, long after the child has left the special treatment unit, the therapists, the social workers, the schoolteachers, the pediatricians, orthopaedic surgeons, neurologists, neurosurgeons, and physiatrists. Orthopaedic surgery in cerebral palsy has been developed and applied in children to prevent serious structural change and decreasing function due to

disabling symptoms in adult life. Progress in orthopaedic surgery in cerebral palsy depends upon the proper analysis of the problem, timing of surgery, and the right surgery in both quantity and quality all of which are subject to many variables both biological and psychological. Whether selective posterior rootlet rhizotomy, intrathecal Baclofen, or repetitive Botulinum myoneural blocks will prevent late disabling pathological changes in the limb joints and spine cannot be ascertained at present. Longer periods of follow-up to assess the outcomes in adults will be necessary. Life does not end at 16. Follow-up and access to care should be available to adults with cerebral palsy.

REFERENCES

Alexander, R. McN. (1984) 'Walking and running.' *American Scientist*, **72**, 348–354.
—— (1988) *Elastic Mechanisms in Animal Movement.* Cambridge: Cambridge University Press.
—— (1989) 'Muscles for the job.' *New Scientist*, **122**, 50–53.
Andersson, C., Mattsson, E. (2001) 'Adults with cerebral palsy: a survey describing problems, needs, and resources, with special emphasis on locomotion.' *Developmental Medicine and Child Neurology*, **43**, 76–82.
Ando, N., Ueda, S. (2000) 'Functional deterioration in adults with cerebral palsy.' *Clinical Rehabilitation*, **14**, 300–306.
Angelini, L., Broggi, G., Nardocci, N., Savoiardo, M. (1982) 'Subacute cervical myelopathy in a child with cerebral palsy. Secondary to torsion dystonia?' *Child's Brain*, **9**, 354–357.
Badell-Ribera, A. (1985) 'Cerebral palsy: postural locomotor prognosis in spastic diplegia.' *Archives of Physical Medicine and Rehabilitation*, **66**, 614–619.
Baumann, J.U. (1972) 'Hip operations in children with cerebral palsy.' *Reconstructive Surgery and Traumatology*, **13**, 68–82.
Bax, M.C.O., Smyth, D.P.L., Thomas, A.P. (1988) 'Health care of physically handicapped young adults.' *British Medical Journal*, **296**, 1153–1155.
Beals, R.K. (1966) 'Spastic paraplegia and diplegia: an evaluation of non-surgical and surgical factors influencing the prognosis for ambulation.' *Journal of Bone and Joint Surgery*, **48A**, 827–846.
—— (1969) 'Developmental changes in the femur and acetabulum in spastic paraplegia and diplegia.' *Developmental Medicine and Child Neurology*, **11**, 303–313.
Beckung, E., Hagberg, G. (2002) 'Neuroimpairment, activity limitations, and participation restrictions in children with cerebral palsy.' *Developmental Medicine and Child Neurology*, **44**, 309–316.
Bennett, G., Bauer, W. (1937) 'Joint changes resulting from patellar displacement and their relation to degenerative hip disease.' *Journal of Bone and Joint Surgery*, **19**, 667–692.
Bleck, E.E. (1968) *Observations and treatment of flexion, internal rotation, and bone deformities of the hip in cerebral palsy.* PhD thesis, American Orthopaedic Association.
—— (1971) 'The hip in cerebral palsy.' *In: Instructional Course Lectures.* American Academy of Orthopaedic Surgeons, St Louis: C.V. Mosby.
—— (1975) 'Locomotor prognosis in cerebral palsy.' *Developmental Medicine and Child Neurology*, **17**, 18–25.
—— (1989) 'Foreword.' *In* Thomas A., Bax, M., Smyth, D. (1989) *The Health and Social Needs of Young Adults with Physical Disabilities. Clinics in Developmental Medicine, No. 106.* London: Mac Keith Press with Blackwell Scientific; Philadelphia: J.B. Lippincott.
—— Koehler, J. P., Dillingham, M., Trimble, S. (1976) 'Histochemical studies of thoracis spinalis and sacrospinalis muscles.' *American Academy of Neurology (Program Abstract).*
—— Nagel, D.A. (1982) *Physically Handicapped Children: A Medical Atlas for Teachers, 2nd edn.* New York: Simon and Schuster.
—— Kleinman, R.G. (1984) 'Special injuries of the musculoskeletal system.' *In* Rockwood, C.A., King, R.E. (Eds) *Fractures. Vol. 3: Fractures in Children.* Philadelphia: Lippincott. C3.
Bobroff, E.D., Chambers, H.G., Sartoris, D.J., Wyatt, M.P., Sutherland, D.H. (1999) 'Femoral anteversion and neck–shaft angle in children with cerebral palsy.' *Clinical Orthopedics and Related Research*, **364**, 194–204.

---

17 Plagiocephaly, from the Greek πλαγιος (oblique) and κεφαλοη (head). In plagiocephaly, the skull is flattened on one side.

Booth, C.M., Cortina-Borja, M.J., Theologis, T.N. (2001) 'Collagen accumulation in muscles of children with cerebral palsy and correlation with severity of spasticity.' *Developmental Medicine and Child Neurology*, **43**, 314–320.

Bose, K., Yeo, K.Q. (1975) 'The locomotor assessment of cerebral palsy.' *Proceedings (Singapore)*, **10**, 21–24.

Bottos, M., Feliciangeli, A., Sciuto, L., Gericke, E., Vianello, A. (2001) 'Functional status of adults with cerebral palsy and implications for treatment of children.' *Developmental Medicine and Child Neurology*, **43**, 516–528.

Brunner, R., Doderlein, L. (1996) 'Pathological fractures in patients with cerebral palsy.' *Journal of Pediatric Orthopaedics*, Part B, **5**, 232–238.

Burke, D. (1983) 'Critical examination of the case for or against fusimotor involvement in disorders of muscle tone.' *Advances in Neurology*, **39**, 133–150.

Cahuzac, M., Nichil, J., Olle, R., Touchard, A., Cahuzac, J. P. (1979) 'Les fractures de fatigue de la rotule chez l'infirme moteur d'origine cérébrale.' *Revue de Chirurgie Orthopédique*, **65**, 87–90.

Campos da Paz Jr, A., Burnett, S.M., Braga, L.W. (1994) 'Walking prognosis in cerebral palsy: a 22-year retrospective analysis.' *Developmental Medicine and Children Neurology*, **36**, 130–134.

Carnack, D.H., Ed. (1987) *Ham's Histology, 9th edn.* Philadelphia: J.B. Lippincott.

Castle, M.E., Reyman, T.A., Schneider, M. (1979) 'Pathology of spastic muscle in cerebral palsy.' *Clinical Orthopaedics and Related Research*, **142**, 223–233.

Cathels, B.A., Reddihough, D.S. (1993) 'The health care of young adults with cerebral palsy.' *Medical Journal of Australia*, **159**, 444–446.

Chaplais, J. de Z., MacFarland, J.A. (1984) 'A review of 404 late walkers.' *Archives of Disease in Childhood*, **59**, 512–516.

Cohen, P., Mustacchi, P. (1966) 'Survival in cerebral palsy.' *Journal of the American Medical Association*, **195**, 642–644.

—— Kohn, J.G. (1979) 'Follow-up study of patients with cerebral palsy.' *Western Journal of Medicine*, **130**, 6–11.

Cooper, R.R. (1972) 'Alterations during immobilization and degeneration of skeletal muscle in cats.' *Journal of Bone and Joint Surgery*, **54A**, 919–953.

Crothers, B., Paine, R.S. (1959) *Natural History of Cerebral Palsy.* Cambridge: Harvard University Press.

Dalen, N., Olsson, K.E. (1974) 'Bone mineral content and physical activity.' *Acta Orthopaedica Scandinavica*, **45**, 170–174.

Delp, S.L., Zajac, F.E. (1992) 'Force- and moment-generating capacity of lower-extremity muscles before and after tendon lengthening.' *Clinical Orthopedics and Related Research*, **284**, 247–259.

Eliasson, A.C., Gordon, A.M., Forssberg, H. (1991) 'Basic coordination of manipulative forces of children with cerebral palsy.' *Developmental Medicine and Child Neurology*, **33**, 661–670.

—— Krumlinde-Sundholm, L., Rosblad, B., Beckung, E., Arner, M., Ohrvall, A.M., Rosenbaum, P. (2000) 'The Manual Ability Classification System (MACS) for children with cerebral palsy: scale development and evidence of validity and reliability.' *Developmental Medicine and Child Neurology*, **48**, 549–554

Enneking, W.F., Horowitz, M. (1972) 'The intra-articular effects of immobilization on the human knee.' *Journal of Bone and Joint Surgery*, **54A**, 973–985.

Evans, E.B., Eggers, G.N.W., Butler, J K., Blumel, D. (1960) 'Experimental immobilization and remobilization of rat knee joint.' *Journal of Bone and Joint Surgery*, **42A**, 737–758.

Eyman, R.K., Olmstead, C.E., Grossman, H.J., Call, T.L. (1993) 'Mortality and the acquisition of basic skills by children and adults with severe disabilities.' *American Journal of Diseases of Children*, **147**, 216–222.

Fabry, G., MacEwen, G.D., Shands, A.R. (1973) 'Torsion of the femur.' *Journal of Bone and Joint Surgery*, **55A**, 1726–1738.

Fedrizzi, E., Facchin, P., Marzaroli, M., Pagliano, E., Botteon, G., Percivalle, L, Fazzi, E. (2000) 'Predictors of independent walking in children with spastic diplegia.' *Journal of Child Neurology*, **15**, 228–34.

Ferguson, A.B. (1934) 'Clinical and roentgenographic interpretation of lumbosacral anomalies.' *Radiology*, **22**, 548–558.

Fiorentino, M.R. (1963) *Reflex Testing Methods for Evaluating Central Nervous System Development.* Springfield, IL: C.C. Thomas.

Forbes, D.B., McIntyre, J.M. (1968) 'A method for evaluating the results of surgery in cerebral palsy.' *Canadian Medical Association Journal,* **98**, 646–648.

Freeman, M.A.R. (1972) *Adult Articular Cartilage.* New York: Grune & Stratton.

Fuji, E., Yonenobu, K., Fujiwara, K., Yamashita, K., Ebara, S., Ono, K., Okada, K. (1987) 'Cervical radiculopathy or myelopathy secondary to athetoid cerebral palsy.' *Journal of Bone and Joint Surgery*, **69A**, 815–821.

Fulford, G.E., Brown, J.K. (1976) 'Position as a cause of deformity in children with cerebral palsy.' *Developmental Medicine and Child Neurology*, **18**, 305–314.

Gamble, J.G. (1988) *The Musculoskeletal System. Physiological Basics.* New York: Raven Press.

Grimby, G., Broberg, C., Krotiewska, I, Krotkiewski, M. (1976) 'Muscle fiber composition in patients with traumatic cord lesion.' *Scandinavian Journal of Rehabilitation Medicine*, **8**, 37–42.

Hensinger, R.N. (1986) *Standards in Pediatric Orthopedics.* New York: Raven Press, pp. 49, 53.

Hill, D.K. (1968) 'Tension due to interaction between the sliding filaments in resting striated muscle. The effect of stimulation.' *Journal of Physiology*, **199**, 637–684.

Hutton, J.L., Pharoah, P.O. (2002) 'Effects of cognitive, motor, and sensory disabilities on survival in cerebral palsy.' *Archives of Disease in Childhood*, **86**, 86–49.

Kleinman, R. G. (1984) 'Special injuries of the musculoskeletal system.' *In* Rockwood, C.A., King, R.E. (Eds) *Fractures, Vol. 3: Fractures in Children.* Philadelphia: Lippincott.

Hall, M.C. (1969) 'Cartilage changes after experimental relief of contact in the knee joint of the mature rat.' *Clinical Orthopaedics and Related Research*, **64**, 64–76.

Harada, T., Ebara, S., Anwar, M.M., Kajiura, I., Oshita, S., Hiroshima, K., Ono, K. (1993), 'The lumbar spine in spastic diplegia. A radiographic study.' *Journal of Bone and Joint Surgery*, **57B**, 534–537.

—— Ebara, S., Answar, M.M., Okawa, A., Kajiura, I., Hiroshima, K., Ono, K. (1996) 'The cervical spine in athetoid cerebral palsy.' *Journal of Bone and Joint Surgery*, **78B**, 613–519.

Henderson, R.C., Lin, P.T., Green, W.B. (1995) 'Bone-mineral density in children and adolescents who have cerebral palsy.' *Journal of Bone and Joint Surgery*, **77A**, 1671–1681.

Hennrikus, W.L., Rosenthal, R.K., Kasser, J.R. (1993) 'Incidence of spondylolisthesis in ambulatory cerebral palsy.' *Journal of Pediatric Orthopaedics*, **13**, 37–40.

Hutton, J.L., Pharoah, P.O. (2002) 'Effective of cognitive, motor, and sensory disabilities on survival in cerebral palsy.' *Archives of Diseases in Childhood*, **86**, 84–89.

Ingelmark, B.E., Saaf, V. (1948) 'Über die Ernährung des Glenkknorpels und die Bildung den Glenkfüssigkeit und der verschiedenen funktionellen Verhätnissen.' *Acta Orthopaedica Scandinavica*, **17**, 303.

Jakobsson, F., Borg, K., Edstrom, L., Grimby, L. (1988) 'Use of motor units in relation to muscle fiber type and size in man.' *Muscle Nerve*, **11**, 1211–1218.

Johnson, A., Goddard, O., Ashurst, H. (1990) 'Is late walking a marker of morbidity? Steering Committee, Oxford Region Child Development Project.' *Archives of Disease in Childhood*, **65**, 486–488.

Kinsman, S.L. (2002) 'Predicting motor function in cerebral palsy.' *Journal of the American Medical Association*, **288**, 1399–1400.

Kottke, F.J. (1966) 'The effects of limitation of activity upon the human body.' *Journal of the American Medical Association*, **196**, 825–830.

Laplaza, F.J., Root, L., Tassanawipas, A., Glasser, D.B. (1993) 'Femoral torsion and neck shaft angles in cerebral palsy.' *Journal of Pediatric Orthopaedics*, **13**, 192–199.

LeDamany, P. (1909) 'La torsion du tibia, normal, pathological, experimental.' *Journal d'Anatomie et Physiologie*, **45**, 589–615.

Lee, J.J., Lyne, E.D. (1990) 'Pathologic fractures in severely handicapped children and young adults.' *Journal of Pediatric Orthopaedics*, **10**, 497–500.

Letts, M., Shapiro, L., Mulder, K., Klassen, O. (1984) 'The windblown hip syndrome in cerebral palsy.' *Journal of Pediatric Orthopaedics*, **4**, 55–62.

Lewis, F.R., Samilson, R.L., Lucas, D.B. (1964) 'Femoral torsion and coxa valga in cerebral palsy—a preliminary report.' *Developmental Medicine and Child Neurology*, **6**, 591–597.

Lottman, D.B. (1976) 'Knee flexion deformity and patella alta in spastic cerebral palsy.' *Developmental Medicine and Child Neurology*, **18**, 315–319.

Maroudas, A., Bullough, P., Swanson, S.A.V., Freeman, M.A.R. (1968) 'The permeability of articular cartilage.' *Journal of Bone and Joint Surgery*, **50B**, 166–177.

Maruishi, M., Mano, Y., Sasaki, T., Shinmyo, N., Sata, H., Ogawa, T. (2001) 'Cerebral palsy in adults: independent effects of muscle strength and muscle tone.' *Archives of Physical Medicine and Rehabilitation*, **82**, 637–641.

McIvor, W.C., Samilson, R.L. (1966) 'Fractures in patients with cerebral palsy.' *Journal of Bone and Joint Surgery*, **48A**, 858–866.

Miwaka, Y., Watanabe, R., Shikata, J. (1997) 'Cervical myelo-radiculopathy in athetoid cerebral palsy.' *Archives of Orthopaedic Trauma and Surgery (Germany)*, **116**, 116–118.

Molnar, G. E., Gordon, S. V. (1974) 'Predictive value of clinical signs for early prognostication of motor function in cerebral palsy.' *Archives of Physical Medicine*, **57**, 153–158.

Moseley, C.L. (1992) 'Physiologic effects of soft-tissue surgery.' *In* Sussman, M.D. (Ed.) *The Diplegic Child*. Rosemont, IL: American Academy of Orthopaedic Surgeons, pp. 259–269.

Murphy, K.P., Molnar, G.E., Lankasky, K. (1995) 'Medical and functional status of adults with cerebral palsy.' *Developmental Medicine and Child Neurology*, **37**, 1075–1084.

Nagashima, T., Karimura, M., Nishimura, M., Tokinobut, H., Kato, S., Kanda, T., Tanabe, H. (1993) 'Late deterioration of functional abilities in adult cerebral palsy.' *Rinsho Shinkeigaku*, **33**, 939–944. (Japanese.)

Nelson, K.B., Ellenberg, J.H. (1982) 'Children who "outgrew" cerebral palsy.' *Pediatrics*, **69**, 529–536.

Nishihara, N., Tanabe, G., Nakahara, S., Imai, T., Murukawa, H. (1984) 'Surgical treatment of cervical spondylitic myelopathy complicating athetoid cerebral palsy.' *Journal of Bone and Joint Surgery*, **66B**, 504–508.

Nwaobi, O.M., Sussman, M.D. (1990) 'Electromyographic force patterns of cerebral palsy patients with windblown hip deformity.' *Journal of Pediatric Orthopaedics*, **10**, 382–328.

O'Dwyer, N.J., Neilson, P.J., Nash, J. (1989) 'Mechanism of muscle growth related to muscle contracture in cerebral palsy.' *Developmental Medicine and Child Neurology*, **31**, 543–547.

Palisano, R.J., Rosenbaum, P.E., Walter, S.D., Russell, D.J., Wood, E.P., Galuppi, B.E. (1997) 'Development and reliability of a system to classify gross motor function in children with cerebral palsy.' *Developmental Medicine and Child Neurology*, **39**, 214–223.

—— Hanna, S.E., Rosenbaum, P.L., Russell, D.J., Walter, S.D., Wood, E.P., Raisa, P.S., Galuppi, B.E. (2000) 'Validation of a model of gross motor function for children with cerebral palsy.' *Physical Therapy*, **80**, 974–985.

Perlman, J.M., Goodman, S., Kreusser, K.L. Volpe, J.J. (1985) 'Reduction in intraventricular hemorrhage by elimination of fluctuating cerebral blood-flow velocity in preterm infants with respiratory distress syndrome.' *New England Journal of Medicine*, **312**, 1353–1357.

Rapp, C.E. Jr, Torres, N.M. (2000) 'The adult with cerebral palsy.' *Archives of Family Medicine*, **9**, 466–472.

Reimers, J. (1972) 'A scoring system for evaluation of ambulation in cerebral palsied patients.' *Developmental Medicine and Child Neurology*, **14**, 155–165.

—— (1980) 'The stability of the hip in children. A radiological study of the results of muscle surgery in cerebral palsy.' *Acta Orthopedica Scandinavica (Suppl.)*, **184**, 1–100.

Romanini, L., Villani, C., Meloni, C., Calvisi, V. (1989) 'Histological and morphological aspects pf muscle in infantile cerebral palsy.' *Italian Journal of Orthopaedic Traumatology*, **15**, 87–93.

Rose, J., Haskell, W.L., Gamble, J.G., Hamilton, R.L., Brown, D.A., Rinsky, L. (1994) 'Muscle pathology and clinical measures of disability in children with cerebral palsy.' *Journal of Orthopaedic Research*, **12**, 758–768.

—— McGill, K.C. (1998) 'The motor unit in cerebral palsy.' *Developmental Medicine and Child Neurology*, **40**, 270–277.

Rosenbaum, P.L., Walter, S.D., Hanna, S.E., Palisano, R.J., Russell, D.J., Raina, P., Wood, E., Bartlett, D.J., Galuppi, B.E. (2002) 'Prognosis for gross motor function in cerebral palsy.' *Journal of the American Medical Association*, **288**, 1357–1363.

Russell, D.J., Rosenbaum, P.L., Cadman, D.T., Gowland, C., Hardy, S., Jarvis, S. (1989) 'The gross motor function measure.' *Developmental Medicine and Child Neurology*, **31**, 341–352.

—— Rosenbaum, P.L., Avery, L., Lane, M. (2002) *Gross Motor Function Measure (GMFM-66 and GMFM-88) User's Manual: Clinics in Developmental Medicine, No. 159*. London: Mac Keith Press; New York: Cambridge University Press.

Ruwe, P.A., Gage, J.R., Ozonoff, M.B., DeLuca, P.A. (1991) 'Clinical determination of femoral anteversion.' *Journal of bone and Joint Surgery*, **74A**, 820–830.

Sala, D., Grant, A.D. (1995) 'Prognosis for ambulation in cerebral palsy.' *Developmental Medicine and Child Neurology*, **37**, 1020–1025.

Saigal, S., Rosenbaum, P., Szatmari, P., Hoult, L., (1992) 'Non-right handedness among ELBW and term children at eight years in relation to cognitive function and school performance. *Developmental Medicine and Child Neurology*, **34**, 425–433.

Salter, R.B. (1993) *Continuous Passive Motion*. Baltimore: Williams and Wilkins.

—— Field, P. (1960) 'The effects of continuous compression in living articular cartilage: an experimental investigation.' *Journal of Bone and Joint Surgery*, **42A**, 31–49.

—— McNeil, R. (1965) 'Pathological change in articular cartilage secondary to persistent deformity.' *Journal of Bone and Joint Surgery*, **47A**, 185–186. (Abstract.)

—— Hamilton, H.W., Wedge, J.H. (1984) 'Clinical application of basic research on continuous passive motion for disorders and injuries of synovial joints: a preliminary report of a feasibility study.' *Journal of Orthopaedic Research*, **1**, 325–342.

Samilson, R.L., Tsou, P., Aamoth, G., Green, W. (1972) 'Dislocation and subluxation of the hip in cerebral palsy.' *Journal of Bone and Joint Surgery*, **54A**, 863–873.

Schlesinger, E.R., Allaway, N.C., Peitin, S. (1959) 'Survivorship in cerebral palsy.' *American Journal of Public Health*, **49**, 343–354.

Shands, A.R., Steele, M.K. (1958) 'Torsion of the femur.' *Journal of Bone and Joint Surgery*, **39**, 803–816.

Shapiro, B.K., Accardo, P.J., Capute, A.J. (1979) 'Factors affecting walking in a profoundly retarded population.' *Developmental Medicine and Child Neurology*, **21**, 369–373.

Shepherd, G.M. (1983) *Neurobiology*. New York and Oxford: Oxford University Press.

Singer, R.B., Strauss, D., Shavelle, R. (1998) Comparative mortality in cerebral palsy patients in California, 1980–1996.' *Journal of Insurance Medicine*, **30**, 240–246.

Somerville, E.W. (1957) 'Persistent foetal alignment of the hip.' *Journal of Bone and Joint Surgery*, **39B**, 106–113.

Sood, S.C. (1971) 'A study of the effects of experimental immobilization on rabbit articular cartilage.' *Journal of Anatomy*, **188**, 497–507.

Strauss, D., Shavelle, R. (1998) 'Life expectancy of adults with cerebral palsy.' *Developmental Medicine and Child Neurology*, **43**, 369–75.

Sutherland, D.H., Olshen, R., Cooper, L., Woo, S.K.-Y. (1980) 'The development of mature gait.' *Journal of Bone and Joint Surgery*, **62A**, 336–353.

Swinyard, C.A., Bleck, E.E. (1985) 'The etiology of arthrogryposis (multiple congenital contracture).' *Clinical Orthopaedics and Related Research*, **194**, 15–29.

Tabary, J.C., Goldspink, G., Tardieu, C., Lombard, M., Chigot, P. (1971) 'Nature de la rétraction musculaire des I.M.C. mesure de l'allongement des sarcomères du muscle étiré.' *Revue de Chirurgie Orthopedique et Reparatrice de l'Appareil Moteur (Paris)*, **57**, 463–470.

Tardieu, C., Tabary, J., Huet de la Tour, E., Tabary, C., Tardieu, G. (1977) 'The relationship between sarcomere length in the soleus and the tibialis anterior and the articular angle of the tibiacalcaneum in cats during growth.' *Journal of Anatomy*, **124**, 581–588.

—— Tardieu, G., Colbeau-Justin, P., Huet de la Tour, E., Lespargot, A. (1979) 'Trophic muscle regulation in children with congenital cerebral lesions.' *Journal of the Neurological Sciences*, **42**, 357–364.

—— Huet de la Tour, E., Bret, M.D., Tardieu, G. (1982) 'Muscle hypoextensibility in children with cerebral palsy: 1. Clinical and experimental observations.' *Archives of Physical Medicine and Rehabilitation*, **63**, 97–102.

Tardieu, G. (1984) *Le Dossier Clinique de L'Infirmité Motrice Cérébrale, 3rd edn.* Paris: Masson.

—— Tabary, J.C., Tardieu, C., Lombard, M. (1971) 'Rétraction, hyper-extensibilité et "faiblesse" de I'I.M.C., expressions apparement opposées d'un même trouble musculaire. Consequences thérapeutiques.' *Revue de Chirurgie Orthopédique et Reparative de l'Appareil Moteur (Paris)*, **57**, 505–516.

—— Tardieu, C., Colbeau-Justin, P., Lespargot, A. (1982) 'Muscle hypoextensibility in children with cerebral palsy: II. Therapeutic implications.' *Archives of Physical Medicine and Rehabilitation*, **63**, 103–107.

Thomas, A., Bax M., Coombes, K. Goldson, E., Smyth, D., Whitmore, K. (1985) 'The health and social needs of physically handicapped young adults: are they being met by the statutory services?' *Developmental Medicine and Child Neurology*, **27** (Suppl. 50), 1–19.

—— Bax, M., Smyth, D. (1989) *The Health and Social Needs of Young Adults with Physical Disabilities. Clinics in Developmental Medicine, No. 106.* London: Mac Keith Press with Blackwell Scientific; Philadelphia: J.B. Lippincott.

van der Dussen, L., Nieuwstraten, W., Roebroeck, M., Stam, H.J. (2001) 'Functional level of young adults with cerebral palsy.' *Clinical Rehabilitation,* **15,** 84–91.

von Lanz, T., Mayet, A.M. (1953), 'Die glenkorper des menschlichen hufgelenkes in der progredienten phase iherer unweigigen ausformung.' *Zeitschrift Anatomie,* **117,** 317–345.

Walsh, E.G. (1992) *Muscles, Masses and Motion. The Physiology of Normality, Hypotonicity, Spasticity and Rigidity. Clinics in Developmental Medicine, No. 125.* London: Mac Keith Press; New York: Cambridge University Press, pp. 166–167.

Watanabe, R.S. (1974) 'Embryology of the human hip.' *Clinical Orthopedics and Related Research,* **98,** 8–26.

Wigglesworth, J. (1984) 'Brain development and its modification by adverse influences.' *In* Stanley, F., Alberman, E. (Eds) *The Epidemiology of the Cerebral Palsies. Clinics in Developmental Medicine, No. 87.* London: Spastics International Medical Publications with Heinemann Medical; Philadelphia: J.B. Lippincott.

Wood, E.P., Rosenbaum, P.L. (2000) 'The gross motor function classification system for cerebral palsy.' *Developmental Medicine and Child Neurology,* **31,** 341–352.

Yamashita, Y., Kuroiwa, Y. (1979) 'Cervical radiculomyelopathy caused by cerebral palsy (dystonic type)-clinical evaluation of our 10 cases.' *Saishin Igaku,* **34,** 293–297. (Japanese.)

Ziv, I., Blackburn, N., Rang, M., Koveska, J. (1984) 'Muscle growth in normal and spastic mice.' *Developmental Medicine and Child Neurology,* **26,** 94–99.

6

GOALS, TREATMENT AND MANAGEMENT

'*The child with cerebral palsy becomes the adult with cerebral palsy.*'

(Terver *et al.* 1981)

In the management of cerebral palsy, we prefer to begin with the goals (or aims) that we wish to achieve for our patients. We hope to assist the patient and family in reaching goals of optimum independence in living a life with dignity, joy and comfort. To 'treat' has several meanings in English derived from the Latin *tractāre*, *tractus* (to drag, handle, draw). We, who deal with patients who have cerebral palsy, might be called 'tractors': we drag them along toward the goal. The American Heritage Dictionary defines 'treatment' as 'the application of remedies with the object of effecting a cure; therapy.'

Is it mere pedantry to dwell on these details? It seems that when we use the term 'treatment' in cerebral palsy it is equated with the treatment of diseases that we can actually now cure, just as we can cure bacterial infections (for example) with the use of antibiotics. Too often the parents of children with cerebral palsy, and sometimes their professional therapists too, expect that they can obtain a 'cure' from physiotherapy, drugs or surgery.

After at least three-quarters of a century of sincere and intense effort by professionals to 'treat' cerebral palsy, most acknowledged in 1984 that these remedial special physical therapy efforts were unsuccessful in achieving function (Bobath and Bobath 1984, Goldkamp 1984, Scrutton 1984), let alone in relieving spastic paralysis and athetosis. Yet it seems that at the beginning of the 21st century some physicians and therapists around the world are continuing to use the special therapy methods, often with an acronym or a proper name (e.g. NDT-neurodevelopmental/ Bobath, Ayres sensorimotor integration, Doman–Delacato/ patterning, Vojta) which may lead parents to expect a cure. If the cure did not seem to be occurring as time passed, then parents were often tempted to pursue a chimerical search for another treatment in the hope of alleviating the disabling brain lesion manifested by the motor disorder. The emotional and financial cost to families and to the child was often not regarded by the treaters as a matter for concern and reflection. With the rise of

'health-care insurance' (both public and private) to pay for the process, parents and patients turned to the legislators to mandate a treatment. The process has become intensely political, as the public increasingly demand the allocation of more economic resources to 'health care'. The legislators were asked to assume the role of arbiters, judges of the efficacy of treatment, and *de facto* certification agents for prescribing. For all of the above reasons, we prefer the term 'management' in helping the patient and family cope and deal with the disability while focusing on goals compatible with the natural history, prognosis, and potential improvement of function.

With the advent of the efficacy of powerful neuropharmacological agents (botulinum toxin and baclofen), and the acceptance of selective posterior rootlet rhizotomy, enthusiasm for special physical therapy systems has waned. The focus has shifted to the goal or aim-oriented approach and increasingly to traditional exercise, sports and play, and assistive technology as an enhancement to lost function. Parallel with this trend is the transfer of many children with cerebral palsy from special schools to integration in the regular school in the United States, and increasingly in other countries. Integrated education of the 'differently able with the able-bodied' has been implemented in some educational institutions in India such as the Amar Jyoti Integrated School in Delhi (Tuli 1998). The teachers are trained to 'inculcate the qualities of a therapist' and play a multi-disciplinary role from primary through secondary education. Required aids and appliances are manufactured at the Amar Jyoti Workshop.

This chapter will delineate the goals, review briefly the many special physical therapy methods that appear to belong to a past age, discuss how the goals might be achieved in the most severely involved patient with assistive technology, review the use of neuropharmacological agents, botulinum toxin, intrathecal baclofen, and selective posterior rootlet rhizotomy, suggest the role and timing of orthopaedic surgery, mention surgery and botulinum toxin injections for drooling, and conclude with the role of the family and its importance in effecting the desired outcome of management.

GOALS

If we can accept the fact that childhood is relatively short, and that adulthood is three or four times longer, then it should be possible to develop goals based upon the needs of adults for optimum independent living. In order of priority, these are as follows.

1. *Communication.* There is an obvious human need to express our wants, thoughts and feelings. We now know that communication need not be exclusively oral or verbal, and that non-oral methods can be equally effective making use of 'inner language'. The use of sign-language by the deaf is the best example of such communication. Non-verbal communication outputs can use writing, symbols or electronic synthetic voice devices.

2. *Activities of daily living.* The basic need is to care for oneself in feeding, toileting, bathing, grooming and dressing. Beyond these elementary activities are meal preparation and household maintenance. In non-industrial societies, daily living tasks might include growing your own food supply, making clothing and constructing shelter. Upper-limb function is essential for the ability to do activities of daily living. Fine-motor skills and general upper-limb capability can be broadly categorized using the Manual Ability Classification System (Eliasson *et al.* 2006), as noted in Chapter 5.

3. *Mobility* is essential for independence, social integration and, if possible, employment. It is particularly important in modern urban mobile environments. If someone cannot walk independently or efficiently, mechanical substitutes are required. Able-bodied persons regularly extend their mobility beyond walking with mechanical devices: bicycles, motor vehicles, trains and aircraft.

4. *Walking*, although often perceived initially as the highest priority for children with cerebral palsy, becomes the last priority as maturation occurs and independence and social integration needs predominate. Walking ability in cerebral palsy was classified in the past as it was for patients with myelomeningocele (Hoffer *et al.* 1973). In cerebral palsy it has been replaced by the *Gross Motor Function Classification System* (GMFCS) as detailed in Chapter 5 (Table 5.II). As can be appreciated by the definition of the five levels of mobility in cerebral palsy, the classification by the Gross Motor Function Measure (GMFM) is more precise, whereas the former system used for spina bifida is broader and more general but is not reflected in any type of scoring system. However, the former classification of 'non-walker' being confined to wheelchair use was subdivided into three to define the function in the chair according to ability to transfer in and out of the chair (Table 6.I, subdivisions a, b and c).

In the GMFCS, which reflects the function of mobility rather than walking (Palisano *et al.* 1997), motor function is divided into five levels. Each level is divided into segments according to the age range: before the 2nd birthday, from age 2 to the 4th birthday, from age 4 to the 6th birthday, and from age 6 to 12 years.

Palisano and associates (1997), with 48 experts in the field, used a nominal group process and a Delphi survey consensus method to achieve a consensus on the validity and revisions of the classification system. Interrater reliability was 0.55 for children less than 2 years old and 0.75 for children from 2 to 12 years. Nordmark *et al.* (1997) confirmed the reliability of the classification in both inter- and intrarater assessment (0.77 and 0.88 at the first and second assessments, respectively).

TABLE 6.I
Gross Motor Function Measure walking classification
(Hoffer *et al.* 1973)

Cerebral palsy	Spina bifida
Level I: walks without restrictions; limitations in more advanced motor skills	*Community walker*: gets about whole community with or without walking aids (e.g. crutches)
Level II: walks without assistive devices; limitation in walking outdoors and community	
Level III: walks with assistive mobility devices; limitation in walking outdoors and community	
Level IV: self-mobility with limitations; children transported or use power mobility	*Physiological walker*: walks in physical therapy department or at home in parallel bars or with assistance of another person; wheelchair required in all other locations
Level V: self-mobility extremely limited even with use of assistive devices	*Non-walker*: wheelchair for all activities: a. independent—in and out of chair without help; b. assistive transfer—needs help of one person; c. dependent—unable to do assistive transfers; must be lifted in and out of chair.

METHODS OF ASSESSMENT, GOAL-SETTING AND RESULTS

Goal-oriented management requires that the child's problem be analyzed consistently with the priorities of needs for independent living. This will depend upon the extent of the physical and mental impairment and the most accurate prognosis possible in the areas of communication, activities of daily living, mobility and walking. This approach demands a careful and detailed examination of the child. As described in Chapter 5, the GMFCS allows a prognosis according to gross motor function score over time with a 95% confidence level (D. Russell, personal communication).

Bax (1995) unequivocally believes that likely outcomes in terms of function can be set early so that time, energy and money is not wasted on chasing impossible therapies to achieve functions. He is convinced that we can make decisions for management based on achievable goals in walking, feeding, speech and communication (Table 6.II): 'If the likely outcome is that the child will never acquire that function, exercise or other treatments designed to promote that function are in fact a waste of time. That sounds heretical, but what I am actually saying is that if we know the child is not going to walk, is not going to be able to feed himself, is not going to develop enough appropriate communication systems, we should be firm in not encouraging therapies which attempt to achieve this unachievable aim, even though sometimes the parents and the child wish to go on trying.'

TABLE 6.II
Predictability of eventual functions (Bax 1995)

Function	Prediction age (yrs)	Alternatives
Walking	By 2	Mobility devices
Oral feeding (inadequate nutrition)	By age 3, 4, or 5	Gastrostomy
Talking	By age 5	Non-verbal communication methods or devices

'If we know the child is not going to walk, is not going to be able to feed himself, is not going to develop enough appropriate communication systems, we should be firm in not encouraging therapies which attempt to achieve this unachievable aim.'

(Bax 1995)

We believe that a reasonably accurate prognosis in the major areas of function can be made based upon reported studies and a knowledge of the natural history. For example, we know that the prognosis for independent function, normal schooling and social integration is generally good for those with spastic diplegia (generally walk independently by age 3–4 years) or spastic hemiplegia (walk independently by 18–21 months if not compromised by severe mental retardation). The natural history study by Crothers and Paine (1959) demonstrated that if a child does not walk functionally by the age of 7 years, it is not likely to occur (see Fig. 5.2). From the examination, the prognosis, and the list of problems of function, we can then try to determine which problems might be eliminated, ameliorated or compensated.

Scrutton (1984) also wisely recommends an analysis of the 'child's situation': where and with whom they are living, the composition of the family and its responsibilities, the status of the child's education and where it occurs, day and night behavior and what activities engage the child beyond schooling. When this comprehensive assessment is completed, a list of practical goals can be made and given priorities. To turn the focus of the parents from the disease to the goal-oriented approach always takes much discussion and time. It is vital that the referring physician, paramedical persons, therapists and teachers have the same perspective.

In order to study the effectiveness of prospective goal-setting in 85 children who had total body involvement, Terver *et al.* (1981) devised a system of numerical scores to record the functional status of the child and to set the goals to be achieved. Table 6.IV defines the numerical score for each function in independence and efficiency. It is always possible to be independent but inefficient in task performance.

Other methods of defining the child's problems have been proposed (Maloney *et al.* 1978). Goldkamp (1984) used a numerical system (PULSES Monitoring System—Table 6.III) to define independence in activities of daily living in a follow-up study on the efficacy of treatment or management in cerebral palsy. Probably no system of assessment of function will satisfy all who work in this field, but at least these methods can

TABLE 6.III
PULSES monitoring system (from Goldkamp 1984)

P = general, systemic or imposed conditions
U = upper limbs
L = lower limbs
S = special senses and speech
E = excretory functions
S = cerebration

Scores

1 = no disorder
2 = disorder with no activities of daily living deficiency
3 = needs some assistance
4 = needs maximum help

(any patient with a score of 3 or 4 is dependent)

Example

P U L S E S
_____
1 2 3 2 1 1

This patient with cerebral palsy has no systemic or other condition and no activities of daily living deficiencies in the upper limb but has deficiencies due to lower-limb impairment, no problems in speech or the special senses and has normal excretory functions and normal intelligence. *This profile seems to describe the person who has spastic diplegia.*

encourage us to think about the needs of the child rather than our own needs in pursuing treatment.

No system of assessment of function will satisfy all who work in this field, but . . . can encourage us to think about the needs of the child rather than our own needs in pursuing treatment.

The Motion Analysis Laboratory of the Gillette Children's Specialty Care, St Paul, Minnesota, has formulated a 10-level walking scale as part of their Gillette Functional Assessment Questionnaire (FAQ) (Novacheck *et al.* 2000). The questionnaire was tested in 41 children with neuromuscular conditions that represented community ambulation levels, 6–10, of a walking scale. Good reliability among parents and caregivers was found. Validity was stated to be high and correlated with standard outcome measures of energy expenditure, and gait analysis data. The authors believe that this scale that is specific to walking should help to document functional change in children who have neuromuscular conditions.

From the University of Texas Medical Branch in Galveston comes another report of functional assessment of 205 children with developmental disabilities using special tests and ratings by parents and teachers on the amount of assistance needed for activities of daily living (Ottenbacher *et al.* 2000). The evaluation tools were the Battelle Developmental Inventory Screening Test, the Vineland Adaptive Behavior Scales, the Functional Independence Measure for Children (WeeFIM instrument), and the Amount of Assistance Questionnaire. The highest correlation was between the WeeFIM[1] total rating and the total amount of assistance rating (r=0.91) given by parents and teachers.

1 FIM=Functional Independence Measure for adults; WeeFIM =Functional Independence Measure for children (Msall *et al.* 1994).

None of the foregoing tests for functional goals can be used for prognosis of a child with cerebral palsy; but they should be helpful in delineating the functional abilities of the child when first examined and subsequently followed with a variety of indicated interventions to maturity. Numerical scores of function are an advantage in outcome studies and might be effective in the individual patient to determine when goals have been met so that no further treatment need be offered. This was the intent of the specialists at McMaster University who devised and proved the validity of the GMFM of 88 items and subsequently, 66 items (see Chapter 5).

The problem and the challenge of the goal-oriented approach are in the total body involved or quadriplegic child (levels IV and V). This group represented approximately 40% of our patients with cerebral palsy at the Children's Hospital at Stanford.[2] The other 60% who had spastic diplegia or hemiplegia generally have a good prognosis for functional goals. For this latter group the needs are mainly educational and social. Orthopaedic surgery for this group can be effective in preventing and correcting deformities of the lower limb so that walking ability will be facilitated and sustained.

A STUDY OF GOAL-ORIENTED MANAGEMENT

MATERIALS AND METHODS
To determine if the goal-oriented approach was successful and to determine at what age goals could be set, at Stanford we conducted a prospective study of 85 children who had total body involvement and spastic quadriplegia (Terver *et al.* 1981). According to the GMFCS all were at levels IV or V. We had two groups of patients: group 1 consisted of 14 children in whom goals were set by age four years and followed for a minimum of 8 years; group 2 comprised 71 children in whom goals were set after age 4 years (mean age, 7 years) and who were followed to an average of 14 years.

The initial and follow-up assessments used the numerical scoring methods as detailed in Table 6.IV. Based upon the initial assessments and prognosis, goals were set and scored.

PROGNOSIS FOR FUNCTIONS
Prognosis for *communication* in the non-verbal child was thought to be good if there was any means of eliciting a 'yes' or 'no' response by any means such as an eye blink, head movement, finger tap etc., by symbol recognition and with psychological tests. There are no published prognostic tests for inner language. The prognosis for *activities of daily living* depended upon voluntary control of at least one hand and upper limb. Assessment of hand function was often deferred until adequate sitting balance could be secured with appropriate seating. *Mobility* prognosis was highly dependent upon the ability to control some part of the body voluntarily—toes, foot, forearm, head, chin or tongue that could be used to control electronic switches of mobility devices.

---

2   The name has been changed to the Lucile Salter Packard Children's Hospital at Stanford.

TABLE 6.IV
Numerical scores for functional assessment (from Terver *et al.* 1981)

Independence

1 = total dependence on others
2 = partial dependence on others
3 = independence from others but dependent on a technical device to accomplish the task
4 = total independence but the activity is not normal in its execution, energy level or appearance

Efficiency
Communication (verbal or non-verbal)

1 = ability to indicate 'yes' or 'no' by any means
2 = ability to express needs only (*e.g.* call for help)
3 = ability to engage in a dialogue of direct questions and answers only
4 = ability to initiate and sustain a conversation, retain information and communicate at a distance

Activities of daily living

1 = ability to assume simple needs of eating, dressing, cleansing face and hands
2 = ability to completely assume all personal needs
3 = ability to assume household activities and needs
4 = ability to assume all of the above and have a social life

Mobility

1 = has mobility but unable to utilize effectively
2 = able to move about household only
3 = able to travel beyond the household within the immediate neighbourhood
4 = able to travel everywhere in the community

Walking

1 = physiological walker, but can transfer in and out of wheelchair
2 = household walker
3 = household and immediate neighbourhood
4 = community walker
0 = no activity, 5 = normal

Walking prognosis, including transfer ability from a wheelchair, was determined by the tests for locomotor prognosis (Bleck 1975) and equilibrium reactions. The findings were as follows.

1. *Communication.* The goal of independent communication was set at 3, which meant the ability to communicate independently with a technical device. It was achieved by all except four total body involved children who were severely mentally retarded. Those who achieved independence in communication also had scores between 4 and 5, which indicated their ability to initiate and sustain a conversation.

2. *Activities of daily living.* Initial scores in this function in both independence and efficiency were 1. The children were totally dependent on others to fulfil basic needs. We set minimal goals of 3 (independent with a technical device and able to do household tasks). Except for those who were mentally retarded (N=4), all achieved this goal at follow-up.

3. *Mobility.* Initially the scores were 2, which meant partial dependence on others for only household mobility. The goal of independence with a technical device (score 3) and the ability to travel beyond the household (score 4 in efficiency) was achieved in all, and in patients over age 18 it included mobility in the community. Again lower scores were achieved by those few who

were mentally retarded, which indicated continued partial dependence on others in the ability to move about the household.

4. *Walking.* In those below 6 years, walking was initially physiological and dependent. Although the goal set was independence with the assistance of a technical aid for household walking only (score 3), walking was not deemed efficient in a final follow-up of those over age 14 years, and they reverted to the physiological dependent walker (GMFM level IV).

Our conclusions were that the major factor in goal achievement in this group of patients was engineering technology and adaptive equipment, including environmental adaptations (e.g. home architectural modifications). Goals could be set as early as age 4 years.

> '*The major factor in goal achievement in a group of 85 children with total body involved cerebral palsy (spastic quadriplegia) was engineering technology, adaptive equipment and environmental adaptations. Goals could be set as early as four years.*'
>
> (Terver *et al.* 1981)

5. *Social, cultural and economic factors* are also undoubtedly responsible for unemployment. Cherpin *et al.* (1985) proposed that the environment defines the extent of the disability. They based their conclusions on a detailed study of function of almost all 500 inhabitants of a small village near Lyon, France. Similar conclusions about mobility and the environmental factors can be found in other countries (Figs 6.1, 6.2).

GOAL-ORIENTED APPROACH IN DEVELOPING COUNTRIES: COMMUNITY-BASED REHABILITATION (CBR)

The World Health Organization classification of function in disabilities adopted in 2001 (World Health Organization 2001) appears to lead the goal-oriented approach. Their training manual for disabled persons is written with only 1600 English words to allow easy translation (Helander *et al.* 1983). Its illustrations demonstrate how to use locally available material for rehabilitation mobility aids to be made on site rather than depending on human carrying capacity (Figs 6.3, 6.4). The recommended techniques for rehabilitation are clearly focused on primary functions: communication, activities of daily living and mobility. These functional goals are combined with education in the community schools with the ultimate goal of employment to assist the family and the community. The community-based rehabilitation (CBR) programs in 1989 were shifted from institutions to the homes and communities of people with disabilities and carried out by minimally trained people and families to reduce cost. A change in the approach was a shift from the exclusively medical model to a social one that added on interventions such as education, vocational training and social rehabilitation. In recent years some successful attempts have been made to integrate the disabled into community development projects, but to do so they need mobility, education and skills. The World Health Organization estimated in 1981 and endorsed again in 1999 that 70% of all those with disabilities could be helped at a

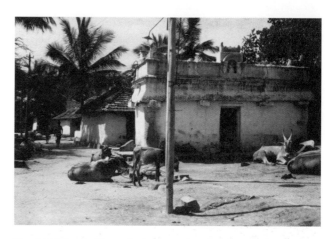

Fig. 6.1. Village in Karnataka State, South India. The only obstruction to mobility would be the cows and their dung-heaps. The monsoon may make the mud too soft for walking or to use mobility aids. From Bleck (1989) *A Study of Mobility of Disabled Persons in Rural Village of Karnataka State, India.* World Rehabilitation Fund, Exchange of Experts and Information in Rehabilitation.

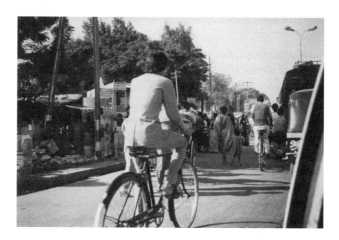

Fig. 6.2. Street scene, Bangalore, India. The street is paved, but no room for a disabled person to use it. The environment often defines the disability. From Bleck (1989) *A Study of Mobility of Disabled Persons in Rural Village of Karnataka State, India.* World Rehabilitation Fund, Exchange of Experts and Information in Rehabilitation.

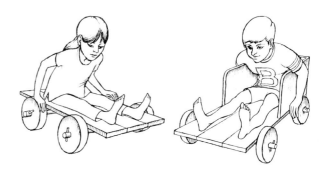

Fig. 6.3. A home-made mobility device and wheelchair comparable to the castor cart innovation by the Ontario Crippled Children's Center (redrawn from Helander *et al.* 1983).

124

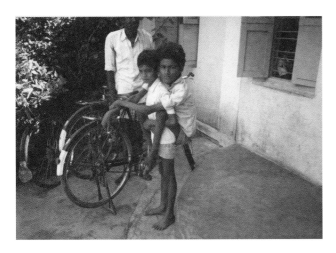

Fig. 6.4. Brother carrying brother when there are no mobility devices (village in Karnataka State, South India).

community level; 30% required specialists who were not available in the community. CBR has been going on for two decades and many believe it is the appropriate approach for people with disabilities. But questions and controversies remain so that additional experience and research will be needed for the coming decade (Thomas and Thomas 2002).

> '*CBR has been going on for two decades and many believe it is the appropriate approach for people with disabilities. But questions and controversies remain so that additional experience and research will be needed for the coming decade.*'
>
> (Thomas and Thomas 2002)

Especially pertinent was the clear statement by the World Health Organization that no more studies of incidence and numbers of disabled people are needed. The drive to register disabled people is totally unjustified unless those who register can immediately receive services. 'Every dollar spent on further investigations is a dollar mis-spent' (*World Health,* May 1984). From this same journal, the quotation of an African might be heeded by those of us in developed countries: 'We disabled people are fed up with being registered, censused, surveyed and photographed. We want services—now!'

Uganda estimates that about 2.1 million persons with disabilities need rehabilitation. In 1989 the Uganda government planned for community based rehabilitation and in 1992 the Norwegian government agreed to implement the first program in three districts and extended to six districts. Because of financial constraints CBR is limited to 10 out of 56 districts in Uganda. A referral system to specialized medical rehabilitation services and hospitals has been integrated into the community-based programs. Primary and adult education makes up part of services (Mpagi 2002).

> '*Governments cannot continue to sit back and leave such heavy work to non-governmental organizations like the Red Cross.*'
>
> (Ndawi 2002)

In Zimbabwe most CBR programs rely on voluntary workers (Ndawi 2002). Programs have been difficult to implement due to scatter of persons with disabilities in rural areas and although free medical care was declared for all at the time of independence in 1980, this proved to be too expensive. Free medical services have been modified so that only certain categories of medical or physical therapy services are available only on payment. Educational, social and vocational rehabilitation are integrated into the Zimbabwe scheme of CBR. However, in 1997 21% of persons with a disability aged 5–24 years had never been to school—yet on a positive note, this means that 79% have attended a school. Ndawi (2002) called for legislation to effect change and to implement it. 'Governments cannot continue to sit back and leave such heavy work to NGOs like the Red Cross.'[3]

Despite the urging of the WHO and general knowledge of prognosis for function in children with cerebral palsy, my experience (EEB) in multiple visits to developing countries such as Indonesia, India and Thailand the goal or aim-oriented approach has been slow in coming. Most care of the child with cerebral palsy is relegated to the physical therapists who have adopted, it seems, the zeal to pursue special therapy systems or methods promoted by Western therapists and some physicians. In general, centers for the care of cerebral palsy were established by groups of parents. In these countries, the cases of cerebral palsy are usually severely involved without the dominance of spastic diplegia seen in developed countries possibly due to lack of survivors of those born too soon or too small. How to shift the focus of therapists and their supervising physicians to realistic goals is the question.

TREATMENT BECOMES MANAGEMENT

> '*Therapeutic choices in locomotor management of the child with cerebral palsy—more luck than judgement?*'
>
> (Patrick *et al.* 2001)

Treatment of cerebral palsy and its manifold manifestations of a central nervous system disorder as a disease to be conquered can be exhausting and depressing. Reorientation to management on goals based upon the needs of the patient is more rewarding. Although Little (1862), founder of the Royal Orthopaedic Hospital, London, was the first to describe in detail the clinical findings in cerebral palsy and attributed them to events in pregnancy and birth, he is not known for treatment. His description of what we know as cerebral palsy was termed as 'Little's Disease' until 1932 when Phelps introduced the term 'cerebral birth injuries'.

Thirty years after Little, Freud (1893), as a neurologist in Vienna, wrote his monograph 'Les diplégies cérébrales infantiles' for *Revue Neurologique*. After its publication, he felt he had reached a dead-end in his studies of cerebral palsy and thought cerebral palsy an intolerable burden: 'I am fully occupied with

---

3 NGO = non-governmental organization.

children's paralysis, in which I am not the least interested' (Accardo 1982). He then founded the new discipline of psychiatry. With the exception of orthopaedic surgery, medicine turned away from cerebral palsy as a 'wastebasket category' (Accardo 1982).

Interest in taking care of children with cerebral palsy was rekindled by Phelps, an orthopaedic surgeon, when he established his famous residential institute for cerebral palsy in Maryland (Slominski 1984). When the success of the poliomyelitis immunization seemed assured in the 1950s, it was perhaps natural for professionals, particularly orthopaedic surgeons, to concentrate their efforts on other disabling conditions in children. Cerebral palsy was and remains the predominant neuromuscular disability in children. Many sincere, serious and often zealous efforts to 'treat' the disease were promoted.

The following paragraphs review the majority of the treatments proposed that might have continuing popularity and others that have been discarded. Descriptions include the rationale of treatments and offer a critique of each based upon reported results or lack of them. In this way the physician who assumes responsibility for the management of the child may become familiar with various methods, and be able to counsel parents on appropriate management.

In a review of treatments of cerebral palsy, Patrick and colleagues (2001) from the famous Robert Jones & Agnes Hunt Orthopaedic Hospital, Oswestry, UK, concluded that 'which treatment the individual child eventually receives is thus often influenced more by factors such as postcode rather than what is clinically optimal.' In this review they called for more objective evaluations of multilevel orthopaedic surgery with instrumented gait analysis and question the long-term benefits of botulinum toxin, long-term outcomes of dorsal rhizotomy, the use of intrathecal baclofen in patients with spastic diplegia who walk, and the efficacy of tone-reducing ankle–foot orthoses. But they believe that contracture correction devices are effective combined with either soft-tissue surgery or botulinum toxin injections, and they conclude: 'Therapeutic dilemma is inevitable in this area of increasing treatment options but in which there is a dearth of guidelines. . . . The whole area is bedeviled by more than a healthy splash of professional prejudice and scepticism.'

NEUROSURGERY

A direct attack on the altered brain function to alleviate the signs of cerebral palsy has obvious appeal (Ramamurthi 2000). Two main types of brain surgery have been preformed, but judging from a literature search from 1987 to 2002, enthusiasm seems to have waned.

STEREOTACTIC BRAIN SURGERY

The methods of locally destroying a region of the brain by electrical current or freezing (cryosurgery) to alleviate the motor disorder of cerebral palsy was popular in times past (Gornall *et al.* 1975, Cooper *et al.* 1976, Vasin *et al.* 1979, Broggi *et al.* 1980, Ohye *et al.* 1983). Broggi *et al.* (1983) and colleagues did

thalamotomy in 33 patients with a 1- to 4-year follow-up in 33 patients. The best results were reported in those who had tremor or hyperkinesia; spasticity tended to recur.

Neurosurgeons in Costa Rica (Trejos and Araya 1990) used stereotactic surgery in 38 patients with cerebral palsy who had spasticity, athetosis, dystonia or tremor. They found varying degrees of improvement in 80% of the patients. From Los Angeles, California, De Salles (1996) appeared enthusiastic from his results using radiofrequency lesions of the basal ganglia in cerebral palsy with rigidity, choreoathetosis and tremor. In Seoul, South Korea, Lee (1997) did 108 thalamotomies with MRI-guided stereotactic surgery in 77 patients who had cerebral palsy and dyskinesia. He reported excellent and good results in 81 patients, and fair in 27 with no complications. However, the dyskinesia returned in six. The Russians (Shabolov *et al.* 1998) seem to persist using stereotactic surgery, CT-guided, in the treatment of a variety dyskinesias including cerebral palsy, but report no details on outcomes and patient selection.

Given the permanence of destroying brain neurons and the complexity of the interneuronal network there may be a natural fear of stereotactic surgery in cerebral palsy with athetosis (dyskinesia). The longest published follow-up study was by Speelman and van Manen of the Netherlands (1989). In a mean follow-up of 21 years (range 12–27) after stereotactic brain lesion creation for hyperkinesia or dystonia of 28 patients, only 18 were available for outcome studies; nine of the 28 had died and one could not be found. Of the 18 surviving patients, eight were said to have had a 'positive' result (44%)—not very good odds on success. The best results were in those who had hyperkinesia, tremor or unilateral dystonia. For spastic paralysis selective posterior rootlet rhizotomy, intramuscular botulinum toxin and intrathecal baclofen seem to have displaced brain surgery.

CEREBELLAR STIMULATION

The principle of electrical stimulation of the cerebellum is derived from Sherrington's observation of decerebrate animals. He noted a decrease in extensor hypertonia with stimulation of the anterior lobe of the cerebellar cortex (Davis et al. 1980). The method of implanting a self-controlled stimulator on the surface of the cerebellum ('cerebellar pacemaker') was introduced by Cooper *et al.* (1976). After a wave of encouraging but short follow-up reports, cerebellar stimulation to reduce spasticity has not regained its initial promise. Davis *et al.* (1980) implanted the device in 262 patients but with only a 6-month follow-up. Robertson *et al.* (1980) observed better phonation and improvement of dysarthria.

Even though no significant benefit from cerebellar stimulation was ascertained by Bensman and Szegho (1978), Whittaker (1980), and Ivan *et al.* (1981), Davis and his neurosurgical colleagues (1987) of Augusta, Maine, persisted in their use of chronic cerebellar stimulation using an implantable pulse generator in 20 patients with cerebral palsy. The study was double-blind using physical therapists as evaluators of joint angle measurements and motor performance testing. After the preoperative tests, repeat postoperative testing was done at intervals with the switch to the stimulator on and off. Sixteen patients were left to comprise the outcome study. Improvement in the parameters measured with the stimulator on in 13 of the patients was 30%–50% in 10, 10%–20% in one, and none in three. Since this trial, no further reports of cerebellar stimulation appeared until a study by Harris *et al.* (1993) who reported 13 children with cerebral palsy who received chronic cerebellar stimulation. The spasticity appeared reduced immediately postoperatively, but this good effect did not persist after a 3- to 5-year follow-up. After this report of outcomes, it seemed as if cerebellar stimulation belonged to the past historical efforts in the treatment of cerebral palsy.

However, Davis (2000) of the Neural Engineering Clinic, Augusta, Maine reported on the use of implanted controlled-current stimulators applied to the superior-medial cortex of the cerebellum in 600 cases of cerebral palsy from 18 clinics. The report by Davis suggests glowing results: 85% had their spasticity reduced, had improvements in speech, drooling, respiration, gait, joint range of motion and mood. A double-blind study of 20 patients was stated to have shown a 60% improvement in motor performance. In a 17-year follow-up of 19 patients, 85% were either seizure free or reduced seizures. The conclusion was that 'chronic cerebellar stimulation (CCS) should be given by a totally implanted controlled current stimulator applied intermittently to the superior-medial cerebellar cortex for safe, effective, and continuous results.' Will some other center try to reproduce these results with a double-blind controlled study? Does it do any harm permanently to the neurons?

SPINAL-CORD ELECTRICAL STIMULATION

Epidural spinal-cord electrical stimulation was tried in 15 patients who had cerebral palsy with either spasticity or dyskinesia in the Netherlands (Speelman 1990). Of the 15 studied, 12 did not continue treatment after the study was completed. None of the patients had measurable improvements in activities of daily living or in the level of disability. As a result of their experience, Speelman could not recommend this method of treatment.

Another method of alleviating athetosis and dystonia was by electrical stimulation of the cervical spinal cord (Waltz and Davis 1983), but after this nothing more has been published about this clinical experiment.

CEREBRAL ELECTRICAL STIMULATION

The fascination with electricity to alleviate motor disorders led Russian investigators to use ultra-high-frequency transcerebral stimulation in 33 patients who had 'hyperkinetic' cerebral palsy. The stimulation was done in a resort sanatorium and combined with physical therapy directed exercise and massage (Burygina *et al.* 1993). The theory behind the method was to improve the vestibular apparatus. The results implied a 70.8% 'effect on

the motor disorder'. Whether the improvement reported was due to the effect of electricity on the brain or due to the general ambience of more relaxed living and exercises in a resort cannot be discerned. Whether ultra-high frequency damages cortical neurons is the question. It seems as if this experimental method has not been tried in the rest of the world probably because of a lack of a theoretical model that promises both efficacy and safety to justify it.

SELECTIVE POSTERIOR ROOTLET RHIZOTOMY

FROM THEORY TO PRACTICE

Sherrington (1898) described abolition of muscle spasticity in decerebrate cats with cutting of the spinal cord posterior roots. To explain this phenomenon the hypothesis formed was that the basis for motor control and muscle tone is due to the balance of two opposing forces on the anterior horn cell (alpha motor neuron): (1) facilitation of muscle contraction via the afferent sensory fibers (type Ia and type II) from the muscle spindle that enter the spinal cord through the posterior roots; (2) inhibition of the muscle contraction via the descending tracts from the brain. Central neuron damage reduces this higher level of inhibition to cause excessive activity of the anterior horn cell with resultant spasticity of the limb muscles. Thus cutting the posterior spinal roots diminishes the inhibitory influences on the motor neuron with the result of reduced spasticity of the muscles (Fig. 6.5).

Almost 100 years ago Foerster applied the work of Sherrington in cats to humans. He published in the American journal *Surgery, Gynecology and Obstetrics*, the results of posterior rhizotomy from the 2nd lumbar to the 2nd sacral nerve roots sparing the 4th lumbar root to preserve quadriceps strength for

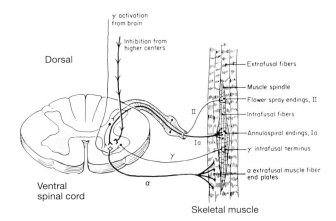

Fig. 6.5. Neurophysiological basis for posterior rootlet rhizotomy: type II and type Ia afferent fibres that originate from the annulospiral endings and the intrafusal γ fibers in the muscle spindle. These occupy the dorsal roots and are facilitory for the alpha motor neuron. In cerebral palsy the inhibition from the brain centers on the anterior horn cell is diminished. The balance between facilitation and inhibition is lost. Cutting the dorsal roots is presumed to restore the imbalance and thus reduce the spasticity of the muscles. (From Oppenheim 1990, by permission of *Clinical Orthopedics and Related Research*, 22.)

standing (Foerster 1913).[4] Of his 150 cases he termed 88 as 'congenital spastic paraplegia' and eight as 'infantile spastic paraplegia'. Although he did not document all his results, the photographs in his paper depict dramatic improvement in limb posture and function. As in the contemporary practice of rhizotomy in cerebral palsy he emphasized that a long exercise program was needed postoperatively and that the patients often required orthopaedic surgery.

Foerster's posterior rhizotomy technique lay fallow through World War I and II, it seems, because of the postoperative sensory loss in the limbs or recurrence of the spasticity.

RESURRECTION

The rebirth of rhizotomy seems to have been instituted by Gros and colleagues of Montpellier, France. They cut four-fifths of the rootlets from the 1st lumbar to the 1st sacral level (Gros *et al.* 1967). Thirty-two years later Gros published the results of 62 cases with an 18-year follow-up (Gros 1979). The failure rate was 25%, and 22 had a relative hypoesthesia in some limb areas. Of the 25 patients who had cerebral palsy he observed improved speech and upper-limb function as well.

In parallel with Gros in France, Privat *et al.* (1976) in Austria and Fasano and colleagues (1976, 1978) in Torino, Italy, adopted 'selective posterior rootlet rhizotomy' in cerebral palsy.[5] Fasano's refinement was to use intraoperative stimulation of the rootlets and the electromyographic (EMG) responses to decide which roots should be cut to reduce the spasticity (Fasano and Zeme 1988). The challenge of directly altering spastic paralysis was also embraced by Beneditti and Columbo (1981, 1982) who reported good results in 18 patients, three of whom with quadriplegia had first to third cervical rhizotomies and 15 with spastic paraplegia who had lumbar rhizotomies. The follow-up ranged from 4 months to 3.5 years.

In South Africa, Peacock modified the Fasano technique by exposing the cauda equina rather than the spinal cord (Peacock and Arens 1982). After Peacock presented his results in North America, and despite a stinging critique by two well-known neurologists, Landau and Hunt (1990), who questioned its efficacy and the neurophysiological rationale, the operation was enthusiastically accepted by neurosurgeons worldwide. As a new and seemingly effective quiver in the armamentarium of the neurosurgeon, the procedure has spread faster and perhaps further than the Four Gospels to all nations. It has created a flood of outcome reports that have at least three co-authors and some as many as six or eight! All attested to its efficacy in reduction of spasticity in the lower limbs (often referred to as 'tone') primarily as estimated by the pre- and postoperative Ashworth scale. We

shall spare the reader a tedious detailing of the results in all of these studies. The authors of the initial papers reported no mortality and few complications (Cahan *et al.* 1987, Arens *et al.* 1989, Peacock and Staudt 1990, Lazareff *et al.* 1990, 1999, Peacock and Staudt 1991, Vaughan *et al.* 1991, Gaskill *et al.* 1992, Purohit and Dinakar 1992, Steinbok *et al.* 1992, Abbott *et al.* 1993, Boscarino *et al.* 1993, Park *et al.* 1993, Peter and Arens 1993, Schijman *et al.* 1993, Xu *et al.* 1993, Dudgeon *et al.* 1994, Kaufman 1994, Lang *et al.* 1994, McLaughlin *et al.* 1994, Morota *et al.* 1995, Nishida *et al.* 1995, Steinbok *et al.* 1995, Shevelev *et al.* 1996, Thomas *et al.* 1996, 1997, Buckon *et al.* 1997, Hodgkinson *et al.* 1997, Engsberg *et al.* 1998, Vaughan *et al.* 1998, Wright *et al.* 1998, Gul *et al.* 1999, Engsberg *et al.* 1999, Yam *et al.* 1999, Smyth and Peacock 2000.

OPERATIVE PROCEDURE

The surgeon exposes the posterior elements of the lumbar vertebral from the 2nd to the 5th lumbar level, removes the lamina while preserving the facets (laminectomy) or hinges them laterally at their base (laminoplasty), opens the dura mater, isolates the posterior roots, separates them into the five to ten rootlets, electrically stimulates the rootlet to identify the particular muscle supplied by it, and cuts 25%–50% of the rootlets. The contraction of the particular muscle when the rootlet is stimulated is observed through sterile clear plastic drapes. Most surgeons appear to have accepted the quality of the EMG response to rootlet stimulation to further localize the rootlet that caused the spasticity of the muscle (Newberg *et al.* 1991, Oppenheim *et al.* 1992, Steinbok *et al.* 1994).

Some surgeons have questioned the selectivity of rootlet rhizotomy using the EMG responses. When Cohen and Webster (1991) stimulated the rootlets in 22 of their cases, they reported normal responses. Lazareff and colleagues (1990, 1999) in Mexico raised some doubt on the selectivity of the procedure. They did a comparative study comprised of the usual 2nd lumbar to 1st sacral rootlet rhizotomy in one group children with cerebral palsy and only the 4th lumbar to the 1st sacral rootlets in a another group randomly selected. They reported a comparable reduction of spasticity in the lower limbs and functional ambulation in both groups.

Adding doubt to the need for electrophysiological monitoring of the rootlets to be cut were the studies of Pollack (1994) and Logigian *et al.* (1994). The latter concluded that 'the current intraoperative methods for selection of 'abnormal' dorsal rootlets for section may be invalid and may have no bearing on successful outcome, since spasticity improves even with random posterior dorsal rhizotomy (PDR).

Rising to the challenge of the doubtful need for intraoperative EMG monitoring, the initial proponents of the technique published their standard EMG technique (Staudt *et al.* 1995). They noted considerable variations in the electrophysiological technique by 16 centers doing rhizotomies in cerebral palsy as shown in a survey by Steinbok and Kestle (1996).

A study from one of the epicenters of rhizotomy, Seattle, Washington, found that with electrophysiological monitoring of

---

4 The article had originally been published in German 5 years earlier: Förster, O. (1908) 'Über eine neue operative Methode der Behandlung spastischer Lähmungen mittels Resektion hinterer Rückenmarkswurzeln.' *Zeitschrift Orthopaedic Chirgie*, **22**, 203–223.

5 When I was a guest speaker at a conference on cerebral palsy, in Milan, Italy, in 1993, I asked colleagues of Fasano about the follow-up of their patients who had rhizotomies in 1976. They told me that they were unable to follow these patients because they were scattered all over continental Europe—such is the fate of outcome studies (EEB).

92 patients during rhizotomy there was no consistent relationship between the proportion of abnormally responding rootlets to electrical stimulation and the severity of muscle spasticity or the gross motor abnormality (Hays *et al.* 1998). Responses to stimulation of the posterior rootlets were found inconsistent by Warf and Nelson (1996). The conclusion was that the current techniques result in only random partial rhizotomy. It appears that EMG monitoring in the attempt to be 'selective' in sacrificing rootlets is not essential. However, nerve rootlet stimulation seems necessary to make sure you have identified the correct rootlet to the correct muscle you wish to relieve of its spasticity.

POSTOPERATIVE CARE

The lower-limb muscles are very weak initially after rhizotomy. Function is gradually recovered over a period of 6 months. Strength gradually improves. A study using a dynamometer that measured the resistive torque of hamstring muscles before and after rhizotomy revealed that these muscles were stronger after rhizotomy (Engsberg *et al.* 1998). All authors reporting their results emphasize that 'intensive' physical therapy is essential postoperatively. This usually entails an inpatient regimen varying among centers from a week or two to 4–6 weeks. Outpatient therapy supervision goes on during the ensuing months until strength is regained (McLaughlin *et al.* 1994). 'Physical therapy' as used to describe the postoperative care connotes nothing specific. Sometimes it is embellished as 'neurodevelopmental therapy' (NDT).

According to the study by Engsberg and colleagues of St Louis, Missouri, adductor spasticity was reduced following rhizotomy compared with normal controls, but muscle strength did not decrease (Engsberg *et al.* 2002). Buckon and colleagues (2002) of Portland, Oregon, also found no change in muscle strength after rhizotomy in ten children with spastic diplegia compared with eight age-matched controls.

Two neurosurgeons from Vancouver have concluded that intensified physical therapy before rhizotomy in children with spastic diplegia did not improve motor outcomes as measured by the GMFM and was not necessary (Steinbok and McLeod 2002).

From my own (EEB) observations and communication with physicians and therapists, the therapy harks back to the days of poliomyelitis. The predominant goal is muscle strengthening with active assisted exercise of the affected muscles, active and resistive exercises, and supplemented by gradual supported weightbearing, the use of plastic ankle–foot orthoses, sometimes knee splints, progression to walking, and pedaling a tricycle. Although swimming is not mentioned as a postoperative exercise, one might imagine that it could be included in the strengthening program as the ideal active exercise. The benefits of a daily workout apply to those with cerebral palsy just as to those without.

Giuliani (1991) noted that although rhizotomy reduced spasticity and improved the joint ranges of motion, abnormal motor patterns persist. This is not surprising because postoperative dynamic electromyographic studies show no change in the phasic activity of the lower-limb muscles. Giuliani suggested that therapists direct their efforts to assessment of motor control and apply principles of motor learning in their treatments.

COMPLICATIONS

Parents and caregivers need to know the possible complications that might occur after posterior rootlet rhizotomy in order to give informed consent. The most worrisome complication would be loss of bladder or bowel control that would add to the person's disability due to the spastic paralysis of the limbs. One group at the New York University Medical Center revealed that half of the 200 children on whom they did selective posterior rhizotomy had 'serious complications', including bronchospasm, aspiration pneumonia, urinary retention, and sensory loss. The incidence of the latter was 2% (Abbott *et al.* 1993).

SENSORY LOSS IN LOWER LIMBS

Of the 158 children who had the operation at the British Columbia Children's Hospital, Vancouver, complications after 6 months included back pain (10.8%) and sensory changes (13.9%). The sensory changes persisted in only 3.8% (Steinbok and Schrag 1998)

BLADDER, BOWEL AND SEXUAL DYSFUNCTION

The 2nd, 3rd and 4th sacral spinal-cord segments and the nerve roots constitute the efferent fibers of the micturition reflex and contain the preganglionic parasympathetic fibers that innervate the bladder wall with their postganglionic outflow. They also innervate the internal sphincter of the bladder. The external sphincter is innervated by somatic efferent fibers in the pudendal nerve. The internal and external anal sphincter muscles also have their nerve supply via the 2nd to the 3rd sacral segments (Mumenthaler 1990, Mayo Clinic 1991).

Because of this neuroanatomy, postoperative bladder, bowel and sex dysfunction is a concern. Among the 50% of complications reported in 200 children, Abbott and colleagues (1993), at the New York University Medical Center, reported that 7% had urinary retention. Four years later this same center minimized this risk by mapping with intraoperative recordings during rhizotomy of 114 patients the distribution of the pudendal nerve afferent fibers from the 1st sacral to the 3rd sacral nerve roots bilaterally (Huang *et al.* 1997). During the procedure, the 2nd sacral roots were preserved; 56% of these roots had pathological afferent activity. They surmised that preservation of these 2nd sacral posterior roots might be important to obviate bladder, bowel and sexual disturbances postoperatively. They had no such complications in their series.

Adding to the concern of altering bowel function is questionable efficacy of electromyography of the anal sphincter to identify the 3rd to the 5th sacral roots intraoperatively during rhizotomy (Ojemann *et al.* 1997). These neurosurgeons observed anal sphincter activity with stimulation of many of the lumbosacral nerve roots save for those at the 1st lumbar level. Anatomical identification of these important lower sacral nerve roots would be necessary to avoid bowel and bladder dysfunction.

Of 158 patients followed at the British Columbia Children's Hospital, neurogenic bladder and bowel dysfunction occurred in 12.7% longer than 6 months after the operation. However, at their latest follow-up, there were eight patients (5.1%) who had bladder and/or bowel dysfunction, but in only two was this complication considered as a result of the rhizotomy (Steinbok and Schrag 1998). They too recommended monitoring the pudendal nerve during the operation and/or cutting less than 50% of the 2nd sacral rootlets to avoid the urological and proctological complications. A 'pudendal neurogram' was used by the neurosurgeons at the New York Medical Center to discern the proper 2nd sacral nerve rootlets to cut. They made the case for sectioning 2nd sacral nerve roots so that spasticity of the ankle and foot plantarflexors could be reduced (Lang *et al.* 1994). Dorsal penile or clitoral nerve stimulation has also been used intraoperatively to monitor afferent pudendal afferent nerve activity in the 1st–3rd sacral rootlets (Deletis *et al.* 1992).

Sweetser *et al.* (1995) used preoperative and postoperative video urodynamics to assess bladder function. Eight of nine patients with quadriplegia were incontinent preoperatively and none were helped by rhizotomy. Rhizotomy improved bladder control in half of those who had spastic diplegia. Adding to the caveat of possible bladder dysfunction attributed to rhizotomy were the preoperative urodynamic studies of 35 children with spastic ages 5–7 years. Of these, 65.7% had abnormal full bladder resting postures (Houle *et al.* 1998). In their group of children 74% were asymptomatic preoperatively. After surgery, five of seven who were incontinent became continent. These urologists proposed preoperative urodynamics studies in all children who might be selected for rhizotomy. In legalistic United States of America, this advice seems prudent albeit adding to the continuing chorus of complaints about rising costs of medical care.

POSTOPERATIVE RESULTS

REDUCTION OF SPASTICITY AND IMPROVED FUNCTION
All authors report a maintenance of the reduction of the spasticity in the lower limbs as measured with the Ashworth scale. Admittedly, there is an element of subjectivity in using this scale, but it is the only clinical test we have. The degree of spasticity seems to be somewhat in the hands of the beholder.

Beyond the relief of some of the spasticity in the lower limbs, most authors report improved walking and a better range of motion of the joints. Preoperative and postoperative dynamic EMG studies show no change in the primitive and abnormal timing of muscle firing during gait (Cahan *et al.* 1990). In a seeming rush to share the good news, only short-term follow-up studies on functional improvement can be found. Bloom and Nazar (1994) used the Pediatric Evaluation of Disability Inventory (PEDI) to assess 16 children who had the rhizotomy 3–12 months afterwards. They reported improvement in self care, mobility and social skills, and that caregiver assistance was less. Similar results were reported in a 2-year follow-up in 27 patients with quadriplegia after rhizotomies in Buenos Aires,

Argentina (Schijman *et al.* 1993), but generalized as better swallowing, less drooling, easier to manage by the caregivers.

A 6-month and 1-year follow-up study of rhizotomy in 26 children with spastic diplegia noted a decrease in spasticity in 6 months and no further change at 1 year (Buckon *et al.* 1997). The range of motion of the hip and ankle, alignment and stability improved after 6 months. Ability to perform difficult transitional movements occurred after 1 year. The authors surmised that these results were not only due to the rhizotomy, but also to maturation and intensive physical therapy.

Longer-term outcomes were reported in 2002. An outcome study of 71 patients who were beyond 3 years after rhizotomy by neurosurgeons of the Montreal Children's Hospital; they used the GMFM to assess improvement. The mean change was 10.1% at 1 year, 19.9% at 3 years, and 34.4% at 5 years (Mittal *et al.* 2002). The same group evaluated functional outcomes using the PEDI in 41 patients. Significant gains in self-care and mobility were found postoperatively at 1 year and persisted in the 3- and 5-year follow-up examinations (Mittal *et al.* 2002).

Not ones to give up, the group from Seattle, Washington (McLaughlin *et al.* 2002), did a meta-analysis of three randomized clinical trials of dorsal rhizotomy in 82 children under age 8 years with spastic diplegia 65 of whom had a GMFCS of either level II or III. Using the Ashworth scale and the GMFM, these investigators concluded that rhizotomy with physical therapy is effective in reducing spasticity and had a small positive effect on gross motor function related to the percentage of dorsal roots cut.

Selective posterior rhizotomy has spread to the Far East where Kim and colleagues (2001) of Seoul, Korea, reported their happiness with 10-year results in 208 patients who had improved over 95% in spasticity, range of motion and gait patterns. They did note that older patients who had limited ranges of joint motion preoperatively continued to have the same limited motions postoperatively. They concluded that the procedure is best done in young children.

Rhizotomy versus only physical therapy. The need to combine physical therapy supervised exercise programs after rhizotomy has led to disagreement about whether this type of 'intensive' physical therapy alone would account for the improvement in function rather than the rhizotomy alone. A comparative trial of rhizotomy plus physical therapy and physical therapy alone indicated that the GMFM score of the rhizotomy plus physical therapy group increased 11.3% and in the group with physical therapy alone 5.2%. The conclusion was that the improvement is more than can be explained by intensive physical therapy alone (Steinbok *et al.* 1997b).

The rhizotomy group at the Seattle center did an investigator-masked randomized clinical trial of posterior rootlet rhizotomy plus the usual physical therapy regimen postoperatively with physical therapy alone in 38 children who had spastic diplegia. Their assessment included electromechanical torque measurements of the spasticity and the GMFM to assess mobility. Although the spasticity was reduced in the rhizotomy group, outcome measurements of independent mobility were the same in both groups at 24 months postoperatively (McLaughlin *et al.* 1998). These investigators suggested that although rhizotomy was safe, it might not be the treatment of choice in children who have mild spastic diplegia.

Wright and colleagues (1998) in Toronto did a GMFM study of 24 children with spastic diplegia randomly split into two groups of 12: one that had physical and occupational therapy only and 12 that had these therapies plus rhizotomy. They confirmed that rhizotomy combined with physical and occupational therapy had statistically significant greater improvement after 1 year than those with therapy alone.

A comparison of intensive physical therapy with rhizotomy was by Graubert and associates of Seattle (2000). Children with mild spastic diplegia ages 3–18 years had instrumented gait analysis before and 1 year after rhizotomy in both groups. Kinematic changes of considerable variability were noted in both groups. But ankle dorsiflexion, foot-progression angles and hip and knee extension were significantly better in the rhizotomy group compared with the physical therapy group. More importantly, no significant improvements in functional gait parameters of time, distance or ambulatory status could be discerned in either group.

While enthusiasm for rhizotomy has waned over most of North America, the group (Engsberg *et al.* 2006) from St Louis Children's studied 68 children with cerebral palsy who underwent either selective dorsal rhizotomy followed by intensive physical therapy or therapy alone. The SDR group showed more improvement in strength, gait speed and gross motor function as measured by Gross Motor Abilities Estimate Score.

Rhizotomy as a defined specific procedure allows a comparison between physical therapy alone and rhizotomy. But rhizotomy without the assistance of a physical therapist postoperatively is apparently not considered good medical practice because postoperatively the limbs muscles are very weak and take weeks to recover. Probably a totally pure answer will never be forthcoming.

RHIZOTOMY VERSUS ORTHOPAEDIC SURGERY

Marty and colleagues (1995) published the one and only paper to date on rhizotomy in the *Journal of Bone and Joint Surgery*. They tried to compare the results of rhizotomy in 100 children who had spastic diplegia divided equally in two groups: 50 who had rhizotomies and 50 who had only who had soft tissue procedures (Achilles and hamstring lengthenings, adductor and iliopsoas releases) at an average age of 5 years and a follow-up of a mean of 4 years. They found no significant differences between the two groups in ranges of motion of the lower limb joints or the walking quality and ability. Thirty-one patients in the rhizotomy group required orthopaedic surgery later.

A very detailed study by Thomas and group (2004) of the Shriners Hospital, Portland, Oregon, compared 18 children with spastic diplegia who had rhizotomy with 7 who had only orthopaedic surgery of the lower limbs. The study was not random, i.e. the surgeons did not decide for the child and family. Instead the family was given a choice and a detailed informed

consent for either procedure. Using the evaluation tools of the Ashworth Scales, passive ranges of motion, gait analysis and energy cost at a 2-year follow-up they found little difference between the two procedures.

Further reporting on some patients (Buckon *et al.* 2004) showed earlier and greater qualitative changes in movement, improvement in mobility, self-help skills and social function in the SDR group compared to the orthopaedic group.

SENSATION

Sensory disturbances in the lower limb do occur, but are not frequent. Peter and Arens (1994) reported dysesthesia in the legs and feet of five of 26 adolescent and adult patients with spastic diplegia; seven had patchy inconsistent areas of pinprick loss. These sensory changes persisted beyond the 2-year follow-up. Cortical somatosensory-evoked responses, H reflex and F wave studies were done preoperatively and postoperatively in 20 children with spastic cerebral palsy (Cahan *et al.* 1987). Although many children had abnormal cortical somatosensory-evoked responses preoperatively, a loss of these responses was seldom observed. Of interest is that these authors judged that some children had evidence of spinal cord dysfunction preoperatively.

GAIT ANALYSIS

The originators of posterior rootlet rhizotomy were hampered in assessing their results due to lack of instrumented gait analysis. In the subsequent years more surgeons and their teams were able to utilize this tool for more objective outcome assessment. Vaughan, with Berman and Peacock (1988), presented the results of sagittal-plane gait analysis with a digital camera system of 14 children who had the rhizotomy in 1985 at Clemson University, South Carolina, and again in 14 children at the University of Virginia (1991). They reported increased motion of the knee and hip, improved stride length and walking speed. The range of motion of the thigh, i.e. the hip, exceeded the normal ranges after 1 year, but returned to the normal range in 3 years.

Boscarino *et al.* (1993) provided kinematic data in 19 children studied preoperatively and postoperatively. Eleven independent walkers did show statistically positive changes toward normal with the exception of hip extension, hip adduction, pelvic tilt and pelvic rotation. In studying their data, maximum knee flexion during swing phase increased 5% (p=0.0439) and at initial contact changed 4º (p=0.0429). The total range of knee motion increased 8º (p=0.0073). The only highly significant change was maximum ankle dorsiflexion in stance that changed 10º (p=0.0001). From this data the improvements in the joint angles measured during gait were not dramatic. Stride and step length improved after rhizotomy, but walking velocity did not. No change in the phasic action potentials of the muscles could be seen in the dynamic electromyograms.

Subsequent reports of gait analysis before and after rhizotomy confirmed the improvement in passive ranges of lower-limb joint motion, dynamic range of motions during gait, and increased stride length and velocity (Thomas *et al.* 1996). The longest follow-up reported is 10 years, by the group at Cape Town,

South Africa (Subramanian *et al.* 1998). Using age-matched normal controls with 19 children who had spastic diplegia and video computer kinematic analysis they concluded that the ranges of motion of the lower-limb joints improved to approximately the normal midrange after rhizotomy. Figure 6.6 (*a–c*) is an example of preoperative and postoperative kinematics derived from gait analysis of a patient who had a selective posterior rootlet rhizotomy.

UPPER LIMBS

Anecdotal reports of improved function of the upper limbs after posterior rootlet rhizotomy appeared in a rather short time after rhizotomy was introduced. Kinghorn (1992) attempted to assess functional changes in the upper limbs of seven children, 12 months postoperatively. Their data suggested that activities of daily living, play, balance and endurance all improved. Therapists in San Antonio, Texas (Beck *et al.* 1993) used blinded videotape assessments of three preoperative and postoperative tasks (assumption of side-sitting, maintenance of side-sitting and block-building) and concluded that patients improved in all three with statistical significance.

Dudgeon and associates (1994) studied 29 children with either spastic diplegia or quadriplegia for postoperative improvement of function utilizing the PEDI scores. Function in mobility and self-care areas improved in those with spastic diplegia, but not spastic quadriplegia. Upper-limb reach and coordination tasks showed no significant improvement. Most importantly, this study emphasized that improvements should be attributed not necessarily to the rhizotomy or special therapies. Rather continued maturation, setting new goals, and positive belief about progress influenced the outcome.

Another study of 26 children with spastic diplegia did not show demonstrable improvement in upper-limb function (Buckon *et al.* 1996). The significant improvements in toilet and dressing skills were deemed due to the lessened spasticity in the lower limbs postoperatively. So it remains that improvement in upper-limb function after rhizotomy may be only a perception in the eyes of the surgeon and therapists.

Recently a group from Montreal (Mittal *et al.* 2002) used the fine-motor skill section of the Peabody Developmental Motor Scales to assess grasping, hand use, eye–hand coordination and manual dexterity 1, 3 and 5 years after rhizotomy in 70 patients. They found significant and durable improvements in upper-limb function.

SPINAL DEFORMITY

Because laminectomy in children has sometimes been followed with late scoliosis or lordosis, initial fears were that this would occur after rhizotomy in cerebral palsy. Fifty-five children were followed by the pediatric neurosurgical team in Cape Town, South Africa (Peter *et al.* 1990). The majority of spinal deformities (scoliosis 16%, kyphosis 5%, lordosis 7%, spondylolysis/spondylolisthesis 9%) were considered due to cerebral palsy and not the laminectomy. Three years later the same group assessed

radiographs of the lumbar spine of 163 children postoperatively (Peter *et al.* 1993). 20% had an isthmic spondylolysis or grade I spondylolisthesis. It was thought that the combination of laminectomy, lordosis and increased mobility after rhizotomy were causative factors.

Surgeons at the Scottish Rite Hospital for Children, Dallas, Texas, described two children with spastic quadriplegia who developed severe lordosis after rhizotomy (Crawford *et al.* 1996). One of these children was a non-walker and the other a household walker. Most of their day was spent sitting, and this became painful and difficult due to the excessive lordosis. As might be expected, surgical correction was complicated and difficult.[6]

Turi and Kalen (2000) assessed the risk of spinal deformity after rhizotomy in a retrospective study of 43 patients. The average follow-up was 5.3 years (range 2–9 years). Preoperative scoliosis in three patients, hyperkyphosis in one, and hyperlordosis in another was found. Postoperatively 28 spinal deformities developed in 19 patients: scoliosis in 15, lumbar hyperlordosis in seven, thoracic hyperkyphosis in five, and one L4–5 spondylolisthesis. The risk of spinal deformity after rhizotomy was calculated as 36%. 6% of these patients needed operative spinal stabilization.

M.B. Johnson and colleagues of the Shriners Hospital, Portland, Oregon in 2004 reported a study of 34 ambulatory patients with spastic diplegia age 10–19.8 years and a follow-up of 5–11.6 years postoperative selective dorsal rhizotomy specifically addressing spinal deformity (personal communication). 50% developed hyperlordosis, 18% had a grade I spondylolisthesis, and scoliosis occurred *de novo* in 24%.

Spinal stenosis was discovered in two postoperative patients who had cerebral palsy and walked with assistive devices (Gooch and Walker 1996). They attributed this late complication to the marked lateral trunk sway these patients had while walking. When the posterior elements of the spine are stripped and removed in growing children, late new bone formation at the operative site has been observed. So, the finding of spinal stenosis due to bony overgrowth is not too surprising.

Chinese orthopaedic surgeons of Peking University reported the effect on the spine in 197 children with the spastic type of cerebral palsy (Yi *et al.* 2001). Analysis of supine, standing, and lateral dynamic projections of the lumbar spine revealed nine cases of scoliosis, six of spondylolysis, and five with spondylolisthesis in those 10 years or older. They concluded that the lamina 'excided', i.e. removed, healed and the stability of the lumbar spine was not significantly effected.

EFFECT ON THE HIP JOINT

Heim and colleagues (1995) studied the anterior–posterior radiographs of the hips in 45 children (90 hips) with spastic quadriplegia before and after rhizotomy using the migration

6 In 1996 when I visited Johannesburg, South Africa, I (EEB) was shown by Faith Bishop, PT, PhD, several quadriplegic children who had a severe, fixed, lumbar lordosis after rhizotomy at a center. Cape Town, South Africa is where selective posterior rootlet rhizotomy was first introduced to the English-speaking medical world (Peacock and Arens 1982).

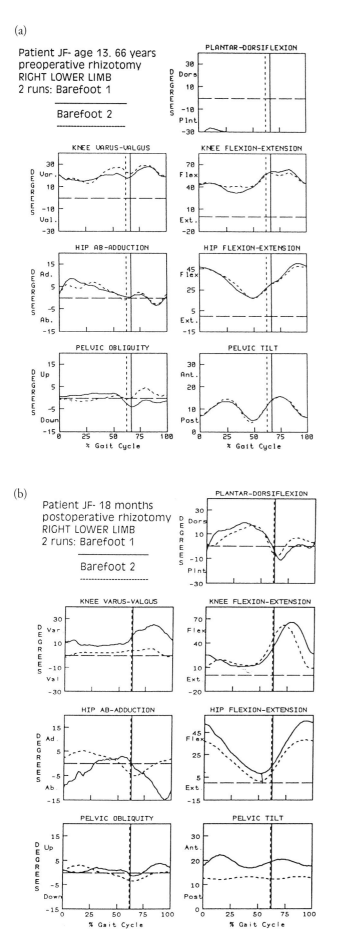

(a)

Patient JF- age 13. 66 years
preoperative rhizotomy
RIGHT LOWER LIMB
2 runs: Barefoot 1

Barefoot 2

(b)

Patient JF- 18 months
postoperative rhizotomy
RIGHT LOWER LIMB
2 runs: Barefoot 1

Barefoot 2

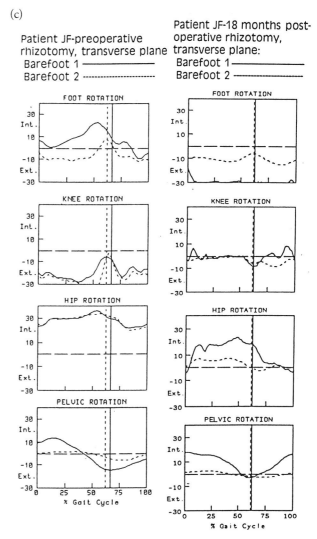

(c)

Patient JF-preoperative
rhizotomy, transverse plane
Barefoot 1 ————
Barefoot 2 - - - - - -

Patient JF-18 months postoperative rhizotomy,
transverse plane:
Barefoot 1 ————
Barefoot 2 - - - - - -

Fig. 6.6. (*a*) Kinematic data, gait analysis, pre-operative selective posterior rootlet rhizotomy, patient JF, spastic diplegia, age 13.66 years: no foot/ankle dorsiflexion; knee in varus throughout gait cycle; flexed knee throughout gait cycle and knee-flexion and extension barely present; hip adducted somewhat in stance; hip remains in flexion; considerable anterior–posterior pelvic tilt. (*b*) Postoperative gait analysis, 18 months, patient JF: foot/ankle now dorsiflex and plantarflex in stance and swing; knee in less varus; hip extension much improved in stance, but not to the normal baseline; hip abduction-adduction on barefoot run 1 (solid line) is not much changed; in run 2 (dotted line) the hip is abducted initially in stance, then adducts, and finally abducts in swing. Which run is the more accurate? (*c*) Pre- and postoperative gait analysis of patient JF of rotational components in lower limbs: internal foot rotation decreased considerably postoperatively; knee rotation was all external preoperatively and came close to neutral postoperatively; hip internal rotation was marked preoperatively in both swing and stance, but diminished postoperatively; pelvic rotation from internal to external during stance and swing was approximately 20° more in swing on run 1, but rotation in either direction in runs 2 preoperatively remained unchanged. (By courtesy of J.R. Gage, MD, Gillette Children's Hospital, St Paul, MN.)

percentage of the femoral head (Reimers 1980). Preoperatively lateral migration of the femoral head was 11%; postoperatively it increased in 18%. The follow-up averaged 20 months (range 7–50 months). Surprisingly, the authors stated that ambulatory status had no bearing on the hip stability. One wonders about this conclusion because none of quadriplegic patients whom we term 'total body involved' are functional walkers. Some therapists and physicians diagnose quadriplegia when they find minimal spasticity in the upper limbs in children who have major involvement in the lower limbs, i.e. spastic diplegia. In addition, an average follow-up of 20 months is not long enough. We have all seen hips go on to dislocation after 3–5 years or longer.

Surgeons at the St Louis Children's Hospital, in a follow-up of 134 hips in 67 children with spastic diplegia, found stability of the hips in 93% after rhizotomy (Park *et al.* 1994). In only 7% did the migration percentage increase and at the time of the report only one required an orthopaedic operation for a persistent hip subluxation. They too did not find any correlation with the ambulatory status of the child. Except for those with spastic diplegia who continually use walkers or crutches, subluxation of the hip is very rare, if ever present (except perhaps in the 1 in 1000 who may have a developmental dislocation of the hip). As a caveat, a surgeon might be guarded in promising rhizotomy as a preventative of subluxation of the hip in a child with spastic diplegia and is dependent on crutches or a walker.

In contrast to the foregoing report, Greene *et al.* (1991) discovered a rapid progression of pre-existing hip subluxation of a 25% migration to 50% in seven hips of six patients 1 year after rhizotomy. Hips with lesser degrees of subluxation had variable outcomes.

ORTHOPAEDIC SURGERY AFTER RHIZOTOMY
When selective posterior rootlet rhizotomy first appeared in North America in about 1985 with videotapes of dramatic results by Peacock, we heard murmurings of veiled anxiety laced with skepticism among some orthopaedic surgeons who imagined that would soon be out of the business of surgery in cerebral palsy. Fifteen years later the widespread adoption of rhizotomy and the outcomes has made these fears unwarranted.

The group at the Shriners Hospital for Children in Portland, Oregon, stated that 66%–75% of their patients required orthopaedic surgery for residual deformities after rhizotomy (Thomas *et al.* 1997). They also found that the improvement in the hip, knee and ankle motions after rhizotomy reached a plateau between 1 and 2 years.

The orthopaedic surgeons at the Primary Children's Medical Center, Salt Lake City, Utah, were able to follow 112 patients who had the rhizotomy between the years 1986 and 1994 (Carroll *et al.* 1998). Seventy-one of these patients needed orthopaedic surgery for correction of deformities and contractures. The most common surgery was for correction of a valgus deformity of the feet with subtalar stabilization (37%) followed by femoral or pelvic osteotomies for hip subluxation in 27 (25%). In all patients muscle tone in the lower limbs had been reduced as measured with the Ashworth scale.

The neurosurgeons at the St Louis Children's Hospital did a data analysis on the need for lower-limb orthopaedic surgery after rhizotomy in 178 children. Those children who had the operation between the ages of 2 and 4 years had a lower orthopaedic surgical rate than those between 5 and 19 years of age. In particular, their data indicated a reduced need for Achilles tendon lengthening, hamstring and adductor releases (Chicoine *et al.* 1997).

Postoperative valgus of the feet with excessive dorsiflexion of the ankle in children with spastic diplegia has been a common deformity that usually requires a subtalar stabilization. Adams *et al.* (1995) suggested sectioning fewer 1st sacral rootlets to preserve plantarflexion strength. In addition these surgeons found persistent knee flexion during gait and significant residual hamstring spasticity. A very detailed follow-up study of 112 post-rhizotomy patients delineated that orthopaedic surgery was required in 65%: 37% needed subtalar stabilization for severe pes valgus, 25% required femoral and/or pelvic osteotomies for hip subluxation. In none did the rhizotomy change the ambulatory status (Carroll *et al.* 1998).

My own experience (EEB) in referral of patients to centers for consideration of rhizotomy is that for the hip internal rotation gait pattern so common in spastic diplegia, femoral derotation osteotomies to correct the femoral torsion have been advised prior to rhizotomy. And some patients with spastic diplegia 2 years post-rhizotomy or longer have had hamstring lengthenings and rectus femoris transfers. However, the argument can be made that rhizotomy by lessening the spasticity makes the orthopaedic operation more effective in restoring more normal gait patterns.

Heterotopic ossification of the hip after rhizotomy appeared in 25% of the 26 spastic quadriplegic patients who had subsequent proximal varus derotation osteotomies compared with none in a similar group of 69 patients who did not have the rhizotomies (Payne and DeLuca 1993). Why this difference in the complication that causes pain and stiffness in the hips defies a scientific explanation. The importance of it, however, is to alert the surgeon to monitor the hips postoperatively if femoral osteotomies are done after rhizotomy. Whether it can be prevented with drugs such as indomethacin opens another avenue for clinical research. Preoperative radiation as prevention would not be indicated in children.

INDICATIONS FOR RHIZOTOMY
The *best candidates* are children with spastic diplegia, age 4–7 years, good voluntary strength and control of muscles, and only moderate contractures (W.J. Peacock, personal communication). In the attempt to find predictors of walking ability after rhizotomy Chicoine and neurosurgical colleagues (1996) at the St Louis Children's Hospital analyzed their 90 children with spastic cerebral palsy who had rhizotomies. They found that the preoperative gait score (p<0.0001) and the diagnosis (p=0.0015) were the best predictors of the ability to walk. Voluntary dorsiflexion of the ankle had some predictive value, but less than the gait score and diagnosis. These data seem to mean that the best candidates

for rhizotomy to ensure postoperative walking ability are those who are able to walk preoperatively, i.e. spastic diplegia.

The best candidates for rhizotomy to ensure postoperative walking ability are those who are able to walk preoperatively, i.e. spastic diplegia.

Unacceptable candidates are those with dystonia, athetosis, rigidity, ataxia, hemiplegia, severe contractures, joint deformities, trunk weakness, prior neurectomy or overlengthening of muscles, fixed spinal deformity, and prior spinal fusion (Oppenheim *et al.* 1992).

Quadriplegia (total body involved) does not seem to be a popular choice as reflected in the current medical literature. Originally, neurosurgeons reported good general results, but without specific measurements of function, and severe spinal deformities seemed to evolve on follow-up. A report from Lyon, France (Hodgkinson *et al.* 1997), on 18 children with spastic quadriplegia indicated a decrease in muscle spasticity, increased range of passive hip abduction and extension, and no hip migration. The GMFM scores, however, increased only 3.2%. These French physicians concluded that orthopaedic problems could not be prevented with rhizotomy.

Intrathecal baclofen appears to have superceded rhizotomy in children and adolescents who have spastic quadriplegia (total body involved).

CURRENT STATUS

Without a doubt, Peacock made a contribution in the much sought for relief of spastic paralysis in cerebral palsy. The patient whom we all wanted to help the most, the total body involved seems to have had the more marginal result. Enthusiasm for selective posterior rootlet rhizotomy seems to have waned, and may be more selective as confined to spastic diplegia.

According to a personal communication from Johannesburg and Pretoria, South Africa, the numbers of children with spastic diplegia or quadriplegia having the procedure has diminished. Physical therapists in this region were 'very keen' on referring patients for rhizotomy, but have become disillusioned with the long-term results (F. Bishop, personal communication). The disillusionment may come from the fact that the patients who needed the relief of spasticity the most—the total body involved—had the least discernible benefit.

Sussman (personal communication) wrote that in the early 1990s the Shriners Hospital for Children, Portland, Oregon, did approximately one selective posterior rootlet rhizotomy per month. In the later 1990s and into the early years of the 21st century he estimated they do one a year.

In the United States some neurosurgeons maintain their enthusiasm for the procedure as reflected in 2003 in the popular press. The reason is probably that almost all the patients selected for the procedure have spastic diplegia that carries a good prognosis for function. However, one wonders if a patient who walks independently with spastic equinus and balanced knee function should have 30%–50% of afferent nerves fibers perma-

nently removed rather than a simple Achilles or gastrocnemius lengthening. If in a independent walking patient the only gait abnormality is a flexed knee gait becoming progressively worse, might hamstring lengthening with a rectus femoris transfer (if the spastic quadriceps is limiting knee flexion in swing more than a physiological range) be safer, have less morbidity, have a relatively short period of postoperative rehabilitation, and be just as effective a solution?

Orthopaedic surgery was required in 60%–75 % of patients after selective posterior rootlet rhizotomy.

Worries about long-term effects on the spine, possible neuropathic joints, and post polio-like syndromes seem reasonable. Unfortunately, the very long-term outcomes (20–30 years) of patients who had selective posterior rootlet rhizotomy in the mid-1970s in Italy are not available for follow-up as they are scattered throughout continental Europe (the International Conference and Updating Course on the Orthopaedic Treatment of Cerebral Palsy, personal communication).

Now that intrathecal baclofen has become established as another way to relieve spastic paralysis, more parents of children and adults seem to opting for it (at least as a trial) before electing surgery that 'cuts nerves'. This seems be true especially in those who have spastic quadriplegia (total body involved).

NEUROPHARMACOLOGY

POSTOPERATIVE ANALGESICS

Relief of pain after orthopaedic surgery or rhizotomy must be assured, particularly during the first 48 hours. All too often inadequate dosages of narcotics are given. Muscle relaxants are no substitute for effective narcotics to relieve pain. We prefer administering narcotics intravenously through the intravenous line inserted by the anaesthesiologist at the time of surgery. Narcotics can be titrated according to the response. Small doses of intravenous narcotics are effective, but need repeating more frequently than if injected subcutaneously or intramuscularly. Anaesthesiologists also use intraoperative regional blocks with a local anesthetic that lasts up to 6 hours.

In patients who have a single-event multilevel surgery of the lower limbs, Nolan and colleagues (2000), from the Royal Children's Hospital, Parkville, Victoria, use epidural administration of bupivacaine 0.125% with clonidine 2.5μg/ml at 0.2–0.3 ml/kg/h and state this combination results in better analgesia, less muscle spasm and less postoperative nausea and vomiting. They insert epidural catheters at two levels according to the level of the incision (usually L1–2) and the second at L4–5. With this system either catheter can be bolused with small volumes to alleviate pain.

Another pain-controlling method is with an epidural catheter that with one injection of a narcotic will last 6 hours; the catheter can be left in place for up to 3 days. Dilaudid is the first choice over morphine because it causes less respiratory depression and itching than occurs with morphine. Repeated injections after the baseline dose is established can be done depending on the response. With either intravenous or epidural analgesia using narcotics respiratory function must be monitored to avoid hypoxia or hypercarbia (A. Hackel, personal communication). Table 6.V gives a guide for postoperative analgesia in children.

Morphine remains the drug of choice for postoperative analgesia in posterior rootlet rhizotomy (Geiduschek *et al.* 1994). At the Children's Hospital and Medical Center in Seattle, a large number of rhizotomies in cerebral palsy have been done. The majority of patients received continuous morphine infusion (20–40 µg/kg/h). A few patients used a patient-controlled system. Occasionally epidural morphine was successful. Ketorolac was an adjunct to morphine. For muscle spasm, intravenous diazepam (0.1 mg/kg or midazolam infusion at 10–30 µg/kg/h) was effective. The authors advised continuous cardiorespiratory monitoring and frequent nursing assessment while receiving these analgesics and/or muscle relaxants.

Botulinum toxin A injections preoperatively into the hip-adductor muscles was found an effective supplement to analgesia after adductor-release surgery in a double-blind controlled study. (Barwood *et al.* 2000).

ORAL MEDICATIONS FOR SPASTICITY

A characteristic that distinguishes humans from other animals is that humans like to ingest pills. In our culture most patients want to take a pill as a cure. Doctors usually accommodate by writing

TABLE 6.V
Postoperative analgesia for children*,**

Meperidine   0.25–0.5mg/kg. IV
  Give slowly over 2–3 min

  After initial dose, attempt to leave the child without stimulation in order to monitor effect on state of consciousness and respirations

  If child still very agitated and crying after 10 mins has elapsed from the initial dose, repeat 0.25 mg/kg IV and wait another 10 mins without stimulation

  Dose can be repeated to a maximum of 1 mg per kg per hour

Morphine   0.025–0.05 mg/kg IV
  Titration of administration the same as with meperidine

Diazepam   Oral administration preferred. Poorly absorbed intramuscularly

  Oral dose 0.1–0.2 mg/kg

  Intravenous dose 0.05–0.1 mg/kg *very* slowly—duration of IV dose: 5–10 minutes

  Danger: respiratory depression with rapid IV administration especially if in combination with a narcotic

  Oral dose can be repeated if child is very agitated and has spasm. *Make sure you have given adequate narcotic if the child is in pain.*

Naloxone   For overdose of narcotic and respiratory depression

  First stimulate patient. If no improvement, start assisted ventilation with a bag and mask and 100% oxygen

  When ventilation is assisted, give naloxone IV in dosage of 0.005–0.01mg/kg

*Prepared by Michael Flynn MD, former assistant professor of anesthesiology, Department of Anesthesia, Stanford University School of Medicine, Stanford, CA.
**Hydromorphone hydrochloride preferred by some—less respiratory impairment and itching (Hackel 2000).

a prescription. Clinicians may find the way to end the interview with the patient is to write a prescription for a medication rather than answer in detail the patient's concerns or to explain why a drug is not needed as well as the risks of ingesting the pill.

Oral medications to reduce spasticity have had only minor benefits in cerebral palsy. All have the side-effect of lethargy because their effects are spread throughout the brain and are not specific to the muscle or its innervation. Some commonly tried drugs are detailed below (Albright 1995).

BENZODIAZEPINES

Diazepam is rapidly absorbed after ingestion. Peak serum concentrations are reached in 15–30 minutes, but the half-life is approximately 36 hours. Usual maintenance doses are from 0.1 to 0.8mg/kg/day. Diazepam acts on the GABA$_A$ receptors distributed throughout the central nervous system so it affects more than muscle spasticity. Depression of the reticular activating system causes lethargy. Lethargy is not much liked by children or parents. Consequently most of our patients discontinued its regular use long ago. Diazepam can be useful occasionally for severe anxiety and some patients with athetosis found it helped them relax, lessened anxiety and the startle response. Postoperatively it is useful in cases of moderate spasticity associated with pain.

Diazepam continues to be a popular muscle relaxant, although there have been no objective assessment methods to demonstrate reduction of muscle spasticity (Hamilton 1984). Its action is central. Schoolchildren usually discontinued it because it seemed to interfere with their ability to learn new subjects. Its effect is cumulative, so there is still an effect 24–36 hours after withdrawal of the medication.

One double-blind study used an intramuscular injection of benzodiazepine clonazepam, a drug primarily for seizure disorders, at low doses to children with spastic hemiplegia or diplegia (Dahlin *et al.* 1993). Electromyographic and dynamometer assessments revealed a significant reduction is spasticity compared with a placebo (p<0.001). But it too causes central nervous system depression and can interfere with cognitive and motor performance.

DANTROLENE SODIUM

Dantrolene sodium was first released for use in 1974. It reduces muscle contraction by blocking the intracellular release of calcium from the muscle sarcoplasmic reticulum (Fig. 6.7). After a flurry of high hopes that this medication would relieve spasticity or decrease muscle tone in dystonic and tension athetosis, its use seems to have gradually diminished. Our experience and study with dantrolene in cerebral palsy was reported by Ford *et al.* (1976). Even though Ford and colleagues found some objective improvement in the gait of hemiplegic and diplegic children, no child in the original study continued its use: partly because of the resultant mental dullness, and the need to monitor liver function for toxicity with SGOT blood-levels every 3–4 months. A random clinical study indicated only slight reduction in spasticity (Joynt and Leonard 1980).

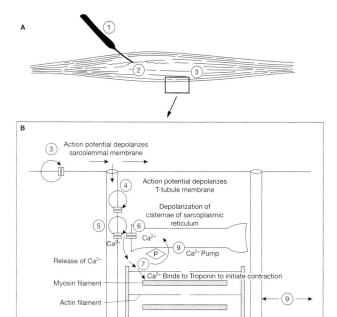

Fig. 6.7. Steps in excitation–contraction coupling in skeletal muscle. (*A*) Overview of the muscle and its nerve supply. The nerve action potential (1) invades the nerve terminals, activating the neuromuscular junction to release acetylcholine and set up the endplate potential (EPP) (2). Thus triggers the muscle action potential (3). (*B*) Steps in the muscle include depolarization of T-tubules (4), activating voltage-sensitive channels (5) that activate Ca^{2+} channels in the sarcoplasmic reticulum (6). This increases Ca^{2+} flux into the sarcoplasm, where it binds to troponin (7) to initiate contraction (8), with pumping of Ca^{2+} back into the sarcoplasmic reticulum (9). (Reproduced from Shepherd 1994, Fig. 17.4, p.187, by permission.)

In four trials dantrolene was considered superior to a placebo in treating children with cerebral palsy, with improvement in the ranges of motion (Krach 2001). Dantrolene combined with diazepam in children has been preferred to the use of either drug alone, and it has been thought better than baclofen in reducing spasticity (Badell 1991).

Dantrolene has occasionally been prescribed postoperatively short term in children who had a severe muscle spasticity unrelieved by diazepam and adequate narcotics. It was taken orally, in an initial dose of 0.5 mg/kg bodyweight for each dose four times a day. The dose can be increased to 3 mg/kg bodyweight for each dose.

A fascinating and effective use of oral dantrolene sodium was found in the prevention of malignant hyperthermia in swine and humans who have a genetic trait for its onset during surgical procedures. Intravenous dantrolene is effective in stopping this life threatening complication through its action on blocking calcium ion release from the skeletal muscle sarcoplasmic reticulum. The hypothesis is that malignant hyperthermia is due to a triggering event, such as general anesthesia, that causes a change in the muscle cell that elevates calcium levels in the myoplasm. This elevation incites an acute cellular catabolic process that goes forward to cause a hyperthermic crisis (Proctor & Gamble Pharmaceuticals 2000).

GABAPENTIN

This drug, widely used in neuralgic pain syndromes, is an anticonvulsant similar in structure to GABA. It crosses the blood–brain barrier. In trials in patients with multiple sclerosis Ashworth scores were reduced when compared to a placebo. No reports of its use in children have been forthcoming (Krach 2001).

ALPHA2-ADRENERGIC AGONISTS: CLONIDINE AND TIZANIDINE

These chemical agents are thought to decrease muscle tone by hyperpolarizing motornuerons due to a decrease in the release of excitatory amino acids. The result is decreased motoneuron excitability. Both drugs have been used in adults with spasticity of spine cord origin or multiple sclerosis (Krach 2001). Clonidine has been used in adults with spinal-cord injury to reduced spasticity and improve gait velocity. It has also been combined with intrathecal baclofen for treatment of spinal cord origin spasticity and neuropathic pain after injury. The side-effects of hypotension, nausea and vomiting, as well as frequent sedation may not be acceptable in children with cerebral palsy.

BACLOFEN

Baclofen is an agonist of gamma amino butyric acid (4-chlorophenyl-GABA) that is an inhibitory neurotransmitter throughout the gray matter of the brain and spinal cord. It is stored in the terminals of the axons. GABA receptors are of two types: GABA$_A$ and GABA$_B$. Price *et al.* (1984) discovered GABA$_B$ receptors in laminae 2 and 3 (substantia gelatinosa) in the rat spinal cord. In the human, the substantia gelatinosa is only 1 mm from the surface. The receptors bind to baclofen to decrease the excitability of the neuron. The result is a reduction in muscle spasticity (Fig. 6.8).

Orally administered baclofen has been used in cerebral palsy for some time, but due to its 30% binding to protein and low lipid solubility transport across the blood–brain barrier its effectiveness is limited (Fig. 6.9). Its oral effectiveness on spasticity is minor. If given in a large enough dose to reduce spasticity, the undesirable side-effect is lethargy. A randomized trial in 20 children who had cerebral palsy with spastic paralysis found that at a dosage of 2 mg/kg/day had no significant effect on muscle tone (McKinlay *et al.* 1980). The usual pediatric oral dose has been 5–10 mg/day with increases of 20–60 mg/day in divided dose. In a review article, Albright (1996) cited 16 European trials of oral baclofen in 315 patients with cerebral origin spasticity. In 10 trials, 80% had a reduction in spasticity.

Before a physician takes the easy way out to terminate the interview with the parents of the child by writing a prescription for an oral drug to reduce spasticity, he or she needs to be aware of the side-effects and toxicity of the drug. This information needs to be transmitted to the parents of the child and preferably in writing, at least in the litigious culture of the USA.

INTRATHECAL BACLOFEN

When baclofen is injected into the cerebral spinal fluid, its concentration is more than 10 times that found with oral

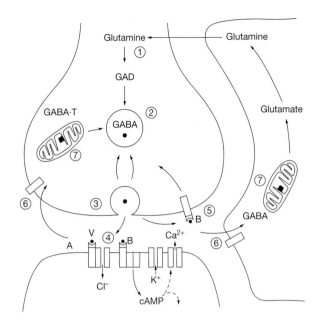

Fig. 6.8. Molecular mechanisms of GABAergic synapses: sites of binding of benzodiazepines, diazepam and blockage by baclofen. (1) Synthesis of γ-aminobutyric acid (GABA) catalyzed by glutamic acid decarboxylase (GAD). (2) Transport and storage of GABA. (3) Release of GABA by exocytosis (co-release with a neuropeptide, e.g. enkephalin or somatostatin). (4) Two types of GABA receptors: $GABA_A$ = site for binding Valium; $GABA_B$ = linked via G protein and/or cAMP to K^+ and Ca^{++} site of block by baclofen. (5) Binding to presynaptic receptors. (6) Reuptake in presynaptic terminals and uptake by glia. (7) Transamination of GABA to α-ketoglutarate catalyzed by GABA transaminase to regenerate glutamate and glutamine; glial glutamine then reenters the neuron. (Modified from Shepherd 1994, Fig. 7.8, p.143, by permission.)

administration. Its action on the $GABA_B$ receptors in the spinal cord is greatly enhanced to make it an attractive drug in the management of spastic paralysis. Intrathecal infusions were first used for treatment of spasticity of spinal-cord origin (spinal-cord injury and multiple sclerosis); investigators reported good results with few side-effects (Penn and Kroin 1985, 1987, Lazorthes *et al.* 1990, Penn 1992). Coffey *et al.* (1993) led a trial of 15 centers using intrathecal baclofen in intractable spasticity of spinal cord origin encompassing 93 adults. At the mean follow-up of 19 months the team concluded that in patients who responded to a test dose up to 100g it may be the treatment of choice.

Albright and colleagues (1991) began testing intrathecal baclofen with a placebo injection in spastic cerebral palsy. The randomized double blind study showed that baclofen was just as effective in reducing spasticity of cerebral origin as it is in spinal cord origins.

With the development of the subcutaneous programmable pump (Medtronic, Inc., Minneapolis, Minnesota) to deliver the drug through an intrathecal catheter, it did not take very long to discover its use and effectiveness in cerebral palsy (Albright *et al.* 1991, 1993).

PATIENT SELECTION
Two groups of patients with cerebral palsy have been selected for intrathecal baclofen: (1) spastic diplegia or ambulatory spastic quadriplegia who use spasticity to stand and walk that would be lost if they had a rhizotomy; (2) non-ambulatory total body involved. All should have 'severe' spasticity (Ashworth scale ≥3, i.e. marked increase in muscle tone with movement of limb in flexion or extension and difficult passive movements). They should be aged ≥4 years, and have sufficient body mass to support a subcutaneous pump (Medtronic 1997). Albright (1996)

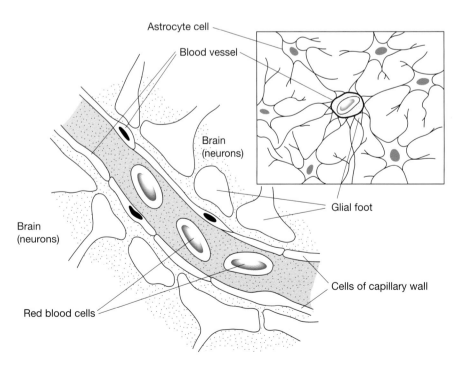

Fig. 6.9. Schematic representation of the blood–brain barrier. A type of glial cell (astrocytes) extends 'feet' that form a continuous layer around blood vessels in the brain, thus creating a fatty barrier that prevents substances not soluble in fat from passing from the blood into the brain. (Reproduced from Thompson 2000, by permission.)

reported that dystonia was 'markedly improved'. Athetosis has not responded.

Oppenheim, who has had considerable experience with patient selection for both selective posterior rootlet rhizotomy and intrathecal baclofen in cerebral palsy, found that parents prefer the baclofen course initially because it is reversible (W.L. Oppenheim, personal communication). Rhizotomy is not reversible.

PROTOCOL

The following is a general description of the technique for intrathecal baclofen. It should not be used as a detailed instruction on its application (Figs 6.10, 6.11). Those who wish to use it should consult the instructions of Medtronic as well as consult the literature referenced.[7] The steps to be taken that have been formulated are as follows (Albright 1996, B. Mandac, personal communication).

(1) The child is admitted to the hospital as early as possible in the morning. An evaluation is done. The child is sedated and has a lumbar puncture to give a test dose of baclofen (usually 50 µg) by bolus.

(2) After the test dose or doses a physician and/or a physical and occupational therapist observes the child and the responses every 2 hours. A positive response is a drop of 1 point on the Ashworth scale. If so, the child is discharged. If the response is not positive, the trial is repeated using higher doses of 75 µg on day 2 and if still no response, a 100 µg dose on day 3. If the response is negative, the patient is deemed ineligible for the implant.

(3) With a positive test dose bolus, implantation of the pump is scheduled and an intrathecal silastic catheter is passed

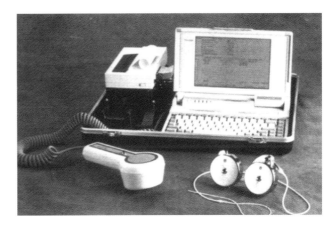

Fig. 6.11. Intrathecal baclofen system set-up with programmable pumps and computer. (By courtesy of Medtronic, Inc., Clinical Reference Guide for Spasticity Management, 1997.)

subcutaneously to the level of the 10th thoracic vertebra. Baclofen is instilled via the infusion pump usually 100–300 µg/day at a rate of 4.2–12.5 µg/hour. The response is assessed by the physical and occupational therapist. Doses can be increased every 8 hours at 50 µg increments per day for a maximum of usually 900 µg/day. If the response is positive, the patient is scheduled for pump implantation.

(4) The programmable pump, about the size of a hockey puck (7.5 cm diameter and 2.8 cm thick), powered with a lithium thionyl-chloride battery (life of 3.5 years) is inserted under the abdominal muscular fascia and filled with saline during surgery. On recovery the saline is replaced with baclofen solution and the infusion started. Neurological and vital signs are checked every 4 hours for 24 hours, and then every 8 hours. An oxygen saturation monitor is used for the first 24 hours. Blood pressure is checked every 8 hours. An abdominal binder is worn for 2–3 weeks.

(5) After 2–3 weeks the physical therapy begins. The physician adjusts the dosage of baclofen and empties and refills the pump every 60–90 days. The reservoir is refilled by percutaneous puncture of its septum with a 22 gauge needle; the septum can be punctured 500 times (Medtronic 1996). The physician addresses complications such as infection, cerebral spinal fluid leaks, system failure, catheter complications, battery depletion, pump replacement and inadvertent baclofen overdosage. To counteract the toxic effects on the central nervous system or heart physostigmine iv should be on hand (pediatric dose 0.02/kg, maximum: 2 mg) infused at a rate of no more than 0.5 mg/minute; adult 1–2 mg iv for 5–10 minutes).

COST ANALYSIS RHIZOTOMY VERSUS INTRATHECAL BACLOFEN

The foregoing details have been written to indicate that although intrathecal baclofen treatment is seemingly simple, it demands special equipment, and most importantly, is highly labor-intensive using medical-care professionals. Consequently, it is not inexpensive. Steinbok *et al.* (1995), of British Columbia, Canada, did a cost analysis of selective posterior rootlet rhizotomy compared

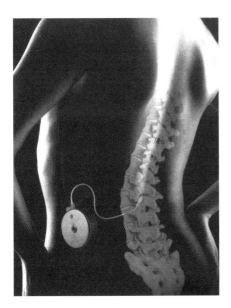

Fig. 6.10. Intrathecal baclofen schematic of catheter and pump in a subcutaneous pocket in the abdominal wall. (By courtesy of Medtronic, Inc., Clinical Reference Guide for Spasticity Management, 1997.)

7 Medtronic, Inc., Neurological Division, 800 53rd Avenue, NW, Minneapolis, MN 55421, USA; www.medtronic.com

with intrathecal baclofen in 10 children with spastic quadriplegia. In Canadian dollars the cost of intrathecal baclofen treatment per patient after 1 year was approximately four times that of rhizotomy. The higher cost of the latter was related to the cost of screening children who did not go on to have the implantable pump.

RESULTS IN CEREBRAL PALSY

Müller (1992) in Germany headed a multicenter trial of 72 patients who had spasticity of cerebral origin and 139 with spastic paralysis of spinal-cord origin. Spasticity was reduced 90%–95% in all; the results in children less than 10 years old were not reported separately. Upper-limb function was improved.

Albright and colleagues (1993) were the first to report intrathecal baclofen infusion for 37 patients who had cerebral palsy with spastic quadriplegia, seven with mixed athetosis and spasticity, three who had traumatic spastic quadriplegia and one who was postencephalitic. Of these patients 25 were considered functional despite moderately severe quadriplegia, and 12 were non-functional and incapable of self-care. Six and 12 months after baclofen, mean muscle tone was reduced in the upper and lower limbs. The functional group improved knee extension by reduction of spasticity in the hamstring muscles. Upper-limb function and activities of daily living functions improved in 25. Only one child who was non-ambulatory pre-intrathecal baclofen became ambulatory with a walker after the intrathecal infusion. The non-functional group all had reduced muscle spasticity, but did not improve in the range of motion of the limb joints, position transfers, or activities of daily living. Caregivers and patients stated they had increased ease of care, although two found that transfers in and out of bed and chair were more difficult due to less lower-limb spasticity, i.e. they had used their extensor thrust for supportive weightbearing on transfers. Anecdotes from physicians have told of a similar loss of transfer function in some total body involved patients who had posterior rootlet rhizotomy. An important advantage of intrathecal baclofen is that the result is reversible by removing the catheter and pump.

An important advantage of intrathecal baclofen is that the result is reversible by removing the catheter and pump.

Since Albright's report of the efficacy of intrathecal baclofen, the method spread throughout the world undoubtedly because spastic quadriplegia (total body involved) has not responded to traditional therapy methods or orthopaedic surgery. The literature on the subject giving testimonials to its efficacy proliferated.

Armstrong *et al.* (1997) did a double-blind controlled study in 19 children who had spasticity of cerebral origin, 10 of whom had spastic quadriplegia. Of these 19 children, seven were withdrawn because of excessive sedation or a poor response. Good reduction in muscle spasticity occurred during the follow-up period of 1–5 years. But one child who had a reduction in spasticity in the lower limbs found transfers from bed to chair more difficult. The price of the results was significant complications in nine patients (hypotension, bradycardia, apnea, and

sedation). Mechanical complications occurred in ten. These authors concluded that more experience and longer follow-up would be necessary to assess the long term efficacy of this new method of spasticity reduction.

Rawicki (1999) of Australia assessed the long-term benefits of intrathecal baclofen with an implantable pump in 18 patients who had cerebral palsy with severe spasticity. Follow-up ranged from 12 months to 9 years. Of the 18 patients, 17 had a reduction in tone with resultant benefits in reduced nursing care and/or increased function.

Van Schaeybroeck *et al.* (2000) of Belgium reported a double-blind placebo study. The Ashworth score, spasms, pain, and functional abilities were measured in 11 patients. Interestingly, they noted a placebo effect with the bolus test injections. But eight of their patients had functional improvement with the continuous infusion of baclofen. These author advised double-blind screening with the initial test bolus injection for each patient.

A multicenter trial by Gilmartin *et al.* (2000) of 51 patients randomized and screened with intrathecal baclofen and a placebo had a decrease in their spasticity of the lower limbs from an Ashworth score of 3.64–1.90. Adverse effects occurred in 42 patients, most commonly hypotonia, seizures (without a new onset), somnolence, nausea or vomiting. 59% had procedural or system-related events.

EFFECT ON AMBULATORY PATIENTS

Intrathecal baclofen has been tried in ambulatory patients with cerebral palsy and lower limb spasticity (Gerszten *et al.* 1997). Twenty-one patients with spastic cerebral palsy and three with traumatic brain injury with a mean age of 18 months had a mean dose of 200µg/day via the implantable pump. At a mean follow-up of 52 months, ambulation was improved one functional level in nine; did not change in 12, and was worse in three. Twenty of 24 patients and their families thought the gait was improved. The authors concluded that this study indicated there was no contraindication to using baclofen in patients who used their spasticity for support when walking.

EFFECT ON UPPER-LIMB FUNCTION

Albright and colleagues (1995) using the Ashworth scale compared upper-limb muscle tone in 36 patients who had continuous intrathecal baclofen infusion with 38 who had selective posterior rootlet rhizotomies. At 6 months a paired follow-up study revealed no significant difference in the reduction of muscle tone between the two procedures. Joint ranges of motion in the upper limbs did not improve in either group at 6 and 12 months. But upper limb function was thought improved.

NEED FOR ORTHOPAEDIC SURGERY

Gerszten and colleagues (1998) from the University of Pittsburgh reported a 24- to 94-month follow-up of 40 patients who had spastic quadriplegia and eight with spastic diplegia with reference to the subsequent need for orthopaedic surgery. Prior to pump implantation, 28 patients (58%) had planned orthopaedic surgery. Eight of these patients had lower-limb orthopaedic surgery prior to intrathecal baclofen. After intrathecal baclofen only 10 (21%) had surgery due to reduction in their lower-limb spasticity. The most common post-baclofen operation was femoral osteotomy that might be expected because no method to relieve spasticity could be expected to change the pathological bone structure of the femur or the hip in cerebral palsy. The authors were quick to point out that no historical controls exist for the rate of orthopaedic surgery in cerebral palsy.

Measurement of plasma concentrations of continuous intrathecal baclofen in six children who had cerebral palsy indicated little systemic effect (Albright and Shultz 1999). These children received the drug at rates of 77–400 µg per day. Plasma levels of baclofen were below the limit of quantification (10 ng/mL).

Albright *et al.* (1993) reported no adverse effects in their first 37 patients who had spastic quadriplegia. Urinary hesitancy occurred in four and resolved with a lower baclofen dosage. Infection occurred in the first 16 patients leading the authors to give all subsequent patients prophylactic antibiotics. Pumps had to be removed because of infection in four, recurrent cerebrospinal fluid leaks in two, and no therapeutic benefits in two.

An alarming and potentially serious complication is withdrawal of intrathecal baclofen that simulates a neuroepileptic malignant syndrome (Samson-Fang *et al.* 2000). The report concerns a 9-year-old boy with cerebral palsy and quadriplegia. When the intrathecal baclofen was withdrawn he had unexplained multiorgan system dysfunction that can be accompanied by rhabdomyolysis. Caregivers should be advised seek urgent medical consultation if a child has a fever or acute illness while receiving intrathecal baclofen.

BOTULINUM TOXIN

'One man's poison is another man's potion.'
(Anderson *et al.* 1995)

The feared botulism from food contamination due to the neurotoxin of the bacterium, *Clostridia botulinum*, has remained a food-borne infection (Lund 1990). The serious and life-threatening neurological effects of ingestion of the bacterium are due to the impaired release of acetylcholine from the calcium-dependent vesicles at the neuromuscular junctions of the nerves. This gram positive bacillus elaborates seven types of neurotoxins, four of which affect humans: types A, B, E, and occasionally F. Type A toxin occurs predominantly in the United States, west of the Mississippi River, type B in the eastern states, and type E in Alaska and the Great Lakes Region (Beers and Berkow 1999).

Botulism can also occur as the result of wound contamination. Infant botulism is due to the ingestion of the spores of the bacillus. Most infantile cases are idiopathic, but are thought to be derived from honey in some cases and possibly the ingestion of microscopic dust particles.

As with botulism the toxin impairs the release of acetylcholine from the vesicles at the neuromuscular junction to cause a local paralysis of the muscle (Fig. 6.12). The effects of botulinum-A toxin have been studied in laboratory mice and rat muscles. Four days after injection, no action potentials were recorded with single-fiber electromyography of the biceps femoris muscle. Fourteen days later jitter in the muscle was measurable. Progressive atrophy of the extrafusal and intrafusal fibers began on the fourth day. Histological evidence of increased neuromuscular terminals was found from the 14th day onward (Rosales *et al.* 1996). After injection of the toxin, increasing nerve terminal sprouting and arborization was observed in the mouse levator auris longus muscle (Juzans *et al.* 1996).

In the mouse sternocleidomastoid injected with botulinum-A toxin, extensive sprouting of nerve terminals was observed. After 28 days vesicles of acetylcholine were evident in the sprouts, but not in the parent nerve terminals. Later on the superfluous sprouts were eliminated and the vesicle turnover returned to the original terminals (de Pavia *et al.* 1999). These animal studies explain the biological reason why botulinum toxin intramuscular injections are usually effective in reducing muscle contractions shortly after injection and the return of spasticity in 3–6 months. A permanent effect has not been observed; the process is biologically reversible.

Cosgrove and colleagues (1994) did a controlled study using the toxin and saline injections into the gastrocnemius muscle of spastic mice. In the spastic mice injection with the toxin the tendon length to tibial length in growth of 1 month was reduced 12% compared to growth of 83% in those injected with saline. The toxin injected muscles developed no contractures after 65–70 days.

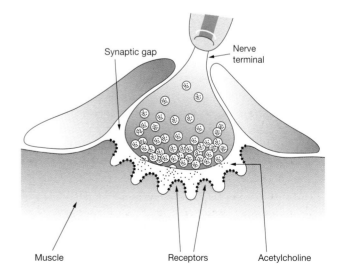

Fig. 6.12. Vertebrate neuromuscular junction. Nerve terminal releases acetylcholine through the synaptic cleft or gap to the acetylcholine receptors in the muscle. Botulinum-A impairs this release of acetylcholine. (Reproduced from Shepherd 1994, by permission.)

Purified Botulinum toxin, Type A (Botox®, Allergan, Inc., USA; Dysport®, Porton Products, UK) for local injection has found uses well beyond the confines of cerebral palsy. A Medline (USA National Library of Medicine) search of the literature became a journey through exotic neurological diseases and not so exotic dermatological and gastrointestinal conditions in the process of spewing forth 2402 references to the use of the toxin from 1990 to July 2000. Some articles have catchy titles: 'Botulinum beyond wrinkles' (Heckman *et al.* 1997), 'Chemical brow lifts' (Frankel and Kramer 1998), '"Toxic" facelifts' (Harvard Women's Health Watch 1998), 'One man's poison' (Hallett 1999). In the culture of 'forever young' the plastic surgeons and dermatologists have been kept very busy injecting facial muscles to erase the passage of time.

Even if the use (and sales) of botulinum toxin for intra-muscular injection in the spastic type of cerebral palsy reaches a plateau, it will continue to boom in cosmetic enhancement of the face. The duration of its effect on facial muscles for the elimination of wrinkles and lines seems to be between 3 and 6 months. Repeat facial injections are needed to stem the toll of aging. Being proximate to a plastic surgical clinic has lowered the cost of botulinum toxin injections for some of the children with cerebral palsy (W.L. Oppenheim, personal communication). It would be possible to use the left-over toxin for injection in the spastic muscles of children at a low cost. Left-over toxin refrigerated at $+4^oC$ or refrozen at -20^oC was found to be just as effective as the reconstituted fresh Botox (Sloop *et al.* 1997). The only possible problem in using left-over toxin is the risk of bacterial contamination drawing multiple doses from a single vial. In personal communication, Dr Oppenheim states that he never uses left-over toxin.

Being proximate to a plastic surgical clinic has lowered the cost of botulinum toxin injections for some of the children with cerebral palsy.

Injectable purified botulinum-A toxin has opened therapeutic interventions for not only for orthopaedic surgeons and dermatologists, but also for neurologists and physiatrists-rehabilitationists, anesthesiologists, gastroenterologists and proctologists. In the literature one encounters unfamiliar medical diagnostic territory such as Frey syndrome,[8] Meige syndrome,[9] achalasia,[10] sphincter of Oddi (also known as Glisson's),[11] and convulsing breast muscle flap—a process of continuing medical education for an orthopaedic surgeon.

The toxin's first clinical use was in the treatment of strabismus. Rayner and associates (1999) in London reported on its efficacy in strabismus of 237 children from 1985 to 1995. Its

clinical applications have extended to a host of rather intractable conditions: fissure-in-ano, anismus (involuntary contraction of anal sphincters), bruxism, cervical dystonia, tardive dystonia, writer's cramp (focal dystonia), inherited benign cramp–fasciculation syndrome, spasmodic dysphonia, spasmodic torticollis, detrusor sphincter dysynergia (spinal cord injuries), drooling saliva in Parkinson's disease, crocodile tears, childhood myoclonus, tics, tension headache, whip-lash injuries of the neck, irreducible shoulder dislocation with pectoralis major spasm, palmar and axillary hyperhidrosis, facial lines and wrinkles, crow's feet, glabellar furrows, the aging face and neck, and facial rejuvenation.[12]

The last but not least application is in cerebral palsy, primarily spasticity, but it is apparently effective in dystonic patterns (dyskinesia) encountered occasionally in children with cerebral palsy. In adults who have idiopathic or tardive extension truncal dystonia injections into the lumbar paravertebral muscles have been effective in relieving this distressful condition (Comella *et al.* 1998).

BOTULINUM TOXIN AS A THERAPY IN CEREBRAL PALSY

Koman and colleagues (1993) were among the first to introduce botulinum-A toxin injections for spastic dynamic equinus in children. Spasticity was reduced in 12–72 hours after injection and lasted 3–6 months. A double-blind control established its safety and efficacy (Koman *et al.* 1994). By 1996 Koman and his colleagues had done 1200 injections of botulinum-A toxin into upper and lower limb muscles in spastic paralysis (Koman *et al.* 1996). As in their initial reports, no complications were encountered. Again they reported a 3- to 6-month duration of the effects and concluded that a positive response could be anticipated in 70% of the patients.

Since 1994 the use of botulinum-A toxin as reflected in the flood of references in the medical literature has spread world-wide from the United States and the United Kingdom to the continents of Africa, Asia, and Australia, Europe, North America, South America, and the island nations of Japan, Singapore, Taiwan and New Zealand. All reports have attested to its efficacy in reducing the spasticity in the particular muscle injected. The major muscles injected have been the heads of the gastrocnemius, posterior tibialis, adductor longus, proximal hamstrings, biceps brachii, pronator teres, flexion digitorum profundus and superficialis, and flexor carpi ulnaris (Table 6.VI).

Lower-limb muscles. Enthusiasm for the use of the toxin injections in lower limb spastic muscles seems to have tempered a bit. The Clinical Trials Unit, Walton Centre for Neurology and Neurosurgery, Liverpool, UK, reviewed the medical reports on the efficacy of botulinum-A toxin in lower-limb spasticity in cerebral palsy (Ade-Hall and Moore 2000). Their systematic review of

---

8 Frey's syndrome is characterized by gustatory sweating, localized flushing and sweating of the pinna of the ear and cheek after eating hot, bitter, spicy substances and chocolate.

9 Meige's syndrome: involuntary blinking, jaw grinding and grimacing. Blepharospasm: ocular mandibular dystonia.

10 Achalasia: neurogenic esophageal impairment of peristalsis and spasm of the lower esophageal sphincter.

11 Sphincter of Oddi (Glisson): sphincter of the hepatopancreatic ampulla.

12 Rather than listing all the references, the reader can find them on Medline via the internet at www.nlm.nih.gov (at no cost).

TABLE 6.VI
Selected reports of botulinum-A toxin in cerebral palsy

Authors	Year	Muscles injected	N	Follow-up	Results
Wall *et al.*	1993	Thumb in palm	5	7.6 months	Improved function; sustained
Calderon-Gonzales *et al.*	1994	Hip adductor, gastroc. hamstrings	15	6 months	All improved
Cosgrove *et al.*	1994	Gastroc–soleus Hamstrings, Post.tibial	26	18 months	Improved; 7 sustained improvement
Chutorian and Root	1994	Gastrocnemius	7	3 months	3 ankle equinus to normal
Denislic and Meh	1995	Foot and hand	13	3.1 months	Improved function
O'Brien	1995	Lower limb	14	26 weeks	Popliteal angle reduced
Garcia-Ruiz *et al.*	2000	Gastrocnemius	8	33 months	All improved
Heinen *et al.*	1997	Hip adductor, gastroc. cervical dystonia, focal	28	12–64 months	Improved; 1 non-response
Pascual-Pascual *et al.*	1997	Upper limbs, gastroc. hamstrings, hip adductors	39	12 months	Improved; highly effective
Sanchez-Carpintero and Narbona	1997	Hip adductors, hamstrings, gastroc., posterior tibialis	27	5–17 months	All improved. Stabilized at 4–6 months
Zelnik *et al.*	1997	Gastroc–soleus	14	6.7 months	Improved gait, 9; no change, 4
Wong	1998	Lower limb	17	10 months	Improved function
Corry *et al.*	1998	Gastroc–soleus	20	12 weeks	Improved ankle kinematics; casts relapsed
Thompson *et al.*	1998	Hamstrings	10	2 weeks	Crouch gait; muscles lengthened.
Corry *et al.*	1999	Hamstrings	10	3 months	Knee extension, stance, improved 8°; Relapsed 12 weeks. Energy cost unchanged in 6 of 10 patients
Eames *et al.*	1999	Gastrocnemius	39	12 months	Pre-injection dynamic component strongly correlated with the response
Massin and Allington	1999	Lower limb	13	6 months	Energy cost variable; improved endurance
Yang *et al.*	1999	Hip adductors &/or gastrocnemius	28	3 months	Ashworth scale improved; GMFM improved
Boyd *et al.*	2000	Gastroc–soleus	25	6 months	Ankle kinetics improved Some also serial casts
Friedman *et al.*	2000	Upper limb	32	4 months	Spasticity elbow and wrist declined. Responses not predictable
Koman *et al.*	2000	Gastrocnemius–soleus	114	3 months	Improved
Mall *et al.*	2000	Hip adductors	18	Not stated	GMFM and Ashworth scale: improve in GMFM level III and IV. Only 1 in 5 in level V improved.
Autti-Ramo *et al.*	2001	Upper and lower limb	49	Not stated	23 or 27 functional improvement 8 for presurgical planning 6 to improve posture and care; 4 benefitted.
Linder *et al.*	2001	Adductor spasm & equinus	25	1 year	Range of motion and Ashworth scale Improved; GMFM gain 6 %.
Boyd *et al.*	2001	Adductors/ hamstrings	35	1 year	GMFM gains: w/BTX-A & orthosis 6%; BTX-A without orthosis 6.1%. progressive hip migration >40%
Molenaers *et al.*	2001	Lower limb-multilevel	29	1 year	BTX-A 29 compare with 23 surgery Gait analysis
Desloovere *et al.*	2001	Lower limb-multilevel	34	2 months	Multilevel injections: 17 with pre-op casting and 17 with post-op casting; 3D gait analysis; slightly more improvement if casts after surgery.

reports did not reveal strong evidence to support or refute the use of the toxin. They called for controlled randomized studies to address the longer-term use of the injections, and outcome measures that would assess function and disability.

The orthopaedic department of the Royal Children's Hospital, Melbourne, Australia, convened a group of 15 clinicians and scientists to formulate a treatment protocol for botulinum-A toxin (Graham *et al.* 2000). They arrived at a consensus on patient selection, assessment, dosage, injection techniques and outcome measurement. They also stressed the importance of physiotherapy, orthoses and casting.[13] At the same institution

Boyd and colleagues (2000) reported their prospective trial in 15 children with spastic diplegia and 10 with hemiplegia who had injections of the *gastrocnemius–soleus muscle.* Using kinematic gait analysis, improvement in ankle kinetics were documented 12 and 24 weeks after injection.

Koman *et al.* (2000) of North Carolina, USA, did a double-blind, placebo-controlled trial of Botox in 114 children with *spastic dynamic equinus.* Each child had 4 units of botulinum toxin type A (BTX) per kg of body weight diluted, divided and injected into the proximal medial and lateral gastrocnemius of each involved leg. The placebo group had injections of the same amount (4cc per leg) of sterile saline. The results measured with observational gait analysis, ankle range of motion measurements and nerve conduction studies to quantify muscle denervation

13 www.unimelb.edu.au

showed improved gait function and partial denervation. They reported no serious adverse effects. Sutherland *et al.* (1999) also verified with gait analysis the efficacy of botulinum-A toxin injections into the gastrocnemius of 20 patients in a double-blind study with saline as a control.

Koman and 12 co-investigators (2001) conducted a prospective, multi-center clinical trial to evaluate the long-term safety and efficacy of repeated intramuscular injections of the equinus gait in 207 children in nine centers. 75% completed at least a year of treatment. Gait patterns improved in 46% and were maintained in 41%–58%, 2 years after the injections. There were no serious adverse effects and only 6% developed antibodies to cause failure of treatment.

Investigators in other countries have joined the bandwagon to tout the efficacy of botulinum-A intramuscular injections of the gastrocnemius in spastic equinus deformities in children (Boyd *et al.* 2001, Australia; Zurcher *et al.* 2001, Belgium; Metaxiotis *et al.* 2002, Germany; Baker *et al.* 2002, Northern Ireland; Carrelet *et al.* 2002, France; Bang *et al.* 2002, Korea; Sal'kov *et al.* 2002, Russia; Polak *et al.* 2002, Derbyshire, UK).

Mall and colleagues (2000) of the University of Freiburg, Germany, issued a positive effect of botulinum-A toxin injections of the *hip-adductors* in 18 patients who were classified as levels III, IV or V with the GMFCS. All had reduction of spasticity on the Ashworth Scale, the range of motion improved, and the gross-motor function improved except in those at level V, the most severe.

Boyd *et al.* (2001) reported the use of botulinum-A toxin injections of the hip adductors and hamstrings with a variable hip abduction orthosis (N=19) and a control group that had only physical therapy (N=20). The outcomes on the GMFM scores were the same at a mean of 6% gain on gross-motor function. After 1 year two children who had botulinum toxin injections of the hip adductors and the orthosis and seven who had only physical therapy had a progressive hip migration greater than 40% necessitating surgery.

Botulinum toxin A (Dysport) was injected into the hip adductor muscles in 11 children at a mean age of 5 years, 9 months with spastic quadriplegia by Delplanque *et al.* (2002). Seven had a unilateral migration of the hip greater than 40%. Although spasticity decreased one point on the modified Ashworth scale, three improved in function from a GMFCS level IV to level III and three had pain relief, *five of the seven children had progression of the hip migration so that surgery was required (failure rate 71%).* Follow-up was 12 months. The reduction of spasticity faded from the 6th to the 12th month.

That the iliopsoas was not included in the injections of the hip adductor muscles (Boyd *et al.* 2001, Delplanque *et al.* 2002) appears significant because of its effect in the evolution of spastic paralytic hip subluxation. Subluxation of the hip progressed despite the botulinum toxin induced reduction of adductor spasticity in both studies.

The iliopsoas was not included in the injections of the hip adductor muscles (Boyd et al. 2001, Delplanque et al. 2002).

Subluxation of the hip progressed despite the botulinum toxin induced reduction of adductor spasticity.

According to Willenborg *et al.* (2002), the *iliacus or psoas* was successfully injected the aid of ultrasound guidance for needle placement in 28 patients (53 hips). These investigators used active electromyographic stimulation to verify needle position. The authors reported no measurements of pre- or postoperative hip extension lack measured either clinically or by instrumented gait analysis. However, they state that the technique is 'a safe, reliable adjunct to surgical intervention in the treatment of dynamic hip-flexor spasticity in cerebral palsy'.

Multilevel lower-limb muscle botulinum injections have been tried in 23 patients with spastic diplegia (mean age 6 years 2 months) and compared with multilevel orthopaedic surgery in 29 patients (mean age 13 years 5 months) as a single event by Belgian orthopaedic surgeons (Molenaers *et al.* 2001). The muscles injected were mainly the gastrocnemius, medial hamstrings, adductors, and iliopsoas. The surgery was varied, but primarily lengthening of the same muscles with the addition of bone surgery, e.g. most often was varus derotation osteotomy. Post-treatment evaluation for the botulinum group was at 2 months and 12 months for the surgery group. After exceptional detailed assessment of results that included 3D gait analysis, they reported that gait was significantly improved in both treatment groups, but improvements were more numerous in the surgical group. 50% of the children in the surgery group had prior surgery. They cautioned that the two groups were not comparable in age and pre-treatment condition. The orthopaedic surgical group had more gait abnormalities in the transverse plane, i.e. rotation and more complications. botulinum toxin A and orthopaedic surgery were deemed complimentary rather than mutually exclusive. The complimentary aspect of the botulinum toxin injections was the temporary effect of the toxin on the muscle that enabled an assessment of the possible effects of surgery of the muscle. Whether repeated multilevel lower-limb muscle botulinum toxin injections over a period of years beyond puberty will be necessary to sustain improved gait function is unknown.

Whether repeated multilevel lower-limb muscle botulinum toxin injections over a period of years beyond puberty will be necessary to sustain improved gait function is unknown.

The same Belgian group (Desloovere *et al.* 2001) used 3D gait analysis to demonstrate the effects of botulinum toxin A injections with prior casting of the foot and ankle and with casting immediately after the injections at multilevels in the lower-limb muscles of 34 children with cerebral palsy. The combination of the injections with casting showed the most improvement at the ankle joint. They advised that multilevel treatment should start at an early age to prevent joint contractures. Of note is that only two gait studies were done on each: one prior to the treatment and then 2 months after.

Functional outcomes after botulinum toxin injections in 49 children age 22–80 months were randomly assigned to two groups: one with the injections plus physiotherapy and the other with physiotherapy alone by a group from Melbourne, Australia (Reddihough *et al.* 2002). Using the assessment tools of the GMFM, the Modified Ashworth Scale, the Vulpe Assessment Battery, joint ranges of motion and a parental questionnaire they found sustained gains in gross-motor function in both groups. Those in the group that had injections and physiotherapy had a trend for improvement in fine-motor ratings of the Vulpe Assessment Battery. This testing was included to ascertain if there is an overflow benefit to the upper-limb skills from treatment of the lower extremities. The parents gave a high rating to the benefits of treatment. This discrepancy from the objective measurements was explained that assessment at 3 and 6 months post-injection was too late to demonstrate peak gross-motor function and most importantly 'that changes in GMFM are not sustained over six months with a single dose'. Further studies were suggested.

Upper-limb muscles. Enthusiasm for the use of botulinum-A toxin injections in spastic upper-limb muscles does not match that of the reports of use in the lower limbs, especially in the gastrocnemius and soleus muscles. A double-blind study of botulinum-A toxin in the hemiplegic upper limb noted that the most improvement was in elbow and thumb extension due to reduction in tone of the injected muscles and was judged to be a cosmetic benefit (Corry *et al.* 1997). Fine-motor function did not improve and temporarily deteriorated in some patients.

The effects of injections into the upper-limb muscles in 32 children with hemiplegia or quadriplegia were assessed in a prospective study of 4 months' duration (Friedman *et al.* 2000). They found that spasticity in the elbow and wrist muscles declined as measured by the Ashworth scores. But the patient response to botulinum-A toxin injections was unpredictable and they concluded that further research was necessary.

Fehlings *et al.* (2001) used a Quality of Upper Extremity Skills Test (QUEST) and the PEDI to define the characteristics of children with spastic hemiplegia who would have a good outcome from botulinum-A toxin injections in the upper-limb muscles. They divided the children into positive functional responders and non-responders. Grip strength was higher in responders (p=0.0001) and a young age was somewhat significant in the outcome (p=0.05). They found that grip strength was reduced after the injections in those children who had weak grip prior to the injection.

From Helsinki, Finland, Autti-Ramo and co-authors (2001) reported the effects of botulinum-A toxin injections in the upper limbs in 27 children with spastic upper limb muscles. Of these, 23 had improved function. They caution that the injection treatments may not be an appropriate treatment option for those with severe upper-limb spasticity due to acquired brain injury (seven children) because of the shorter duration of its effects and the potential reduction of functional abilities. They recommended that the dose of the toxin should not be more than 1.5U/kg per forearm muscle.

Pediatricians from Hong Kong, People's Republic of China (Wong *et al.* 2002), did an open label study of botulinum toxin injections into upper limb muscles of 11 children with cerebral palsy. In those assessed with the Jebson Hand Function Test improvement was found in five cases (45 %) with a 1-, 4- and 16-week assessment.

An Australian Botox battle seems to have occurred concerning the reported efficacy of the intramuscular injections in the upper limbs of patients with spastic hemiplegia. Wasiak and co-workers (2002) of the Centre for Clinical Effectiveness, of the Southern Health/Monash Institute of Public Health reviewed the literature and found only the studies of Corry *et al.* (1997) and Fehlings *et al.* (2001) qualified as randomized controlled trials. The Institute representatives concluded that they could not confirm or refute the efficacy of botulinum toxin A in improving the upper-limb function. Therefore it should remain as part of a clinical trial. In response Graham and colleagues (2003) wrote that the conclusions of Wasiak *et al.* (2002) were incorrect. They stated that the study by Corry *et al.* (1997) did not qualify as evidence-based, did not use a validated outcome measure for function and was a pilot study, whereas the study by Fehlings *et al.* (2001) was evidenced based and used a functional outcome test (QUEST). In reply, Wasiak *et al.* (2003) stood by their conclusion that they could not support or refute the efficacy of botulinum toxin injections in the upper limb in improving function. They noted that in the study by Fehlings *et al.* (2001), the significant improvement on the QUEST assessment was weightbearing.

This little Australian conflict concerning the outcome of botulinum toxin injections in the spastic muscles of the upper limbs exemplifies a major problem of the specific test used for outcome assessment; all those who assess results ought to be using the same test. The most important question is whether over a period of 2 years and longer after repeated intramuscular injections of the toxin the improvement is sustained compared with orthopaedic surgery of the spastic upper limb in hemiplegia. The need to repeat injections every 4–6 months in maintaining a more youthful face suggests it may not be the case. At issue in Australia and like countries that have a national health insurance scheme or in the USA that has Federal and State funds for care of the disabled is who pays? Thus the need for government sponsored assessments of the evidence of efficacy.

The issue in the Botox battles on efficacy might be not the cost, but who pays?

Botulinum-A toxin injections may be more useful in *dystonic postures of the hand* in cerebral palsy. The surgical techniques used in the spastic hand deformities are not effective in dystonia. The experience of Denislic and Meh (1995) of Ljubljana, Slovenia, indicated good results in improving skilled movements of the hand after intramuscular injections in the arm and forearm of 13 patients with dystonia.

Treatment of *paralytic scoliosis* with injections of the toxin has been tried in 12 patients who had a short-term follow-up (Nuzzo *et al.* 1997). All had a reduction of curvatures that were greater than 50º. The trial was done to delay surgical treatment because of complicating additional diseases.

An innovative use of toxin injections was preoperatively in two patients with cerebral palsy and *cervical dystonia* (Racette *et al.* 1998). These surgeons injected the cervical muscles prior to the application of halo fixation and spinal fusion for a spondylitic myelopathy. This seems to be a very good idea given the difficulty of immobilizing the cervical spine in patients who have incessant movement of the neck with dystonia.

INJECTION TECHNIQUE AND DOSAGE
(BOTOX® ALLERGEN, INC.)

The vacuum dried purified toxin in 100 unit vials is reconstituted immediately with normal saline solution (0.9% sodium chloride *without preservative*), and the proper dose calculated. The reconstituted toxin can be stored in a refrigerator (2°–8°C) and used within four hours. For the gastrocnemius the dose is 1–2 u/kg of body weight. No dose should be greater than 6 u/kg of body weight (Koman *et al* 1996). The optimum volume for injection is unknown; the advice is that it should not be greater than 20% of the muscle mass (Table 6.VII). A needle injection is done directly into the muscle. For deep muscles a teflon-coated hollow electrode needle is used to localize the injection site with dynamic electromyography, for example, the posterior tibialis (Koman *et al.* 1996) (Fig. 6.13*a*, *b*).

Other than the slight pain from the injection needle puncturing the skin, the toxin is not painful when injected. Local anesthesia is not necessary. Frightened children may need to be sedated a bit. The relative painless injection of the toxin compared to alcohol is a distinct advantage. Electrical stimulation through the hollow injection needle to identify the specific muscle should be useful in patients who are unresponsive or sedated (O'Brien 1997).

Investigators from Duisburg, Germany, use an elegant technique of sonography-guided injections to assure accurate placement of the needle in the targeted muscle. They believe the additional cost of this technology is 'more than offset by the improved reliability in correct needle placement' (Berweck *et al.* 2002). For deep muscles such as the iliopsoas and the posterior tibialis they may be correct.

Although systemic spread of the toxin is apparently rare, respiratory support should be readily available when doing the injections. Antitoxin from the Center for Disease Control, Atlanta, Georgia, USA, should be on hand.

TABLE 6.VII
Dilution table for Botox® injection

Diluent added, 0.9% sodium chloride injection	Resulting dose in units/0.1 ml.
1.0 ml	10.0 U
2.0 ml	5.0 U
4.0 ml	2.5 U
8.0 ml	1.25 U

Dilutions are calculated for an injection volume of 0.1 ml. A decrease or increase in Botox dose is possible by administering in smaller or larger injection volume—from 0.05 ml (50% decrease in dose) to 0.15 ml (50% increase in dose). (Allergan, Inc. *Physician's Desk Reference 2003*. Montvale, NJ, USA: Medical Economics Co., p. 554).

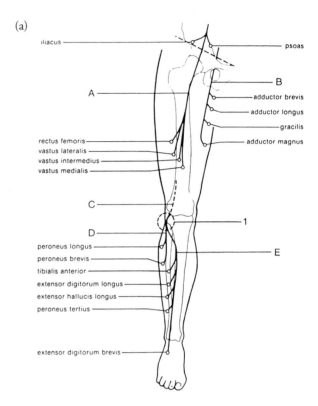

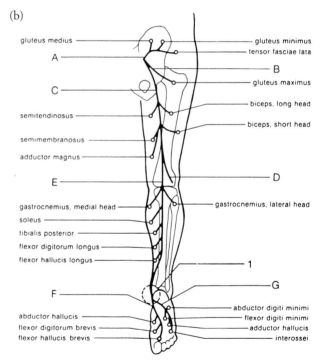

Fig. 6.13. (*a*) Schematic of anterior lower-limb peripheral nerves and motor points. A, femoral nerve; B, obturator nerve; C, common peroneal nerve; D, superficial peroneal nerve; E, deep peroneal nerve; 1, head of fibula. (*b*) Schematic of posterior lower limb peripheral nerves and motor points. A, superior gluteal nerve; B, inferior gluteal nerve; C, sciatic nerve; D, common peroneal nerve; E, tibial nerve; F, medial plantar nerve; G, lateral plantar nerve. (Reproduced by permission from Kimura, J. (1989) *Electrodiagnosis in Disease of Nerve and Muscle: Principles and Practice, 2nd edn*. New York: Oxford University Press; Kimura, J. (1986) *Guarantors of the Brain: Aids to the Examination of the Peripheral Nervous System*. East Sussex, England: Baillière-Tindall.)

Neurologists at Innsbruck, Austria, found that a dose of 200 units of Botox per leg was superior to 100 units of Botox in a study of 33 children and teenagers with cerebral palsy. In addition they reported that children younger than age seven years had a better functional result than those who were older (Wissel *et al.* 1999).

Dysport® injections in patients with various dystonias in 107 patients using doses 50%–70% lower than usually reported and found to be effective (Van den Bergh *et al.* 1995). The group at Karolinska Hospital, Stockholm, did a double-blind, randomized, parallel study to investigate the dose equivalence of Dysport® and Botox® in patients who had cervical dystonia (Odergren *et al.* 1998). They found that the effectiveness and adverse effects were similar with either product. The average dose of Dysport (mean 477 units) was three times that of Botox (mean 152 units).

Portuguese investigators found that the results with either Dysport or Botox were the same with virtually the same adverse effects when the dose of Dysport to Botox was 4:1 in patients with blepharospasm or hemifacial spasm (Sampaio *et al.* 1997).

TOXICITY

Toxicity is expressed as LD_{50} that is equal to 1 unit of botulinum-A toxin (Botox®) when injected into the peritoneum of an 18–20 g female Swiss-Webster mice and is lethal to 50%. Dysport® is available in the United Kingdom as the trade name for botulinum-A toxin. Dysport has different characteristics of diffusion and is not interchangeable with Botox (O'Brien 1995). One vial of Botox (100 units) is below the systemic toxicity of humans weighing 6 kg or more. A 39 units/kg parenteral dose was lethal in the monkey so it was assumed that 3000 units would be lethal in the human (Chutorian and Root 1994). Contraindications are practically non-existent. The manufacturer, Allergan Inc., advises that adverse effects may occur in patients taking aminoglycoside antibiotics because of their possible interference with neuromuscular transmission.[14] Persons who have neuromuscular transmission defects such as myasthenia gravis should be excluded (Chutorian and Root 1994).The manufacturer also advises that as with all biological products anaphylactic reactions can occur so that epinephrine and other precautions should be available.

Electrophysiological studies have indicated effects on distant muscles from the local botulinum-A toxin injections in one case of cervical dystonia and two of hemidystonia (Ansved *et al.* 1997). Percutaneous muscle biopsies of the vastus lateralis in 11 patients who had toxin injections for cervical dystonia were compared with age-matched healthy controls. The histological findings revealed an increased frequency of angular atrophic type IIB fibers which were significantly smaller (p<0.5). The authors called for further studies on the long term effect of treatment.

A multicenter retrospective study to assess the risk/benefit of botulinum-A toxin (Dysport) was done at the University of Plymouth, UK, by Bakheit *et al.* (2001). Data from the

treatments of 758 patients with chronic muscle spasticity (mean age 7.2 years) was analysed retrospectively. If total dosage exceeded 1000 IU, 22% had adverse events. This was about three times higher than adverse events noted with lower doses. Most frequently noted was focal muscle weakness adjacent to the injection site. Higher doses than 1000 IU also showed fewer therapeutic results. A good overall response occurred in 82%.

Three patients with dystonia developed systemic generalized muscle weakness compatible with mild botulism. The authors suggest that patients who have symptomatic dystonia may be more prone to have this side-effect (Bhatia *et al.* 1999).

The worry of a direct injection of Botox into a peripheral nerve was dispelled by the study of Lu *et al.* 1998). Direct intraneural injection of Botox in rats revealed no histological changes compared with phenol that caused severe damage, but with signs of regeneration at 7 weeks.

ANTIBODIES AND IMMUNORESISTANCE TO BOTULINUM-A TOXIN

Antibody formation and resistance to the effects of the toxin has been reported using mouse lethality assay as occurring in 3%– 10% of the patients treated (Brin 1997). Unresponsive patients who had cervical dystonia developed resistance after several months of treatment. Some reversal of their immune response occurred in 10–78 months. Botulinum-B and F toxins were effective substitutes (Sahkhla *et al.* 1998). Another study of botulinum toxin type B compared with type A reported that the type B muscle paralysis was not as complete or long-lasting as that of type A (with B maximal paralysis with 320–480 units was 50–75%; with A maximal paralysis with 7.5–10 units was 70%–80%) (Sloop *et al.* 1997). Limiting the dose has been suggested to reduce antigen exposure and immunoresistance (Borodic *et al.* 1996).

Type B (NeuroBloc®) has been tested in cervical dystonia in a multicenter, randomized, double-blind, placebo-controlled trial (Brashear *et al.* 1999). If was found to be effective and safe at doses of 5,000 and 10,000 units. Following this report is the effectiveness of type B in type A resistant cervical dystonia (Brin *et al.* 1999).

SUMMARY

It appears that botulinum-A toxin injections are safe and effective for short-term reduction of spasticity in specific muscles in the upper and lower limbs. The question is its effectiveness and practicality as a long-term regimen. A detailed sampling of follow-up studies as delineated in Table 6.V reveals mainly short-term follow-ups in small numbers of patients who have cerebral palsy. Reasonable follow-up time for orthopaedic surgical procedures acceptable for publication is a minimum of 2 years. Botulinum toxin has only been used in cerebral palsy since the early 1990s. Five-year outcomes would be excellent to have and we hope these will be forthcoming.

It appears that botulinum-A toxin injections are safe and effective for short-term reduction of spasticity in specific muscles in the upper and lower limbs.

---

14 Allergan, Inc., Product Information, Botox, *Physicians' Desk Reference, 2000,* 495.

The question is its effectiveness and practicality as a long-term regimen.

How many years of injections every 3–6 months will be tolerated? Gormley *et al.* (2001) of St Paul, Minnesota, did a retrospective chart review of 270 children with cerebral palsy in a 2-year follow-up after botulinum toxin injections. The average age at injection was 6.2 years and the average interval between injections ranged from 134 to 199 days. In 2 years, it can be expected that a child will have injections three or four times a year; one wonders if the child will grow weary of injections and if the child wonders when it will end? Will there be muscle weakness due to atrophy and limited restoration of the neuromuscular junctions?

It is clear that short-term use is effective and useful as a preoperative test for orthopaedic surgery of the upper and lower limbs, and to 'buy time' in dynamic equinus in young children with the hope of stemming a shortening of the muscle and the need for surgical lengthening. It might be useful in borderline cases whether or not to surgically weaken the hip adductors by myotenotomy, to lengthen the iliopsoas or the hamstrings, to transfer the rectus femoris tendon, and to decide on a posterior tibialis by split transfer or lengthening. The intramuscular injections of the toxin seems particularly useful in dystonic posturing of the neck and the upper and lower limbs for which there has been no good solution either with orthopaedic surgery or oral medications.

As might be expected in the ongoing anxiety about costs of medical care, a preliminary report on cost analysis of ankle equinus management in cerebral palsy was read at the annual meeting of the American Academy of Orthopaedic Surgeons in 1999. Borschneck and Smith (1999) assessed retrospectively the cost of surgical treatment of spastic equinus compared to Botox® in 56 patients who had 73 surgeries. They noted that the effects of botulinum-A injections in 28 patients had significant short-term effects but a 100% recurrence rate in 2–12 months. The recurrence rate of equinus after surgery was 15% in an average follow-up of 5 years. The preliminary conclusion was that the use of Botox® was cost additive if the patient eventually required an Achilles tendon or gastrocnemius–soleus lengthening. The authors decided not to publish this study in a scientific journal (J.T. Smith, personal communication). We only reference it to lend a perspective to the clinical application of botulinum toxin injections in the management of cerebral palsy.

The cost of Botox A injections compared with serial casting for spastic equinus was calculated by the Physical Therapy Department of the Royal Children's Hospital, Melbourne (Corry *et al.* 1998). A series of three casts was approximately A\$300. A 100 u vial of Botox was A\$450 (the physician time for the pre-injection physical examination and for the injection does not appear to be included in the cost analysis). In this study by physicians from Belfast (Northern Ireland) and Melbourne (Australia) there were few differences between the Botox and the group who had serial casting as measured by clinical examination and instrumented gait analysis. By 12 weeks the tone had relapsed

in both groups. The Botox group had a more prolonged improvement in passive ankle dorsiflexion.

Based on the published reports of botulinum toxin injections compared with serial casts (Corry *et al.* 1998, Flett *et al.* 1999) a study of costs was done by Houltram *et al.* (2001) of Sydney, Australia as an 'evidenced-based economic evaluation' of botulinum-A toxin injections compared with serial casting. The conclusion was that botulinum-A toxin treatment was A\$160 more for one episode than with serial casting for spastic equinus in hemiplegia and A\$175 in diplegia. The overall treatment duration was stated as 3.7 years with an average of 5.4 treatments. The intent of the study was to recommend that 'Botox should attract a full Government subsidy in Australia.'

Overall, however, the use of botulinum toxin in the treatment of cerebral palsy continues to be refined. The reader should consult various websites for continued updates on its use. These include the Americna Academy for Cerebral Palsy and Developmental Medicine (AACPDM) at www.aacpdm.org, and the Neurotoxin Institute (NTI) at www.neurotoxininstitute.com

PHYSICAL THERAPY

'We need to prune physical therapy. We need play, not play therapy.'

(Milani-Comparetti 1979)

ORIGINS AND PURPOSES OF PHYSICAL THERAPY—HISTORICAL PERSPECTIVE
By the mid-1990s it appears that abstract and mystifying neurological theories to justify various therapy 'systems' has reverted physiotherapy in cerebral palsy to its origins in World War I—therapeutic exercise and muscle training for function. Fetters (1991) shared the perception of 'a need for a shift in our therapeutic strategies for patients with cerebral palsy. Changes in function abilities must be stressed in therapy.' In the same year and in the same issue of the same journal Giuliani (1991) perceptively observed: 'The results from selective dorsal rhizotomy research suggest that therapists need to question some common clinical assumptions about movement dysfunction. Abnormal movement patterns persist after the spasticity is reduced. I believe we can maximize the functional potential of children with cerebral palsy by identifying problems related to motor control and applying sound principles of motor learning to treatment.'

It seems that a bit of history of physical therapy might lend a perspective on the past half century of dedicated and zealous attempts to overcome the effects of the motor disorder that originate in the brain. To counter American hubris, we have to acknowledge that rehabilitation efforts were originally established in some European countries and in England. In the United States this foundation was laid by Marguerite Sanderson and also by Mary McMillan, who became the first physical therapist on February 23 1918. On that date she was assigned to the Reconstruction Aides program by the Surgeon General of the United States, Major General William C. Gorgas (Davies 1976a).

The physician founders, Frank B. Granger (a primary-care physician and neurologist, and instructor in physical therapeutics at the Harvard Graduate Medical College), and two orthopaedic surgeons, Elliott G. Brackett and Joel E. Goldthwait of Boston and Harvard, were strong advocates of good body mechanics and posture and used corrective exercises in their practices. Miss Marguerite Sanderson with Dr Goldthwait organized the Reconstruction Aides program and went to Europe with the American Expeditionary Force during the World War I. Miss McMillan was an American whose formation as a physical therapist began with Sir Robert Jones who used physical therapy extensively in England. She returned to the United States in 1915 and became the first American physical therapist on February 23, 1918, appointed by the Surgeon General of the Army. She subsequently taught at Reed College (Portland, Oregon) in a program for reconstruction aides (Davies 1976a). Her book *Massage and Therapeutic Exercise* confirms the early focus of physical therapy on exercise (McMillan 1921).

But even prior to World War I, Robert Lovett, an orthopaedic surgeon of Boston, became the leading proponent and activator of muscle training for the residuals of infantile paralysis (poliomyelitis) in 1914. He established special clinics in Vermont during the poliomyelitis epidemics. He was skeptical of massage and electricity in the treatment of these patients, but stated that muscle training was of 'undoubted value' (Lovett 1924). His junior gymnasium assistant in Boston, Alice Lou Plastridge, became the first director of physical therapy at the Georgia Warm Springs Foundation for the care of poliomyelitis patients (Davies 1976b). She was the physical therapist for Franklin D. Roosevelt before he became President of the United States. Dr Lovett was his physician and with Miss Plastridge devised the first manual muscle test we all use even today when Roosevelt went to the Meriweather Inn at Warm Springs, Georgia, for exercise of his paralyzed lower limbs in the pool.

The result of botulinum-A toxin injections into spastic muscles has changed physical therapy regimens to exercise and functional training. 'The weakness brought on by botulinum toxin treatment provides important opportunities for functional retraining' (Leach 1997). The same statement could be made for the effects of selective posterior rootlet rhizotomy and intrathecal baclofen. The advance of the science of engineering and the resultant technology has created a boom in assistive technology for the severely disabled. Compensation rather than remediation has become the modus operandi. The disease-oriented treatment has been replaced by the goal-oriented approach that focuses on function.

The advance of the science of engineering and the resultant technology has created a boom in assistive technology for the severely disabled. Compensation rather than remediation has become the modus operandi.

Although we find pockets of physical therapists in some countries, especially less developed ones, still trying to carry on with passive movement systems and stimulation of various sorts, generally the therapists have changed their approach. The problem it seems is 'not with the stars', but with the physicians who have not paid much attention or applied their knowledge of biomedical science in prescribing and guiding physical therapy and the therapists.

HISTORY OF PHYSICAL THERAPY SYSTEMS IN CEREBRAL PALSY

Thompson (1977) provided a review of the past history of physical therapy 'methods' in cerebral palsy. He surveyed 233 cerebral-palsy treatment units in the United States by questionnaire. The responses indicated that most therapists used a combination of 'methods' or 'systems' (Gillette 1969). The most commonly used methods were Ayres sensory integration (Ayres 1971, 1972, 1977, 1978, Sellick and Over 1980) and the Bobath neurodevelopmental treatment (Bobath 1954, 1966, 1967, 1980, Bobath and Bobath 1958, 1984). Other methods were those of Rood (1954), Phelps (Slominski 1984), Knott (1953), Kabat (1977), Fay (1958, 1977), Doman *et al.* (1960), Doman-Delacato (Cohen *et al.* 1970, Sparrow and Zigler 1978, Holm 1983), Vojta (Jones 1975, Kanda *et al.* 1984, Vojta 1981, 1984), and Rolfing (Perry *et al.* 1981).

In North America these systems of therapy appear to have fallen by the wayside as physical and occupational therapists became more sophisticated, scientific, and critical of their outcomes. For example, a study by Sellick and Over (1980) reported negative results of vestibular stimulation on motor development in cerebral palsy in a controlled study adjusted for normal maturation of the child.

Polatajko (1985) stated that based on the evidence the concept of vestibular dysfunction in the learning-disabled child should be abandoned.

A survey of 406 occupational therapists (response rate of 74.1%) in four south-western states of the USA revealed a use of motor and visual perception tests but a decreased use of sensory integration methods and *an increase in function-based assessments* (Burtner *et al.* 2002).

It seems as if physiotherapy directed toward function has been adopted in some places in Europe. At a center in Utrecht, the Netherlands, a randomized study of 55 children with cerebral palsy age 2–7 years compared practicing functional activities with physiotherapy based on normalization of the quality of movement (Ketelaar *et al.* 2001). Assessments with the GMFM and the PEDI showed that children in the functional group improved more.

In a search of the medical literature since the first edition of this book (1987–2005), these former methods appear sporadically in countries beyond the shores of the US and the UK. Bumin and Kayihan (2001) of Ankara, Turkey, reported sensory integration programs for spastic diplegia and thought to be effective. However, they used the evaluation tests devised by the originator, Ayres Southern California Sensory Integration and Physical

Ability Tests, to show improvement. Also from Ankara is a study of 34 children with spastic diplegia who had Bobath's neurodevelopmental therapy alone in 17 and Johnstone pressure splints with neurodevelopmental therapy in 17 in the age range of 36–82 months (Kerem *et al.* 2001).[15] The treatment regimen was 5 days a week for 3 months. Ashworth scale scores, ranges of motion of the lower limbs were improved and somatosensory evoked potentials from the posterior tibial nerve stimulation in both groups were improved, but significantly more in those who had the Johnstone splints.

The Finnish neurologists, Salokorpi and associates (2002), prospectively studied the effects of sensory integration and neurodevelopmental therapy given by occupational therapists in 126 extremely low-birthweight infants on neurological development. At age 4 years, the Miller assessment for preschoolers showed that neither therapy method had a detectable effect on long-term neurological development compared to the untreated case controls.

Maurer (2002) of Gräz, Austria, in a review paper of the management of preterm infants with birthweights less than 1500g, listed 'established classical treatment methods' that included the therapies of Bobath, Vojta and Castillo-Morales, hippotherapy, sensory integration, and other 'therapeutical concepts' of Petö, Affolter and Frostig.

A few reports on the Vojta method appear in a search of papers published since 1987. Kovac *et al.* (2002) from Serbia-Croatia attributed the recovery of one 8-year-old boy from a head injury and coma to the Vojta 'neural stimulation' and 'sclerodermal message'. From Yokahama, Japan, Hayashi (1995) indicated that he treated all children with cerebral palsy with the Vojta method and concluded that early treatment of 'risky babies' at age 4 months should have Vojta treatment at age 6 months at the latest. The criterion used was ability to walk. Of the 90 cases, all 11 children with hemiplegia walked; 41 with quadriplegia did not walk; 84.6% of those treated before 6 months walked and 40.4% treated after 7 months walked.[16] Hayashi and Arizono (1999) reported on the efficacy of the Vojta in two infants at age 2 months and 1 month. They stated that these two infants evolved without evidence of paresis or mental retardation. Hayashi, Uehara and Saito (2001) reported their use of 'reflex rolling I of Vojta' as 'physical training for infants' in their consultations of 666 infants at risk ages 1–56 months.

Bobath neurodevelopmental therapy seemed to be still favored at the Bobath Hospital in Osaka, Japan (Okawa *et al.* 1990). However, that team combines the therapy program with orthopaedic surgery. Law *et al.* (1991) of McMaster University,

Ontario, Canada, incorporated neurodevelopmental therapy with upper-extremity inhibitive casting. They concluded that the quality of upper-extremity movement and range of motion improved.[17]

From Munich, Germany, Bauer *et al.* (1992) published extensive indications for the Vojta method as a 'neurophysiologic facilitation system for the whole CNS and neuromuscular apparatus'. Candidates for the treatment included those with cerebral palsy, myelomeningocele, myopathies, peripheral nerve paralysis, congenital malformations, and orthopaedic problems. In Göttingen, Germany, Vojta physiotherapy was found more stressful in the mother–child relationship, but only at the beginning of therapy, compared with the Bobath therapy regimen (Ludewig and Mahler 1999).

More unusual forms of therapy reported have been 'mud therapy' (Kvashnik *et al.* 1978), 'rhythmic psychomotor music therapy' (Gollnitz and Schulz-Wulf 1973), 'Der Dudelsack' (bagpipe) as a practical aid (Kirsch and Lange 1969), and 'Adeli-92', the Russian spacesuit (Semonova 1997). Skinnerian behavioral modification was suggested as an occupational therapy method for cerebral palsy (Skinner 1971, Hollis 1974). An unusual reward of listening to the dishwasher was reported as successful in promoting independent walking in a child who had mental retardation and cerebral palsy (Horton and Taylor 1989). For a while some therapists used M & Ms (coated chocolate lozenges) as a reward for task completion. But fears of inducing dental decay caused them to shift to Cheerios (a breakfast cereal). Such are the fads that come and go in child development.

Chinese physicians at Zhejian Medical University, Hangzhou, used acupuncture, acupressure and functional training. They reported a positive effect on 75 children with cerebral palsy (Zhou *et al.* 1993). The children were treated with a 'comprehensive meridian therapy' that included scalp and body acupuncture, acupoint injection, auriculo-point stimulation, acupressure, massage and functional training for a minimum of 120 days per year. Acupuncture in cerebral palsy is apparently in use in Vienna, Austria. Stockert (1998) compared acupuncture with Vojta therapy and concluded that Vojta uses 'more or less' the identical muscle chains for manual pressure of 'trigger points' as acupuncture.

Two structured educational methods have become well known: 'conductive education' (Cotton 1974) and the 'Portage Project Model' (Jesien 1984). These systems seem to combine therapeutic efforts with goal-oriented approaches.

'Early intervention' was the primary emphasis and byword with most proponents of therapy methods or systems because the best results in alleviating the condition were to be with very

---

15 Margaret Johnstone developed transparent inflatable plastic pressure splints in 1967 applied to adult patients with hemiplegia. These are inflated with neutral heat with air expired from the lungs, The theory is to stimulate proprioceptive and cutaneous receptors by deep pressure to give support for extremity stabilization during exercise, to control motion patterns and to inhibit pathological reflexes (Johnstone 1983).

16 The results from the study by Hayashi (1995) based on walking ability only did not included prognostic testing (not possible with reasonable accuracy

before the age of 10–12 months). We have known for a long time that 100% of those with spastic hemiplegia usually walk by age 18 months.

17 Of note is that Law and colleagues (1991) were from the same Canadian group that subsequently devised and validated the now widely used GMFM. If they had this measure available prior to 1991 undoubtedly they would have used it to judge the efficacy of the Johnstone pressure splints.

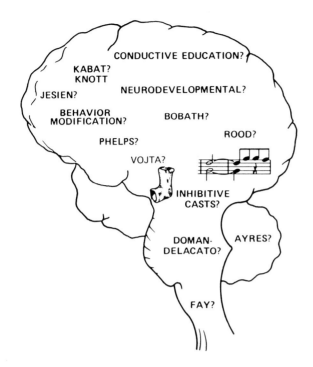

Fig. 6.14. Which area of the brain do you select for treatment of cerebral palsy?

The advice of Golden (1980) still seems apt. The burden of proof is on the proponents of the treatment. Critics need not prove ineffectiveness, but can insist on positive data. Ethically, controlled studies are demanded. Golden quotes Bronowski (1978): 'Magic is a technology, technology without science.' But critics did rise to the challenge to demonstrate the lack of efficacy of special therapy methods. The polemic about the efficacy of physical therapy treatment versus no treatment in cerebral palsy goes back 40 years (Bobath and Bobath 1961).

The debate continued after Taft (1972) raised the question: 'Are we handicapping the handicapped?' with the subsequent flow of letters to the editor expressing shock, indignation, and dismay (Taft 1973a) and a defense by Taft in the same year (1973b). Belief in the efficacy of infant therapy methods were strong enough to make a Swedish physical therapist (whose doll, Lisa, she used to demonstrate reflex inhibiting postures) say that she wanted to 'punch Dr Bleck in the nose' at a seminar in Atlanta, Georgia in the mid-1970s. I had the temerity to question whether she had a controlled study of her claimed (actually hoped-for) results. Now at the beginning of the millennium the belief systems and rhetoric seem to be muted.

EVALUATION OF THERAPY METHODS

'The advantage of one treatment over another can be proved only by careful clinical evaluation. Knowledge of the neurophysiological mechanisms that could be involved is irrelevant to this process.'

(McLellan 1984)

EARLY INTERVENTION OF INFANTS AT RISK

Early intervention of 'high-risk' infants with various therapies became the paradigm of the 1970s and 80s. This concept of 'reprogramming' the assumed 'plasticity' of the infant brain gave rise to the identification of infants at risk. In questioning the efficacy of early-intervention programs, Ferry (1981) wrote: 'Premature infants in neonatal intensive care units are being cuddled, patted, stroked with vibrators, and rocked in water

early treatment (*i.e.* under the age of 6 or 8 months) under the theory of restoring neuronal damage in the brain (6.14).

Rather than consume more pages of print and the reader's time, I have eliminated the detailed description of the various intended remedial methods used in children who have cerebral palsy. Table 6.VIII is a brief summary of the main features of the past and dedicated efforts to alleviate the impairments imposed by cerebral palsy. How could these special physical therapy methods have persisted for so many years? The answer may be in the 'belief engine' common to the human race. 'The belief engine credits the treatment with any improvement that follows. It is the common logical fallacy *post hoc, ergo proper hoc*—after it, therefore because of it' (Park 2000).

TABLE 6.VIII
Historical physical therapy systems and methods

Author	Theory	Methods
Ayres (1972), White (1984)	Cerebral palsy lacks integration of sensory inputs	Passive and active tactile stimulation
Bobath (1980), Bobath and Bobath (1984)	Defect interferes with normal postural control	Passive positioning in Neurodevelopmental, NDT against gravity posture to reduce spasticity.
Fay (1958, 1977)	Brain evolution from amphibian to primate	Passive patterning exercise
Doman *et al.* (1960)	Brain organized in evolutionary layers	
Hagbarth and Eklund (1977)	Vibration relieved motor neuron pools of excessive excitation and excessive inhibition by stimulation of muscle spindles, Golgi tendon organ, spindle endings.	Muscle vibrator
Kabat and Knott (1953)	Summation of facilitation of motor centers	Active mass movement exercise patterns
Phelps (1932, 1956)	Residential, Children's Rehabilitation Institute	Eclectic, assisted motion, orthopaedic surgery.
Slominski (1984)	MD, founded 1936. Directed toward needs relaxation, exercise, braces, of the child	Self-help skills, education.
Rood (1954)	Active contraction of antagonistic muscles	Heat, cold, brushing
Vojta (1984)	Movements have common neurogenic pattern in subcortex, not in motor cortex	Patterns of reflex motion by manual pressure of 'trigger zones'

151

beds and motorized hammocks; they are exposed to flashing lights, dangling birds and toys, piped-in heart-beat sounds and music ("This old man"). We have home-based parent-oriented programs, home-based child-oriented programs, center-based child-oriented programs, and center-based parent and child-oriented ones. Infant stimulation and developmental therapy programs became a major industry' (Fig. 6.15).

Do these programs unwittingly convey to parents that the brain cells will grow or reform with this sort of special intervention? Tizard (1980) took to task those who screen alleged infants-at-risk because more parental misery is caused by uncertainty than when the diagnosis is certain. The effect of much early treatment has been to enhance its reputation. Tizard was correct in criticizing the role of the popular press in promoting therapies 'mostly in periodicals intended, sometimes rather insultingly, for a female readership'.

The Bobaths (1984) recognized that very early treatment presents a problem because the diagnosis of cerebral palsy is usually impossible under the age of 4 months and often under the age of 8 months. Parmelee and Cohen (1985) have also found it impossible to predict outcomes of suspected infants at risk, except those with immediate and catastrophic neurological problems. Their studies showed no correlation between perinatal factors and later development. Michaelis *et al.* (1985) studied infants who had serious abnormal findings during the first year of life but did not show any developmental abnormalities later in childhood. Amiel-Tison (1985) also noted that most cases of perinatal origin had mild cerebral palsy that mimicked spastic hemiplegia or diplegia, and that these signs often disappeared by age 6–8 months. This neurologist thought that brain plasticity was overrated; normalization was related more to maturation.

Weber (1983) discussed the inevitability of treating a considerable number of unaffected infants when the diagnosis is in doubt. He posed a pertinent and often disregarded question: are there adverse psychological effects from treatments such as that promulgated by Vojta? That there may be adverse physiological effects is suggested by the studies in mice by Sanes and

Constantine-Paton (1983) of Princeton University. Eight-day-old mice were exposed to repetitive clicks at the rate of 20 per second from an overhead speaker for 19–24 days after birth. The study of neurons in the central nucleus of the inferior colliculus showed that the normal frequency of tuning neurons was prevented or delayed.

Adding to this phenomenon were Zhang and colleagues of the University of California, San Francisco (2001, 2002). In the study, distorted acoustic environments in mice significantly altered the bandwidths of tuning curves in the developing inferior colliculus of mice. They cited research that the topographic representations of the spatial locations of sound sources within the superior colliculus could be altered by modifying sensory experiences via manipulation of auditory or visual inputs in ferrets and owls. Their experiment involved 9-day-old rats which were exposed to pulsed white noise in a sound shield chamber to age 28 postnatal days. When they were returned to a normal environment, and their auditory cortex examined at 80 postnatal days, the neurons that are organized into tonotopic maps were disrupted in tonotopicity and had degraded tonal frequency selectivity. The neuroscientists who conducted the studies asked whether or not the marked plasticity induced by passive stimuli in the environment applies to human infants, and what is the window of this plasticity in the human fetus and infant. If the child is born preterm (as so many of the children with cerebral palsy are), is the child at greater risk for environmental distortion of its primary auditory cortical representations?

These results of neurobiological experiments in animals (Zhang *et al.* 2001, 2002) ought to make therapists and their presumed supervising physicians cautious in using excessive auditory and visual stimulation of infants, particularly those thought to be 'at-risk' because of preterm birth—the phenomenon of unintended consequences. Put away the tambourines, bells, whistles, and castanets; silence may be golden after all. As with any proposed 'treatment' of hoped-for brain manipulation informed consent of the parents might be appropriate comparable to what is required for invasive procedures such as surgery or drug therapy.

The results of neurobiological experiments in animals ought to make therapists and their presumed supervising physicians cautious in using excessive auditory and visual stimulation of infants.

Early treatment was sometimes thought to raise the intelligence quotient (Köng 1966), but others have disputed this (Bobath 1967). Intelligence might be related to gains from therapeutic intervention programs (Parette and Hourcade 1983, 1984a). Scherzer *et al.* (1976) also noted a trend towards positive change in children who had higher intelligence.

While perinatal asphyxia with low Apgar scores might predict neurological disability later in childhood, data on 49,000 infants who did not achieve a score higher than 8 at 5 minutes (Ellenberg and Nelson 1981) do not make us certain of identifying all infants at risk for cerebral palsy. In this study of infants who

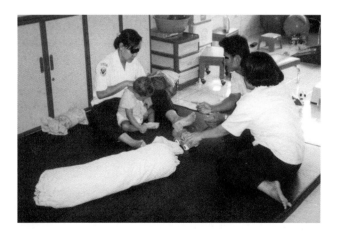

Fig. 6.15. Typical infant stimulation of one infant with three therapists at a cerebral palsy center in Jakarta, Indonesia.

survived severe asphyxia, three-quarters had no apparent neurological problem at age 7 years. In another prospective study of 51,285 pregnancies and births of babies weighing more than 2500 g (Nelson and Ellenberg 1984), there was no increased risk of cerebral palsy after obstetric complications in those with high 5-minute Apgar scores. The final capstone to early identification of infants who might have cerebral palsy is the study of 32,000 infants assessed for risk factors at 4 months and then again at age 7 years. The majority 'outgrew' their presumed cerebral palsy (Nelson and Ellenberg 1982).

Despite the impossibility of clearly identifying infants who will later have serious disabilities, is early intervention effective? Denhoff (1981) reviewed the data on 1000 infants in the United Cerebral Palsy Association collaborative study. These infants had intensive therapy and enrichment programs. The only parameter to show significant improvement on test–retest was the measurement of social–emotional interaction.

Probably the study that had the most impact on physical therapy and infant stimulation programs was by Palmer *et al.* (1988). These investigators from the Kennedy Institute for Handicapped Children studied 48 infants, age 12–19 months, with mild to severe spastic diplegia. Two groups were randomly assigned: group A to receive 6 months of physical therapy and group B to have 6 months of infant stimulation and 6 months of physical therapy. There were no significant differences in the incidence of contractures, the need for bracing or orthopaedic surgery. The preliminary conclusion was that physical therapy was not better than infant stimulation and that further study was needed.

Pediatricians in Johannesburg, South Africa, found no benefit in 80 children followed to a mean age of 6 years (Rothberg *et al.* 1991). Physiotherapy had no influence on locomotor development on either normal or at-risk very low-birthweight children at 1 year or 6 years. The physiotherapy, however, did predict a risk for cerebral palsy or 'soft' neurological problems. Turnbull (1993) of Edinburgh, Scotland, echoed the same opinion of ineffectiveness of therapeutic early intervention for infants and young children at risk of a motor disability based on well-conducted scientific studies. This kind of data should enable health planners to simplify management and costs of the 'at-risk infant' interventions programs and shift money to research and measures for prevention.

McCormick and colleagues of Boston (1993) did a follow-up study of cognitive development, behavioral competence, health status and functional status of 280 infants born with very low birthweight. The infants were randomly assigned to a day-care center program; one-third had intervention with home visits and center-based educational interventions until the age of 36 months. Two-thirds had follow-up only with no interventions. Cognitive scores were 7.2 points higher (p=0.002) in the intervention group, and 9.4 points higher when the 29 children who had severe cerebral palsy were removed from the database. No differences in behavior, serious morbidity, functional ratings or health ratings were evident between the two groups. The study, while not stating so, indicates that early intervention caused no change in the motor manifestations of cerebral palsy.

Despite the questionable results, primarily negative, of infant stimulation, some centers continue to promote it. Garcia-Navarro *et al.* (2000) of Havana, Cuba, studied 20 children aged 9 and 41 months with cerebral palsy and retardation of psychomotor development who were treated for 1–3 months. They concluded that there was 'better performance' and an 'accelerated rate of development in all'.

Palisano *et al.* (1995) found that the Peabody Gross Motor Scale was unresponsive to measuring change in infants with cerebral palsy after a 6-month trial of physical therapy. It was suggested that this test be used only in large clinical trials. Amiel-Tison (1985) perhaps offered the best perspective about these infant programs. She suggested that any attempt to help parents to accept their infant and reinforce interaction is also early intervention. Anastasiow (1985) suggested that these programs are primarily interventions with the parents; the objective should be to raise parents to the level of adult functioning. Bax (1983) surmised that if such programs decreased child abuse they would be worthwhile. It seems that prudence dictates avoidance of an overelaborate infant program, particularly one that projects resolution of the neurological problem by a system of passive physical or occupational therapy. In the third 'Infant At-Risk' Workshop in Israel in 1991 (Anastasiow and Harel 1993) early intervention appears to have focused on communication and language, vision, learning, neuronal and brain development, and families. Discussions on the effects of early intervention with physical therapy on cerebral palsy were not evident.

When early therapy is labeled with a name or an abbreviation (e.g. NDT), something more than parent support and education is connoted. In our population (San Mateo County, California), about 60% of the infants enrolled in these programs evolved with mild cerebral palsy (spastic hemiplegia or diplegia), walked, and went on to regular school. The other 40% were the severely involved children. Then their parents either demanded more therapy to achieve the 'cure' observed in the milder involved, felt guilty because they did not do the 'home' program exercises, or accused the therapy or therapist of being inadequate.

The real value of preschool nursery programs (Bleck and Headley 1961) seems to be the opportunity for sorting out the children according to their potential and directing them and the parents to the appropriate next step, where they can best achieve their potential. The major part of the process is parent education and counseling, with appropriate referral to the community educational resources (Fig. 6.16). Whether this needs to be accomplished in a school-like setting with a team of professionals, or only in the home with one professional visitor–counselor as in the Portage Project (Jesien 1984), depends primarily on the parents' needs, and secondarily on the size, location and resources of the community.

A parent-centered home program for children with cerebral palsy in sparsely populated northern Sweden was deemed successful by 21 of the 26 families who responded to a questionnaire. But five of these families (25%) thought that there were too many exercises, and another five thought that the exercises were inadequate (Von Wendt *et al.* 1984). The question of use

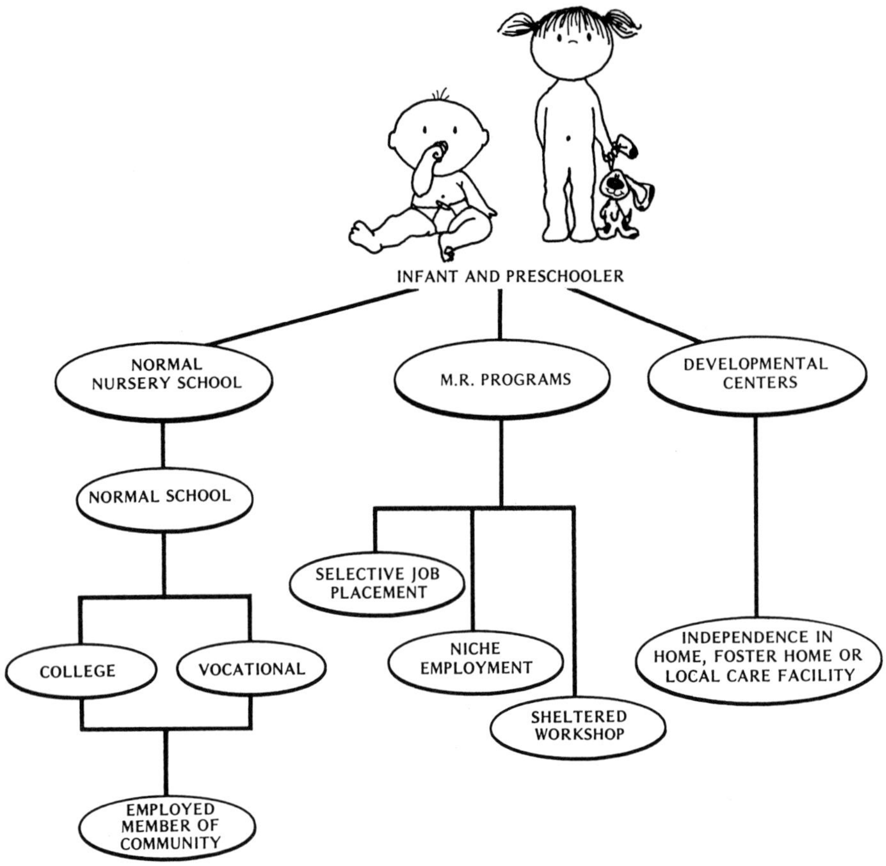

Fig. 6.16. One real advantage of early education programs is to help the parents define the child's abilities so that the next step in maturation can be taken 'maturely'.

of home programs was raised in small database of eight mothers who had previously participated in or attempted to use a home program and were not doing so at the time of the follow-up study (Hinojosa and Anderson 1991). The mothers did selective activities that were doable and could be integrated into their daily routines.

Graves (1995) of Melbourne, Australia, reviewed the literature on therapy methods in cerebral palsy and compared this with the literature on early intervention for children with intellectual disabilities. He concluded that the claims for functional improvement from therapy methods could not be substantiated. In contrast, the literature on early intervention for children with cognitive impairments indicated a shift to the whole child, the family and wider community. He opined that demands for more and better therapy were 'at best, simplistic' and detracted from the real needs of the child and family. Perhaps this opinion based upon the results of therapies in cerebral palsy will be considered by medical and paramedical persons in developing countries who can ill afford to adopt the failed therapy methods of the Western developed countries in rehabilitation programs for children with cerebral palsy. Nutrition, shelter, education, preventative medicine and health-care support should take precedence.

So there you have it. If every man's home is his hassle, should we make daily life more of a hassle with systems of physical or occupational therapy that have equivocal or negative outcomes in the treatment of cerebral palsy? Should the treatment prescribed as a home program be more burdensome to the family and child than the chronic neurological disease?

Should the treatment prescribed as a home program be more burdensome to the family and child than the chronic neurological disease?

Schowalter (1977) in a discussion of behavior modification cautioned that 'child-rearing is a trendy, cyclical business'. Beware of behavioral modification management that hound the child such as forced sitting in the reverse tailor position on the theory that it might reduce hip internal rotation so common in cerebral palsy (Bragg *et al.* 1975). Schedules and home-therapy programs may be so energy-consuming that they may destroy the parent–child relationship through the busy work recommended by the therapist. The busy work may absorb the parent's anger, or the hostility may be increased (Schowalter 1977). If there are no scientifically conducted valid studies that prove the efficacy of home programs in the alleviation of the motor disorder of cerebral palsy, why take a chance on experiments to be done by the parents?

STUDIES ON THE EFFECTIVENESS OF PHYSICAL THERAPY IN CEREBRAL PALSY

'Therapists should not make claims regarding the therapeutic effects of physical therapy in cerebral palsy.'

(Campbell 1990)

'Systems of therapy' have been described in books (Gillette 1969) and published in journals, and they have been the subject of many conferences and seminars. It might seem that after at least 40 years of intensive trials, at least some data on the effectiveness would be forthcoming. Other than generalizations to confirm hypotheses, most clinical studies have been either negative or at best inconclusive—always calling for 'more research'. Perhaps it is time to give up trying to 'cure' the neurological deficits by remedial methods, to stop looking for positive studies, and get on with the task of helping children and their parents in the management of the motor disorder to allow optimum function for independent living.

Over 40 years ago, Paine (1962) questioned the value of treatment in cerebral palsy by comparing a group of 74 patients who had no therapy with 103 children who had intensive physical therapy, bracing and orthopaedic surgery. He found that those who had mild spastic hemiplegia improved both with and without treatment. More severely involved patients with spasticity, who had various forms of treatment, did have a better gait and fewer contractures. But physical therapy did not reduce the need for orthopaedic surgery and made no difference in patients with athetosis.

Bobath neurodevelopmental therapy had one good clinical study by Wright and Nicholson (1973), who conducted a prospective controlled study in two groups of children. They found no significant differences after 12 months between treated and untreated children, when analyzed with regard to motor function, range of movement or joints, and loss of primitive reflexes.

Goldkamp (1984), in a study of 53 children rated according to an ADL scoring system, found no significant improvement as the result of therapy (more than 50% had Bobath treatment), surgery or time. He concluded that 'management' would be a more appropriate term than 'treatment', and 'adaptation' more acceptable than 'improvement'. Adaptation could be facilitated by assistive devices, environmental modifications, and even practice.

The Bobaths (1984) admitted that they grossly overrated the tonic reflexes in explaining abnormal patterns in the spastic child and no longer included them in their assessments. They also reported the inadequacy of concentrating on automatic righting reactions, and the detrimental effects of absent or insufficient balance reactions which remain 'one of our greatest problems' (p. 8). They continued that 'indeed it was wrong to try to follow the normal developmental sequence too closely'. They admitted that children do not need to go rigidly through a developmental sequence of rolling over, sitting, kneeling and half-kneeling before progressing to standing.

Finally, the Bobaths observed that their treatment program had not carried over into activities of daily life as they had expected. Their treatment 'now incorporates systematic preparation for specific functions. There is no time to waste on unspecific, general, developmental treatment, for we cannot expect that such treatment will automatically carry over into functional skills later on' (p. 11). These honest, intelligent and dedicated professionals, who lived only for the improvement of care of the child with cerebral palsy, deserve our gratitude for having the temerity to admit the limitations of their treatment and their desire to learn from their experience.

'There is no time to waste on unspecific, general, developmental treatment, for we cannot expect that such treatment will automatically carry over into functional skills later on.'

(Bobath and Bobath 1984)

Many critiques of physiotherapy interventions have appeared since Wright and Nicholson's study in 1973. A review by Parette and Hourcade (1984b) of 18 published studies on the effects of early intervention using physical and/or occupational therapy found that as research paradigms became more vigorous the support for these interventions decreased. Tirosh and Rabino (1989) found flawed methodological and reporting criteria in 11 of 14 studies; in the three other studies where statistical analysis was used, two had negative results and one positive using clinical analysis only.

Hur (1995) did an exhaustive analysis of 37 studies published since 1966 on the outcomes of physiotherapy in cerebral palsy. In general, the studies lacked scientific rigor using small numbers of participants for short durations, poorly controlled experimental conditions, and no follow-ups. No clinical scientifically based studies in a literature review since Hur's report to August 2000 have produced evidence that physical therapy changed the nature of the motor disorder or eliminated muscle contractures or joint deformities. If this had been the case, the indications for the use of selective posterior rootlet rhizotomy, intrathecal baclofen, and intramuscular injections of botulinum toxin would not have been found, nor would orthopaedic surgery continue to be used to correct muscle contractures, joint deformities, or scoliosis.

In the new millennium, Butler and Darrah (2001)—on behalf of the American Academy for Cerebral Palsy and Developmental Medicine (AACPDM) Outcomes Committee Review Panel—did an exhaustive study of published reports on the effectiveness of neurodevelopmental treatment (NDT). They carefully examined 65 citations in the literature excluded 41 because they were descriptive or review articles, data contained children with diagnoses other than cerebral palsy, or the intervention did not appear to be primarily 'NDT'. Twenty-one studies met the inclusion criteria. Reports were classified according to the dimensions of disability (Table 6.IX) and 'levels of evidence' I–V (Table 6.X).

The details of the 21 reports can be perused in the paper by Butler and Darrah (2001). The conclusions were as follows. (1) The evidence of improvement in motor responses was incon-

TABLE 6.IX
Dimensions of disability

Dimension	Description
Pathophysiology	Interruption or interference of normal physiology and developmental processes or structures
Impairment	Loss or abnormality of body structure or function
Functional limitation/activity	Restriction of ability to perform activities
Disability/participation	Restricted participation in typical societal tests
Social limitation/context factors	Barriers to full participation imposed by societal attitudes, architectural barriers, social policies and other external factors

From Butler and Darrah (2001).

TABLE 6.X
Levels of evidence. Maximum level of evidence is determined by research design; conduct of study may result in reduction of level of evidence by one level

Level	Criteria
I	*Group research*: randomized control trial; all-or-none case series *Single subject research*: N-of-1 randomized controlled trial
II	*Group research*: non-randomized controlled trial. Prospective cohort study with concurrent control group. *Outcomes research*: Analytic survey *Single subject research*: ABABA design. Alternating treatments. Multiple baseline across participants
III	*Group research*: case control study. Cohort study with historical control group *Single subject research*: ABA design
IV	*Group research*: before and after case series without control group *Single subject research*: AB design
V	*Non-empirical*: descriptive case series/case reports. Anecdotes. Expert opinion. Theories base on physiology, bench, or animal research. Common sense/first principles

Adapted from Butler and Darrah (2001), Table II

sistent in eight studies and in five were either not different or were improved in the control treatment children. (2) Joint range of motion was improved immediately after a 20- to 25-minute session in two studies (levels II and III) and after 6 weeks in one study at level IV. One study at level IV reported improved static measurements after 6 weeks of treatment. When assessed after 12 months of treatment, no difference between treatments was detected in six other studies at level II. (3) Motor development, as measured by motor age eight times in five studies, found no advantage conferred by NDT. Two studies at level II favored NDT and two others at level I favored the controls. In one level I study showed that the group with lesser exposure to NDT made greater gains in overall motor development. (4) No findings bestowed an advantage to NDT in cognitive, language, social or emotional domains. (5) The quantity of therapy did not demonstrate a statistically significant change when the amount of therapy per week or when then number of months was extended. (6) Functional limitations/activity failed to reveal a

gain; one study at level IV increased motor function, but included no attempt to differentiate the gain from maturation of the child. (7) Only one of 14 reports confirmed expectation that NDT improved mother–child interaction. (8) No report presented evidence that NDT effected a change in the pathophysiology of cerebral palsy.

Luckily for therapists and their prescribing physicians, an increasing prevalence of spastic diplegia due to survivorship of preterm births has given approbation to the therapy as effecting change. It is luck because in general children with spastic diplegia and hemiplegia have a natural history of a good outcome for locomotor function and cognitive skills.

In summary, the study of Butler and Darrah (2001) casts a negative light on NDT as a method to improve the physiological or functional status of the children subjected to it. As pointed out by the authors, the problem with all studies is the small sample size and above all, the heterogeneity of the children in the studies. They suggest that the use of NDT could be as a control intervention in the evaluation of new approaches.

The Neurodevelopmental Treatment Association (Sharkey *et al.* 2002) struck back at the negative report by Butler and Darrah (2001). First of all, they wrote that 'NDT is not a "treatment" for CP. It is an approach used to assess and to assist children with CP to perform functional tasks sooner and better with minimal negative effect on future functional abilities.' Second, they made the point that cerebral palsy population is not homogeneous and that it is nearly impossible to recruit a homogeneous population of sufficient size. The methodology was questioned, and it was stated that it had omitted the data contained in a table in one study reviewed (later admitted as a typographical error in the response by Richard Adams, MD, Chairperson of the AACPDM Treatment Outcomes Committee, 2002). The operative statement from the Neurodevelopmental Treatment Association was that 'trying to evaluate the effectiveness of NDT for CP, as was done in this report, is neither useful nor appropriate'. It is not a treatment, as stated by the NDT Association representatives, but rather an '*approach*'. 'This is new information for the field and is counterintuitive since the name remains neurodevelopmental treatment' (Adams 2002). If terminology is important, then perhaps the name of the regimen and association ought to be changed, e.g. neurodevelopmental assessment or management to avoid therapeutic implications.[18]

> '*NDT is not a "treatment" for CP. It is an approach used to assess and to assist children with CP to perform functional tasks sooner and better and with minimal negative effect on future functional abilities.*'
>
> (Sharkey *et al.* 2002)

18 As I (EEB) write on March 24, 2003 I happened to enter our local hospital, Mills-Peninsula, San Mateo, California. In the lobby was a sign with an arrow to the auditorium. The sign read 'NDT'. I entered the room and noted about 25 physical therapists taking a course in NDT. So over a year after the study by Butler and Darrah and 9 months since the NDT defensive letter, promulgation of the method continues—a demonstration of the limitations of the printed word in scientific journals.

It seems time to make peace, and for professionals who care for children with cerebral palsy and their families to accept the negative studies. More studies on the efficacy of therapy methods will probably not be forthcoming given the complexity of the neurological condition and the small sample sizes. The cost and professional time of doing more and more clinical studies to prove the efficacy of physical or occupational therapy paradigms seems hardly worth the benefit to the patient and community. Rather money should be spent on research on causation and prevention. It is time to move onto other more promising roles for physical therapists in the management of cerebral palsy as delineated in the following paragraphs.

EXERCISE

The contemporary popularity of 'working-out' (taking physical exercise) seems to have sparked interest in exercise for those with neuromuscular diseases, particularly cerebral palsy. Machines and measuring devices have probably taken the boredom out of ordinary exercise regimens, especially when accompanied by music and television screens.

The histochemical studies of muscle biopsies in spastic diplegia by Rose and colleagues (Rose *et al.* 1994, Rose and McGill 1998), describing a preponderance of type-1 fibers similar to myopathies and genetic dystrophies, suggest that the exercise of limb muscles may be beneficial for those with cerebral palsy (see Chapter 5). J. Rose (personal communication) opined that this data makes the case for resistance exercises in patients with cerebral palsy. To do so would depend on voluntary control of the limb muscles that most children with spastic diplegia and hemiplegia have completely or to some degree.

Because spastic muscles seemed too strong, therapists were reluctant to strengthen them more and risk increasing the spasticity. This perception has been disproved. Fowler *et al.* (2001) studied the effects of quadriceps femoris muscle strengthening exercises in 24 persons with spastic diplegia. Using the pendulum test to assess the degree of spasticity, they found no evidence of increased spasticity with maximum-effort exercise.

Anaerobic endurance and peak muscle power with the Wingate Anaerobic Test of the upper and lower limbs in spastic cerebral palsy were measured in 29 boys and 20 girls, age 6–14 years (Parker *et al.* 1992) Those who had spastic quadriplegia had performance values of 3–4 SD below normal controls and in spastic diplegia and hemiplegia the values were below two standard deviations. In an elegant study of 15 children with spastic diplegia and 15 with spastic hemiplegia maximum voluntary contraction of eight muscle groups in the lower extremity were tested with a hand-held dynamometer and matched with normal controls (Wiley and Damiano 1998). Results were expressed in Newtons/kg of body weight. The study confirmed quantifiable weakness of the lower-limb muscles in the cerebral palsy group. The most pronounced weakness was in the hip-extensors, ankle-dorsiflexors and plantarflexors.

The Wingate Anaerobic Test devised in Israel has been widely used to determine muscle power and endurance. It is described as an 'all-out' 30-second cycling or arm-cranking test. In 66 girls and boys aged 5–18 years old who had cerebral palsy it was found to be feasible, reliable and reproducible (Tirosh *et al.* 1990). Ayalon and colleagues (2000) at the Wingate Institute, Israel, established the reliability of isokinetic testing of knee-flexors and extensors in 12 children who had cerebral palsy.

The GMFM scores and muscle performance of 15 boys and eight girls with spastic cerebral palsy correlated well with aerobic and anaerobic power in the lower limbs, but not the upper limbs. The measure was deemed an unsuitable tool to measure aerobic fitness in children with cerebral palsy or anaerobic power of the arms (Parker *et al.* 1993).

Quadriceps and hamstring weakness were found in 14 children with spastic diplegia and crouch gait. Strength training using heavy resistance exercise of the muscles three times a week for 6 weeks using ankle weights resulted in increased quadriceps femoris strength. Improvement in the degree of crouch at foot contact, and increased stride length was the result (Damiano *et al.* 1995a, b). Six children with spastic diplegia had less than 50% normal strength and five with spastic hemiplegia had a 20% strength asymmetry in at least two muscles (Damiano and Abel 1998). After specific strength training, the muscles gained strength, gait velocity increased with a greater capacity to walk faster. Isokinetic strength testing of the knee musculature in 12 children with cerebral palsy showed that it was only reliable at 30° of knee flexion compared with 39 healthy controls (van den Berg-Emons *et al.* 1996). After an 8-week isokinetic training of knee-extensors and flexors of 17 mildly involved adolescents with cerebral palsy, strength gains were found in the range of 21%–25%. These gains were similar to those found in able-bodied individuals. Walking velocity and efficiency were unchanged (MacPhail and Kramer 1995).

Industrial engineers at Wichita State University, Kansas, found that the physical work capacity of seven ambulatory individuals with cerebral palsy increased significantly in an 8-week simulated task training program (Fernandez and Pitetti 1993). The objective was to increase their ability to work an 8-hour day before experiencing fatigue.

Engineers at the University of Utah designed a tricycle to exercise the hip extensors (Howell *et al.* 1993, Bloswick *et al.* 1994). They used the tricycle in five children with cerebral palsy. Although gait patterns were observed as improved in four, the results of strength testing were inconclusive. Nevertheless the children enjoyed the exercise and the parents thought it improved their general physical condition, coordination and self-esteem.

Even pediatric wheelchair users have had muscle progressive resistance training with a trend toward improvement of strength (O'Connell *et al.* 1992, O'Connell and Barnhart 1995). Another study (Bhambhani *et al.* 1993) measured anaerobic thresholds using blood lactate levels and respiratory gas exchange criteria in 11 wheelchair athletes with spastic cerebral palsy using cycle ergometry with inconclusive results. Inadequate hip flexion due to spasticity was thought to be the primary limiting factor in cycle ergometry.

Because of the effects of botulinum toxin, rhizotomy and baclofen on muscles, exercise has returned as the traditional treatment arm of physical therapy. There is now something more than an x–y–z method and a more substantial and time-tested physical therapy to prescribe for patients with cerebral palsy.

Because of the effects of botulinum toxin, rhizotomy and baclofen on muscles, exercise has returned as the traditional treatment arm of physical therapy.

BALANCE TRAINING

Deficient balance in patients with spastic diplegia was among the central nervous system defects other than spasticity that affected walking as recognized by Rab (1992). A consensus statement from the participants of a symposium on the diplegic child in Charlottesville, Virginia, in 1991 reiterated the problem (Sussman 1992): 'Balance is extremely important for the ultimate function of the child with spastic diplegia and may influence the outcome following surgery.' Lack of balance does not necessarily preclude surgery and having more stable lower limbs might possibly help overcome some of the effects of its lack.

Technological advances in the measurement of balance using instrumented force plates and computer programs have allowed some objective assessment of balance (equilibrium). Data on measured normal balance in 92 children was published by Wolff *et al.* (1998) and reviewed in Chapter 3. Cherng and colleagues in Taiwan (1999) measured static balance using a force platform in 7 children with spastic diplegia against 14 age-matched normal children. When there was fixed foot support, no significant difference in stance stability between the children and the matched controls was found. When there was a 'compliant foot support', stance stability was significantly affected in the children with spastic diplegia when the eyes were closed or unreliable (referenced to sway). Also from Taiwan is a study of sitting balance measured with the dispersion index provided by the Chattecx Balance System in 17 children before and 3 months after selective posterior rootlet rhizotomy (Yang *et al.* 1996). Dynamic sitting balance improved postoperatively except in the non-visual testing conditions. Their balance with dynamic testing was significantly higher than with static testing.

A number of investigators have addressed the lack of balance reactions in cerebral palsy and have suggested ways to improve equilibrium. Liao and colleagues in Taipei, Taiwan (1997), studied eight children who had cerebral palsy compared with normal children. They confirmed that the children with cerebral palsy had worse static balance stability and rhythmic shifting ability that correlated significantly with walking function. Weight-shifting exercises were recommended.

The group at the Robert Jones and Agnes Hunt Orthopaedic Hospital (Butler *et al.* 1992) studied the effect of fixed ankle–foot orthoses to control the ground reaction force in relation to the knees. Balance training was targeted to the knees in six children with spastic diplegia and showed a decrease in the knee extension moment when barefoot.

Japanese investigators used a progressively inclined platform to measure postural alignment and geometric models to determine the maximal stretch of the gastrocnemii and hamstring muscles in 11 children with cerebral palsy and 10 normal controls (Suzuki *et al.* 1998). They found that the gastrocnemii began to be strained when the trunk inclined forward at the hip joints simultaneously. The children who had cerebral palsy had more gastrocnemii strain than in the normal children and by lesser degrees of inclination of the platform (one child also had strain on the hamstrings). What these results mean practically in attempts to treat lack of postural control cannot be discerned.

Of possible practical application is the study of head stability in children with cerebral palsy compared with normals and normal adults when walking on a treadmill (Holt *et al.* 1999). The mean fluctuation of the head in period and amplitude was greater in children with cerebral palsy. Two possible applications of this data might be: (1) use head motion when walking on a treadmill to define the amount of postural instability, and (2) when observing a child with spastic diplegia who walk with a marked body sway, you can walk behind the child holding your hands on their head as they progress forward. When the ungainly gait becomes much less with this head stabilization, the effect of deficient balance reactions on the lower limbs and trunk becomes evident.

Lending support to the benefits of horse-riding is a study of 25 children with cerebral palsy in Poland, where an artificial saddle was used as a training method, twice a week for 3 months (20 minute microprocessor-controlled) (Kuczynski and Slonka 1999). Their data derived from center-of-pressure analysis of postural sway indicated a decrease in sway and an increase in ankle-joint stiffness as the explanation for the improvement in balance.

In the 1990s the literature reflected instrumental measurement of balance using force plate analysis that measures the radial deviation of the center of pressure and its path length of sway per unit of time. The majority of studies have been done in adults with neurological and otological conditions and in the elderly. One study used somatosensory training in 12 subjects age 65–90 years and reported improvement after 4 weeks (Hu and Woollacott 1994). A clue to improving balance in cerebral palsy may come from a study of nursing-home residents in Connecticut that indicated a strong relationship between lower-extremity muscle strength, balance and gait (Wolfson *et al.* 1995). As might be expected walking sticks improved peripheral vestibular balance disorders when measured with and without the sticks in 25 adult patients (Nandapalan *et al.* 1995). Hormone replacement with transdermal estrogen improved measured balance reactions in 19 postmenopausal women in Linköping, Sweden (Hammer *et al.* 1996). From Uppsala, Sweden, Naessen *et al.* (1997) reported the same results in women who had implanted estradiol. The available technology of force-plate platforms and computer programs has made balance training by physical therapists objective and feasible with auditory or visual feedback (Nichols 1997).

Tai Chi Chuan (see below) was found to be no better than exercise when measurements from platform balance measurements in 24 subjects were made. This may seem unfortunate because Tai Chi Chuan (also spelled Quan) seems exotic, of low impact, and in tune not just with the times but also with the large Asian community in the United States (Wolf *et al.* 1997).

Of some pertinence to ambulatory children with spastic diplegia who want to dress 'Western' is a Seattle-based study of relative balance measured by forward acceleration on a balance platform in 27 women, ages 18–40 years old that compared wearing cowboy boots to tennis shoes. Cowboy boots decreased balance performance compared with tennis shoes (Brecht *et al.* 1995). That women wear cowboy boots in Seattle should not be surprising given its reputation for outlandish dress styles.[19]

PRESCRIBING PHYSICAL AND OCCUPATIONAL THERAPY

After this review of questionably effective methods, it is obvious that a special method of therapy is impossible to prescribe or approve for the 'treatment' of cerebral palsy. Despite the lack of data to support the efficacy of physical and occupational therapy in cerebral palsy in a survey of 197 physicians who dealt with cerebral palsy by the American Academy of Pediatrics and the AACPDM, physicians continued to believe in the value of therapy for children with cerebral palsy. Their 'belief engine' led 82% to expect improvement in parents' capability to mange the disability and cope emotionally and 69% believed that contractures and deformities would be prevented. Only 17% believed that physical therapy would not improve motor skills beyond natural maturation (Campbell 1992).

A quarter of a century ago the official position of the American Association of Occupational Therapists (1981) was that 'the philosophical core of occupational therapy education-related service is in the purposeful use of activities to increase the functional performance of independent living skills'. In other words the association does not claim that occupational therapists have a function in attempting to improve fine motor-skill defects in cerebral palsy or enhance learning through methods such as 'sensory integration'.

It is difficult for us to accept that orthopaedic surgeons who regularly dealt with children with cerebral palsy would have these positive beliefs that physical therapy prevented deformity. Any orthopaedic surgeon who has examined hundreds of children with cerebral palsy who were exposed to physical therapy programs since infancy cannot escape the obvious evolution of contractures and deformities (e.g. subluxation and dislocation of the hip, scoliosis, knee-flexion contracture) and abnormal gait patterns. Perhaps their beliefs were skewed by so many children with spastic diplegia and hemiplegia who functioned quite well without taking into account the natural history of their growth and development. It may be that the positive reporting physicians did not take the time to examine and reexamine their patients

and explain to the parents the prognosis and reasonable goals that could be achieved. It is much easier and less time consuming to simply refer to the therapist and state: 'Evaluate and treat'—a common practice of open-ended prescriptions for a variety of adult musculoskeletal conditions such as neck and low back pain. The question 'Who guides the therapist?' was raised 35 years ago by the late Ronnie Mac Keith (1970).

In an effort to improve the communication between physician and therapist, Levine and Kliebhan (1981) suggest that this communication be written (called a 'prescription' in the USA), including the diagnosis, the family picture, the motor abnormalities, the functional goals, the precautions and the intensity (e.g. for maintenance, 1 hour per month; moderately active intensity, 1 hour per month to half an hour per week; active, 1–2 hours per week; intensive, more than 2 hours per week).

The intensity of the physical therapy was addressed in a study by Trahan and Malouin of Quebec City, Canada (2002). With five children severely involved with cerebral palsy, they compared a program of intensive therapy periods (four times a week for 4 weeks) with periods without therapy (8 weeks) in a 6-month period. Assessments were by the GMFM. Motor functions improved (mean 9.2%) in three children, and were maintained in the 8-week rest periods. This is good news for children. It seems that we can easily stop therapy and give children a 2-month vacation without loss of function.

This sort of precision in measuring time seems unrealistic because it presumes a result. It does not seem that merely going to the therapist for 'treatment' 1–2 hours per week or even for more than 2 hours would be more than a physician assistant visit and counseling of the parents. Some parents do need regular visits with some professional who can assess the progress or lack of it, give a prognosis, be aware of structural changes, and always direct the parents toward functional goals that are within the child's capabilities. These authors then advise that much depends on the 'faithfulness with which the family carries out the home program'. Their statement seemed to accept the Bobath neurodevelopmental therapy as the standard.

Levine and Kliebhan (1981, p. 209) highlighted the dilemma of the physician who wants to be rational in this matter: 'We recognize that therapy services are being provided even though uncertainty exists about the efficacy of some of the specific therapy techniques. However, therapy will continue because it is mandated by law (in the USA).' Mandating and enshrining any medical treatment by law surely could not have been the intention of our legislators.

> *'We recognize that therapy services are being provided even though uncertainty exists about the efficacy of some of the specific therapy techniques. However, therapy will continue because it is mandated by law.'*
>
> (Levine and Kliebhan 1981)

The way out of this dilemma is to change the terms. We do not 'treat' cerebral palsy, any more than we treat spina bifida or a host of other musculoskeletal diseases; we manage them. We manage

---

19 'Seattle grunge,' for instance: a disheveled look, with tattered, faded and mismatched clothing.

them to allow optimum fulfilment of that child's potential for adult living. This means the goal- or aim-oriented approach as recommended by us and Scrutton (1984).

In the aim-oriented management, Scrutton's (1984) guidelines are the best. In 1985 the Committee on Children's Disabilities of the American Academy of Pediatrics advised that the proper therapy prescription should meet the functional needs of the child and include necessary adaptive equipment. The essential features of Scrutton's (1984) program are: (1) achieving the most accurate possible prognosis in all areas; (2) assessing the problems which might be eliminated or alleviated; (3) assessing the child's daily life situation; (4) using this assessment to form the framework for listing a priority of aims and how these might be accomplished; and (5) setting a time-frame and review date.

In this new framework, which calls for management rather than treatment, no hourly or weekly 'therapy' sessions should need to be specified. The therapist and parents decide on how to accomplish the tasks for function and how much time need be spent. This will often entail special positioning, seating and adaptive equipment for the child with total body involvement.

THE ROLE OF THE MODERN THERAPIST

'The therapist discusses functions of everyday life instead of mystifying neurophysiological problems avoiding mysterious and irrelevant concepts such as muscle tone, reflexes, and spasticity.'
(Milani Comparetti 1979)

Rather than just following a cookbook of therapy recipes, the modern therapist has a much more demanding role as analyst, catalyst and family adviser. Management involves the home and the family. The modern therapist needs training and skill in interpersonal relationships, and must not inadvertently disturb the delicate relationships that exist within most families. 'Physical therapists and occupational therapists who serve children can assist children and their families in understanding the lifespan issues of CP' (Gajdosik and Ciricello 2001).

The modern therapist is a professional, with a knowledge of normal and abnormal motor and psychological behavior, the entire range of compensatory devices from the fields of science and technology, and the realities of life in both urban and rural communities. The therapist works with the physician towards the common goal of all rehabilitation—independence consistent with the extent of the disability. The modern therapist is the physician's assistant for musculoskeletal disease and trauma. The therapist is the physician's *alter ego* who is in more frequent contact with the patient and the family. The relationship between the therapist and the physician can be strained if neither has formed a consensus on the goals and methods and no regular personal contact.

After orthopaedic surgery, intensive short-term therapeutic exercise, gait restoration and confidence-building are invaluable. It need not continue indefinitely, just to the point of the maximum improvement anticipated. Usually, after major orthopaedic lower-limb surgery in ambulatory patients, this intensive program is no longer than 6 months; often 3 months is sufficient. The physical therapist is deemed essential in restoring muscle weakness of the lower limbs after selective posterior rootlet rhizotomy and may be with the patient as long as a year postoperatively. The same probably holds true after intrathecal baclofen. The therapists also assess the effects of baclofen in the test dose and after the subsequent insertion of the intrathecal catheter and pump.

STOPPING THERAPY

When to stop seeing the therapist? When the child is outdoors playing with his/her peers, then *this is the therapy* and it is time to halt. Some parents and children like to visit the therapist once a week or once a month. This is not really a therapeutic session but a physician assistant's check-up and perhaps a psychological help. Each patient's and family's needs in this regard have to be ascertained. If they perceive no need, then no physical or occupational check-up is necessary.

In order to integrate the child with cerebral-palsy into regular school (providing intellectual functioning is satisfactory), it is usually essential for the physician and therapist to state that optimum benefits of 'therapy' have been obtained. Certainly by the age of 7 years, motor improvement of children with spastic diplegia levels off (Beals 1966) (Fig. 6.17). Walking patterns in unaffected children are normally mature by the age of 7; Burnett and Johnson (1971) showed that the adult walking pattern is achieved 55 weeks after walking begins. The elegant instrumented gait analysis of children by Sutherland *et al.* (1980) confirms that adult gait patterns are fixed by age 7 years.

More severely involved children who do not walk can have goals set by the age of 4 years (Terver *et al.* 1981). Goal achievement entails the cooperation of the therapist and rehabilitation engineers and orthotists to achieve communication, optimum self-care and mobility. Much of this program can be accomplished by the age of 8 years. Its success depends on the extent of the motor disability, and especially on the intellectual function of the child.

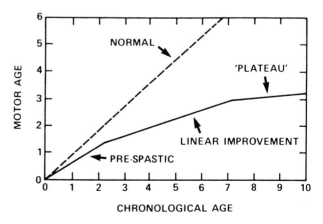

Fig. 6.17. Motor development and maturation in a child with spastic diplegia. Improvement reaches a plateau at age 7 years. (Redrawn from Beals 1966.)

CONDUCTIVE EDUCATION

Hari and Tillemans (1984) admitted that conductive education is 'difficult to understand'. After a visit in July 2000 to a non-residential private conductive education center in Millbrae, California, I believe I do understand it (EEB). It is an educational and rehabilitation system for children who have cerebral palsy. At the Petö Institute, Budapest, the 'conductor' trains in a 4-year college program encompassing medical specialties, psychology, education, physical and occupational and speech therapy in the education and management of physically disabled children. The conductor is a special education teacher, counselor, physical and occupational therapist, and speech therapist all wrapped into one. This seemingly structured and intensive inpatient program, founded by Dr Petö in Budapest over 55 years ago, is located in the Institute for the Motor Disabled in Budapest and administered by the Ministry of Education of Hungary.

The system is basically educational and goal-oriented towards maximum independence. They have no special techniques, but there are principles: e.g. 'rhythmic intention', which means involving the children in their own learning directed by their 'inner voice'; all learning must be relevant to that particular child, who obtains feedback on his performance so that the brain can 'restructure' itself; in learning tasks, the child finds the most efficacious way to learn (this is called 'orthofunction'). The old adage on education is practiced: *repetitio mater est studiorum*.[20]

Equipment often pictured in demonstrating Petö's methods is a 'plinth' which consists of a platform of slotted boards around which the children can fit their hands and grab to transfer, turn over and adjust their posture (Hari and Tillemans 1984). Old-fashioned iron or brass-rail bedsteads have been used to assist self-transfer into and out of bed (Cotton 1977). The toilets in the Millbrae school consisted of white potties with arm- and back-rests. At the time of my visit children who could not navigate to the toilet downstairs sat on the potty chairs behind cardboard screens. In the room were wood ladders with smooth rounded rungs supported on firm bases to be used for standing practice. Stools were made of smooth hardwood slats onto which the child could grab when transferring from floor to stool. Everything needed was located in one large well-lit room, a third of which was carpeted for body and motion control exercises done prone and supine. The room had the usual accoutrements of children's schoolrooms.

The 12 children, all of whom appeared to have total body involved cerebral palsy, were with the one conductor and three assistant conductors for all of the 6-hour day. All staff were paid a salary as full-time employees. Some children needed assistance when turning from supine to prone. All posture changes were controlled and done slowly to the count of five, usually with a chant, e.g. 'Then kneel-up, I kneel-up, I kneel-up.' The children seemed quite composed; none cried or fussed. I heard none of the rattles, tambourines, bells or whistles that I've seen in therapy units around the world under the rubric of 'sensory stimulation'.

20 Repetition is the mother of studies. From the *Ratio Studiorum*, Ignatius Loyola, 1599.

TABLE 6.XI
Daily schedule: Conductive Education Center of Millbrae §

Time	Activity
9:00–9:15	Transportation skills: transportation to and from the classroom
9:15–10:05	Academic skills and gross motor skills *Learning ways to change places and posture from the lying position*
10:05–10:20	Self-help skills *Toileting activities*
10:20–10:50	Self-help skills *Self-cleaning (hand-washing) and self-feeding (snack)*
10:50–11:00	Transportation skills *Transportation to the carpet*
11:00–11:30	Academic skills and gross motor skills and self-help skills *Group standing and walking program and dressing*
11:30–11:40	Transportation skills *Transportation to the school program areas*
11:40–12:20	Academic skills and fine Motor skills *K & 1st grade program & pre-school program (speech and computer program as Augmentative and Alternative Communication (AAC) as needed.*
12:20–12:45	Self-help skills *Self-cleaning (hand-washing and tooth-brushing) and self-feeding (lunch) and toileting*
1:25–1:40	Transportation skills *Transportation to the library*
1:40–2:10	Story and playtime
2:10–2:25	Transportation skills *Transportation to the program area*
2:25–3:00	Academic skills, gross-motor skills and fine-motor skills (Monday and Wednesday) *Sitting program and application*
2:10–3:00	Academic skills, gross-motor skills and fine-motor skills (Tuesday and Thursday) *Individual program*

*Transportation skills =when students change their place from one activity to another as independent as possible by crawling, rolling, walking with or without canes or ladderback chairs etc.

§Prepared by Kinga É. Czégeni, Director/Conductor–Teacher, Conductive Education Center of Millbrae, California, USA, Calvary Lutheran Church, Santa Lucia & Cypress Avenues, Millbrae, CA 94030, USA. julielu@pacbell.net or balogh.e@worldnet.att.net

The director and conductor–teacher gave me the daily schedule (Table 6.XI). Although it seems rigid, the schedule notes that between activities students have the opportunity for 'free choice', and that the speech program includes a computer program and assistive technology as needed. Wheelchairs and constricting seat inserts are not used in the classroom and only to transport the children to and from the school to their residences. For non-verbal communication the conductor used simple symbol language communication boards, but she said she is quite willing and interested in using more sophisticated communication devices.

The conductor was a young, calm and composed, knowledgeable, not too zealous woman, and a keen observer. She told me that in contrast to the children who had cerebral palsy at the Petö Institute in Budapest, her students in California had more severe cerebral palsy. She surmised the reason was that in Hungary at the time she was a student at the Petö Institute the very low-birthweight children did not survive, but in California they do;

so, her students all have total body involved cerebral palsy (GMFCS levels IV and V). In California the majority of children with cerebral palsy have spastic diplegia and are in integrated into the regular schools. Some parents of the more severely involved total body involved child are apt to seek educational and treatment programs they think are more appropriate for their child.

The 12 children ranged in age from 5 to 9 years. The conductor told me that most are placed in regular school by age 7–8 years. By law in the USA a child must be placed in the 'least restrictive environment'. After the child leaves the conductive education center, they offer supportive services. The school functions throughout the year in 6-hour days, 5 days a week. The tuition was $2000 a month. Of the nine full-time students, seven are recipients of the public tuition grant program. Private pay students are provided partial scholarships from fund raising by the center.

Conductive education continues to have its advocates and enthusiasts as it has spread from Hungary to Germany, Belgium, Norway, the UK, Australia, New Zealand, Canada, the United States and Mexico (Calderon-Gonzalez *et al.* 1989). Currently there are three conductive education centers in California. The American Association for Conductive Education lists over 50 centers, although some are currently not operating (K.E. Czégeni, personal communication).

Conductive education has precipitated controversy as a treatment for cerebral palsy primarily, it seems, because of parental demands for its support with public funds comparable to the traditional physical therapy programs. First of all, one has to concur that the Petö method is 'an educational system and *not* a therapeutic one' (Bax 1991) If so, politically, these demands probably translate into the concept of freedom of choice in education with tuition supported by tax funds for education at the school of your choice. The parents then share in the responsibility to assess the results.

But if conductive education is projected as therapeutic, then public and private insurance funding demands a judgement by a commission or study group in what constitutes reasonable and effective treatment. Public tax money can support approved experimental treatment via government grants if the grant proposal meets the criteria for scientific studies. It is not clear that it is therapeutic because no claims are made as a treatment. It is primarily a special education regimen for children disabled with cerebral palsy who are taught self-control as much as possible.

In 1989 a team from East Sussex, UK, spent a week at the Petö Institute in Budapest in order to assess whether it could be considered a true treatment of cerebral palsy, as widely (but incorrectly) publicized (Robinson *et al.* 1989). They concluded that a minority of carefully selected children with cerebral palsy and spina bifida had education that was carried out with appropriate medical, surgical and orthotic interventions. They also thought that the children probably functioned better than in facilities in Britain where facilities were scarce. However, they emphasized that their findings did not justify spending public funds to send self-selected families for a visit to Budapest. Instead, the British team commented that the integration of the programs

in the classroom and the role of the conductor had much to recommend it.

Because of media attention to the Petö Institute after the Second World War, some parents from the UK took their disabled children to Budapest. Hill (1990) sent a questionnaire to eight families who had gone to Budapest. Six responded that rather than adopt 'wholesale' introduction of this kind of facility into Northern Ireland their hope was improved existing local services.

In Britain, a parent-led drive in the late 1980s established The Foundation for Conductive Education. This culminated in the transfer of the system from Hungary to the Birmingham Institute and subsequent funding by the UK Government (Bairstow *et al.* 1991).

A study by Bairstow *et al.* (1991) at the Birmingham Institute found that only approximately 35% of the children who had cerebral palsy were accepted as suitable for conductive education; that the majority of parents whose children were deemed suitable did not seek this special educational program. The 'conductor' who screened the children for admission judged children unsuitable if they had conditions that precluded participation, e.g. 'mental problem', epilepsy, 'poor contact', visual problem, fixed orthopaedic deformities (conductive education does not exclude orthopaedic surgery as part of a management program), and children whose cerebral palsy was so mild that they did not need this special regimen. Bax (1991) commented on this study and lamented that although 'there is an array of methodological problems' with assessment, such should be attempted. Otherwise, 'we shall never know what are the advantages and disadvantages of the Petö system'.

Reddihough and colleagues (1998) at the Royal Children's Hospital, Melbourne, Australia, compared 34 children with cerebral palsy at a mean age of 22 months who were randomly selected for conductive education or traditional neurodevelopmental therapy. The result indicated no difference in the outcomes of the two groups following 6 months of intervention. A similar study in Mexico (Calderon-Gonzalez 1989) compared the outcomes after 12 and 16 months of 10 preschool and school-age children and 12 infants. The authors stated that children given conductive education had a 'definite advantage' in all areas compared with the physiotherapy control group. The best summary of this in the literature has been produced by Darrah *et al.* (2004) in the AACPDM evidence report. Their review of the literature elegantly concludes that while children made progress with conductive education that they did not fare any better than children who took part in more conventional types of therapy in educational programs. Cost and availability need to be factored in pursuing this line of treatment for an individual child. Reddihough *et al.* (1998), in a randomized controlled study (and perhaps the most elegant of all studies on conductive education), compared children in a conductive education program to youngsters in a neurodevelopmental program. The children were matched by age (12–36 months), motor ability and cognitive levels. They concluded that both groups made similar progress.

Fortunately, the majority of children whom we have followed during the past 40 years have spastic diplegia and hemiplegia that have a good prognosis for reasonably independent function as adults providing they had the opportunity for regular school at the appropriate age, and occasional surgical, orthotic and physical therapy interventions. I have had a handful of adolescent patients with spastic diplegia or hemiplegia who never saw the inside of a special school or physiotherapy unit and who have been able to function beautifully, well educated and well integrated (EEB). In a medicalized culture there may be too few patients like this for a comparative study, and too few parents who are willing to accept the children as is and nurture them as children growing up in a family.

THE PORTAGE PROJECT

The Portage Project (Jesien 1984) derives its name from the town of founding, Portage, Wisconsin. It is a home educational program, directed and encouraged by a home teacher who visits the family weekly. An initial assessment is based upon 580 developmentally sequenced skills which occur from birth to 6 years. This assessment is used as a guide for an individual curriculum, in which one can select four to seven possible ways to teach the 580 skills. Despite the seeming rigidity of the skill-learning lists, they are not applied in this way for every child, and require modification depending upon the child's motor and intellectual involvement.

After the teacher has collected the baseline data from the assessment and demonstrated the activity to be performed (called 'modeling'), parents are taught to become educators. The teacher regularly reviews the activity with the parents during the weekly home visit. The method insists on weekly progress, if not, the objectives are modified. The teacher or 'home visitor' acts as a counselor and supporter of the family. The originator of this program insists that the program must be flexible and easily suited to the family's needs.

The home visitor sees 10–15 families per week; visits range from 60 to 90 minutes each. The visitor's role is reinforced by weekly half-day conferences with the supervisor, to discuss problems and plan the following week's activities. The visitor also assists the family in arranging clinic visits to evaluate the child.

The Portage Project system was translated into 12 languages and implemented in 20 countries (Jesien 1984). To be successful, Jesien insists on 'strict adherence' to the model, while still adapting the specific procedures to the needs of the child and the parents. Maximum involvement of the parents seemed to be the essential ingredient in this early childhood educational method. No reports of the outcomes of this home educational system have been found since 1984. The increasing 'home schooling' of children by parents has gained considerable momentum in the United States. The Portage project may seem as an educational model for the disabled as well. It seems probable that the 'home schooling' movement which has spread across the USA with reported excellent academic achievement is comparable to the Portage Project.

PLASTER OR FIBERGLASS CASTING

The focus on dynamic equinus (so common in children with spastic diplegia and hemiplegia) as a crucial determinant of walking ability led to a wave of popularity for plaster-cast immobilization in the late 1970s through the 1980s. Why the foot is considered all important to the exclusion of the rest of the human body seems to rest on a timeless notion put forward by footwear manufacturers: 'You are what your feet are. When your feet hurt, you hurt all over.'

It was tempting to give plaster-casting for dynamic equinus short shrift in this text because it has waned with the emergence of intramuscular blockade using botulinum-A toxin. But on the premise that others around the world may decide to give it a try, we decided to include details on its use and outcomes.

Plaster immobilization to reduce muscle hypertonicity may have been first suggested by Australian therapists (Hayes and Burns 1970). But it was Yates and Mott (1977), working in the United States Northwest region, who ignited a wave of enthusiasm by therapists and some physicians for treatment of dynamic spastic equinus with plaster immobilization of the foot and ankle. Yates and Mott reported their results in the application of bilateral short-leg walking plasters that extended under the toes in 49 children with cerebral palsy. They coined the term 'inhibitive casts' because 100% of their patients exhibited changes in 'tone', and all but four walking patients improved their gait. The posture and movement of non-walkers improved, and it was said that upper-limb tone was reduced as well. The unexplained neurological mechanism responsible for the change towards relaxation of the muscles was called 'inhibition'. Mott and Yates (1981) later developed removable bivalved plaster–polymer short-leg casts that were fastened with Velcro straps and worn several hours a day for an average of 10 months. Only three of their original 49 patients required Achilles tendon lengthenings. For some unspecified reason, six had plantar fasciotomies, a procedure usually reserved for progressive cavus deformities, and unusual in young children with cerebral palsy.

Sussman and Cusik (1979) joined in the enthusiasm for 'inhibitive casts' reporting that in 99 patients with cerebral palsy had 'tone reduction' and increased postural stability, and were useful in improving walking. Sussman (1983) later recanted and suggested that the plaster casts were not inhibitive, but acted more like a rigid plastic ankle foot orthosis that were worn after casting for an unspecified duration. Duncan and Mott (1983) in an analysis of their results of the cast treatment for dynamic equinus in 111 children in an 8-year mean follow-up proposed a theory to explain the 'inhibition' of spasticity of the lower limbs, trunk and upper limbs.

The theory was that inhibitive casts controlled reflex-induced foot deformities by reduction of the spasticity of the co-contracting muscles. It was based Duncan's (1960) hypothesis and on experiments that early balance of the infant was facilitated by inborn supporting reflexes, righting reactions and four superficial plantar foot reflexes that could be elicited in the first year of life in normal infants. The four areas were the head of the first metatarsal, the head of the fifth metatarsal, the ball of the foot, and the plantar aspect of the heel. If the center of gravity is displaced forward, then pressure on the ball of the foot evokes the toe grasp reflex with contraction of the toe-flexors, the triceps, hamstrings, gluteal muscles, and spine musculature in a proximal cascade to counteract the continuing displacement. The casts blocked the plantarflexion and pressure on the ball of the foot to prevent the toe-grasp reflex that elicited the contraction of the proximal limb muscles.

Watt *et al.* (1984) used the same casts to immobilize the foot and ankle in 34 children with dynamic equinus. A prospective study reported statistically significant improved ankle dorsiflexion 5 weeks post-casting. Deterioration, however, occurred to the pre-casting range in 6 months.

After 'inhibitive casts' were first introduced in 1977, they were recommended and applied by specially trained therapists to increasing numbers of infants and toddlers who had spastic paralysis and equinus, as a 'method' for reducing 'tone' through-out the body and to obtain improved function, particularly in children who had not yet begun walking and had no actual shortening of the triceps surae (i.e. no contracture). For a few years inhibitive casts seemed to displace 'neurodevelopmental therapy' as a treatment of choice in many young children: so much so, that in the late 1980s the majority of new patients with their often frazzled and conscientious mothers referred for consultation brought not just one set of bivalved plasters but two, as well as plastic ankle–foot orthoses.

There was nothing really new in attempting to control equinus with plaster cast immobilization. It had been done by Westin in Los Angeles over a period of 27 years (1952–79). The plasters were changed throughout the growth of the child. Of 194 patients, 61% were treated by plaster alone and 23% had plaster and surgery (Westin and Dye 1983). Westin pointed out that one disadvantage of plaster was 'problems with atrophy'.

This observation of induced muscle atrophy after plaster immobilization is probably one explanation why inhibitive or any other immobilization reduces 'tone'. Any physician who has treated fractures of the tibiae of children or adults with lower-limb plasters knows that calf atrophy with weakness of the triceps surae is an inevitable result. Cooper (1972), in a landmark paper on the effects of immobilization on muscle in cats, clearly demonstrated distinct degeneration of muscle fibers which began to regenerate 1 week after immobilization was discontinued. Other investigators documented the histological effects of immobilization on experimental immobilization of limb muscles in animals (Tabary *et al.* 1972, Herbison *et al.* 1978). Lower energy metabolites were found in rabbit limb muscle immobilized in plaster for 1–6 weeks (Sziklai and Grof 1981). In humans, Rosemeyer and Stürz (1977) described mechanical and electrical changes in the quadriceps muscles of 40 patients in whom one lower limb was immobilized in plaster in periods from 3 to 12 weeks. Mechanical and electrical investigations of the quadriceps muscles showed changes after immobilization. After 12 and 24 weeks of remobilization, the muscle mass remained diminished.

Although short-leg walking plaster casts have been successfully used in reversing the gait pattern of habitual toe-walkers (Griffin *et al.* 1977), we might not be able to transfer this experience to that of spastic paralysis. Habitual toe-walkers have no clinical or electromyographic evidence of spastic paralysis. We have not used plaster-cast treatment in children with cerebral palsy. The method seems tedious and time-consuming, and has the usual risks of skin pressure sores and blisters (Westin and Dye 1983).

Yet plaster casts for spastic equinus and idiopathic toe-walking were once again resurrected. Brouwer and associates (1998) carried on with serial plaster casts in seven children with spastic equinus. After 6 weeks of casting dorsiflexion of the ankle increased and peak tension in the length-tension curve was gained in dorsiflexion rather than plantarflexion (p<0.001). The gains were stated to be present at the 6-week follow-up, 'although generally to a lesser extent'. These short-term results may be indicative of eventual recurrence of the equinus. In a subsequent study at Queen's University, Kingston, Ontario, Canada (Brouwer *et al.* 2000), eight children who had spastic cerebral palsy and eight idiopathic toe-walkers at about the same age of 7 years had casts applied for 3–6 weeks. Immediately after cast removal the range of ankle dorsiflexion increased and no child toe-walked. Two of the children with cerebral palsy resumed their former equinus gait pattern. The gait velocity and stride length did not change. These authors surmised that serial casting may be longer lasting in idiopathic toe-walking.

Physicians at the University of Saint-Étienne, France (Cottalorda *et al.* 2000), retrospectively analyzed the results of serial resin casting of 30 feet in 20 children with either spastic hemiplegia or diplegia who toe-walked at a mean age of 4 years 1 month. Their static contracture of the gastrocnemius–soleus was no greater than 10º of fixed equinus with the knee extended. Follow-up was at 3 years, 1 month. At this time all had improved their gait toward normal. Half of the feet could be passively dorsiflexed beyond neutral and half were below, i.e. equinus. At the latest follow-up, equinus had returned in 15 feet that could be dorsiflexed beyond neutral and 22 feet had reverted to toe-walking. This failure of long-term success with serial casting was rationalized by the concept that the goal of treatment was not to avoid surgery, but to allow eventual surgery through an unscarred Achilles tendon.

Corry and colleagues (1998) of Belfast, Northern Ireland, compared botulinum-A toxin injections with stretching casts in 20 children at a mean age of 4.6 years with cerebral palsy and dynamic equinus in a randomized study. At a 12-week assessment, gastronemius muscle tone was decreased significantly in those who had had botulinum-A toxin injections; it had also decreased, but not significantly, in the casted limbs. In both groups tone relapsed but there was more prolonged improvement in passive dorsiflexion of the foot in the botulinum injected cases. 3D gait analysis confirmed maintenance of improvement in the botu-linum injection group and relapse in the cast group. The ankle range of motion in the gait cycle was not changed in either group. The hope was that the more prolonged effect of the botulinum toxin injections would induce an increase in muscle length.

Not surprisingly, given the considerable inconvenience of casts on limbs (bathing etc.), parents in Adelaide, Australia, consistently favored botulinum toxin over serial casting for dynamic equinus in a comparative study of 10 children who had cerebral palsy in each group (Flett *et al.* 1999).

Is there a neurological explanation for the claimed results? Conrad *et al.* (1983) used electromyographic gait analysis, and found that bilateral local anaesthetic blocks of the plantar nerves had no effect on the normal electromyographic pattern of the gastrocnemii. The conclusion was that afferent nerve fibers have no effect on the gait pattern itself, and the central nervous system stabilizes balance at the expense of walking speed.

In children who have dynamic equinus, we prefer to use rigid plaster ankle–foot orthoses. If the orthosis could not resist the degree of spasticity, in the past myoneural blocks using 45% alcohol into the gastrocnemius muscle were helpful; currently, botulinum-A toxin blocks appears better and longer-lasting. As the child develops better equilibrium reactions, improvement in foot equinus can occur. If the hamstring muscles are very spastic, posterior stability is threatened and balance is achieved by tiptoe posture which brings the anterior to the base of support between the ankle joints. The effect of hamstring spasticity on dynamic equinus could be tested with a myoneural block with botulinum-A toxin.

If we accept that muscle length growth occurs parallel with the bone as sarcomeres are added at the musculo-tendinous junction, then keeping the spastic muscle on a stretch during growth does provide a rationale for the short leg cast treatment for spastic calf muscles (see Chapter 5, muscle contracture). But the casts would have to be worn almost continuously throughout the growth of the child. This hardly seems acceptable management as the casts on the legs would thwart most activities that should be part of child development: playing outdoor games, bike-riding, hiking in the woods etc., let alone inducing atrophy and weakness. It is apparent that cast immobilization to alleviate the effects of a spastic muscle is practical only for the accessible foot and ankle. It would not be rational or practical to do the same for the hamstrings, hip-adductors and flexors, or the spastic muscles of the upper limb.

For a fixed contracture of the triceps surae, most orthopaedic surgeons now prefer a sliding Achilles tendon or gastrocnemius lengthening rather than inducing atrophy by immobilization and stretching in plaster.

UPPER-LIMB CASTING

Because forced use or constraint induced movement had shown some improvement in the upper limbs in persons who had hemiparesis due to stroke, the concept has been extended to children with cerebral palsy. Restraint of the unimpaired upper limb with a plaster cast was tried in 12 children aged 1–8 years with hemiplegia and compared with 13 hemiplegic children whose upper limbs were not immobilized (Willis *et al.* 2002).

Using the Peabody Development Motor Scales the children whose unimpaired limbs were restrained by the casts improved 12.6 points after one month compared with a 2.5 point improvement in those not casted. Seven children returned for follow-up after 6 months; the improvement in their upper-limb functions improved.

ELECTRICAL STIMULATION

De Veribus Electricitatis in Motu Musculari Commentarius[21]
(Aloysio Luigi Galvani 1791)

Galvani's spark that caused muscular contraction in the frog ignited the interest and use of electrotherapy in the 19th century and into the first quarter of the 20th century. Duchenne used Michael Faraday's (1791–1867) discovery of direct current induction in his monumental study of the limb motion and muscles by combining electrical stimulation with clinical observations that formed our basic knowledge of skeletal muscle functions (Duchenne 1866, English translation by Kaplan 1959).

Electrotherapy became the vogue for many aches and pains in the limbs and spine in the first quarter of the 20th century. The 1927 catalogue of the Betz Company, Hammond, Indiana, offering physician supplies depicts electrical stimulators under the title 'physiotherapy': a Light Office Model High Frequency Set ($13.50); a 'New' Galvanic Set stated to be useful for relieving pain, stopping bleeding, and stimulating circulation; the Betzo Quatremod ($45)—'A simple, durable and practical electro-therapy cabinet designed for the physician who is starting to use physiotherapy in his practice.' Under the heading of 'Physiotherapy', the company cited a resolution passed by the American Hospital Association favoring complete electro-therapeutic equipment in every American hospital (p. 81) (Fig. 6.18). It is not surprising that long after 'electro-therapy' disappeared from common use in medical practice it has been sporadically resurrected as a treatment modality.

Electrical stimulation today is used as a means to gain strength and improve motor function. Two types of electrical stimulation are commonly used in cerebral palsy, neuromuscular electrical stimulation (NMES) and threshold electrical stimulation (TES). NMES applies electric current to elicit muscle contraction by placing electrodes on the skin and thereby stimulating intramuscular nerve branches. The stimulation is of high intensity but short duration. It can be used for task specificity to produce a functional activity, functional electrical stimulation (FES).

TES applies a low-amplitude electrical current that is insufficient to cause muscle contraction. Typically this is used throughout sleeping hours.

Kerr *et al.* (2004) reviewed the scientific literature regarding the benefits of electrical stimulation. In a number of studies there is a level of evidence in the measurements in levels one and two. At least three studies have shown no significant difference

---

21 'The Effects of Artificial Electricity on Muscular Motion'; see Bick 1972.

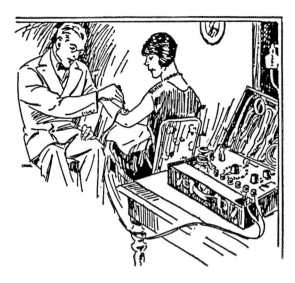

Fig. 6.18. Nothing new about electrical stimulation. Drawing from the Betz Catalogue, 1927, advertising electrical stimulators for the physician's office under the title of 'physiotherapy'.

in the use of electrical stimulation (Sommerfelt 2001, Dali 2002, van der Linden 2003). On the other hand Steinbok (1997) studied children with diplegia who had had dorsal rhizotomies, and found improvement in the GMFM score without significant differences in other measures. Hazlewood *et al.* (1994) studied 10 patients with hemiplegia with matched controls and found improvement in passive ankle range of motion and strength when the anterior tibialis was stimulated with electrical stimulation. In a randomized controlled study (Park *et al.* 2001), infants aged 8–16 months with spastic diplegia and poor trunk control had physical therapy with or without electrical stimulation to abdominal and back muscles. They showed that the group with the electrical stimulation had decreased kyphotic angle and increased GMFM compared to infants without the electrical stimulation. While there was a decreased Cobb angle in those with electrical stimulation this was not significant. Sommerfelt *et al.* (2001) studied 12 children with diplegia in a randomized controlled double-crossover study using physical therapy plus electrical stimulation for 12 out of months. Eleven of 24 parents noted that TES helped significantly but objective measures of motor function and video studies did not confirm this. In a double blinded placebo controlled study of 57 children with cerebral palsy (ages 5–18 years), Dali *et al.* (2002) found no evidence of improved motor skills following 12 months of electrical stimulation to the tibialis anterior and the quadriceps and showed no significant difference in their outcome compared to the control group. Van der Linden and group (2003) studied 22 children, seven with hemiplegia, 14 with diplegia, and one with quadriplegia who underwent neuromuscular electrical stimulation to the gluteus maximus plus the usual physical therapy and compared them with a control group with just therapy. After 8 weeks of treatment there was no significant difference in evaluating all measures. Interestingly, seven of 11 parents felt that their children had improved in spite of a lack of

quantitative validation of that. Many other articles showing ongoing enthusiasm for this modality indicating its value may be a matter of obtaining the optimal amount, timing and placement of electrical stimulation.

ALTERNATIVE MEDICINE AND METHODS

Just in case a therapist, physician or organization promotes an 'alternative' method of treatment for cerebral palsy, we mention three that may possibly be sought by parents of a child with cerebral palsy; though as Bax (1992) has remarked, 'There is a huge range of "alternatives" and it is difficult to keep up with them all.'[22]

Three methods that might come to the attention of parents and the physician are: (1) the *Feldenkrais method* for 'movement coordination learning' (Baniel 1999/2000); (2) Tai Chi Chuan; and (3) hyperbaric oxygen. The first two have some appeal as a way to control movement. The Feldenkrais method was devised by Dr Moshe Feldenkrais (1904–84). He was a mechanical engineer, physicist and judo master. Due to a severe knee injury he developed his method to acquire new ways to move and continue to function. His student, Anat Baniel, established a Movement Coordination Learning center in Marin County, California. The method focuses on the 'rapid and easy acquisition of new movement skill and their integration into daily life'. It is projected as beneficial for anyone who needs coordinated movement ranging from performing artists to elderly persons and includes '*children with developmental difficulties*' (emphasis added).

The method has been tested in multiple sclerosis (Johnson *et al.* 1999). There were non-significant trends toward high self-sufficiency after both Feldenkrais and sham sessions. Levels of functional ability and upper extremity performance were unaffected with either type of session. Another report on the use of Feldenkrais for the elderly in a controlled 6-week study of residents in retirement housing failed to show any differences with the group that did not have the exercises of Feldenkrais (Gutman *et al.* 1977). Beyond these two negative studies none can be found in the medical literature that pertain to cerebral palsy or developmental disabilities in the past 30+ years. Whether it will be tried and studied in children who have cerebral palsy is questionable—anyone for 'informed consent'?

Tai Chi Chuan is a 300-year-old art-form, religious ritual, relaxation technique and method of self-defense for people of all ages. It is popular in China where large groups of people stand in public areas doing slow controlled body movements. Uncontrolled studies report improvement in balance, endurance and muscular strength in the elderly (Hong *et al.* 2000, Lau *et al.* 2000). Its potential benefit in cerebral palsy has not been established.

---

22 According to a detailed review in the *Wall Street Journal* (March 27 2003), alternative health programs have become a service in major medical school centers from the east (University of Maryland) to the west (Stanford University and the University of California, San Francisco).

Hyperbaric oxygen (HBO) is an alternative therapy used with some current popularity to treat children with cerebral palsy. The theory is that adding oxygen under pressure into the body to stimulate impaired areas of brain tissue. The most definitive study of this came from Montreal with Hardy and Collet's group (2002) studying 25 children who underwent 40 sessions of HBO treatment or treatment with 1.3 atmospheres of room air. While both groups improved, there was no statistical difference found between the two treatments. The groups improved in self-control and auditory attention and visual working memory. The changes persisted for 3 months. No changes were seen in either group in verbal span, visual attention, or processing speed. Essex (2003) pointed out potential hazards of hyperbaric treatments. This includes at least 88 deaths worldwide from fires in HBO chambers, and ear problems such as perforated ear drums or middle-ear bleeding. Drs Pierre Marois and Michel Vanasse (2003) took issue with Dr Essex's views, pointing out that most complications from HBO treatment is related to pressures over 2 ATA. Nevertheless in view of the lack of sufficient evidence showing that HBO therapy is helpful with children with cerebral palsy, the Hyperbaric Medical Society position statement from November 2003 does not support the use of HBO therapy in cerebral palsy. They do however support clinical trials that are prospective, randomized and controlled. Due to its current non-demonstrated efficacy, the authors are in concurrence with the Hyperbaric Medical Society regarding this use for children with cerebral palsy.

CONCERNS REGARDING ALTERNATIVE THERAPIES

There would be no argument about the use of these methods if the persons wanting to do so paid out of their own pocket, and the public could be reasonably assured as a matter of public health information that they do no harm, either physical or psychological. The controversy usually arises when demands for payment out of the public purse are made for 'health care' entitlements either through public or private insurance schemes. The Congress of the United States spearheaded by Senator Tom Harkin (Democrat, Iowa) formed within the National Institutes of Health an Office of Alternative Medicine in 1992. What advice and approval they give to alternative treatments will be interesting. We have to remember that the placebo effect is always operative: 'Once we are convinced of the healing power of a doctor or a treatment, something remarkable happens; a sham treatment induces *real* biological improvement.' Scientific evidence suggests that the complex interaction between the brain and the endocrine system gives rise to the placebo effect (Park 2000). Continued investigation into new modalities for treatment should include thinking out of the box so we do not overlook potential benefits.

ORTHOPAEDIC SURGERY

'Today the orthopaedic surgeons seem to have got it just about right.'

(Tizard 1980)

Whether Tizard's opinion on the effectiveness of orthopaedic surgery still pertains in the second millennium might be questioned in this era of neuropharmacological and neurosurgical treatments. It does appear probable that orthopaedic surgery will continue as a treatment arm of cerebral palsy. The evidence is that orthopaedic surgery and other interventions to relieve spasticity are not mutually exclusive.

We accept Tizard's compliments despite a negative comment in Goldkamp's (1984) paper on treatment effectiveness in cerebral palsy. He studied the functional outcomes of 53 children with cerebral palsy who began treatment at age 3.9 years and were followed to the age of 18.8 years. Physical therapy treatments (mainly neurodevelopmental) did not improve function for activities of daily living, and the surgery results were reported as 'less than good' in 24%. But even in this small sample, 76% seem to have had good results from surgery.

The perception of the failures of orthopaedic surgery was operative over 40 years ago. 'For years medical students and physicians were told of disastrous results of tenotomies with increased disability due to overcorrection. The fact is, of course, that complete tenotomy, in cerebral palsy, is almost unheard of in these days. Skilful tendon lengthening, partial myotomies or neurectomies and readjustment of the origin or insertion of muscles, fasciotomy, or stabilization of joints have taken its place' (Crothers and Paine 1959). The latter undoubtedly made their observations on the results of surgery by one of the leaders in orthopaedic surgery for cerebral palsy in those days, the late William T. Green, Henry Banks and orthopaedic colleagues at the Boston Children's Medical Center.

With careful preoperative analysis, instrumented gait analysis in those who walk, correct selection of surgical procedure, proper surgical technique and follow-up care, and when the aims of surgery are clearly defined, good results should be greater than 80% and probably 90%. A pioneer in orthopaedic surgery for cerebral palsy, Dr Lenox D. Baker of Duke University, published a review of 3522 orthopaedic procedures in 606 cerebral-palsied patients selected from a group of 3200 based on 31 years' experience. Results according to the specific procedure could only be assessed as improved or unimproved. The one standard for improved was: 'Did the results justify the surgery having been done?' (Baker *et al.* 1970). Some of the operations have been discarded over the years. However, Baker and his colleagues pointed out their study was based 'on a long trial and error experience'.

It must be realized that when orthopaedic surgeons embarked on greater volumes of surgery in cerebral palsy they applied their knowledge and massive experience with surgery for deformities due to the flaccid paralysis of poliomyelitis. The deformities in spastic paralysis and the deforming muscle forces are not the same as in flaccid paralysis; the contracture in flaccid paralysis is in the epimysium and fascia with preservation of central motor control; in spastic paralysis the muscle is short and central motor control is altered.

For example, the Yount-Ober fasciotomy for the contracture of the iliotibial band of poliomyelitis failed to correct the hip-flexion contracture in spastic cerebral palsy; transfer of the posterior tibial and peroneal tendons to restore dorsiflexion resulted in overcorrection to excessive dorsiflexion; transfer of the origin of the tensor fascia femoris muscle from its anterior iliac insertion to further posteriorly did not correct the hip internal rotation gait pattern; transfer of the iliopsoas to through a hole in the ilium to the greater trochanter of the femur to restore abductor muscle strength as was done in flaccid paralysis of the gluteus medius also failed.

In those early days of intensive surgery orthopaedic surgeons were hampered by lack of knowledge of muscle function with dynamic electromyography and gait analysis to understand the normal kinematics, and relate their physical examinations to the abnormal movements. Additionally, the precision in reporting results of surgery were not as demanding by refereed journals as they have been in the past 30 years. Other than the genetic spastic mouse, and Sherrington's decerebrate cat, there are no animal models in which to test the effects of spasticity on skeletal structures or surgery. George Orwell's pigs who walked on their hind legs, declaring themselves better than pigs on four legs, have not been cloned.

A very candid paper by Phelps (1957) of 422 operations in patients with cerebral palsy from 1902 to 1950 with careful personal follow-up from 5 to 43 years records many failures and his reasons why could have been published in a 'Journal of Negative Results' (Table 6.XII). Of all procedures, osteotomies primarily for rotational deformities and triple arthrodesis were successful in correcting the deformity in 90%—still true in our era of practice.

We can sum up the lessons we have learned from Phelps as follows.

(1) Except for bone deformities, surgery should be confined to spastic paralysis, and not done in athetosis. Tension athetosis and dystonia have been mistaken for spasticity. Careful examination will differentiate. Muscle and tendon surgery in athetosis or dystonia can result in the 'athetoid shift', i.e. the reverse deformity.

(2) Muscle and tendon transplantation frequently fails in cerebral palsy because 'the injury in cerebral palsy does not involve individual muscles' as in poliomyelitis.

(3) Bone surgery (osteotomies and arthrodesis) is successful in correcting deformities.

(4) Neurectomies such as popliteal neurectomy and obturator neurectomy frequently fail and should be done with caution, and are not required in the majority of patients with spastic paralysis. Phelps thought that neurectomies failed because nerve regeneration accounted for a recurrence of the deformity. Whether this is true or not has not been shown, but is unlikely. Some have claimed that obturator neurectomy paralyzes the muscle that causes muscle fibrosis, a contracture, and recurrence (M. Tachdjian, personal communication). Popliteal neurectomy causes muscle atrophy and marked weakness of the gastrocnemius and only denervates the gastrocnemius while sparing the soleus muscle that is also spastic.

In a study of 3460 records of patients who had surgery for cerebral palsy from 1966 to 1983 in Brasilia, Brazil (Campos da Paz *et al.* 1984), 274 post-surgical patients were found for follow-up study. The relapse rate of deformity, after soft-tissue procedures such as hamstring lengthening, varied from 40% to 67%. Interestingly, adductor tenotomies had good results up to four years in the follow-up study. They speculated that a complex interaction occurs between the deformity, altered perception and brain processing. Theoretically, new mechanisms of compensation could be triggered due to operative treatment. Their question was

TABLE 6.XII
Results of orthopaedic surgery (Phelps 1957)

Operative procedure	N	% failed	Reasons for failure
Heelcord lengthening	121	75%	Tendon growth lagged at the bone; spastic dorsiflexors; lack of power of Ankle-dorsiflexors; athetoid 'shift'; imbalance of lateral muscles; helpless patient who could not benefit.
Popliteal neurectomy	59	90%	Spastic dorsiflexors, calcaneus; muscle imbalance to valgus or varus; athetoid 'shift' to toe-flexors; severity of the general condition.
Adductor tenotomy	43	76%	Lack of abductor power to maintain correction; substitution of internal rotators of hip; persistence of deformity due to athetoid 'shift'; bone changes; general severity.
Obturator neurectomy	46	76%	All of the above plus flexion deformity of hip, athetoid 'shift', recurrence due to nerve regeneration.
Durham procedure (transfer of tensor fascia femoris origin) rotators, femoral torsion, recurrence of internal rotation from contracture or substitution.	8	88%	Absence of power in hip external
Hip subluxation/dislocation	59	66%	Only 60% shelf procedures successful: shelf absorption in children or inadequate in adults.

how far we should go in interfering with 'the natural course' of the condition.

At the risk of generalizing, our own follow-up studies make me more optimistic about the effects of orthopaedic surgery. From 1955 to 1979 we had 693 patients who were being followed. This group included patients who had orthopaedic surgery. By 1984 we had follow-ups of surgery that ranged from 8 to 18 years (mean 12 years). The recurrence rates for specific surgeries and over corrections are delineated in Table 6.XIII.

In the study from Brasilia by Campos da Paz *et al.* (1984), 40% developed *genu recurvatum* after hamstring transfer. I (EEB) did not need a series of 100 patients, but only two who had hamstring transfer to realize that transferring too many of the hamstrings might cause over activity of the spastic quadriceps and a non-functional gait—a straight but stiff knee. This means that outcome studies depend not only upon the type of surgery chosen, but also on the indications for surgery, the preoperative analysis for decision-making, and the type of patient (45% were quadriplegic in the 1984 report by Campos da Paz *et al.*) Campos da Paz may be correct when he opined that sudden alteration of a long-standing deformity does disturb the person's self-perception.

Studies and writings on the development of body-image strongly suggest that it is not fully developed in normal children until late childhood (Eiser and Patterson 1983, van der Velde 1985). Body-image may have important clinical implications (Bauman 1981). Apparently its importance in paediatric orthopaedic surgical procedures has been recognized by at least one orthopaedic service in a children's hospital (Letts *et al.* 1983). They implemented a program of preoperative play with puppets and dolls, to prepare the child for loss of part of a limb or its sudden alteration by surgery. If at all possible, orthopaedic surgery should not be delayed in cerebral palsy until skeletal maturity has

been reached and adolescent body-image and concern is at its height. Body-image studies have not been reported in children with cerebral palsy.

The progression of structural changes in the joints, despite assiduous therapy and bracing, has been evident when patients have been followed for long periods. If a child is followed only to age 15 or 16 years, physicians and therapists might have an illusion that structural changes in childhood and early adolescence are not significant. Those who have followed patients for longer periods know that a painless subluxation of the hip in a crutch-walking child may not jeopardize mobility due to the pain of degenerative arthritis until after age 18 years. Similarly, a dislocated hip may not be painful until after age 15 years. Orthopaedic surgery deferred until later adolescence is more difficult, more complicated and has a greater incidence of postoperative psychological problems (Williams 1977).

If a child is followed only to age 15 or 16 years, physicians and therapists might have an illusion that structural changes in childhood and early adolescence are not significant.

In Goldkamp's follow-up study (1984), 17 of the 53 patients with cerebral palsy needed psychiatric assistance (32%). The reason for this high incidence of psychiatric problems with and without surgery in adolescent patients is not explained. It may be that overemphasis on the disease-oriented and ineffective treatments in their childhood years has thwarted their psychological development. Reality occurs when the cerebral-palsied child becomes an adult with the same cerebral palsy. The struggle to overcome the disease may then be recognized as time wasted.

TIMING OF ORTHOPAEDIC SURGERY

THE PRESCHOOL CHILD
In general, surgery for intended functional improvement of gait should be deferred until the child with a good prognosis for walking is actually walking independently or with walking aids. Samilson and Hoffer (1975) made the valid point of deferring surgery in the first 3–4 years because it was difficult to know what the main problem would be. They also advised against upper-limb surgery until age 5 or 6 years, so that selective control and sensation could be ascertained.

If the child has a good prognosis for ambulation, surgery will not hasten its development: although if one fortuitously performs the operation just when central nervous system maturation occurs, walking may begin very shortly after the surgery. If the surgeon wants to be a 'miracle-worker', this is the time to do surgery. For example almost all children with spastic hemiplegia walk by age 18–21 months.

The preschool child may need surgery, however, if structural changes develop especially in the hip. Early subluxation can be prevented in most cases from developing into persistent subluxation and secondary acetabular dysplasia or dislocation (almost always in children who are non-walkers) if surgery is done before the age of 3 or 4 years.

TABLE 6. XIII
Recurrence and overcorrection of deformities after orthopaedic surgery, 8- to 18-year follow-up (mean 12 years). Spastic diplegia—ambulatory

Type of surgery	N	Recurrence	Overcorrection
Adductor longus and gracilis myotomy, anterior branch obturator neurectomy	92	0 (< 20º abduction*)	1 (>10º abduction during stance **) = 1 %
Hamstring lengthening	79	4 (>15º flexion during stance)=4 %	5 (> 10º recurvatum of knee)=6 %
Achilles tendon sliding lengthening (Hoke)	50	5=9 %	1 (calcaneus)=2 %
Iliopsoas recession §	25	1 = 4 %†	0

*Passive range of hip abduction with hip extended. **Stance phase of the gait cycle.

†One had no correction of the hip-flexion deformity: 60º preoperatively and post-operatively.

§After 1987, iliopsoas recession not done; iliopsoas tendon lengthening had results comparable to recession. Current practice is iliopsoas tenotomy at the pelvic brim (Novacheck 2001).

The locomotor prognosis has to be kept in mind when considering the type of surgery in subluxation of the hip. If the child has a good prognosis, an iliopsoas lengthening or tenotomy at the pelvic brim might be preferable to an iliopsoas tenotomy at the lesser trochanter which could permanently weaken hip flexion. But if the prognosis is poor, then iliopsoas tenotomy through the same incision used for an adductor longus myotenotomy could be the best choice because possible hip-flexion weakness may have no long-term functional significance in a child who will be dependent upon a wheelchair.

THE SCHOOL-AGE CHILD
The major *indication* for orthopaedic surgery in children with cerebral palsy is to prevent structural changes of the limbs and trunk which may become disabling in later life. The indications for surgery to improve function need more discernment. For those who walk either independently or with aids, surgery for functional improvement is usually in the hip, knee and foot. For those who do not walk, the functional goal will be to maintain or improve the ability for either assistive or self-transfer from the wheelchair. Straightening a knee-flexion contracture is justifiable in these cases, as is a corrective arthrodesis of a severe foot deformity. The patient who can only sit in a wheelchair also needs to maintain this function, which can be destroyed by an uncorrected hip dislocation or scoliosis.

Orthopaedic surgery is also needed to correct structural deformities of the joints and spine when these are present, painful or reduce independence before and after skeletal maturity. The decision to recommend a posterior rootlet rhizotomy in a child with spastic diplegia is a choice on the extent and permanence of the rhizotomy versus an orthopaedic procedure. For example, it the only functional complaint is knee flexion during stance phase, then a simple fractional hamstring lengthening would seem to be the correct decision. Or, if the major joint deformity is fixed ankle equinus with mild of moderate spasticity of the knee and hips, then a sliding Achilles tendon lengthening (or gastronemius lengthening that some surgeons prefer) might be more appealing as a simpler and effective intervention.

Orthopaedic surgery for upper-limb dysfunction due to spasticity is limited, but can be effective in restoring some function such as relief of the thumb-in-palm, or a fisted hand. However, we have to inform the patient and the family that the goals of surgery are limited and will not make the hand 'normal'. Appearance can be improved. But generally function will always be compromised because of the sensory defect in the hands so that visual feedback is necessary in hand function.

The optimum time for lower-limb surgery in the ambulatory child seems to be between the ages of 5 and 7 years although Russman (2000) of the Portland, Oregon Shriners Hospital stated 5–10 years; Gage (1991) recommended 8–10 years as the best time. At these times the gait pattern can be analyzed and decisions made on the basis of desired functional improvement. For example, a passive stretch test may indicate contracted hamstring muscles. But when the child walks, knee flexion during stance phase may be less than 10° due to the counterbalancing

effect of the spastic quadriceps. As a result of such observations, hamstring lengthening need not be considered unless combined with rectus femoris transfer or distal release to improve the range of knee flexion on swing phase.

With careful and repeated analysis by examinations and recognition of potential structural skeletal changes, most soft-tissue surgery can be performed at one time and at as many levels as required (Norlin and Tkaczuk 1985, 1992) (Fig. 6.19). Fabry and fellow orthopaedic surgeons (1999) from Belgium monitored 15 patients with spastic diplegia 9.5 years after staged surgery. Using gait analysis and clinical evaluations of joint ranges of motion they reported that staging operative procedures gave unpredictable results. As a result these Belgian surgeons have changed to a multilevel simultaneous procedure. Other surgeons have confirmed the efficacy of multilevel orthopaedic surgery in spastic diplegia (Zwick *et al.* 2001, Germany; Desloovere *et al.* 2001, Belgium; Saraph *et al.* 2002, Austria).

When the postoperative immobilization entails limited time in a plaster (usually 3–6 weeks), and early mobilization even in plaster within 2–5 days postoperatively, postoperative rehabilitation has not been unduly prolonged (Sussman and Cusick 1981). Often 3–6 months of supervision by a physical therapist is all that is necessary. Short-term intensive supervised therapeutic exercise and functional training by the therapist is more effective than long-term rehabilitative training sessions once a week.

THE ADOLESCENT AND ADULT
In skeletally mature persons, fixed contracture and permanent skeletal changes are the most frequent indications for surgery. We and others have found good responses to soft-tissue surgery in adults with spastic cerebral palsy, particularly for improved gait function (J.L. Goldner, personal communication). The principles and practice of surgery in these cases are identical to that used in

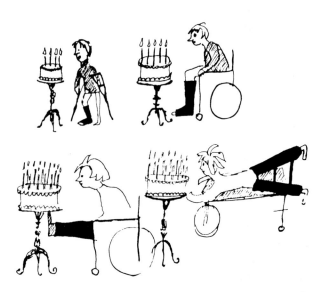

Fig. 6.19. Orthopaedic surgery birthday syndrome: birthdays in the life of the cerebral-palsied child. When possible surgery should be done at one sitting. (Reproduced by courtesy of the artist, Mercer Rang MD, Toronto.)

children. Adults who have no flexion contracture of the knee beyond 10° are amazed at the functional improvement in their gait due to increasing stride-length following fractional hamstring lengthening. The same has held true for adductor myotomy. Adults who have flexion contractures of the hip, resultant compensatory anterior inclination of the pelvis and constant low back pain due to the lumbar lordosis, have obtained relief of the back pain after iliopsoas tendon lengthening.

Severe skeletal changes in adults (e.g. subluxation of the hip with degenerative arthritis or degenerative arthritis of the knee due to flexion contracture of the knee beyond 15° and a painful patellar–femoral arthritis) need bone surgery combined with tendon lengthenings or tenotomies to restore function. In a small study referred to in a publication by Thomas *et al.* (1985) on the needs of physically disabled adults, 11% required orthopaedic surgery. You have to live a fairly long time, be willing to accept adults with cerebral palsy as your patient, and have a stable location in order to appreciate the long-term results of structural joint changes.

Although not conforming to a scientific study, and dependent on memory, the following personal vignettes of adult patients might dramatize the need to consider outcomes in adults who had continuing structural changes in their joints.

A 42-year-old fully employed bookkeeper who always needed crutches for walking and eventually was rendered wheelchair bound due to a painful hip from a long-standing subluxation and degenerative joint disease.

An active 46-year-old man, an immigrant from Pakistan with spastic diplegia and flexed knees, developed severe retropatellar pain in both knees as a first stage degenerative joint disease. The successful outcome was hamstring lengthening and supracondylar extension osteotomy.

A 48-year-old man with total body tension athetosis had always been wheelchair-bound and found his livelihood as a rehabilitation coordinator jeopardized by severe pain in his subluxated right hip. After hip arthrodesis he was pain free and continued to hold down his job very effectively as well as promoting assisted speech in a telephone voice communication program.

A 62-year-old grandmother with spastic diplegia who was forced into virtual immobility because of continuing and severe pain in her left knee due to the years of flexed knee posture and progressive degenerative joint disease. A patellectomy and a supracondylar extension osteotomy combined with hamstring lengthening eliminated the pain so she once again could walk with crutches.

PREPARATION OF THE CHILD AND PARENTS FOR SURGERY

The basis of all human relationships is trust. Above all, the child and parents must feel secure with the surgeon. Distrust and anxiety will complicate the postoperative course and can compromise the result by placing the surgeon on the defensive. Defensive attitudes can cause errors in judgement. One does not go to a surgeon (or any physician for that matter) in order to dictate the procedure or method of management. If the surgeon discerns distrust and anxiety, it is better not to do the surgery—or at least to defer it until more conducive attitudes prevail.

If possible, it is best for the child to become familiar with the physical therapist for 3–6 months prior to surgery. The therapist will need the full cooperation of the child in the period of postoperative rehabilitation. The therapist can also assist the surgeon in a preoperative analysis of the many-faceted aspects of the motor disorder: the gait pattern, ranges of motion of joints, the behavior of the child and the attitude of the parents. The therapist can supplement the physician's task by explaining the reasons for surgery to the child and parents. Ideally the therapist would be familiar with the general surgical plan, the operative procedures and the postoperative rehabilitation plan (whether crutches, walker or wheelchair will be necessary), and the duration of non-weightbearing if this will be required.

Preoperative preparation of the child takes time, but is rewarding in decreasing postoperative psychological complications and hospital stay (Ferguson 1979, Wolfer and Visintainer 1979). At Children's Hospital at Stanford we had a special preoperative program with illustrated material, video and hospital play. Barring physiological complications (e.g. postoperative infection), postoperative recovery was smooth with very little persistent pain or spasm beyond the first 48 hours after surgery in the majority of the children.

If we always practiced what we preached in adequately preparing children for surgery, they ought to be admitted to the hospital 1–2 days in advance. In this way the children would be able to integrate the radical change in their lives, especially in the modern and highly complex hospital organization (Sylvester 1977). Due to steady progress in the application of biomedical science to the practice of surgery, hospital stays have steadily dropped in paediatric orthopaedic surgery. By 1984 our average hospital stay had decreased to a mean of 4.6 days. Today, stays are much shorter and outpatient surgery in cerebral palsy or a same-day admission with an overnight stay is usual.

The limited ability of the child to adjust to the myriad of personnel and procedures within 8–10 hours before a major operation must be considered. Because professional personnel are always so busy, there is considerable merit in Sylvester's (1977) suggestion that the patient should have a 'best friend' in the hospital. At Guy's Hospital in London, a 'best friend'-type person was employed (Parks 1977). This non-medical person was able to establish a supportive relationship with the child and parents, interpret and advise on hospital procedures, and tell them what was likely to happen next. We cannot forget that surgery is unique; instantly it sets in motion an irreversible biological change, and in cerebral palsy, a sudden structural change as well. In this third millennium with the drive to keep hospital costs 'contained', it is not likely that children will be admitted a day early for surgery.

The surgeon can help prepare the child for surgery by talking directly to him or her and answering all questions by both parent and child. The child must be told: (1) that it is going to hurt, but medicines will be given to relieve the discomfort which usually lasts about 48 hours; (2) where the incisions will be made in the skin; (3) that a plaster will be applied, and what part of the limb will be enclosed; and (4) how long the plaster will be on the limb, when walking will be permitted, whether crutches or a wheelchair will be necessary and the duration of non-weightbearing if this is required.

INFORMED CONSENT

The USA claims that its democracy is based on 'the rule of law'. Accordingly, we have more lawyers per head of population than any nation in the world. So it is not surprising that we have litigation that claims injury to patients as the result of medical interventions, particularly surgery. While such claims are usually dismissed and poor results that occur in cerebral palsy are not grounds for a lawsuit (providing that the interventions are consistent with the standards of the community), a new reason for a claim is lack of informed consent on expected outcomes of orthopaedic surgery pertaining to the function of walking. It has arisen when a procedure is done to correct a specific deformity such as a severe pes valgus in a GMFCS level III or IV pre-adolescent or adolescent patient and their limited walking ability usually with a walker ceases postoperatively. The giving-up of walking by patients in this level of function is usual in the natural history of their cerebral palsy. As they approach adulthood these patients often find that their struggle to walk consumes too much energy; they gain weight and settle down to the wheelchair for living with the disability. When after surgery this happens, suits are filed on the basis of lack of informed consent that did not include postoperative walking limitations.

It takes considerable time to explain to the parents or guardians the objectives of the orthopaedic surgery, what it entails, and the risks. Such discussions should include that function of walking might not be the same as when the child was 7 years old and appear more limited after surgery, particularly on the feet. As tedious at it seems, all of this information should be conveyed in writing.

ORAL SURGERY AND BOTULINUM-A TOXIN FOR DROOLING

Other than orthopaedic and ophthalmic surgery, oral surgery has a role in cerebral palsy in the treatment of sialorrhoea (drooling or excessive salivation). We mention this here because parents expect the orthopaedic surgeon to have knowledge of surgical treatment in general.

Drooling is common in babies and young children. When it persists into mid-childhood and beyond, it becomes distressing for parents and sometimes the aware child. Approximately 10% of the population with cerebral palsy have persistent drooling (Koheil *et al.* 1985) and more than 58% of those with more severely involved cerebral palsy (Tahmassebi and Curzon 2003b). Drooling decreased with dentition age. Those with permanent teeth drooled less. Studies show that drooling is associated with poor motor control and poor swallowing rather than due to excessive amounts of saliva being produced (Tahmassebi and Curzon 2003a). Drooling that requires the constant use of a bib is a hindrance to social integration. Head control is important in achieving a good result from the procedures designed to reduce salivation.

Biofeedback methods have been reported as promising in relieving drooling. Eleven of 12 patients treated with biofeedback techniques were improved (Koheil *et al.* 1985). Tympanic neurectomy and chorda tympanectomy were proposed as a method of alleviating the condition. However, Pariser *et al.* (1978) found an unacceptable recurrence of the drooling with these procedures.

Parotid duct relocation to the tonsillar fossa, originally described by Wilke (1967), has had reasonably good results. Messingill (1978) observed decreased salivation in six of eight patients who had the parotid duct relocation. Tongue function during swallowing, as visualized by cinefluorography, was helpful in prognosis when correlated with the postoperative results. The age when the procedure was performed varied from 6 to 22 years (mean 12.6 years).

Better results seem to be achieved with parotid duct transplantation and submandibular salivary gland excision (Chait and Kessler 1979, Morgan *et al.* 1981). Surgical treatment continues to be effective. One group of surgeons from Taiwan reported good results using an yttrium aluminum garnet laser intraductal on the parotid gland ducts (Wong *et al.* 1997). O'Dwyer and Conlon of Dublin, Ireland (1997) had very good results with very few complications in submandibular duct rerouting to the posterior tonsillar fossa.

Botulinum-A toxin has found a use in reduction of drooling in children with cerebral palsy (Jongerius *et al.* 2004). Physicians at Nijmegen, the Netherlands, tried injections of the submandibular glands in 45 patients with cerebral palsy who had severe drooling. Injections into the glands were guided by ultrasound. In a 24-week trial drooling was reduced by 69% at 2 weeks and 49% at 24 weeks. Side-effects were minimal. This compared favorably with results noted from scopolamine treatment, which resulted in a mean baseline reduction of 25% compared with a mean reduction of 42% with botulinum neurotoxin A.

Comparable results in Nova Scotia, Canada, were found in with injections of five units of the toxin into the parotid gland in nine patients, ages 4–17 years and followed for a minimum of 16 weeks. A favorable response of 55% occurred (Bothwell *et al.* 2002). Suskind and Tilton (2002) of New Orleans, Louisiana, reported that injections of the toxin into either the parotid glands or into both the submandibular and parotid glands was safe and 'promising' treatment for sialorrhea in 22 subjects with cerebral palsy.[23]

---

23 Sialorrhea=excessive drooling (another word you can add to your medical lexicon).

SPORTS

'If horseback riding and swimming are good for the athetoid, this does not make the horse a therapist or the swimming pool a medical appliance.'

(Milani-Comparetti 1979)

Even though for several generations medicine took a dim view of anything that might be fun, sports programs for the disabled have proliferated and have been rapidly advanced in North America, Europe and Asia. In Brasilia, after 10 years of passive physical therapy to effect change in the motor disorder of cerebral palsy in 2000 patients, this approach was abandoned in favour of fun and games (Campos da Paz Jr 1980). Perhaps the study (van den Berg-Emons *et al.* 1995) that reported significantly lower total daily energy expenditure and the sleeping metabolic rate in five boys with spastic diplegia compared with five unaffected controls reinforces the need for fun and games. From the data the authors concluded that children with spastic diplegia are considerably less active than their healthy peers and made the case for special physical activity programs, also known as 'adaptive physical education'.

HIPPOTHERAPY AND THERAPEUTIC HORSE-RIDING

Therapeutic horse-riding develops riding skills with people with disabilities while hippotherapy uses the movement of a horse to improve gross motor function including walking. Both of these therapies seem effective in improving the skills of children with cerebral palsy. McGibbon (1998), reporting on 5 children with spastic cerebral palsy, compared their GMFM scores after hippotherapy compared to themselves doing therapy on an 'A'-frame barrel. The original study was extended to 15 children in a report in a 2003 study. The 2003 study showed improved symmetry and muscle activity following hippotherapy with no change noted while sitting astride a barrel. Children involved in hippotherapy enjoy this type of therapy more and see it as fun and game time activity: a feeling they do not see in the usual more clinical setting. Notably, children enjoyed mastering skills which their peers did not have. Sterba *et al.* (2002) reported similar improvement in gross motor function in a study of 17 children with cerebral palsy participating in an 18-week therapeutic horse-riding program. Improvements of 7.6% were noted in dimensions A–E of GMFM total score after 18 weeks of therapy and returned to control level 6 weeks following conclusion of the therapy. Other improvements were noted on the GMFM dimension E (walking, running, and jumping) with an 8.7% improvement after 12 weeks, and 8.5% after 18 weeks of therapy. There was continued elevation over the baseline at 6 weeks following conclusion of the hippotherapy. Although they call for larger studies, the conclusion was that 'horseback riding should be considered for sports therapy in children with CP'.

Bertoti in 1998 also noted improvement in posture and muscle tone and balance with improved functional skills following therapeutic horse-riding. Early reports noted the therapeutic value of 'hippotherapy' (Tauffkirchen 1978) and 'therapeutic horseback riding for cerebral-palsied children' (Hengst 1976, Feldkamp 1979.)

We have found these therapy modalities useful as they are both therapeutic and fun for children with cerebral palsy. Larger numbers of children, both with cerebral palsy and normal controls would be needed to demonstrate the efficacy of 'hippotherapy'. Perhaps the therapist will turn out to be the horse. What is the best breed of horse for riding therapy? Will the horse be paid by public or private insurance funds? It may be that horses will find a role in retirement rather than going to the proverbial fox farm.

AQUATIC SPORTS

An experienced physical therapist gave the best reason for the efficacy of immersion in water for exercise. The water displaces the body weight to give an anti-gravity effect so that the limbs move more easily and freely. At the same time the water offers resistance to the muscles and strengthens them. What could be better? So, for children and adults with cerebral palsy, swimming and pool exercises are one of the best activities. Although there is a little science to support the efficacy of immersion in water, we have a great deal of history of its perceived health benefits since Roman times. Public baths were the environment of the medieval surgeon (Lyons and Petrucelli 1987). And there are famous resorts such Bath in England, Baden-Baden in Germany, the bath-houses of Budapest, Turkey, Aix-les-Bains and Évian-les-Bains, France, and the boiling hot-water baths of Japan. The French can use their spa resorts a *vacances santé*, a health vacation, approved by the French health-care system. The belief in the curative power of water in the United States dates back to the 18th century. Resorts are still operative in such as Hot Springs, Virginia and Calistoga in the Napa Valley of California.

Water displaces the body weight; the limbs move easily in an anti-gravity condition while the water offers resistance to the muscles—the ideal exercise.

A twice-weekly swimming program and a once a week group physical activity gym program for 5- to 7-year-old children who had cerebral palsy were compared with a control group who had Bobath therapy in Israel (Hutzler *et al.* 1998). Those who had the swimming and exercise program improved their baseline vital capacities by 65% while the control group of therapy only improved 23%. Children who have total body involvement with spastic quadriplegia seem to get more relaxation from a heated whirlpool spa or tub than any other modality or medication.

Swimming aids, flotation devices, swim wear, amphibious wheelchairs, adaptive water skis, canoes, kayaks and sail-boats can be found in the abledata website. No less than 19 organizations are devoted to adaptive water sports such as the US Wheelchair Swimming, Physically Challenged Swimmers, the US Rowing Association and the US Sailing Association (see www.abledata. com).

WINTER SNOW SPORTS

Alpine and cross-country skiing is another sport well suited to many children and adults who have cerebral palsy. As might be expected from 'God's frozen people', Canadians have been among those in the forefront promoting snow play for the disabled—'There's no play like snow play' (Arnoff 1973). In the USA the alpine skiing program for disabled children was founded under the auspices of the Children's Hospital Medical Center, Denver, Colorado (Messner 1976). As a result, other winter sport programs for the disabled have continued to go forward in locales that have snowy winters.

BALL GAMES AND OTHER SPORTS

Soccer is a popular sport for young people who have spastic diplegia or hemiplegia and are independent walkers. For children with spastic diplegia or hemiplegia another sport is golf, and tennis may be possible with proper instruction. The wheelchair Olympics and the Special Olympics for the disabled are now national institutions in most nations and regions in the world. The *Exceptional Parent Resource Guide*, 2000,[24] lists 53 organizations devoted to adaptive recreation from archery to wheelchair tennis. In addition to mailing addresses, phone and fax numbers, most have websites. The Far East and South Pacific Games for the Disabled (under the acronym, FESPIC, originally denoting 'Far East South Pacific International Competition') were held in December 1998 in Bangkok. Over 2000 disabled representing 32 countries participated in these games. Wheelchair racing is the most popular sport, but basketball, volleyball and fencing have been adapted for the disabled (R.A. Brennan, personal communication).

Given the growing recognition and success of sports for the disabled, physicians and therapists have every reason to encourage and assist children with cerebral palsy in learning and preparing for a lifelong sporting activity rather than a life of passive manipulation and medicalization. Hebestreit and Bar-Or (2001) of Germany made a plea to promote exercise and sports in children born preterm. If adults who have normal motor control want to exercise at a health club regularly, why not a health club for the disabled rather than a recurring prescription for physical therapy at a medical rehabilitation unit or hospital?

ASSISTIVE TECHNOLOGY (REHABILITATION ENGINEERING)

Welcome to the electronic warehouse: www.abledata.com[25]
(no charge for service)

HISTORY AND RESOURCES

The seed for the growth of assistive technology in the United States was rehabilitation engineering for the physically disabled developed at the Ontario Crippled Children's Center, Toronto, Canada, under the leadership of Dr Colin McLaren, an engineer. A national workshop of orthopaedic surgeons at Annapolis, Maryland, in 1972 on 'The Child with an Orthopaedic Disability: His Orthotic Needs and How to Meet Them' gave the stimulus for the establishment of Rehabilitation Engineering Centers in 1973 (Committee on Prosthetics Research and Development 1973). With a large private foundation grant we began the Rehabilitation Engineering Center at the Children's Hospital at Stanford in 1973 (Bleck 1978). After a good deal of skepticism, particularly from physical therapists who had dedicated their lives to overcoming the disabilities of children with severe cerebral palsy, and some hand wringing over costs by public funding agencies, it soon became evident that science and technology in the service of the physically disabled was more effective in compensating for lost function than therapeutic attempts at remediation (Berkowitz 1976).

Since the last edition of this book two decades ago, 'assistive technology' has replaced the term 'rehabilitation engineering', and the availability of assistive technology products has exploded. So much so, that there is no need to specify all that is commercially available other than list them generically. The abledata internet base has information on more than 25,000 products from 'white canes to voice output programs.' Online assistive technology products and information are also available from this website of most of the fifty States.

> *'The abledata internet base has information on more than 25,000 products from 'white canes to voice output programs.'*
> (www.abledata.com)

Other countries may have similar on-line services. A comprehensive collection of eight books from communication technology to sports is available in England.[26] For some patients, simple adaptive equipment designed and recommended by a physical or occupational therapist or communication specialist will be sufficient. Ideally the therapist or the communication specialist should be able to test the equipment before purchase, and measure the child or adult for the appropriate size In the more severely disabled, a team of electrical and mechanical engineers or special rehabilitation engineers, occupational therapists, speech pathologists, and orthotists are required to analyze the patient's functional capacity and the ability to utilize various standard commercially available devices and the necessity to custom-design appropriate interfaces and controls (Bleck 1977a, b, 1978, 1982, 1984, 1985). Included in assistive technology are the old devices of orthotics, walking aids, canes, and crutches.

---

24 *Exceptional Parent* offers a free resource guide for cerebral palsy and a host of many other diseases (555 Kinderkamack Road, Oradell, NJ, 07649-1517, USA; www.eparent.com).

25 Website sponsored by the USA National Institute on Disability and Rehabilitation Research (NIDDR).

26 The Disability Information Trust, Mary Marlborough Centre, Nuffield Orthopaedic Centre, Headington, Oxford OX3 7LD, UK. T: (44) (01865) 227592; F: (44) (01865) 227596; www.dlf.org.uk (similar to abledata).

ORTHOTICS

HISTORY FROM SPLINTS TO BRACES TO ORTHOSES (RANG 2000)

Non-surgical devices to correct limb and spinal deformities date back five centuries. Turnbuckle splints to correct joint deformities were described by Hans von Gersdoff in 1517. Ambrose Paré used fabricators of armor sheet metal in 1564 to brace the spine and foot. Braces must have been very popular for treatment in the 16th century. In 1592, Heironymus Fabricius published a treatise, *Hoplomochlion*, encompassing every type of brace. For three centuries brace treatment of orthopaedic deformities held sway. James Knight, founder of the Hospital for Ruptured and Crippled in New York (later became the Hospital for Special Surgery), as a strong advocate of braces forbade surgical interventions (Rang 2000).

With the development of thermoplastic molding (polypropylene) in the 1950s braces became orthoses stimulated by the Committee on Prosthetics and Orthotics of the National Academy of Sciences. The committee devised the current terminology for an orthosis depending on the joint or joints immobilized, e.g. AFO=ankle–foot orthosis (short leg brace), AFKO=ankle foot knee orthosis (long leg brace).[27] The term 'orthotic' soon became popular in podiatry and orthopaedic practices concentrating on sports medicine, particularly runners. 'Orthotic' in these circles describes a molded thermoplastic shoe insert usually with a small heel that can be wedged medially or laterally. Runners seem to become dependent, if not addicted, to wearing these for various aches and pains in the lower limbs and back.

> *Are orthotics useful or necessary in cerebral palsy?*
> *'I will be glad to give any lecture except braces in cerebral palsy.'*
> (Alice Garrett MD)

Full-control bracing was popular 30 years ago (Stamp 1973). It has been abandoned by most experienced professionals in cerebral palsy. Although it was hoped that the child with cerebral palsy would eventually 'learn' how to walk correctly in the brace, no carry-over was ever noticed or reported. Nor did bracing prevent serious structural change. Hips dislocated even though the hip-control brace was worn all day (and presumably at night too, when this was the fashion) (Figs 6.20, 6.21).

Lee (1982) reviewed 204 children with cerebral palsy and classified them according to the motor disorder and the extent of involvement. Regardless of spastic hemiplegia, diplegia or athetosis, bracing versus non-bracing was ineffective in preventing the need for surgery to correct deformities, in preventing recurrences after surgery, or improving the gait. Very few, if any, adults continue with orthoses—especially in the case of athetosis, in which an orthosis seemed logical to control involuntary movements, but confining (Sharrard 1976). We had the identical

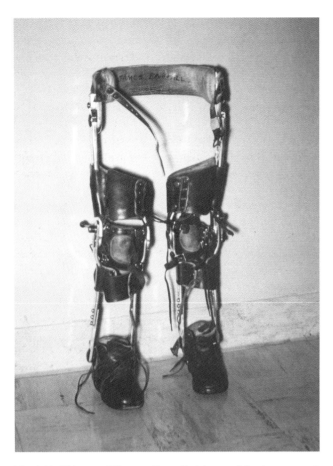

Fig. 6.20. Old empty full-control lower-limb braces of aluminum or steel, locked knee and ankle joints intended to control joint motion, now relics from the not too distant past in cerebral palsy management.

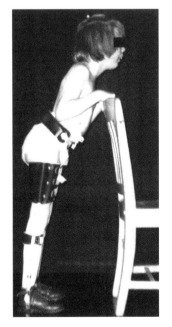
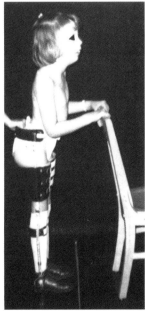

Fig. 6.21. *Left*: Girl with spastic diplegia and wearing long leg braces with the hip joints unlocked. Her trunk leans forward to accommodate hip-flexor spasticity and contracture. *Right*: with hip-joint locked, posture adapted to the hip-flexion contracture by increased anterior inclination of pelvis and lumbar lordosis.

---

27 Abbreviations in can obfuscate understanding, but these orthotic descriptors are so common, that they are used in this section.

experience as Sharrard when full-control and extensive bracing was imposed on children.

When the parents were assured of our non-punitive attitudes, the majority removed the braces after school so that the child 'could play and run about'. We have not used night splinting in an attempt to prevent structural change (e.g. contracture of the triceps surae or hamstrings). Our analysis of recurrence of the triceps surae contracture after Achilles tendon lengthening, in patients in whom we did not use day or night splinting post-operatively, is convincing evidence that this added management is not often necessary (Lee and Bleck 1980). Our recurrence rate of 9% after Achilles tendon lengthening compared favourably with others (usually stated to be about 6%). This means that if we had enforced night splinting we would have imposed unnecessary management 91% of the time!

Another tool to help overcome equinus was a sort of short aluminum ski attached to the plantar aspect of the shoe with French leather ski bindings. It appeared to be successful in stretching contractures of the triceps surae (Hanks and MacFarlane 1969). So why not try cross-country skis, or Swedish roll skis when there is no snow, and practice on paved roads or fiberglass tracks through the forest?

HIP-KNEE-ANKLE–FOOT ORTHOSIS (HKAFO)

In contemporary orthopaedic management, hip–knee–ankle–foot orthoses are almost never applied in cerebral palsy. On one or two occasions in 25 years we used a Garrett temporary hip-abduction orthosis in an infant or toddler, in whom the signs of spasticity seemed to be diminishing and who had no contracture but only dynamic adduction (Garrett *et al.* 1966). The 'abduction pants' described by Hare (1977) seem adequate for this purpose; the pants are a large H-shaped diaper with a foam center of maximum width to obtain abduction of the hips. This appears similar to the Friejka pillow splint, which was used for congenital dysplasia of the hips. No data on results has ever been published.

Hip-flexion contracture has not been controlled with hip–knee–ankle orthoses which can be locked at the hip and knee in extension. The only change this orthosis will make is on the pelvis, as it is forced into anterior inclination, and concomitant lumbar lordosis to compensate for the hip-flexion contracture (Fig. 6.22).

Cable twister orthotics have not corrected a hip internal-rotation deformity in cerebral palsy (or for that matter in a non-paralytic hip internal-rotation gait due to excessive femoral anteversion). Instead the orthosis may only reinforce the development of compensatory excessive external (lateral) tibial fibular torsion (Fig. 6.23). Lining up the lower limbs often requires osteotomies, not bracing.

KNEE-ANKLE–FOOT ORTHOSIS (KAFO)

The knee–ankle–foot orthosis with a drop-lock at the knee joint is occasionally useful in a child who has just begun to walk and whose knees are flexed more than 15° during the stance phase of gait, and in whom the hamstring spasticity and contracture can

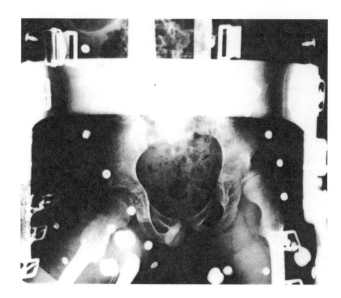

Fig. 6.22. Spastic paralytic dislocation of hip occurs despite restrictive full control bracing—useless to prevent hip subluxation or dislocation.

possibly be tolerated for function and counterbalanced by increasing spasticity of the quadriceps.

After hamstring lengthening and posterior capsulotomy of the knee joint in older children, knee orthoses are useful to control excessive flexion: particularly if little quadriceps spasticity seems to be present. An orthosis like this is usually used from 6 to 12 months postoperatively until the patient regains quadriceps strength and confidence during gait. Once walking can be done with the knee unlocked, and extension of the joint occurs in the stance phase, the orthosis is no longer required.

Knee hyperextension deformity (*genu recurvatum*) can sometimes be managed with a rigid plastic ankle–foot orthosis with the foot dorsiflexed, providing the ankle does have a sufficient range of dorsiflexion (at least 5° or more measured

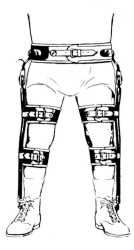

Fig. 6.23. Outmoded cable twister orthosis. A truck speedometer cable generated a constant external torque on the lower limb. It does not control or correct hip internal rotation deformities. Instead, if anything, it forces compensatory external torsion of the tibia and fibula.

with the knee extended and the foot held in varus; Rosenthal *et al.* 1975).

ANKLE–FOOT ORTHOSIS (AFO)

The plastic molded ankle–foot orthosis is the most widely used in cerebral palsy (Staros and LeBlanc 1975, Hoffer and Koffman 1980, Rosenthal 1984, Taylor and Kling 1984). The modern plastic orthosis is so useful because all motions of the foot and ankle can be controlled; and if the spasticity is not too great, equinus, varus and valgus can be controlled providing passive motion corrects the deformity. The orthotist makes the orthosis from a negative plaster shell made with the foot held in the corrected position. A positive plaster mold is made from this, and the heat-softened plastic sheet is drawn over it by vacuum and then trimmed to the finished product. It can be worn over a stocking in an ordinary shoe.

The AFO is the most commonly used orthosis in cerebral palsy to control dynamic spastic equinus. With the increasing use of botulinum toxin it may become redundant. Some have combined botulinum toxin injections with the AFO in hope that muscle length will be maintained during growth. Several modifications of the plastic AFO have been used (Fisk and Supam 1997).

(1) The *solid ankle orthosis* is rigid, to control dynamic equinus and the subtalar joint (Fig. 6.24). Abel and colleagues (1998) used motion analysis techniques to study the effects of the rigid AFO in 35 children who had spastic diplegia. Equinus control was the objective in 18 and pes planovalgus and crouch

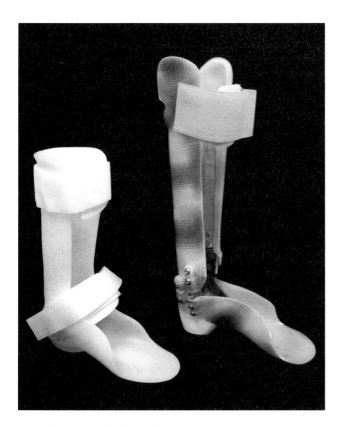

Fig. 6.24. Solid ankle and articulated AFOs.

control in 17. Compared with barefoot gait, the AFOs improved gait function by limiting premature plantarflexion, but had no effect on the knee or hip joints. A decade ago studies appeared to confirm the efficacy of the bilateral AFOs on energy expenditure at self-selected walking speeds by children who had spastic diplegia (Mossberg *et al.* 1990).

Compared with no AFO and a dynamic AFO when stance balance was perturbed, the solid AFO resulted in decreased action of the gastrocnemii, disorganized muscle response patterns, decreased use of ankle strategies and increased joint velocity angles at the knee in four children with spastic cerebral palsy (Burtner *et al.* 1999). Anther comparative study of rigid AFOs with dynamic hinged ankle with a plantarflexion stop AFOs, and no AFOs in ten children with cerebral palsy, showed improvement in gait parameters with both types of AFOs (Ratka *et al.* 1997).

The literature and our own experience does not support prevention or correct of a spastic paralytic valgus deformity of the foot with plastic ankle–foot orthosis or any other orthosis or shoe modifications. The single medial metal upright short leg brace proposed by Bolkert (1979) mechanically should bring the foot from valgus to a more varus position in a sturdy shoe. There are no data supporting its effectiveness in correcting the valgus foot in cerebral palsy.

(2) The *floor reaction AFO*. The addition is an anterior shell grasping the proximal third of the tibia to minimize flexion through the floor reaction force. Fixed AFOs adjusted to control the position of the ground reaction force in relation to the knee in six children with spastic diplegia and hyperextension of the knee were tested. Three improved the foot–ground reaction contact and three improved their stance-phase posture after 6 months use of the AFO (Butler *et al.* 1992).

(3) The *articulated AFO*. A flexible toe plate allows forefoot dorsiflexion at the third rocker of gait by limiting plantarflexion in the early swing phase of the gait cycle (the first rocker is at heel contact, the second at flat foot in stance, and the third is heel off at beginning of the swing phase, Gage 1991).

In a study of children aged 2–5 years with spastic diplegia and dynamic equinus their sit-to-stand times were significantly improved with the articulated AFO compared to bare foot (Wilson *et al.* 1997).

Investigators at the Motion Analysis Laboratory of the Children's Hospital of Los Angeles used gait analysis in 21 children with spastic diplegia who wore fixed AFOs, articulated ankle–foot orthoses (AAFOs) and walked barefoot (Rethlefsen *et al.* 1999). They found that dorsiflexion at terminal stance was greatest with the AAFO and that plantarflexion power in pre-swing was preserved as well. The conclusion was that the AAFO was satisfactory with varying degrees of calf muscle spasticity and if an adequate range of passive motion was present. But the orthosis could not be used in patients who had a tendency to crouch.

(4) The *articulated floor reaction AFO* has an adjustable ankle joint and is used to prevent forward progression of the tibia over the talus. It is used to prevent knee flexion in the stance phase.

(5) The *thermoplastic elastomer AFO* has a spring like function that assists dorsiflexion during gait. It is used if the

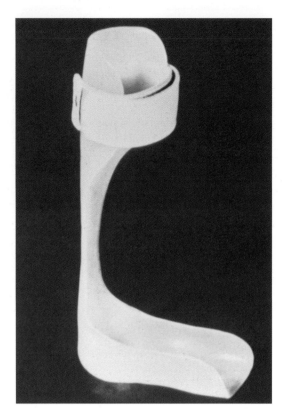

Fig. 6.25. Posterior spring leaf AFO for drop foot of flaccid paralysis—not very useful in spastic paralysis. It puts the calf muscles on a stretch inducing more spasticity.

ankle dorsiflexor muscles are weak (also called 'posterior leaf spring orthosis', PLSAFO) (Fig. 6.25). Because it stretches the gastrocnemius–soleus muscles, it will create more spasticity of these muscles in cerebral palsy. But Õunpuu and colleagues (1996) did a computer-assisted gait analysis in 31 children with cerebral palsy who were tested both barefoot and with the PLSAFO. They found that the orthosis reduced ankle equinus in swing, but did not improve the mechanical, or spring energy in terminal stance.

(6) The *thermoplastic elastomer articulated AFO* has an adjustable ankle joint that can be set at the desired angle to limit dorsiflexion and/or plantarflexion.

(7) The *tone inhibitive AFO* (also called 'tone-inhibiting AFO' or TRAFO). The origin of this one is from the 'inhibitive cast' experience that kept the toes dorsiflexed. The plantar sole rest piece is molded to apply pressure to the metatarsal arch with relief under the metatarsal heads, applies pressure under the sustentaculum tali and the peroneal arch, and has an extension that is built-up to keep the toes in dorsiflexion. The modifications have been included in the articulated AFO.

Another modification of the idea of inhibition of tone with an orthosis is the supramalleolar orthosis (SMO) that extends only to 5 cm above the tip of the malleoli and curved down on the posterior aspect to allow full dorsiflexion and plantarflexion. The tone reducing feature is the 0.5 cm elevation at the toes to reduce tone, decreased toe grasp, and improve roll over in terminal stance.

Kinematic and kinetic gait analysis studies in eight children who had spastic diplegia compared the tone reducing AFOs with the standard articulated AFO (Crenshaw *et al.* 2000). No clinical or statistical differences were found between the AFO and the TRAFO. Most refreshing for many of us who appreciate all-too-rare negative results, there were no differences between shoes-only and the SMO. The data strongly suggests that more elaborate orthoses than the old AFO to limit plantarflexion are not necessary.

FOOT ORTHOSES (FO)

Plastic, felt or metal arch supports have not been useful in correcting either valgus or varus deformities in spastic or athetoid types of cerebral palsy. The University of California Biomechanics Laboratory (UCBL) plastic shoe insert has not been successful in correcting spastic valgus deformities (Bleck and Berzins 1977). The popular sports medicine type of 'orthotic' has not been useful in children with cerebral palsy, although we have seen a few children who had these prescribed by foot-problem practitioners.

SHOES

> '*If you don't see it, it's not there.*'
>
> (Jacqueline Perry, on the theory of the corrective orthopaedic shoe; Fig. 6.26)

Bleck (1971) and presumably other orthopaedic surgeons have found no use for 'corrective orthopaedic shoes' in the past 30 years. We are indebted to the late Berta Bobath who visited our special therapy unit for cerebral palsy in San Mateo, California, circa 1956. She gave us the courage to eliminate on all children the heavy stiff so-called 'orthopaedic shoes' often prescribed with a Thomas heel and a stiff heel counter (Fig. 6.27). We began taking off these 'clown shoes' (the children's name for them) and recommended sneakers (tennis shoes or sport shoes) much to the joy of the children. After a while the grandparents and parents

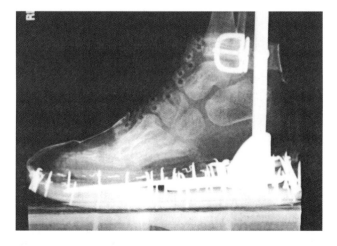

Fig. 6.26. Lateral radiograph of foot and ankle in a child with spastic equinus and wearing a double upright tubular steel brace with a 90° ankle stop to dorsiflexion attached to a high top leather shoe. The equinus inside is nicely hidden.

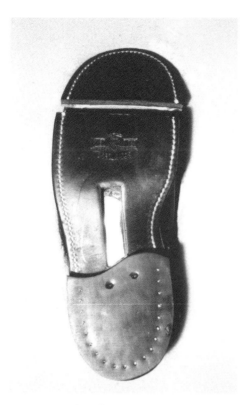

Fig. 6.27. Another relic: the 'corrective' orthopaedic shoe with a stiff sole and steel shank and a Thomas heel used to treat and prevent 'flat feet' in growing children.

came around to accept this seemingly radical change. They were wedded to the idea that 'you are what your feet are'. We overcame their perceptions that the foot was the seat of the soul by comparing shoes to gloves, i.e. only a protection from the stones, glass and other objects that damage the skin of the foot. Sneakers (performance shoes, 'trainers' or jogging shoes) provide good ground-contact and possibly force more muscle coordination. There is also a place for hiking-boots with crepe or heavy rubber soles that seem to help ankle stability, possibly by decreasing the range of ankle plantar and dorsiflexion so that postural adaptation and control by the anterior tibial and the gastrocnemius–soleus muscles need not be as great; boots also add a bit of weight, and might help control balance. I noted that the 'conductor' of a local conductive education school does not allow the children to wear anything but sturdy high-quality leather laced high top or three-quarter top shoes—very European (EEB).

What is so bad about children with cerebral palsy going barefoot? Quite a few children with cerebral palsy had never gone without shoes, even in the home on thick pile carpets! As a result, these children's feet were super-sensitive to touch; they often complained of painful feet when barefoot, and the plantar skin was devoid of callous. The soles of their feet were like a baby's buttocks. When the ground environment is safe, going barefoot in the home, in the sand at the beach and on the lawn, seems a rational and natural way to stress the plantar skin and fat so that hypertrophy occurs and sensitivity decreases. European grandmothers may not like such advice, even though it would seem unnecessary and obvious to people in South-East Asia and Polynesia. Standing and walking barefoot does not cause 'fallen arches'!

BIOFEEDBACK DEVICES

Biofeedback means that the patient by some mechanical–electrical device is able to monitor the action performed. Auditory feedback is more correctly called augmented feedback. In the past decade the technique has captured the imagination of professionals who deal with locomotor system disorders (Russell *et al.* 1976, Harrison 1977). Biofeedback devices have been used for a variety of problems in children with cerebral palsy. The Ontario Crippled Children's Centre was at the forefront of clinical investigations of biofeedback for head and joint position, jaw closure and postural alignment (Woolridge and McLaurin 1976). It was thought that the majority of patients could be trained with this technique, and that in some cases it carried over for sustained performance. Long-term clinical results have been lacking.

Conrad and Bleck (1980) reported their results with auditory augmented feedback for dynamic equinus. The device was a pressure-sensitive on/off switch inside the shoe and under the heel. The switch was connected to a battery-powered beeper. When the beep was heard, the child knew that heel contact occurred.[28] The device was used 3 hours per day for 3 months at home. This regimen appeared more effective than daily visits to a physical therapist for 'stretching' and 'gait training', or nagging by parents. All patients had dynamic equinus, i.e. no contracture of the triceps surae so that the ankle could be dorsiflexed with the foot in varus at least to neutral. The results in eight children (six with cerebral palsy, two idiopathic toe-walkers) were carefully analyzed with time and event counters, pedographs, and measured ranges of motion. Immediate and follow-up study at 3 months showed improvement in all when compared with the untreated foot; the range of dorsiflexion improved ($p<0.001$), the total accumulated heel-down position was 90% ($p<0.001$) and the total heel strikes increased ($p<0.01$). At longer follow-up of 3 months to 1 year (mean 5.7 months) without the auditory signal, the total heel-down time improved 45% from the pretreatment status. We thought that this method might be worthwhile in patients over 4 years of age, who have mild spasticity of the triceps surae and no contracture of the muscle—a highly selected group to be sure.

Seeger *et al.* (1981) reported a practically identical auditory feedback device for dynamic equinus in four girls with spastic hemiplegia. All had good results. But Seeger and Caudry (1983) reported on the long-term efficacy of this method, and found that the results were not maintained after 24–28 months. Kassover *et al.* (1984) used essentially the same method in four patients with spastic diplegia and equinus. They reported significant and dramatic improvement within 3 weeks of this treatment.

Unless there are more clinical outcome studies than have been published to date, we can conclude that biofeedback methods

---

28 Similar ready-made shoes for small children were made in Japan ('nightingale' shoes) so you could hear them walking. 'Nightingale floors' were installed in old Japanese houses and inns-the polished wood planking squeaked so you could hear thieves in the house.

have not fulfilled their initial promise in motor behavioral modification of cerebral palsy. No reports on augmented feedback for equinus gait have appeared in the medical literature of the Medline files for the past 16 years. In the authors' experience, biofeedback is of limited benefit.

NON-VERBAL COMMUNICATION

Communication is a basic human need. How can you make your wishes, thoughts and feelings known? In those individuals who cannot verbalize, the solution has been the rapid development of non-oral methods of communication.

SIGN LANGUAGE

The simplest method of non-oral communication has been with American sign-language developed for the deaf. However, most non-verbal children with cerebral palsy do not have the finger dexterity necessary to use sign-language.

SYMBOL LANGUAGE

Credit goes to Mrs Shirley McNaughton for demonstrating that non-verbal children had inner language to be tapped by the use of symbol language devised by Bliss (1965) and modified by McNaughton and her group at the Ontario Crippled Children's Centre in Toronto, Canada (McNaughton 1977, 1982) (Fig. 6.28). Bliss symbols have been adapted to many languages. Non-electronic communication boards have been used in India, for example, as simple and cost-effective devices to transmit and receive messages to and from non-verbal persons. These vary from simple alphabet to word/picture boards (Fig. 6.29). No

Fig. 6.28. Example of Bliss symbol language. (Reproduced by permission from McNaughton 1982.)

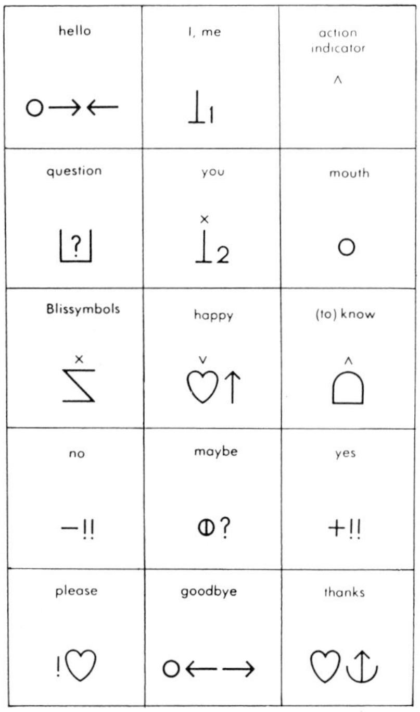

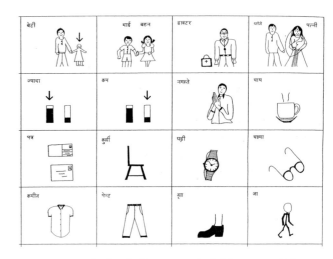

Fig. 6.29. Example of symbol language in Hindi (Bhatnagar and Silverman 1999). (Reproduced from the *Asia Pacific Disability Rehabilitation Journal*, by permission.)

Hindi vowel 'mantras' have been included in the board to keep it simple. Electronic communication devices are too costly for the majority of disabled in India unless paid for by charitable or government agencies (Bhatnagar and Silverman 1999).

The Eye-gaze E-tran Communication Board consists of a transparent plastic on which the letters or complete messages are printed. The partner holds the board to that the letters are visible to the disabled person who will be reading the letters backwards. As the disabled person gazes through the plastic chart, the eyes will appear in the center of the board to the partner. Six sequences of gaze are needed. The partner says the word for correctness. Whole messages on the board for Medical, Daily Needs, Family/People, and Feelings are more efficient (Bhatnagar and Silverman 1999) (Fig. 6.30). Morse code symbols can also be used

अ. **Medical** 1. मैं ठीक नहीं हूँ । 2. डाक्टर को बुलाओ । 3. मुझे दवा दो । 4. मुझे सिर दर्द है ।	इ. **Daily Needs** 1. मुझे पलट दो । 2. मुझे गमा लग रही है । 3. मुझे भूख/प्यास लगी है । 4. मुझे शौचालय जाना है ।
उ. **Family/People** 1. नमस्ते । 2. मैं ठीक हूँ । 3. आप कैसे हैं ? 4. पति/पत्नी को बुलाइये ।	ए. **Feelings** 1. मुझे अच्छा लगा, फिर आइये । 2. मुझे बहुत खेद है । 3. माफ करिये मैं थका हूँ । 4. मुझे आराम करना है/ नींद आरही है ।

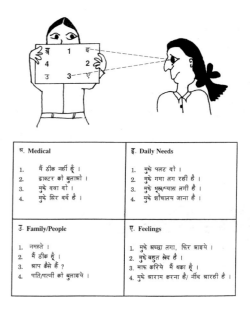

Fig. 6.30. E-gaze E-tran Communication with whole messages in Hindi. (From Bhatnagar and Silverman 1999; reproduced by permission from *Asia Pacific Disability Rehabilitation Journal*).

if the disabled person has the cognition to activate a muscle gesture, e.g. blinking the eyes once for a dot and blinking longer for a dash (Bhatnagar and Silverman 1999).

ELECTRONIC COMMUNICATION DEVICES

The first electronic communication device, the IBM electric typewriter with an overlay template, for written communication by persons with compromised hand function due to cerebral palsy was noted half a century ago by Crothers and Paine (1959). Many communication aids are now commercially available. The abledata website lists 24 alternative and augmentative communication systems. These can be categorized as providing (1) visual outputs, (2) printed outputs, and (3) speech outputs. The latter is a synthetic voice which satisfies the psychological needs of many non-verbal children and adults (LeBlanc 1982) (Figs 6.31–6.33). The computer has revolutionized the ability of children to communicate their thoughts and feelings; some have also exercised their latent artistic talents using computer graphics programs. Any time a non-verbal student is able to communicate using a computer-enhanced communication system, the quality of life is remarkably improved.

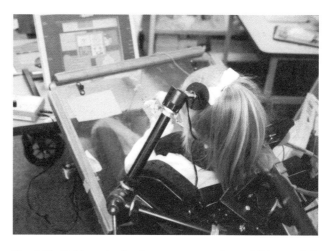

Fig. 6.32. Child uses her head movements to activate a jellybean switch on a mount to access a *DynaVox 3100*® voice-output device (DynaVox, Division of Sunrise Medical, 2100 Wharton Street, Pittsburgh, PA 15203, USA). (By permission of the Bridge School, Hillsborough, CA, and parents; www.bridgeschool.org.)

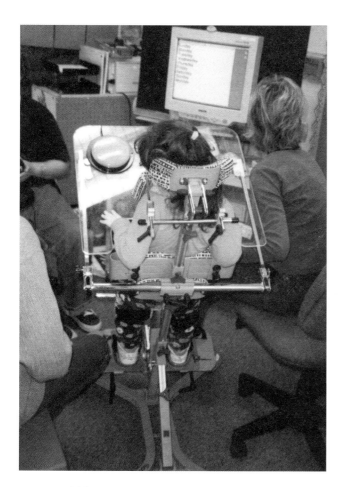

Fig. 6.31. Child uses jellybean switch interfaced with *IntelliKeys* expanded keyboard and a talking 60 word-processing program, *IntelliTalk* word-processing software (IntelliTools, Inc., 55 Leveroni Court, Suite 9, Novato, CA 94949, USA). (By permission of the Bridge School, Hillsborough, CA, and parents; www.bridgeschool.org.)

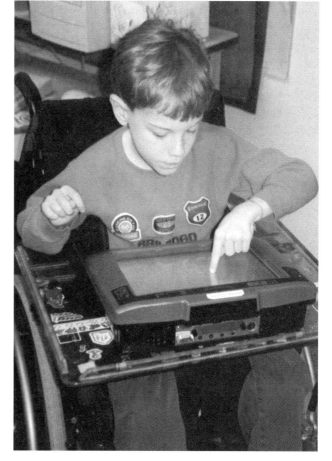

Fig. 6.33. Boy uses his finger to activate a *Vanguard*® voice-output communication device (Prentke Romich Company, 1022 Heyl Road, Wooster, OH 44691, USA). (By permission of the Bridge School, Hillsborough, CA, and parents; www.bridgeschool.org.)

SPEECH TO SPEECH RELAY

Speech to Speech (STS) is a service that allows persons who have a speech disability to communicate by telephone.[29] Although there are many augmentative and assistive communication devices that speech-impaired persons can use to communicate, and text telephone (TTY) relay has been mandated by the Federal Communication Commission since 1992 and available in all 50 States in the Union, many persons with speech impairment do not have the manual dexterity or type very slowly so that it takes too much time. The speech to speech call is a relay call in which the speech of one person is relayed to the other. In the case of the person who has poor articulation due to the disability the relay is to a communication assistant who has been trained to understand the particular disabled person's speech. The communication assistant restates verbatim the speech of the disabled—known as 'revoicing' (Keller 2001a, b).

This innovative and needed service for the speech impaired was founded in 1996 by Bob Segalman, PhD, who has total body involved cerebral palsy, poorly understood oral communication, and is fully employed by the California State Department of Rehabilitation. By January 2001 it was expected that ten more States would be added to the 30 that have offered the service since December 2000 (R. Segalman, personal communication). Training of communication assistants for 'revoicing' does not seem to be long or difficult (Keller 2001b). Australia has implemented the same service for the disabled. Sweden did so before the United States, but has discontinued providing it.

MOBILITY

WALKERS

Four-post aluminum frames, usually with small wheels in the front, are most commonly used in children who have dysequilibrium in all four planes (see Chapter 5), and who can grasp the top sides of the frame. Most children prefer to have the opening of the walker in front (Fig. 6.34). Two studies demonstrated the superior walking postures and performance in children who used the posterior walker. Both studies used gait analysis to prove the point (Logan *et al.* 1990, Greiner *et al.* 1993).

Holm *et al.* (1983) cautioned against the use of the walker in 'high-risk infants', because theoretically it might interfere with the development of more mature balance reactions and should be deferred until such are established. They also worried that the walker might threaten success with the neurodevelopmental therapy (Bobath) by not allowing inhibition of abnormal reflexes (though as we have learned, the Bobaths were no longer worried about such inhibition). We know that developmentally children want to move and need to move to explore their environment. So why hold back on providing a walker for toddlers and young children with cerebral palsy who do not have their balance reactions developed or intact? Other than accidents due to infant walkers (Kavanagh and Banco 1982), no clinical data exist that indicates walkers do harm to posture or lower-limb joint development.

29 For information: www.stsnews.com or bob.segalman@worldnet.att.net

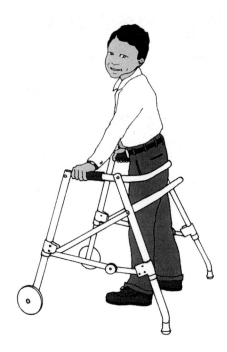

Fig. 6.34. Front open aluminum walker preferred by the majority of children with spastic diplegia and dysequilibrium.

In countries where manufactured walkers are not available, they can be made from locally available materials, so that another person does not have to carry an individual who has an impairment that precludes walking (Figs 6.35, 6.36).

Gait trainers and mobility devices
Gait trainers consist of a wide-based steel frame on four casters that include a trunk support for children who cannot use an ordinary walker because of poor trunk balance. Some take advantage of the forward leaning position of the child with and anterior trunk support (e.g. PONY by Snug Seat, Inc.) (Fig. 6.37). The various devices are intended to teach reciprocal stepping patterns with the assessment and the aid of the physical therapist. A curriculum called MOVE (Mobility Opportunities Via

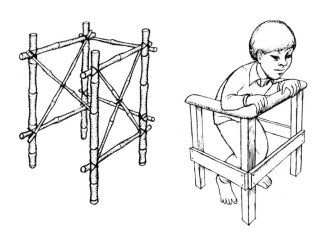

Fig. 6.35. Simple walkers can be constructed at home with locally available materials (redrawn from Helander *et al.* 1983).

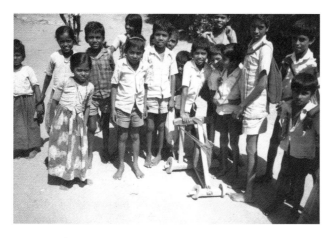

Fig. 6.36. This 8-year-old boy who used a wood frame walker constructed by his father was the star among his classmates in a village in Karnataka State, South India, 1989.

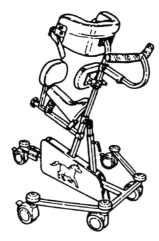

Fig. 6.37. Pony gait trainer (by Snug Seat).

Education) was developed at the Hospital for Sick Children in Washington DC and certifies MOVE instructors in the United States.[30] Seven gait trainers available in the United States (others are made in Europe) were evaluated for their various features as a guide for therapists and parents (Paleg 1997). All should be available for testing in a therapy unit before purchase. The therapist does a side-by-side evaluation by walking alongside the child who uses the trainer.

The weight-relieving walker, first designed by Wally Motloch at the Rehabilitation Engineering Center at Stanford, was used for children with osteogenesis imperfecta. We subsequently found that it was very useful to provide hands-free walking in children who had minimal athetosis or spasticity and mainly ataxia (Figs 6.38–6.40). The concept design has been modified and commercially available (Walkabout by Mulholland Positioning Systems, Inc.)

Mobility is vital for community integration. For play and exercise, special devices are useful for some children who have

insufficient balance mechanisms and require compensation for this deficit (Letts *et al.* 1976). Steerable walkers and special backward pedaling tricycles that make use of the dominant extensor pattern, may be practical for some children. All sorts of innovative mobility play equipment have been designed and are commercially available. Bicycles with training wheels are the most common adaptation for children who can pedal but lack adequate postural balance.[31]

MECHANICAL SUPPORT SYSTEMS FOR WALKING

Attempts to construct a total mechanical support system to enable severely disabled persons to walk have captured the imagination of orthotists and engineers over the past years. It can be done, but these systems are so confining that the disabled person's quality of life seems quite compromised. The pneumatic space suit was heralded at one time, but apparently it never came into practical use. In Australia, the country that brought the world Speedo bathing suits, Blair *et al.* (1995) studied use of a suit (the 'UPsuit') fabricated of Lycra to provide proximal stability and reduction of involuntary movements of children with cerebral palsy . Their study showed immediate improvement in a posture and reduced involuntary movement. They concluded that Lycra splinting rather than the suit they had devised could be useful for less intrusive splints. They also support continued investigation into adjunctive use of these types of modalities. Issues concerning its use included compromised respiratory function, 'limited capacity for purposeful intent' (i.e. function to carry out an action), and a negative attitude.

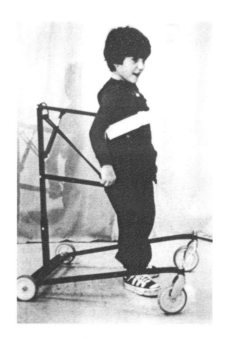

Fig. 6.38. Stanford weight-relieving walker, prototype designed by W. Motloch, B.S., C.O., Rehabilitation Engineering Center, Children's Hospital at Stanford. Hands free walking for children primarily with ataxia.

---

30 For information on MOVE curriculum: telephone number 800-397-MOVE. Address: The Hospital for Sick Children, 1731 Bunker Hill Road NE, Washington, DC, 20017, USA.

31 *Exceptional Parent* magazine (see footnote 25, above) has many advertisements for many different types of mobility devices.

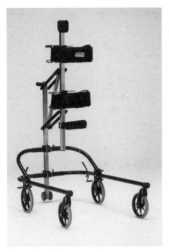

Fig. 6.39. Weight-relieving walker, Walkabout, by Mulholland Positioning Systems, Inc., PO Box 391, 215 N. 12th Street, Santa Paula, CA 93060, USA.

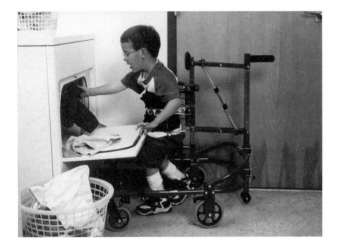

Fig. 6.40. Mulholland Walkabout enables the child to use his upper limbs freely.

Rennie and colleagues (2000) from Derby, UK, studied the use of whole body garments in eight children (seven with cerebral palsy and one muscular dystrophy) using gait analysis. Stability around the pelvis improved in five and distally in three. Although five children improved in at least one aspect of the PEDI scale as noted by the parents, the disadvantage of wearing the suit for 6 hours are day were such that only one of the eight families continued using the garment. Pneumatic suits and space suits that encase the body appear to have had their day as well.

The Polish suit or Adeli suit—a modification of a suit originally used by Soviet cosmonauts—provides resistance with motion and is therefore supposed to improve muscle strength. This suit, which is marketed by EuroMed, is used in conjunction with a comprehensive physical therapy program for 5–7 hours a day, 5–6 days a week for 4 weeks. Russian literature points to its improvements in 70% of patients with spastic diplegia due to cerebral palsy in areas of walking and self-care (Semenova 1998).

The Orthotic Research Unit in Oswestry, UK, designed and tried a prototype a special walking-frame with thoracic, abdominal and sacral level supports, castor steering and upper-

limb supports and lower-limb orthotics for those who have total body involved cerebral palsy (Stallard *et al.* 1996). It could be used only indoors.

With modern power chairs and interfaces and controls using any part of the body under voluntary control to operate them (tongue, breath puffs, a finger, a toe) and the freedom of mobility these provide, body suits comparable to a medieval knight's armor and other walking contraptions are probably not worth pursuing. Perhaps these efforts to make a disabled person walk with elaborate mechanical supports ought to be abandoned as an example of a technology that reached its end-point. These negative reports of encasing the body in space suits to control limb movements and provide trunk and limb support in cerebral palsy will not tempt professionals to try them again. The contemporary cliché, 'been there, done that', seems appropriate.

CRUTCHES AND CANES

Crutches are essential for children with cerebral palsy who have good lateral equilibrium reactions but deficient anterior and posterior ones (see Chapter 5). *Crutches are used not so much for weightbearing as to compensate for lack of balance.* Because the need for balance is primary, the usual axillary crutches used by patients for non-weightbearing (as in a limb fracture) are not necessary in cerebral palsy. Most use either a triceps cuff crutch with a hand support, or the Lofstrand-type crutch. The abledata base retrieved 26 different kinds of crutches. A unique one, LaCome Flipski®, allows walking on icy or snowy areas using a ski attachment that can be flipped into the vertical position by pulling on a hand-grip cord.

Quad canes have great stability and stand alone because of the four-post base. Patients generally walk more slowly with quad canes, but these are useful in those who seem to be borderline on balance ability. Rose *et al.* (1985) studied the energy requirements in children with spastic diplegia and quadriplegia using either a walker or quad canes. By monitoring the heart rate, they found the mean heart-rate while walking with walkers was 164 beats per minute, and with quad canes 157 beats per minute (compared to 114 beats per minute in normal children without assistive devices). With this measure of energy requirements, some of the children were more efficient with walkers and others with quad canes. The heart-rate was closely correlated with the energy cost as measured with oxygen consumption.

The children in the heart-rate study had slower mean walking-speeds (27 m per minute with walkers and 20 m per minute with canes, compared to the normal mean of 70 m per minute). These slow walking-speeds and high heart-rates suggest a high physiological workload. These data indicate how impractical it is to encourage (or force) disabled children to walk long distances with assistive devices. They need to avoid undue fatigue in order to accomplish other tasks of daily living as well as schoolwork, learning, social life and community integration.

WHEELCHAIRS

'It makes a big change in the life of the people who receive these wheelchairs and also a big change for us, the producer. A miracle. A small miracle that we have already more than 40,000 in Cambodia. Really, for me this wheelchair is a sacrament.'

(Fr Enrique Figaredo, SJ)[32]

Due to the growing awareness of the disabled as part of our society and humanity, and their need for mobility in order to achieve social integration, there has been a rapid increase in the acceptability of the wheelchair in not only Western countries, but in much of the world (Fig. 6.41). Urbanization and concrete paving have also made the wheelchair easier to use. And there are special power driven chairs that are all-terrain—even at the beach.

MANUAL WHEELCHAIRS

Wheelchairs can be either hand-driven or power-driven. Hand-driven types are for children who have good function in both upper limbs and can move the chair with efficiency and speed. Many children who use walkers or crutches for household and neighbourhood mobility find wheelchairs essential for traveling longer distances. A wheelchair conserves energy; crutches use it (Campbell and Ball 1978, Fisher and Patterson 1981). The energy expended when using a manual wheelchair is comparable to that used by normal persons when walking on level surfaces (Cerny 1978).

Depending on personal needs, a great choice of manual wheelchairs is available There are lightweight sport chairs for play and games, and heavy-duty chairs for large-bodied people who are very active. Two chairs are often desirable: one for sport and quick transport into an automobile, and the other for everyday school or work. Use of only one upper limb is a contraindication for a manual wheelchair. The adaptive chair for one-hand operators (a 'hemiplegic' chair) was complex, cumbersome and generally not optimally functional. For these individuals we unequivocally recommend an electrically powered wheelchair.

POWERED WHEELCHAIRS

Electric-powered wheelchairs are available in a variety of designs and sizes. Portable electric wheelchairs for children were first produced by ABEC®, and were responsible for giving independence and mobility to total body involved children with cerebral palsy (Fig. 6.42). All children learn control of the chair with minimal coaching and not over-direction by the parents. All chairs come with joystick controls. Those who cannot use a joystick can have pressure-sensitive hand- or finger-control switches. In fact any part of the body that the patient can move voluntarily can be linked to a control of the powered chair (and also to control communication devices).

Children learned to use the chair within six 1-hour sessions. One group of therapists used a Piagetian-based assessment tool

32 Director, Banteay Prieb (*House of the Dove*), Jesuit Relief Services in Cambodia (in *Company*, Summer 1999, p.8–10).

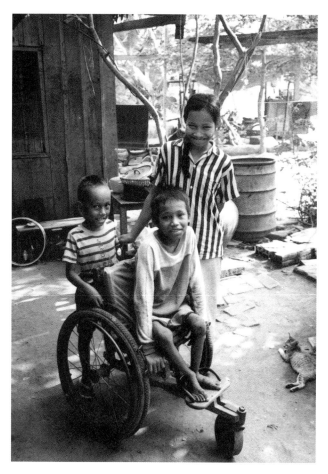

Fig. 6.41. Khaung, age 10, poliomyelitis; locally made wheelchair at the House of the Dove, Jesuit Refugee Service, Cambodia. (Reproduced by permission of *Company*, Chicago, IL, Summer 1999.)

followed by a Powered Mobility Program that consisted of 34 tasks representing a hierarchy of motor skills. Cognitive development, spatial relationship and problem solving skills are important factors in considering a powered wheelchair. Tefft *et al.* (1999) developed a Powered Wheelchair Screening test at the Rancho Los Amigos Medical Center, Downey, California.

Improvements in powered chairs continue apace (Fig. 6.43). The abledata base contains hundreds of powered wheelchairs with various controls ranging from joysticks to voice and puff command controls. Alternative power chairs and scooters with three or four wheels with joystick, tiller or arm rest controls comparable to golf carts numbered 93.

That the power chair makes a difference in employment of non-ambulatory adults with cerebral palsy is the outcome study data by Murphy and colleagues (2000). Of the 28 persons who held a competitive job, 24 used a power wheelchair, and four a manual chair.

TRANSITIONAL POWERED MOBILITY AIDS

We originally introduced a custom-made powered cart for little children who needed mobility. It was amazing that a 2-year-old with cerebral palsy and poor upper-limb use could learn to use a joystick control within an hour or two. These battery operated

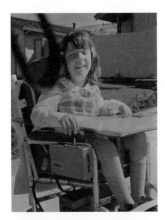
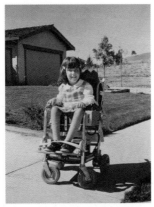
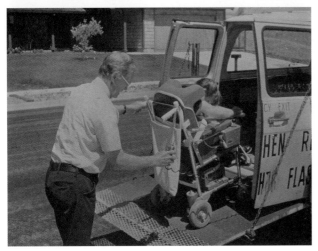

Fig. 6.42. ABEC electric powered wheelchair, one of the first used for children circa 1987.

carts have been developed over the years and tested and many are available (Wright-Ott and Egilson 1996). The Rehabilitation Engineering Center at the Lucile Salter Packard Children's Hospital at Stanford had a 'mobility camp' for 37 children, 32 of whom had cerebral palsy, to test and learn how to use the devices for children who had no independent mobility; the average age was 2 years 10 months (range 15 months to 6 years). A pediatric occupational therapist directed the program and participated with the technical staff in the development of a transitional power mobility aid (GOBOT®) in 1991 (Wright-Ott and Egilson 1997) (Fig. 6.44).

These are termed 'transitional' because of their use by children much earlier than the usual age of 10 years when powered wheelchairs usually have been prescribed and considered much too late for optimum child development. The theoretical basis for early powered mobility is that the child's social and psychological development is linked with motor ability, control and independent exploration of their environment (Butler *et al.* 1983). Usually these will be compatible with a child up to age 8 years. One manufacturer states the limit in height of the child is 43 inches. When the prognosis for functional walking is poor, the recommendation and testing of a power cart for mobility opens a new horizon for the parents of a severely disabled child. They can see a future of independence. The child becomes a person

early on controlling their mobility. As the child grows, he or she graduates to a power wheelchair.

SEATING

Children who have no trunk control must constantly use their upper limbs for balance; this necessity precludes the functional use of their hands. Seat-inserts for wheelchairs have become an accepted technology for children and adults with cerebral palsy. Rang *et al.* (1981) delineated grades of sitting ability and the appropriate seat that could be used: (1) no-hands sitters need a foam cushion and removable arm supports; (2) hand dependent and propped sitters require more support of their torso and sometimes their head. Many different designs and methods of construction have been developed (Cristarella 1975, Motloch 1977, Barber 1978, Carlson and Winter 1978, Carrington 1978, Ring *et al.* 1978, Trefler *et al.* 1978, Holte 1980, Fulford *et al.* 1982, Nwaobi *et al.* 1983, Craig *et al.* 1984). Three types of seating surfaces are: planar, contoured and custom-molded. Contoured seating consists of layers of varying densities of foam that can be shaped around the torso and pelvis to conform to spinal curvatures and pelvic obliquity. Assessment for the proper seating can be done manually by the therapist holding the patient in various positions such as the angle of hip flexion and the posture of the child in orientation in space.

The therapist and seating specialist can also use seating simulators to assist in design of the seat (Wight-Ott and Egilson

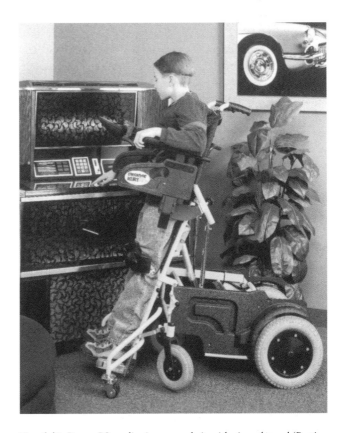

Fig. 6.43. Pogon PS, pediatric power chair with sit and stand 'Putting activities within reach'. (By courtesy of Theradyne, Division of KURT, 395 Irvin Industrial Drive, Jordan, MN 53352, USA, www.theradyne.com)

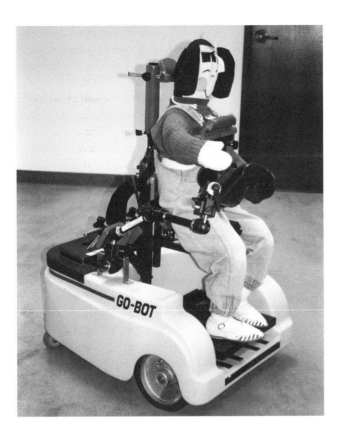

Fig. 6.44. GO-BOT®, transitional electric powered mobility aide for children from 12 months to 6 years (Courtesy of Christine Wright-Ott, MPA, OTR, Rehabilitation Engineering Center, Lucile Salter Packard Children's Hospital at Stanford, Stanford, CA, 1999. Manufactured by Innovative Products, Inc., 830 South 48th Street, Grand Forks, ND, USA.)

1996). The Mattrix system of interlocking plastic components from Edinburgh was tested in 25 severely disabled children for 12 months (Trail and Galasko 1990). In 21 the subjective assessment by the guardian and/or physical therapist was that this system was satisfactory or good. Three children did not like it—two because of pain and one for no apparent reason. Alterations were necessary a mean of 4.6 times per chair. The system was also used as a seat orthosis for scoliosis. Of eight patients in this study who had radiographs depicting scoliosis, six had not deteriorated while using the Mattrix seat. However, the duration of follow-up was only 12 months. And as might be expected in total body involved children, hip dislocation was not prevented.

We preferred a modular plastic seat-insert, padded with foam material carved to fit the patient's trunk contour, and upholstered with fabric. The objective was trunk stabilization and above all, comfort. A wide choice of seating systems is commercially available, and some can be custom made. Finding the right technical person to help select, design if necessary, and modify the seat for the particular person is probably the most important factor for a successful outcome (P. Trudeau, personal communication) (Fig. 6.45). In 1981, Mercer Rang of Toronto posed the question: 'Do you make the seat fit the child or the child to fit the seat?' By this he meant correct the scoliosis and pelvic obliquity first and then construct the seat.

'Do you make the seat to fit the child or the child to fit the seat?'
(Mercer Rang)

A few studies have been done to show the effectiveness of special seating to provide truncal stability and improvement in upper-limb function. Formerly most seats were constructed to flex the hips beyond 90º in varying slopes, to reduce the extensor pattern in total body involved children and thus improve hand function. Seeger and O'Mara (1984), in a sophisticated analysis of hand function by the ability to control a joystick and target an object, found that the hip-flexion position made no significant difference. Myhr and von Wendt (1991) tested six positions. A forward-tipped seat, a firm backrest that supported the pelvis and arm against a table while allowing the feet to move backwards resulted in the best arm and hand function. These investigators from Gotheburg, Sweden, used surface electromyograms from four leg muscles to measure various seat inclinations and an abductor orthosis while doing upper limb tasks (Myhr and von Wendt 1993). Their results indicated that horizontal and forward-leaning seats decreased low-limb muscle-firing and surmised that this might portend improved upper limb function. Another study by Myhr and colleagues (1995) was a 5-year follow-up assessment of functional sitting positions using videotapes. They concluded that eight children had 'slight but significant improvement' in their upper-limb functions, while in two it had deteriorated.

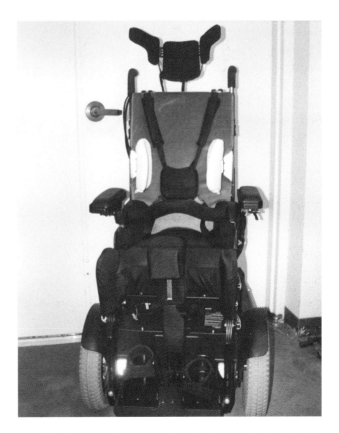

Fig. 6.45. Custom seat insert mounted on electric powered wheelchair. (By courtesy of Paul Trudeau, Seating Specialist, Rehabilitation Engineering Center, Lucile Salter Packard Children's Hospital at Stanford, CA, 2000.)

187

Trefler and Angelo (1997) reported no difference in upper limb function in four anterior trunk supports in 17 children with mild to moderate spastic or athetoid cerebral palsy tested by pressing a switch to activate a computer software program. Trunk supports should be chosen based on the patient preferences, ease of removal, cost and aesthetics.

COSTS

The cost of a powered wheelchair and seating system for severely disabled persons were analyzed by Kohn *et al.* (1983). The mean use time was 10 hours per day for 30.9 months. The cost per patient was $1.50 per day (1983 dollars need adjusting for inflation from 1983 to 2005). The system provided was judged optimal by 79% of the 196 patients in the study; and the remaining 21% who thought the effectiveness was suboptimal could think of no other choice to accomplish the mobility desired. The cost-effectiveness of their mobility and seating was assessed in human terms and cannot be ignored: 'Family enjoys more social life' (81%); 'more contact with peers' (67%); and 'allows more normal function' (62%). These costs have to be weighed against the costs of long-term therapies which hoped somehow to reprogram the brain and stimulate the child to walk.

The cost to a parent who has to attend the child day-in and day-out (including weekends when the medical team is off) is another calculation missing in cost considerations by fiscal administrators. If, by use of comfortable and effective seating and mobility equipment, a child can remain at home or in an independent living situation in a community proximate to families and friends rather than in a distant State long-term care institution, the argument about cost should become moot.

TRAVEL AND TRANSPORTATION

Of all the factors that limit adult independence and employment, the inability to get out of the home is the most important (Bachman 1972) (Fig. 6.46). Root (1977) found that only 16% of the total body involved persons with cerebral palsy had the capability or means for independent travel.

Public transport presents many obstacles for the severely disabled (Bourgeois *et al.* 1977). Even though there has been much pressure to improve access to public transport, the cost will probably always preclude widespread alterations of public systems to accommodate all disabled persons. In small villages the powered electric wheelchair with all terrain capabilities and all sorts of small alternative electric-powered vehicles may provide all the local transportation necessary for the individual person. In this regard, it is probably true that the environment does determine the extent of the disability (Cherpin *et al.* 1985).

We have found that modern autovans and buses equipped with ramps or hydraulic lifts are the best mode of travel for urban and inter-urban transportation. Not all persons with cerebral palsy will be able to operate a motor vehicle independently. Special testing for depth perception, direction sense and motor control are required and need to be done in special motor-vehicle operation assessment centers. If the tests confirm a person's potential to operate a vehicle, special instruction is essential. Persons who have major spastic involvement of the lower limbs but minor motor incoordination in the upper limbs (spastic diplegia or hemiplegia) can usually be successful and safe drivers using hand controls that can be adapted to any automobile. Such adaptations are usual and customary for persons who have traumatic spinal paraplegia or quadriplegia, various types of flaccid paralysis, rheumatoid arthritis and osteogenesis imperfecta.

ACTIVITIES OF DAILY LIVING AIDS

Adaptive equipment and devices have proliferated for eating, toileting and bathing. Commercially available devices can be found in catalogues, trade literature and central databases. Some simple aids can be made at home or in the local community by almost anyone with a minimum of manual skills (Fig. 6.47). One can find toilet seats that automatically wash-off and dry your bottom (some have called this 'the American bidet'). Electric toothbrushes help ensure dental hygiene. Ledgeless shower stalls with stools facilitate bathing of the wheelchair-confined.

Robotic feeding devices have captured the imagination of engineers and three, Beeson, Handy 1, and Winsford have been tested (Hermann *et al.* 1999). The response was positive from the subjects and their feeding attendants; they felt they would use a feeding device on a daily basis. An attendant is still necessary to

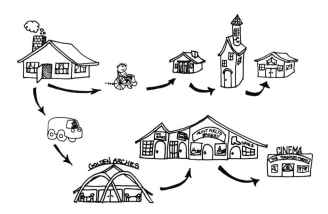

Fig. 6.46. Mobility needed for living a full life in the neighborhood and community.

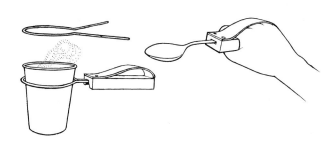

Fig. 6.47. Simple adapted eating utensils which can be made by almost anyone from locally available materials. Spoon and mug holder. (Redrawn from Helander *et al.* 1983.)

set up the device and if the person has a propensity to choke, an attendant should be present. Feeding devices have not been as popular as one might think probably because of the perspective shared by W.M. Motloch (personal communication). He observed that the only time when the disabled person had close human contact was at mealtimes.

Architectural and community barriers (e.g. curb street crossings without curbs) continue to be eliminated in North America and European countries. Patients just need the expertise of a physical and occupational therapist to advise them on appropriate equipment, to make required adaptations by a rehabilitation engineering expert, and (of great importance) to advise them on financial considerations (McCollough 1985). Architectural barriers have come down in most public buildings in the United States. Resources are available for architectural adaptations to houses and apartments and special kitchen designs for wheelchair use (Barrett *et al.* 1995; www.abledata.com, architectural elements, home management, personal care).

IMPACT AND OUTCOMES OF ASSISTIVE TECHNOLOGY

It seems evident that assistive technology has had a tremendous impact on compensating for lost function of the disabled person's impairments. But formal long-term outcome studies are lacking and may never be done because of the complex interaction of the clinical aspects of the disability, the instruments required to assess various functions, the psychosocial aspects, and the culture. Attempts have been outlined to measure outcomes within this framework, but none have been done within the context of total rehabilitation (Jutai *et al.* 1996).

In a large study of the causes of excess mortality in cerebral palsy, included were the functional characteristics of 14,655 persons with severe cerebral palsy out of a total of 45,992 in California surveyed in the years 1986–95 (Strauss *et al.* 1999). This data indicates the need for assistance to compensate for functional loss in this group. Delineated were the following: 80.3% could not walk; 29.1% had no hand use; 54.9% could not feed themselves; 64.4% were unable to put on their clothes; 64.4% could make no oral sounds or babbled with no words; severe and profound mental retardation in 54.4%.

The retrospective study by Terver and co-authors at Stanford University (1981) was an attempt to show that in the total body involved child with cerebral palsy, goals could be set as early as age 4 years, and that engineering technology was the major factor in achieving independence in functions primarily in communication and mobility.

A number of publications are surveys that attempt to define the need for technology in the service of the disabled and urge implementation. Finnish rehabilitation experts (Korpela *et al.* 1992) surveyed the need for technical aids in activities of daily living of 204 children with disability. They found that although parents were ready to accept technical aids, they needed more information about the possibilities, benefits and therapeutic aspects. This latter perception that somehow assistive technology

be therapeutic (other than enhancing education, social life) possibly reflects a lack of understanding of the permanence of the central nervous system pathology that caused the impairment of function, and probably points out the need for parent education.

Specific technologies have been assessed for efficacy in sporadic reports. Australians surveyed 82 people with disability, eight of whom had cerebral palsy, in the Brisbane area for computer use (Pell *et al.* 1999). 60% used a computer, but only 15% used assistive devices. The authors suggested that there needs to be more training in computer use and assistive devices need to be provided. Another study from Brisbane (Pell *et al.* 1997) demonstrated that of 82 individuals with disability contacted, 46 were employed. Gender, education and the level of computer skill and training were significant predictors of employment.

The Communication Aids Centre, London, presented a study of nine children and the length of time they would have to wait for the provision of a communication aid in the UK. They urged better training of the children and their communication partners (Jolleff *et al.* 1992). Better integration of communication aids and environmental controls in powered wheelchair users was urged by Nisbet (1996) of Edinburgh. From England came a 2-year study of 93 adolescent and adult Augmentative Alternative Communication systems (Murphy *et al.* 1996). The obstacles for effective use of these systems were listed as lack of availability and accessibility, the communicator's partner's lack of knowledge about the system, insufficient therapy, and the type of vocabulary in the system. McCall and colleagues (1997) from Scotland studied augmentative and alternative communication users, their strategies, and advantages and disadvantages. Formal communication partners thought that more vocabulary for social purposes was actually available to users and were less aware of daily routines in day and residential environments. The importance of the study was thought to be the contributions of the users based on their experiences.

ATTITUDES AMONG DIFFERENT CULTURES AFFECT THE USE AND VALUE OF ASSISTIVE TECHNOLOGY.

Attitudes among different cultures affect the use and value of assistive technology. In Japan, Shigenari (1998) called for more use of technical aids in the activities of daily living for the rehabilitation of children with cerebral palsy. However, Nakamura (1998) found that in Japan negative attitudes toward thc usc of technical aids persisted in parents, therapists, physicians and teachers despite the effectiveness of communication aids.

ADULT LIVING AND PARENT COUNSELING

It may seem strange that an orthopaedic surgeon would even attempt to supplement the counseling role which may be the turf of the paediatrician, physiatrist or social-worker. Nevertheless parents and patients consider the orthopaedic surgeon to be a physician and not a technician just following orders. Those surgeons who perform more than an occasional surgery in cerebral palsy have found themselves to be inextricably bound with the patient and the family. The one who cuts also counsels. The surgeon wields a powerful therapeutic tool which the patient almost never forgets. Therefore the surgeon needs some knowledge gained from the experience of others who have dealt with children who have long-term orthopaedic impairments.

The one who cuts also counsels.

BEHAVIORAL AND PSYCHOLOGICAL PROBLEMS
What happens to children with cerebral palsy when they become adults? Are there social and psychological as well as medical problems that evolve? In order to counsel parents on the management of cerebral palsy, one needs to know what lies beyond childhood—beyond the curly-headed smiling child in braces on posters and fund-raising brochures. The focus must be on the longer lifespan: adulthood. In the goal-oriented approach, the direction is always towards optimum independent adult living and community integration, and away from the disease. We can prevent structural changes and late disability with appropriate orthopaedic surgery, combined with the talents of the physical and occupational therapist. We need to look ahead with the parents, and also prevent behavioral and psychiatric problems in late adolescence and early adulthood. In the few studies that are available, the family is the key ingredient upon which one has to rely. No substitute for the nuclear family has been found (Davis 1976).

Behavioral and psychiatric problems were reviewed by Thomas *et al.* (1985). We know that studies of children with disability suggest a much higher incidence of psychiatric disorders than expected in normal children (Heller *et al.* 1985). Not surprisingly, those with marked disabilities are more likely to have psychological problems. Girls had more anxiety and depression than boys in one study quoted by Thomas *et al.* (1985). Our own observations on children with cerebral palsy followed to young adulthood (age 21–30 years) suggest that serious emotional breakdown is more likely after age 18 years.

In the patients we have known, there was no relationship with the severity of the disability and psychological breakdown. Adolescents and young adults with spastic diplegia seem more vulnerable; here, too, young women seem to comprise the majority. In our experience, most have stable families (often they were the only child) who always want to do the right and best thing (be it physical therapy, special education or surgery) for their child, usually a daughter, in the hope that they will somehow become 'normal'. The constant over-direction of the child by parents, physicians and therapists may have set the stage for the emotional crisis.

Reality strikes when you realize that childhood is over. Overachieving in school, in the attempt to prove that innate intellectual defects can be overcome, can create anxiety which is more decorticating than any of the cerebral damage. A belief in 'The Little Engine That Could' fairy-tale syndrome may be destructive: 'I think I can, I think I can, I think I can' (Bettelheim 1977).

Parents then need to know what can happen by slavishly adopting the disease-oriented approach. It may take years to judge its emotional cost.

A follow-up of a 27-year-old young lady who had spastic diplegia and completed college and weathered a serious psychiatric breakdown, possibly said it best: 'I was pissed off at everybody.' She attributed her recovery to finding Christian faith. Another young lady who also had spastic diplegia, and had eventually recovered from a severe anxiety neurosis after consultation and psychotherapy, said to me: 'If only people would look at the person behind the handicap.' It was her psychiatrist who diagnosed her severe anxiety and attributed it to overachieving. He opined that the anxiety was more 'decorticating' than her organic brain pathology.

Awareness of psychiatric problems, their prevention and psychiatric consultation, should be obvious to the physicians who assume primary responsibility for the care of the child with cerebral palsy (Freeman 1970). Orthopaedic surgeons often must assume the primary role as it is forced upon them by default and parental expectations.

AWARENESS OF SEXUAL FUNCTIONS
Not to be ignored are sexual problems of individuals with disability (Thomas *et al.* 1985). The sexual knowledge of people with disability is said to be very poor. Sex education and counseling services have been established and should be recommended, but in a study of 101 adults with cerebral palsy by Murphy *et al.* (2000) 90% desired more sexual education. Personal accounts of sexual concerns and encounters by the physically handicapped have been published (Bullard and Knight 1981). In sexual practices, other perspectives beyond mere knowledge need to be developed by the disabled person.

The sexual functioning of 1,150 young adult women who had physical disabilities (11% had cerebral palsy) and those who had no disabilities was assessed by questionnaire from investigators in Houston, Texas (Nosek *et al.* 1996). The major findings were highly significant differences in sexual activity, response, and satisfaction between women with and without disabilities. The severity of the disability was not related to the level of sexual activity and there were no differences between the groups in sexual desire. The authors prudently state that there were no interventions.

'The severity of the disability was not related to the level of sexual activity and there were no differences between the groups in sexual desire.'

(Nosek *et al.* 1996)

THE FAMILY (Figs. 6.48, 6.49)
The vital role of families in health status has received scant attention in the medical literature (Somers 1979, Stein and Jessof 1984). Currently in the USA 'the family' has become a focal point for political rhetoric and concern. The primary role of the

family in developing countries was emphasized by Bose (1980) in a discussion about the management of cerebral palsy in Singapore. A study by Agosta and Bradley (1985) focuses on the significance of the family and the care of persons with developmental disabilities. The contribution of the family was confirmed in a study of 106 children with cerebral palsy under age 18 years: 90% were living at home, 2% were in a foster home, and 8% were in a nursing home.

In 1977 we studied 71 children with severe mental and physical disability; and 4 years later we added another 89 such children who were in special day-care development centers in San Mateo County, California. These studies confirmed the importance of the family, because most children were living at home with their biological parents. The role of the mother in caring for the child was particularly significant (E.E. Bleck *et al.*, unpublished observations) (Table 6.XIV). In the 1977 study, mothers who worked outside the home comprised only 16.3% in contrast to the estimate of over 50% of the mothers who worked at outside jobs in the United States. The contribution of these caregiving mothers to the society, and the resultant reduction in institutional costs, has not become a major issue of public knowledge or concern.

Mothers of 50 children with disability, aged 6–11 years, were examined for the mother's perceived role restriction and ability to pursue her own interests due to her responsibilities in raising a disabled child in Alabama (Wallander and Venters 1995). Perceived role restriction was variable in their adjustment beyond the objective parameters of the child's disability or the level of problem behaviors. These two factors did not predict the perception of restriction, but social support did. The authors recommend more attention to 'intrapersonal processes' as a

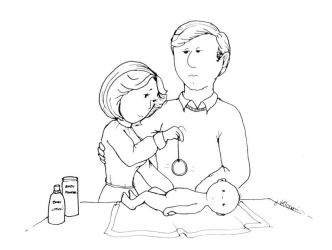

Fig. 6.49. Pre-diagnosis: worried parents, baby does not seem normal. (From Bleck and Nagel 1982, pp. 182–192; by permission of Judy Howard, MD.)

'component of a multidimensional model of adjustment' in these mothers whose children have chronic physical disabilities.

A study of 139 two-parent families that had either a child with diabetes, a non-visible disability or cerebral palsy, a visible disability did not impact on family functioning regardless of the severity of the disability. These families had a high level of functioning comparable to the controls (Saddler *et al.* 1993).

Something must have been right in families who had an adolescent at home (90%) with either cerebral palsy or spina bifida as reflected in a study of 102 youths (Blum *et al.* 1991). 'Almost without exception parental relationships were defined as positive.' But out-of-school social contacts were very limited. Only 28.3% of those with cerebral palsy had been on a date. Both groups had low levels of responsibility at home and lacked discussions about sexuality and menstruation.

A recent study of the relationship between the mother's resolution or non-resolution of the child's diagnosis gave evidence that 'resolved' mothers had lower levels of parenting stress than the unresolved, i.e. not accepting, mothers (Sheeran *et al.* 1997). The results were deemed to predict a greater potential to disrupt the child–parent interaction. Unresolved mothers may use a defensive process by developing elaborate and heterogeneous strategies to cope with the trauma of the diagnosis as grieving 'the loss of the perfect child'. A report from Munich, Germany, appears to confirm one strategy that entailed intensive physical therapy by the mother using the Vojta method. The authors suggested that the treatment regimen provided a coping mechanism so that they were overprotective in ambiguous everyday life situations (Sarimski and Hoffmann 1993). Experienced physicians who have dealt with parents of children who have cerebral palsy are undoubtedly aware of these attitudes and resultant problems in relationships not only within the family but also within the professional community.

That the stress of parenting is universal with children who have cerebral palsy is reflected in a study of Malaysian children (Ong *et al.* 1998). In the Malaysian study maternal education

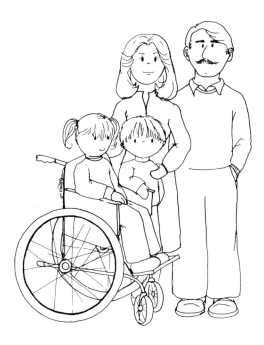

Fig. 6.48. Family unit includes the child with disability. (From Bleck and Nagel 1982, pp. 182–192; by permission of Judy Howard, MD.)

TABLE 6.XIV
Living environment of children and adolescents with severe mental retardation and physical disability in La Esperanza
Development Centers. San Mateo County, California, 1977 and 1981 (from Bleck *et al.* 1981)

1977	%	N	Age range	Mean (years)	Mothers	%
Home	66	71	3–19	9.6	At home, no other job	77
Foster home	16				Work full-time outside	16
Custodial care	18					
1981 (two centers, San Mateo County, California)						
North Center						
Home	77	43	4–22	11	At home, no other job	46
Foster home	2				Work full-time, outside	48
South Center						
Home	91	46	4–33	13	At home, no other job	64
Foster home	0				Work full-time, outside	25
Custodial care	9					

was inversely related to stress. Low economic status, low levels of parent education and negative attitudes with poor coping ability have been noted in Asian, African, and Caucasian populations cited in this study. Ethnic Chinese mothers appeared to have greater stress than their Indian or Malay counterparts.

In Japan 'burnout' was more frequent in the families who cared for children with developmental disabilities (Horiguchi *et al.* 1999). The families who had help from unrelated persons were also in better mental health. In Nigeria, the impact on mental health of the caregiver was noted in a General Health Questionnaire study of caregivers of 68 disabled children compared with 40 who had only minor ailments (Amosun *et al.* 1995). In England one study reported that early physiotherapy intervention had no effect on the prevalence of depression in mothers whose children were at risk for cerebral palsy (Lambrenos *et al.* 1996). This observation does put the damper on the zeal for and presumed efficacy of very early 'infant-at-risk' physio-therapy programs termed 'early intervention'. It seems that such programs would need therapists who had 'prognostic awareness' (Milani-Comparetti 1979) and education in family counseling.

Fifteen years ago Palmer and colleagues (1990) at the Kennedy Institute, Baltimore, Maryland, assessed the effects of either 6 months of infant stimulation followed by 6 months of physical therapy or 12 months of neurodevelopmental physical therapy in 28 infants, age 12–19 months, with spastic diplegia. No short-term effect on the temperament, mother–infant interaction, or home environment was found in those who had the infant stimulation program. But the mothers in the 12-month neurodevelopmental regimen had greater improvement in emotion and verbal responsiveness. Thus it seems probable that the therapists who worked with the mother and child consistently were quite adept at charting the motor progress of the child, giving encouragement, addressing questions and providing support to the mothers.

The family set-up is changed irreversibly when a disabled child enters its circle.

The family set-up is changed irreversibly when a child with disability enters its circle. Life does become more complex. Physicians and paramedics who care for these children and their families might also remember the role of the father, and not make life more difficult for them by needless treatments and home programs. Although some physicians might feel that life would be easier without parents and families, the fact is that they exist. We need to appreciate them and listen (Bax 1985). One study has produced convincing evidence that parental estimates of a child's developmental level (when applied to a child who was already defined as developmentally delayed) was quite accurate when compared with formal developmental tests (Coplan 1982).

SUMMARY OF COUNSELING POINTS FOR PHYSICIANS

Mercer Rang (1982) has encapsulated the best guidelines for counseling parents who have children with chronic disabling conditions quoted directly from his booklet (Rang 1982, pp. 71–72).

PROBLEMS OF CHILDREN WITH CHRONIC DISABILITY

The chief problem is that the difficulties of the chronically disabled never go away. The physical difficulties impede emotional development, and the problems remain a lifetime preoccupation of the entire family.

CRISIS TIMES
- Prediagnosis (the worry that the child is not normal)
- Diagnosis

  - this is often late; parents blame themselves or their doctor
  - difficulty of explaining the disease to the parents
  - difficulty that parents have, in understanding and accepting coindition
  - parental need for ongoing support

- 'treatment' is not easy and is not curative
- worry often increases after a few weeks when the full impact sinks in

- School entry—intellectual impairment may have to be faced?
- Adolescence—lack of independence must be faced
- Parents' middle age—arrangements for future care must be made.

PARENTS

Parents usually feel that they lack information; they misunderstand and misquote. Their lives are disrupted; there are implications for their housing, work and finances. Even the apparently successful ones are stressed. They may go through a grief reaction. At each stage the doctor has a special role.

- Denial—parents hide disability; MD suggests investigation
- Disbelief—parents shop around for cure; MD puts cranks into perspective
- Anger—parents quarrel with people who try to help; MD is patient
- Apathy—parents leave it all to others; MD plans for them
- Acceptance—the sensible attitude; MD's reward
- Helping others—organizing groups, building residences; MD cooperates.

TEENAGERS AND YOUNG ADULTS WITH DISABILITY

Teenagers and young adults with disability face many problems:

- at this age they comprehend their future
- they recognize their own social insecurity and lack interpersonal skills—the change from being protected to being a social reject.

PHYSICIANS

Physicians have difficulty relating to individuals with chronic disability but can follow many helpful approaches:

- make a thorough assessment on suspicion and without delay
- explanations should be slow, complete and repeated several times
- group therapy is important
- establish a management plan
- avoid a 'try this, try that' approach
- avoid pinning hopes on tomorrow being better than today
- emphasize care rather than cure
- examine repeatedly, looking for an opportunity to offer medical help
- turn pity into action by

  - suggesting books to read[33]
  - giving advice on groups to join

33 *Exceptional Parent* magazine has a large catalog of books for sale; the United Cerebral Palsy Associations also have reading materials, www.ucpa.org.

- recommending where to go for treatment
- giving advice on selection of schools
- suggesting helpful toys
- organizing recreation
- suggesting holiday relief
- suggesting baby-sitting.

OUTCOME STUDIES

'There is no problem so great that you can't walk away from it.'
(Charles Schulz)

All studies have been retrospective, but very valuable in the data produced and the perspectives needed to have a prognosis encompassing more than merely the ability to walk and the effectiveness of treatment. The oldest and most complete study was published by Crothers and Paine (1959) of the Boston Children's Medical Center, Harvard University. They found records of 1821 children who had been admitted to the neurological ward of the hospital from 1930 to 1950. Of this group 467 with cerebral palsy were re-examined at the Medical Center or at their homes. Ninety-four were reexamined in institutions. Successful follow-up was obtained by letter in 746 patients. Of these 183 had died, 118 were in institutions, and 445 were still at home. The remained 420 were written to but not contacted.

Of considerable importance to those who are calling for outcome studies that are comprehensive such as the one by Crothers and Paine (1959) is that their study was financed by grants from the United Cerebral Palsy Association and the National Institute of Neurological Disease and Blindness of the United States Public Health Service. There were a number of important findings and recommendations. (1) Clinic directors should ensure that 'the existence of an elaborate team of associates should not involve the patient in confusion' (p. 33). (2) 'We do not believe that rigid, prolonged, and closely supervised physical therapy is always necessary, but we are not asserting that it does not have a place. *Certainly we believe that the skillful physical therapist is indispensable*' (emphasis added) (p. 208). (3) The number of patients who learned to walk past the age of 6 years was relatively small (p. 126). (4) Patients with hemiplegia are the most frequently employable; 27 of 94 adults were either working or occupied as housewives and the range of employment generally parallels those available to non-disabled persons of comparable intelligence (p. 183). (5) Of the 57 surviving adults with extrapyramidal cerebral palsy personally examined, 14 were employed (p. 183). (6) None of the 49 adults with spastic tetraplegia and none of the 38 with the mixed-type personally examined were employed (p. 183). (7) Only 13 were classified as spastic paraplegia. Spastic diplegia was not used as a classification at this time. Crothers and Paine used the term 'bilateral spastic cerebral palsy', and termed Osler's 'bilateral hemiplegia' and 'spastic diplegia' as tetraplegia (p. 107). (8) 'It is a disturbing fact that volumes are written about treatment and almost no suggestion can be found to indicate that termination of treatment

193

is ever desirable.' (p. 209). 'Unless we accept the idea of permanent care, it is essential to consider seriously, and repeatedly, the advantages of the abdication of the therapists.' (p. 210). (9) 'It is generally accepted that motor development depends, to a very large extent, on maturation rather than training.' 'It is evident, however, that training was not effective in accelerating walking.' (p. 8).

'It is a disturbing fact that volumes are written about treatment and almost no suggestion can be found to indicate that termination of treatment is ever desirable.'

(Crothers and Paine 1959)

EMPLOYMENT AND INDEPENDENCE

Various positive indicators for employment and independence have been reported: (1) regular schooling and completion of high school (Bachman 1972, O'Reilly 1975); (2) independence in mobility with ability to travel beyond the home, p=0.01 (1972); (3) good hand-function and skills, p=0.05 (Bachman 1972); (4) niche employment for the disabled, which was best found in small towns rather than large cities (Ingram *et al.* 1964); (5) spastic paralysis was more favourable for employment than athetosis (O'Reilly 1975). Not surprisingly, spastic hemiplegia and diplegia were most often associated with full-time employment (Ingram *et al.* 1964, Hassakis 1974, Soboloff 1981).

OUTCOME STUDIES: CHILD TO ADULT

Subsequent outcome studies of children with cerebral palsy who have reached adulthood were published in 1975 and 1981. In O'Reilly's (1975) study of 336 adult patients 28% who had normal cognition were sufficient in self-care; one-third were mentally retarded and totally dependent. The outlook for employment was best in those who had spastic paralysis and had attended regular school. In the whole group, 35.4% had a chance of having an occupation. Institutional care was necessary for 11% of those severely involved; 17% had died; 39% had no organized activity, were unable to obtain employment, or were sitting at home with nothing to do.

A study of 119 adolescents and young adults with spastic diplegia followed at the Children's Hospital at Stanford confirmed the good prognosis of this group for independence in all areas (S. Miranda, personal communication). None were in a day-care center, only 3% were in a sheltered workshop, and 97% were either still in high school, more advanced education or working. Of the 30% over age 21 years and working, the jobs varied: some were housewives and mothers, computer programers, bankers or salesmen, and one became the mayor of his California town, Antelope Valley. Twenty years later only anecdotal follow-up of these 119 persons is possible. The majority appear to have finished college and some have university degrees in primary education and one is an attorney.

Soboloff (1981) investigated the status of 248 adults with cerebral palsy (age range 20–50 years). He found that 48% were self-sufficient community walkers; 30% had part-time care and used the wheelchair except for household walking; 22% were totally dependent. Full-time employment was documented in 31% and, as reported in other studies, the majority had spastic diplegia or hemiplegia. About one-third were homebound or institutionalized. Of the 24 (8%) who had married, only three had married another person with cerebral palsy. The causes of some of the 15 deaths are tragic but possibly instructive: three respiratory arrests, two cardiac arrests, two suicides, one murdered by his mother who then killed herself, one choked on a hot dog, one fell down a staircase and another off a ramp.

Social outcomes of 48 adults age 19–25 years who had cerebral palsy (half had hemiplegia) and four with spina bifida and compared with age-matched controls consumed the interest of investigators in Oulu, Finland (Kokkonen *et al.* 1991). Forty of the group with disability had completed elementary education, 10 had finished high school, and 11 had gone on to advanced education. The group with disability had twice as much unemployment as the controls. 58% still lived with their parents versus 35% of the controls. Half of those with disability received a disability pension, and 46% felt they were independent of the parents for income. The authors make the point that this data might change with the changing etiology and resultant disability of cerebral palsy. That half of those who had cerebral palsy had hemiplegia was probably responsible for a more favorable educational and employment status. A main finding in this study was delayed social maturation in the disabled group and was not related to the severity of the disability. The authors thought that the environment influenced later development more than the disability.

'Delayed social maturation of the disabled, age 19-25 years, compared with normal matched controls was unrelated to the disability.'

(Kokkonen *et al.* 1991)

Another retrospective study was done of 810 patients seen at the University of California, San Francisco, from 1951 to 1974 (O'Grady *et al.* 1995). Patients from this base were contacted either through the California Department of Developmental Disabilities as probably needing ongoing support services or from the Department of Motor Vehicles registration list. Seventy-one were interviewed at a follow-up and 46 completed an anonymous questionnaire. The follow-up ranged from 13 to 36 years after their initial evaluation in childhood. The motor involvement was spasticity in 71.5%, athetosis and mixed in 21.1%; only 1.4% were ataxic. In the interviewed group 22.5% were non-ambulatory, 9.8% had non-functional use of their hands, and 33.8% had no oral ability or were difficult to understand.

Of the 71 interviewed, 36 had competitive employment, 22 were in sheltered employment, and only four never worked. Prediction for employment was 90% accurate, and predictions of no employment were 100% accurate. About half of them lived independently of their parents, a third with their parents, and the remainder were in boarding and care institutions. The message of this study was that caution should be exercised in predicting employment of children with cerebral palsy. Some exceeded expectations that were considered due to family support and sense of self-confidence that may be as important as any technological interventions. The Irish film, *My Left Foot*, illustrates this point.

The health status of women with cerebral palsy living in the area of Syracuse, New York, was ascertained with a questionnaire (Turk *et al.* 1997). The majority of women considered themselves healthy; 83% engaged in common physical activities and 43% did stretching and aerobic exercises. 68% were able to walk and over 50% required no assistance in activities of daily living. Hip and back deformities were commonly reported (59%). Beyond orthopaedic concerns were bladder and bowel problems (56% and 43%), poor dental health (43%) and gastroesophageal reflux (28%). There was no significant association among the variables reported.

Tobimatsu and Nakamura (2000) of Sendai, Japan, did a non-randomized retrospective study of 99 persons with cerebral palsy with a mean age of 19.9 years enrolled in vocational training after graduation from high school. They concluded that the ability to get a job in Japan was mainly determined by the ability to walk and having had education in a regular school.

Murphy and colleagues (2000) of Duluth, Minnesota, presented a report that reflects progress compared to those cited published 20–25 years ago. These investigators contacted 101 persons, ages 27–74 years who lived independently in the community of Duluth, Minnesota, and volunteered to be studied. The PULTIBEC system was used as a modified measure of function (Lindon 1963). It was derived from Pulheems system used to evaluate functional capacities in Her Majesty's Forces published in 1949. As a guide for those who wish to do outcome studies in cerebral palsy, it may be useful.[34] The data are encouraging; 67% lived independently, and of these 34% had an attendant while 33% did not; 53% had competitive employment, 22% earned a high enough income that threatened loss of disability benefits if it became higher. Speech deficits compromised verbal communication in 50% and correlated more with cognition than with the physical or communicative impairments. Educational achievement was outstanding with 64 of the 101 completing college. Among the 12 who had severe dyskinesia, two had doctoral degrees and one had a master's degree in social sciences. On the emotional and interpersonal relationships front, 84% felt they had overprotective parents in childhood; 90% wanted more sexual education.

This recent study of Murphy *et al.* (2000) of patients who had reached the age of 33.5 to 48.8 years is in contrast to the one by Crothers and Paine in which only 22 had the diagnosis of spastic diplegia and a mean age of 37.8 years at follow-up, and

only 10 had hemiplegia. Ninety had varying degrees of quadriplegia or dyskinesia. The study has some important messages for those promoting and planning CBR. *The greatly improved lot of the adult with cerebral palsy can be attributed to advances in rehabilitation technology, better home support services, legal mandates in education, and environmental access.*

NEGATIVE FACTORS FOR INDEPENDENCE AND EMPLOYMENT

Negative factors include intellectual retardation (Ingram *et al.* 1964, Hassakis 1974, O'Reilly 1975, Cohen and Kohn 1979), and severity of the disability (Ingram *et al.* 1964, Cohen and Kohn 1979).

Prolonged treatment programs have not been effective in achieving maximum independence (Cohen and Kohn 1979, Goldkamp 1984). Indeed, prolonged treatment programs and special schools may have been detrimental in permanently segregating the disabled from the rest of the community (Taft 1972). To demonstrate the action behind the rhetoric, Milani-Comparetti (1979) was instrumental in closing some 13 special schools in Florence, Italy. Finally, the family could act as a barrier to achievement by not accepting the child's disability and allowing the child to accept responsibility (Cohen and Kohn 1979, Soboloff 1981).

OUTCOMES RESEARCH IN CEREBRAL PALSY

In the new millennium health care policy is focused on 'outcomes research', meaning 'acceptance of measures for patient perceptions, functional status, emotional health, and quality of life as indicators of the effectiveness of treatment' (Winter 1999). All the rhetoric and urging to do something about outcomes stems from the desire to control costs of medical care and not pay for ineffective or questionable treatment. It is relatively easy to do a prospective study of total joint replacements with several years of follow-up in stable populations. Can it be done in cerebral palsy?

Torner (1992) detailed the design of outcome studies in cerebral palsy; he too stated that 'outcomes must focus on the goal. Improvement of performance, function and the quality of life are primary objectives'. Barry (1996) called for more study on the effects of physical therapy with goals of communication, self-care and mobility to prepare a child for independent adult life. Lepage *et al.* (2000) in their study from Quebec City, Canada, of the 'handicap situation' of 98 children aged 5–17.8 years (mean, 10.5; SD 3.5) had results that suggested that locomotion might influence 'life habits' (i.e. activities of daily living and social roles). This is an inkling of how one function would be linked to other functions and roles in life, but it is not an outcome study.

Novacheck and associates (2000) used the Gillette FAQ for community ambulation levels.[35] It is a 10-level parent-report

---

34 *Physical Qualities:* P, physical capacity (endurance and general health); U, upper limbs, right and left hand and arm; L, locomotion; T, toilet. *and communication:* I, intelligence; B, behavior; E, vision (eyes); C, communication, hearing and speech. Grade 1, normal; grades 2–5, progressively poorer function; grade 6, virtually absent.

35 Motion Analysis Laboratory of Gillette Children's Specialty Healthcare, St Paul, MN 55101, USA.

walking scale. They concluded that this was a reliable and valid scale when tested for community ambulation levels, 6–10, in the 41 individuals with neuromuscular conditions and assessed by standard functional outcome measures, gait analysis, and energy expenditure. It's another way to measure one locomotor outcome function. These foregoing studies currently seem to be 'as good as it gets'.

Goldberg (1991) clearly delineated three components that would comprise outcome studies in cerebral palsy: technical outcomes, e.g. increased range of joint motion, decreased spasticity; (2) functional health assessment: what the patient is doing e.g. lifting, walking, working, roles (student, shopkeeper, pilot etc.)—the quality of life; (3) patient satisfaction. Goldberg concluded that 'as pediatric orthopaedists invested in the lifelong well-being of children, we must be in the forefront by providing accurate and precise outcome studies and documentation of the value of what we do.' The forefront is here, but more than a decade has passed since Goldberg's editorial, and no such comprehensive long term studies of orthopaedic surgery have appeared. By 'long term' in children, we would have to follow them through skeletal maturity to over the age of 18 years and preferably older.

Unless there is a dramatic change in funding such careful long-term studies, one can doubt that it's going to happen. It will take a great deal of professional time in many disciplines to study the effect of orthopaedic surgery in cerebral palsy, rhizotomy, intrathecal baclofen or botulinum toxin. Compounding the study would be efficacy of physical therapy done in parallel with surgical interventions, neuropharmacological drugs, family and social factors, the culture and the environment. Furthermore, studies of long-term outcomes will depend on a relatively stable population. It is estimated that 50% of the US population moves every year. Additionally, such studies depend on the longevity and stability of the research team who might be as peripatetic as the patients (even more so if the physician is an academic). Confirming this opinion is the 1995 study of 810 adults with cerebral palsy who had been seen at the clinics at the University of California, San Francisco. Finding these former patients entailed searching the files of the State motor vehicle registration department where the investigators found 196 patient addresses, but 112 of these persons never responded to the letter of inquiry. Of the 308 registered with the Department of Developmental Services 99 were found, but 27 had moved out of the State, five were deceased and seven were institutionalized (O'Grady et al. 1995).

Questions could be answered such as: does an 8° increase in knee flexion on swing phase make any difference in the quality of life of the patient? What are the family, cultural and environmental conditions that have determined the restriction in participation as the result of the disability? The list goes on. Long term outcomes research could be done but it will take time, money and dedicated professionals with stamina to do it prospectively or retrospectively. And then the problem of matching the intervention against no intervention would be considerable. Could such control subjects be found in the

contemporary society or would one have to look at wherever primitive societies still exist? Furthermore, if they do, it must be asked whether these societies would have survivors of birth events that cause cerebral palsy (e.g. preterm birth, perinatal hypoxia).

Does an eight degree increase in knee flexion on swing phase make any difference in the quality of life of the patient?

Judging from the follow-up studies on specific surgical procedures, even an 8- to 10-year study would be a break through. Again, who is going to carefully follow his or her patient from the day of surgery and for the succeeding 8–10 years and get all the data desired? What surgeon or institution will have the time and finances to have nothing but follow-up patients in the clinic? Doctors, therapists, and social workers 'burn-out' too, like Freud, from too much cerebral palsy. More importantly, can the patients be found for follow-up? If we really want such studies, then someone will have to pay for them. Finally, if the results are equivocal or negative, then who is going to say so and who is going to protest having their fiscal nourishment taken away?

Evidence-based outcome studies have come into fruition with the development of 'levels of evidence' from published results for specific treatments by Butler *et al.* (1999) adopted by the American Academy for Cerebral Palsy and Developmental Medicine. As noted previously, results are classified according to the 'dimensions of disablement' of the subjects studied (see Table 6.IX). Evidence of the efficacy of a treatment is based on five levels the study represents (see Table 6.X). Level I studies present the strongest evidence; level II studies have tentative conclusions; levels III and IV only suggest causation. The lowest level, V, indicates that no conclusion can be drawn from the evidence in the published study.

Butler and Campbell (2000) applied the foregoing guidelines in 17 studies of the effects of *intrathecal baclofen in spastic and dystonic cerebral palsy* found via the Medline database from 1956 to March 2000. They identified 17 studies of intrathecal baclofen in spasticity, three of which did not meet the criteria for inclusion because no results were reported. Fourteen studies were subjected to scrutiny for the levels of evidence of efficacy. Of these only two were level I: Albright *et al.* (1991) and Gilmartin *et al.* (2000). Only two were considered having level II evidence: Almeida *et al.* (1997)[36] and Van Schaeybroeck *et al.* (2000). The remaining published studies fell into either level III, IV or V. The conclusion was that 'the research methodology of the overall body of evidence is relatively weak for several reasons'. Among the reasons was that only half of the 14 studies used statistical analysis to remove the possibility of chance affecting the result.

Despite the limitations of the studies published intrathecal baclofen did reduce the spasticity in the lower limbs, but the

---

36 The study by Almeida *et al.* (1997) of Sao Paulo, Brazil, was considered 'exemplary' although it concerned only one child, age 11 years, with spastic diplegia. The authors found that after 2 years, the range of joint motion was worse than at baseline and there was concern about subluxation of the hip.

effect on the upper limbs remained unclear. The authors called for studies in greater numbers of patients within a group, randomized, and with more detailed assessment of function in the outcome, e.g. improvement in motor control, functional skills and participation in social roles of daily life.

Using the same principles of evidence, intrathecal baclofen in dystonic cerebral palsy only 15 individuals with cerebral palsy who had dystonia were found in the published studies (Narayan *et al.* 1991, Silbert and Stewart-Wynne 1992, Albright *et al.* 1996). Twelve of these patients notably improved in initial screening, and 10 continued longer term, but the maintenance of this improvement occurred in only eight. In two, body positioning was better, but no other results referable to the dimensions of disablement could be found. One patient became worse after a bolus injection (Silbert and Stewart-Wynne 1992). Again the authors recommended more investigations, but made the point that first a description and assessment of dystonia in cerebral palsy needs development.

This long report by Butler and Campbell (2000) should be read in its entirety for a more details of the analysis of the published papers on intrathecal baclofen. There is no doubt that intrathecal baclofen as well as selective posterior rootlet rhizotomy and botulinum toxin reduces muscle spasticity in cerebral palsy. How this result translates into improved function by overcoming the dimensions of disablement has yet to be shown in controlled studies.

SUMMARY OF GOALS, TREATMENT AND MANAGEMENT

The goals for children including those with cerebral palsy and other disabling conditions should be for optimum independence in adult life. Major goals are communication, activities of daily living, and mobility. Goals can be set as early as age 4 years given prognostic awareness. To achieve the goals the main management/treatment techniques available are physical and occupational therapy, orthotics, orthopaedic surgery, posterior selective rootlet rhizotomy, intramuscular botulinum toxin, intrathecal baclofen, and assistive technology. Special physical therapy 'methods or systems' have been scrutinized with evidence-based studies and found wanting. Occupational therapy roles are to facilitate activities of daily living. Non-verbal communication methods and technological advances have helped to overcome the lack of verbal ability.

Studies have indicated short-term effects of reducing spasticity of muscles and dystonia. Whether these effects will persist with repeated injections over a period of years remains questionable. Orthopaedic surgery remains as effective in prevention and correction of structural deformities of the limbs and spine. Selective posterior rootlet rhizotomy has had a wave of popularity and many studies at first seemed to demonstrate efficacy. However, in limited studies its effects on function, structural change, and spasticity compared with orthopaedic surgery alone are problematical at this time. Intrathecal baclofen appears to have a place primarily in the total body involved patient with cerebral palsy. Assistive technology has become established and accepted as an effective way to overcome restrictions primarily in mobility as a compensation for inability to walk functionally. Other than the plastic ankle–foot orthosis, orthotics (braces) are usually not effective in preventing or overcoming deformities of the limbs.

REFERENCES

Abbott, R., Johann-Murphy, M., Shiminski-Maher, T., Quartermain, D., Forem, S.L., Gold, J.T., Epstein, F.J. (1993) 'Selective dorsal rhizotomy: outcome and complications in treating spastic cerebral palsy.' *Neurosurgery*, **33**, 851–857.

Abel, M.R., John, G.A., Vaughan, D.L., Damiano, D.L. (1998) 'Gait assessment of fixed ankle–foot orthoses in children with spastic diplegia.' *Archives of Physical Medicine and Rehabilitation*, **79**, 126–133.

Accardo, P.J. (1982) 'Freud on diplegia—commentary and translation.' *American Journal of Diseases of Children*, **136**, 452–456.

Adams, J.M., Perry, J., Beeler, L.M. (1990) 'Instrumented gait analysis after selective dorsal rhizotomy.' *Developmental Medicine and Child Neurology*, **32**, 1037–1043.

—— Cahan, L.D., Perry, J., Beeler, L.M. (1995) 'Foot contact pattern following selective dorsal rhizotomy.' *Pediatric Neurosurgery*, **23**, 76–81.

Adams, R. (2002) 'Letter to the editor.' *Developmental Medicine and Child Neurology*, **44**, 431–432.

Ade-Hall, R.A., Moore, A.P. (2000) 'Botulinum toxin type A in the treatment of lower limb spasticity in cerebral palsy.' *Cochrane Database System Review 2000*, **2**, CD001408.

Agosta, J.M., Bradley, V.J. (1985) *Family Care for Persons with Developmental Disabilities: A Growing Commitment.* Boston, MA: Human Services Research Institute.

Albright, A.L. (1995) 'Spastic cerebral palsy. Approaches to drug treatment.' *CNS Drugs*, **4**, 17–27.

—— (1996) 'Baclofen in the treatment of cerebral palsy.' *Journal of Child Neurology*, **11**, 77–83.

—— Cervi, A., Singletary, J. (1991) 'Intrathecal baclofen for spasticity in cerebral palsy.' *Journal of the American Medical Association*, **265**, 1418–1422.

—— Barron, W.B., Fasick, M.P., Polinko, P., Janosky, J. (1993) 'Continuous intrathecal baclofen infusion for spasticity of cerebral origin.' *Journal of the American Medical Association*, **270**, 2475–2477.

—— Barry, M.J., Fasick, M.P., Janosky, J. (1995) 'Effects of continuous intrathecal baclofen infusion and selective posterior rhizotomy on upper extremity spasticity.' *Pediatric Neurosurgery*, **23**, 82–85.

—— —— Fasick, P., Barron, W., Shultz, B. (1996) 'Continuous intrathecal baclofen infusion for symptomatic generalized dystonia.' *Neurosurgery*, **38**, 934–939.

—— Shultz, B.L. (1999) 'Plasma baclofen levels in children receiving continuous intrathecal baclofen infusion.' *Journal of Child Neurology*, **14**, 408–409.

Almeida, G.L., Campbell, S.K., Girolami, G.L., Penn, R.D., Corcos, D.M. (1997) 'Multidimensional assessment of motor function in a child with cerebral palsy following intrathecal administration of baclofen.' *Physical Therapy*, **77**, 751–764.

American Association of Occupational Therapists (1981) 'The role of occupational therapy as an education-related service: official position paper.' *American Journal of Occupational Therapy*, **35**, 811.

Amiel-Tison, C. (1985) 'Neurological assessment from birth to 7 years of age.' *In* Harel, S., Anastasiow, N.J. (Eds) *The At-Risk Infant.* Baltimore and London: Paul H. Brookes, pp. 239–251.

Amosun, S.L., Ikuesan, B.A., Oloyede, I.J. (1995) 'Rehabilitation of the handicapped child—what about the caregiver? *PNG (Papua and New Guinea) Medical Journal*, **38**, 208–214.

Anastasiow, N.J. (1985) 'Parent training as adult development.' *In* Harel, S., Anastasiow, N.J. (Eds) *The At-Risk Infant.* Baltimore and London: Paul H. Brookes, pp. 5–12.

—— Harel, S. (1993) *At-Risk Infants.* Baltimore and London: Paul H. Brookes.

Anderson, T.J., Donaldson, I. MacG. (1995) 'Botulinum toxin: one man's poison is another man's potion.' *New Zealand Medical Journal*, **108**, 307–308.

Ansved, T., Odergren, T., Borg, K. (1997) 'Muscle fiber atrophy in leg muscles after botulinum toxin type A treatment of cervical dystonia.' *Neurology*, **48**, 1440–1442.

Arens, L.J., Peacock, W.J., Peter, J. (1989) 'Selective posterior rhizotomy: a long term follow-up study.' *Childs Nervous System*, **5**, 148–152.

Armstrong, R.W., Steinbok, P., Cochrane, D.D., Kube, S.D., Fife, S.E., Farrell, K. (1997) 'Intrathecally administered baclofen for treatment of children with spasticity of cerebral origin.' *Journal of Neurosurgery*, **87**, 409–414.

Arnoff, G. (1973) 'There's no play like snow play.' *Canadian Journal of Occupational Therapy*, **40**, 79–82.

Autti-Ramo, I, Larsen, A., Taimo, A., von Wendt, L. (2001) 'Management of the upper limb with botulinum toxin type A in children with spastic type cerebral palsy and acquired brain injury: clinical implications.' *European Journal of Neurology*, **8** (Suppl. 5), 136–144.

Ayalon, M., Ben-Sira, D., Hutzler, Y., Gilad, T. (2000) 'Reliability of isokinetic strength measurements in children with cerebral palsy.' *Developmental Medicine and Child Neurology*, **42**, 398–402.

Ayres, A.J. (1971) 'Characteristics of types of sensory integrative dysfunction.' *American Journal of Occupation Therapy*, **7**, 329–334.

—— (1972) 'Improving academic scores through sensory integration.' *Journal of Learning Disabilities*, **5**, 336–343.

—— (1977) 'Effect of sensory integrative therapy on the coordination of children with choreoathetoid movements.' *American Journal of Occupational Therapy*, **31**, 291–293.

—— (1978) 'Learning disabilities and the vestibular system.' *American Journal of Learning Disabilities*, **2**, 18–29.

Bachman, W.H. (1972) 'Variables affecting post-school economic adaptation of orthopaedically handicapped and other health impaired students.' *Rehabilitation Literatures*, **33**, 98–114.

Badell, A. (1991) 'The effects of medications that reduce spasticity in the management of spastic cerebral palsy.' *Journal of Neurologic Rehabilitation*, **5** (Suppl. 1), S13–S14.

Bairstow, P., Cochrane, R., Rusk, I. (1991) 'Selection of children with cerebral palsy for conductive education and the characteristics of children judged suitable and unsuitable.' *Developmental Medicine and Child Neurology*, **33**, 984–992.

Baker, L.D., Bassett, F.H., Dyas, E.C. (1970) 'Surgery in the rehabilitation of cerebral palsied patients.' *Developmental Medicine and Child Neurology*, **12**, 330–342.

Baker, R., Jasinski, M., Maciag-Tymecka, I., Michalowska-Mrozek, J., Bonikowski, M., Carr, L., MacLean, J., Lin, J.P., Lynch, B., Theologis, T., Wendorff, J., Eunson, P., Cosgrove, A. (2002) 'Botulinum toxin treatment of spasticity in diplegic cerebral palsy: a randomized, double-blind, placebo-controlled, dose-ranging study.' *Developmental Medicine and Child Neurology*, **44**, 666–675.

Bakheit, A.M., Severa, S., Cosgrove, A., Morton, R., Roussounis, S.H., Doderlein, L., Lin, J.P., Roussounis, S.H. (2001) 'Safety profile and efficacy of botulinum toxin A (Dysport) in children with muscle spasticity.' *Developmental Medicine and Child Neurology*, **43**, 234–238.

Bang, M.S., Change, S.G., Kim, S.B., Kim, S.J. (2002) 'Change of dynamic gastrocnemius and soleus muscle length after block of spastic calf muscle in cerebral palsy.' *American Journal of Physical Medicine and Rehabilitation*, **81**, 760–764.

Baniel, A. (1999–2000) *Anat Baniel's Movement Coordination Learning and Feldenkrais Method*. Greenbrae, CA: Movement Coordination Learning.

Barber, E. (1978) 'Modifications of a MacLaren Buggy Major for orthopaedic seat inserts.' *Orthotics and Prosthetics*, **32**, 6–9.

Barrett, J., Herriotts, P., Houghton, R.H., Cochrane, G.M. (1995) *Home Management and Housing*. Oxford: Disability Information Trust.

Barry, M.J. (1996) 'Physical therapy interventions for patients with movement disorders due to cerebral palsy.' *Journal of Child Neurology*, **11** (Suppl. 1), S51–60.

Barwood, S., Baillieu, C., Boyd, R., Brereton, D., Low, J., Nattrass, G., Graham, H.K. (2000) 'Analgesic effects of botulinum toxin A: a randomized, placebo-controlled clinical trial.' *Developmental Medicine and Child Neurology*, **42**, 116–121.

Bauer, H., Appaji, G., Mundt, D. (1992) 'Vojta neurophysiologic therapy.' *Indian Journal of Pediatrics*, **59**, 37–51.

Bauman, S. (1981) 'Physical aspects of the self. A review of some aspects of body image development in childhood.' *Psychiatric Clinics of North America*, **4**, 455–470.

Bax, M. (1983) 'Abuse and cerebral palsy.' *Developmental Medicine and Child Neurology*, **25**, 141–142.

—— (1985) 'Meeting the parents' needs.' *Developmental Medicine and Child Neurology*, **27**, 139–140.

—— (1991) 'Conductive education assessed.' *Developmental Medicine and Child Neurology*, **35**, 659–660. (Editorial.)

—— (1992) 'Alternative methods.' *Developmental Medicine and Child Neurology*, **34**, 471–472.

—— (1995) 'Predicting outcome and planning management.' *Developmental Medicine and Child Neurology*, **37**, 941–942.

Beals, R.K. (1966) 'Spastic paraplegia and diplegia: an evaluation of non-surgical and surgical factors influencing prognosis for ambulation.' *Journal of Bone and Joint Surgery*, **48A**, 827–846.

Beck, A.J., Gaskill, S.J., Marlin, A.E. (1993) 'Improvement in upper extremity function and trunk control after selective posterior rhizotomy.' *American Journal of Occupational Therapy*, **47**, 704–707.

Beers, M.H., Berkow, R., Eds. (1999) *The Merck Manual of Diagnosis and Therapy, 17th edn*. Whitehouse Station, NJ: Merck Research Laboratories.

Benedetti, A., Colombo, F. (1981) 'Spinal surgery for spasticity.' *Neurochirurgia*, **24**, 195–198.

—— Alexander, A., Pellegri, A. (1982) 'Posterior rhizotomies for spasticity in children affected by cerebral palsy.' *Journal of Neurosurgical Science*, **26**, 179–184.

Bensman, A.S., Szegho, M. (1978) 'Cerebellar electrical stimulation: a critique.' *Archives of Physical Medicine and Rehabilitation*, **59**, 485–487.

Berkowitz, M. (1976) 'Public policy towards disability—the number, the programs, and some economic problems.' *In: Science and Technology in the Service of the Physically Handicapped*. PB 261–451, Springfield, VA: National Technical Information Service, US Department of Commerce, pp. 42–63.

Bertoti, D.B. (1988) 'Effect of therapeutic horseback riding on posture in children with cerebral palsy.' *Physical Therapy*, **68**, 1505–1512.

Berweck, S., Feldkamp, A., Francke, A., Nehles, J., Schwerin, A., Heinen, F. (2002) 'Sonography-guided injection of botulinum toxin A in children with cerebral palsy.' *Neuropediatrics*, **9**, 928–933.

Bettelheim, B. (1977) *The Uses of Enchantment*. New York: Vintage Books.

Bhambhani, Y.N., Holland, L.J., Steadward, R.D. (1993) 'Anaerobic threshold in wheelchair athletes with cerebral palsy: validity and reliability.' *Archives of Physical Medicine and Rehabilitation*, **74**, 305–311.

Bhatia, K.P., Munchau, A., Thompson, P.D., Houser, M., Chauhan, V.S., Hutchinson, M., Shapira, A.H., Marsden, C.D. (1999) 'Generalized muscular weakness after botulinum toxin injections for dystonia: a report of three cases.' *Journal of Neurology, Neurosurgery and Psychiatry*, **67**, 90–93.

Bhatnagar, S.C., Silverman, F. (1999) 'Communicating with non-verbal persons in India: inexpensive augmentative communication devices.' *Asia Pacific Disability Rehabilitation Journal*, **10**, 52–58.

Bick, E.M. (1972) 'The classic. The effects of artificial electricity on muscular motion. Aloysio Luigi Galvani.' *Clinical Orthopaedics and Related Research*, **88**, 2–10.

Blair, E., Ballantyne, J., Horsman, S., Chauvel, P. (1995) 'A study of a dynamic proximal stability splint in the management of children with cerebral palsy.' *Developmental Medicine and Child Neurology*, **37**, 544–554.

Bleck, E.E. (1971) 'The shoeing of children: sham or science?' *Developmental Medicine and Child Neurology*, **13**, 188–195.

—— (1975) 'Locomotor prognosis in cerebral palsy.' *Developmental Medicine and Child Neurology*, **17**, 18–25.

—— (1977a) 'Rehabilitation engineering for severely handicapped children.' *In* Ahstrom, J.P. Jr (Ed.) *Current Management in Orthopaedic Surgery*. St Louis: C.V. Mosby.

—— (1977b) 'Severe orthopaedic disability in childhood: solutions provided by rehabilitation engineering.' *Orthopaedic Clinics of North America*, **9**, 509–527.

—— (1978) 'Integrating the care of multiply handicapped children.' *Developmental Medicine and Child Neurology*, **20**, 10–13.

—— (1982) 'Cerebral palsy.' *In* Bleck, E.E., Nagel, D.A. (Eds) *Physically Handicapped Children: A Medical Atlas for Teachers, 2nd edn*. Orlando, FL: Grune & Stratton.

—— (1984) 'Where have all the CP children gone? The needs of adults.' *Developmental Medicine and Child Neurology*, **26**, 674–676.

—— (1985) 'L'enfant paralysé et son appareillage—concepts de base.'

(Translation by Dimeglio, A.) *In: L'Enfant Paralysé. Rééducation et Appareillage.* Paris: Masson, pp. 180–190.

—— Headley, L. (1961) 'Treatment and parent counseling for the pre-school child with cerebral palsy.' *Pediatrics*, **27**, 1025–1032.

—— Berzins, U.J. (1977) 'Conservative management of pes va1gus with plantar flexed talus flexible.' *Clinical Orthopaedics and Related Research*, **122**, 85–94.

Bliss, C.K. (1965) *Semantography/Blissymbolics*. Sydney: Sematography Publications.

Bloom, K.K., Nazar, G.B. (1994) 'Functional assessment following selective posterior rootlet rhizotomy in spastic cerebral palsy.' *Child's Nervous System*, **10**, 84–85.

Bloswick, D.S., King, E.M., Brown, D., Gooch, J.R., Peters, M. (1994) 'Evaluation of a device to exercise hip extensor muscles in children with cerebral palsy: a clinical and field study.' *Assistive Technology*, **6**, 147–151.

Blum, R.W., Resnick, M.D., Nelson, R., St Germaine, A. (1991) 'Family and peer issues among adolescents with spina bifida and cerebral palsy.' *Pediatrics*, **88**, 280–285.

Bobath, B. (1954) 'A study of abnormal postural reflex activity in patients with lesions of the central nervous system.' *Physiotherapy*, **40**, 9–12.

—— Bobath, K. (1961) 'Is treatment really necessary?' *Cerebral Palsy Bulletin*, **3**, 613–614.

—— (1967) 'The very early treatment of cerebral palsy.' *Developmental Medicine and Child Neurology*, **9**, 373–390.

—— (1966) *The Motor Deficit in Patients with Cerebral Palsy. Clinics in Developmental Medicine, No. 23.* London: Spastics International Medical Publications with Heinemann Medical; Philadelphia: J.B. Lippincott.

—— (1980) *A Neurophysiological Basis for the Treatment of Cerebral Palsy. Clinics in Developmental Medicine, No. 75.* London: Spastics International Medical Publications with Heinemann Medical; Philadelphia: J.B. Lippincott.

—— Bobath, B. (1958) 'An assessment of motor handicap of children with cerebral palsy and their response to treatment.' *Occupational Therapy Journal*, **21**, 1–16.

—— —— (1984) 'The neuro-developmental treatment.' *In* Scrutton, D. (Ed.) *Management of the Motor Disorders in Children with Cerebral Palsy. Clinics in Developmental Medicine, No. 90.* London: Spastics International Medical Publications with Heinemann Medical; Philadelphia: J.B. Lippincott.

Bolkert, R. (1979) 'Medial uprights for valgus feet, spastic.' *Orthotics and Prosthetics*, **33**, 54–62.

Borodic, G., Johnson, E., Goodnough, M., Schantz, E. (1996) 'Botulinum toxin therapy, immunologic resistance, and problems with available materials.' *Neurology*, **46**, 26–29.

Borschneck, D., Smith, J.T. (1999) 'Cost analysis of equinus contracture management in the patient with cerebral palsy.' *Paper read at the Annual Meeting American Academy of Orthopaedic Surgeons, Anaheim, CA.*

Boscarino, L.F., Õunpuu, M.S., Davis, R.B. III, Gage, J.R., DeLuca, P.A. (1993) 'Effects of selective dorsal rhizotomy on gait in children with cerebral palsy.' *Journal of Pediatric Orthopaedics*, **13**, 174–179.

Bose, K. (1980) 'Management of cerebral palsy in a developing country.' *Orthopaedic Transactions*, **4**, 75.

Bothwell, J.E., Clarke, K., Dooley, J.M., Gordon, K.E., Anderson, R., Wood, E.P., Camfield, C.S., Camfield, P.R. (2002) 'Botulinum toxin A as a treatment for excessive drooling in children.' *Pediatric Neurology*, **27**, 18–22.

Boyd, R.N., Pliatsios, V., Starr, R., Wolfe, R., Graham, H.K. (2000) 'Biomechanical transformation of the gastroc–soleus muscle with botulinum toxin A in children with cerebral palsy.' *Developmental Medicine and Child Neurology*, **42**, 32–41.

—— Dobson, F., Parrott, J., Love, S., Oates, J., Larson, A., Burchall, G., Chondros, P., Carlin, J., Nattrass, G., Graham, H.K. (2001) 'The effect of botulinum toxin type A and a variable hip abduction orthosis on gross motor function: a randomized controlled trial.' *European Journal of Neurology*, **8** (Suppl. 5), 109–119.

Bourgeois, O., Chaigne, M.O., Cherpin, J., Minaire, P., Weber, D. (1977) *Diminues Physiques et Transports Collectifs.* Born, France: Institut de Récherche des Transports, Centre d'Evaluation et de Récherche des Nuisances.

Bragg, J.H., Houser, C., Shumaker, J. (1975) 'Behavior modification: effects on reverse tailor sitting in children with cerebral palsy.' *Physical Therapy*, **55**, 860–868.

Brashear, A., Lew, M.F., Dykstra, D.D., Comella, C.L., Factor, S.A., Rodnitzky,

R.L., Trosch, R., Singer, C., Brin, M.F., Murray, J.J., Wallace, J.D., Wilmer-Hulme, A., Koller, M. (1999) 'Safety and efficacy of NeuroBloc (botulinum toxin type B) in type A-responsive cervical dystonia.' *Neurology*, **53**, 1439–1436.

Brecht, J.S., Chang, M.W., Price, R., Lehmann, J. (1995) 'Decreased balance performance in cowboy boots compared with tennis shoes.' *Archives of Physical Medicine and Rehabilitation*, **76**, 940–946.

Brin, M.F. (1997) 'Botulinum toxin: chemistry, pharmacology, toxicity, and immunology.' *Muscle Nerve* (Suppl.), S146–148.

—— Lew, M.F., Adler, C.H., Comella, C.L., Factor, S.A., Jankovic, J., O'Brien, D., Murray, J.J., Wallace, J.D., Wilmer-Hulme, A., Koller, M. (1999) 'Safety and efficacy of NeuroBloc (botulinum toxin type B) in type A-resistant cervical dystonia.' *Neurology*, **53**, 1431–1438.

Broggi, G., Angelim, L., Giorgi, C. (1980) 'Neurological and psychological side effects after stereotactic thalamotomy in patients with cerebral palsy.' *Neurosurgery*, **7**, 127–134.

—— Bono, R., Giorgi, C., Nardocci, N., Franzini, A. (1983) 'Long term results of stereotactic thalarnotomy for cerebral palsy.' *Neurosurgery*, **12**, 195–202.

Bronowski, J. (1978) *Magic, Science and Civilization.* New York: Columbia University Press.

Brouwer, B., Wheeldon, R.K., Stradiotto-Parker, N., Allum, J. (1998) 'Reflex excitability and isometric force production in cerebral palsy: the effect of serial casting.' *Developmental Medicine and Child Neurology*, **40**, 168–175.

—— Davidson, L.K., Olney, S.J. (2000) 'Serial casting in idiopathic toe-walkers and children with spastic cerebral palsy.' *Journal of Pediatric Orthopaedics*, **20**, 221–225.

Buckon, C.E., Thomas, S.S., Aiona, M.D., Piatt, J.H. (1996) 'Assessment of upper-extremity function in children with spastic diplegia before and after selective dorsal rhizotomy.' *Developmental Medicine and Child Neurology*, **38**, 967–975.

—— —— Harris, G.E., Piatt, J.H. Jr, Aiona, M.D., Sussman, M.D. (2002) 'Objective measurement of muscle strength in children with spastic diplegia after selective dorsal rhizotomy.' *Archives of Physical Medicine and Rehabilitation*, **83**, 454–460.

—— —— Pierce, R., Piatt, J. H. Jr, Aiona, M.D. (1997) 'Developmental skills of children with spastic diplegia: functional and qualitative changes after selective dorsal rhizotomy.' *Archives of Physical Medicine and Rehabilitation*, **78**, 946–951.

—— —— Piatt, J.H., Jr, Aiona, M.D., Sussman, M.D. (2004) 'Selective dorsal rhizotomy versus orthopedic surgery: a multidimensional assessment of outcome efficacy: *Archives of Physical Medicine and Rehabilitation*, **85**, 457–465.

Bullard, D.C., Knight, S.E. (Eds) (1981) *Sexuality and Physical Disability.* St Louis: C.V. Mosby.

Bumin, G., Kayihan, H. (2001) 'Effectiveness of two different sensory-integration programmes for children with spastic diplegia.' *Disability Rehabilitation*, **15**, 394–399.

Burnett, C.N., Johnson, E.W. (1971) 'Development of gait in childhood. Parts I and II.' *Developmental Medicine and Child Neurology*, **13**, 196–206, 297–315.

Burtner, P.A., Woollacott, M.H., Qualls, C. (1999) 'Stance balance control with orthoses in a group of children with spastic cerebral palsy.' *Developmental Medicine and Child Neurology*, **41**, 748–575.

—— McMain, M.P., Crowe, T.K. (2002) 'Survey of occupational therapy practitioners in southwestern schools: assessments used and preparation of students for school-based practice.' *Physical and Occupational Therapy in Pediatrics*, **22**, 25–39.

Burygina, A.D., Andreev, M.K., Kukhnina, T.M., Bogdanova, L.A. (1993) 'Changes in the clinical electromyographic indices of patients with hyperkinetic form of infantile cerebral palsy and their dynamics during combined sanatorium-health resort treatment including transcerebral exposure to an ultra high-frequency electrical field.' *Voprosy Kurtologii, Fizioterapii I Lechebnoi Fizicheskoi Kultury*, **5**, 42–46. (Russian.)

Butler, C. (1998) *AACPDM Methodology for Developing Evidence Tables and Reviewing Treatment Outcomes.* http://www.aacpdm.org

—— Okamoto, G., McKay, T. (1983) 'Powered mobility for very young disabled children.' *Developmental Medicine and Child Neurology*, **25**, 472–474.

—— Goldstein, M., Chambers, H., Harris, S., Adams, R., Darrah, J. (1999) 'Evaluating research in developmental disabilities: a conceptual framework for review treatment outcomes.' *Developmental Medicine and Child Neurology*, **41**, 55–59.

—— Campbell, S. (2000) 'Evidence of the effects of intrathecal baclofen for spastic and dystonic cerebral palsy.' *Developmental Medicine and Child Neurology*, 42, 634–645.

—— Darrah, J. (2001) 'Effects of neurodevelopmental treatment (NDT) for cerebral palsy: an AACPDM evidence report.' *Developmental Medicine and Child Neurology*, 43, 778–790.

Butler, P.B., Thompson, N., Major, R.E. (1992) 'Improvement in walking performance of children with cerebral palsy: preliminary results.' *Developmental Medicine and Child Neurology*, 34, 567–576.

Cahan, L.D., Kundi, M.S., McPherson, D., Starr, A., Peacock, W. (1987) 'Electrophysiologic studies in selective dorsal rhizotomy for spasticity in children with cerebral palsy.' *Applied Neurophysiology*, 50, 459–462.

—— Adams, J.M., Perry, J., Beeler, L.M. (1990) 'Instrumented gait analysis after selective dorsal rhizotomy.' *Developmental Medicine and Child Neurology*, 32, 1037–1043.

Calderon-Gonzalez, R., Tijerina-Cantu, E., Maldonado-Rodriguez, C. (1989) 'Conductive education in integral rehabilitation of patients with cerebral palsy.' *Boletin Medico del Hospital Infantil de Mexico*, 46, 265–271. (Spanish.)

—— Calderon-Sepulveda, R., Rincon-Reyes, M., Garcia-Ramierez, J., Mino-Arango, E. (1994) 'Botulinum toxin A in management of cerebral palsy.' *Pediatric Neurology*, 10, 284–288.

Campbell, J., Ball, J. (1978) 'Energetics of walking in cerebral palsy.' *Orthopedic Clinics of North America*, 9, 374–377.

Campbell, S.K. (1990) 'Proceedings of the consensus conference on the efficacy of physical therapy in the management of cerebral palsy.' *Pediatric Physical Therapy*, 2, 125, 176.

—— (1992) 'Expected outcomes of physical therapy for children with cerebral palsy: the evidence and the challenge.' *In* Sussman, M.D. (Ed.) *The Diplegic Child.* Rosemont, IL: American Academy of Orthopaedic Surgeons, pp. 221–227.

Campos da Paz Jr, A. (1980) 'Management of cerebral palsy in Brazil.' *Lecture, Children's Hospital at Stanford, Palo Alto, CA.*

—— Nomura, A.N., Braga, L.W., Burnett, S.M. (1984) 'Speculations on cerebral palsy.' *Journal of Bone and Joint Surgery*, 2, 283. (Abstract.)

Carlsen, P.N. (1975) 'Comparison of two occupational therapy approaches for treating the young cerebral-palsied child.' *American Journal of Occupational Therapy*, 29, 267–272.

Carlson, J.M., Winter, R. (1978) 'The Gillette sitting support orthosis.' *Orthotics and Prosthetics*, 4, 35–45.

Carmick, J. (1993 a) 'Clinical use of neuromuscular electrical stimulation for children with cerebral palsy, part I: lower extremity.' *Physical Therapy*, 73, 505–513.

—— (1993 b) 'Clinical use of neuromuscular electrical stimulation for children with cerebral palsy, part 2: upper extremity.' *Physical Therapy*, 73, 514–522.

Carrelet, P., Bollini, G., Mancini, J., Chabrol, B. (2002) 'Treatment of the motor cerebral palsy child with botulinum toxin A: mode of action, injection places in management.' *Archives de Pédiatrie*, 9, 928–933. (French.)

Carrington, E. (1978) 'A seating position for a cerebral-palsied child.' *American Journal of Occupational Therapy*, 32, 179–181.

Carroll, K.L., Moore, K.R., Stevens, P.M. (1998) 'Orthopedic procedures after rhizotomy.' *Journal of Pediatric Orthopaedics*, 18, 69–74.

Cerny, K. (1978) 'Energetics of walking and wheelchair propulsion in paraplegic patients.' *Orthopedic Clinics of North America*, 9, 370–372.

Chait, L.A., Kessler, E. (1979) 'An antidrooling operation in cerebral palsy.' *South African Medical Journal*, 56, 676–678.

Cherng, R.J., Su, F.C., Chen, J.J., Kuan, T.S. (1999) 'Performance of static balance in children with spastic diplegic cerebral palsy under altered sensory environments.' *American Journal of Physical Medicine and Rehabilitation*, 78, 336–343.

Cherpin, J., Minaire, P., Flores, J.L., Weber, D. (1985) *Approche Fonctionelle de la Population Française. Phase Exploratoire et Construction du Protocols Experimental. Rapport final.'* Paris, France: Institute de Réchreche des Transports.

Chicoine, M.R., Park, T.S., Vogler, G.P., Kaufman, B.A. (1996) 'Predictors of the ability to walk after selective dorsal rhizotomy in children with cerebral palsy.' *Neurosurgery*, 38, 711–714.

—— —— Kaufman, B.A. (1997) 'Selective dorsal rhizotomy and rates of orthopedic surgery in children with spastic cerebral palsy.' *Journal of Neurosurgery*, 86, 34–39.

Chutorian, A.B., Root, L. (1994) 'Management of spasticity in children with botulinum-A toxin.' *International Pediatrics*, 9 (Suppl. 1), 35–43.

Coffey, R.J., Cahill, D., Steers, W., Park, T.S. and 16 others (1993) 'Intrathecal baclofen for intractable spasticity of spinal origin: results of long-term multicenter study.' *Journal of Neurosurgery*, 78, 226–232.

Cohen, A.R., Webster, H.C. (1991) 'How selective is selective posterior rhizotomy?' *Surgical Neurology*, 35, 267–272.

Cohen, M.J., Brick, H.G., Taft, L.T. (1970) 'Some considerations for evaluating the Doman–Delacato "patterning" method.' *Pediatrics*, 45, 302–314.

Cohen, P., Mustacchi, P. (1966) 'Survival in cerebral palsy.' *Journal of the American Medical Association*, 195, 642–644.

—— Kohn, J.G. (1979) 'Follow-up study of patients with cerebral palsy.' *Western Journal of Medicine*, 130, 6–11.

Comella, C.L., Shannon, K.M., Jaglin, J. (1998) 'Extensor truncal dystonia: successful treatment with botulinum toxin injections.' *Movement Disorders*, 13, 552–555.

Committee on Prosthetic Research and Development, National Research Council (1973) '*The child with an orthopaedic disability: his orthotic needs and how to meet them.*' Report of a Workshop, Washington, DC: National Academy of Sciences.

Conrad, L., Bleck, E.E. (1980) 'Augmented auditory feedback in the treatment of equinus gait in children.' *Developmental Medicine and Child Neurology*, 22, 713–718.

—— Benick, R., Carnehl, J.H., Hohne, J., Meinck, H.M. (1983) 'Pathophysiological aspects of human locomotion.' *Advances in Neurology*, 39, 717–726.

Cooper, I.S., Riklan, M., Amin, I., Waltz, J.M., Cullinan, T. (1976) 'Chronic cerebellar stimulation in cerebral palsy.' *Neurology*, 26, 744–753.

Cooper, R.R. (1972) 'Alterations during immobilization and degeneration of skeletal muscle in cats.' *Journal of Bone and Joint Surgery*, 54A, 919–953.

Coplan, J. (1982) 'Parental estimate of child's developmental level in a high-risk population.' *American Journal Diseases of Children*, 136, 101–104.

Corry, I.S., Cosgrove, A.P., Walsh, E.G., McClean, D., Graham, H.K. (1997) 'Botulinum toxin A in the hemiplegic upper limb: a double-blind trial.' *Developmental Medicine and Child Neurology*, 39, 491–492.

—— —— Duffy, C.M., McNeill, S., Taylor, T.C., Graham, H.K. (1998) 'Botulinum toxin A compared with stretching casts in the treatment of spastic equinus: a randomized clinical trial.' *Journal of Pediatric Orthopaedics*, 18, 304–311.

—— Taylor, T.C., Graham, H.K. (1999) 'Botulinum toxin A in hamstring spasticity.' *Gait Posture*, 10, 206–210.

Cosgrove, A.P., Graham, H.K. (1994) 'Botulinum toxin A prevents the development of contractures in the hereditary spastic mouse.' *Developmental Medicine and Child Neurology*, 36, 379–385.

—— Corry, I.S., Graham, H.K. (1994) 'Botulinum toxin in the management of lower limb in cerebral palsy.' *Developmental Medicine and Child Neurology*, 36, 386–396.

Cottalorda, J., Gautheron, V., Metton, G., Charmet, E., Chavier, Y. (2000) 'Toe-walking in children younger than six years with cerebral palsy. The contribution of serial corrective casts.' *Journal of Bone and Joint Surgery*, 82B, 541–544.

Cotton, E. (1974) 'Improvement in motor function with the use of conductive education.' *Developmental Medicine and Child Neurology*, 16, 637–643.

—— (1977) 'A bedroom routine for the cerebral palsied child.' *Study Group on Integrating Multiply Handicapped Children, St Mary's College, Durham, England.* London: Spastics Society Medical Education and Information Unit.

Craig, C.L., Sosnoff, F., Zimbler, S. (1984) 'Seating in cerebral palsy—a possible advance.' *Orthopaedic Transactions*, 8, 456. (Abstract.)

Craig, J.J., Mathias, A. (1977) 'Forest Town boot.' *Physical Therapy*, 57, 918–920.

Crenshaw, S., Herzog, R., Castagono, P., Richards, J., Miller, F., Michaloski, D. Ped., Moran, E. (2000) 'The efficacy of tone-reducing features in orthotics on the gait of children with spastic diplegia.' *Journal of Pediatric Orthopaedics*, 20, 210–216.

Crawford, K., Karol, L.A., Herring, J.A. (1996) 'Severe lumbar lordosis after dorsal rhizotomy.' *Journal of Pediatric Orthopaedics*, 16, 336–339.

Cristarella, M.C. (1975) 'Comparison of straddling and sitting apparatus for the spastic cerebral palsied child.' *American Journal of Occupational Therapy*, 29, 273–276.

Crothers, B., Paine, R.S. (1959) *The Natural History of Cerebral Palsy.* Cambridge, MA: Harvard University Press.

Dahlin, M., Knutsson, E., Nergardh, A. (1993) 'Treatment of spasticity in children with low dose benzodiazepine.' *Journal of Neurological Science*, **117**, 54–60.

Dali, C., Hansen, F.J., Pedersen, S.A., Skov, L., Hilden, J., Bjornskov I., Strandberg, C., Christensen J., Haugsted, U., Herbst, G., Lyskjaer, U. (2002) 'Threshold electrical stimulation (TES) in ambulant children with CP: a randomized double-blind placebo-controlled clinical trial.' *Developmental Medicine and Child Neurology*, **44**, 364–369.

Damiano, D.L., Vaughn, C.L., Abel, M.F. (1995a) 'Muscle response to heavy resistance exercise in children with spastic cerebral palsy.' *Developmental Medicine and Child Neurology*, **37**, 731–739.

—— Kelly, L.E., Vaughn, C.L. (1995b) 'Effects of quadriceps femoris muscle strengthening on crouch gait in children with spastic diplegia.' *Physical Therapy*, **75**, 658–667.

—— Abel, M.F. (1998) 'Functional outcomes of strength training in spastic cerebral palsy.' *Archives of Physical Medicine and Rehabilitation*, **79**, 119–125.

Davies, E. (Ed.) (1976a) 'The beginning of "modern physiotherapy".' *Physical Therapy*, **56**, 15–21.

—— (Ed.) (1976b) 'Infantile paralysis: pioneers in treatment.' *Physical Therapy*, **56**, 42–49.

Davis, K. (1976) 'The changing family in industrial societies.' Reprint from Jackson, R.C., Morton, J. (Eds.) *Family Health Care: Health Promotion and Illness Care*. Berkeley, CA: School of Public Health, University of California.

Davis, R. (2000) 'Cerebellar stimulation for cerebral palsy spasticity, function, and seizures.' *Archives of Medical Research*, **31**, 290–299.

—— Barolat-Romana, G., Engle, H. (1980) 'Chronic cerebellar stimulation for cerebral palsy—5 year study.' *Acta Neurochirurgica* (Suppl. 30), 317–322.

—— Schulman, J., Delehanty, A. (1987) 'Cerebellar stimulation in cerebral palsy—a double blind study.' *Acta Neurochirugia Supplement (Wein)*, **39**, 126–128.

Deletis, V., Vodusek, D.B., Abbott, R., Epstein, F.J., Turnoff, H. (1992) 'Intraoperative monitoring of the dorsal sacral roots: minimizing the risk of iatrogenic micturition disorders.' *Neurosurgery*, **30**, 72–75.

Delplanque, B., Lagueny, A., Flurin, A., Arnaud, C., Pedespan, J.J., Fontan, D., Pontallier, J.R. (2002) 'Botulinum toxin in the management of spastic hip adductors in non-ambulatory cerebral palsy children.' *Revue de Chirurge Orthopédique Réparatrice de l'Appareil Moteur*, **88**, 279–285.

Denhoff, E. (1981) 'Current status of infant stimulation or enrichment programs for children with developmental disabilities.' *Pediatrics*, **67**, 32–37.

Denislic, M., Meh, D. (1995) 'Botulinum toxin in the treatment of cerebral palsy.' *Neuropediatrics*, **26**, 249–252.

de Pavia, A., Meunier, F.A., Molgo, J., Aoki, K.R., Dolly, J.O. (1999) 'Functional repair of motor endplates after botulinum neurotoxin type A poisoning: biphasic switch of synaptic activity between nerve sprouts and their parent terminals.' *Proceedings of the National Academy of Sciences of the USA*, **96**, 3200–3205.

De Salles, A.A. (1996) 'Role of stereotaxis in the treatment of cerebral palsy.' *Journal of Child Neurology*, **11** (Suppl. 1), S43–50.

Desloovere, K., Molenaers, G., Jonkers, I., De Cat, J., De Borre, L., Nijs, J., Eyssen, M., Pauwels, P., De Cock, P. (2001) 'A randomized study of combined botulinum toxin type A and casting in the ambulant child with cerebral palsy using objective outcome measures.' *European Journal of Neurology*, **8** (Suppl. 5), 75–87.

Detrembleur, C., Lejeune, T.M., Renders, A., Van Den Bergh, P.Y. (2002) 'Botulinum toxin and short-term electrical stimulation in the treatment of equinus in cerebral palsy.' *Movement Disorders*, **17**, 162–169.

Doman, R.J., Spitz, E.B., Zucman, E., Delacato, C., Doman, G. (1960) 'Children with severe brain injuries—results of treatment.' *Journal of the American Medical Association*, **174**, 257–262.

Duchenne, G. B. (1866) *Physiology of Motion*. (Translated by Kaplan, E.B., 1959.) Philadelphia: W.B. Saunders.

Dudgeon, B. J., Libby, A. K., McLaughlin, J. F., Hays, R. M., Bjornson, K. F., Roberts, T. S. (1994) 'Prospective measurement of functional changes after selective dorsal rhizotomy.' *Archives of Physical Medicine and Rehabilitation*, **75**, 46–53.

Duncan, W.R. (1960) 'Tonic reflexes of the foot.' *Journal of Bone and Joint Surgery*, **42A**, 859–868.

—— Mott, D.H. (1983) 'Foot reflexes and use of the "inhibitive cast".' *Foot and Ankle*, **4**, 145–148.

Eames, N. W., Baker, R., Hill, N., Graham, K., Taylor, T., Cosgrove, A. (1999)

'The effect of botulinum toxin A on gastrocnemius length: magnitude and duration of response.' *Developmental Medicine and Child Neurology*, **41**, 226–232.

Eiser, C., Patterson, D. (1983) '"Slugs and snails and puppy-dog tails"—children's ideas about the inside of their bodies.' *Child Care Health Development*, **4**, 233–240.

Eliasson, A.C., Krumlinde-Sundholm, L., Rosblad, B., Beckung, E. Arner, M., Ohrvall, A.M., Rosenbaum, P. (2006) 'The Manual Ability Classification System (MACS) for children with cerebral palsy: scale development and evidence of validity and reliability.' *Developmental Medicine and Child Neurology*, **48**, 549–554.

Ellenberg, J.H., Nelson, K.B. (1981) 'Early recognition of infants at high risk for cerebral palsy: examination at four months.' *Developmental Medicine and Child Neurology*, **23**, 705–716.

Engsberg, J.R., Olree, K.S., Ross, R.A., Park, T.S. (1998) 'Spasticity and strength changes as a function of selective dorsal rhizotomy.' *Journal of Neurosurgery*, **88**, 1020–1026.

—— Ross, S.A., Park, T.S. (1999) 'Changes in ankle spasticity and strength following selective dorsal rhizotomy and physical therapy for spastic cerebral palsy.' *Journal of Neurosurgery*, **91**, 727–732.

—— Wagner, J.M., Park, T.S. (2002) 'Changes in hip spasticity and strength following selective dorsal rhizotomy and physical therapy for spastic cerebral palsy.' *Developmental Medicine and Child Neurology*, **44**, 220–226.

—— Ross, S.A., Collins, D.R., Park, T.S. (2006) 'Effect of selective dorsal rhizotomy in the treatment of children with cerebral palsy.' *Journal of Neurosurgery*, **105** (suppl. 1), 8–15.

Fabry, G., Liu, X.C., Molenaers, G. (1999) 'Gait pattern in patients with spastic diplegic cerebral palsy who underwent staged operations.' *Journal of Pediatric Orthopaedics B*, **8**, 33–38.

Fasano, V.A., Barolat-Romana, G., Ivaldi, A., Sguazzi, A. (1976) 'La radiotomie postérieure fonctionelle dans le traitement de la spasticité cérébrale. Premières observations sur la stimulation electrique peroperatorie des raciens postérieures, et leur utilisation dans le choix des racines à sectionner.' *Neurochirurgie*, **22**, 23–34.

—— Broggi, G., Barolat-Romano, G., Sguazzi, A. (1978) 'Surgical treatment of spasticity in cerebral palsy.' *Childs Brain*, **4**, 289–305.

—— Zeme, S. (1988) 'Intraoperative electrical stimulation for functional posterior rhizotomy.' *Scandinavian Journal of Rehabilitation Medicine (Suppl.)*, **17**, 149–154.

Fay, T. (1958) 'Neuromuscular reflex therapy for spastic disorders.' *Journal of Florida Medical Association*, **44**, 1234–1240.

—— (1977) 'The neurophysical aspects of therapy in cerebral palsy.' *In* Payton, O.D., Hirt, S., Newton, R.A. (Eds) *Neurophysiological Approaches to Therapeutic Exercise*. Philadelphia: F.A. Davis, pp. 237–246.

Fehlings, D., Rang, M., Glazier, J., Steele, C. (2001) 'Botulinum toxin type A injections in the spastic upper extremity of children with hemiplegia: child characteristics that predict a positive outcome.' *European Journal of Neurology*, **8** (Suppl. 5), 145–159.

Feldkamp, M. (1979) 'Motor goals of therapeutic horseback riding for cerebral palsied children.' *Rehabilitation*, **18**, 56–61.

Ferguson, B.F. (1979) 'Preparing young children for hospitalization: a comparison of two methods.' *Pediatrics*, **64**, 656–664.

Fernandez, J.E., Pitetti, K.H. (1993) 'Training of ambulatory individuals with cerebral palsy.' *Archives of Physical Medicine and Rehabilitation*, **74**, 468–472.

Ferry, P.C. (1981) 'On growing new neurons. Are early intervention programs effective?' *Pediatrics*, **67**, 38–44.

Fetters, L. (1991) 'Measurement and treatment in cerebral palsy: an argument for a new approach.' *Physical Therapy*, **71**, 244–247.

Fisher, S.V., Patterson, R.P. (1981) 'Energy cost of ambulation with crutches.' *Archives of Physical Medicine and Rehabilitation*, **62**, 250–256.

Fisk, J.R., Supam, T.J. (1997) 'Cerebral palsy.' *In* Goldberg, B., Hsu, J.D. (Eds) *Atlas of Orthoses and Assistive Devices, 3rd edn*. St Louis, Mosby-Year Book, pp. 536–538.

Flett, P.J., Stern, L.M., Waddy, H., Connell, T.M., Seeger, J.D., Gibson, S.K. (1999) 'Botulinum toxin A versus fixed cast stretching for dynamic tightness in cerebral palsy.' *Journal of Pediatrics and Child Health*, **35**, 71–77.

Foerster, O. (1913) 'On the indications and results of excision of the posterior spinal roots in men.' *Surgery Gynecology and Obstetrics*, **16**, 463–474.

Ford, L.F., Bleck, E.E., Aptekar, R.G., Collins, F.J., Stevick, D. (1976) 'Efficacy of dantrolene sodium in the treatment of spastic cerebral palsy.' *Developmental Medicine and Child Neurology*, **18**, 770–783.

Fowler, E.G., Ho, T.W., Nwigwe, A.I, Dorey, F.J. (2001) 'The effect of quadriceps femoris muscle strengthening exercises on spasticity in children with cerebral palsy.' *Physical Therapy*, **81**, 1215–1223.

Frankel, A.S., Kramer, F.M. (1998) 'Chemical browlift.' *Archives of Otolaryngology, Head and Neck Surgery*, **124**, 321–323.

Freeman, R.D. (1970) 'Psychiatric problems in adolescents with cerebral palsy.' *Developmental Medicine and Child Neurology*, **12**, 64–70.

Freud, S. (1893) 'Les diplégies cérébrales infantiles.' *Revue Neurologique*, **1**, 177–183.

Friedman, A., Diamond, M., Johnston, M.V., Daffner, C. (2000) 'Effects of botulinum toxin A on upper limb spasticity in children with cerebral palsy.' *American Journal of Physical Medicine and Rehabilitation*, **79**, 53–59.

Fulford, G.E., Cairns, T.P., Sloan, Y. (1982) 'Sitting problems of children with cerebral palsy.' *Developmental Medicine and Child Neurology*, **24**, 48–53.

Gage, J.R. (1991) *Gait Analysis in Cerebral Palsy*. London: Mac Keith Press with Blackwell Scientific Publications; New York, Cambridge University Press, p. 82.

Gajdosik, C., Circirello, N. (2001) 'Secondary conditions of the musculoskeletal system in adolescents and adults with cerebral palsy.' *Physical and Occupational Therapy in Pediatrics*, **21**, 49–68.

Garcia-Navarro, M.E., Tacoronte, M., Sarduy, I., Abdo, A., Galvizu, R., Torres, A., Leal, E. (2000) 'Influence of early stimulation in cerebral palsy.' *Revista de Neurologia*, **31**, 716–719. (Spanish.)

Garcia-Ruiz, P.J., Pascual-Pascual, I., Sanchez-Bernardos, V. (2000) 'Progressive response ot botulinum A toxin in cerebral palsy.' *European Journal of Neurology*, **7**, 191–193.

Garrett, A.L., Lister, M., Drennan, J. (1966) 'New concept in bracing for cerebral palsy.' *Physical Therapy*, **46**, 728–733.

Gaskill, S.J., Wilkins, K, Marlin, A.E. (1992) 'Selective posterior rhizotomy to treat spasticity associated with cerebral palsy: a critical review.' *Texas Medicine*, **88**, 68–71.

Geiduscheck, J.M., Haberkern, C.M.N., McLaughlin, J.F., Jacobson, L.E., Hays, R.M., Roberts, T.S. (1994) 'Pain management for children following selective dorsal rhizotomy.' *Canadian Journal of Anesthesia*, **41**, 492–496.

Gerszten, P.C., Albright, A.L., Barry, M.D. (1997) 'Effect on ambulation of continuous intrathecal baclofen infusion.' *Pediatric Neurosurgery*, **27**, 40–44.

—— —— Johnstone, G.F. (1998) 'Intrathecal baclofen infusion and subsequent orthopedic surgery in patients with spastic cerebral palsy.' *Journal of Neurosurgery*, **88**, 1009–1013.

Gibson, J.N., Smith, K. Renni, M.J. (1988) 'Prevention of disuse muscle atrophy by means of electrical stimulation: maintenance of protein synthesis.' *Lancet*, **ii (8614)**, 767–770.

Gillette, H. (1969) *Systems of Therapy in Cerebral Palsy*. Springfield, Ill.: C.C. Thomas.

Gilmartin, R., Bruce, D., Storrs, B.B., Abbott, R., Krach, L., Ward, J., Bloom, K., Brooks, W.H., Johnson, D.L., Madsen, J.R., McLaughlin, J.F., Nadell, J. (2000), 'Intrathecal baclofen for management of spastic cerebral palsy: multicenter trial.' *Journal of Child Neurology*, **15**, 71–77.

Giuliani, C.A. (1991) 'Dorsal rhizotomy for children with cerebral palsy: support for concepts of motor control.' *Physical Therapy*, **71**, 248–259.

Goldberg, M.J. (1991) 'Measuring outcomes in cerebral palsy.' *Journal of Pediatric Orthopaedics*, **5**, 683–685.

Golden, G.S. (1980) 'Nonstandard therapies in the developmental disabilities.' *American Journal of Diseases of Children*, **134**, 487–491.

Goldkamp, O. (1984) 'Treatment effectiveness in cerebral palsy.' *Archives of Physical Medicine and Rehabilitation*, **65**, 232–234.

Gollnitz, G., Schulz-Wulf, G. (1973) 'Rhythmisch-pscyhomotrische Musiktherapie. Eine gezielter Behgandrung entwicklungsgeschadigeter Kinder und Jungendlicher.' *Sammiung Zwangloser Abhandlungen auz dem Gebiete der Psychiatrie und Neurologie*, **44**, 1–112.

Gooch, J.L., Walker, M.L. (1996) 'Spinal stenosis after total lumbar laminectomy for selective dorsal rhizotomy.' *Pediatric Neurosurgery*, **25**, 28–30.

Gormley, M.E., Gaebler-Spira, D., Delgado, M.R. (2001) 'Use of botulinum toxin type A in pediatric patients with cerebral palsy: a three-center retrospective chart review.' *Journal of Neurology*, **16**, 113–118.

Gornall, P., Hitchcock, E., Kirkland, I.S. (1975) 'Stereotaxic neurosurgery in the management of cerebral palsy.' *Developmental Medicine and Child Neurology*, **17**, 279–286.

Graham, H.K., Aoki, K.R., Autti-Ramo, I., Boyd, R.N., Delgado, M.R., Gaebler-Spira, D.J., Gormley, M.E., Guyer, B.M., Heinen, F.,Holton, A.F., Matthews, D., Molenaers, G., Mottoa, F., Garcia Ruiz, J., Wissel, J.

(2000) 'Recommendations for the use of botulinum toxin type A in the management of cerebral palsy.' *Gait Posture*, **11**, 67–79.

—— Boyd, R.N., Fehlings, D. (2003) Letter to the editor re Wasiak *et al.* (2002) 'Does intramuscular botulinum toxin A injection improve upper-limb function in children with hemiplegic cerebral palsy?' *Medical Journal of Australia*, **178**, 95.

Graubert, C., Song, K.M., McLaughlin, J.F., Bjornson, K.F. (2000) 'Changes in gait at 1 year post-selective dorsal rhizotomy: results of a prospective randomized study.' *Journal of Pediatric Orthopaedics*, **20**, 496–500.

Graves, P. (1995) 'Therapy methods for cerebral palsy.' *Journal of Paediatrics and Child Health*, **31**, 24–28.

Greene, W.B., Dietz, F.R., Goldberg, M.J., Gross, R.H., Miller, F., Sussman, M.D. (1991) 'Rapid progression of hip subluxation in cerebral palsy after selective posterior rhizotomy.' *Journal of Pediatric Orthopaedics*, **11**, 494–497.

Greiner, B.M., Czerniecki, J.M., Deitz, J.C. (1993) 'Gait parameters of children with spastic diplegia: a comparison of effects of posterior and anterior walkers.' *Archives of Physical Medicine and Rehabilitation*, **74**, 381–385.

Griffin, P.P., Wheelhouse, W.W., Shiavi, R., Bass, W. (1977) 'Habitual toe-walkers.' *Journal of Bone and Joint Surgery*, **59A**, 97–101.

Gros, C. (1979) 'Spasticity: clinical classification and surgical treatment.' *Advances and Technical Standards in Neurosurgery*, **6**, 55–97.

—— Ouknine, G., Vlahovitch, B., Frerebeau, P. (1967) 'La radiotomie sélective postérieure dans le traitement neurochiurgical de l'hypertonie pyramidale.' *Neurochiurgie*, **13**, 505–518.

Gul, S.M., Steinbok, P., McLeod, K. (1999) 'Long-term outcome after selective posterior rhizotomy in children with spastic cerebral palsy.' *Pediatric Neurosurgery (Switzerland)*, **31**, 84–95.

Gutman, G.M., Herbert, C.P., Brown, S.R. (1977) 'Feldenkrais versus convential exercises for the elderly.' *Journal of Gerontology*, **32**, 562–572.

Hagbarth, K.E., Eklund, G. (1977) 'The muscle vibrators—a useful tool in neurological therapeutic work.' *In* Payton, O.D., Hirt, S., Newton, R.A. (Eds) *Scientific Basis for Neurophysiologic Approaches to Therapeutic Exercise*. Philadelphia: F.A. Davis, pp. 133–145.

Hallett, M. (1999) 'One man's poison—clinical applications of botulinum toxin.' *New England Journal of Medicine*, **8**, 118–120.

Hamilton, M.S. (1984) 'Centrally acting muscle relaxants.' *Drug Information News Letter*. Stanford, California: Stanford University Hospital.

Hammer, M.L., Lindgren, R., Berg, G.E., Moller, C.G., Niklasson, M.K. (1996) 'Effects of hormonal replacement therapy on the postural balance among postmenopausal women.' *Obstetrics and Gynecology*, **88**, 955–960.

Hanks, S.B., MacFarlane, D.W. (1969) 'Device for heel-cord stretching and gait training.' *Physical Therapy*, **49**, 380–381.

Hare, N. (1977) 'Abduction pants.' *Physiotherapy*, **63**, 227.

Hari, M., Tillemans, T. (1984) 'Conductive education.' *In* Scrutton, D. (Ed.) *Management of the Motor Disorders of Children with Cerebral Palsy. Clinics in Developmental Medicine, No. 90*. London: Spastics International Medical Publications with Blackwell Scientific; Philadelphia: J.B. Lippincott.

Harris, G.F., Millar, E.A., Hemmy, D.C., Lochner, R.C. (1993) 'Neuroelectric stimulation in cerebral palsy: long-term quantitative assessment.' *Stereotactic Functional Neurosurgery*, **61**, 49–59.

Harrison, A. (1977) 'Augmented feedback training of motor control in cerebral palsy.' *Developmental Medicine and Child Neurology*, **19**, 75–78.

Harryman, S. (1992) 'Rationale of physical therapy in the management of children with spastic diplegia.' *In* Sussman, M.D. (Ed.) *The Diplegic Child*. Rosemont, IL: American Academy of Orthopaedic Surgeons, pp. 209–220.

Harvard Women's Health Watch (1998) '"Toxic" facelifts.' *Harvard Women's Health Watch*, **6**, 7.

Hassakis, P.C. (1974) 'Outcomes of cerebral palsy patients.' *Paper presented at the Annual Meeting of the American Academy for Cerebral Palsy, Denver, CO.*

Hayashi, M. (1995) 'The effect of early treatment for children with cerebral palsy in cooperation with city health welfare offices.' *No To Hattatsu*, **27**, 480–486. (Japanese.)

—— Arizono, Y. (1999) 'Experience of very early Vojta therapy in two infants with severe perinatal hypoxic encephalopathy.' *No To Hattatsu*, **31**, 535–541. (Japanese.)

—— Uehara, S., Saito, K. (2001) 'Developmental consultation conducted by Yokohama Rehabilitation Center at health welfare offices—combination of early impairment detection and support nursing.' *No To Hattatsu*, **33**, 505–510. (Japanese.)

Hayes, N.K., Burns, Y.R. (1970) 'Discussion on use of weight-bearing plasters in reduction of hypertonicity.' *Australian Journal of Physiotherapy*, **16**, 108–117.

Hays, R.M., McLaughlin, J.F., Bjornson, K.F., Stephens, K., Roberts, T.S., Price, R. (1998) 'Electrophysiological monitoring during selective dorsal rhizotomy, and spasticity and GMFM performance.' *Developmental Medicine and Child Neurology*, **40**, 233–238.

Hazlewood, M.E., Brown, J.K. Rowe, P.J. Salter, P.M. (1994) 'The use of therapeutic electrical stimulation in the treatment of hemiplegic cerebral palsy.' *Developmental Medicine and Child Neurology*, **36**, 661–673.

Hebestreit, H., Bar-Or, O. (2001) 'Exercise and the child born prematurely.' *Sports Medicine*, **31**, 591–599.

Heckman, M., Schaller, M., Ceballos-Baumran, A., Plewig, G. (1997) 'Botulinum beyond wrinkles.' *Dermatological Surgery*, **23**, 1221–1222.

Heim, R.C., Park, T.S., Vogler, G.P., Kaufman, B.A., Noetzel, M.J., Ortman, M.R. (1995) 'Changes in hip migration after selective dorsal rhizotomy for spastic quadriplegia in cerebral palsy.' *Journal of Neurosurgery*, **82**, 567–571.

Heinen, F., Wissel, J., Philipsen, A., Mall, V., Leititis, J.U., Schenkel, A., Stucker, R., Korinthenberg, R. (1997), 'Interventional neuropediatrics: treatment of dystonia and spastic muscular activity with botulinum toxin A.' *Neuropediatrics*, **28**, 307–313.

Helander, E., Mendis, P., Nelson, G. (1983) *Training Disabled People in the Community*. Geneva: World Health Organization.

Heller, A., Rafman, S., Zvagulis, I., Pless, I. V. (1985) 'Birth defects and psychosocial adjustment.' *American Journal of Diseases of Children*, **139**, 257–263.

Hengst, C. (1976) 'Sport therapy and rehabilitation—especially riding therapy.' *Zeitschrift für Orthopädie*, **114**, 690–691. (German.)

Herbison, B.J., Jaweed, M.M., Ditunno, J.F. (1978) 'Muscle fiber atrophy after cast immobilization in the rat.' *Archives of Physical Medicine and Rehabilitation*, **59**, 301–305.

Hermann, R.P., Phalangas, A.C., Mahoney, R.M., Alexander, M.A. (1999) 'Powered feeding devices: an evaluation of three models.' *Archives of Physical Medicine and Rehabilitation*, **80**, 1237–1242.

Hill, A.E. (1990) 'Conductive education for physically handicapped children: parental expectations and experience.' *Ulster Medical Journal*, **59**, 41–45.

Hinojosa, J., Anderson, J. (1991) 'Mothers' perceptions of home treatment programs for their preschool children with cerebral palsy.' *American Journal of Occupational Therapy*, **45**, 273–279.

Hodgkinson, I., Berard, C., Jindrich, M.L., Sindou, M., Mertens, P., Berard, J. (1997) 'Selective dorsal rhizotomy in children with cerebral palsy. Results in 18 cases at one year postoperatively.' *Stereotactic and Functional Neurosurgery*, **69**, 268–273.

Hoffer, M.M., Feiwell, E., Perry, J., Bonnett, C. (1973) 'Functional ambulation in patients with myelomeningocele.' *Journal of Bone and Joint Surgery*, **55A**, 137–148.

—— Koffman, M. (1980) 'Cerebral palsy: the first three years.' *Clinical Orthopaedics and Related Research*, **151**, 222–227.

Hollis, L.I. (1974) 'Skinnerian occupational therapy.' *American Journal of Occupational Therapy*, **28**, 208–213.

Holm, V.A. (1983) 'A western version of the Doman–Delacato treatment of patterning for developmental disabilities.' *Western Journal of Medicine*, **139**, 553–556.

—— Harthun-Smith, L., Tada, W.L. (1983) 'Infant walkers and cerebral palsy.' *American Journal of Diseases of Children*, **137**, 1189–1190.

Holt, K.G., Ratcliffe, R., Jeng, S.F. (1999) 'Head stability in walking in children with cerebral palsy and in children and adults without neurological impairment.' *Physical Therapy*, **79**, 1153–1162.

Holte, R.N. (1980) *Final Report: A Modular System for Seating the Multiply Handicapped Child*. Project 6607-1181-51, National Health Research and Development Program, Ottawa, Canada: Health and Welfare.

Hong, Y., Li, J.X., Robinson, P.D. (2000) 'Balance control, flexibility, and cardiorespiratory fitness among older Tai Chi practitioners.' *British Journal of Sports Medicine*, **34**, 29–34.

Horiguchi, T., Kaga, M., Uno, A., Inagaki, M., Akiyama, C. (1999) 'Mental health of families caring for people with developmental disabilities: the present situation and strategies for improvement.' *No To Hattatsu*, **31**, 349–354. (Japanese.)

Horton, S.V., Taylor, D.C. (1989) 'The use of behavior modification therapy and physical therapy to promote independent ambulation in a preschooler with mental retardation and cerebral palsy.' *Research in Developmental Disabilities*, **10**, 363–375.

Houle, A.M., Vernet, O., Jednak, R., Pippi Salle, J.L., Famer, J.P. (1998) 'Bladder function before and after selective dorsal rhizotomy in children with cerebral palsy.' *Journal of Urology*, **160**, 1088–1091.

Houltram, J., Noble, I., Boyd, R.N., Corry, I., Flett, P., Graham, H.K. (2001) 'Botulinum toxin type A in the management of equinus in children with cerebral palsy: an evidence-based economic evaluation.' *European Journal of Neurology*, **8** (Suppl. 5), 194–202.

Howell, G.H., Brown, D.R., Bloswick, D.S., Bean, J., Gooch, J.L. (1993) 'Design of a device to exercise hip extensor muscles in children with cerebral palsy.' *Assistive Technology*, **5**, 119–129.

Hu, M.H., Woollacott, M.H. (1994) 'Multisensory training of standing balance in older adults: I. Postural stability and one-leg stance balance.' *Journal of Gerontology*, **49**, M52–61.

Huang, J.C., Deletis, V., Vodusek, D.B., Abbot, R. (1997) 'Preservation of pudendal afferents in sacral rhizotomies.' *Neurosurgery*, **41**, 411–415.

Hur, J.J. (1995) 'Review of research on therapeutic interventions for children with cerebral palsy.' *Acta Neurologica Scandinavica*, **91**, 423–432.

Hutzler, Y., Chacham, A., Bergman, U., Szeinberg, A. (1998) 'Effects of a movement and swimming program on vital capacity and water orientation skills of children with cerebral palsy.' *Developmental Medicine and Child Neurology*, **40**, 176–181.

Ingram, T.T.S., Jameson, S., Errington, J., Mitchell, R.G. (1964) *Living with Cerebral Palsy. Clinics in Developmental Medicine, No. 14*. London: Spastics Society Medical Education and Information Unit with Heinemann Medical.

Ivan, L.P., Ventureyra, E.C., Wiley, J., Doyle, D., Pressman, E., Knights, R., Guzman, C., Uttley, D. (1981) 'Chronic cerebellar stimulation in cerebral palsy.' *Surgical Neurology*, **15**, 81–84.

Jesien, G. (1984) 'Home-based early intervention: a description of the Portage Project model.' *In* Scrutton, D. (Ed.) *Management of Motor Disorders of Children with Cerebral Palsy. Clinics in Developmental Medicine, No. 90*. London: Spastics International Medical Publications with Blackwell Scientific; Philadelphia: J.B. Lippincott, pp. 36–48.

Johnson, M.B., Goldstein, L., Thomas, S.S., Piatt, J., Aiona, M., Sussman, M. (2004) 'Spinal deformity after selective dorsal rhizotomy in ambulatory patients with cerebral palsy.' *Journal of Paediatric Orthopaedics*, **24**, 529–536.

Johnson, S.K., Frederick, J., Kaufman, M., Mountjoy, B. (1999) 'A controlled investigation of bodywork in multiple sclerosis.' *Journal of Alternative and Complementary Medicine*, **5**, 237–243.

Johnstone, M. (1983) *Restoration of Motor Function in the Stroke Patient*. New York: Churchill Livingstone.

Jolleff, N., McConachie, H., Winwyard, S., Jones, S., Wisbeach, A., Clayton, C. (1992) 'Communication aids for children: procedures and problems.' *Developmental Medicine and Child Neurology*, **34**, 719–730.

Jones, R.B. (1975) 'The Vojta method of treatment of cerebral palsy.' *Physiotherapy*, **61**, 112–113.

Jongerius, P.H., Rottevell, J.J., van den Hoogen, F., Joosten, F., van Hulst, K., Gabreels, F.J. (2001) 'Botulinum toxin A: a new option for treatment of drooling in children with cerebral palsy. Presentation of a case series.' *European Journal of Pediatrics*, **160**, 509–512.

Joynt, R.L., Leonard R.A. Jr (1980) 'Dantrolene sodium suspension in treatment of spastic cerebral palsy.' *Developmental Medicine and Child Neurology*, **22**, 755–767.

Jutai, J., Ladak, N., Schuller, R., Naumann, S., Wright, V. (1996) 'Outcomes measurement of assistive technology: an institutional case study.' *Assistive Technology*, **8**, 110–120.

Juzans, P., Comella, J.X., Molgo, J., Faille, L., Angaut-Petit, D. (1996) 'Nerve terminal sprouting in botulinum type-A treated mouse levator auris longus muscle.' *Neuromuscular Disorders*, **6**, 177–185.

Kabat, H. (1977) 'Studies on neuromuscular dysfunction.' *In* Payton, O.D., Hirt, S., Newton, R. A. (Eds) *Scientific Basis for Neurophysiologic Approaches to Therapeutic Exercise*. Philadelphia: F.A. Davis, pp. 219–235.

—— Knott, M. (1953) 'Proprioceptive facilitation techniques for treatment of paralysis.' *Physical Therapy Review*, **33**, 53–64.

Kanda, T., Yuge, M., Yamori, Y., Suzuki, J., Fukase, H. (1984) 'Early physiotherapy in the treatment of spastic diplegia.' *Developmental Medicine and Child Neurology*, **26**, 438–444.

Kanter, R.M., Clark, D.C., Allen, L.C., Chase, M.A. (1976) 'Effects of vestibular stimulation on nystagmus response and motor performance in the developmentally disabled infam.' *Physical Therapy*, **156**, 414–421.

Kassover, M., Tauber, C., Oau, J., Johnson, S., Pugh, J. (1984) 'Auditory feedback in spastic diplegia: gait analysis.' *Transactions of Orthopaedic Research Society, 30th Annual Meeting, Atlanta, GA*.

Kaufman, H.H., Bodensteiner, J., Durkart, B., Gutman, L., Kopitnick, T., Hochberg, V., Loy, N., Cox-Ganser, J., Hobbs, G. (1994) 'Treatment of spastic gait in cerebral palsy.' *West Virginia Medical Journal*, **90**, 190–192.

Kavanagh, C.A., Banco, L. (1982) 'The infant walker: a previously unrecognized health hazard.' *American Journal of Diseases of Children*, **135**, 205–206.

Keller, K. (2001a) *STSNews*, 2: 1 (http:\\www.stsnews.com).

—— (2001b) 'Conversations with Bob Segalman, Ph.D.' *Interview*, December 29, 2000.

Kerem, M., Livanelioglu, A., Topeu, A. (2001) 'Effects of Johnstone pressure splints combined with neurodevelopmental therapy on spasticity and cutaneous sensory inputs in spastic cerebral palsy.' *Developmental Medicine and Child Neurology*, **43**, 307–313.

Kerr, C., McDowell B., McDonough S. (2004) 'Electrical stimulation in cerebral palsy: a review of effects on strength and motor function.' *Developmental Medicine and Child Neurology*, **46**, 205–213.

Ketelaar, M., Vermeer, A., Hart, H., van Petegem-van Beek, E., Helders, P.J. (2001) 'Effects of a functional therapy program on motor abilities of children with cerebral palsy.' *Physical Therapy*, **81**, 1534–1545.

Kim, D.S., Choi, J.U., Yang, K.H., Park, C.I. (2001) 'Selective posterior rhizotomy in children with cerebral palsy: a 10 year experience.' *Child's Nervous System*, **17**, 556–562,

Kinghorn, J. (1992) 'Upper extremity functional changes following selective posterior rhizotomy in children with cerebral palsy.' *American Journal of Occupational Therapy*, **46**, 502–507.

Kirsch, M., Lange. E. (1969) 'Der "Dudelsack"—eine Ubungshilfe bei der Behandlung cerbralpparetischer Kinder.' *Psychiatrie, Neurologie und medizinishe Psychologie (Leipzig)*, **21**, 67–70.

Knight, S.E. (Ed.) (1981) *Sexuality and Physical Disability.* St Louis: C.V. Mosby

Knott, M. (1953) 'Proprioceptive facilitation techniques for treatment of paralysis.' *Physical Therapy Review*, **33**, 53–64.

Koheil, R., Sochaniwskyj, A., Bablich, K., Kenny, D., Milner, M. (1985) 'Biofeedback techniques and behaviour modification in the conservative remediation of drooling in children with cerebral palsy.' *Scientific Program, American Academy for Cerebral Palsy and Developmental Medicine, Seattle.*

Kohn, J. (1982) 'Multiply handicapped child.' *In* Bleck, E.E., Nagel, D.A. (Eds) *Physically Handicapped Children: A Medical Atlas for Teachers, 2nd edn.* Orlando, FL: Grune & Stratton.

—— Enders, S., Preston, J., Motloch, W.O. (1983) 'Provision of assistive equipment for handicapped persons.' *Archives of Physical Medicine and Rehabilitation*, **64**, 378–381.

Kokkonen, J., Saukkonen, A.L., Timonen, E., Serlo, W., Kinnunen, P. (1991) 'Social outcome of handicapped children as adults.' *Developmental Medicine and Child Neurology*, **33**, 1095–1100.

Koman, L.A., Mooney, J.F. 3rd, Smith, B., Goodman, A. Mulvaney, T. (1993) 'Management of cerebral palsy with botulinum-A toxin: preliminary investigation.' *Journal of Pediatric Orthopaedics*, **13**, 489–495.

—— —— —— —— —— (1994) 'Management of spasticity in cerebral palsy with botulinum-A toxin: report of a preliminary, randomized, double-blind control.' *Journal of Pediatric Orthopaedics*, **14**, 299303.

—— —— —— (1996) 'Neuromuscular blockade in the management of cerebral palsy.' **11** (Suppl. 1), S23–S28.

—— —— Walker, F., Leon, J.M. (2000) 'Botulinum toxin type A neuromuscular blockade in the treatment of lower extremity spasticity in cerebral palsy: a randomized, double-blind, placebo-controlled trial.' *Journal of Pediatric Orthopaedics*, **20**, 108–115.

—— Brashear, A., Rosenfeld, S., Chambers, H., Russman, B., Rang, M., Root, L., Ferrari, E., Garcia de Yebenes Prous, J., Smith, B.P., Turkel, C., Walcott, J.M., Molloy, P.T. (2001) 'Botulinum toxin type a neuromuscular blockade in the treatment of equinus foot deformity in cerebral palsy: a multicenter, open-label clinical trial.' *Pediatrics*, **108**, 1062–1071.

Köng, E. (1966) 'Very early treatment of cerebral palsy.' *Developmental Medicine and Child Neurology*, **8**, 198–202.

Korpela, R., Seppanen, R.L., Koivikko, M. (1992) 'Technical aids for daily activities: a regional survey of 204 disabled children.' *Developmental Medicine and Child Neurology*, **34**, 985–998.

Kovac, M., Serpak D., Vucinic, J., Borovcanin, D., Krstic, T. (2002) 'Case presentation.' *Medicinski Pregled*, **55**, 427–430. (Serbo–Croatian/Roman.)

Krach, L.E. (2001) 'Pharmacotherapy of spasticity: oral medications and intrathecal baclofen.' *Journal of Child Neurology*, **16**, 31–36,

Kuczynski, M., Slonka, K. (1999) 'Influence of artificial saddle riding on postural stability in children with cerebral palsy.' *Gait and Posture*, **10**, 154–160.

Kvashnik, B.L., Pelevin, V.V., Deniskina, L.N. (1978) 'Opyt griaxelech eniia na lechebnorn pliazhe sanatoriia.' *Voprosy Kurotologii, Fizioterapii Lechebnoi Fizicheskoi Kultury (Moskova)*, 4, 82.

Lambrenos, K., Weindling, A.M., Calam, R., Cox, A.D. (1996) 'The effect of a child's disability on mother's mental health.' *Archives of Disease in Childhood*, 74, 115–120.

Landau, W.M., Hunt, C.C. (1990) 'Dorsal rhizotomy, a treatment of unproven efficacy.' *Journal of Child Neurology*, 5, 174–178.

Lang, F.F., Deletis, V., Cohen, N.W., Velasquea, L., Abbott, R. (1994) 'Inclusion of the S2 dorsal rootlets in functional posterior rhizotomy for spasticity in children with cerebral palsy.' *Neurosurgery*, 34, 847–853.

Lau, C., Lai, J.S., Chen, S.Y., Wong, M.K. (2000) 'Tai Chi Chuan to improve muscular strength and endurance in elderly individuals: a pilot study.' *Archives of Physical Medicine and Rehabilitation*, 81, 604–607.

Law, M., Cadman, D., Rosenbaum, P., Walter S., Russell, D., DeMatteo, C. (1991) 'Neurodevelopmental therapy and upper-extremity inhibitive casting for children with cerebral palsy.' *Developmental Medicine and Child Neurology*, 33, 377–378.

Lazareff, J.A., Mata-Acosta, A.M., Garcia-Mendez, M.A. (1990) 'Limited selective posterior rhizotomy for the treatment of spasticity secondary to infantile cerebral palsy: a preliminary report.' *Neurosurgery*, 27, 535–538.

—— Garcia-Mendez, M.A., DeRosa, R., Olmstead, C. (1999) 'Limited (L4–S1, L5–S1) selective dorsal rhizotomy for reducing spasticity in cerebral palsy.' *Acta Neurochiurgie*, 141, 743–751.

Lazorthes, Y., Sallerin-Caute, B., Verdie, J.C., Bastide, R., Carillo, J.P. (1990) 'Chronic intrathecal baclofen administration for control of severe spasticity.' *Journal of Neurosurgery*, 72, 393–402.

Leach, J. (1997) 'Children undergoing treatment with botulinum toxin: the role of the physical therapist.' *Muscle and Nerve Supplement*, 6, S194–207.

LeBlanc, M. (1982) 'Systems and devices for nonoral communication.' *In* Bleck, E.E., Nagel, D.A. (Eds) *Physically Handicapped Children: A Medical Atlas for Teachers.* Orlando, FL: Grune & Stratton, pp. 159–169.

Lee, C.L. (1982) 'Role of lower extremity bracing in cerebral palsy.' *Developmental Medicine and Child Neurology*, 24, 250–251. (Abstract.)

—— Bleck, E.E. (1980) 'Surgical correction of equinus deformity in cerebral palsy.' *Developmental Medicine and Child Neurology*, 22, 287–292.

Lee, K.H. (1997) 'MRI-guided stereotactic thalamotomy for cerebral palsy patients with mixed dyskinesia.' *Stereotactic Functional Neurosurgery*, 69, 300–310.

Lepage, C., Noreau, L., Bernard, P.M. (1998) 'Association between characteristics of locomotion and accomplishment of life habits in children with cerebral palsy.' *Physical Therapy*, 78, 458–469.

Letts, M., Stevens, L., Coleman, J., Kenner, R. (1983) 'Puppetry and doll play as an adjunct to pediatric orthopaedics.' *Journal of Pediatric Orthopaedics*, 3, 605–609.

Letts, R.M., Fulford, R., Eng, B., Hobson, D.A. (1976) 'Mobility aids for the paraplegic child.' *Journal of Bone and Joint Surgery*, 58A, 38–41.

Levine, M.S., Kliebhan, L. (1981) 'Communication between physician and physical and occupational therapists: a neurodevelopmentally based prescription.' *Pediatrics*, 68, 208–214.

Liao, H.F., Jeng, S.F., Lai, J.S., Cheng, C.K., Hu, M.H. (1997) 'The relation between standing balance and walking function in children with spastic diplegic cerebral palsy.' *Developmental Medicine and Child Neurology*, 39, 106–112.

Linder, M., Schindler, G., Michaelis, U., Stein, S., Kirschner, J., Mall, V., Berweck, S., Korinthenberg, R. Heinen, F. (2001) 'Medium-term functional benefits in children with cerebral palsy treated with botulinum toxin type A: 1-year follow-up using gross motor function measure.' *European Journal of Neurology*, 8 (Suppl. 5), 120–126.

Lindon, R.L. (1963) 'The Pultibec system for the medical assessment of handicapped children.' *Developmental Medicine and Child Neurology*, 5, 125–145.

Little, W.J. (1862) 'On the influence of abnormal parturition, difficult labours, premature birth, and asphyxia neonatorum, on the mental and physical condition of the child, especially in relation to deformities.' *Transactions of the Obstetrical Society of London*, 3, 253–293.

Logan, L., Byers-Hinkley, K., Ciccone, C.D. (1990) 'Anterior versus posterior walkers: a gait analysis study.' *Developmental Medicine and Child Neurology*, 32, 1044–1048.

Logigian, E.L., Wolinsky, J.S., Soriano, S.G., Madsen, J.R., Scott, R.M. (1994) 'H reflex studies in cerebral palsy patients undergoing partial dorsal rhizotomy.' *Muscle Nerve*, 17, 539–549.

Love, S.C., Valentine, J.P., Blair, E.M., Price, C.J., Cole, J.H., Chauvel, P.J. (2001) 'The effect of botulinum toxin type A on the functional ability of the child with spastic hemiplegia a randomized controlled trial.' *European Journal of Neurology*, **8** (Suppl. 5), 50–58.

Lovett, R.W. (1924) 'The treatment of infantile paralysis: preliminary report based on a study of the Vermont epidemic of 1914. *In Infantile Paralysis in Vermont, 1894–1922*. Battleboro, VT: State Department of Public Health; Vermont Printing Co., p. 201.

Lu, L., Atchabahian, A., Mackinnon, S.E., Hunter, D.A. (1998) 'Nerve injection injury with botulinum toxin.' *Plastic and Reconstructive Surgery*, **101**, 1875–1880.

Ludewig, A., Mahler, C. (1999) 'Early Vojta or Bobath physiotherapy: what is the effect on mother–child relationship?' *Praxis der Kinderpyschologie und Kinderpsychiatrie*, **48**, 326–339.

Lund, B.M. (1990) 'Foodborne disease due to Bacillus and Clostridium species.' *Lancet*, **336**, 982–986.

Lyons, A.S., Petrucelli, R.J. (1987) *Medicine. An Illustrated History.* New York: Abradale Press, Harry N. Adams, pp. 362–365.

Mac Keith, R. (1970) 'Who guides the therapist?' *Developmental Medicine and Child Neurology*, **12**, 518–519.

MacPhail, H.E., Kramer, J.F. (1995) 'Effect of isokinetic strength-training on functional ability and walking efficiency in adolescents with cerebral palsy.' *Developmental Medicine and Child Neurology*, **37**, 763–765.

Mall, V., Heinen, F., Kirschner, J., Linder, M., Stein, S., Michaelis, U., Bernius, P., Lane, M., Korinthenberg, R. (2000) 'Evaluation of botulinum toxin A therapy in children with adductor spasm by gross motor function measures.' *Journal of Child Neurology*, **15**, 214–217.

Maloney, F.P., Mirrett, P., Brooks, C., Johannes, K. (1978) 'Use of the goal attainment scale in the treatment and ongoing evaluation of neurologically handicapped children.' *American Journal of Occupational Therapy*, **32**, 505–510.

Marois, P., Vanasse, M. (2003) 'Hyperbaric oxygen therapy and cerebral palsy.' *Developmental Medicine and Child Neurology*, **45**, 646–647. (Letter.)

Marty, G.R., Dias, L.S., Gaebler-Spira, D. (1995) 'Selective posterior rhizotomy and soft-tissue procedures for the treatment of cerebral diplegia.' *Journal of Bone and Joint Surgery*, **77A**, 713–718.

Massin, W., Allington, N. (1999) 'Role of exercise testing in functional assessment of cerebral palsy after botulinum A toxin injection.' *Journal of Pediatric Orthopaedics*, **19**, 362–365.

Maurer, U. (2002) 'Etiologies of cerebral palsy and classical treatment possibilities.' *Weiner Medizinische Wochenschrift*, **152**, 14–18. (German.)

Mayo Clinic, Department of Neurology (1991) *Clinical Examination in Neurology*. St Louis: Mosby Year Book, pp. 284–285.

McCall, F., Markova, I., Murphy, J., Moodie, E., Collins, S. (1997) 'Perspectives on AAC systems by users and their communication partners.' *European Journal of Disorders of Communication*, **32**, 235–256.

McCollough, N.C. III (1985) *Critical Needs of the Child with Long Term Orthopaedic Impairment Conference Report, October 18–20, 1984.* Washington, DC: American Academy of Orthopaedic Surgeons.

McCormick, M.C., McCarton, C., Tonascia, J., Brooks-Gunn, J. (1993) 'Early educational intervention for very low birth weight infants: results from the Infant Health and Development Program.' *Journal of Pediatrics*, **123**, 527–533.

McGibbon, N.H., Andrade, C.K., Widener, G., Cintas, H.L. (1998) 'Effect of an equine-movement therapy program on gait, energy expenditure, and motor function in children with spastic cerebral palsy: a pilot study.' *Developmental Medicine and Child Neurology*, **40**, 754–762.

McKinlay, I. Hyde, E., Gordon, N. (1980) 'Baclofen: a team approach to drug evaluation of spasticity in childhood.' *Scottish Medical Journal*, **25**, S26–28.

McLaughlin, J.F., Bjornson, K.F., Astley, S.J., Hays, R.M., Hoffinger, S.A., Armantrout, E.A., Roberts, T.S. (1994) 'The role of selective dorsal rhizotomy in cerebral palsy: critical evaluation of a prospective clinical series.' *Developmental Medicine and Child Neurology*, **36**, 755–769.

—— Bjornson, K.F., Astley, S.J., Graubert, C., Hays, R.M., Roberts, T.S., Price, R., Temkin, N. (1998) 'Selective dorsal rhizotomy: efficacy and safety in an investigator-masked randomized clinical trial.' *Developmental Medicine and Child Neurology*, **40**, 220–232.

—— —— Temkin, N., Steinbok, P., Wright, V., Reiner, A., Roberts, T., Drake, J., O'Donnell, M., Rosenbaum, P., Barber, J., Ferrel, A. (2002) 'Selective dorsal rhizotomy: meta-analysis of three randomized controlled trials.' *Developmental Medicine and Child Neurology*, **44**, 17–25.

McLellan, L. (1984) 'Therapeutic possibilities in cerebral palsy: a neurologist's view.' *In* Scrutton, D. (Ed.) *Management of the Motors Disorders of Children with Cerebral Palsy. Clinics in Developmental Medicine, No. 90.* London: Spastics International Medical Publications with Blackwell Scientific; Philadelphia: J.B. Lippincott.

McMillan, M. (1921) *Massage and Therapeutic Exercise*. Philadelphia: W.B. Saunders.

McNaughton, S. (1977) 'Blissymbolics and technology.' *Proceedings of the Workshop on Communication Aids for the Handicapped*. Ottawa, Canada: Peter Nelson, National Research Council.

—— (1982) 'Augmentative communication system: Blissymbolics.' *In* Bleck, E.E., Nagel, D.A. (Eds) *Physically Handicapped Children: A Medical Atlas for Teachers, 2nd edn.* Orlando, FL: Grune & Stratton, pp. 146–154.

Medtronic, Inc. (1996, 1997) *Patient Selection Algorithm: Intrathecal Baclofen (ITB ᵀᴹ) Therapy for Spasticity of Cerebral and Spinal Origin.*

Messingill, R. (1978) 'Follow-up investigation of patients who have had parotid duct transplantation surgery to control drooling.' *Annals of Plastic Surgery*, **2**, 205–208.

Messner, D. (1976) *The Mountain Does it for Me*. Denver, Colorado: Children's Hospital Medical Center. (16 mm film.)

Metaxiotis, D., Siebel, A., Doederlien, L. (2002) 'Repeated botulinum toxin A injections in the treatment of spastic equinus foot.' *Clinical Orthopedics and Related Research*, **394**, 177–185.

Michaelis, R., Haas, G., Buchwald-Saal, M. (1985) 'Neurological development and assessment in infants at risk.' *In* Harel, S., Anastasiow, N.J. (Eds) *The At-Risk Infant*. Baltimore and London: Paul H. Brookes, pp. 269–273.

Milani-Comparetti, A. (1979) 'Priorities in rehabilitation: a progress report on a community program.' *Presented as the 1979 Mary Elaine Meyer O'Neal Award Lectureship in Developmental Pediatrics, Omaha, Nebraska.*

Miller, T.G., Goldberg, K. (1975) 'Sensorimotor integration: an interdisciplinary approach.' *Physical Therapy*, **55**, 501–504.

Mittal, S., Farmer, J.P., Al-Atassi, B., Gibis, J., Kennedy, E., Galli, C., Courchesnes, G., Poulin, C., Cantin, M.A., Benaroch, T.E. (2002) 'Long-term functional outcome after selective posterior rhizotomy.' *Journal of Neurosurgery*, **97**, 315–325.

—— —— —— Montpetit, K., Gervais, N., Poulin, C., Benaroch, T.E., Cantin, M.A. (2002) 'Functional performance following selective posterior rhizotomy: long-term results determined using a validated evaluative measure.' *Journal of Neurosurgery*, **97**, 510–518.

—— —— —— —— —— —— C., Cantin, M.A., Benaroch, T.E. (2002) 'Impact of selective posterior rhizotomy on fine motor skills. Long-term results using a validated evaluative measure.' *Pediatric Neurosurgery*, **36**, 133–141.

Molenaers, G., Desloovere, K., De Cat, J., Jonkers, I., De Borre, L., Pauwels, P., Nijs, J., Fabry, G., De Cock, P. (2001) 'Single event multilevel botulinum toxin type A treatment and surgery: similarities and differences.' *European Journal of Neurology*, **8** (Suppl. 5), 88–97.

Montgomery, P., Richter, E. (1977) 'Effect of sensory integrative therapy on the neuromotor development of retarded children.' *Physical Therapy*, **57**, 799–806.

Morgan, R.F., Hansen, F.C., Wells, J.H., Hoopes, J.E. (1981) 'The treatment of drooling in the child with cerebral palsy.' *Maryland State Medical Journal*, **30**, 79–80.

Morota, N., Abbott, R., Kofler, M., Epstein, F.J., Cohen, H. (1995) 'Residual spasticity after selective posterior rhizotomy.' *Childs Nervous System*, **11**, 161–165.

Mossberg, K.A., Linton, K.A., Friske, K. (1990) 'Ankle foot orthoses: effect on energy expenditure of gait in cerebral spastic diplegic children.' *Archives of Physical Medicine and Rehabilitation*, **71**, 490–494.

Motloch, W.M. (1977) 'Seating and positioning for the physically impaired.' *Orthotics and Prosthetics*, **31**, 11–21.

Mott, D.H., Yates, L. (1981) 'An appraisal of inhibitive casting as an adjunct to the total management of the child with cerebral palsy.' *Proceedings of the American Academy for Cerebral Palsy and Developmental Medicine Annual Meeting, Detroit.*

Mounsy, M., Allington, N. (1999) 'La toxine botulinique A dans le traitement de la spasticité dynamique en equin chez les enfants porteurs d'infirmité motrice d'origine cérébrale. Etude preliminaire.' *Revue de Chirurgie Orthopédique et Réparative de l'Appareil Moteur (France)*, **85**, 156–163.

Mpagi, J.S. (2002) 'Government's role in CBR.' *In* Hardy, S. (Ed.) *CRB—A Participatory Strategy in Africa*. London: University College London, Centre for International Child Health, pp. 86–96.

Msall, M.E., DiGaudio, K., Rogers, B.T., LaForest, S., Catanzaro, N.L., Campbell, J., Wilczenski, F., Duffy, L.C. (1994) 'The Functional Independence Measure for Children (WeeFIM). Conceptual basis and pilot use in children with developmental disabilities.' *Clinical Pediatrics*, 7, 421–430.

Müller, H. (1992) 'Treatment of severe spasticity: results of a multicenter trial conducted in Germany involving the intrathecal infusion of baclofen by an implantable drug delivery system.' *Developmental Medicine and Child Neurology*, 34, 739–745.

Mumenthaler, M. (1990) *Neurology, 3rd edn.* New York: Theime Medical, p. 194.

Murphy, J., Markova, I., Collins, S., Moodie, E. (1996) 'AAC systems: obstacles to effective use.' *European Journal of Disorders of Communication*, 31, 31–44.

Murphy, K.P., Molnar, G.E., Landkasky, K. (2000) 'Employment and social issues in adults with cerebral palsy.' *Archives of Physical Medicine and Rehabilitation*, 81, 807–811.

Myhr, U., von Wendt, L. (1991) 'Improvement of functional sitting positions for children with cerebral palsy.' *Developmental Medicine and Child Neurology*, 33, 246–256.

—— —— (1993) 'Influence of different sitting positions and abduction orthoses on leg muscle activity in children with cerebral palsy.' *Developmental Medicine and Child Neurology*, 35, 870–880.

—— —— Norrlin, S., Radell, U. (1995) 'Five-year follow-up of functional sitting position in children cerebral palsy.' *Developmental Medicine and Child Neurology*, 37, 587–596.

Naessen, T., Lindmark, B., Larsen, H.C. (1997) 'Better postural balance in elderly women receiving estrogens.' *American Journal of Obstetrics and Gynecology*, 177, 412–416.

Nakamura, K. (1998) 'Development of communication method.' *No To Hattatsu*, 30, 220–226. (Japanese.)

Nandapalan, V., Smith, C.A., Jones, A.S., Lesser, T.H. (1995) 'Objective measurement of the benefit of walking sticks in peripheral vestibular balance disorders, using the Sway Weigh balance platform.' *Journal of Laryngology and Otology*, 109, 836–840.

Narayan, R.K., Loubser, P.G., Jankovic, J., Donovan, W.H., Bontke, C.F. (1991) 'Intrathecal baclofen for intractable axial dystonia.' *Neurology*, 42, 1141–1142.

Ndawi, O.P. (2002) 'The role of legislation in facilitating CRB in Zimbabwe.' *In* Hardy, S. (Ed.) *CRB—A Participatory Strategy in Africa,* London: University College London, Centre for International Child Health, pp. 97–105.

Nelson, K.B., Ellenberg, J.H. (1981) 'Apgar scores as predictors of chronic neurologic disability.' *Pediatrics,* 68, 36–44.

—— —— (1982) 'Children who "outgrew" cerebral palsy.' *Pediatrics,* 69, 529–536.

—— —— (1984) 'Obstetric complications as risk factors for cerebral palsy or seizure disorders.' *Journal of the American Medical Association*, 251, 1843–1848.

Newberg, N.L., Gooch, J.L., Walker, M.D. (1991) 'Intraoperative monitoring in selective dorsal rhizotomy.' *Pediatric Neurosurgery*, 17, 124–127.

Nichols, D.S. (1997) 'Balance retraining after stroke using force platform biofeedback.' *Physical Therapy*, 77, 553–558.

Nisbet, P. (1996) 'Integrating assistive technologies: current practice and future possibilities.' *Medical Engineering and Physics*, 18, 193–202.

Nishida, T., Thatcher, S.W., Marty, G.R. (1995) 'Selective posterior rhizotomy for children with cerebral palsy: a 7-year experience.' *Child's Nervous System*, 7, 374–380.

Nolan, J., Chalkiadis, G.A., Low, J., Olesch, C.A., Brown, T.C.K. (2000) 'Anesthesia and pain management in cerebral palsy.' *Anaesthesia*, 55, 32–41.

Nordmark, E., Hagglund, G., Jarnlo, G.B. (1997) 'Reliability of the gross motor function measure in cerebral palsy.' *Scandinavian Journal of Rehabilitation Medicine*, 29, 25–28.

Norlin, R., Tkaczuk, A. (1985) 'One-session surgery for correction of lower extremity deformities in children with cerebral palsy.' *Journal of Pediatric Orthopaedics*, 5, 208–211.

—— —— (1992) 'One session surgery on the lower limb in children with cerebral palsy. A five year follow-up.' *International Orthopaedics*, 16, 291–293.

Nosek, M.A., Rintala, D.H., Young, Y.E., Howland, C.A., Foley, C.C., Rossi, Dr., Chanpong, G. (1996) 'Sexual functioning among women with physical disabilities.' *Archives of Physical Medicine and Rehabilitation*, 77, 107–115.

Novacheck, T.F., Stout, J.L., Tervo, R. (2000) 'Reliability and validity of the Gillette Functional Assessment Questionnaire as an outcome measure in children with walking disabilities.' *Journal of Pediatric Orthopaedics*, 20, 75–81.

—— Trost, J.P., Schwartz, M.H. (2002) 'Intramuscular psoas lengthening improves dynamic hip function in children with cerebral palsy.' *Journal of Pediatric Orthopaedics*, 22, 158–169.

Nuzzo, R.M., Walsh, S., Boucherit, T., Massoud, S. (1997) 'Counterparalysis for treatment of paralytic scoliosis with botulinum toxin type A.' *American Journal of Orthopedics*, 26, 201–207.

Nwaobi, O.M., Brubaker, C.E., Cuskick, B., Sussman, M.D. (1983) 'Electromyographic investigation of extensor activity in cerebral palsied children in different seating positions.' *Developmental Medicine and Child Neurology*, 25, 175–183.

O'Brien, C. (1995) 'Clinical issues in the management of spasticity with Botulinum toxin.' *In* O'Brien, C., Yablon, S. (Eds) *Management of Spasticity with Botulinum Toxin. Proceedings of the 12th World Congress of International Federation of Physical Medicine and Rehabilitation, March 27–31, Sydney, Australia.* Littleton, CO: Postgraduate Institute for Medicine, pp. 17–13.

—— (1997) 'Injection techniques for botulinum toxin using electromyography or electrical stimulation.' *Muscle Nerve* (Suppl. 6), S176–180.

O'Connell, D.G., Barnhart, R., Parks, L. (1992) 'Muscular endurance and wheelchair propulsion in children with cerebral palsy or myelomeningocoele.' *Archives of Physical Medicine and Rehabilitation*, 73, 709–711.

—— —— (1995) 'Improvement in wheelchair propulsion in pediatric wheelchair users through resistance training: a pilot study.' *Archives of Physical Medicine and Rehabilitation*, 76, 368–372.

Odergren, T., Hjaltason, H., Kaakkola, S., Solders, G., Hanko, J., Fehling, C., Martilla, R.J., Lundh, H., Gedin, S., Westergren, I., Richardson, A., Dott, C., Cohen, H. (1998) 'A double blind, randomized, parallel group study to investigate the dose equivalence of Dysport and Botox in the treatment of cervical dystonia.' *Journal of Neurology, Neurosurgery, and Psychiatry*, 64, 6–12.

O'Dwyer, T.P., Conlon, B.J. (1997) 'The surgical management of drooling— a 15 year follow-up.' *Clinical Otolaryngology*, 22, 284–287.

O'Grady, R.S., Crain, L.S., Kohn, J. (1995) 'The prediction of long-term functional outcomes of children with cerebral palsy.' *Developmental Medicine and Child Neurology*, 37, 997–1005.

Ohye, C., Miyazaki, M., Hirai, T., Shibazaki, T., Nagaseki, Y. (1983) 'Stereotactic selective thalamotomy for the treatment of tremor type of cerebral palsy in adolescence.' *Child's Brain*, 10, 157–167.

Ojemann, J.G., Parks, T.S., Komanetsky, R., Day, R.A., Kaufman, B.A. (1997) 'Lack of specificity in electrophysiological identification of lower sacral roots during selective dorsal rhizotomy.' *Journal of Neurosurgery*, 86, 28–33.

Okawa, A., Kajiura, I., Hiroshima, K. (1990) 'Physical therapeutic and surgical management in spastic diplegia. A Japanese experience.' *Clinical Orthopedics and Related Research*, 253, 38–44.

Ong, L.C., Afifah, I., Sofiah, A., Lye, M.S. (1998) 'Parenting stress among mothers of Malaysian children with cerebral palsy: predictors of child- and parent-related stress.' *Annals of Tropical Pediatrics*, 18, 301–307.

Oppenheim, W.L. (1990) 'Selective posterior rhizotomy for spastic cerebral palsy.' *Clinical Orthopedics and Related Research*, 253, 20–29.

—— Staudt, L.A., Peacock, W.J. (1992) 'The rationale for rhizotomy.' *In* Sussman, M.D. (Ed.) *The Diplegic Child.* Rosemont, IL: American Academy of Orthopaedic Surgeons, pp. 271–285.

O'Reilly, E.D. (1975) 'Care of the cerebral palsied: outcomes of the past and needs for the future.' *Developmental Medicine and Child Neurology*, 17, 141–149.

Ottenbacher, K.J., Msall, M.E., Duffy, L.C., Ziviani, J., Granger, C.V., Braun, S. (2000) 'Functional assessment and care of children with neurodevelopmental disabilities.' *American Journal of Physical Medicine and Rehabilitation*, 79, 114–123.

Ōunpuu, S., Bell, K.J., Davis, R.B. 3rd, DeLuca, P.A. (1996) 'An evaluation of the posterior spring leaf orthosis using joint kinematics and kinetics.' *Journal of Pediatric Orthopaedics*, 16, 378–384.

Paine, R. S. (1962) 'On the treatment of cerebral palsy: the outcome of 177 patients, 74 totally untreated.' *Pediatrics*, 29, 605–616.

Paleg, G. (1997) 'Made for walking—a comparison of gait trainers.' *Team Rehab Report*, July, 41–45.

Palisano, R.J., Kolbe T.N., Halry, S.M., Lowes, L.P., Jones, Q. (1995) 'Validity of the Peabody Developmental Gross Motor Scale as an evaluative measure of infants receiving physical therapy.' *Physical Therapy*, 75, 939–951.

—— Rosenbaum, P., Walter, S., Russell, D., Wood, E., Galuppi, B. (1997) 'Development and reliability of a system to classify gross motor function in children with cerebral palsy.' *Developmental Medicine and Child Neurology*, 39, 214–223.

Palmer, F. B., Shapiro, B. K., Wachtel, R. C., Allen, M.C., Hiller, J.E., Harryman, S.F. (1988) 'The effects of physical therapy on cerebral palsy: a controlled trial in infants with spastic diplegia.' *New England Journal of Medicine*, 318, 803–808.

—— —— Allen, M.C., Mosher, B.S., Bilker, S.A., Harryman, S. E., Meinert, C.L., Capute, A.J. (1990) 'Infant stimulation curriculum for infants with cerebral palsy: effects on infant temper-infant interaction, and home environment.' *Pediatrics*, 85, 411–415. CHECK TITLE

Pape, K.E., Kirsch, S.E., Galil, A., Boulton, J.E., White, A., Chipman, M. (1993) 'Neuromuscular approach to the motor deficits of cerebral palsy: a pilot study.' *Journal of Pediatric Orthopaedics*, 13, 628–633.

Parette, H.P. Jr, Hourcade, J.J. (1983) 'Early intervention: a conflict of therapist and educator.' *Perceptual and Motor Skills*, 57, 1056–1058.

—— —— (1984a) 'A review of therapeutic intervention research on gross and fine motor progress in young children with cerebral palsy.' *American Journal of Occupational Therapy*, 38, 462–468.

—— —— (1984b) 'How effective are physiotherapeutic programmes with young mentally retarded children who have cerebral palsy.' *Journal of Mental Deficiency Research*, 28, 167–175.

Pariser, S.C., Blitzer, A., Binder, W.J., Friedman, W.F., Marovitz, W.F. (1978) 'Evaluation of tympanic neurectomy and chorda tympanectomy surgery.' *Otolaryngology*, 86, 308–321.

Park, E.S., Park, C.I., Lee, H.J., Cho, Y.S. (2001) 'The effect of electrical stimulation on the trunk control in young children with spastic diplegic cerebral palsy.' *Journal of Korean Medical Science*, 16, 347–350.

Park, R.L. (2000) *Voodoo Science. The Road from Foolishness to Fraud.* Oxford and New York: Oxford University Press, p. 50.

Park, T.S., Gaffney, P.E., Kaufman, B.A., Molleston, M.C. (1993) 'Selective lumbosacral dorsal rhizotomy immediately caudal to the conus medullaris for cerebral palsy spasticity.' *Neurosurgery*, 33, 929–933.

—— Vogler, G.P., Phillips, L.H. 2nd, Kaufman, B.A., Ortman, M.R., McClure, S.M., Gaffney, P.E. (1994) 'Effects of selective dorsal rhizotomy for spastic diplegia on hip migration in cerebral palsy.' *Journal of Pediatric Neurosurgery*, 20, 43–49.

Parker, D.F., Carriere, L., Hebstreit, H., Salsberg, A., Bar-Or, O. (1992) 'Anaerobic endurance and peak muscle power in children with spastic cerebral palsy.' *American Journal of Diseases of Childhood*, 146, 1069–1073.

—— —— —— —— (1993) 'Muscle performance and gross motor function of children with spastic cerebral palsy.' *Developmental Medicine and Child Neurology*, 35, 17–23.

Parks, L. (1977) 'The need for "someone with nothing to do".' *Paper presented at the Study Group on Integrating the Care of Multiply Handicapped Children, St Mary's College, Durham, England.* Spastics Society Medical Education and Information Unit.

Parmelee, A.H., Cohen, S.E. (1985) 'Neonatal follow-up for infants at risk.' *In* Harel, S., Anastasiow, N.J. (Eds) *The At-Risk Infant.* Baltimore and London: Paul H. Brookes, pp. 269–273.

Pascual-Pascual, S.I., Sanchez de Muniain, P., Roche, M.C., Pascual-Castroviejo, I. (1997) 'La toxina botulinica como tratamiento de la paralisis cerebral infantile.' *Revisita de Neurologia*, 25, 1369–1375.

Patrick, J.H., Roberts, A.P., Cole, G.F. (2001) 'Therapeutic choices in the locomotor management of the child with cerebral palsy.' *Archives of Disease in Childhood*, 85, 275–279.

Payne, L.Z., DeLuca, P.A. (1993) 'Heterotopic ossification after rhizotomy and femoral osteotomy.' *Journal of Pediatric Orthopaedics*, 13, 733–738.

Peacock W.J., Arens, L.J. (1982) 'Selective posterior rhizotomy for relief of spasticity in cerebral palsy.' *South African Medical Journal*, 62, 119–124.

—— Staudt, L.A. (1990) 'Spasticity in cerebral palsy and the selective posterior rhizotomy procedure.' *Journal of Child Neurology*, 5, 179–185.

—— (1991) 'Functional outcomes following selective posterior rhizotomy in children with cerebral palsy.' *Journal of Neurosurgery*, 74, 380–385.

Pell, S.D., Gillies, R.M., Carss, M. (1997) 'Relationship between use of technology and employment rates for people with physical disabilities in Australia: implications for education and training programmes.' *Disability and Rehabilitation*, 19, 332–338.

—— —— —— (1999) 'Use of technology by people with physical disabilities in Australia.' *Disability and Rehabilitation*, 21, 56–60.

Penn, R.D. (1992) 'Intrathecal baclofen for spasticity of spinal origin: seven years experience.' *Journal of Neurosurgery*, 77, 236–240.

—— Kroin, J.S. (1985) 'Continuous intrathecal baclofen for severe spasticity.' *Lancet*, 2, 125–127.

—— —— (1987) 'Long-term intrathecal baclofen infusion for treatment of spasticity.' *Journal of Neurosurgery*, 66, 181–185.

Perry, J., Jones, M.H., Thomas, L. (1981) 'Functional evaluation of Rolfing in cerebral palsy.' *Developmental Medicine and Child Neurology*, 23, 719–729.

Peter, J.C. (1994) 'Selective posterior lumbosacral rhizotomy in teenagers and young adults with spastic cerebral palsy.' *British Journal of Neurosurgery*, 8, 135–139.

—— Hoffman, E.B., Arens, L.J., Peacock, W.J. (1990) 'Incidence of spinal deformity in children after multiple level laminectomy for selective posterior rhizotomy.' *Child's Nervous System*, 6, 30–32.

—— Arens, L.J. (1993) 'Selective posterior lumbosacral rhizotomy for the management of cerebral palsy spasticity. A 10-year experience.' *South African Medical Journal*, 83, 745–747.

—— Hoffman, E.B., Arens, L.J. (1993) 'Spondylolysis and spondylolisthesis after five-level lumbosacral laminectomy for selective posterior rhizotomy in cerebral palsy.' *Child's Nervous System*, 9, 285–287.

Phelps, W.M. (1932) 'Cerebral birth injuries: their orthopaedic classification and subsequent treatment.' *Journal of Bone and Joint Surgery*, 14, 773–782.

—— (1956) 'The infantile cerebral palsies and their non-operative treatment.' *American Academy of Orthopaedic Surgeons Instructional Course Lectures, vol. XIII.* J.W. Edwards, p. 79.

—— (1957) 'Long term results of orthopedic surgery in cerebral palsy.' *Journal of Bone and Joint Surgery*, 39A, 53–59.

Polak, F., Morton, R., Ward, C., Wallace, W.A., Doderlein, L., Siebel, A. (2002) 'Double-blind comparison study of two doses of botulinum toxin A injected into calf muscles in children with hemiplegic cerebral palsy.' *Developmental Medicine and Child Neurology*, 44, 551–555.

Polatajko, H.J. (1985) 'A critical look at vestibular dysfunction in learning-disabled children.' *Developmental Medicine and Child Neurology*, 27, 283–292.

Pollack, M.A. (1994) 'Limited benefit of electrophysiological studies during dorsal rhizotomy.' *Muscle Nerve*, 17, 553–555.

Price, G.W., Wilkin, G.P., Turnbull, M.J., Bowery, N.G. (1984) 'Are baclofen sensitive GABA$_B$ receptors present on primary afferent terminals of the spinal cord? *Nature*, 307, 71–74.

Privat, J.M., Benezech, J., Frerebeau, P., Gros, C. (1976) 'Sectorial posterior rhizotomy, a new technique of surgical treatment for spasticity.' *Acta Neurochirurgica (Wein)*, 35, 181–195.

Proctor & Gamble Pharmaceuticals (2000) 'Dantrium intravenous.' Product Information, *Physicians' Desk Reference, 54th edn.* Montvale, NJ: Medical Economics Co.

Purohit, A.K., Dinakar, I. (1992) 'Neurosurgical intervention during resistant phase of motor development of cerebral palsied.' *Indian Journal of Pediatrics*, 59, 707–717.

Rab, G.T. (1992) 'Diplegic gait: is there more than spasticity?' *In* Sussman, M.D. (Ed.) *The Diplegic Child.* Rosemont, IL: American Academy of Orthopaedic Surgeons, pp. 103, 111.

Racette, B.A., Lauryssen, C., Perlmutter, J.S. (1998) 'Preoperative treatment with botulinum toxin to facilitate cervical fusion in dystonic cerebral palsy. Report of two cases.' *Journal of Neurosurgery*, 88, 328–330.

Ramamurthi, B. (2000) 'Stereotactic surgery in India: the past, present and the future.' *Neurology India*, 48, 1–7.

Rang, M., Douglas, G., Bennet, G.C., Koreska, J. (1981) 'Seating for children with cerebral palsy.' *Journal of Pediatric Orthopaedics*, 1, 279–287.

—— (1982) *The Easter Seal Guide to Children's Orthopaedics.* Ontario, Canada: Easter Seal Society.

—— (2000) *The Story of Orthopaedics.* Philadelphia: W.B. Saunders, pp. 227–228.

Ratka, S.A., Skinner, S.R., Dixon, D.M., Johanson, M.E. (1997) 'A comparison of gait with solid, dynamic, and no ankle–foot orthoses in children with spastic cerebral palsy.' *Physical Therapy*, 78, 222–241.

Rawicki, B. (1999) 'Treatment of cerebral origin spasticity with continuous intrathecal baclofen delivered via an implantable pump: long-term follow-up of 18 patients.' *Journal of Neurosurgery*, 91, 733–736.

Rayner, S.A., Hollick, E.J., Lee, J.P. (1999) 'Botulinum toxin in childhood strabismus.' *Strabismus*, 7, 103–111.

Reddihough, D.S., King, J.A, Coleman, G.J, Catanese, T. (1998) 'Efficacy of programmes based on Conductive Education for your children with cerebral palsy.' *Developmental Medicine and Child Neurology*, 40, 763–770.

—— —— —— (2002) 'Functional outcome of botulinum toxin A injections to the lower limb muscles in cerebral palsy.' *Developmental Medicine and Child Neurology*, 44, 820–827.

Reimers, J. (1980) 'The stability of the hip in children. A radiological study of the results of muscle surgery in cerebral palsy.' *Acta Orthopaedica Scandinavica (Suppl.)*, 184, 1–97.

Rennie, D.J., Atfield, S.F., Morton, R.E., Polak, F.J., Nicholson, J. (2000) 'An evaluation of lycra garments in the lower limb using 3-D gait analysis and functional assessment (PEDI).' *Gait and Posture*, 12, 1–6.

Rethlefsen, S., Kay, R., Dennis, S., Forstein, M., Tolo, V. (1999) 'The effects of fixed and articulated ankle–foot orthoses on gait patterns in subjects with cerebral palsy.' *Journal of Pediatric Orthopaedics*, 19, 470–474.

Ring, N.D., Nelham, R.L., Pearson, D.A. (1978) 'Molded supportive seating for the disabled.' *Prosthetics and Orthotics International*, 2, 30–34.

Robertson, L.T., Meek, M., Smith, W.L. (1980) 'Speech changes in cerebral palsied patients after cerebellar stimulation.' *Developmental Medicine and Child Neurology*, 22, 608–617.

Robinson, R.O., McCarthy, G.T., Little, T.M. (1989) 'Conductive education at the Petö Institute, Budapest.' *British Medical Journal*, 299, 1145–1149.

Rood, M.S. (1954) 'Neurophysiologic reactions as a basis for physical therapy.' *Physical Therapy Review*, 34, 444–449.

Root, L. (1977) 'The total body involved cerebral palsy patient.' *Instructional course lectures, Annual Meeting, American Academy of Orthopaedic Surgeons*, Las Vegas, Nevada.

Rosales, R.L., Arimura, K., Takenaga, S., Osame, M. (1996) 'Extrafusal and intrafusal muscle effects in experimental botulinum toxin-A injection.' *Muscle Nerve*, 19, 488–496.

Rose, J., Mederios, J.M., Parker, R. (1985) 'Energy cost index as an estimate of energy expenditure of cerebral-palsied children during assisted ambulation.' *Developmental Medicine and Child Neurology*, 27, 485–490.

—— Haskell, W.L., Gamble, J.G., Hamilton, R.L., Brown, D.A., Rinsky, L. (1994) 'Muscle pathology and clinical measures of disability in children with cerebral palsy.' *Journal of Orthopaedic Research*, 12, 758–768.

—— McGill, K.C. (1998) 'The motor unit in cerebral palsy.' *Developmental Medicine and Child Neurology*, 40, 270–277.

Rosemeyer, B., Stürz, H. (1977) 'Musculus quadriceps femoris bei Immobilization und remobilisation.' *Zeitschrift für Orthopädie*, 115, 182–188.

Rosenthal, R.K. (1984) 'The use of orthotics in foot and ankle problems in cerebral palsy.' *Foot and Ankle*, 4, 195–200.

—— Deutsch, S.D., Miller, W., Schumann, W., Hall, J.E. (1975) 'A fixed ankle below-the-knee orthosis for the management of genu recurvatum in spastic cerebral palsy.' *Journal of Bone and Joint Surgery*, 57A, 545–549.

Rothberg, A.D., Goodman, M., Jacklin, L.A., Cooper, P.A. (1991) 'Six-year follow-up of early physiotherapy intervention in very low birth weight infants.' *Pediatrics*, 88, 547–552.

Russell, G., Sharp, E., Iles, G. (1976) 'Clinical biofeedback applications in pediatric rehabilitation.' *Inter-Clinics Information Bulletin*, 15, 1–6.

Russman, B.S. (2000) 'Cerebral palsy.' *Current Treatment Options in Neurology*, 2, 97–108.

Saddler, A. L., Hillman, S. B., Benjamin, D. (1993) 'The influence of disability condition visibility on family functioning.' *Journal of Pediatric Psychology*, 18, 425–439.

Sahkhla, C., Jankovic, J., Duane, D. (1998) 'Variability of the immunologic and clinical response in dystonic patients immunoresistant to botulinum toxin injections.' *Movement Disorders*, 13, 150–154.

Sal'kov, V.N., Lil'in, E.T., Stepanchenko, A.V., Stepanchenko, O.V., Malanchenko, E.A. (2002) 'Botox in children with cerebral palsy and triceps syndrome.' *Zhural Nevrologii i Psikhiartrii Imeni S. S. Korsakova*, 102, 24–25. (Russian.)

Salokorpi, T., Rautio, T., Kajantie, E., Van Wendt, L. (2002) 'Is occupational therapy in extremely preterm infants of benefit in the long run?' *Pediatric Rehabilitation*, 5, 91–98.

Samilson, R.L., Hoffer, M.M. (1975) 'Problems and complications in orthopaedic management of cerebral palsy.' *In* Samilson, R.L. (Ed.) *Orthopaedic Aspects of Cerebral Palsy. Clinics in Developmental Medicine, Nos 52/53*. London: Spastics International Medical Publications with Heinemann Medical; Philadelphia: J.B. Lippincott, pp. 258–274.

Sampaio, C, Ferreira, J.J., Simoes, F., Rosas, M.J., Magalhaes, M., Correia, A.P., Bastos-Lima, A., Martins, R., Castro-Caldes, A. (1997) 'DYSBOT: a single-blind randomized parallel study to determine whether an differences can be detected in the efficacy and tolerability of two formations of botulinum toxin type A—Dysport and Botox—assuming a ration of 4:1.' *Movement Disorders*, 12, 1013–1018.

Samson-Fang, G., Gooch, J., Norlin, C. (2000) 'Intrathecal baclofen withdrawal simulating neuroepileptic malignant syndrome in a child with cerebral palsy.' *Developmental Medicine and Child Neurology*, 42, 561–565.

Sanchez-Carpintero, P., Narbona, J. (1997) 'Toxina botulinica en paralisis cerebral infantil: resultados en 27 sujetos a lo largo de un año.' *Revista de Neurologia*, 25, 531–535.

Sanes, D.H., Constatine-Paton, M. (1983) 'Altered activity patterns during development reduce neural timing.' *Science*, 221, 1183–1185.

Saraph, V., Zwick, E.B., Zwick, F., Steinwender, C., Steinwender, G., Linhart, W. (2002) 'Multilevel surgery in spastic diplegia: evaluation by physical examination and gait analysis in 25 children.' *Journal of Pediatric Orthopaedics*, 22, 150–157.

Sarimski, K., Hoffmann, I.W. (1993) ('Overprotectiveness as a coping reaction in intensive physical therapy') 'Uberfursorglichkeith als Bewaltigungsreaktion bei der Durchfuhrung intensiver Krankengymnastik.' *Zeitschrift für Kinder-und Jugendpsychiatrie und Psychotherapie*, 21, 109–114.

Scherzer, A.L. Mike, V., Ilson, J. (1976) 'Physical therapy as a determinant of change in the cerebral palsied infant.' *Pediatrics*, 58, 47–51.

Schijman, E., Erro, M.G., Meana, N.V. (1993) 'Selective posterior rhizotomy: experience with 30 cases.' *Childs Nervous System*, 9, 474–477.

Schowalter, J.E. (1977) 'The modification of behavior modification.' *Pediatrics*, 59, 130–131.

Scrutton, D. (1984) 'Aim-oriented management.' *In* Scrutton, D. (Ed.) *The Management of Motors Disorders of Children with Cerebral Palsy. Clinics in Developmental Medicine, No. 90*. London: Spastics International Medical Publications with Blackwell Scientific; Philadelphia: J.B. Lippincott, pp. 49–58.

Seeger, B.R., Caudry, D.J., Scholes, J.R. (1981) 'Biofeedback therapy to achieve symmetrical gait in heiniplegic cerebral palsied children.' *Archives of Physical Medicine and Rehabilitation*, 62, 364–368.

—— —— (1983) 'Biofeedback therapy to achieve symmetrical gait in children with hemiplegic cerebral palsy: long-term efficacy.' *Archives of Physical Medicine and Rehabilitation*, 64, 160–162.

—— O'Mara, N.A. (1984) 'Hand function in cerebral palsy—the effect of hip-flexion angle.' *Developmental Medicine and Child Neurology*, 26, 601–606.

Sellick, K.J., Over, R. (1980) 'Effects of vestibular stimulation on motor development of cerebral-palsied children.' *Developmental Medicine and Child Neurology*, 22, 476–483.

Semenova, K.A. (1997) 'Basis for a method of dynamic proprioceptive correction in the restorative treatment of patients with residual-stage infantile cerebral palsy.' *Neuroscience and Behavioral Physiology*, 27, 639–643.

Shabalov, V.A., Melikian, A.G., Kadin, A.L., Arutiunov, N.V., Golanov, A.V., Shtok, A.V., Sharkey, M.A., Banaitis, D.A., Giuffrida, C., Mullens, P.A., Rast, M., Pratt, B. (2002) 'Letter to the Editor.' *Developmental Medicine and Child Neurology*, 44, 430–441.

Sharrard, W.J.W. (1976) 'Indications for bracing in cerebral palsy.' *In* Murdoch, G. (Ed.) *The Advance in Orthotics*. London: Edward Arnold, pp. 453–461.

Shcherbina, IuI. (1998) 'The use of computed tomography in stereotaxic operations in dyskinesia patients.' *Zhurnal Voprosy Neirokhirurgii Imeni N.N. Burdenko*, 3, 3–6. (Russian.)

Sheeran, T., Marvin, R.S., Pianta, R.C. (1997) 'Mothers' resolution of their child's diagnosis and self-reported measures of parenting stress, marital relations, and social support.' *Journal of Pediatric Psychology*, 22, 197–212.

Shepherd, G.M. (1994) *Neurobiology, 3rd edn*. Oxford: Oxford University Press.

Sherrington, C.S. (1898) 'Decerebrate rigidity and reflex coordination of movements.' *Journal of Physiology (London)*, 22, 319–337.

Shevelev, I. N., Shabolov, V.A., Artarian, A.A., Safronov, V.A., Stepanenko, A.Iu. (1996) 'The use of selective dorsal rhizotomy for treating spasticity in patients with infantile cerebral palsy.' *Zhurnal Voprosy Neirokhirurgii Imeni N. N. Burdenko*, 3, 19–22. (Russian.)

Shigenari, T. (1998) 'Technical aids for children with cerebral palsy.' *No To Hattatsu*, 30, 227–232. (Japanese.)

Silbert, P.T., Stewart-Wynne, E.G. (1992) 'Increased dystonia after intrathecal baclofen.' *Neurology*, 42, 1639–1640.

Skinner, B.F. (1971) *Beyond Freedom and Dignity*. New York: Knopf.

Slominski, A.H. (1984) 'Winthrop Phelps and the Children's Rehabilitation Institute.' *In* Scrutton, D. (Ed.) *Management of the Motor Disorders of*

Children with Cerebral Palsy. Clinics in Developmental Medicine No. 90. London: Spastics International Medical Publications with Blackwell Scientific; Philadelphia: J.B. Lippincott, pp. 59–74.

Sloop, R.R., Cole, B.A., Escutin, R.O. (1997) 'Reconstituted botulinum toxin type A does not lose potency in humans if it is refrozen or refrigerated for 2 weeks before us.' *Neurology*, **48**, 249–253.

—— —— —— (1997) 'Human response to botulinum toxin injection: type B compared with type A.' *Neurology*, **48**, 189–194.

Soboloff, H.R. (1981) 'Long term follow-up of handicapped children.' *Paper read at the Eighth World Congress of Social Psychiatry, Zagreb, Yugoslavia.*

Somers, A.R. (1979) 'Marital status, health, and the use of health services.' *Journal of the American Medical Association*, **241**, 1818–1822.

Sommerfelt, K., Markestad, R., Berg, K., Saetesdal, I. (2001) 'Therapeutic electrical stimulation in cerebral palsy: a randomized, controlled, crossover trial.' *Developmental Medicine and Child Neurology*, **43**, 609–613.

Smyth, M.D., Peacock, W.J. (2000) 'The surgical treatment of spasticity.' *Muscle Nerve*, **23**, 153–163.

Snyder-Mackler, L., Delitto, A., Bailey, S.L., Stralka, S.W. (1995) 'Strength of the quadriceps femoris muscle and functional recovery after reconstruction of the anterior cruciate ligament. A prospective, randomize clinical trial of electrical stimulation.' *Journal of Bone and Joint Surgery*, 77A, 1166–1173.

Sommerfelt, K., Markestatd, R., Berg, K., Saetesdal, I. (2002) 'Therapeutic electrical stimulation in cerebral palsy: a randomized, controlled, crossover trial.' *Developmental Medicine and Child Neurology*, **44**, 609–613.

Sparrow, S., Zigler, E. (1978) 'Evaluation of patterning treatment for retarded children.' *Pediatrics*, **62**, 137–150.

Speelman, J.D. (1990) 'Cervical epidural spinal cord stimulation in infantile encephalopathy.' *Nederlands Tijdschrift voor Geneeskunde*, **134**, 1732–1735. (Dutch.)

—— van Manen, J. (1989) 'Cerebral palsy and stereotactic neurosurgery.' *Journal of Neurology Neurosurgery and Psychiatry*, **52**, 23–30.

Stallard, J., Major, E.E., Farmer, S.E. (1996) 'The potential for ambulation by severely handicapped cerebral palsy patients.' *Prosthetics and Orthotics International*, **20**, 122–128.

Stamp, W.G. (1973) 'Bracing in cerebral palsy.' *Instructional Course Lectures, American Academy of Orthopaedic Surgeons*, **18**, 286–306.

Staros, A., LeBlanc, M. (1975) 'Orthotic components and systems.' *In* American Academy of Orthopaedic Surgeons (Eds) *Atlas of Orthotics—Biomechanical Principles and Applications.* St Louis: C.V. Mosby.

Staudt, L.A., Nuwer, M.R., Peacock, W.J. (1995) 'Intraoperative monitoring during selective posterior rhizotomy: technique and patient outcome.' *Electroencephalography and Clinical Neurophysiology*, **97**, 296–309.

Stein, R.E.K., Jessof, D.J. (1984) 'Relationship between health status and psychological adjustment among children with chronic conditions.' *Pediatrics*, **73**, 169–174.

Steinbok, P., Reiner, A., Beauchamp, R.D., Cochrane, D.D., Keyes, R. (1992) 'Selective functional posterior rhizotomy for treatment of spastic cerebral palsy in children. Review of 50 consecutive cases.' *Pediatric Neurosurgery*, **18**, 34–42.

—— Kestle, J.R. (1996) 'Variation between centers in electrophysiological techniques used in lumbosacral selective dorsal rhizotomy for spastic cerebral palsy.' *Pediatric Neurosurgery*, **25**, 233–239.

—— Reiner, A.M., Kestle, J.R., Armstrong, R.W., Beauchamp, R.D., Cochrane, D. (1996) 'Therapeutic electrical stimulation (TES) following selective posterior rhizotomy in children with spastic diplegia due to cerebral palsy: a randomized clinical trial.' *Developmental Medicine and Child Neurology*, **38** (Suppl. 74), 32–33.

—— —— —— (1997a) 'Therapeutic electrical stimulation following selective posterior rhizotomy in children with spastic diplegic cerebral palsy: a randomized clinical trial.' *Developmental Medicine and Child Neurology*, **39**, 515–520.

—— —— Beauchamp, R., Armstrong, R.W., Cochrane, D.D., Kestle, J.R. (1997b) 'A randomized clinical trial to compare selective posterior rhizotomy plus physiotherapy with physiotherapy alone in children with spastic diplegic cerebral palsy.' *Developmental Medicine and Child Neurology*, **39**, 178–184.

—— Keyes, R., Langill, L., Cochrane, D.D. (1994) 'The validity of electrophysiological criteria used in selective posterior rhizotomy for treatment of spastic cerebral palsy.' *Journal of Neurosurgery*, **81**, 354–361.

—— Daneshvar, H., Evans, D., Kestle, J.R. (1995) 'Cost analysis of continuous intrathecal baclofen versus selective functional posterior rhizotomy in the treatment of spastic quadriplegia associated with cerebral palsy.' *Pediatric Neurosurgery (Switzerland)*, **22**, 255–264.

—— Gustavsson, B., Kestle, J.R., Reiner, A., Cochrane, D.D. (1995) 'Relationship of intraoperative electrophysiological criteria to outcome after selective functional posterior rhizotomy.' *Journal of Neurosurgery*, **83**, 18–26.

—— Schrag, C. (1998) 'Complications after selective posterior rhizotomy for spasticity in children with cerebral palsy.' *Pediatric Neurosurgery*, **28**, 300–313.

—— McLeod, K. (2002) 'Comparisons of motor outcomes after selective dorsal rhizotomy with and without postoperative intensified physiotherapy in children with spastic diplegic cerebral palsy.' *Pediatric Neurosurgery*, **36**, 142–147.

Sterba, J.A., Roders, B.T., France, A.P., Vokes, D.A. (2002) 'Horseback riding in children with cerebral palsy: effect on gross motor function.' *Developmental Medicine and Child Neurology*, **44**, 301–308.

Stockert, K. (1998) 'Acupuncture and Vojta therapy in infantile cerebral palsy—a comparison of the effects.' *Weiner Medizinische Wochenschrift*, **148**, 434–438.

Strauss, D.J., Shavelle, R.M., Anderson, T.W. (1998) 'Life expectancy in children with cerebral palsy.' *Pediatric Neurology*, **18**, 143–149.

—— Shavelle, R.M. (1998) 'Life expectancy of adults with cerebral palsy.' *Developmental Medicine and Child Neurology*, **40**, 369–375.

—— Cable, W., Shavelle, R. (1999) 'Causes of excess mortality in cerebral palsy.' *Developmental Medicine and Child Neurology*, **41**, 580–585.

Subramanian, N., Vaughan, C.L., Peter, J.C., Arens, L.J. (1998) 'Gait before and 10 years after rhizotomy in children with cerebral palsy.' *Journal of Neurosurgery*, **88**, 1014–1019.

Suskind, D.L., Tilton, A. (2002) 'Clinical study of botulinum-A toxin in the treatment of sialorrhea in children with cerebral palsy.' *Laryngoscope*, **112**, 73–81.

Sussman, M.D. (1983) 'Casting as an adjunct to neurodevelopmental therapy in cerebral palsy.' *Developmental Medicine and Child Neurology*, **25**, 804–805.

—— (1992) *The Diplegic Child.* Rosemont, IL: American Academy of Orthopaedic Surgeons.

—— Cusick, B. (1979) 'Preliminary report: the role of short-leg, tone-reducing casts as an adjunct to physical therapy of patients with cerebral palsy.' *Johns Hopkins Medical Journal*, **145**, 112–114.

—— —— (1981) 'Early mobilization of patients with cerebral palsy following muscle release surgery.' *Orthopaedic Transactions*, **5**, 193.

Sutherland, D.H., Olshen, R., Cooper, L., Woo, S.K. (1980) 'The development of mature gait.' *Journal of Bone and Joint Surgery*, 62A, 336–353.

—— Kaufman, K.R., Wyatt, M.P., Chambers, H.G., Mubarak, S.J. (1999) 'Double-blind study of botulinum A toxin injections into the gastrocnemius muscle in patients with cerebral palsy.' *Gait and Posture*, **10**, 1–9.

Suzuki, N., Mita, K., Watakabe, M., Akataki, K., Okagawa, T., Kimizuka, M. (1998) *Bulletin Hospital for Joint Diseases*, **57**, 208–215.

Sweetser, P.M., Badell, A., Schneider, S., Badlani, G.M. (1995) 'Effects of sacral dorsal rhizotomy on bladder function in patients with spastic cerebral palsy.' *Neurourology and Urodynamics*, **14**, 57–64.

Sylvester, E. (1977) 'Psychological problems in pediatric orthopaedic patients.' *Lecture at Children's Hospital at Stanford, Palo Alto, CA.*

Sziklai, I., Grof, J. (1981) 'Effect of immobilization by plaster on the level of various energy metabolites in skeletal muscle.' *Acta Physiologica Academiae Scientirarum Hungaricae*, **58**, 47–51.

Tabary, J.C., Tabary, C., Tardieu, C., Tardieu, G., Goldspink, G. (1972) 'Physiological and structural changes in the cat's soleus muscle due to immobilization at different lengths by plaster casts.' *Journal of Physiology*, **224**, 231–244.

Taft, L.T. (1972) 'Are we handicapping the handicapped?' *Developmental Medicine and Child Neurology*, **14**, 703–704.

—— (1973a) 'Are we handicapping the handicapped?' *Developmental Medicine and Child Neurology*, **15**, 113–116. (Letter.)

—— (1973b) 'Are we handicapping the handicapped?' *Developmental Medicine and Child Neurology*, **15**, 401–402. (Letter.)

Tauffkirchen, E. (1978) 'Hippotherapy—a supplementary treatment for motion disturbance caused by cerebral palsy.' *Pädiatrie und Pädologie*, **13**, 405–411. (German.)

Taylor, S., Kling, T.F. (1984) 'An improved system of orthotic management in neuromuscular disease.' *Orthopaedic Transactions*, **8**, 105.

Tefft, D., Guerette, P., Furumasu, J. (1999) 'Cognitive predictors of young children's readiness for powered mobility.' *Developmental Medicine and Child Neurology*, 41, 665–670.

Terver, S., Levai, J.P., Bleck, E.E. (1981) 'Motricité cérébrale réadaption neurologique du développement.' *Motricité Cérébrale*, 2, 55–68.

Thomas, A., Bax, M., Coombes, K., Goldson, E., Smyth, D., Whitmore, K. (1985) 'The health and social needs of physically handicapped young adults: are they being met by statutory services?' *Developmental Medicine and Child Neurology*, Supplement No. 50.

Thomas, M., Thomas, M.J. (2002) 'Some controversies in community based rehabilitation.' *In* Hardy, S. (Ed.) *CRB—A Participatory Strategy in Africa*. London: University College London, Centre for International Child Health, pp. 13–25.

Thomas, S.S., Aiona, M.D., Pierce R., Piatt, J.H. II (1996) 'Gait changes in children with spastic diplegia after selective dorsal rhizotomy.' *Journal of Pediatric Orthopaedics*, 16, 747–752.

—— Aiona, M.D., Buckon, C.E., Piatt, J.H. Jr (1997) 'Does gait continue to improve 2 years after selective dorsal rhizotomy?' *Journal of Pediatric Orthopaedics*, 17, 387–389.

—— Buckon, C.E., Piatt, J.H., Aiona, M.D., Sussman, M.D. (2004) 'A 2-year follow-up of outcomes following orthopaedic surgery or selective dorsal rhizotomy in children with spastic diplegia.' *Journal of Pediatric Orthopaedics*, 13, 358–366.

Thompson, N.S., Baker, R.J., Cosgrove, A.P., Corry, I.S., Graham, H.K. (1998) 'Musculoskeletal modeling in determining the effect of botulinum toxin on the hamstrings of patients with crouch gait.' *Developmental Medicine and Child Neurology*, 40, 622–625.

Thompson, R.F. (2000) *The Brain: A Neuroscience Primer, 3rd edn.* New York: Worth.

Thompson, S. (1977) 'Results of questionnaire on therapy.' *Regional Course, American Academy for Cerebral Palsy and Developmental Medicine, New Orleans, LA.*

Tirosh, E., Rabino, S. (1989) 'Physiotherapy for children with cerebral palsy—evidence for its efficacy.' *American Journal of Diseases of Childhood*, 143, 552–555.

—— Bar-Or, O., Rosenbaum, P. (1990) 'New muscle power test in neuromuscular disease. Feasibility and reliability.' *American Journal of Diseases of Childhood*, 144, 1083–1087.

Tizard, J.P. (1980) 'Cerebral palsies: treatment and prevention. The Croonian Lecture 1978.' *Journal of the Royal College of Physicians, London*, 14, 72–77.

Tobimatsu, Y., Nakamura, R. (2000) 'Retrospective study of factors affecting employability of individuals with cerebral palsy in Japan.' *Tohoku Journal of Experimental Medicine*, 192, 291–299.

Torner, J.C. (1992) 'Designing outcome studies in cerebral palsy.' *In* Sussman, M.D. (Ed.) *The Diplegic Child*. Rosemont, IL: American Academy of Orthopaedic Surgeons, pp. 117–123.

Trahan, J., Malouin, F. (2002) 'Intermittent intensive physiotherapy in children with cerebral palsy: a pilot study.' *Developmental Medicine and Child Neurology*, 44, 233–239.

Trail, I.A., Galasko, C.S.B. (1990) 'The Matrix seating system.' *Journal of Bone and Joint Surgery*, 72B, 666–669.

Trefler, E., Hanks, S., Huggins, P., Chiarizzo, S., Hobson, D.A. (1978) 'A modular seating system for cerebral palsied children.' *Developmental Medicine and Child Neurology*, 20, 199–204.

—— Angelo, J. (1997) 'Comparison of anterior trunk supports for children with cerebral palsy.' *Assistive Technology*, 9, 15–21.

Trejos, H., Araya, R. (1990) 'Stereotactic surgery in cerebral palsy.' *Stereotactic Functional Neurosurgery*, 54–55, 130–135.

Tuli, U. (1998) 'Integrated education–teacher as therapist.' *ActionAid Disability News*, 9, 26–27.

Turi, M., Kalen, V. (2000) 'The risk of spinal deformity after selective dorsal rhizotomy.' *Journal of Pediatric Orthopaedics*, 20, 104–107.

Turk, M.A., Geremski, C.A., Rosenbaum, P.T., Weber, R.J. (1997) 'The health status of women with cerebral palsy.' *Archives of Physical Medicine and Rehabilitation*, 78 (12 Suppl. 5), S10–17.

Turnbull, J.D. (1993) 'Early intervention for children with or at risk of cerebral palsy.' *American Journal of Disease of Childhood*, 147, 54–59.

Van den Bergh, P., Francart, J., Mourin, S., Kollmann, P., Laterre, P. (1995) 'Five-year experience in the treatment of focal movement disorders with a low-dose Dysport botulinum toxin.' *Muscle Nerve*, 18, 720–729.

van den Berg-Emons, H.J., Saris, W.H., de Barbanson, D.C., Westerterp, K.R., Huson, A., van Baak, M.A. (1995) 'Daily physical activity of schoolchildren with spastic diplegia and of healthy control subjects.' *Journal of Pediatrics*, 127, 578–584.

—— van Baak, M.A., de Barbanson, D.C., Speth, L., Saris, W.H. (1996) 'Reliability of tests to determine peak aerobic power, anaerobic power and isokinetic muscle strength in children with spastic cerebral palsy.' *Developmental Medicine and Child Neurology*, 38, 1117–1125.

Van der Linden, M.L., Hazlewood, M.E., Aitchison, A.M., Hillman, S.J. Robb, J.E. (2003) 'Electrical stimulation of gluteus maximus in children with cerebral palsy: effects on gait characteristics and muscle strength.' *Developmental Medicine and Child Neurology*, 45, 385–390.

Van der Velde, C.D. (1985) 'Body images of one's self and of others: developmental and clinical significance.' *American Journal of Psychiatry*, 142, 527–537.

Van Schaeybroeck, P., Nuttin, B., Lagae, L., Schrijvers, E., Borghgraef, D., Feys, P. (2000) 'Intrathecal baclofen for intractable cerebral spasticity: a prospective placebo-controlled, double-blind study.' *Neurosurgery*, 46, 603–609.

Vasin, N.L, Nodvornik, P., Lesnov, N., Kadin, A.L., Shramka, M. (1979) 'Stereotaxic combined dentate-thalamotomy in the treatment of spastic-hyperkinetic forms of subcortical dyskinesias.' *Zhurnal Voprosy Neirokhirurgii Imeni N.N. Burdenko (Moskova)*, 6, 23–28.

Vaughan, C.L., Berman, B., Peacock, W.J. (1988) 'Gait analysis of cerebral palsy children before and after rhizotomy.' *Pediatric Neuroscience*, 14, 297–300.

—— —— —— (1991) 'Cerebral palsy and rhizotomy. A 3-year follow-up evaluation with gait analysis.' *Journal of Neurosurgery*, 74, 178–184.

—— Subramanian, N., Basse, M.E. (1998) 'Selective dorsal rhizotomy as a treatment option for children with spastic cerebral palsy.' *Gait and Posture*, 8, 43–59.

Vojta, V. (1981) *Die zerebralen Bewegunstrorungen im Sduglingsalter, Früdiagnose und Frütherapie, 3rd edn.* Stuttgart: F. Enke, pp. 183–189.

Von Wendt, L., Ekenberg, L., Dagis, D., Janlert, U. (1984) 'A parent-centered approach to physiotherapy for their handicapped children.' *Developmental Medicine and Child Neurology*, 26, 445–448.

—— (1984) 'The basic elements of treatment according to Vojta.' *In* Scrutton, D. (Ed.) *The Management of the Motor Disorders of Children with Cerebral Palsy. Clinics in Developmental Medicine, No. 90.* London: Spastics International Medical Publications with Blackwell Scientific; Philadelphia: J.B. Lippincott, pp. 75–85.

Wall, S.A., Chait, L.A., Temlett, J.A., Perkins, B., Hillen, G., Becker, P. (1993) 'Botulinum A chemodenevation: a new modality in cerebral palsied hands.' *British Journal of Plastic Surgery*, 46, 703–706.

Wallander J.L., Venters, T.L. (1995) 'Perceived role restriction and adjustment of mothers of children with chronic physical disability.' *Journal of Pediatric Psychology*, 20, 619–632.

Waltz, J.M., Davis, J.A. (1983) 'Cervical cord stimulation in the treatment of athetosis and dystonia.' *Advances in Neurology*, 37, 225–237.

Warf, B.C., Nelson, K.R. (1996) 'The electromyographic responses to dorsal rootlet stimulation during partial dorsal rhizotomy are inconsistent.' *Pediatric Neurosurgery*, 25, 13–19.

Wasiak, J., Hoare, B.J., Hender, K.M. (2002) 'Does intramuscular botulinum toxin A injection improve upper-limb function in children with hemiplegic cerebral palsy?' *Medical Journal of Australia*, 177, 158.

—— —— —— (2003) 'Letter to the editor re reply to letter of Graham *et al.* (2003).' *Medical Journal of Australia*, 178, 96.

Watt, J., Sims, D., Harckham, F., Schmidt, L., McMillan, A., Hamilton, J. (1984) 'A prospective study of inhibitive casting as an adjunct to physiotherapy in the cerebral palsied child.' *Orthopaedic Transactions*, 8, 110.

Weber, S. (1983) 'Indication for exercise therapy in infancy in prevention of childhood cerebral palsy.' *Klinische Pädiatrie*, 195, 347–350.

Westin, G.W., Dye, S. (1983) 'Conservative management of cerebral palsy in the growing child.' *Foot and Ankle*, 4, 160–163.

White, R. (1984) 'Sensory-integrative therapy for the cerebral-palsied child.' *In* Scrutton, D. (Ed.) *Management of the Motor Disorders of Children with Cerebral Palsy. Clinics in Developmental Medicine, No. 90.* Spastics International Medical Publications with Blackwell Scientific; Philadelphia: J.B. Lippincott, pp. 86–95.

Whittaker, C.K. (1980) 'Cerebellar stimulation in cerebral palsy.' *Journal of Neurosurgery*, 52, 648–653.

Wiley, M.E., Damiano, D.L. (1998) 'Lower-extremity strength profiles in spastic cerebral palsy.' *Developmental Medicine and Child Neurology*, 40, 100–107.

Wilke, T.F. (1967) 'The problem of drooling in cerebral palsy: a surgical approach.' *Canadian Journal of Surgery*, **10**, 60–67.

Willenborg, M.J., Shilt, J.S., Smith, B.P., Estrada, R.L., Castle, J.A., Koman, L.A. (2002) 'Technique for iliopsoas ultrasound-guided active electromyography-directed botulinum A toxin injection in cerebral palsy.' *Journal of Pediatric Orthopaedics*, **22**, 165–168.

Williams, I. (1977) 'The consequences of orthopaedic surgery in the adolescent cerebral palsied: medical education and parental attitudes.' *Paper read at the Study Group on Integrating the Care of Multiply Handicapped Children, St Mary's College, Durham, England.* London: The Spastics Society Medical Education and Information Unit.

Willis, J.K., Morello, A., Davie, A., Rice, J.C., Bennett, J.T. (2002) 'Forced use treatment of childhood hemiparesis.' *Pediatrics*, **110**, 94–96.

Wilson, H., Haideri, N., Song, K., Telford, D. (1997) 'Ankle–foot orthoses for preambulatory children with spastic diplegia.' *Journal of Pediatric Orthopaedics*, **17**, 370–376,

Winter, R.B. (1999) 'The fallacy of short-term outcomes analysis in pediatric orthopaedics.' *Journal of Bone and Joint Surgery*, **81A**, 1499–1500.

Wissel, J., Heinen, F., Schenkel, A., Doll, B., Eberbach, G., Muller, J., Poewe, W. (1999) 'Botulinum toxin A in the management of spastic gait disorders in children and young adults with cerebral palsy: a randomized, double-blind study of "high dose" versus "low dose" treatment.' *Neuropediatrics*, **30**, 120–124.

Wolf, S.L., Coogler, C., Xu, T. (1997) 'Exploring the basis for Tai Chi Chuan as a therapeutic exercise approach.' *Archives of Physical Medicine and Rehabilitation*, **78**, 886–892.

Wolfer, J.A., Visintainer, M.A. (1979) 'Prehospital psychological preparation for tonsillectomy patients: effects on children's and parents' adjustment.' *Pediatrics*, **64**, 646–655.

Wolff, D.R., Rose, J., Jones, V.K., Bloch, D.A.,Oehlert, J.W., Gamble, J.G. (1998) 'Postural balance measurements for children and adolescents.' *Journal of Orthopaedic Research*, **16**, 271–275.

Wong, A.M., Chang, C.J., Chen, L.R., Chen, M.M. (1997) 'Laser intraductal photocoagulation of bilateral parotid ducts for reducing drooling of cerebral palsied children: a preliminary report.' *Journal of Clinical Laser Medicine and Surgery*, **15**, 65–69.

Wong, V. (1998) 'Use of botulinum toxin injection in 17 children with spastic cerebral palsy.' *Pediatric Neurology*, **18**, 124–131.

—— Ng, A., Sit, P. (2002) 'Open-label study of botulinum toxin for upper limb spasticity in cerebral palsy.' *Journal of Child Neurology*, **17**, 138–142.

Woolridge, C.P., McLaurin, C. (1976) 'Biofeedback—background and applications to physical rehabilitation.' *Bulletin of Prosthetic Research*, **Spring**, 25–37.

World Health (1984) May, 4, 5, 20, 25.

World Health Organization (2001) *International Classifications of Functioning Disability and Health (ICF)*. Geneva: World Health Organization (http://www3.who.int/icf/icftemplate.cfm)

Wright, F.V., Sheil, E.M., Drake, J.M., Wedge, J.H., Nauman, S. (1998) 'Evaluation of selective dorsal rhizotomy for the reduction of spasticity in cerebral palsy: a randomized controlled trial.' *Developmental Medicine and Child Neurology*, **40**, 239–247.

Wright-Ott, C., Egilson, S. (1996), 'Mobility' *In* Case-Smith, J., Allen, A.S., Pratt, P.N. (Eds) *Occupational Therapy for Children, 3rd edn.* St Louis: C.V. Mosby, pp. 562–580.

—— —— (1997) 'The transitional powered mobility aid: a new concept and tool for early mobility.' *In* Furamasu, J. (Ed.) *Pediatric Powered Mobility: Developmental Perspectives, Technical Issues, and Clinical Approaches.* Arlington, Virginia: Rehabilitation Engineering and Assistive Technology Society of North America, pp. 58–69.

Wright, T., Nicholson, J. (1973) 'Physiotherapy for the spastic child: an evaluation.' *Developmental Medicine and Child Neurology*, **15**, 146–163.

Xu, L., Hong, Y., Wang, A.Q., Wang, Z.X., Tang, T. (1993) 'Hyperselective posterior rhizotomy in treatment of spasticity of paralytic limbs.' *Chinese Medical Journal*, **106**, 671–673.

Yam, K.Y., Fong D, Kwong, K. Yiu, B. (1999) 'Selective posterior rhizotomy. Results of five pilot cases.' *Hong Kong Medical Journal*, **5**, 287–290.

Yang, T.F., Chan, R.C.,Wong, T.T., Bair, W.N., Kao, C.C., Chuang, T.Y., Hsu, T.C. (1996) 'Qualitative measurement of improvement in sitting balance in children with spastic cerebral palsy after selective posterior rhizotomy.' *American Journal of Physical Medicine and Rehabilitation*, **75**, 348–352.

—— —— Chuang, T.Y., Liu, T.J., Chiu, J.W. (1999) 'Treatment of cerebral palsy with botulinum toxin: evaluation with gross motor function measure.' *Journal of Formosa Medical Association*, **12**, 832–836.

Yates, H., Mott, D.H. (1977) 'Inhibitive casting.' *Paper read at the First William C. Duncan Seminar on Cerebral Palsy.* Seattle: Children's Orthopaedic Hospital and Medical Center and the University of Washington.

Yi, B., Xu, L., Hong, Y. (2001) 'Lumbar structural observation of children with cerebral palsy after selective posterior rhizotomy.' *Zhonghua Yi Xue Za Zhi*, **81**, 983–987. (Chinese).

Zelnik, N., Giladi, N., Goikhman, I., Karen, G., Moris, R., Honigman, S. (1997) 'The role of botulinum toxin in the treatment of lower limb spasticity in children with cerebral palsy—a pilot study.' *Israel Journal of Medical Science*, **33**, 129–133.

Zhang, L.I., Bao, S., Merzenich, M.M. (2001) 'Persistent and specific influences of early acoustic environments on primary auditory cortex.' *Nature Neuroscience*, **4**, 1123–1130.

—— —— —— (2002) 'Disruption of primary auditory cortex by synchronous auditory inputs during a critical period.' *Proceedings of the National Academy of Sciences of the USA*, **99**, 2309–2314.

Zhou, X.J., Chen, T., Chen, J.T. (1993) '75 infantile palsy children treated with acupuncture, acupressure and functional training.' *Zhongguo Zhon Xi Yi He Za Zhi*, **13**, 220–222. (Chinese.)

Zurcher, A.W., Molenaers, G., Desloovere, K., Fabry, G. (2001) 'Kinematic and kinetic evaluation of the ankle after intramuscular injection of botulinum toxin A in children with cerebral palsy.' *Acta Orthopaedica Belgica*, **67**, 475–480.

Zwick, E.B., Saraphy, V., Strobl, W., Steinwender, G. (2001) 'Single event multilevel surgery to improve gait in diplegic cerebral palsy—a prospective clinical trial.' *Zeitschrift für Orthopadie und ihre Grenzgebiete*, **139**, 485–489.

7
SPASTIC HEMIPLEGIA

SNAPSHOT: SPASTIC HEMIPLEGIA

- **Communication**: generally good oral language
- **Mobility**: level I; neighborhood and community
- **Activities of daily living**: no problem; spastic upper limb as a helper

CHARACTERISTICS AND NATURAL HISTORY

The typical posture of the child with spastic hemiplegia is equinus of the foot and ankle, flexion of the elbow, wrist and fingers, and an adducted thumb (Fig. 7.1). Variations of this pattern will be found whether the spastic paralysis is barely discernible or severe. In mild forms of hemiplegia, the upper-limb involvement is not noticed until the child runs and 'stresses' the central nervous system. Varus of the foot is usual; pes valgus does occur, but not nearly as often as in spastic diplegia.

Most of these children begin independent walking between the ages of 18 and 21 months, gain independence in activities of daily living, are able to talk, can participate in peer-group activities and attend regular school. Their greatest disability can be mental retardation, behavioral problems, and late-onset convulsive disorder (Perlstein and Hood 1956, Jones 1976, Cioni *et al.* 1999, Yude and Goodman 1999).

GENERAL MANAGEMENT

PHYSICAL AND OCCUPATIONAL THERAPY

Because children who have spastic hemiplegia have an intact unilateral sensory and motor system, the management of their motor problems to achieve function for independent living is not difficult. They need only short-term supervision, if any, by a physical or occupational therapist. The therapist can be of great help in analyzing the functional capacity of the hand, the sensibility, the active and passive ranges of motion of the fingers

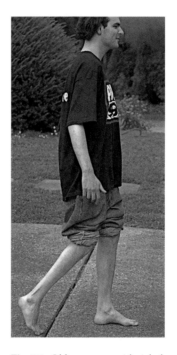

Fig. 7.1. Older teenager with right hemiplegia, thin right calf, fixed right equinus.

and wrist, and the strength of the controlling muscles. The therapist can also suggest ways to practice and to use adaptive devices for efficiency in bimanual skills. Whether specific resistance exercises of the ankle dorsiflexors done daily will improve function and lessen equinus is not known. To enforce daily exercise is a bore for children. Visiting a therapist once a week or once a month will probably not help to 'treat' the condition. Learning to play games, ride a bike, and participate in the same sports as other children is probably the best management.

A new therapy that promises the restoration of function of the affected limb in spastic hemiplegia due to stroke is 'constraint-induced movement therapy' (CI therapy) reported by Taub and colleagues of Birmingham, Alabama (1999). The therapy consisted of constraining movements of the less affected arm in

Orthopaedic problems:

- Upper limb: flexion spasticity of wrist and fingers and elbow; thumb-in-palm
- Lower limb: equinus, varus, occasional hip internal rotation, flexed knee gait.

Physiotherapy: monitoring, encouragement of parents and patient, little need after age 7 and some never need see a physiotherapist—usually rural children in remote areas.

Occupational therapy: test hand function and sensation. Suggest and test adaptive tools and utensils for the involved helping hand for two-handed tasks.

Orthoses: early dynamic equinus; AFO probably worth a trial.

Neurosurgery: rhizotomy not indicated.

Intrathecal baclofen not indicated.

Botulinum toxin: useful for dynamic equinus– gastrocnemius. Might be helpful in dynamic wrist flexion, primarily flexor carpi ulnaris and elbow-flexors short term; long-term effect not established.

Orthopaedic surgery:

- Upper limb spasticity and contracture—selective surgery
- Fixed equinus—sliding Achilles tendon lengthening, or aponeurotic gastrocnemius lengthening
- Dynamic varus—split posterior tibial-tendon transfer; supramalleolar posterior tibial lengthening; some need split anterior tibial-tendon transfer
- Fixed varus—triple arthrodesis
- Upper limb—thumb-in-palm correction; tendon transfers and lengthening; pronator teres release
- Helping hand only; cosmetic improvement.

a sling for 90% of the waking hours for 2 weeks and intensive training of the affected arm. Taub *et al.* (1999) reported successful improvement in the upper limbs of chronic stroke patients, patients with chronic traumatic brain injury and even in the lower limbs of patients following cerebral vascular accidents, incomplete spinal-cord injury and fractured hips. This approach has been extended to focal hand dystonia of musicians.

The basis of restriction of the non-affected limb in hemiplegia appears to be the experimental section of the dorsal root afferent nerves of only one upper limb in monkeys. When the opposite limb was restricted in movement, recovery of the deafferented limb was enhanced (Taub *et al.* 1973).

Liepert *et al.* (1998) of the University of Jena, Germany, spatially mapped the motor cortex with transcranial magnetic stimulation before and after 2 weeks of treatment in chronic stroke patients, all of whom improved after constraint of the unaffected upper limb. They found that the reduced motor cortex representations of the affected body part could be enlarged and increased in the level of excitability by the rehabilitation procedure. Kunkel *et al.* (1999) of Berlin, Germany, also found constraint-induced movement therapy was effective in five chronic stroke patients with a follow-up of 3 months. The therapy entailed restraint of the unaffected upper limb in a sling for 14 days combined with 6 hours of training per weekday of the affected limb.

Taub *et al.* (2002), reporting from the Department of Psychology of the University of Birmingham, Alabama, had maintained their enthusiasm for 'new therapies in rehabilitation' that promises 'substantial enhancement of extremity use' and 'linguistic function by behavioral therapy'. Constraint-induced movement therapy has found its way into the treatment of chronic hemiparesis in childhood through Willis *et al.* (2002) of the Department of Psychiatry and Neurology of Tulane University, New Orleans, Louisiana. Twelve hemiparetic children, aged between 1 and 8 years, had their unimpaired arm immobilized in a plaster cast for 1 month; they were then compared with 13 children with hemiplegia who had not been casted, and who served as controls. Using the Peabody Developmental Motor Scales before and after treatment revealed improved scores of 12.6 in the casted children in 2.5 points in the controls. The scores persisted in seven children who returned after 6 months. In a crossover trial in which ten of the control children were casted, parents reported improvement in function. Children in both groups had physical/occupational therapy with the treatment children having 1.4 visits per week and the controls somewhat more, at 2.1 visits per week. What is meant by physical/occupational therapy is not clearly defined—properly these sessions are termed 'visits'.

Gordon and Charles (2003) tried CI therapy in 18 children with spastic hemiplegia. These children were randomized to nine in the treatment group and nine in the group with treatment. The treatment consisted of keeping the non-involved upper limb in a sling, 6 hours a day for 14 days. Hand function was tested with an array of assessment tools: Jebsen–Taylor, Bruininks–Oseretsky, Melbourne Assessment, and a Children's Motor Activity Log. Tests were done prior to treatment and again after 1 week, 4 weeks and 6 months.

The results indicated that the greatest changes occurred immediately after invention; there was modest improvement in the spastic upper limb, according to the tests. The authors suggested that impairment of sensorimotor control in children with hemiplegia may be partly attributed to non-use.

ORTHOTICS

'Functional hand bracing is a joke.'

(Mercer Rang, 1993)

Orthotic use is minimal, and usually consists of the plastic ankle–foot orthosis at an early age in an attempt to control ankle equinus and prevent contractures, although we have little evidence that this occurs (see Chapter 6). Upper-limb orthoses are temporary expedients, and do not seem to be effective in encouraging function or in correcting contractures. Most of us have used the opponens-type splint to keep the thumb out of the palm in young children while their nervous system is maturing. Currie and Mendiola (1987) reported the only use of a thumb orthosis to improve the thumb-in-palm of five children (aged 20–26 months) and stated it was effective, but with no follow-up.

Similar use has been made of plastic volar wrist-extension splints. Both are used only part of the day because they seem to interfere with the child's hand function and attempts to adapt. Möberg (1984) made the good point that the usual volar hand and finger splint covers the area where tactile gnosis is important in order to grasp. He suggested replacing this part of the splint with soft non-elastic straps.

Although night splinting of the hand and fingers is often recommended to prevent contractures, no data exist to confirm their efficacy. The hand and wrist are usually relaxed during sleep. Splinting, however, is regarded as being 'something to do', and cannot be entirely condemned if it satisfies the needs and perceptions of the parents, physician and therapist in the management of the very young hemiplegic child. But it would be better to be honest about its long-term efficacy.

MANAGEMENT

Surgical management of the lower limb is mainly for equinus due to contractures of the triceps surae, and to prevent fixed varus deformities when dynamic inversion of the foot occurs during gait. Surgery of the hand and upper limb is highly selective. While surgery can improve upper-limb function and appearance, it never restores hand function to normal—mainly because of the almost universal defect in stereognostic sensation in the involved limb.

While surgery can improve upper-limb function and appearance, it never restores hand function to normal.

The major thrust of the management program is educational and behavioral, to allow as normal a maturation as possible so that independent function and community integration can be achieved.

UPPER-LIMB SURGERY

EVALUATION OF THE HAND FOR SURGERY
The following factors need to be considered and examinations conducted in the assessment of the hand and upper limb.

1. TYPE OF SPASTIC DISORDER: DYSTONIC OR ATHETOID
Dystonic posturing of the hand and upper limb is often confused with that of spastic paralysis especially in patients with hemidystonia. Dystonia is differentiated from spasticity when relaxation of the patient restores the hand to a normal posture, when there are no contractures or increased stretch reflexes and when the deep tendon reflexes are either normal or hypoactive (see Fig. 1.2). Tendon lengthenings or transfers in dystonic hands either fail to relieve the flexed posture of the wrist or fingers, or cause a reversal to an extension posture.

2. BEHAVIORAL STATUS AND INTELLECTUAL FUNCTION
The patient must have sufficient intellectual function and emotional stability to comprehend the goals of surgery and to cooperate in the optimum restoration of hand function postoperatively (Zancolli and Zancolli 1981).

3. HAND SENSATION
Most patients with hemiplegia have deficient stereognosis (tactile gnosis). The tests for shape recognition are done with the eyes occluded and using the normal hand as a control (see Fig. 2.28). Goldner and Ferlic (1966) long ago recognized the importance of good sensation in the prognosis for function in cerebral-palsied hands. If tactile gnostic sensation is deficient, patients and parents need to be informed that while this deficiency is not an absolute contraindication to surgery, it always does limit the functional result. No 'therapy' has been discovered to restore defective sensation even by 'early intervention'.

In contrast to the poor prognosis for regaining sensation, Dahlin *et al.* (1998) of Malmö, Sweden, reported a significant

---

> **WARNING**
>
> Spastic hands must be differentiated from those with dystonic posturing. This error in diagnosis seems to be prevalent. The dystonic hand will be completely relaxed during sleep, with sedation and voluntarily. There are no contractures and no increased stretch reflexes. The deep-tendon reflexes are normal or hypoactive in dystonia.

improvement in stereognosis 18 months postoperatively upper limb surgery in 36 patients with spastic hemiplegia. They used various objects for the patient, presumably blinded but not so stated, to identify (square block, ball, pencil, coin, matchbox, tuft, toothbrush, button and other non-specified objects pre-operatively). However, the same four objects were not used at follow-up. They did a variety of standard orthopaedic operations on the hand, wrist, forearm and elbow.

The results in improvement of sensation after upper-limb surgery in spastic hemiplegia, as reported by Dahlin and colleagues, represents 'neuroplasticity'. The hand is represented in the cerebral cortex as shown in the experimental studies in primates (squirrel and owl monkey) by Blake *et al.* (2002). In these animals, trained behavior using somatosensory stimuli increased digit representation in the cortical cells 1.5 to 3-fold. The enlargement of the receptive field in the cerebral cortex and a breakdown of the columnar architecture of the cells give evidence of plasticity. These cellular dedifferentiated hand representations in the cortex were observed in repetitive voluntary hand movement in the animals. The repetitive tasks with the digits has been considered the etiology of focal dystonia as a cause of writer's cramp.

For patients who can articulate or indicate the difference between one and two points, Möberg's (1962) two-point discrimination test with a paper-clip may be more useful (Fig. 2.29), especially in those patients who have a bilateral motor involvement. The test must be carefully performed by stabilizing the patient's and the examiner's fingers, so that the skin does not blanch from the pressure applied through the tips of the clip. The pressure should not exceed 10 g (Möberg 1976, 1984). The distance between the ends of the clip should be approximately 5 mm.

Bolanos *et al.* (1989) compared Möberg's paper-clip test to shape recognition in our patients with cerebral palsy. Our results indicated that it is probably as accurate as shape recognition and simpler to perform. Verbal ability to describe the object is not necessary. All the patient has to do is indicate one or two points with a 'yes' or 'no'. The two-point discrimination test had a sensitivity of 62.7% (at a cut-off of one incorrect answer) and a specificity of 80.6%[1]. The stereognosis test had a maximum sensitivity of 39.2% (at a cut-off of no incorrect answers), with a specificity of 94.1%. All patients with spasticity had defects in two-point discrimination and stereognosis: respectively in hemiplegia 50% and 40%, in diplegia 40% and 25%, in quadriplegia 87% and 53%. Möberg (personal communication) emphasized the importance of tactile gnosis as the highest quality of sensibility; it puts 'eyes' on the fingertips (Fig. 7.2). Without it, visual feedback is necessary and this can provide control of only one hand at a time.

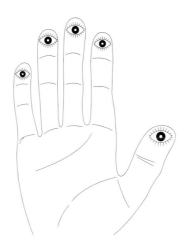

Fig. 7.2. The fingertips are the eyes of the hand (Eric Möberg).

Lesny *et al.* (1993) tested two-point discrimination in the hands of 220 children with cerebral palsy. They found that two-point discrimination decreased in all cases including those with diplegia and hemiplegia (on the involved side), while there was less loss of discrimination for those with athetosis. In 40 children with spastic hemiplegia Van Heest and colleagues (1993) also found deficient stereognosis in 97%, two-point discrimination in 90%, and proprioception in 46%. Yekutiel *et al.* (1994) of Israel confirmed similar sensory impairment in 51% of 55 children with cerebral palsy compared to 15 children who were post-poliomyelitis.

Sensory tests involving pins, touching or testing temperatures have no relevance in the evaluation for hand surgery. More sophisticated sensory tests of finger and thumb pulp have been described. The 'pulp-writing' test was found to be more indicative of higher functions than the two-point discrimination test after sensory-nerve reconstructive surgery (Hirasawa *et al.* 1985). In this test, the patient's eyes are closed and the examiner writes letters with a blunt rod on the pulp of the patient's finger. The patient then draws his impressions of the letters on a prepared outline of the thumb pulp. This test might give more information about sensibility and prognosis in cerebral-palsied hands than other tests. The results would depend very much on the intelligence and age of the patient.

4. HAND FUNCTION IN ACTIVITIES OF DAILY LIVING

How the patient manages such actions as turning on a light-switch and faucets, dressing, toileting, bathing and grooming should be part of the examination. Möberg (1962) suggested various tasks to test precision grip: (1) screw on a bolt, (2) wind a wristwatch, (3) sew with a needle, (4) knot a piece of string, (5) lift a teacup with the thumb and forefinger, and (6) button and unbutton. Gross grip can be functionally assessed by the ability to (1) work with a heavy handled object like a wheelbarrow, (2) use a spade, (3) manipulate a doorknob, (4) hold a bottle and (5) carry a basket.

Elliott and Connolly's (1984) classification of manipulative hand movements as intrinsic movement patterns of the digits

---

1 Cut-off is defined as the upper limit of number of incorrect answers expected from control patients; errors exceeding this limit are not acceptable as normal. Sensitivity= the proportion of positive test results (*i.e.* tests exceeding cut-off) among actually positive cerebral palsy cases. Specificity = the proportion of negative test results among actually negative (control) cases.

seemed to be a better method of analysis of preoperative and postoperative results. Alas, it does not appear much used, let alone by our own staff. Another test for hand function known as the Jebsen-Taylor Hand Function Test was published by Jebsen *et al.* (1969) and refined by Taylor *et al.* (1973). This involves broad sampling of timed simple hand functions including writing, card turning, picking up small objects, simulated feeding, stacking checkers, and picking up light and heavy objects (Table 7.I) While used not infrequently in assessing hand function in stroke or arthritis patients, it is used in only a few reports regarding patients with cerebral palsy (Noronha *et al.* 1989, Gordon *et al.* 2006). These simple tests are useful in quantifying changes preoperatively to postoperatively. They are presented here just in case some surgeon and an evaluation team would want to do a prospective outcome study as they are easily duplicated assessment tools.

Elliott and Connolly subdivided the intrinsic movements of the hand into simultaneous patterns as simple synergies of pinch, dynamic tripod (e.g. holding a pencil) and squeeze; the reciprocal synergies of thumb function are twiddle, rock, radial roll, index roll and full roll. Sequential patterns are those in which movement is step-like: rotary step (e.g. moving a circular object with the fingertips), interdigital step (*e.g.* a pen or chopstick is turned from one end to the other), and linear step (where the fingers are repositioned along the linear axis of an object, as in playing a violin). The palmar slide is the action of the thumb against the index finger, while the other fingers grasp an object (e.g. when uncapping a fountain pen) (Fig. 7.3 *a–l*).

(a)

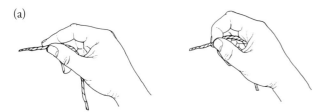

Fig. 7.3. (*a*) Pinch. *Left*: key pinch. *Right*: pulp pinch. Terminal positions for digits when executing this pattern of movement. (Reproduced by permission from Elliot and Connolly 1984.)

(b)

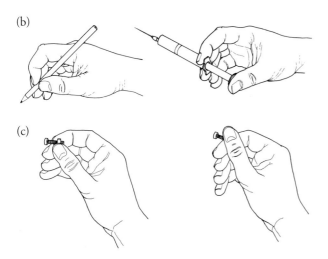

(c)

Fig. 7.3 (*b*) *Left*: dynamic tripod. *Right*: squeeze. (*c*) Twiddle. *Left*: thumb in full abduction. *Right*: thumb in partial adduction.

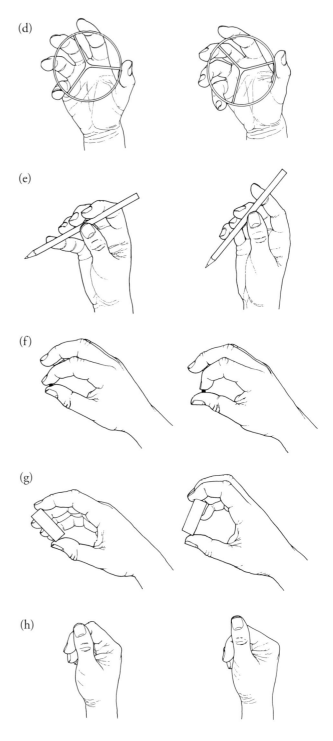

(d)

(e)

(f)

(g)

(h)

Fig. 7.3 (*d*) Rock: ventral view with a petri dish. *Left*: thumb in partial abduction. *Right*: thumb in partial adduction. (Reproduced by permission from Elliot and Connolly 1984.) (*e*) Rock: illustrated with pencil held transversely in radial–ulnar axis. Movements of thumb and digit 3 are much reduced compared with movements of other digits. *Left*: ulnar digits relatively extended. *Right*: ulnar digits relatively flexed. (*f*) Index roll. *Top left*: slight reciprocal flexion of thumb and extension of index, and *top right*: the reverse. (*g*) Full roll (*bottom left and right*) as for index roll, but with involvement of additional digits. The object rocks about the radio-ulnar axis as a result of movement between the positions illustrated. (*h*) Radial roll. In this example the thumb is abducted throughout; in other instances it may be partially adducted, consequently operating radial index more distally. *Left*: index less flexed. *Right*: index more flexed. (Reproduced by permission from Elliot and Connolly 1984.)

(i)

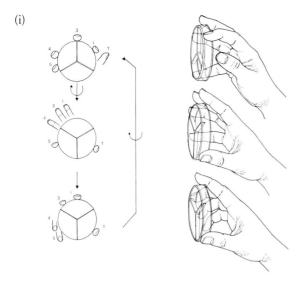

Fig. 7.3 (*i*) Rotary step. A schematic representation of positions in which the digits are placed (*left*) and successive postures of the hand (*right*). Sequence (*right, top to bottom*) shows successive phases in clockwise rotation totaling approximately 120° of object rotation. This occurs between transitions top to *center and bottom to top*, as indicated by the rotary arrows. (Reproduced by permission from Elliot and Connolly 1984.)

(j)

(k)

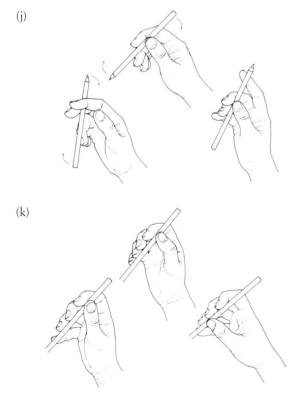

Fig. 7.3 (*j*) Interdigital step: from *center to left* the object is rotated by extension of ulnar digits, especially digit 3. Flexed thumb passes under rotating object to assume its position shown left. From *left to right*, thumb and ulnar digits flex to grasp object and index extends and may lose contact with it. From *right to center*, index flexes to preserve position of object against thumb, while ulnar digits flex to reposition below object in readiness for next cycle. (*k*) Linear step: from *center to left*, ulnar digits extend interphalangeally, but flex at carpo–metacarpal joints, sliding along object. From *left to right*, thumb abducts to oppose ulnar digits. From *right to center*, index flexes to restore initial posture. (Reproduced by permission from Elliot and Connolly 1984.)

(l)

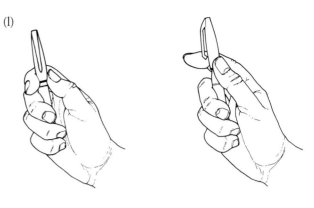

Fig. 7.3 (*l*) Palmar slide: the movement, illustrated in change from *left to right*, involves extension of thumb and radial deviation of index, with some extension. (Reproduced by permission from Elliot and Connolly 1984.)

TABLE 7.I
Jebsen-Taylor test of hand function

Subtest	Hand task	Description
1	Writing	24-letter sentence
2	Turning over cards	3 × 5 cards to simulate turning pages
3	Picking up small objects	Pennies, bottle caps, paperclips
4	Simulated feeding	Spoon five dried beans into coffee can
5	Stacking checkers	Four checkers
6	Picking up light objects	Empty cans
7	Picking up heavy objects	Full cans (1 lb)

5. VOLUNTARY GRASP AND RELEASE PATTERNS

Voluntary grasp and release patterns have been classified into three types by Zancolli *et al.* (1983). In *pattern I*, the fingers actively extend with the wrist in less than 20° of flexion. Surgery is indicated. In *pattern II*, the wrist and fingers are constantly in flexion. Active finger extension occurs only when the wrist is flexed more than 20°. This pattern has been subdivided into two groups. In *pattern IIa*, when the wrist and fingers are flexed, active extension of the wrist is possible because the wrist extensors exert good voluntary control; while in *pattern IIb*, when the fingers are flexed, wrist extension is not possible because the wrist extensors are weak or lack voluntary control. In these patients the hand can open only by wrist flexion, which creates a tenodesis effect on the finger-extensors. Surgery can improve function. Finally, *pattern III* is a severe flexion deformity of the hand, without finger extension even with maximum wrist flexion, and with no active wrist extension with the fingers flexed. Passive extension of the fingers and thumb is possible when the wrist is flexed. Function will not improve much with surgery, but appearance may be greatly improved.

In an earlier publication, Zancolli and Zancolli (1981) presented a more refined classification of cerebral palsy hand dysfunction and deformity (Table 7.II). In the examination, the effect of wrist position on finger extension should be observed. Very often finger extension occurs not by active extension, but by the tenodesis effect of the extensor digitorum communis as the wrist drops into flexion. In these cases wrist stabilization or an extension contracture of the wrist will preclude opening the hand for release from the grasp.

217

*Very often finger extension occurs not by active extension, but by
the tenodesis effect of the extensor digitorum communis as the
wrist drops into flexion.*

Goldner's original classification (1975) is useful and
straightforward. (1) Minimal involvement. The patient's hand has
pinch, grasp and release, but lacks dexterity and speed. No surgery
is indicated. (2) Thumb-in-palm, wrist flexed moderately; to
extend the fingers the wrist must be dropped into full flexion
(tenodesis effect on the finger extensors) (Fig. 7.4). (3) Thumb-
in-palm, wrist and fingers completely flexed; the patient is unable
to extend the fingers (Fig. 7.5). Surgery is indicated to improve
appearance and hand hygiene.

To the above classification the following observations may
assist in decision-making for surgery. (1) Voluntary control. (2)
No voluntary control; mirror movements by the opposite hand
are the controlling mechanism. Mirror movements are probably
normal up to the age of 6 or 7 years in some children. These can
be ascertained by asking the child to place his hands on the

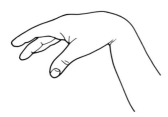

Fig. 7.4. Spastic hand pattern II. To open the fingers, wrist must flex,
exerting a tenodesis effect on the finger-extensor tendons.

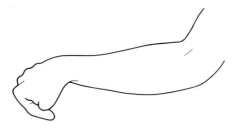

Fig. 7.5. Spastic hand pattern III. Complete flexion of the wrist and
fingers, thumb-in-palm.

tabletop and perform alternating movements (e.g. finger tapping
or rapid pronation and supination) with one hand alone, and then
the other hand. (3) No voluntary or mirror movement control.
Surgery may be indicated in the first two patterns. In the third,
restoration of any function cannot be promised; surgery is
indicated for appearance, hygiene and comfort.

Although the above patterns are useful to organize thinking,
examining and reporting results, they are only general guides and
cannot be slavishly applied in decisions for specific surgery. Only
examination, repeat examination and repeat examination of the
patient's hand and upper limb will create a reasonably correct plan
for surgical treatment.

*Only examination, repeat examination and repeat examination
. . . will create a reasonably correct plan for surgical treatment.*

ELECTROMYOGRAPHIC EVALUATION

Electromyography (EMG) of the spastic muscle to be lengthened
or transferred has been used as an additional method of analysis
for many years (Samilson and Morris 1964, Feldkamp and Güth
1980, Hoffer *et al.* 1983, Mowery *et al.* 1985).

Hoffer and colleagues (Hoffer *et al.* 1979, Hoffer 1993)
used the EMG information preoperatively in the finger-flexed
hand. They transferred the tendons of muscles only when these
muscles showed isolated electrical activity in grasp in those with
weak grasp, and only muscles that had isolated activity on release
in hands with a poor release. The flexor carpi ulnaris and the
brachioradialis were the most commonly selected for transfer to
open the hand. Based on the EMG data, less than half of these
two muscles were deemed suitable for transfer.

Dynamic EMG with fine wires into the selected muscle has
to be correlated with the clinical examination and myoneural
blocks in some cases.

MYONEURAL BLOCKS

Infiltration of the muscle bellies of the flexor muscles of the wrist
and fingers with lidocaine (either 0.5 or 1%[2]) is useful to
determine whether the spastic flexor muscles of the wrist or
fingers are preventing voluntary extension of the wrist or fingers
(Goldner 1983, E. Möberg, personal communication). In con-

---

2 The dose of lidocaine should not exceed 4.5mg/kg in children over 10 years
and in adults; in children under age 10, the dosage should be adjusted
downward according to the usual pediatric drug dose rules.

trast to a local anesthetic block of the median nerve, a myoneural block obviates the loss of finger sensation which occurs over a fairly large area of the palm and fingers. This loss of sensation might alter the functional evaluation considerably because Möberg's study (1976) demonstrated the important role of cutaneous sensory endings in providing feedback of joint-position sense: 'There is no *muscle sense* in man' (p. 34).

Infiltration of the biceps muscle with the local anesthetic may help to decide the effect of muscle release in flexion deformities of the elbow. In two patients who had severe, painful and disabling contraction of the elbow flexor muscles in hemidystonia, Bleck infiltrated the biceps brachii with 45% alcohol. This gave the surgeon, the patient and the family 2–4 weeks to decide on the effects of denervating the biceps brachii in order to reduce the severe elbow-flexion posture. Injections of forearm muscles with alcohol should not be done. Its effects can be very destructive on the adjacent peripheral nerves, and the resultant paralysis might last a distressing 3–4 months.

In lieu of lidocaine or alcohol blocks, botulinum-A toxin may be used. However, the duration of its effect will be from 3 to 6 months. This may be too long a time-span to be useful to the surgeon and patient as to the effects of the proposed surgery. For dystonic posturing of the elbow in flexion, botulinum toxin injections appear to be better choice. As described in Chapter 6, botulinum toxin has been used in spastic forearm muscles as a treatment of flexion spasticity. It seems unlikely that the result of relief of the spasticity will be long-term. If the muscle is contracted, i.e. shortened, then this injection will not be effective. Surgery will probably be necessary if improvement in appearance and some function of the hand is the goal.

PREREQUISITES FOR SURGERY
Judging from reports of the number of patients with cerebral palsy who had hand surgery compared with the whole of the cerebral palsy population, the surgical indications have restricted the number of patients operated on (Goldner 1955, Chait *et al.* 1980, Zancolli and Zancolli 1981, Hoffer *et al.* 1983, Mowery *et al.* 1985).

1. SPASTIC PARALYSIS
Although a satisfactory surgical result may be possible when the spastic hand has a minor degree of athetosis (*e.g.* chorea), the best results are achieved only in those with spastic paralysis, and most of these have hemiplegia. In one study of results of 87 spastic hands, only two had quadriplegia; all the others had hemiplegia (Zancolli and Zancolli 1981).

2. AGE OF THE PATIENT
Most experienced surgeons in this field recommend deferring surgery until age 5 years or older. By this time the child can cooperate in the preoperative analysis and the postoperative regimen. An exception to this advice is that of Goldner (1983). He will lengthen a wrist tendon (usually the flexor carpi ulnaris) in a 3-year-old if it is deforming and contracted. This procedure is always followed by prolonged splinting. Lipp and Jones (1984)

strongly recommended that this procedure could and should be done at age 3 years, based upon their results of transfer of the flexor carpi ulnaris to correct the flexion–pronation deformity of the wrist. But if the pronator teres is contracted this transfer will not give the intended active supination unless the pronator teres tendon is released and the patient has voluntary control.

3. SENSATION
Although stereognosis is absent in the majority of patients with spastic hemiplegia, this is not a contraindication to surgery. If tactile gnosis is normal (a rare occurrence), then the result will be better.

4. MENTAL STATUS
The mental status obviously will affect the result. Children with severe mental retardation and adults will not obtain the desired functional result. Of more importance is their behaviour. Emotional instability with increased spasticity in response to stimuli will compromise the function (Zancolli *et al.* 1983).

5. VOLUNTARY CONTROL
This is most important for function after reconstructive surgery. Some ability to extend the fingers with active wrist flexion assures a better result. The best candidates for surgery are those who have either patterns I or II (Zancolli *et al.* 1983) or Goldner group 2 (1975).

GOALS OF SURGERY
The goals are to improve the function of grasp, release, and pinch, and appearance of the hand. The patient and the parents must be told that the hand will never be normal—it will be a helping hand. *It is wise to not only say it, but also put it in writing* (Goldner 1983). Those who pursued conservative methods of splinting, stretching or special therapies have not reported objective changes. Adaptive utensils, tools tested and recommended by the therapist can assist in creating a satisfactory helping hand.

> *The patient and the parents must be told that the hand will never be normal—it will be a helping hand.*

When discussing the proposed plan of surgery with the parents and child, the surgeon should reiterate that additional surgery may be necessary to accomplish the goal. This will be true even though most of us now try to do multiple surgical procedures at one stage. The preoperative analysis and planning, while very good, is not perfect.

Appearance of the hand will usually be improved with surgery. Appearance often outweighs the functional result; after all, the hand is a highly visible part of the human anatomy. In the analysis of results, authors often comment on the improved appearance as an important parameter of the outcome (Chait *et al.* 1980, Zancolli and Zancolli 1981, Mowery *et al.* 1985).

Improvement of appearance is often termed 'cosmetic'. However, to deny the human need of looking one's best is to deprive the person with spastic hemiplegia and a deformed hand the opportunity to overcome just one obstacle for acceptance. While it is true that we should strive to look at the person behind the disability, it is also true that this is a process which takes time and understanding by others. Rather than hide the deformed hand in the pocket or explain it in detail to the other person, it seems that a more normal-appearing hand will help to improve initial relationships and increase chances in a job interview. So surgery to improve the appearance of the hand can be a most important functional as well as psychological goal.

Bleck observed that patients with hemiplegia over age 18 years wanted their hands to be 'fixed' without any regard for function (unpublished observations). They readily accept arthrodesis of the wrist, finger-flexor tendon lengthenings and thumb reconstructive surgery. With people spending billions of dollars a year worldwide on grooming aids, cosmetics and wrinkle reduction with botulinum toxin injections, is it irrational and unwarranted to want the best possible appearance of your hands?

SURGICAL PROCEDURES FOR THE UPPER LIMB

It must be realized that no single procedure offers the complete reconstruction of the spastic hand and wrist. The procedures described are reliable, but must be combined according to the preoperative analysis; multiple procedures at one stage are usually necessary to achieve the desired result. House *et al.* (1981) gave an example of the need for multiple procedures; they performed 165 different procedures for the thumb-in-palm deformity in 56 patients.

The best way of assessing the results is to use a preoperative and postoperative functional classification. An elaborate and precise method of evaluation of the results of surgery was published by Swanson (1982) and Zancolli *et al.* (1983) (Table 7.II). The classification of House *et al.* is also included in preoperative and postoperative assessments of the hand with cerebral palsy and is more functionally based (Table7.I). The classification by Mowery (Table 7.III) is less complicated than that of House but also less sensitive to changes in hand function. In assessing patients using these classifications, Waters and colleagues (2004) compared the House and Mowery classifications in the observation of 10 videotaped patient examinations by three examiners. They noted interobserver and intraobserver reliability using these tests with the best reliability in the consolidated House classification system (Table 7.IV). The consolidated House classification system batches the levels into: unable to use (level 0); passive assist (levels 1, 2, 3); active assist (levels 4, 5, 6); spontaneous use (levels 7, 8). In the paper by Mowery *et al.* (1985), the functional grade after tendon transfers about the hand improved by at least one level in all patients. Of the 12 patients reported, results were evenly divided into excellent, good and fair. They used videotaping, muscle grading and EMGs to evaluate their results.

TABLE 7.III
Functional classification (from Mowery *et al.* 1985)

Poor	Paperweight, absent grasp and release
Fair control	Helper hand, no effective use, moderate grasp and release, fair
Good	Helper hand, effective grasp and release, some voluntary control
Excellent	Good use of hand, effective grasp and release, voluntary control

TABLE 7.IV
Classification of upper extremity function (House *et al.* 1981)

Level	Category	Description
0	Does not use	Does not use
1	Poor passive assist	Uses as stabilizer
2	Fair passive assist	Holds object placed in hand
3	Good passive assist	Holds object & stabilize for use by other hand
4	Poor active assist	Actively grasps object and hold weakly
5	Fair active assist	Actively grasps object and stabilize
6	Good active assist	Actively grasps object and manipulate
7	Spontaneous use, partial	Bimanual activities & occasionally use spontaneously
8	Spontaneous use, complete	Uses hand independent of other hand

THUMB DEFORMITIES

In the upper limb, the thumb is as much of the focus of surgery as is the equinus in the lower limb. Whether the thumb is only adducted (either a dynamic or a fixed deformity) due to contracture, or is a thumb-in-palm deformity, the objective is to get the thumb out of the palm and to restore pinch. True opposition by pulp pinch cannot be achieved in most. This is not a functional pinch. A 'key' pinch will suffice (Figs 7.6, 7.7). Smith (1982) reported improved grasp in seven patients, but manipulation of small objects was not improved.

SPASTIC DYNAMIC ADDUCTION
This deformity is due to spasticity of the adductor pollicis muscle, with the metacarpal and interphalangeal joints maintained in extension. If the deformity is only dynamic, passive abduction of the thumb is possible, and the adducted position interferes with the release of the side pinch to the index finger. In this case, a simple release of the adductor insertion through an ulnar incision over the metacarpal–phalangeal joint is sufficient. Goldner (1983) sutures this insertion to the annular ligament of the metacarpal–phalangeal joint. Arthrodesis of this joint is not necessary. If arthrodesis is required, then the adductor pollicis insertion is sutured more proximally.

Hoffer *et al.* (1983) advised more selectivity in tenotomy of the adductor pollicis based upon the dynamic electromyogram. If the adductor muscle demonstrates selective control during grasp and release, then only myotomy of the transverse fibers is needed. If there is non-selective control (a patterned type of

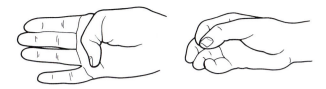

Fig. 7.6. *Left:* thumb-in-palm deformity due to spastic adductor pollicis and flexor pollicis longus. *Right:* normal pinch.

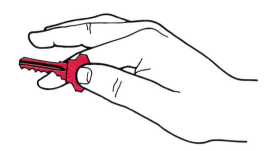

Fig. 7.7. Key pinch: the thumb pulp opposes the radial side of the index finger.

contraction with continuous firing of the muscle), a complete myotomy that includes the oblique head of the adductor pollicis muscle was recommended. These procedures were done through a z-plasty incision in the web space. The thumb procedures were always combined with tendon transfers at the wrist or fingers, and in some with a capsulodesis of the first metacarpal–phalangeal joint.

ADDUCTION CONTRACTURE

When a severe adduction contracture of the thumb occurs (which is very rare in children), then a release of the origin of the adductor pollicis is necessary. This procedure, introduced by Matev (1963, 1991), uses a palmar incision. Goldner (1983) found the palmar approach unnecessary; the origin release from the third and second metacarpals can be done through a dorsal incision. The first dorsal interosseus muscle aggravates these severe adduction deformities, and can be released from the first and second metacarpals (Goldner 1955, 1975, 1983, Silver *et al.* 1976, House *et al.* 1981).

SKIN WEB-SPACE CONTRACTURE

A z-plasty of the web space is almost never required in children with cerebral palsy. If needed in long standing contractures, Goldner (1983) advised that the flap of skin on the thumb side of the incision be made larger so that with undermining the dorsal skin advancement of both flaps and a loose closure can be accomplished. The various techniques of z-plasty of the thumb web space have been described in detail by Meyer *et al.* (1981). If in severe skin contractures the web-space skin cannot be completely closed even with z-plasty, then a full-thickness skin graft from the elbow flexor crease is a solution (Goldner 1983).

THUMB-IN-PALM

This is the commonest thumb deformity; as well as the adduction spasticity and eventual contracture there is a flexion spasticity and contracture of the flexor pollicis longus, and at times also the flexor pollicis brevis and the abductor pollicis brevis (Goldner 1983). Several procedures are required to alleviate the untenable position of the thumb so that grasp can occur, and if possible to restore lateral or key pinch. (1) Release of the adductor pollicis insertion, and (depending upon the degree of the dynamic deformity and contracture) a release of the first dorsal interosseus. (2) Release of the flexor pollicis brevis and abductor pollicis brevis insertions from the thumb sesamoid bones and resuturing of the insertions proximally after arthrodesis of the metacarpal–phalangeal joint (Goldner 1983). (3) Arthrodesis of the metacarpal–phalangeal joint if unstable (excessive motion) in both flexion and extension, or capsulodesis of the joint if hyperextendable (Zancolli *et al.* 1983) (Fig. 7.8). (4) Lengthening of the flexor pollicis longus and reinforcement if it has weak muscle power (Goldner 1983), or transfer of this tendon to the radial side of the proximal phalanx with arthrodesis of the interphalangeal joint of the thumb in 15º of flexion (Smith 1982). (5) Rerouting of the extensor pollicis longus (Goldner 1983, Manske 1985, Ryan and Saccone 1996). (6) Reinforcement of the abductor and extensor pollicis longus with the brachioradialis or the flexor digitorum superficialis from the long or ring finger. (7) Shortening by placation of the tendon of the abductor pollicis longus.

Matev (1991) did essentially the same procedures for the spastic thumb-in-palm in 56 patients with correction in 82%; he did not do any bone-stabilizing operations.

A classification of the thumb-in-palm deformity was proposed by Sakellarides and colleagues (1995) to help in selecting options for treatment by assortment into four types: I, weak or paralyzed extensor pollicis longus; II, spastic adductor pollicis and flexor pollicis longus and brevis with or without first dorsal interosseus involvement; III, weak or paralyzed

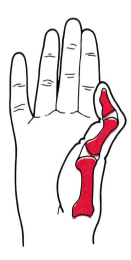

Fig. 7.8. Common posture of the thumb with instability in extension at the metacarpal–phalangeal joint.

abductor pollicis longus; and IV, spastic or contracted flexor pollicis longus.

To add a bit of confusion to the surgical management of what we call 'thumb-in-palm' deformity, Matsuo (2002) recommended section of the oblique head of the adductor pollicis in 'mild thumb adduction deformity' and the entire proximal origin of the oblique head in 'moderate and severe deformities of the thumb-in-flexion' and in hyperextension of the metacarpal–phalangeal joint section of the entire proximal origins of the transverse and oblique heads of the adductor pollicis. A sliding and intramuscular lengthening of the flexor pollicis longus is always included: 2–3 cm for a moderate flexion contracture, 3–4 cm for a 'severe' deformity. The only problem is how do you define 'moderate' or 'severe'. Our guess is that this is a matter of the canard, 'surgical judgement'.

ARTHRODESIS OF THE METACARPAL–PHALANGEAL JOINT

This procedure can be done in children who have open epiphyses (Goldner 1975, 1983, Zancolli *et al.* 1983, Goldner *et al.* 1990), but *very carefully* to avoid fusion of the physis and a resultant short thumb. Through a midlateral ulnar incision over the joint, the lateral band is retracted dorsally, the ulnar collateral ligament and capsule cut, the joint opened and the articular cartilage on both surfaces removed. In children it is safer to 'nibble' away the cartilage with a rongeur. The joint surfaces are coapted manually in 5° of flexion. Using a motorized drill, a single smooth pin is drilled through the center of the proximal phalanx in line with the center of the nail. Then with the joint flexed 5°, the pin is drilled in retrograde manner into the first metacarpal. The phalanx is rotated so that the palmar thumb-pad coincides with the radial aspect of the index finger. Smooth pins are inserted at a 45° angle across the joint to secure the arthrodesis. Small bone chips can be added to any gaps in the arthrodesis site (Fig. 7.9).

The ends of the pins are clipped off beneath the skin and removed when the arthrodesis is solid (8–12 weeks). A plaster holds the thumb and wrist in position while healing occurs.

In skeletally mature patients a small (3.5 mm) screw provides for more secure fixation. After the joint surfaces are denuded, the joint is manually compressed and held in the proper position. A 3.5 mm hole (the same diameter as the screw) is bored with an air-powered drill in the distal end of the dorsal surface of the metacarpal neck through the cortex. Through this hole the 2.5 mm drill is directed obliquely into the center of the proximal phalanx through the cortex. The entry hole in the metacarpal is enlarged so that the screw-head can be countersunk slightly. The screw is then inserted and the joint surfaces compressed (Fig. 7.10). With this rigid fixation, it is possible to remove the postoperative plaster or fiberglass cast in 3–4 weeks so that early motion of the hand and wrist can commence. If the screw-hole in the metacarpal breaks during the procedure, all is not lost. The joint can always be secured with multiple crossed threaded pins.

CAPSULODESIS OF THE METACARPAL–PHALANGEAL JOINT

This operation has been recommended if the metacarpal–phalangeal joint is unstable in hyperextension but not flexion (Filler *et at.* 1976, Zancolli 1979, Zancolli *et al.* 1983). It consists of detachment of the volar capsule of the metacarpal–phalangeal joint from the first metacarpal and advancement of the capsular attachment proximally into a groove in the metacarpal shaft. Fixation is with a pullout suture, threaded first through the capsule and then through two drill holes directed dorsally in the neck of the metacarpal, and tied over a button on the dorsum of the first metacarpal (Fig. 7.11); 30° of flexion is recommended by advocates of the procedure. Plaster immobilization is 6 weeks postoperatively. This procedure creates a flexion contracture of the joint.

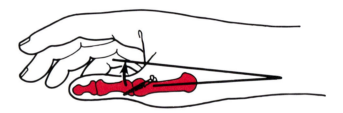

Fig. 7.10. Arthrodesis of the metacarpal–phalangeal joint of the thumb with small screw fixation. The joint is flexed 5°–10° for optimum function.

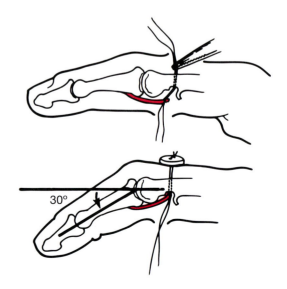

30°

Fig. 7.11. Technique for volar capsule advancement to stabilize the metacarpal–phalangeal joint of the thumb.

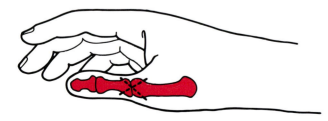

Fig. 7.9. Arthrodesis of the metacarpal–phalangeal joint of the thumb with crossed fixation pins.

This should be done if the distal phalanx of the thumb is
persistently flexed. Contracture of the flexor pollicis longus
contributes to the thumb-in-palm. A weak muscle decreases
endurance of grasp and pinch (Goldner 1983). Lengthening is
not indicated if there is no flexion contracture found on 30° of
wrist extension and passive hyperextension of the thumb is
possible. Reinforcement would not be indicated if the extensor
muscles are half normal strength or better, or if reinforcement of
the extensor and abductor pollicis longus is not done. The
indications to reinforce the flexor pollicis longus muscle are
probably uncommon.

Lengthening can be done through an incision over the volar
radial surface of the wrist and forearm. To determine the amount
of lengthening, the wrist is placed in 15° extension with the
thumb held in full abduction and the proximal phalanx held in
neutral extension. The resultant amount of flexion at the distal
joint is measured, and the flexor pollicis longus tendon is
lengthened 0.5 mm per degree (Goldner 1983). The lengthening
is done above the transverse carpal ligament so that the suture line
will not impinge on this ligament.

Reinforcement of the flexor pollicis longus is with the
brachioradialis (which must be extensively mobilized) or a flexor
digitorum superficialis tendon. The pronator teres is said to be
usable as well (Goldner 1983) (Fig. 7.12). If the flexor superficialis
is selected, it is adjusted to one-half its resting length for the suture
to the flexor pollicis longus tendon.

REROUTING OF THE EXTENSOR POLLICIS
LONGUS TENDON

This procedure is almost always performed in conjunction with
other techniques for correction of the thumb-in-palm. Through
a lazy-s incision from the metacarpal–phalangeal joint of the
thumb to about 4 cm proximal to the wrist, the extensor pollicis
longus tendon is dissected from its dorsal hood insertion to its
musculotendinous junction. The tendon is lifted out of its fibro-
osseus tunnel in the radial styloid and shifted to the radial side
of the wrist. It is held in its new location by fashioning a flap of
subcutaneous fascia and fat to make a tunnel 3–4 cm long (Figs
7.12, 7.13).

Manske (1984) observed in spastic thumb deformities that
the distal phalanx extended during finger extension (indicating
in-phase muscle function of the extensor pollicis longus) and
also that the extensor pollicis longus acted as a thumb adductor
(noted as well by other surgeons). His procedure in 17 patients
was to detach the extensor pollicis longus at the extensor
hood, withdraw the tendon into the forearm, reroute it through
the first extensor compartment and suture it to the first
metacarpal–phalangeal joint capsule and extensor hood. The
procedure was done in conjunction with the usual myotomies
of the spastic intrinsic thumb muscles. His results were good
after an average follow-up of 28 months.

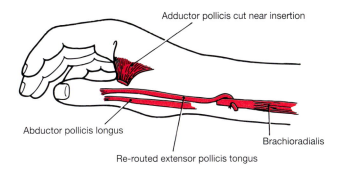

Fig. 7.12. Technique for reinforcement of thumb abduction by transfer
of the brachioradialis to the rerouted extensor pollicis longus. The abductor
pollicis longus can be shortened and advanced.

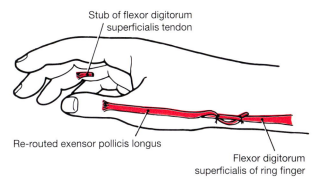

Fig. 7.13. Technique for reinforcement of thumb abduction by transfer
of the flexor digitorum superficialis to the rerouted extensor pollicis longus.

REINFORCEMENT OF THE REROUTED EXTENSOR
POLLICIS LONGUS

Two muscle-tendon units can be used: the flexor digitorum
superficialis of the long or ring finger or the brachioradialis. The
superficialis tendon is cut at the proximal phalanx of the finger,
pulled out through a separate incision 8–10 cm above the wrist
and rerouted subcutaneously to the extensor pollicis longus
(Fig. 7.12). The brachioradialis is detached at its insertion on the
radius, and the muscle mobilized to the junction of the upper and
middle thirds of its belly. The tendons of either are woven into
the extensor pollicis longus tendon after the thumb has been
repositioned (Fig. 7.13). To determine the proper tension of the
transferred tendon, a temporary anchoring suture is used so that
the thumb can move passively to the index finger with the wrist
in the neutral position, and to allow passive extension of the
thumb about 2.5 cm from the index finger. It is not necessary to
detach the extensor pollicis tendon from its muscle belly, because
keeping it in continuity will help prevent volar displacement of
the rerouted tendon (Goldner 1983).

ARTHRODESIS OF THE DISTAL INTERPHALANGEAL
JOINT OF THE THUMB

Arthrodesis of this joint is indicated if it is hypermobile in
extension, flexion, radial or ulnar deviation. It is not indicated if

the distal phalangeal flexion and extension are controlled by the muscle–tendon unit (Goldner 1983).

The operative technique consists of removing the articular surfaces of the joint, and securing it in 5º–10º of flexion with threaded pins cut off beneath the skin.

WRIST- AND FINGER-FLEXION DEFORMITIES

A spastic wrist-flexion deformity is often due to a combination of both wrist- and finger-flexor spasticity. Only a careful and repeat examination allows discernment if one or the other or both predominate. The possibility that the flexor muscle spasticity prevents active extension of the wrist can be determined by infiltration of the flexor muscle bellies in the proximal forearm with 0.5% or 1% lidocaine.

TENDON LENGTHENING

To avoid overlengthening of the finger-flexor tendons, a controlled lengthening is used to retain the 'normal' tension so that when the hand is relaxed and the wrist in neutral position, the fingers assume their normal flexed position (as it is with your own hand when relaxed on a desktop with the forearm supinated). When lengthening a contracted wrist-flexor muscle–tendon unit, enough elongation of the tendon should permit about 20º of wrist extension.

One way to estimate the amount of z-lengthening of a tendon, to restore its resting length and preserve the proper tension for function, is to lengthen it approximately one-half of the contracted resting state of the muscle. One way to do this is to incise and split the tendon longitudinally for a distance of double the estimated amount of lengthening needed (in general plan to lengthen a tendon 0.5 mm. for every degree of flexion contracture; e.g. 40º of contracture = 20 mm of lengthening).

Plan to lengthen a tendon 0.5 mm for every degree of flexion contracture, e.g. 40º contracture = 20 mm of lengthening.

A 2 cm lengthening would require a 4cm split in the tendon; a suture is placed in the distal end of one of the splits in the tendon, which is then cut distal to the suture. Next, this distal end is brought proximally 2 cm and sutured to the adjacent intact split tendon, which is then cut proximally. The two slips

of tendon are sutured side by side. Handling dangling tendon ends is avoided by this method (Goldner 1983, 1987, 1998). The suture should be temporary until the proper resting position of the fingers is observed (Fig.7.14). It is safer to underlengthen, since overlengthening results in too much loss of muscle strength. Matsuo (2002) advocates sliding lengthening of almost all tendons. He isolates the tendon with two plastic tubes under it, places a zig-zag suture in the middle, then cuts half the tendon proximally and distally. The tendon is slid to the desired length and then the suture is tied.

In young children, Goldner advised lengthening of the flexor carpi radialis ('the heel cord of the hand') when it appears to be the major deforming force. In other cases it may be the flexor carpi ulnaris. Zancolli and Zancolli (1981) found tenotomy to be a satisfactory solution only in cases of mild flexion deformities. Bleck found few children who were candidates for wrist-flexor tendon lengthening (unpublished observations). In any case, overlengthening and/or lengthening of both wrist-flexor tendons should be avoided.

Lengthening of the finger-flexor tendons is performed in the forearm (Koman *et al.* 1990). When necessary to overcome severe flexion of the digits when the wrist is dorsiflexed to neutral, the flexor digitorum superficialis tendons can be lengthened by the z-method or sliding method described above. Simultaneous lengthening of the flexor digitorum profundus tendons is not advised.

Another procedure to relieve the flexion deformities of the fingers was proposed by Braun *et al.* (1974). The profundus tendons are sectioned above the wrist, and their proximal ends are sutured to the distal ends of the cut superficialis tendons. The procedure (as in lengthening of both superficialis and profundus tendons) can result in pronounced weakness of finger flexion and the subsequent development of an intrinsic-plus deformity with the fingers practically fixed in extension. Braun had this kind of result initially, and in subsequent patients recommended post-operative splinting of the fingers in 45º of flexion. Bleck had patients who had this operation referred to him with resultant very stiff intrinsic-plus fingers (unpublished observations). Koman *et al.* (1990) also imposed a limit on using the procedure: 'Superficialis-to-profundus transfer should be reserved for patients who have problems with hygiene and in whom functional

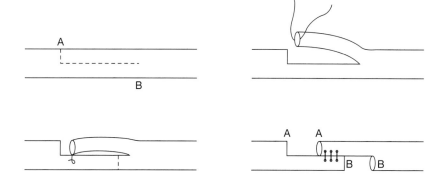

Fig. 7.14. Technique of controlled lengthening of finger-flexor tendons in the forearm (Goldner 1983, 1987, 1988).

224

recovery is not an issue' (p.69). Presumably the 'problem with hygiene' is the tight-fisted hand precluding adequate hand-washing or nail care.

RELEASE (DETACHMENT) OF THE WRIST AND FINGER-FLEXOR ORIGINS

Other methods to lengthen spastic and contracted finger and wrist flexors are variations of release of the flexor muscle origins at the elbow. The variations depend upon the range of finger extension possible when the wrist is flexed.

1. If finger extension is possible with the wrist flexed less than 50º, Zancolli and Zancolli (1981) recommended section of the aponeurosis of the origin of the flexor muscles at the medial epicondyle of the humerus.

2. If finger extension is possible only with the wrist flexed more than 50º, then the entire flexor origin is detached from the humerus (Zancolli and Zancolli 1981). This 'flexor slide' operation, in which the origins are detached and allowed to slide distally, was reported by Inglis and Cooper (1966). It was reviewed as the operation first described by Max Page in 1923 in a report by White (1972), who had 11 failures with this operation in 21 patients. To ensure a complete relief of the flexion contracture of the wrist and fingers, Haddad (1977) added the release of the origins of the flexor digitorum profundus muscles. But it seems as if this extensive and non-selective release of the flexor-muscle origins results in loss of flexion power, while with a more limited release, the problem is a failure of correction. Selective lengthening and/or transfer of tendons is probably a better solution.

Flexor slide at the elbow: extensive release of the flexor muscle origins results in loss of flexion power . . . a more limited release results in failure of correction.

A better solution: lengthen and/or transfer the tendons.

Matsuo *et al.* (1990) were pleased with their results in a combined 'release' of the flexor digitorum profundus, flexor digitorum sublimis, and extensor digitorum communis muscles in 19 patients with cerebral palsy. These authors thought that the simultaneous release of the co-contracting muscles facilitated the voluntary use of the intrinsic muscles of the hand for better function.

FINGER-HYPEREXTENSION DEFORMITY (SWAN-NECK)

The 'swan-neck' deformity of the fingers is so-called because it more or less resembles a swan's neck. A more precise description is a hyperextension of the proximal interphalangeal joint and flexion of the distal interphalangeal joint. It is caused by a persistent flexed posture of the wrist; spasticity of the intrinsic muscles is secondary. The flexion of the wrist results in pulling of the extensor tendons across the dorsum of the proximal interphalangeal joints with stretching of the volar capsules.

Surgical treatment is indicated only when the fingers lock in extension and cannot be actively flexed. The wrist-flexion deformity must also be corrected in all cases. Two surgical procedures to correct the deformity have been described. Bleck (unpublished observations) combined both because of unwelcome recurrences of the deformity in some patients who had congenital generalized increased ligamentous laxity. The five signs of ligamentous laxity might be included in the preoperative evaluation: (1) hyperextension more than 10º of the uninvolved elbow; (2) thumb tip can be approximated to the wrist on the uninvolved side; (3) in the uninvolved hand with the wrist held in neutral flexion-extension the fingers can be extended at the metacarpal–phalangeal joints so they lie parallel to the forearm; (4) again on the uninvolved side, hyperextension of the knees more than 10º; (5) dorsiflexion of the foot/ankle more than 45º on the uninvolved side (Wynn-Davies 1970).

VOLAR CAPSULODESIS

Radial and ulnar midlateral incisions over the proximal interphalangeal joint expose the retinacula which are incised (Goldner 1975, 1983). The volar joint capsule is detached from the distal end of the proximal phalanx and pulled proximally to flex the joint 45º. The capsule is anchored to its new attachment with sutures passed through the bone and tied to a dorsal button. The retinacula are sutured by overlapping the dorsal leaf distally and the volar leaf proximally (Fig. 7.15*a*).

FLEXOR SUPERFICIALIS TENODESIS

The flexor tendons are exposed through a midlateral incision over the proximal joint, and the sheath is then opened; the tendons are retracted volar-ward (Swanson *et al.* 1960). The volar aspect of the proximal phalanx is stripped of its periosteum. The superficialis tendon is then sutured to the distal end of the proximal phalanx through two drill-holes directed dorsally in the distal end of the phalanx. The suture is tied over a button on the dorsum of the finger (Fig. 7.15*b*). The proximal phalanx should be flexed about 45º. Koman *et al.* (1990) did the

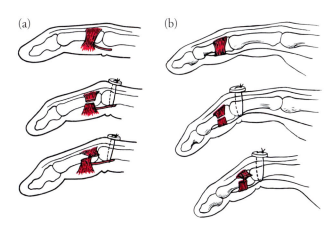

Fig. 7.15. (a) Technique for advancement of volar capsule of proximal interphalangeal joint and retinacular overlap to correct hyperextension locking of the proximal joint ('swan-neck' deformity). (b) Technique for tenodesis of flexor digitorum superficialis to correct hyperextension deformity of the proximal interphalangeal joint. This can be combined with volar capsular advancement.

superficialis tenodesis by splitting the cut tendon in half and looping each half around the posterior aspect of the proximal phalanx where it was sutured.

In both reconstructions, a fine smooth pin driven from the proximal end of the middle phalanx through to the distal end of the proximal phalanx prevents disruption of the capsule and tendon while healing occurs. The pin can be removed in 3–4 weeks. The postoperative immobilization consists of a plaster with the wrist in neutral position and the fingers flexed for 6 weeks.

SUMMARY OF SURGICAL TREATMENT OF WRIST- AND FINGER-FLEXION DEFORMITIES

Although it is impossible to offer a recipe for what is to be done, the trinity of Zancolli, Goldner and Swanson (Zancolli *et al.* 1983) did attempt to give some recommendations which depend upon which of the three hand patterns occur.

Pattern I. Mild flexion spasticity, especially of the flexor carpi ulnaris and the finger-flexors. Perform tenotomy of the flexor carpi ulnaris and musculoaponeurotic release of the flexor origins.

Pattern II. If wrist-extensors are weak or absent, transfer the flexor carpi ulnaris to the extensor carpi radialis brevis.

If finger extension is possible with less than 50° of wrist flexion, perform musculoaponeurotic release of the origins of the flexor muscles.

If finger extension is possible only with more than 50° of wrist flexion, do the more extensive release of the flexor muscle origin with a pronator teres release if desired.

Pattern III. Severe flexion of the fingers and inability to extend with full wrist flexion. Do multiple tendon lengthenings in the forearm.

In all patterns, the adducted thumb or the thumb-in-palm is treated as described in the preceding section.

POSTOPERATIVE CARE OF TENDON LENGTHENINGS AND TRANSFERS

Four weeks of immobilization in dressings and splints are usually followed by 6–8 weeks of intermittent daytime splinting and all-night splinting with the wrist in neutral position and the fingers extended. During these latter 8 weeks the splint can be removed three to four times a day, for periods of up to an hour, for guided functional activities and restoration of motion. Flexible action splints can be used, but excessive pulling by the elastic should not be so great as to elicit a stretch reflex to cause hyperextension of the wrist or preclude flexion of the fingers. This protection is necessary while the collagen fibers mature and recontracture is a risk.

This postoperative regimen undoubtedly varies with the experience of the surgeon, the type of motor disorder and the cooperation of the patient and parents. Therefore these recommendations are only a general guide for a postoperative plan. Some patients may need months of postoperative splinting. All need functional hand activities to obtain the best postoperative result (washing dishes, for instance, can be good home occu-pational therapy). Bimanual activities should be chosen. But remember, the usual defective sensory input from the operated hand will demand visual feedback for function.

WRIST ARTHRODESIS

Wrist arthrodesis is rarely indicated. It should be reserved for when the goal is mainly a normal appearance and a paperweight (stabilizing) function, and when there is deformity of the carpal bones due to the long-standing flexion contracture of the wrist and fingers. In adults who had an average of 85° of a flexion deformity restored to a 15° flexed position with arthrodesis, Rayan and Young (1999) reported very satisfied patients and caregivers with the improved wrist position.

CONTRAINDICATIONS AND INDICATIONS

Arthrodesis should *not* be done if: (1) the fingers can extend only by flexing the wrist; (2) the fingers can flex only by extending the wrist; (3) tendon transfers are feasible to improve the wrist position.

Wrist arthrodesis is a satisfactory solution for a severe wrist flexion deformity if: (1) there is general poor muscle control and strength that precludes active flexion and extension; (2) there is a severe fixed deformity that precludes correction by tendon lengthenings and transfer; (3) tendon transfers have been done and the wrist position is either not corrected or hyperextended.

OPERATIVE TECHNIQUE

A dorsal longitudinal incision exposes the extensor tendons, which are then retracted. The dorsal capsule of the joint is opened and the navicular and lunate bones excised; the articular surfaces of the carpal bones and distal radius are denuded of cartilage. The denuded articular surface of the capitate is fixed to the saucer-like depression in the denuded articular surface of the radius. A Steinman pin is introduced at the distal end of the third metacarpal in the web space between the third and fourth metacarpal heads. The pin is driven straight through the base of the third metacarpal, across the carpal bones, through the capitate and into the center of the distal radial epiphysis into the shaft of the radius. Iliac bone grafts are added. A plaster cast is used until fusion is solid—usually 3–4 months.

POSITION OF THE WRIST IN ARTHRODESIS

The best position is with the wrist extended to the point where the first metacarpal is in alignment with the shaft of the radius (Figs 7.9, 7.10). The contracted wrist and finger-flexor tendons are lengthened the proper amount. To prevent an intrinsic-plus hand with no finger flexion, overlengthening of the flexor digitorum profundus should be avoided. A sliding bone graft from the distal radius and a dynamic compression plate as reported by Sorial *et al.* (1994) resulted in successful fusions in an average of 16° extension and 7° ulnar deviation.

PRONATION DEFORMITY
OF THE FOREARM

Pronation spasticity and early contracture are common. Posterior subluxation of the radial head occurs early in life, and often accounts for a fixed deformity that limits elbow extension. Posterior dislocation of the radial head occurs as the child matures. Pletcher *et al.* (1976) found this deformity in 2.4% of 384 elbows, in 184 patients with cerebral palsy. A radiographic study of wrists and elbows in cerebral palsy by Nishioka *et al.* (2000) of Fukuoka, Japan, found bilateral dislocations of the radial head in two patients among 96 (2%).

Aitken (1952) described these identical changes in the elbow in a study of children with Erb's obstetric paralysis. He described subtle early signs of posterior subluxation of the radial head and increased posterior bowing of the ulna. Dislocation of the radial head occurred between the ages of 5 and 8 years. The mechanism of the gradual displacement of the radial head was thought to be due to the pull of the pronator teres when forced supination was imposed by treatment, and contracture of the interosseus membrane was the deforming force on the ulna.

Although Keats (1974) reported success with bilateral radial head-excision in a 7-year-old with cerebral palsy, Bleck (unpublished observations) and Aitken (1952) had poor results long ago in two adolescents who were skeletally mature. Excision of the radial head as every surgeon probably knows is ill-advised in growing children.

INDICATIONS FOR SURGERY

Prevention of subluxation of the radial head seems possible if the pronation contracture is relieved early enough, probably before the age of 3 years. In older children who have a pronation contracture and some evidence of active voluntary supination, pronator teres tenotomy has improved active supination. In children who have spastic hemiplegia, the ability to supinate is crucial for participation in ball-games. It is not easy to catch a ball when one hand is supinated and the other pronated.

Pronator teres tenotomy can be performed alone or in combination with a flexor carpi ulnaris transfer to the distal radius (Green and Banks 1962). Bleck (unpublished observations) has not found it necessary to do the flexor carpi ulnaris transfer merely to improve active supination. Sakellarides *et al.* (1981) had disappointing results with this procedure, and had much better results when he performed a transfer of the pronator teres insertion. In their 17-year experience with transfer of the flexor carpi ulnaris to the extensor carpi radialis or brevis, Beach and associates (1991) found that 'supination improved markedly', but only when this transfer included the pronator release.

In Bleck's experience (unpublished observations), simple tenotomy of the pronator teres with resection of its tendon to the muscle belly was sufficient. House (1975) was of the same opinion. Good results have also been reported with more complex procedures, such as transfer of the pronator teres posteriorly to the anterolateral border of the radius (Sakellarides *et al.* 1981) or

to the extensor carpi radialis brevis (Colton *et al.* 1976, Patella and Martucci 1980). One can doubt this extra step is necessary. In fact, a reliable report on the transfer of the flexor carpi ulnaris to the extensor carpi radialis brevis observed that it resulted in extension contracture of the wrist and consequent limitation of finger flexion and extension (Hoffer *et al.* 1986).

Gschwind and Tonkin (1992) classified the pronation deformity into four groups to help the decision for the proper procedure. Group 1 patients can supinate actively to beyond neutral and no treatment is necessary. Group 2 subjects can supinate to neutral, and may be candidates for a pronator quadratus release and possible flexor aponeurotic release at the elbow. Group 3 have no active supination, but complete passively (advised pronator teres transfer). Group 4 have no active supination (advised a flexor aponeurotic and pronator quadratus release). This paper was listed as 'Part 1'. In the paper to follow in the same issue of the journal and stated as 'Part 2', no results of the surgery for a pronation deformity appear. It seems as if a pronator quadratus release entails much more surgical dissection than a simple tenotomy of its insertion on the radius. Absent confirming studies of the results of pronator quadratus dissection a surgeon would be reluctant to try it for the rather functional insignificance of this forearm deformity.

The *operative technique* of pronator teres tenotomy is simple. A straight incision is made over the insertion of the tendon on the volar aspect of the proximal shaft of the radius. The tendon is detached from its insertion and excised up to its muscle. Immobilization of the forearm in supination for 3 weeks, followed by active supination exercises, has been sufficient. Supination function activities such as opening doorknobs and catching a large ball appear effective in achieving the desired result.

Complete active supination is rarely achieved. No active supination is ever achieved in those patients who have no evidence of active voluntary control of supination, which is highly dependent upon the activity of the biceps brachii muscle. In the report of the procedure by Sakellarides *et al.* (1981), 82% were judged to have good or excellent results, with an average gain of 46º of active supination. A bit of perspective on forearm position and function of the hand seem warranted to temper surgical zeal. Most daily activities are done with the forearm in pronation so much so that in congenital radio–ulnar synostosis the objective of surgery is to provide a more functional position from various degrees of fixed supination to pronation, although the results of such surgery have not resulted necessarily in improved function (Cleary and Omer 1985).

Most daily activities are done with the forearm in pronation.

Congenital radioulnar synostosis with fixed supination is corrected by osteotomy to place the hand in a more functional position of pronation.

ELBOW-FLEXION DEFORMITY

INDICATIONS FOR SURGERY

If the elbow extension lacks only 30°–40°, the problem is probably not worth treating. The most frequent need to correct the flexed elbow is in spastic hemiplegia, although Mital (1979) did surgery on patients with spastic quadriplegia to gain elbow extension in order to facilitate walking with crutches in six patients; all became independent in walking with crutch support.

Despite some informal pessimism on the results of surgery for the spastic elbow flexion contracture, Goldner *et al.* (1977) reported 32 cases followed from one to 22 years; the flexion contracture recurred in only three patients, and four had a slow recovery of flexion strength. Mital (1979) performed a surgical release in 32 elbows (26 patients), with good results on follow-up of 25 patients.

To ascertain the effect of surgically decreasing the spastic elbow flexion, Goldner's (1983) recommendation to infiltrate the biceps and brachialis muscles with lidocaine has merit. Botulinum toxin injection into both the biceps, and brachialis muscles might also be used for a longer time to observe the effect.

OPERATIVE TECHNIQUES

Mital (1979) used a lazy-s incision, beginning on the anterolateral aspect of the distal third of the arm and crossing the elbow crease to end on the anteromedial aspect of the forearm. The lacertus fibrosis was excised, the biceps tendon z-lengthened and the brachialis aponeurosis incised transversely in two or three locations so that the muscle could be stretched on extension of the elbow. Anterior capsulotomy was rarely done, but it is obviously necessary in severe contractures. The anatomy of the nerves and vessels needs to be remembered in the dissection.

Goldner (1983) used a curved incision anterior to the medial epicondyle of the humerus. The ulnar nerve was isolated and the origins of the flexor carpi ulnaris, radialis brevis and pronator teres were detached from the proximal ulna. The lacertus fibrosis was incised and the biceps tendon and the brachialis were z-lengthened at their insertions. If more extension is needed, the anterior capsule was incised. The ulnar nerve was mobilized and transferred anteriorly. If the brachioradialis was very spastic and contracted, it too was released from its origin on the humerus.

Matsuo (2002) does an intramuscular lengthening of the brachialis with a transverse cut through its musculotendinous junction and a sliding lengthening of the biceps tendon. He too sections the brachioradialis tendon if the flexion contracture is severe.

POSTOPERATIVE CARE

It seems wise to use splinting with heavily padded dressing in just enough extension to obviate excessive stretch on the nerves and vessels. Intermittent supervised flexion and extension exercise with extension splinting can be started within a week. The day-splinting continues for 3 weeks, and night-splinting in extension for 3 months. Because the elbow joint is extremely prone to arthrofibrosis and stiffness, postoperative care and encouragement of early motion is important to achieving a good result. Bleck's experience in elbow-joint arthrotomy and capsulotomy, in cases other than cerebral palsy, has shown the value of continuous passive motion (CPM) machines for the first 7–14 days post-operatively (unpublished observations). Perhaps this might be considered after the release of the elbow-flexion contracture in spastic hemiplegia—CPM can be considered a mechanical physiotherapist without time off (Breen *et al.* 1988, Salter 1993).

Complications of elbow-flexor release (other than what might be expected from over stretching of the nerves and vessels, hematoma and infection) can include a fixed elbow-extension posture and contracture. This position of constant elbow extension is much worse than a flexion contracture. Bleck has seen it in only one patient, who had tension athetosis that had been confused with spasticity (unpublished observations). Only awareness of the peculiarities of the motor disorders in cerebral palsy preoperatively can prevent this kind of distressing result.

Elbow-flexion posturing in hemidystonia is not accompanied by any contracture or skeletal change. In some patients, the hyperflexed posture of the elbow during waking hours is quite uncomfortable (it disappears during sleep). Such patients ask for relief.

To assess the effect of surgery in this kind of problem, infiltration of the biceps muscle with 1% lidocaine solution is helpful. If this provides significant relaxation of the hyperflexed posture, a neurectomy of the musculocutaneous nerve has effected sustained relief in two patients followed up for 11 and 12 years. The brachialis muscle continued to function for active flexion of the elbow; the dystonic flexion posture was reduced to tolerance and comfort. Current practice may be to infiltrate the biceps muscle with Botulinum toxin.

Recently, neurosurgeons from Hyderabad, India, described their results in an Austrian journal of neurosurgery of 'selective musculocutaneous fasciulotomy' in 52 patients (75 elbows) in children with the average age of 9.5 years (Purohit *et al.* 1998). With electrical stimulation of the fascicles of the musculo-cutaneous nerve and ablation of those deemed responsible for the spastic elbow flexion, they stated that total relief of spasticity occurred in 47 of these elbows (62.66%). There were no recurrences.

Denervation of the brachioradialis muscle in three adolescent boys after a traumatic intracranial hematoma in one, and a mycotic cerebral aneurysm in two was successful in relieving elbow-flexion spasticity (Meals 1988). The diagnostic test was a block of the radial nerve with lidocaine. The surgery exposed the radial nerve at the elbow and the single branch to the brachioradialis was cut. This might be a good procedure to remember in the occasional patient who has intractable elbow flexion after a head injury or cerebral hemorrhage. Clearly, the brain pathology in such cases is more localized rather than the diffuse brain damage found in cerebral palsy as we define it.

INTERNAL ROTATION CONTRACTURE OF THE SHOULDER

Very rarely, a spastic contracture of the pectoralis major and subscapularis preclude the neutral or slightly externally rotated position of the shoulder and thus interferes with function of the hand. This dysfunctional position may be more common in athetosis or mixed types of cerebral palsy (Goldner 1983). A logical solution is lengthening of the pectoralis major tendon and subscapularis myotomy (Goldner 1983). Bleck performed shoulder surgery in a 6-year-old with spastic quadriplegia and satisfactory hand function (unpublished observations). He had a severe forward cupping of the shoulders as well as restriction of external rotation. Shoulder position was improved by bilateral pectoralis major lengthening, subscapularis myotomy and especially pectoralis minor tenotomy.

SURGERY OF THE LOWER LIMB

EQUINUS DEFORMITY

A little equinus is better than calcaneus.

In all the spastic types of cerebral palsy, the equinus position of the foot receives the most attention. It is the most visible of the abnormal postures. Consequently, treatment efforts are often directed zealously to correcting it, either with passive stretching by the parents and the physical therapist, or with plaster immobilization, or with a variety of surgical techniques. Conservative methods of management with plaster, myoneural blocks and orthotics are discussed in Chapter 6. The welter of reports in the literature attests to the continuing churning of the subject of equinus in cerebral palsy.

In hemiplegia, even minor degrees of equinus are noticeable because of the obvious comparison with the normal side. Although the description of the surgical management of equinus is described in this chapter on hemiplegia, the same procedures are applicable to equinus in spastic diplegia and the total body involved. The role of the spastic hamstring muscles in dynamic equinus sometimes found in spastic diplegia can be found in Chapter 8.

INDICATIONS FOR SURGERY

Is the plantarflexed position of the ankle and foot detrimental to achieving functional walking? We know that patients with cerebral palsy will walk despite equinus if their neurological status permits. We also know that the lack of normal equilibrium reactions cannot be compensated for by the plantigrade foot. Patients who only have ataxia do not usually have equinus, yet their ability to balance can be so poor that a four-post walker is necessary. Normal people run (as opposed to jog) in equinus. Ballet artistes seem to have perfect postural control on tiptoe. Women who wear high-heeled shoes walk in equinus all day. So what is so bad about having an equinus deformity throughout life? Even though no reports are found in the literature on the

effects of long-term equinus, William John Little (1810–94) himself visited Georg Stromeyer in Hanover, Germany, and subsequently in London. On February 20 1837, Stromeyer did an Achilles tenotomy for Little's fixed equinovarus of one foot due to poliomyelitis, referred to as 'talipes' in Little's own description (perhaps meaning 'club foot') (Rang 1993, 2000). So if equinus distressed Little enough to seek surgery, then all other persons with the same deformity are probably intuitively correct in accepting surgery for relief of equinus.

In hemiplegia, unilateral equinus creates a relative lengthening of the limb, a pelvic obliquity and compensatory postural lumbar scoliosis. The result is a limp. Furthermore, persistent equinus necessitates a greater degree of knee and hip flexion during the swing phase of gait in order for the foot to clear the ground; or if the quadriceps is spastic, the constant extension of the knee causes the patient to circumduct the limb in order for the foot to clear in swing phase. A slight degree of equinus (5°) can compensate for shortness of the limb which occurs frequently in hemiplegia (usually no more than 1.5 cm). Unlike equinus due to flaccid paralysis of the ankle dorsiflexors or congenital club foot, the long-standing equinus in spastic cerebral palsy is not usually accompanied by a contracture of the posterior capsule of the ankle joint.

It is important to understand that the soleus in gait contributes 40%–50% of the force needed for erect posture during gait (Õunpuu *et al.* 1991). Furthermore, the hip-extensors (gluteus medius and maximus) and vasti each contribute 20%–30 % of force to maintain upright posture during gait mainly in the initial third of stance phase. Ground reaction force is countered by the stabilizing force of the gastrocsoleus which decelerate the forward motion of the tibia through the lever arm of the forefoot pushing the knee into extension (Gage 2004).

Gait patterns in spastic hemiplegia in children and young adults were studied in great detail with gait analysis by Winters *et al.* (1987). The intent was to move from purely empirical treatment to a more scientific approach. The four gait patterns were: group I, drop foot in swing phase with an adequate range of dorsiflexion of the ankle; group II, plantarflexion throughout the gait cycle and full or hyperextension of the knee in the stance phase, hyperflexion of the hip and increased lumbar lordosis; group III, equinus and more limited flexion of the knee in swing phase; total flexion–extension was less than 45°; and group IV equinus, limited knee motion and total flexion–extension of the hip during gait was less than 35° and increased pelvic lordosis during terminal stance.

Lin and Brown (1992) introduced an intriguing concept to explain the equinus gait in cerebral palsy. According to their clinical examination of 24 children with hemiplegia, toe-strike during forward progression of gait can be independent of spasticity or a fixed equinus. Their contention was that gait equinus was not merely a paralytic foot drop, but rather is due to an abnormal 'kick' at toe-strike, and a 'hemiplegic engram' that exists normally. The intriguing proposition is that this engram emerges physiologically and normally when running or after a loss of cortical inhibition. Accordingly, an ankle–foot orthosis was suggested as correcting the central nervous system engram and neutralizing the 'kick'. This might be all well and good in dynamic equinus, but what do you do when it is fixed due to the muscle shortening?

Rodda and Graham (2001) of Melbourne, Australia, refined the classification of spastic hemiplegia gait patterns and included the recommended management as an algorithm which we have modified (Table 7.V). However, it is evident this is only a guide because of obvious variables that have to be considered in the individual patient. For example, is the problem mainly with spasticity and no contracture of the muscle? Or is there a fixed shortening of the muscle? Only careful clinical examination and reexamination coupled with observational gait analysis using video-recordings (Rodda and Graham 2001), and instrumented gait analysis will give the answer and decision. Hullin and colleagues (1996) described similar gait patterns derived from three-dimensional gait analysis, but divided them into five groups.

EXAMINATION FOR CONTRACTURE

Surgery is indicated for a contracture of the triceps surae. If the foot can be dorsiflexed to the neutral (zero) position when measured with the plantar aspect of the heel and *the foot inverted* (to lock the talonavicular joint and prevent false dorsiflexion at the midtarsal joint) and with the knee extended, surgery is not indicated (Fig. 7.16).

To differentiate a contracture from spasticity alone demands a very slow and careful dorsiflexion of the ankle, with the knee first flexed and then extended. Truscelli *et al.* (1979) separated the contracture from the spasticity by creating ischemia of the limb with a pneumatic tourniquet inflated to 200 mmHg pressure for 20 minutes; then they determined the true shortening

of the muscle with the usual measurements of the range of passive dorsiflexion of the ankle. It seems problematic that children would tolerate the pain with the duration of tourniquet inflation.

The examination should also include the ability of the patient to dorsiflex the ankle voluntarily with the knee extended. Often this is not possible, and dorsiflexion will occur only with simultaneous hip and knee flexion against resistance. This is a reflex motion found in upper motor-neuron disorders. It accounts for the observation that patients who have only this flexor withdrawal reflex (or 'confusion' reflex) will walk with a steppage gait in order for the foot to clear the floor on swing phase.

FUNCTION OF THE GASTROCNEMIUS AND SOLEUS MUSCLE

Electromyographic gait studies have demonstrated that the gastrocnemius and soleus muscles become active at heel strike and continue their activity through the mid-stance phase of gait. The function of the calf muscles is to reduce forward acceleration of the tibia during the stance phase. Through stance phase the gastrocnemius and soleus contract eccentrically, i.e. they lengthen. The terminus of the stance phase is mechanical when the foot action consists of a passive 'roll-off' motion (Perry *et al.* 1992). Gage disagrees that this is a 'roll-off' noting that at terminal stance the gastroc-soleus contraction changes from eccentric lengthening, decelerators of mid-stance to concentric contracting accelerators of terminal stance. The posterior calf muscles provide an acceleration or 'push off' which is about 50% of the propulsive force required for normal walking (Gage 2004).

There is no disagreement on the disabling effects of a weak soleus which can easily occur with excess or unneeded lengthening of the soleus when it was not contracted. Sutherland *et al.* (1980),

TABLE 7.V
Common postural/gait patterns in spastic hemiplegia

Type	Characteristics	Management
1	Drop foot in swing phase No contracture	Orthosis: leaf spring or hinged AFO
2a	Equinus during stance phase Variable degree of drop foot Knee in neutral and extended hip	Botox injection younger children Cast if mild contracture Hinged AFO with plantarflexion
2b	Equinus fixed contracture Recurvatum knee and extended hip Equinovarus Equinovalgus (rare)	Achilles or gastrocnemius tendon lengthening Strayer-type lengthening if only gastrocnemius contracted Solid ankle AFO in 5° dorsiflexion Botox injection posterior tibial Split posterior and/or posterior tendon transfer Botox injection in gastrocnemius and AFO Older children, brace intolerant, require bone surgery
3	Gastroc–soleus spasticity or contracture Impaired ankle dorsiflexion in swing andLater stage: flexed knee, 'stiff knee gait' due to hamstring/quadriceps contraction	Botox injections in calf and hamstrings Gastrocnemius lengthening hamstring lengthening with rectus femoris tendon transfer to semitendinosus or gracilis Solid or hinged AFO
4	Equinus, flexed stiff knee gait, flexed hip, anterior pelvic tilt, hip adduction and internal rotation (comparable to spastic	Spasticity only: multilevel Botox injections 4U/kg/muscle; total dose 12–16 mg/kg body weight. Lengthening gastroc–soleus, hamstrings, distal rectus femoris transfer (if indicated), adductor longus myotenotomy, iliopsoas tenotomy at the pelvic brim or lengthening; Femoral derotation osteotomy Solid or hinged AFO (depends on Plantar Flexion–knee extension couple (Chapter 8).

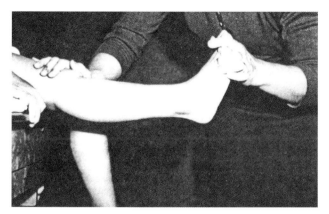

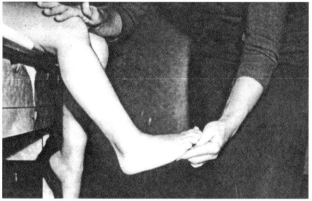

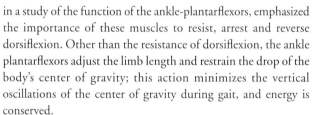

Fig. 7.16. *Top*: with knee extended and foot in varus, limited passive dorsiflexion of the ankle demonstrates contracture of gastrocnemius–soleus muscles. *Bottom*: with knee flexed, passive dorsiflexion of ankle is easily accomplished. This indicates more contracture in gastrocnemius muscle.

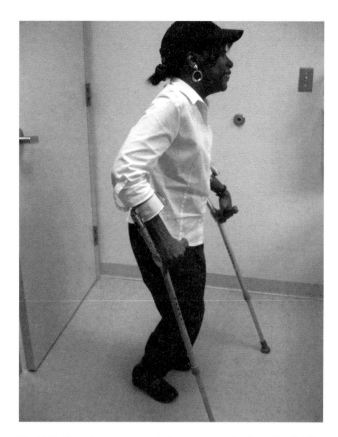

Fig. 7.17. Crouch posture and gait due to overlengthening of the Achilles tendon and resultant loss of muscle strength of the gastrocnemius–soleus which normally prevents forward acceleration of the tibia.

in a study of the function of the ankle-plantarflexors, emphasized the importance of these muscles to resist, arrest and reverse dorsiflexion. Other than the resistance of dorsiflexion, the ankle plantarflexors adjust the limb length and restrain the drop of the body's center of gravity; this action minimizes the vertical oscillations of the center of gravity during gait, and energy is conserved.

Constant contraction of the calf muscles (as occurs in spastic paralysis, and especially with a fixed equinus due to contracture) eliminates the 'roll-off'; the patient vaults over his foot, raises the vertical oscillation of the center of gravity and thus expends more energy. A paralysis of these muscles induced by a local anesthetic block of the tibial nerve demonstrated drastic changes in the gait variables: ankle dorsiflexion increased during stance, and the opposite heel did not leave the floor until weight was transferred to the opposite foot. The result was to shorten the step length, reduce the gait velocity, increase the vertical and forward velocities of the center of gravity (center of mass) and increase the energy expenditure (Sutherland *et al.* 1980). These accurate measurements on the effect of weakening the calf muscles should be a sufficiently strong reason to avoid a surgical procedure which would overcorrect the contracture. A calcaneus deformity is functionally worse than a moderate degree of equinus. It is the main cause of the crouch posture in spastic diplegia (Fig. 7.17).

MECHANISM OF THE CONTRACTURE

In a normal person the ankle plantarflexors have 17 times the potential torque of the ankle dorsiflexors, and yet there is no calf-muscle contracture (J. Perry, personal communication). This is because when normal people walk, passive dorsiflexion of the ankle occurs in stance phase so that periodic elongation of the calf muscles prevents excessive shortening. The dorsiflexors lift the foot in the swing phase and decelerate plantarflexion during heel strike until the foot is flat. Their strength requirements are much less than those of the plantarflexors.

In spastic paralysis, constant contraction of the calf muscles and insufficient central control of ankle dorsiflexion fails to preserve the elasticity of the calf muscles. As skeletal growth occurs, the muscle length fails to keep up with the bone length. At the microscopic level, Tardieu *et al.* (1977) found in cats that the sarcomere length of the calf-muscle fibers was the same, regardless of the angle of dorsiflexion of the ankle. This mechanism was thought to explain why muscles adapt to skeletal growth, and in some cases of cerebral palsy this mechanism was absent with a resultant contracture. Another explanation came from the experimental data of Huet de la Tour *et al.* (1979), who observed a reduction of sarcomeres in the muscle fiber as well as a loss of extensibility after prolonged and sustained contractions in experimental tetany resembling spastic paralysis.

In a unique experiment which studied the growth of the gastrocnemius muscle in hereditary spastic mice, Ziv *et al.* (1984) confirmed the view that muscle growth was not interstitial but was appositional at the musculotendinous junction. The cells here added sarcomeres to the end of the muscle fiber. In these spastic mice, growth of the muscle was definitely reduced and contractures ensued. The authors concluded that the contracture of the muscle in children is due to the failure of its growth, which in turn is the result of a spastic muscle's inability to stretch to its full length.

The velocity of muscle growth is greatest from birth to age 4 years, when muscles double in length; from then until skeletal maturity they double in length again (Rang *et al.* 1986). This phenomenon of early rapid growth explains the observation that recurrence of contracture after Achilles tendon lengthening is more common when done in early childhood. Lee and Bleck (1980) had a 75% recurrence rate in children at age 2 years, 25% at 4 years, 14% at 7 years and none (N = 31) at 8 years and older. Unlike in children, adult muscle contractures are accompanied by loss of sarcomeres; there is no growth, and therefore, few recurrences after lengthenings.

The experiment in which springs were attached to the wings of chickens, so that constant stretch was applied to the wing muscles, did demonstrate an increase in length of the muscles (Barnett *et al.* 1980). Perhaps this provides a rationale for keeping a child's ankle constantly dorsiflexed in plasters ('inhibitive' or ordinary) or orthotics (AFOS—ankle–foot orthoses) to restrain the muscle contracture. However, muscle atrophy due to disuse will also occur. And is constant use of a plaster cast or a plastic orthotic practical for everyday living and functioning?

SURGICAL PROCEDURES: WHAT TO CHOOSE IN HEMIPLEGIA

What surgical procedure do you perform to correct an equinus deformity? Many have been proposed: neurectomy of the gastrocnemius and/or soleus muscles, gastrocnemius lengthening, gastrocnemius origin recession, Achilles tendon lengthening and Achilles tendon translocation. All are designed to reduce the increased stretch reflex and to lengthen the muscle. All weaken the muscle. Which one strikes the best compromise between relieving the contracture and preserving the strength?

This dilemma is physiologically based. The excursion of muscles is determined by the length of their fibers (the number of sarcomeres); the strength is determined by the number of fibers. The strongest force at any joint during anytime at any point in the gait cycle is the ankle plantarflexion moment at the end of stance. Joint power measured in watts/kg is greatest by the ankle-plantarflexors (85% of the kinetic energy in normal walking) compared with the hip-extensor, hip-flexor, and the knee-extensor muscles (Gage 1991). Both equinus and overstretched plantarflexor muscles dramatically reduce the plantarflexion moment so that the primary source of the momentum of gait is lost.

Delp and colleagues (1995) used computer modeling to analyze the effect of lengthening the aponeurosis of the gastrocnemius (Strayer 1950, 1958, Baker 1954) and the Achilles tendon. The computer model was constructed to represent isolated contracture of the gastrocnemius and contracture of both the gastrocnemius and soleus. The effects of lengthening the gastrocnemius aponeurosis and the Achilles tendon were simulated. The computer program simulations showed that nearly normal moment generating characteristics were preserved with lengthening the gastrocnemius aponeurosis. Lengthening of the Achilles tendon reduced greatly the moment-generating capacity of the plantarflexors.

Simulated aponeurotic lengthening did not decrease the excessive passive moment generated by the soleus (Delp *et al.* 1995). But Achilles tendon lengthening did restore the passive range of ankle dorsiflexion, but substantially reduced the active force-generating capacity of the muscles. Achilles tendon lengthening reduces the excursion of the gastrocnemius–soleus muscle, but this excursion that dorsiflexes the ankle actively remains in the same range as before; only passive dorsiflexion is increased; lengthening weakens the muscle. In 95% of the patients with spastic equinus, both muscles are firing abnormally (J. Perry, personal communication).

Borton and colleagues (2001) of the Royal Children's Hospital, Melbourne, Australia, compared percutaneous lengthening of the Achilles tendon with open Z-lengthening and gastrocnemius aponeurotic lengthening in children with hemiplegia (N=45), diplegia (N=65), and quadriplegia (N=24). The surgery was done at a mean age of 7.6 years with a mean follow-up of 6.9 years. Outcomes were assessed with 3D gait analysis for kinematics and kinetics, observational gait analysis, and with lateral projection radiographs of the foot and ankle. In hemiplegia 56% had a good outcome, 38% had a recurrent equinus, and only two (4%) had a calcaneus gait pattern. The study suggested it might be worthwhile to postpone surgery until age 7–8 years with a trial with physiotherapy, orthoses, and intramuscular injections of botulinum-A toxin. There were no data that indicated orthoses or night splints affected the rate of recurrence, but controls are lacking. The risk factor for calcaneus was percutaneous lengthening of the Achilles tendon and for recurrence was surgery before 8 years of age. Any of the three methods of calf lengthening in hemiplegia were deemed to have few risks and acceptable results.

There is reluctance to weaken the plantarflexors of the ankle too much. In children 50% of power for walking comes from the plantarflexors (Gage 2004). The larger muscle is the soleus so that Achilles tendon lengthening weakens this muscle as well as the gastrocnemius and risks a calcaneus gait. Computer simulation by Delp and Zajac (1992) calculated that with a 1.2 cm Achilles tendon lengthening, soleus power diminished 50% compared with much less loss of strength of plantarflexor power with gastrocnemius lengthening alone.

Consequently, the Strayer gastrocnemius aponeurotic lengthening (Strayer 1950, 1958), or Baker's aponeurotic tongue-in-groove lengthening (Baker 1954, 1956), or the Vulpius gastrocnemius lengthening modified by sectioning the soleus aponeurosis through the same incision is favored (Rosenthal and

Simon 1992) or Bauman's modification (Saraph *et al.* 2000). Matsuo (2002) was so discouraged by Achilles tendon lengthening results that he abandoned it even though he is a strong advocate of sliding tendon lengthenings. Instead he chooses gastrocnemius aponeurosis lengthening (termed 'recession'). But the risk for recurrence of the equinus is greater than with Achilles tendon lengthening. Even so, Matsuo (2002) believes that recurrence of equinus should not be a criterion of the efficacy of the operation—better to lengthen again.

The rather poor results from Achilles tendon lengthening as reported by Borton *et al.* (2001) might well be attributed to the open Z-lengthenings that were done in their institution. Z-lengthening and then resuturing places the burden on the surgeon to keep the tension on the muscle–tendon unit just right. Once the tendon is separated, it is difficult to estimate and restore the correct tension in the muscle—there are no measuring instruments or methods to do this.

Z-lengthening of the Achilles tendon and then resuturing places the burden on the surgeon to keep the tension on the muscle–tendon unit just right—there are no measuring instruments or methods to do this.

Simon and Ryan (1992) used sagittal-plane kinematics in gait analysis to make a decision on which procedure to do—either the Achilles tendon lengthening or the gastrocnemius–soleus calf lengthening. They described three types of patterns of ankle motion and recommendations for one or the other surgical procedures dependent on the graphic pattern from gait analysis. However, no clinical results from adoption of this decision process were delineated. We can hear the late Dr Arthur Steindler whispering in our ear: 'What is practically right, can't be theoretically wrong.'

The latest advice on what procedure to do for equinus is in a paper presented by Westwell-O'Connor and associates (2002) from the Connecticut Children's Medical Centre, Hartford. They compared the effectiveness of percutaneous Achilles tendon lengthening with gastrocnemius lengthenings in 18 patients evenly divided between the two procedures. They obtained data using clinical measurements, kinematic and kinetic data in a follow-up of ambulation at a mean of 1 year (SD 3 months). The measured results were the same in both procedures. The percutaneous lengthenings did not cause plantarflexion weakness. The conclusion was that percutaneous Achilles tendon lengthening might be the preferable procedure for equinus because it was less invasive and less time-consuming, and resulted in less scarring.

Fifteen years ago Graham and Fixsen of London (1988) gave approbation to the White sliding Achilles tendon lengthening for equinus in spastic hemiplegia with a mean follow-up of 13 years. No patient developed a calcaneus deformity, but 17% required another surgery for recurrence. Recurrence was higher in those who had the first operation at age 4 years, 5 months compared with non-recurrence when surgery was at a mean age of 7 years, 7 months.

Borton and colleagues (2002) that included Graham of Melbourne, Australia, concluded in their study of options for the treatment of equinus that percutaneous lengthenings had unpredictable results. They favored Baker's tongue-in-groove gastrocnemius–soleus lengthening because of low incidence of calcaneus deformity and a slightly higher incidence of recurrence.

The solution to the dilemma of decision appears to do an open sliding lengthening of the Achilles tendon by the Hoke method. This method controls the lengthening and avoids over-lengthening. But you have to temper your zeal and muscle power and *stop yourself and/or your strong assistants from pushing the foot beyond the neutral position of ankle plantar and dorsiflexion, i.e. don't overdo it* (Fig. 7.18)!

GASTROCNEMIUS NEURECTOMY

It seemed that neurectomy of the gastrocnemius heads and recession of them as done in the past has dropped out of sight in contemporary practice (Silfverskiöld 1923–24, Silver and Simon 1959, Silver 1977). But no, the late 1990s brought a return of neurectomy of the calf muscle by the orthopaedic surgeons at Johns Hopkins University. Doute *et al.* (1997) did *soleus* neurectomies for ankle clonus along with Achilles tendon or gastrocnemius lengthenings and stated this to be beneficial in 19 of 21 children (38 legs). These surgeons added that the greatest improvement was seen in the children who did not have contractures, i.e. dynamic equinus. The question that arises is whether the relief of clonus is outweighed by the resultant permanent weakness of the soleus and loss of function by this important muscle in gait. We rather doubt that contemporary orthopaedic surgeons will do neurectomies or lengthenings of the calf muscles for *dynamic equinus.*

Camacho and colleagues of Mexico (1996) also continued with gastrocnemius neurectomies combined with Achilles tendon lengthening in six of 12 children that had ankle clonus and equinus and compared the results with six that had Achilles tendon lengthening alone. In all the equinus deformity persisted,

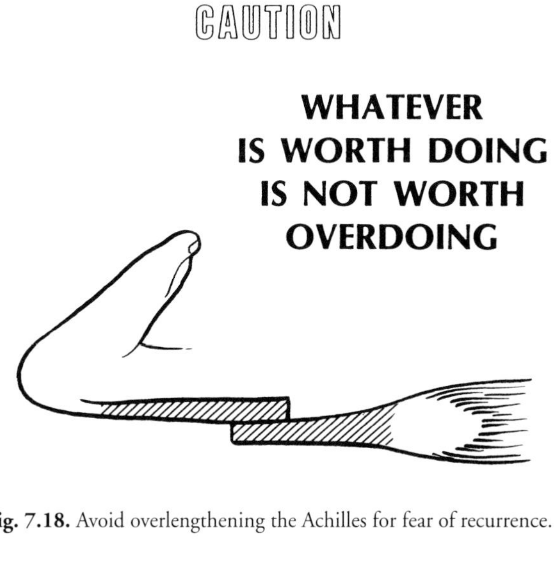

CAUTION

WHATEVER IS WORTH DOING IS NOT WORTH OVERDOING

Fig. 7.18. Avoid overlengthening the Achilles for fear of recurrence.

but the clonus subsided in 50% of those who had the neurectomy versus 27% in those who did not. That the equinus persisted is not a good recommendation for adoption of this procedure.

GASTROCNEMIUS APONEUROSIS LENGTHENING

Vulpius is credited with the operation designed to lengthen the gastrocnemius only and thereby spare the soleus muscle (Vulpius and Stoffel 1913). This operation consists of an inverted V incision in the gastrocnemius tendinous aponeurosis and forcing the ankle into dorsiflexion, followed by plaster immobilization. This procedure was modified by Strayer (1950, 1958) and then by Baker (1954, 1956). In the Strayer procedure the gastrocnemius aponeurosis is sectioned transversely, the muscle bellies dissected free of the underlying soleus muscle, the foot dorsiflexed and a plaster applied. Baker's modification was a tongue-in-groove incision in the aponeurosis and section of the median raphe of the soleus muscle, foot dorsiflexion and plaster immobilization.

The latest is Baumann's modification that cuts the fascia in several horizontal slices over the anterior aspect of the gastrocnemius and the adjacent fascia over the soleus muscles ('intramuscular lengthening') (Saraph *et al.* 2000). The cutting of the fascia does not address the pathology of the contracture which is a shortening of the muscle. As can be observed in fractional lengthening of the semimembranosus and short head of the biceps, cutting the enveloping fascia and aponeurosis over the muscle fibers and then extending the knee, the muscle fibers tear apart. Detailed gait analysis studies in 22 children demonstrated that the procedure did not weaken the plantarflexion significantly, the work during push-off was increased, and there were no recurrences or calcaneus deformities. Rose and colleagues (1995) using kinetic evaluations of 29 walking patients after gastrocnemius aponeurotic lengthening reported the same results of increased energy generation at push-off. But neither study could state the result as a comparison with Achilles tendon lengthening.

The basis for the Vulpius, Strayer and Baker procedures was the positive Silfverskiöld test, in which ankle dorsiflexion was greater with the knee flexed than extended (Fig. 7.26). However, Perry *et al.* (1974) clearly demonstrated with electromyograms that the test is unreliable. Usually when the ankle was dorsiflexed 90º, electrical activity was recorded in *both* the gastrocnemius and soleus muscles. Indeed, in two patients with a positive Silfverskiöld test, the gait electromyograms showed premature contraction of the soleus and the gastrocnemius muscles on swing phase.

The Strayer–Baker type of gastrocnemius lengthening has lost its popularity with many surgeons probably because of a high recurrence rate, the resultant sometimes ugly and crooked long mid-calf surgical scar, and the longer surgery time. Recurrences in follow-up studies of 2 years or longer were 29% (Lee and Bleck 1980), 41% (Schwartz *et al.* 1977), 48% (Olney *et al.* 1988), and 38% (Borton *et al.* 2001). The recurrence rate of equinus was balanced by the rare case of postoperative calcaneus gait (4%, Borton *et al.* 2001).

In fact this type of surgery for correction of equinus has regained popularity in the last decade because of its ability to correct equinus while maintaining strength of the soleus. About 50% of the force needed to maintain stance is generated through the soleus (Õunpuu *et al.* 1991, Winter 1991). When the gastrocnemius is contracted but not the soleus as in most cases of equinus in cerebral palsy, it only makes sense to correct the offender and lengthen the gastrocnemius aponeurosis. This can be differentiated in part by the Silfverskiöld test under anesthesia. Delp (1995) has shown in computer-modeled muscles that lengthening of the soleus by 1 cm causes a 50% loss of moment-generating capacity. The Gillette group has been especially influential in alerting orthopaedic surgeons to the merits of aponeurotic gastrocnemius lengthening. In hemiplegia the soleus is more likely to be contracted than in diplegia. If the soleus needs lengthening this can approached through the gastrocnemius.

Craig and Van Voren (1976) measured the proximal migration of the gastrocnemius muscle bellies after gastrocnemius muscle lengthening and Achilles tendon lengthening with metallic markers and radiographic examinations. The postoperative radiographs showed a proximal shift of just 0.8 cm of the gastrocnemius muscle after the Achilles lengthening, and a 4.7 cm shift after the Strayer gastrocnemius lengthening. Based upon this data they recommended both operations at the same time. Equinus recurred in 9% of their cases.

To add a bit more complexity to this discussion, Reimers (1990) combined his 39 cases of 'z-plasty' lengthening of the Achilles with 13 who had a gastrocnemius 'aponeurotomy'. Reimers found increased strength in the ankle dorsiflexors of more than 200% by 14 months postoperatively. Equinus recurred in two of the 13 cases of Achilles lengthening.

A gait electromyogram does not offer much assistance in making the decision because surface electrodes do not discriminate gastrocnemius firing from the soleus. Only plastic-coated wire electrodes inserted into the soleus muscle belly can do this. And since we know that both muscles are firing in spastic paralysis of cerebral palsy, the extra time and trouble to subject children to this test does not seem justified to decide on surgery for the contracture.

But why continue with these aponeurotic lengthenings when there are so many recurrences necessitating re-operation which may be an Achilles tendon lengthening? Of grave concern to the orthopaedic surgeon who deals with long-term outcomes is the weakness caused by Achilles tendon lengthening. However, lending support to sticking with the Achilles tendon is a study by Etnyre *et al.* (1993) who determined with gait analysis no differences between surgical methods for correction of spastic equinus. Another comparison study was of 22 Vulpius procedures and 27 Achilles tendon z-lengthenings in 33 patients (who also had hip and knee operations to compound the analysis). With gait analysis all had 'satisfactory' results after 1 year (Yngve and Chambers 1996). Recurrences may also be related to hamstring contracture postoperatively as observed by Sala *et al.* (1997). They noted that their 22.4% recurrence rate occurred in those patients who had a greater popliteal angle postoperatively and had a significantly small angle preoperatively.

ACHILLES TENDON LENGTHENING

Achilles tendon lengthening is still an acceptable way to correct equinus, especially in spastic hemiplegia when both the gastrocnemius and the soleus are contracted, provided the lengthening is not overdone. The z-lengthening method may cause overcorrection, although it has its adherents (Gräbe and Thompson 1979, Rattey *et al.* 1993). Gaines and Ford (1984) tried to titrate the amount of Achilles tendon lengthening needed according to three grades of spasticity, voluntary control and strength of the muscle. According to their system the ankle was placed at neutral, 10° or 20° of dorsiflexion after lengthening and immobilization in a cast. Given the risk of overlengthening the soleus, the authors generally recommend a Strayer–Baker lengthening so that there can be differential lengthening dependent on a contracture of each muscle.

OPEN VERSUS PERCUTANEOUS SLIDING LENGTHENING

Most surgeons today have found the sliding method of lengthening, either by the White or the Hoke techniques, more controlled and very satisfactory (White 1943, Graham and Fixsen 1988, J.L. Goldner and W.M. Roberts, personal communications). Many surgeons seem to prefer the percutaneous method to the open method of Achilles tendon lengthening (Coleman 1983, Lake *et al.* 1985, Greene 1987, Moreau and Lake 1987, Cheng 1993). Whether the tendon is exposed and lengthened or cut in the two sites of the White method or in three sites of the Hoke way by the blind percutaneous technique, the principle is the same (White 1943, Crenshaw 1963). The advantage of the percutaneous method is that it can be an outpatient procedure and the operative scars are tiny and barely visible. But Borton *et al.* (2001) found the results unpredictable and furthermore, there is a chance to inadvertently cut the whole tendon in two with loss of the tension on the muscle that is needed to preserve strength and reduce the risk of a calcaneus gait.

Based on White's observation that the tendon rotated 9° on its longitudinal axis between its origin and insertion from medial to lateral, two cuts are made: one in the anterior two-thirds of the tendon distally near the insertion and the other in the medial two-thirds 5–7 cm proximal to the distal cut. Because of the variations in the twist of the tendon (Crenshaw 1963), and the ankle dorsiflexion force necessary to produce the lengthening with the White percutaneous method,[3] Bleck preferred the Hoke open method where he could see the tendon slide and cut a tiny fiber or two when necessary to facilitate sliding without undue force (unpublished observations). Rang *et al.* (1986) make the point that with the percutaneous method, the opportunity to

lengthen the toe-flexor tendons is lost; in the open method, these can be easily lengthened if acute flexion of the great and/or lesser toes is evident after Achilles tendon lengthening when the ankle is dorsiflexed to neutral.

The successful results of sliding Achilles tendon lengthenings have been reported by Banks and Green (1958), Banks (1977), Lee and Bleck (1980), Banks (1983), Graham and Fixsen (1988) with recurrence rates of 2%–9%. Our regimen (Lee and Bleck 1980) differed from that of Banks and Green in that we did not use physical therapy and definite exercises, daytime orthosis or night splints postoperatively. The difference in the recurrence rate of 2% does not appear significant.

POSTOPERATIVE IMMOBILIZATION IN PLASTER AND ORTHOSES

Our experience shows that an elaborate postoperative regime of splints and exercises is usually superfluous (the children aged 5 years and older wore only sneakers after plaster removal, and there was only one recurrence). Two cases developed postoperative calcaneus (4%). In the 15 lengthenings age 4 years or younger the recurrence rate was 33%. Given the greater velocity of growth which doubles the length of the limb up to age 4 years, we doubt that exercises, physical therapy, night splints and orthoses would have made much difference to this recurrence rate. Borton and colleagues (2001) found no convincing data that suggested orthoses or night splints affected the recurrence rate. However, controlled trials are lacking.

Sharrard and Bernstein (1972) also found that postoperative bracing did not affect the result or the recurrence rate. They also opined that the success rate of the operation should not be related exclusively to the recurrence of equinus, because a small amount of equinus was much more desirable for a functional gait than excessive weakness of the triceps surae produced by too much fear of recurrence (Figs 7.18, 7.19). It is better to perform a second operation to relieve unacceptable equinus than to risk an intractable calcaneus deformity.

POSTOPERATIVE CALCANEUS DEFORMITY

In one very detailed gait analysis study, Segal *et al.* (1989) defined, calcaneal gait as ≥1 SD from the normal mean at weight acceptance, midstance and weight release (midstance was the most specific). The mean dorsiflexion at weight acceptance was + 1.45°, midstance + 10.7°, and weight release + 5.9° (the standard deviations in all three were wide ranging from 19.4°–23.1°). Using these criteria, six children, three of whom had percutaneous Achilles lengthening and three who had open z-lengthenings had a calcaneal gait. Perhaps this study is important in that the three patients who had the open sliding lengthening, calcaneal gait did not occur. With z-lengthening, control of the length is uncertain; with percutaneous techniques it seems easier to overlengthen because the tendon is not seen and forced dorsiflexion of the ankle may separate the segments too much.

---

3 The foot was dorsiflexed forcefully until a snap was heard' (Lake *et al.* 1985). Tibiae have been fractured when dorsiflexing the foot in total body involved patients who have osteoporotic bones (R.L. Samilson, personal communication).

A different procedure to alleviate equinus is a translocation of the Achilles tendon (Throop *et al.* 1975). The Achilles tendon was moved to a more anterior insertion on the calcaneus and held with a pull-out suture over a padded button on the plantar surface of the heel. The rationale for this procedure in 79 cases was to preserve the strength of the triceps surae muscle; they estimated that the plantarflexion strength was reduced by 50%. Their correction rate was 89.9%. These results do not seem to be appreciably different from those reported with sliding Achilles tendon lengthening. The translocation procedure is more complicated than lengthening, and although the authors reported no increased morbidity with this procedure, Achilles tendon lengthening seems simpler. Why not do the least complex procedure if the results are similar?

It is hard to argue with the success of anterior transposition of the Achilles tendon when authors present a huge number of cases, 612 in 8 years (Strecker *et al.* 1990). But of this large group only 100 were randomly selected that had at least a 30-month follow-up. If the foot could not be dorsiflexed to neutral or beyond after the transposition of the tendon, these surgeons added a 'judicious' Vulpius procedure. Cast immobilization was for 6 weeks followed by an ankle–foot orthosis for 6 months. The study was retrospective and one wonders about the 512 patients that were not included for study.

CAST TREATMENT OF EQUINUS

The prolonged plaster immobilization for equinus has some theoretical merit, based upon the observations of appositional muscle growth in spastic mice. The muscle grows along with the bone as long as it is kept stretched to is resting length (Rang *et al.* 1986).

Westin and Dye (1983) have persisted in the conservative management of spastic equinus, using plasters over a period of three decades. In a retrospective review of 1194 patients, 61% had plaster alone, 23% had both plaster and surgery, and 16% were not treated but only observed. They concluded that their decreasing incidence of surgery for equinus (from 33 operations in 1952–61, to 19 operations in the period 1970–79) is a reflection of their belief that a major cause of the equinus is hamstring muscle spasticity rather than spasticity primarily of the gastrocnemius–soleus muscles. This observation has validity, particularly when considering the surgical treatment of equinus in young children with spastic diplegia.

Other than Westin of Los Angeles only Cottalorda *et al.* (1997) of Saint-Etienne, France, used successive plaster casts in 20 children (28 legs) to elongate the gastrocnemius–soleus muscles in children age 2 years 4 months to 8 years. They considered cast treatment a 'quick, safe, complication-free, and a simple technique'. Pre-casting, the range of ankle dorsiflexion was in ranges from 0º to 20º with the knees in extension; post-casting after a 21–40 month follow-up the ranges increased from 10º to 30º. But the authors did admit that if recurrence of

equinus is probable, the surgical procedure could be done on an 'operative-free tendon.' Generally, in the use of language, if something is 'probable', then it seems as if cast treatment was proposed as a temporizing measure in the expectation that surgery would eventually be done.

We have been reluctant to tie up children in walking casts during their development by restricting their ability to run and play. In addition, having casts repetitively applied over a period of weeks and months seems to make the treatment more burdensome than the disease, especially for the mother and father. French children and parents may be more patient and compliant than ours.

HOKE ACHILLES TENDON LENGTHENING OPERATIVE TECHNIQUE

Through a longitudinal posterior medial incision (5–7 cm), the posterior portion of the Achilles tendon is exposed and (if possible) its sheath preserved. Three cuts are made in the tendon: (1) one half medially and distally; (2) half medially and proximally; and (3) one half is cut laterally between the two medial cuts. The ankle is dorsiflexed just to the neutral (zero) position with the foot in varus; the tendon ends slide apart, leaving a lateral splice in between. No tendon sutures are necessary (Fig. 7.19). Dorsiflexion of the foot should be possible without force: the pressure of two fingers is all that is necessary. If the tendon does not slide apart easily, a few additional fibers may be cut.

In mild contractures (< 10º of equinus), a transverse incision can be used; the resultant incisional scar is barely visible. Bleck has used two separate transverse incisions 3–4 cm apart in more severe contractures, but it is necessary to undermine the skin in order to see the tendon (unpublished observations). Bleck

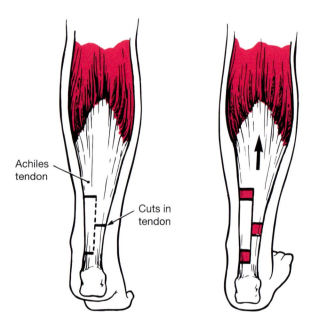

Achiles
tendon

Cuts in
tendon

Fig. 7.19. Technique of Hoke Achilles tendon lengthening. The tendon cuts are allowed to slide only to the point where the ankle is dorsiflexed to neutral and no more.

continued to use the open Hoke method because it was reliable. Even in a teaching institution it has produced overcorrection in only two lengthenings in some 175 cases in the past 14 years; there have been few complications and the results have been quite satisfactory. In a teaching program it might be better to see first what you are doing to the tendon before adopting the blind percutaneous approach.

In the application of the postoperative plaster it is vital that the foot is not forced into more than neutral dorsiflexion; otherwise the tendon will be overlengthened and strength impossible to restore. Generally we used a long-leg plaster for 6 weeks, though we did reduce the plaster to a short leg (below-the-knee) in 3 weeks, if it was convenient for the patient to return. Patients are allowed to walk the first day postoperatively with weightbearing to tolerance. Most children do so within 2 days. Crutches and walkers are necessary only if the child needs them for postural stability. Magnetic resonance imaging at intervals after percutaneous Achilles tendon lengthening in seven children demonstrated that 3 weeks' immobilization is safe and did not lead to rupture of the tendon (Blasier and Wood 1998).

After plaster removal, ordinary low quarter shoes or tennis shoes are adequate (Lee and Bleck 1980). In the rare cases which require repeat surgery, we use plastic ankle–foot orthoses for 6 months.

A similar early weightbearing program in short-leg casts after 1–2 days postoperatively has been successfully used by Sirna and Sussman (1985). They applied Buck's traction immediately after surgery to overcome the flexed-knee posture and then applied the casts.

WHITE TECHNIQUE OF SLIDING ACHILLES TENDON LENGTHENING
Banks and Green (1958) used the White technique. Half the tendon is cut proximally in its posterior–lateral segment, and half distally in its anterior–medial segment. The ankle is dorsiflexed to neutral and plaster immobilization is used as with the Hoke method described above.

PERCUTANEOUS SLIDING ACHILLES TENDON LENGTHENING
Through a skin stab wound, the surgeon makes three cuts in the tendon: a distal and proximal cut laterally, and a medial cut between these two (Coleman 1983). Moreau and Lake (1987) did percutaneous lengthening with two stab wounds 3 cm apart: one half of the medial side distally and one half the lateral side proximally. Immobilization of the dorsiflexed ankle in plaster and immediate ambulation were implemented.

GASTROCNEMIUS-LENGTHENING: OPERATIVE TECHNIQUE
A 5–7 cm longitudinal incision is made at the junction of the proximal and middle thirds of the calf, where the muscle bellies of the gastrocnemius join to form the broad gastrocnemius aponeurosis overlying the soleus muscle (Strayer 1950, Baker 1956). The sural vein and nerve are retracted. One end of the gastrocnemius aponeurosis is identified and separated from the underlying soleus. The aponeurosis is cut transversely (a 1–2 cm segment can be removed). The muscle bellies of the gastrocnemius are easily separated from the soleus. The knee is then extended and the ankle dorsiflexed. A long-leg walking cast is used for 6 weeks postoperatively.

The Baker modification of the Strayer procedure is a proximally directed 'tongue' cut in the aponeurosis. The base of the 'tongue' is distal. When the ankle is dorsiflexed with the knee extended, the 'tongue' slides distally to effect the lengthening. Most often the median fibrous raphe of the soleus was cut and when insufficient lengthening occurred, the surgeon stripped the soleus muscle fibers from the emerging Achilles tendon. This extensive muscle-stripping possibly caused more scar tissue formation and accounted for the high recurrence rate of contracture reported.

Rosenthal and Simon (1992) created another modification of the Vulpius procedure in 87 patients. They made the first cut in the gastrocnemius aponeurosis just distal to the muscle belly. Then they dorsiflexed the foot to separate the cut ends. Next the soleus fascia was cut, the foot dorsiflexed and the last horizontal cut was made a bit distally through the aponeurosis remaining in between the two cuts (Fig. 7.20). Only 15% of their patients required a repeat operation. Gait analysis in 26 of their patients documented that the lengthening did not weaken the muscles and the force of contraction was lessened due to better ankle position at heel strike.

POSTOPERATIVE CALCANEUS
Postoperative calcaneus deformities after surgical procedures to overcome equinus are usually due to overlengthening of the Achilles tendon. Although this complication is rare (about 1% of cases in our experience) there are multiple factors that may produce the unwanted result in the best of surgical hands.

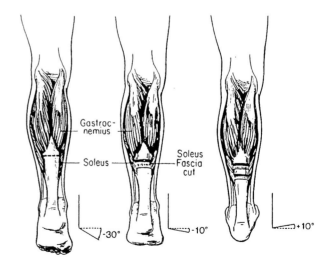

Fig. 7.20. Modified Vulpius method of gastrocnemius and soleus aponeurotic lengthening. (Reproduced from Rosenthal and Simon 1992, Fig. 2, p. 358, by permission.)

Postoperative calcaneus occurred most often after surgical correction of severe pes valgus, with either extra-articular subtalar or triple arthrodesis in total body involved patients. In pes valgus it is practically always necessary to lengthen the Achilles tendon and allow it to slide so that the foot can be manipulated into the corrected position. These partly ambulatory patients usually have severe spasticity, so that when the plantarflexor muscles are weakened the antagonist dorsiflexor muscles become predominant.

Operative shortening of the Achilles tendon has not been successful in correcting this distressing postoperative complication. If the anterior tibial muscle is spastic, it may be transferred through the interosseus membrane to the os calcis at the insertion of the Achilles tendon. To prevent further deformity due to the resulting imbalanced spasticity of the peroneal muscles, subtalar arthrodesis or triple arthrodesis of the foot might be considered (depending on age). If arthrodesis has been done, then lengthening of the anterior tibial tendon will at least reduce the force of ankle dorsiflexion.

The most satisfactory solution, with or without anterior tibial-tendon transfer, has been to stop all ankle motion with a rigid plastic ankle–foot orthosis (floor reaction brace) which holds the foot in slight equinus. Foot–ankle function can be restored with the addition of a rocker-sole and a cushion heel to the shoe. The principle applied is the same one used in lower-limb prosthetics with the solid ankle cushion heel (SACH) foot.

DYNAMIC EQUINUS DEFORMITY IN HEMIDYSTONIA

Bleck performed neurectomy of both gastrocnemius muscle heads in three patients who had severe and disabling dystonic equinus deformity (unpublished observations). When relaxed, all patients had a full range of passive dorsiflexion of the ankle well above the neutral position. All were over 13 years of age and had long and extensive trials of various physical therapy methods, muscle-relaxing drugs and restrictive ankle orthoses. The preoperative assessment in all was with 45% alcohol myoneural blocks of the gastrocnemius muscle heads. These blocks resulted in improvement of the equinus for a period of 2–6 weeks. Most importantly, no 'athetoid shift' to the opposite dystonic pattern occurred. In all three patients, a neurectomy of the medial and lateral heads of the gastrocnemius was performed through a transverse incision just distal to the popliteal crease. A long-leg walking plaster was used for 3 weeks postoperatively to ensure wound healing.

Follow-up observation for 8 years confirmed no recurrence of the severe disabling dynamic equinus posturing of the foot. In these patients the weakening of the gastrocnemius did not relieve all the equinus posturing or convert the gait into the normal heel–toe pattern, but it did allow the use of a plastic ankle–foot orthosis. The gait, while not normal, was at least more functional. Calcaneus deformities have not occurred.

Currently, botulinum toxin intramuscular injections might be the first choice in attempting to control dystonic equinus. But long term results are not known or reported. If the injections had to be repeated only every 6 months it might be worthwhile management of this difficult problem.

SUMMARY OF TREATMENT OF EQUINUS

'When change is not necessary, it is not necessary to change.'
(Lord Melbourne, 1779–1848)

It is apparent that surgeons can become fully invested in an operative procedure that seems to work for them. We can be grateful to them for continuing to analyze their results and publish them so we might make informed choices for our patients. How is the neophyte surgeon going to decide what is best for the patient? Perhaps it will help to recall the three principles of the scientific method: simplicity, reproducibility and predictability. Of all the interventions for spastic equinus, the sliding Achilles tendon lengthening seems to qualify as first choice. But with the proviso that the gastrocnemius–soleus is actually contracted, and the lengthening is not overdone, i.e. dorsiflex the ankle just to the neutral position at the time of lengthening and immobilize it exactly in the same position.

How is the neophyte surgeon going to decide what is best for the patient?

Principles of the scientific method: simplicity, reproducibility, predictability.

If gastrocnemius aponeurotic lengthening gives the same result, but with a longer scar in the mid-calf, and higher recurrence rate, should this not be a consideration? Neurectomy of either the gastrocnemius or soleus would appear not too physiological if we believe the kinetic data from gait analysis studies and wish to preserve the major energy generation muscles during level walking.

Anterior transposition of the Achilles insertion also apparently gives a result equal to Achilles lengthening, and perhaps with less risk of a calcaneus gait or deformity. But the procedure seems more complicated and may demand longer immobilization than the 3 weeks usual with lengthening.

SPASTIC PES VARUS

'Thou shalt not varus.'
(Old orthopaedic adage)

The etiology of varus deformity of the foot in cerebral palsy is not complex. It is due to spastic muscle imbalance where the force of the spastic foot invertor muscles exceeds that of the spastic evertors. In this respect the cause of the varus deformity is different from flaccid paralysis, where the imbalance is due to weakness or absence of the evertor muscles. Our electromyographic gait analyses of cases of spastic varus deformities, in which we recorded the simultaneous electrical activity of the posterior tibial, anterior tibial and peroneal muscles, clearly indicated that all these muscles fired during gait—albeit often out of phase. This is why underneath every varus there is a valgus. If the invertor spasticity is decreased too much, the evertor spasticity predominates and the foot which was formerly in varus ends up in valgus.

Spastic pes varus or valgus. . . . Underneath every varus there is a valgus and visa versa.

Only two muscles account for the varus deformity: the posterior tibial, which causes hindfoot varus, and the anterior tibial which causes mid-foot varus. Either or both may be responsible. Judging from the literature, most surgeons in recent years have concentrated on the posterior tibial muscle.

Spasticity and contracture of the gastrocnemius–soleus accounts for some varus, but this is in the ankle and positional due to the obliquity of the ankle axis of dorsi–plantarflexion (Inman 1976). This axis is in the line constructed through the tips of the ankle malleoli—it slopes downward obliquely from lateral to medial. Because of the oblique axis of the ankle joint, the foot is directed medially on plantarflexion and laterally on dorsiflexion. However, this anatomical construction does not cause inversion at the subtalar joint or the mid-tarsal joints of the

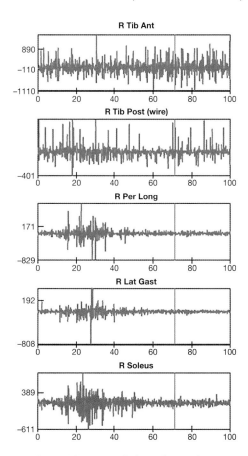

Fig. 7.21. Gait EMG: spastic right hemiplegic with equinovarus. Anterior tibialis very active and posterior tibialis moderately active throughout gait cycle. Peroneals contracting appropriately during stance. This is why under every varus there is a potential for valgus. (EMG courtesy of Alberto Esquenazi, MD.)

foot. If we recognize these aspects of varus, then the surgeon will not be disappointed by the failure of Achilles tendon lengthening to correct a dynamic pes varus.

INDICATIONS FOR SURGERY

Surgical treatment is generally indicated in a child more than 4 years old, when the deforming force of the spastic muscle persists and cannot be controlled with an orthosis and/or botulinum toxin injections. If surgery is delayed, skeletal changes in the direction of the dynamic deformity will result. Early surgery on the tendons is indicated to prevent late fixed bony deformities that can be corrected only with surgery of the bones and joints, and the attendant loss of foot mobility and greater morbidity.

A varus foot is an uncomfortable foot. Walking on the outer border of the foot eventually causes a painful callous over the base of the fifth metatarsal. When severe, shoes or sandals can no longer be worn and recurrent ankle sprains occur. Participation in sport becomes almost impossible; rigid ski boots do not fit.

The selection of the patient for surgery of the posterior tibial tendon is based upon the clinical examination of gait observation of the foot position during the stance phase, and the passive correction of the foot to the neutral position. Soft-tissue surgery alone will not correct a fixed skeletal deformity.

The gait electromyogram is useful in making a decision (Hoffer 1976, Perry and Hoffer 1977, Barto *et al.* 1984, Adler *et al.* 1985). Continuous activity of the posterior tibial muscle indicated lengthening; if this muscle had activity in swing phase, then transfer was selected (Fig. 7.21). If the anterior tibial shows continuous and out-of-phase activity, a split anterior tibial-tendon transfer was considered.

SURGICAL PROCEDURES FOR PES VARUS

The choice of operative interventions to correct pes varus is very wide (Fig. 7.22). It seems inconceivable that any more operations could be devised for the poor spastic posterior tibial muscle and its tendon. According to reports, and the excellent results on follow-up examinations, the surgeon can lengthen the tendon, cut it at its musculotendinous junction in the calf, transfer it anteriorly through the interosseus membrane, reroute it anterior to the medial malleolus, or split it in two and transfer its lateral half to the peroneus brevis tendon. Since the introduction of the split posterior tibial-tendon transfer in the mid-1980s, it seems to be favored above all others.

Supramalleolar lengthening of the posterior tibial tendon was my choice for correction of varus of the hindfoot (Fig. 7.23*b*). It had been the preference of Banks and Panagakos (1966), Tachdjian (1972) and Coleman (1983). In 21 patients, Root and Kirz (1982) reported poor results in nine and good in 12. The only poor results Bleck had were in those patients in whom the hindfoot varus was corrected but mid-foot varus persisted due to the concomitant spasticity of the anterior tibial muscle; these required a split transfer of the anterior tibial tendon (unpublished observations). Spastic metatarsus adductus cannot be alleviated with either posterior tibial or anterior tibial-tendon procedures.

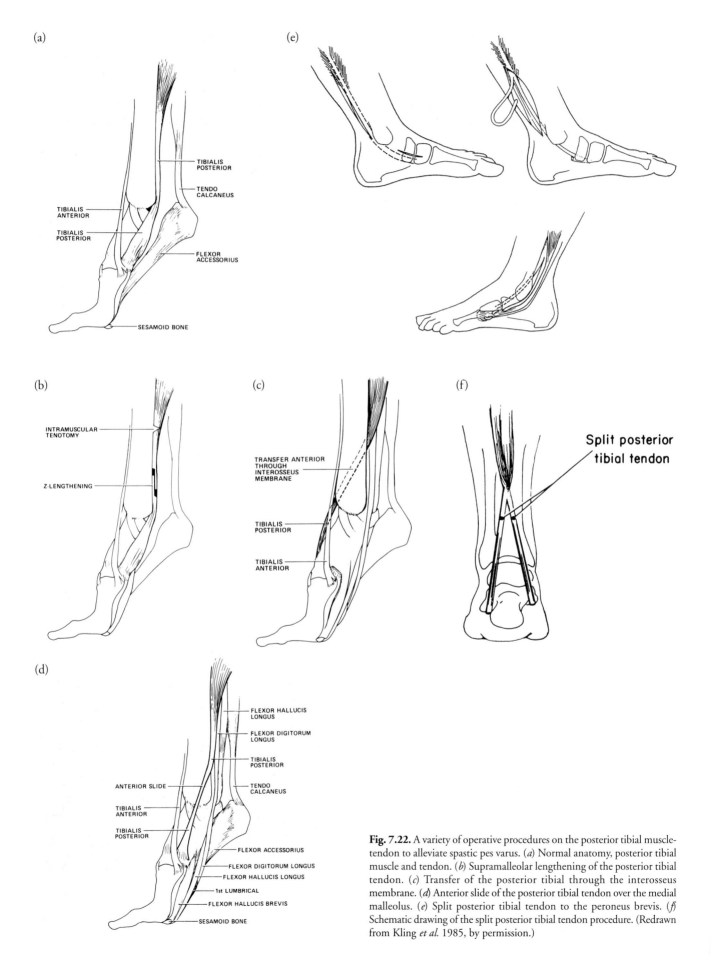

(a)

TIBIALIS
POSTERIOR

TENDO
CALCANEUS

TIBIALIS
ANTERIOR

TIBIALIS
POSTERIOR

FLEXOR
ACCESSORIUS

SESAMOID BONE

(b)

INTRAMUSCULAR
TENOTOMY

Z-LENGTHENING

(c)

TRANSFER ANTERIOR
THROUGH
INTEROSSEUS
MEMBRANE

TIBIALIS
POSTERIOR

TIBIALIS
ANTERIOR

(d)

FLEXOR HALLUCIS
LONGUS

FLEXOR DIGITORUM
LONGUS

TIBIALIS
POSTERIOR

ANTERIOR SLIDE

TENDO
CALCANEUS

TIBIALIS
ANTERIOR

TIBIALIS
POSTERIOR

FLEXOR ACCESSORIUS

FLEXOR DIGITORUM LONGUS

FLEXOR HALLUCIS LONGUS

1st LUMBRICAL

FLEXOR HALLUCIS BREVIS

SESAMOID BONE

(e)

(f)

Split posterior
tibial tendon

Fig. 7.22. A variety of operative procedures on the posterior tibial muscle-tendon to alleviate spastic pes varus. (*a*) Normal anatomy, posterior tibial muscle and tendon. (*b*) Supramalleolar lengthening of the posterior tibial tendon. (*c*) Transfer of the posterior tibial through the interosseus membrane. (*d*) Anterior slide of the posterior tibial tendon over the medial malleolus. (*e*) Split posterior tibial tendon to the peroneus brevis. (*f*) Schematic drawing of the split posterior tibial tendon procedure. (Redrawn from Kling *et al.* 1985, by permission.)

240

This should be obvious, but sometimes we tend to overgeneralize in the definition of pes varus.

Intramuscular tenotomy of the posterior tibial tendon in the middle third of the calf was described by Ruda and Frost (1971). No plaster immobilization was used; the patients walked soon after surgery. Matsuo (2002) also describes intramuscular lengthening of the posterior tibial-tendon muscle unit through a medial supramalleolar incision. Nather *et al.* (1984), in experimental intramuscular lengthenings in rabbits, confirmed that without plaster immobilization this type of lengthening did not change while healing occurred. The gap in the tendon remained the same. In the 29 cases of Ruda and Frost there were no failures and only two recurrences and was recommended in children younger than age 6 years.

Tenotomy of the posterior tibial tendon at its insertion on the navicular bone is not recommended because of the great risk of a late valgus deformity. Collapse of the longitudinal arch in disruptions of the posterior tibial tendon at its insertion in adults has been reported (Kettlekamp and Alexander 1969, Goldner *et al.* 1974, Jahss 1980, Mann and Soecht 1982, Johnson 1983, Funk *et al.* 1986). Overlengthening of the posterior tibial tendon can theoretically result in the same reverse deformity.

Transfer of the posterior tibial tendon to the dorsum of the foot through the interosseous membrane has had its adherents and detractors (Fig. 7.22c). In reviewing the literature, one is struck by the recurring reports of transfer of the posterior tibial tendon to the dorsum of the foot. The operation is at least 50 years old (Mayer 1937). Some reports praised the procedure as being the best for a spastic pes varus (Gritzka *et al.* 1972, Bisla *et al.* 1976, Williams 1976), while others reflect disappointment—particularly with the later valgus and calcaneus deformities. Williams (1976) advised anchoring the tendon to the mid-dorsum of the foot. Often it is necessary to correct the equinus at the same time, and overlengthening of the Achilles tendon would be more detrimental when the spastic posterior tibial tendon is transferred anteriorly under tension; it can then act as too strong a dorsiflexion force. This transfer of tendon of a spastic muscle probably is not the best operation for spastic pes varus.

Bisla *et al.* (1976) reported good results in 13 of 19 cases; Turner and Cooper (1972) had poor results in 10 of 14 patients, in whom reversal from varus to valgus occurred. Banks (1975) had only moderate success. Schneider and Balon (1977) reported poor results; within 1 year 68% of the feet were either in valgus or calcaneus. Root and Kirz (1982) performed 67 transfers in 59 patients, and had better results: 22 excellent, 25 good and 12 poor (18%). These 12 developed valgus, which was not deemed severe enough to merit further corrective surgery. Five years later, Root and colleagues (1987) reported better results in 51 patients who had a mean follow-up of 9.3 years (range 5–26 years). Only four developed postoperative valgus deformities attributed to placing the new insertion of the tendon into the cuboid, rather than in alignment with the third metatarsal.

Miller *et al.* (1982) transferred the posterior tibial tendon through the interosseus membrane to the dorsolateral aspect of the foot in seven patients (nine feet) who had cerebrospastic

paralysis (two were post-head injury). They had a 56% failure rate, with four overcorrections to valgus and one undercorrection (Fig. 7.23). These orthopaedists recommended that a posterior tibial-tendon transfer anteriorly should be done in cerebral palsy only if confirmation of its swing-phase activity is found on gait electromyography—a rare circumstance, if indeed it ever happens at all.

Transfer of the posterior tibial tendon anteriorly through the interosseous membrane was originally used successfully in cases of flaccid and spastic paralysis of the dorsiflexor muscles of the ankle. Watkins *et al.* (1954) performed the transfer in seven patients with spastic paralysis; the results were excellent in two, good in three and fair in one (one patient was lost to follow-up). In one patient (presumably the fair result) a valgus deformity occurred. These original authors cautioned against transferring the tendon too far laterally in the foot in spastic paralysis. Twelve of their 29 patients had a triple arthrodesis combined with the transfer. Arthrodesis of the talo-navicular joint will nullify the valgus producing effect of a total transfer of a spastic posterior tibial tendon.

Parsch and Rubsaamen (1992) reporting from Stuttgart, Germany, transferred the anterior tibial tendon in 24 feet (19 children) and the posterior tibial tendon in 20 feet (19 patients). Additional surgery was either an Achilles tendon lengthening or a Vulpius procedure. Although they had good results in 75%, they did note overcorrections to calcaneal–valgus deformities in 25%, i.e. one out of every four patients had this result. What if your first four patients happened to have this poor outcome? Your poor results would be 100%, and as always, 100% for the individual patient.

Transposition of the posterior tibial tendon anterior to the medial malleolus was devised by Baker and Hill (1964) (Fig. 7.22d). In this simple procedure, the posterior tibial tendon was removed from its sheath through two incisions proximal and distal to the medial malleolus, and then allowed to slide anteriorly to act as a dorsiflexor of the ankle. Bisla *et al.* (1976) had poor results with this procedure. In 1985 Lester and Johnson reviewed the 'Baker slide operation' in 28 patients (35 feet) who had an average

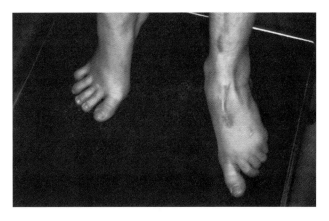

Fig. 7.23. Postoperative pes valgus after transfer of the posterior tibial tendon through the interosseus membrane to the dorsum of the foot. Solution: cut the posterior tibial tendon and subtalar extraarticular arthrodesis.

follow-up of 10.4 years and stated that the results were very good in 30 of the 35 feet. Two feet that had simultaneous Achilles tendon lengthening had continued hindfoot varus and three developed a calcaneocavus deformity, a very difficult if not impossible deformity to correct satisfactorily. If the posterior tibial muscle is spastic and transferred, it continues the spastic pattern that pulls the foot into excessive dorsiflexion. The operation has fallen out of favor.

SPLIT POSTERIOR TIBIAL-TENDON TRANSFER

Half of the posterior tibial tendon is transferred to the peroneus brevis tendon to correct the spastic hindfoot varus (Fig. 7.22*e, f*). Green *et al.* (1983) had excellent results in all 16 patients who had this operation. They had no valgus or calcaneus deformities in a minimum 2-year follow-up. Kling *et al.* (1985) were also enthusiastic with their results, which were excellent in 35 of 37 feet with spastic equinovarus deformities. Achilles tendon lengthening was usually done in combination with the transfer. The incision was modified to one posterior ankle horizontal incision (the Cincinnati) by Townsend *et al.* (1990). If you were also going to do an Achilles tendon lengthening this might pose a problem.

Medina *et al.* (1989) modified the operation slightly by attaching the split end of the posterior tibial tendon proximally to the peroneus brevis. They had good results with this simplification that avoids more extensive dissection on the lateral aspect of the foot. Whether other surgeons can confirm that this modification is successful or not cannot be confirmed from reports in the literature.

It seems probable that we have exhausted all the possibilities with this tendon in cerebral palsy. The split posterior tibial transfer for the spastic varus deformity of the foot has become the first choice by many pediatric orthopaedic surgeons (Kagaya *et al.* 1996, Renshaw *et al.* 1996).

The split posterior tibial transfer for the spastic varus deformity of the foot has become the first choice.

What we do not know in split-tendon transfers is whether the tension on each half of the tendon is equal, or whether one half has weaker tension that merely removes the deforming force of the spastic muscle. The only data I have seen on this question come from an anatomical study of tension of the split anterior tibial tendon in various insertion sites by colleagues from the National University of Singapore (Hui *et al.* 1998). Insertion of the split tendon on the fourth metatarsal produced maximum dorsiflexion with minimal supination and pronation. The third metatarsal axis was the ideal site for insertion of the whole tendon.

Leggio and Kruse (2001) of the A.I. duPont Institute, Wilmington, DE, had the temerity to report that combining an external rotation osteotomy with the split posterior tibial-tendon transfer had bad results. Only 27% had excellent results; 13% had a rigid equinovarus deformity and 40% had severe planovalgus deformities. The latter reverse deformity is not so surprising given the anatomical effect of derotation of the tibia externally. Through the mitered hinge effect on the subtalar joint, external rotation of the tibia is translated through the joint to cause the valgus of the foot; conversely internal rotation of the tibia causes varus of the foot (Inman and Mann 1978).

POSTERIOR TIBIAL-TENDON LENGTHENING

To confirm my impression of the efficacy of the posterior tibial-tendon lengthening, Bleck (unpublished observations) reviewed the operative notes and charts of patients who had only this procedure for spastic pes varus, usually in combination with a sliding Achilles tendon lengthening for the equinus (Table 7.VI). While admitting the defects of retrospective review, it appears that posterior tibial-tendon lengthening has been successful

TABLE 7.VI
Retrospective review of posterior tibial-tendon lengthening with and without transfer of anterior tibial tendon and with transfer of anterior tibial tendon alone for spastic pes varus 1956–1982

	N	Follow-up	Recurrence	Late valgus (mean years)
Posterior tibial-tendon lengthening only (supramalleolar-Z type)				
Spastic hemiplegia	23	7.0	2	2
Spastic diplegia	16	7.5	2	
Spastic quadriplegia	4	8.5		
Total patients	43			
Total feet	47	7.5	4 (8%)	2 (4%)
Posterior tibial-tendon lengthening with anterior tibial-tendon transfer				
Spastic hemiplegia	9	7.0		2§
Spastic diplegia	12	8.0		1§
Spastic quadriplegia	1	10.0		
Total patients (all unilateral)	22	8.0	0	3 (13%)

§Whole tendon transferred to mid-foot in these three patients; all others had split transfers.

Split anterior tendon transfer alone				
Spastic hemiplegia	6	8.0		
Spastic diplegia	2	4.0		
Total patients (all unilateral)	8	6.0	0	0

in correcting the deformity. Two of the 47 feet developed late valgus; this was probably due to overlengthening of the tendon. Four feet had a recurrence of the varus but it was in the mid-foot; a split anterior tibial-tendon transfer corrected it nicely. No attempt was made to assess the preoperative or postoperative strength of plantarflexion, being satisfied preoperatively with a passively correctable foot and postoperatively with a foot in neutral position of the heel and forefoot.

Twenty-two of Bleck's patients had the posterior tibial-tendon lengthening and the anterior tibial-tendon transfer at the same time. Three of these developed late valgus; in these three the entire tendon had been transferred to the mid-dorsum of the foot. All others had a split anterior tibial-tendon transfer.

Since 1977 we have relied on the gait electromyograms and the clinical examination to decide whether to do both the anterior tibial-tendon transfer and the posterior tibial-tendon lengthening. If there is varus of the hindfoot, and the tendon of the posterior tibial is prominent and under obvious tension on passive eversion of the heel, it was lengthened. If in the same patient the mid-foot moved into dynamic varus, especially on the maneuver of resistance against flexion of the hip with the knee flexed (flexor withdrawal or 'confusion' reflex), then the split anterior tibial-tendon transfer is included. Others have done an intramuscular lengthening of the posterior tibial tendon and a split anterior tibial transfer with good results (Barnes and Herring 1991).

Only eight of our patients had a split anterior tibial-tendon transfer alone because they did not have hindfoot varus or resistance to passive eversion of the heel. They did have electromyographic confirmation of continuous activity of the anterior tibial muscle during gait. To repeat: clinical examination must always be combined with the laboratory results, i.e. the electromyographic gait examination.

Green *et al.* (1983) wrote that simple lengthening of the posterior tibial tendon gave the best results. They changed to the split posterior tibial transfer because they felt theoretically that lengthening of the Achilles tendon and the posterior tibial tendon would weaken the plantarflexor muscles too much. They also feared that overlengthening of the posterior tibial tendon would result in a late valgus deformity. Bleck agrees with Green and his colleagues that simple lengthening has been quite satisfactory in correction of the hindfoot varus (unpublished observations). It does not seem possible to gauge accurately the strength of the plantarflexors in cerebral palsy. Standing strength of the gastrocnemius–soleus can only be assessed by rising on tiptoe on one foot. Few patients with cerebral palsy can stand on tiptoe on one leg due to lack of balance reactions. In normal persons this is the recognized clinical test for the strength of the calf muscles. The average adult should be able to rise on one foot at least eight or nine times.

OPERATIVE TECHNIQUE OF POSTERIOR TIBIAL-TENDON LENGTHENING
Through a 3–5 cm incision directly over the posterior tibial tendon *proximal* to the medial malleolus, the tendon is z-lengthened. The heel is everted to the neutral position and the split tendon is sutured side-to-side, with just enough tension to prevent it from wrinkling. A short-leg plaster is worn for 6 weeks. The procedure can be combined with a sliding Achilles tendon lengthening.

Matsuo (2002) is dedicated to sliding tendon lengthenings. For the posterior tibial through a supramalleolar medial incision he isolates the tendon with two plastic tubes under it, places a zig-zag suture in the midpoint between the intended cuts in the tendon, then makes a cut half-way through the tendon—one proximal anterior and the other distal posterior. He slides the tendon apart as the foot is manipulated into the corrected neutral position and the suture is tied to secure the slid part of the tendon.

OPERATIVE TECHNIQUE OF THE SPLIT ANTERIOR TIBIAL-TENDON TRANSFER ('SPLATT')
When gait analysis and EMG monitoring indicate that there is continuous and out-of-phase activity of the anterior tibialis which is contributing to dynamic varus foot deformity, a split anterior tendon transfer may be indicated (Fig. 7.24). The technique is as follows. Three incisions are required. The first is over the dorsal–medial aspect of the first cuneiform bone and the base of

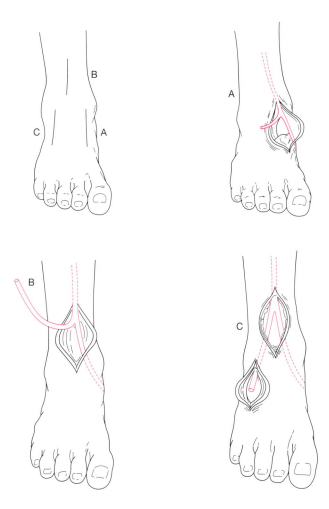

Fig. 7.24. Split anterior tibial tendon transfer.

the first metatarsal. The lateral half of the anterior tibial tendon is cut at its insertion and the tendon slit in half proximally. A thick (0) nonabsorbable suture is placed through the distal tendon in a secure manner (Strickland 1999). A long hemostat is used to pass the suture subcutaneously under the inferior and superior extensor retinaculum in line with the anterior tibialis tendon proximally. The second incision is made just lateral to the tibial crest of the musculotendinous junction of the anterior tibial at about the level of the distal and middle thirds of the leg. The fascial envelope over the muscle is incised and the lateral half of the tendon brought out through this wound. The third longitudinal incision is made over the dorsum of the cuboid, and the tendon suture passed subcutaneously under the superior and inferior extensor retinaculum from the incision to the cuboid region. Two convergent drill holes ($7/_{64}$ or $9/_{64}$ inch) are drilled in the cuboid and curetted to make them large enough for the tendon. The lateral half of the transferred tendon is passed through these holes and sutured to itself under tension with the foot slightly dorsiflexed and the hindfoot in eversion (Hoffer et al. 1974, 1985). A short-leg walking plaster is worn for 6 weeks. Hoffer and colleagues advised use of an orthosis for 6 months postoperatively.

It can be difficult to maintain the drill hole in the cuboid (the roof breaks) in some cases, especially in young children whose bones are small and cartilaginous. In these instances, the results seem just as good when the tendon is anchored with strong sutures to the peroneus tertius tendon and the thick periosteum of the cuboid. To prepare for this contingency, the periosteum of the cuboid should be carefully preserved when exposing the bone prior to making the drill holes. Alternatively the suture through the split tendon can be passed through a hole drilled through the cuboid to the plantar surface of the foot using long Keith needles. The tendon is pulled taut, balancing the medial insertion. The suture ends on the needles are run through a felt pad and secured on a button with a knot on the plantar surface of the foot. The foot is casted with a short leg cast for 6 weeks. Full weightbearing is allowed at 3 weeks. Upon cast removal the button is cut off, the suture is pulled through the plantar skin and cut short.

Hoffer et al. (1985) combined the SPLATT with an intra-muscular posterior tibial lengthening when there was a relatively fixed hindfoot varus and continuous firing of the posterior tibial tendon on gait electromyograms. All cases had an Achilles tendon lengthening to correct the equinus. The posterior tibial tendon was lengthened in eight of their 27 feet reported. The split anterior tibial-tendon transfer alone was performed when the electromyogram showed continuous activity of the muscle. Their results were quite satisfactory; only two had a recurrent equinus and one had a recurrence of a mild dynamic varus. Given the 10-year follow-up and results like these, who can argue about their approach to the treatment of dynamic pes varus? Vogt (1998), reporting from Strasbourg, France, gave similar approbation to this transfer in a review of 73 feet in 69 patients.

As usual with orthopaedic surgeons a modification of this operation was done by Belgian surgeons who transferred the

split portion through the interosseous membrane to the dorsum of the foot (Mulier et al. 1995). The idea was to restore active dorsiflexion of the ankle. They had only two poor results in 21 procedures; the two poor results were attributed to 'technical errors'. Although these orthopaedic surgeons thought their anterior tibial-tendon transfer was unique, the identical transfer was reported by Saji and colleagues from Hong Kong with good results (Saji et al. 1993). This modification of Hoffer's original procedure appears to entail more dissection and a bit more time and trouble to obtain the same result.

OPERATIVE TECHNIQUE SPLIT POSTERIOR TIBIAL-TENDON TRANSFER

Sage (1992) delineated Kaufer's technique for a split posterior tibial-tendon transfer using large open incisions. This operation is however amenable to smaller incisions. Initially a small (3 cm) incision is made over the insertion of the posterior tibialis tendon. The distal tendon is divided longitudinally. A strong suture, e.g. 0 Ethibond, is put into the anterior half of the distal tendon using a Bunnell, Tajima or similar suture technique (Strickland 1999). Using a long curved hemostat or tendon passer, the ends of the suture are passed through the tendon sheath proximally to the musculotendinous junction. The sheath is left intact. A small incision is made proximally over the tip of the hemostat. The sutures are released from the hemostat and pulled through the proximal wound. The tendon is pulled gently yet firmly through the tendon sheath proximally into the proximal wound. This allows the tendon to be split longitudinally along the tendon fiber lines.

Similarly the sutures and tendon are passed behind the tibia and fibula to the lateral compartment leading bluntly while hugging the posterior cortex of the bones and avoiding the neurovascular structures. A small incision is made over the peroneal sheath to pull the suture and split tendon laterally and into the peroneal sheath. The tendon is then weaved through the peroneus brevis in the manner of Pulvertaft (Schneider 1999) while the foot is held in slight valgus to ensure adequate tension. The tendon ends and weave are sutured into place. At closure the foot should be in a neutral to slight valgus position. A short leg-splint is followed by a short leg cast for 6–8 weeks postoperatively. A short leg cast can be used for 6–12 months postoperatively. Leggio and Kruse (2001) reported on the combination of a split posterior tibialis transfer with distal tibial rotation osteotomy. Disappointing results included 40% severe planovalgus and 13% rigid equinovarus at a follow-up of 15 equinovarus feet in nine children who mostly with diplegic involvement.

'*Warning: don't combine the transfer with rotation osteotomy of the tibia—40% severe planovalgus; 13% rigid equinovarus.*'
(Leggio & Kruse 2001)

TWO UNIQUE PROCEDURES FOR SPASTIC EQUINOVARUS DEFORMITIES

Orthopaedic surgeons from Osaka, Japan (Hiroshima et al. 1988), transferred the long toe-flexors through the interosseous membrane to the fourth metatarsal looping the tendon around it. Both the flexor hallucis longus and flexor digitorum longus tendons were cut and transferred. The transfer was combined with Achilles tendon lengthening and posterior tibial-tendon lengthening in 21 patients with cerebral palsy. Excellent and good results occurred in 57.1%. One wonders if a 42.9% poor result would now be acceptable to a pediatric orthopaedic surgeon.

The 'bridle' procedure derives its name from the harness that fits over a horse's head and was presented as a new procedure for equinovarus deformities in cerebral palsy and other neuromuscular conditions (McCall *et al.* 1991). The bridle is an anastamosis anteriorly of the anterior tibial, the posterior tibial and the peroneus longus tendons as cut from their insertions and woven together. The operation was done through three incisions and seems a bit complicated. Achilles tendon lengthening accompanied the bridle. Of 80 patients who had spastic cerebral palsy, 67% had excellent or good results. Unfortunately 13 of the 107 bridles created had a postoperative calcaneus deformity. This may not be a large percentage, but as the authors state, 'This is a difficult problem to treat.' Apparently, no other surgeon has had the temerity to try the procedure and report the results.

HINDFOOT VARUS, NOT PASSIVELY CORRECTABLE: CLOSED WEDGE OSTEOTOMY OF THE CALCANEUS

If passive correction of the hindfoot varus deformity is not possible, a closed wedge osteotomy of the calcaneus is an effective procedure. It must be combined with a posterior tibial-tendon lengthening and, if required, Achilles tendon lengthening (Silver *et al.* 1967). We have found it useful in a few patients who had fixed varus of the heel after overcorrection of a subtalar extra-articular arthrodesis performed for a pes valgus.

Through a lateral oblique incision, coursing from a point anterior to the Achilles tendon to a distal point almost parallel to the peroneal tendons, the lateral aspect of the calcaneus is exposed subperiosteally. A laterally based wedge of bone is removed from the calcaneus. Sufficient bone is removed to correct the heel varus to neutral when the wedge is closed. A staple, screw or pins maintain the closure (Fig. 7.25).

HINDFOOT AND MIDFOOT VARUS, NOT PASSIVELY CORRECTABLE: TRIPLE ARTHRODESIS

If the varus of the hind- and midfoot cannot be passively corrected, a triple arthrodesis is the time-tested and best procedure in children over the age of 12 years. The deforming force of the spastic muscles should be relieved by lengthening of the posterior tibial and Achilles tendons. If the peroneal muscles are non-functional, the anterior tibial tendon should be transferred to the mid-dorsum of the foot.

In cerebral palsy, triple arthrodesis is not often performed in pes varus, because early muscle lengthenings and tendon transfers to balance the spastic muscle deforming forces are successful. Horstmann and Eilert (1977) reported triple arthrodesis in only 37 patients from a pool of 899 with cerebral palsy. Twenty of these

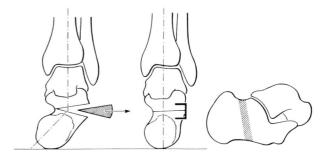

Fig. 7.25. Technique of lateral closing-wedge osteotomy of calcaneus for fixed hindfoot varus deformity.

had equinovarus deformities that were more successfully corrected with triple arthrodesis than occurred in equinovalgus feet.

Ireland and Hoffer (1985) found triple arthrodesis a successful procedure in 18 of 20 patients with cerebral palsy whose mean age was 15.5 years. They did report four talonavicular joint non-unions. Non-union of this joint is fairly common. Perhaps this occurs because of inadequate contact between the head of the talus and the navicular articulating surface. Removal of an excessive amount of talar head is to be avoided, and it should be contoured to fit snugly against the navicular articular surface.

Orthopaedic surgeons have been concerned that after a triple arthrodesis a 'ball and socket' ankle might develop after many years and cause intractable ankle pain. The explanation for the ball and socket joint is the function of the subtalar joint which absorbs the torques between the foot and the floor during the stance phase of gait when the lower limb abruptly changes from internal rotation to external rotation. If these rotational forces cannot be absorbed at the subtalar joint due to arthrodesis, the next proximal joint that may do so is the ankle (Inman 1976).

Not every patient who has a triple arthrodesis will develop a 'ball and socket' ankle joint. This inconsistency might be explained by the great individual variations that occur in the axis of the ankle joint. This axis is oblique, and it corresponds almost exactly to a line drawn just through the tips of the malleoli. When a second line is drawn through the midline of the tibia, the ankle axis has a mean of 82.7º (SD + 3.7º; range 74º–94º) (Inman 1976). It is possible that the more horizontal the axis of the ankle joint, the more rotation is possible; such patients are more likely to develop a late 'ball and socket' ankle after triple arthrodesis.

University of Iowa orthopaedic surgeons who are unique for long-term follow-up studies reported the results of 67 feet in 57 patients who had a triple arthrodesis for a variety of paralytic foot deformities (4% had cerebral palsy) (Saltzman *et al.* 1999). At the average follow-up of 44 years, all had evidence of degenerative changes in the ankle, naviculocuneiform and tarsometatarsal joints; 55% had pain, but apparently not too disabling inasmuch as 95% were satisfied with the result of the operation. So it remains a satisfactory solution to imbalance of the hindfoot in paralytic conditions.

The operative technique of triple arthrodesis is described in so many surgical technique textbooks that the details need not be repeated here. Bleck (unpublished observations) used the technique which is an adaptation of several methods and preferred by the Campbell Clinic (Edmonson and Crenshaw 1980). The skin incision is on the lateral aspect of the foot and courses obliquely from the talar head to the peroneal tendons in a line that bisects the heel. The three joints are resected in the following order: calcanealcuboid, talonavicular and subtalar. A lamina spreader helps to visualize the subtalar articular surfaces. Excessive valgus position of the foot can be avoided by not taking overly generous laterally based wedges from the three joints; it is best to go slowly.

Bleck did not use staples or other forms of internal fixation (unpublished observations). Two Steinman pins, one through the heel across the subtalar joint and one dorsally across the talonavicular joint, permit the application of a heavily padded postoperative plaster. The foot and ankle are sandwiched between dorsal and plantar ABD pads[4] that are secured with rolled cast padding before the plaster is applied (W.M. Roberts, personal communication). This padding accommodates the postoperative swelling, and the plaster seldom needs to be split. Continuous suction drainage of the wound up to 48 hours after surgery has been a useful additional detail that has helped prevent wound breakdown. The long-leg plaster and pins are removed 4 weeks postoperatively. At this point the foot can be manipulated under sedation or anesthesia if the position of the hindfoot or forefoot configuration appear unsatisfactory, i.e. too much varus or valgus. A short-leg walking plaster is used for an additional 4–6 weeks.

PES VALGUS

Although pes valgus occurs in patients with spastic hemiplegia, it is more common in spastic diplegia. In one study of 230 patients with cerebral palsy and foot deformities, pes varus occurred in 38% of spastic hemiplegic patients and 21% of the diplegic/quadriplegic group. Pes equinovalgus was more common in quadriplegics and diplegics (37%) and rare in hemiplegics (2%) (Bennet *et al.* 1982). The management of pes valgus is discussed in Chapter 8.

PES CAVUS—CAVOVARUS OR CALCANEALCAVUS

Pes cavus is only occasionally seen in spastic hemiplegia. In Wilcox and Weiner's (1985) description of their dome osteotomy for cavus, only two of 22 patients reported had cerebral palsy. Although theoretically pes cavus is caused by spasticity of the intrinsic muscles, in Bleck's experience (unpublished observations) it has followed Achilles tendon lengthening—not once but three times in one patient—due to a confusion of forefoot equinus with ankle equinus. In cavus, the primary problem is excessive plantar flexion of the tarsal and metatarsal bones beyond the range of normal. As in flaccid paralysis, weakening the triceps surae creates excessive dorsiflexion of the calcaneus, and the

4 ABD = Army battle dressing.

substitution of the toe-flexor muscles for the gastrocnemius–soleus 'pulls' the forefoot to the hindfoot; the deformity is calcanealcavus (Coleman 1983, Dillin and Samilson 1983). The higher the arch of the foot, the more discomfort ensues due to the excessive pressure of weightbearing on the metatarsal heads and strain on the mid-tarsal joints at the apex of the arch.

MEASUREMENT OF CAVUS

It is useful to have some objective method of determining the degree of cavus. One method used is measurement of the angle made by a line through the first metatarsal shaft and the plantar surface of the heel when weightbearing or when the foot is passively dorsiflexed. On weightbearing, the foot perceived to be normal has an angle between these two landmarks of 25º in a range of 20º–40º. Feet with this angle greater than 40º have excessive forefoot equinus and can be termed cavus deformities (Fig. 7.26). This measurement can be used at the time of surgical correction.

The extent of the calcaneal-cavus deformity is defined by radiographic measurements of the dorsiflexion angle of the calcaneus with the horizontal plane when the patient is standing (Fig. 7.27). The normal upper limit with this measurement is about 25º. If this angle is 30º or more, the deformity called 'calcaneus' is certain.

Barenfeld *et al.* (1971) measured the degree of forefoot equinus on standing lateral radiographs of normal children's feet.

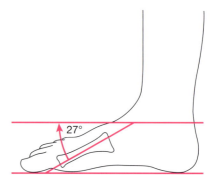

Fig. 7.26. Photograph of foot in weightbearing; measurement to determine clinically the degree of forefoot equinus (cavus).

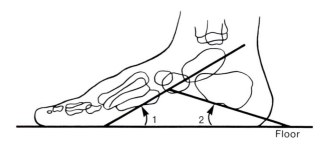

Fig. 7.27. Tracing of weightbearing radiograph of a child's foot. Angle 1 is the talar plantar flexion angle (normal mean 26.5º, SD 5.3). Angle 2 is the calcaneal dorsiflexion angle (normal mean 16.8º, SD 5.6º). A calcaneal dorsiflexion angle >25º indicates a calcaneus deformity (Bleck and Berzins 1977).

The obtuse angle between the horizontal plane of the calcaneus and a line along the shaft of the first metatarsal varied from 140º to 160º. If this angle was less than 140º, the foot was defined as cavus. In 75% of the children with pes cavus, the angle was less than 125º.

MANAGEMENT OF PES CALCANEALCAVUS

No conservative management has been successful and orthotic treatment is useless (Coleman 1983). Surgery is indicated in children under the age of 10 years to prevent the severe and often symptomatic deformity in adolescence. In older children and adolescents, it is probably wise to perform the extensive surgery required in this difficult deformity only if the patient has intolerable foot discomfort.

Pes cavus: it is probably wise to perform the extensive surgery required . . . only if the patient has symptoms of foot discomfort.

Calcanealcavus in children between the ages of 5 and 10 years will require first an extra-articular subtalar arthrodesis to stabilize the hindfoot, followed 6 weeks later by transfer of the peroneal and posterior tibial tendons to the calcaneus in order to substitute for the weak triceps surae muscle (Coleman 1983). In cerebral palsy, the spastic anterior tibial muscle is usually the major deforming force in causing the imbalance. Therefore transfer it to the calcaneus rather than using the peroneals or the posterior tibial which are plantarflexors. In all cavus deformities it is necessary to do a plantar fasciotomy and a myotomy of the origin of the flexor digitorum brevis muscles ('plantar release') as well as the preceding operations. Calcanealcavus in children with the spastic type of cerebral palsy over the age of 12 years will require the 'plantar release', a triple arthrodesis, a crescentric osteotomy of the calcaneus (Samilson 1976), and usually a transfer of the deforming spastic anterior tibial muscle-tendon to the calcaneus (Fig. 7.28).

The problem with triple arthrodesis in correcting a severe forefoot equinus is that removal of the talar head and neck is limited by the tibial articular surface of the talus; excessive dorsiflexion of the forefoot by resection of more and more of the talar neck will compromise the integrity of the ankle joint. It is

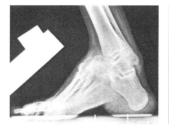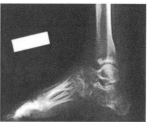

Fig. 7.29. *Left:* severe calcaneus deformity; spastic diplegia. The patient had two Achilles tendon lengthenings and a posterior capsulotomy of the ankle joint in attempts to correct ankle equinus. *Right:* postoperative crescentric calcaneal osteotomy and midtarsal osteotomy arthrodesis to correct the severe deformity shown top.

then necessary to do a form of mid-tarsal osteotomy with the dorsally based wedge. In cerebral palsy the metatarsal–cuneiform osteotomy–arthrodesis described by Jahss (1980) for idiopathic pes cavus and that associated with club foot and flaccid paralysis can be used (Bleck 1984). If the triple arthrodesis and calcaneal osteotomy is done, then in the operating room the degree of forefoot equinus can be measured as described. If it does not exceed the clinical measurement of 30º, then additional mid-tarsal or metatarsal–cuneiform dorsally based wedge osteotomies need not be performed (Fig. 7.29).

The 'Akron midtarsal dome osteotomy' (Wilcox and Weiner 1985) is probably best applied in cavovarus deformities. The V-osteotomy of the mid-tarsus in the coronal plane, with the point of the v in the middle cuneiform bone, is yet another method to correct the forefoot equinus (Japas 1968). It is designed to avoid forefoot shortening that can occur when a large dorsally based wedge of bone is removed from the mid-tarsal joints in order to correct the forefoot equinus. Because of limited experience and technical difficulties with this procedure, Bleck (unpublished observations) has not used it to correct cavus or Swanson's V-type osteotomies at the base of the metatarsals (Swanson *et al.* 1966) in cerebral palsy. Perhaps these procedures could be useful in rigid pes cavus without a hindfoot deformity, *i.e.* neither calcaneus or varus. In cerebral palsy this is hardly ever the case.

MANAGEMENT OF PES CAVOVARUS

If pes cavovarus ever occurs in cerebral palsy, the decision to perform only the plantar release can be made by application of Coleman's block test (Paulos *et al.* 1980). The child stands on a 1-inch block of wood so that the heel rests on it and the foot is diagonally placed to allow the medial half of the forefoot to drop downward on the floor. If the varus of the heel corrects with this maneuver, the deformity is flexible and a plantar release indicated. If it does not correct this way, additional bone surgery will be necessary to correct the fixed hindfoot varus (Coleman 1983). Any equinus component should not be corrected until after healing of the plantar fascial release to allow stretching of the longitudinal arch postoperatively (Paulos 1980, Herring 2002a, b).

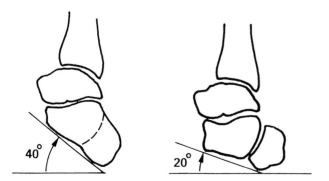

Fig. 7.28. Crescentric osteotomy of the calcaneus to correct a calcaneus deformity.

METATARSUS ADDUCTUS

PATHOGENESIS

The pathogenesis of metatarsus adductus in spastic hemiplegia appears to be the spastic abductor hallucis muscle. In children the deformity is dynamic and later evolves into a fixed skeletal one (Bleck 1967). Unilateral hallux valgus and bunion in spastic hemiplegia on the side of the paralysis has been observed (Fig. 7.30). This seems more prone to occur after Achilles tendon lengthening in some patients who have spasticity of the intrinsic muscles of the foot. These muscles are active during the stance phase of gait, and the abductor hallucis is a major intrinsic muscle of the foot. Probably with weakening of the gastrocnemius–soleus muscle, the intrinsic muscles of the foot act as substitutes during walking and running (Fig. 7.31).

Indications for treatment

The indications for treatment in the young child who has a dynamic spastic metatarsus adductus is the recognition that it will eventually become a fixed deformity. The dynamic forefoot

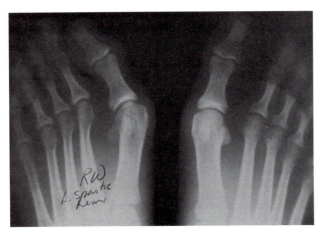

Fig. 7.30. Anterior posterior radiographs of patient with left spastic hemiplegia; metatarsus adductus and hallux valgus of the left foot.

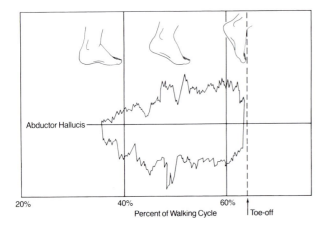

Fig. 7.31. Gait electromyograms confirm that the abductor hallucis is a stance-phase muscle.

adduction deformity can be ascertained as due to the abductor hallucis by infiltration of its muscle belly with 5–10 ml of 1% lidocaine. This injection can be eliminated by comparing an anterior–posterior radiograph of the foot when the child stands with another radiograph taken when the forefoot is manually abducted against the heel (a lead apron and gloves are necessary to protect the physician from radiation). If the radiograph shows passive correction of the metatarsal adduction, abductor hallucis release is indicated. A simple release is not indicated if there is a fixed deformity, particularly of the first metatarsal. In this case it is a fine procedure to produce hallux valgus and a bunion (Fig. 7.32).

If the metatarsals are fixed in adduction and abduction occurs only at the mid-tarsal joints, it is not passively correctable. In these cases more extensive surgery is required. The use of a simple grading system to define the severity of the metatarsus adductus assists in the decision. The heel bisector method visualizes the plantar weightbearing aspect of the heel as an ellipse, the major axis of which bisects the heel and forms the center line of the foot. In what appeared to be normally aligned feet (85% of those studied) this line falls between the second and third toes (Bleck 1971). This center line is through the third toe in mild metatarsus adductus, between the third and fourth toes in moderate and between the fourth and fifth toes in severe cases (Bleck 1983) (Fig. 2.40).

In mild and moderate fixed metatarsus adductus, the surgery does not seem worthwhile. In severe cases the tarsal–metatarsal capsulotomies are satisfactory up to the age of 3 or 4 years (Heyman *et al.* 1958). After that age, metatarsal osteotomies with laterally based wedges at the proximal ends of these bones correct with greater facility than capsulotomies (Berman and Gartland 1971). Be careful to avoid damage to the first metatarsal proximal growth plate. As an alternative to the first metatarsal osteotomy, in a younger child (aged 3–7 years), you could release the capsule at the first metatarsal cuneiform joint (Tachdjian 994). In cerebral palsy an abductor hallucis release should also be done.

Coleman (1983) has used the open-wedge medial cuneiform osteotomy with either a homogenous or an autogenous bone

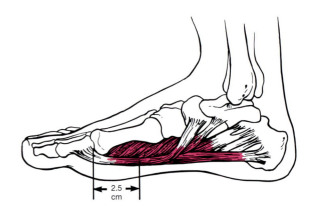

Fig. 7.32. In abductor hallucis tenotomy a 2.5 cm incision is made over the medial aspect of the first metatarsal neck and proximal shaft. A 1 cm section of the abductor hallucis tendon is resected.

graft, and 6 weeks of fixation with a threaded pin to prevent collapse of the osteotomy in cases of residual metatarsus adductus in congenital club foot. This procedure has not been used in cerebral palsy, but Bleck (unpublished observations) did try it in severe metatarsus adductus in children at age 6 years with freeze-dried bone homografts, which failed to incorporate even after 8 weeks. Coleman is correct; a threaded pin seems to be necessary. It seems excessive to keep a child non-weightbearing and in plaster for many weeks while awaiting healing. Therefore an autogenous graft appears preferable to ensure more rapid healing of the osteotomy although in the 1990s synthetic hydroxyapatite blocks seem to work as a spacer in osteotomies.

OPERATIVE TECHNIQUE—ABDUCTOR HALLUCIS RELEASE

A 2.5 cm incision is made over the medial aspect of the first metatarsal, and the tendon of the abductor hallucis is found and grasped with a Kocher hemostat (Fig. 7.32). The tendon is cut distal to the hemostat and the tendon is pulled out of the wound so that a 1 cm piece can be excised. With the forefoot held in abduction and the heel in the neutral position, a short-leg walking plaster is applied and worn for 6 weeks. No special shoes or splints have been necessary after plaster removal. The results of this procedure have been excellent, providing it is done when there is no fixed deformity (Bleck 1967). In two of my patients who had a fixed adduction of the first metatarsal, hallux valgus developed later.

Operative technique: modifications of capsulotomies and osteotomies for metatarsus adductus

The only modification of the description of these operations is to use two longitudinal incisions on the dorsum of the foot: one between the first and second metatarsals and the other over the fourth metatarsal (the single dorsal transverse incision originally described leaves an ugly scar). In performing the osteotomies, a small upbiting rongeur is a convenient and gentle way of removing the laterally based wedge of bone. In both the capsulotomies and osteotomies, Kirschner wires are driven from the medial distal and lateral distal sides of the first and fifth metatarsals through their shafts and into the tarsal bones. These hold the corrections reasonably well in molded padded casts for 4–6 weeks while healing occurs. Another method of pin fixation was described by Tachdjian (1972).

HALLUX VALGUS AND BUNION

The *pathogenesis* of hallux valgus can be a spastic adductor hallucis muscle alone or in combination with excessive adduction of the first metatarsal. In many patients it is secondary to pes valgus, which causes excessive pressure on the medial border of foot. The great toe is forced into progressive abduction (Holstein 1980; Kalen and Brecher 1988) (Fig. 7.33).

The *indications for surgery* are a painful bunion over the head of the first metatarsal, and painful callosities over the medial

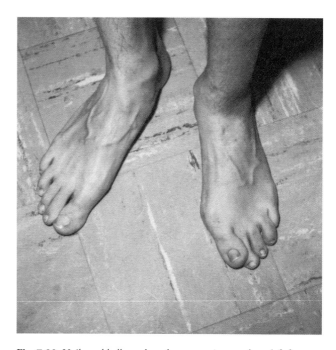

Fig. 7.33. Unilateral hallux valgus due to spastic pes valgus, left foot.

aspect of the great toe or crossover toe. In some patients a recurrent ingrown great toenail results from the pressure on the medial distal end of the great toe, which is not only in valgus but also rotated internally.

Selection of the surgical procedure. If the hallux valgus is secondary to pes valgus, then the foot deformity must also be corrected in addition to correcting the hallux valgus. In children under the age of 12 years, a subtalar extra-articular arthrodesis or the calcaneal lengthening osteotomy (Mosca 1995) are the usual procedures to correct pes valgus (see Chapter 8); in older children and skeletally mature patients, triple arthrodesis is sometimes indicated. Severe hallux valgus can be prevented when it is recognized early in pes valgus in cerebral palsy; in this case a subtalar extra-articular arthrodesis or the calcaneal lengthening osteotomy to bring the foot into a neutral weightbearing position prevents progression of the great toe abduction deformity.

Symptomatic and primary *dynamic hallux valgus* (without pes valgus and/or adduction of the first metatarsal) can be relieved with a tenotomy of the adductor hallucis through a short linear incision in the first web space.

In children whose *fixed hallux valgus* is symptomatic, the correction is possible with adductor hallucis tenotomy, lateral capsulotomy of the metatarsal–phalangeal joint and pin fixation of the great toe to the first metatarsal. In 1977, J.L. Sequist reported success with this method in 20 of 26 patients (personal communication). However, in most of our child patients the hallux valgus is secondary to pes equinovalgus which should be corrected first.

In *adolescents and adults* with cerebral palsy who have a painless metatarsal–phalangeal joint, the preference has been to correct the skeletal deformities in hallux valgus. The adductor hallucis tenotomy is always done. There is a choice of two first metatarsal osteotomies. (1) A chevron osteotomy of the first metatarsal to correct its adduction deformity can be done through the distal metatarsal (Johnson 1979, Kitaoka 2002). (2) The crescentic osteotomy in the *proximal* shaft of the first metatarsal used by Mann and colleagues (Mann *et al.* 1992, Mann and Coughlin 1999) seems preferable to the one through the neck for severe hallux valgus (metatarsal–phalangeal angle greater than 35°). The Mitchell osteotomy is easy to displace dorsally and compromise the result. A distal chevron osteotomy of the first metatarsal is a more stable configuration and can be fixed with percutaneous K wire or an absorbable pin (Gill *et al.* 1997). It is appropriate for mild to moderate hallux valgus with deformity up to 35° first metatarsal phalangeal angle measured off a weightbearing anteroposterior X-ray of the foot. Although we have not seen avascular necrosis in the head of the first metatarsal with the Mitchell procedure, others have reported it. It probably occurs by interfering with the blood supply of the bone on the lateral aspect of the head and neck if capsulotomies and extensive dissection are done with the osteotomy of the neck.

Excessive removal of the prominence on the medial aspect of the first metatarsal head should be avoided, and the osteotomy should not go beyond the sagittal groove which separates the articular cartilage of the metatarsal from the bone (Mann and Coughlin 1999). If the prominence disappears with the realignment of the first metatarsal osteotomy, there is less to remove. Normal feet have a slight medial bulge on the metatarsal head. Look at your own foot—assuming it is perfect!

If the hallux valgus does not correct at the time of the first metatarsal osteotomy, the preference is to correct the great toe valgus with a closed wedge osteotomy at the base of the proximal phalanx (Goldner 1981). This procedure has preserved motion of the metatarsal–phalangeal joint. Attempts to 'reef' the medial capsule of the joint to correct the hallux valgus, seem to create undesirable stiffness of the joint. Goldner (1981) corrected 26 feet in 16 patients with the adductor hallucis tenotomy, proximal shaft metatarsal osteotomy and the osteotomy at the base of the proximal phalanx. In his patients, followed for 2–20 years, none developed a degenerative arthritis of the first metatarsal–phalangeal joint and none needed arthrodesis of the joint.

Jenter *et al.* (1998) assessed their experience with four procedures for hallux valgus in 26 feet of 17 patients with cerebral palsy: proximal first metatarsal osteotomy with distal soft-tissue release and exostectomy, a distal soft-tissue release and exostectomy, osteotomy of the great toe proximal phalanx, metatarsophalangeal soft-tissue release and exosctetomy, and great toe metatarsophalangeal arthrodesis. Only arthrodesis consistently gave excellent results.

ARTHRODESIS OF THE METATARSAL–PHALANGEAL JOINT OF THE GREAT TOE
Because of discouraging results with the Mitchell metatarsal osteotomy and the McBride (1928) adductor hallucis transfer and exostectomy, Renshaw *et al.* (1979) preferred arthrodesis of the metatarsal–phalangeal joint of the great toe and removal of the medial bump (exostosis) on the head of the first metatarsal

(McKeever 1952). Davids et al. (2001) came to the same conclusions in the management of hallux valgus in cerebral palsy with metatars-phalangeal arthrodesis in patients aged 10–21 years. Patient/caregiver/parent satisfaction was in the range of 81–100% after arthrodesis. Arthrodesis is a permanent solution and is indicated in those patients who have degenerative arthritis of the joint. The arthrodesis of the joint should be in varying degrees of dorsiflexion depending upon the metatarsal angle relative to the floor on standing (and presumably the amount of equinus during the stance phase of gait in cerebral palsy); in McKeever's cases the great toe dorsiflexion varied between 15° and 35°. The angle of the arthrodesis should approximate the angle of inclination of the metatarsal on standing (Alexander 2002). Evaluate a standing lateral X-ray to determine this. The desired position on standing postoperatively should allow for the great toe to be elevated off the floor just slightly with no impingement onto the second toe.

With careful observation one can appreciate that much of the hallux valgus occurs at the interphalangeal joint of the great toe in some adolescents and adults. Frequently, the great toe crosses under the second toe. In these cases correction can be accomplished with an osteotomy with a medially based wedge of bone removed through the proximal phalanx and fixation with a threaded pin (Frey 1991, 2002).

OPERATIVE TECHNIQUE FOR BUNION AND HALLUX VALGUS IN ADOLESCENTS WITH CEREBRAL PALSY
The operative technique is as follows: (1) tenotomy of the adductor hallucis insertion on the proximal phalanx of the great toe, or transfer to the distal medial first metatarsal; (2) a crescentic osteotomy of the proximal end of the first metatarsal (Mann 1992, Coughlin 1999, 2002). Do this procedure after closure of the first metatarsal physis. A motorized crescentic shaped saw is used, with the concavity of the crescent proximal and the osteotomy started 1 cm distal to the metatarsocuneiform joint dorsally going further distal and plantarward. The metatarsal is then abducted laterally to correct the wide intermetatarsal angle. The osteotomy is secured with a single longitudinal screw (usually 4 mm by 26 mm), directed dorsal distal to plantar proximal. Fixing the screw is easier if the drill hole and screw is placed in the shaft of the metatarsal distal to the intended osteotomy before the saw cut is made. (3) For residual hallux valgus, an Akin procedure (a medially based closed-wedge osteotomy of the proximal phalanx) may be indicated. Before the bone is cut, two drill holes are placed proximally and distally just beyond the intended osteotomy. Then after the osteotomy is completed and the wedge (usually 2 mm or less) removed, a strong suture (*e.g.* no. 0 Vicryl) is passed through these holes and tied on the medial cortex of the phalanx to secure the osteotomy (Seelenfreund and Fried 1973). Alternatively, percutaneous crossed Kirschner wires will stabilize the osteotomy. Avoid plantar angulation when positioning the toe (Frey 1991).

In these children's feet, 10° of hallux valgus is not likely to cause significant symptoms so that a tenotomy of the insertion of the adductor hallucis muscle is probably sufficient.

PAINFUL HALLUX VALGUS IN ADULTS

In adults with cerebral palsy the preferred operation for painful hallux valgus due to joint cartilage degeneration is arthrodesis of the metatarsal–phalangeal joint. The usual degree of dorsiflexion is 20º–25º and 15º of valgus. After denudation of the articular cartilage a dorsal compression plate and screws provides good fixation and assures a high incidence of fusion (Coughlin 1996).

DORSAL BUNION

The *pathogenesis* of dorsal bunion in cerebral palsy is dorsiflexion of the first metatarsal due to spastic anterior tibial muscles, and acute flexion of the great toe due to spasticity of the flexor digitorum longus and flexor hallucis brevis muscles. It has occurred after triple arthrodesis for severe pes equinovalgus in which the midfoot and forefoot are dorsiflexed and the hindfoot plantarflexed ('rocker bottom') (Fig. 7.34). In cerebral palsy it is not associated with a weak peroneus longus muscle, as it was in cases of poliomyelitis. The dorsal bunion is the prominent head of the first metatarsal on the dorsum of the foot. With shoes it is most uncomfortable.

The *management* of dorsal bunion is surgical. The only conservative management possible is to relieve the pressure on the prominence with extra large toe-box in the shoes or the elimination of enclosing footwear (e.g. sandals, slippers or heavy stockings).

The operative technique is based upon the cause. The first metatarsal must be plantarflexed, the spasm of the anterior tibial relieved and the toe-flexion deformity corrected. To accomplish this, Goldner (1981) transferred the anterior tibial tendon to the second metatarsal, did an osteotomy at the base of the first metatarsal and transferred the flexor hallucis longus to the extensor hallucis longus. In 26 feet of 16 patients it was not necessary to perform an arthrodesis of the metatarsal–phalangeal joint.

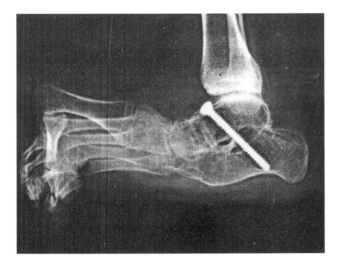

Fig. 7.34. Lateral radiograph of the foot of a 14-year-old male with spastic diplegia postoperative triple arthrodesis. The screw between the talus and calcaneus used to maintain proper alignment between these bones. Dorsal bunion developed, prominent and symptomatic.

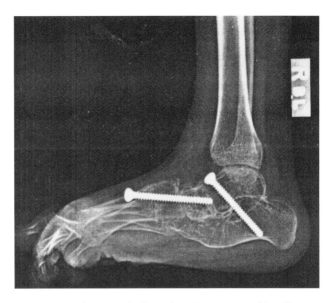

Fig. 7.35. Lateral radiograph of same foot after correction of dorsal bunion with closed wedge osteotomy–arthrodesis of the first metatarsal cuneiform and cuneiform navicular joints. The screw crossing both joints afforded firm fixation of the correction while healing occurred.

The operations performed by Bleck (unpublished observations) in *skeletally mature* patients have followed Goldner's principles (1981): (1) z-lengthening of the anterior tibial tendon; (2) arthrodesis of the metatarsal–cuneiform joint from which a dorsally based wedge of bone was removed and an arthrodesis of the cuneiform–navicular joint. A single screw directed from the shaft of the first metatarsal across both joints gave secure fixation; (3) a z-lengthening of the flexor hallucis longus tendon and if required, a tenotomy of the insertions of the flexor hallucis brevis muscle. With this correction the dorsal bunion disappears. It is not necessary to remove any of the bone from the dorsum of the metatarsal head (Fig. 7.35). Fiberglass cast immobilization is presumed.

If the articular cartilage of the metatarsal–phalangeal joint has degenerative changes, an arthrodesis of the joint (or an excision of the proximal half of the proximal phalanx—the toe will be short) may prevent a painful joint after correction of the dorsal bunion.

FLEXION DEFORMITY OF THE TOES

Flexion deformities of the toes are more common in adolescents and adults than in children. When these cause discomfort, tenotomy of the flexor tendons of the toes at their proximal skin creases usually solves the problem. Menelaus (1984) successfully treated 'curly' and hammer toes in children (not necessarily those who had cerebral palsy) with toe-flexor tenotomy. He made the point to be sure that preoperatively the metatarsal–phalangeal joint could be flexed. If not, then it is a claw toe which is rare in patients with cerebral palsy. Claw-toe correction would need more than a simple flexor tenotomy.

KNEE-FLEXION AND HYPEREXTENSION DEFORMITIES

Knee-flexion deformities in hemiplegia are managed as described in the following chapter on spastic diplegia. The results of surgery are often better in hemiplegia than in diplegia because of normal function in the opposite limb.

Spastic knee hyperextension during gait is more often found in patients whose hemiplegia is due to a cerebral vascular accident or a head injury. Because the knee does not flex sufficiently in swing phase of gait, the lower limb circumducts in order for the foot to clear the ground. The spasticity in the quadriceps can be partly relieved with a distal rectus femoris tendon transfer. Orthotic management of knee hyperextension may be found in the plastic ankle–foot orthosis, in which the ankle is dorsiflexed above the neutral position (Rosenthal *et al.* 1975).

HIP-FLEXION AND INTERNAL ROTATION DEFORMITY

As with the knee deformities, the management of the hip-flexion and internal rotation deformities are the same as in spastic diplegia (Chapter 8). The most common pitfall of femoral derotation osteotomy in the child with spastic hemiplegia is the failure to recognize concomitant excessive compensatory external tibial–fibular torsion (>30º). When only a femoral derotation osteotomy is done in this circumstance, the external rotation of the foot is greatly exaggerated. To prevent this undesirable change in the limb posture and gait, it is necessary to do an internal derotation tibial and fibular osteotomy at the time of the femoral osteotomy. Another less common pitfall of femoral derotation osteotomy is overcorrection so that no internal rotation of the hip is preserved. Then the pelvis cannot externally rotate during gait and remains in an anteriorly rotated position. Therefore, you should try to retain 30º–45º of internal rotation of the hip in femoral derotation osteotomies. Check the range of internal rotation before wound closure.

LEG-LENGTH DISCREPANCY

Stunting of linear growth in the hemiplegic limb is common; however, the discrepancy rarely exceeds 1.5 cm at the time of skeletal maturity. If serial measurements during growth show the discrepancy to be increasing, with a projected shortening of more than 2 cm leg length, equalization by epiphyseal arrest or stapling of the distal femoral (and if need be, proximal tibial) physis is indicated. Limb shortening of less than 2 cm is conceded to have no functional disability and need not be corrected.

Shoe lifts are not necessary. They prevent the child from participating fully in sports and games. Short legs do not cause structural scoliosis. Spinal curvatures in hemiplegia result from unknown causes (idiopathic scoliosis) or are due to congenital anomalies of the vertebrae and are independent of a leg-length discrepancy. The child with spastic hemiplegia is already burdened with an abnormal gait. Why add to the disability by prescribing shoe lifts? If anything, the shoe lift will sometimes prevent a desirable compensation for the inability of the ankle to dorsiflex so that the toes can clear the ground during the swing phase of gait.

A short leg in hemiplegia: 'shoe lifts are unnecessary'.
'A short leg does not cause a structural scoliosis.'
'Why add to the disability by prescribing shoe lifts?'

Treatment of the child and adult with spastic hemiplegia encompasses the spectrum of modalities available to the clinician. Goal-specific therapy and surgery can result in some improvement over the natural history. Surgery to the upper extremity can improve motion and position but never change the deficits involving stereognosis and sensation. Through the lower extremity, surgery can help remove or neutralize deforming forces. Deformities causing gait problems can be improved but spasticity and weakness will continue due to underlying cerebral palsy.

REFERENCES

Adler, N., Bleck, E.E., Rinsky, L.A. (1985) 'Decision making in surgical treatment of paralytic deformities of the foot with gait electromyograms.' *Orthopedic Transactions*, **9**, 90–91.

Aitken, J. (1952) 'Deformity of the elbow joint as a sequel to Erb's obstetrical paralysis.' *Journal of Bone and Joint Surgery*, **34B**, 352–365.

Alexander, I.J. (2002) 'Hallux metatarso–phalangeal arthrodesis.' *In* Kitaoka, H.B. (Ed.) *The Foot and Ankle, 2nd edn.* Philadelphia: J.B. Lippincott, Williams & Wilkins, pp. 45–60.

Baker, L.D. (1954) 'Triceps surae syndrome in cerebral palsy.' *Archives of Surgery*, **68**, 216–221.

—— (1956) 'A rational approach to the surgical needs of the cerebral palsy patient.' *Journal of Bone and Joint Surgery*, **38A**, 313–323.

—— Hill, L.M. (1964) 'Foot alignment in the cerebral palsy patient.' *Journal of Bone and Joint Surgery*, **46A**, 1–15.

Banks, H.H. (1975) 'The foot and ankle in cerebral palsy.' *In* Samilson, R.L. (Ed.) *Orthopaedic Aspects of Cerebral Palsy. Clinics in Developmental Medicine, Nos 52/53.* London: Spastics International Medical Publications with Heinemann Medical; Philadelphia: J.B. Lippincott.

—— (1977) 'The management of spastic deformities of the foot and ankle.' *Clinical Orthopaedics and Related Research*, **122**, 70–76.

—— (1983) 'Equinus and cerebral palsy.' *Foot and Ankle*, **4**, 149–159.

—— Green, W.T. (1958) 'The correction of equinus deformity in cerebral palsy.' *Journal of Bone and Joint Surgery*, **40A**, 1359–1379.

—— Panagakos, P. (1966) 'Orthopaedic evaluation in the lower extremity in cerebral palsy.' *Clinical Orthopaedics and Related Research*, **47**, 117–125.

Barenfeld, P.A., Weseley, M.D., Shea, J.M. (1971) 'The congenital cavus foot.' *Clinical Orthopaedics and Related Research*, **79**, 119–126.

Barnes, M.J., Herring, J.A. (1991) 'Combined split anterior tibial-tendon transfer and intramuscular lengthening of the posterior tibial tendon.' *Journal of Bone and Joint Surgery*, **73A**, 734–738.

Barnett, J.G., Holly, R.G., Ashmore, C.R. (1980) 'Stretch-induced growth in chicken wing muscles: biochemical and morphological characterization.' *American Journal of Physiology*, **239**, C39–C46.

Barto, P.S., Supinski, R.S., Skinner, S.R. (1984) 'Dynamic EMG findings in varus hindfoot deformity and spastic cerebral palsy.' *Developmental Medicine and Child Neurology*, **26**, 88–93.

Beach, W.B., Strecker, W.B., Coe, J., Manske, P.R., Schoenecker, P.L., Daily, L. (1991) 'Use of the Green transfer in treatment of patients with spastic cerebral palsy: 17-year experience.' *Journal of Pediatric Orthopaedics*, **11**, 731–736.

Bennet, G., Rang, M., Jones, D. (1982) 'Varus and valgus deformities of the foot in cerebral palsy.' *Developmental Medicine and Child Neurology*, **24**, 499–503.

Berman, A., Gartland, J.J. (1971) 'Metatarsal osteotomy for the correction of adduction of the forepart of the foot in children.' *Journal of Bone and Joint Surgery*, **53A**, 498–506.

Bisla, R.S., Louis, H.H., Albano, P.S. (1976) 'Transfer of the tibialis posterior tendon in cerebral palsy.' *Journal of Bone and Joint Surgery*, **58A**, 497–500.

Blake, D., Byl, N., Merzenich, M. (2002) 'Representation of the hand in the cerebral cortex.' *Behavioral Brain Research*, **135**, 179–184.

—— —— Cheung, S., Bedenbaugh, P., Nagarajan, S., Lamb, M., Merzenich, M. (2002) 'Sensory representation abnormalities that parallel focal hand dystonia in a primate model.' *Somatosensory and Motor Research*, **19**, 347–357.

Blasier, R.D., White, R. (1998) 'Duration of immobilization after percutaneous sliding heel-cord lengthening.' *Journal of Pediatric Orthopaedics*, **18**, 299–303.

Bleck, E.E. (1967) 'Spastic abductor hallucis.' *Developmental Medicine and Child Neurology*, **9**, 602–608.

—— (1971) 'The shoeing of children: sham or science?' *Developmental Medicine and Child Neurology*, **13**, 188–195.

—— (1983) 'Metatarsus adductus: classification and relationship to outcomes of treatment.' *Journal of Pediatric Orthopedics*, **3**, 2–9.

—— (1984) 'Forefoot problems in cerebral palsy—diagnosis and management.' *Foot and Ankle*, **4**, 188–194.

—— Berzins, U.L. (1977) 'Conservative management of pes valgus with plantar flexed talus flexible.' *Clinical Orthopaedics and Related Research*, **122**, 85–94.

Bolanos, A.A., Bleck, E.E., Firestone, P., Young, L. (1989) 'Comparison of stereognosis and two-point discrimination testing of the hands of children with cerebral palsy.' *Developmental Medicine and Child Neurology*, **31**, 371–376.

Borton, D.C., Walker, K., Pirpiris, M., Nattrass, G.R., Graham, H.K. (2001) 'Isolated calf lengthening in cerebral palsy outcome analysis of risk factors.' *Journal of Bone and Joint Surgery*, **83B**, 364–370.

Braun, R.M., Vise, G.T., Roper, B. (1974) 'Preliminary experience with superficialis-to-profundus tendon transfer in the hemiplegic upper extremity.' *Journal of Bone and Joint Surgery*, **56A**, 466–472.

Breen, T.F., Gelberman, R.H., Ackerman, G.H. (1988) 'Elbow flexion contractures. Treatment by anterior release and continuous passive motion.' *Journal of Hand Surgery*, **13B**, 286–287.

Camacho, F.J., Isunza, A., Coutino, B. (1996) 'Comparison of tendo-Achilles lengthening alone and combined with neurectomy of the gastrocnemius muscle in the treatment of equinus deformity of the foot associated with clonus in children with cerebral palsy.' *Orthopedics*, **19**, 319–322.

Carr, C.R., Boyd, B.M. (1968) 'Correctional osteotomy for metatarsus primus varus and hallux valgus.' *Journal of Bone and Joint Surgery*, **50A**, 1353–1367.

Chait, L.A., Kaplan, I., Stewart-Lord, B., Goodman, M. (1980) 'Early surgical correction in the cerebral palsied hand.' *Journal of Hand Surgery*, **5**, 122–126.

Cheng, J.C. (1993) 'Percutaneous elongation of the Achilles tendon in children with cerebral palsy.' *International Orthopedics*, **17**, 162–165.

Cioni, G., Sales, B., Paolicelli, P.B., Petacchi, E., Scusa, M.F., Canapicchi, R. (1999) 'MRI and clinical characteristics of children with hemiplegic cerebral palsy.' *Neuropediatrics*, **30**, 249–255.

Cleary, J.E., Omer, G.E. Jr (1985) 'Congenital proximal radio-ulnar synostosis. Natural history and functional assessment.' *Journal of Bone and Joint Surgery*, **67A**, 539–545.

Coleman, S.S. (1983) *Complex Foot Deformities in Children*. Philadelphia: Lea & Febiger.

Colton, C.L., Ransford, A.D., Lloyd-Roberts, G.C. (1976) 'Transposition of the tendon of the pronator teres in cerebral palsy.' *Journal of Bone and Joint Surgery*, **58B**, 220–223.

Cottalorda, J., Gautheron, V., Charmet, E., Chavrier, Y. (1997) 'Allongement musculaire due triceps par platres successifs chez l'enfant infirme moteur cerebral.' *Revue d'Orthopédie et du Chirurgie de l'Appareil Moteur*, **83**, 368–371.

Coughlin, M.J. (1996) 'Instructional Course Lectures. The American Academy of Orthopaedic Surgeons. Hallux Valgus.' *Journal of Bone and Joint Surgery*, **78A**, 932–966.

—— (1999) 'Juvenile hallux valgus.' *In* Coughlin, M.J., Mann, R.A. (Eds) *Surgery of the Foot and Ankle, 7th edn*. St Louis: C.V. Mosby, pp. 270–319.

—— (2002) 'Proximal first metatarsal osteotomy.' *In* Kitaoka, H.B. *The Foot and Ankle, 2nd edn*. Philadelphia: J.B. Lippincott, Williams & Wilkins, pp. 71–98.

Craig, J.J., Van Voren, J. (1976) 'The importance of gastrocnemius recession in the correction of equinus deformity in cerebral palsy.' *Journal of Bone and Joint Surgery*, **58B**, 84–87.

Crenshaw, A.H. (1963) *Campbell's Operative Orthopaedics, Vol. 2, 4th edn*. St Louis: C.V. Mosby, p. 1052.

Currie, D.M., Mendiola, A. (1987) 'Cortical thumb orthosis for children with spastic hemiplegic cerebral palsy.' *Archives of Physical Medicine and Rehabilitation*, **68**, 214–216.

Dahlin, L.B., Komodo-Tufvesson, Y., Salgeback, S. (1998) 'Surgery of the spastic hand in cerebral palsy. Improvement in stereognosis and hand function after surgery.' *Journal of Hand Surgery*, **23B**, 334–339.

Davids, J.R., Mason, T.A., Danko, A., Banks, D, Blackhurst, D. (2001) 'Surgical management of hallux valgus deformity in children with cerebral palsy.' *Journal of Pediatric Orthopaedics*, **21**, 89–94.

Delp, A., Zajac, F.E. (1992) 'Force- and moment-generation capacity of lower extremity muscles before and after tendon lengthening.' *Clinical Orthopedics and Related Research*, **284**, 247–259.

Delp, S.L., Statler, K., Carroll, N.C. (1995) 'Preserving plantar flexion strength after surgical treatment for contracture of the triceps surae: a computer simulation study.' *Journal of Orthopaedic Research*, **13**, 96–104.

Dillin, W., Samilson, R.L. (1983) 'Calcaneus deformity in cerebral palsy.' *Foot and Ankle*, **4**, 167–170.

Doute, D.A., Sponseller, P.D., Tolo, V.T., Atkins, E., Silberstein, C.E. (1997) 'Soleus neurectomy for dynamic ankle equinus in children with cerebral palsy.' *American Journal of Orthopedics*, **26**, 613–616.

Dutkowsky, J.P. (1998) 'Cerebral palsy.' *In* Canale, S.T. (Ed.) *Campbell's Operative Orthopaedics, 9th Edn*. St Louis: C.V. Mosby, pp. 3895–3969.

Edmonson, A.S., Crenshaw, A.H. (1980) *Campbell's Operative Orthopaedics, 6th edn, vol. 2*. St Louis: C.V. Mosby, pp. 1426–1428.

Elliott, J.M., Connolly, K.J. (1984) 'A classification of manipulative hand movements.' *Developmental Medicine and Child Neurology*, **26**, 283–296.

Etnyre, B., Chambers, C.S., Scarborough, N.H., Cain, T.E. (1993) 'Preoperative and postoperative assessment of surgical intervention for equinus gait in children with cerebral palsy.' *Journal of Pediatric Orthopaedics*, **13**, 24–31.

Feldkamp, M., Güth, V. (1980) 'Operative Korrekturn an der Hand des Zerebralparetikers.' *Zeitschrift für Orthopedie*, **118**, 256–264.

Filler, B.C., Stark, N.H., Boyes, J.H. (1976) 'Capsulodesis of the metacarpophalangeal joint of the thumb in children with cerebral palsy.' *Journal of Bone and Joint Surgery*, **58A**, 667–670.

Frey, C. (2002) 'Hallux proximal phalanx osteotomy—the Akin procedure.' *In* Kitaoka, H.B. (Ed.) *The Foot and Ankle, 2nd edn*. Philadelphia: J.B. Lippincott, Williams & Wilkins, pp. 61–70.

—— Jahss, M., Kummer, F.J. (1991) 'The Akin procedure: an analysis of results.' *Foot and Ankle*, **12**, 1–6.

Funk, D.A., Cass, J.R., Johnson, K.A. (1986) 'Acquired adult flat foot secondary to posterior tibial-tendon pathology.' *Journal of Bone and Joint Surgery*, **68A**, 95–102.

Gage, J.R. (1991) *Gait Analysis in Cerebral Palsy*. London: Mac Keith Press with Blackwell Scientific Publications; New York: Cambridge University Press, pp. 65–66.

—— (ed.) (2004) *The Treatmemt of Gait Problems in Cerebral Palsy*. London: MacKeith Press with Cambridge University Press.

Gaines, R.W., Ford, T.B. (1984) 'A systematic approach to the amount of Achilles tendon lengthening in cerebal palsy.' *Journal of Pediatric Orthopedics*, **4**, 488–451.

Gill, L.H. Martin, D.F., Coumas, J.M., Kiebzak, G.M. (1997) 'Fixation with bioabsorbable pins in Chevron bunionectomy.' *Journal of Bone and Joint Surgery*, **79A**, 1510–1518.

Goldner, J.L. (1955) 'Reconstructive surgery of the hand in cerebral palsy and spastic paralysis from injury to the spinal cord.' *Journal of Bone and Joint Surgery*, **37A**, 1141–1154.

—— (1975) 'The upper extremity in cerebral palsy.' *In* Samilson, R.L. (Ed.) *Orthopaedic Aspects of Cerebral Palsy. Clinics in Developmental Medicine, Nos 52/53*. London: Spastics International Medical Publications with Heinemann Medical; Philadelphia: J.B. Lippincott, pp. 221–257.

—— (1981) 'Hallux valgus and hallux flexus associated with cerebral palsy: analysis and treatment.' *Clinical Orthopaedics and Related Research*, **157**, 98–104.

—— (1983) 'Surgical treatment for cerebral palsy.' *In* Evarts, C.McC. (Ed.) *Surgery of the Musculoskeletal System, Vol. 2*. Edinburgh: Livingstone, pp. 439–469.

—— (1987) 'Surgical reconstruction of the upper extremity in cerebral palsy.' *Instructional Course Lectures, vol. XXXVI*. Rosemont, IL: American Academy of Orthopaedic Surgeons, pp. 207–235.

—— Ferlic, D.C. (1966) 'Sensory status of the hand as related to reconstructive surgery of the upper extremity in cerebral palsy.' *Clinical Orthopaedics and Related Research*, **46**, 87–92.

—— Keats, P.K., Bassett, F.H. III, Clippinger, F.W. (1974) 'Progressive talipes equinovalgus due to trauma or degeneration of the posterior tibial tendon and medial plantar ligaments.' *Orthopedic Clinics of North America*, **5**, 39–50.

—— Goodman, W.B., Bookman, M. (1977) 'The long term results of soft tissue elbow releases for improved elbow and forearm function in children with cerebral palsy.' *Paper read at Annual meeting, American Academy for Cerebral Palsy and Developmental Medicine, Atlanta.*

—— Koman, L.A., Gelberman, R., Levin, S., Goldner, R.D. (1990) 'Arthrodesis of the metacarpo-phalangeal joint of the thumb in children and adults. Adjunctive treatment of the thumb-in-palm deformity in cerebral palsy.' *Clinical Orthopedics and Related Research*, **253**, 75–89.

—— (1998) 'Thumb-in-palm deformity in cerebral palsy, diagnosis and treatment.' *In* Strickland, J.W. (Ed.) *The Hand*. Philadelphia: Lippincott-Raven, 93–110.

Gordon, A., Charles, J. (2003) 'Constraint-induced movement therapy in children with congenital hemiplegia.' *Developmental Medicine and Child Neurology* (Suppl. 94), 45.

—— Wolf, S.L. (2006) 'Efficacy of constraint-induced movement therapy on involved upper-extremity use in children with hemiplegic cerebral palsy.' *Pediatrics*, **117**, 263–373.

Gräbe, R.P., Thompson, P. (1979) 'Lengthening of the Achilles tendon in cerebral paresis.' *South African Medical Journal*, **56**, 993–996.

Graham, H.K., Fixsen, J.A. (1988) 'Lengthening of the calcaneal tendon in spastic hemiplegia by the White slide technique. A long-term review.' *Journal of Bone and Joint Surgery*, **70B**, 472–475.

Green, N.E., Griffin, P.P., Shiavi, P. (1983) 'Split posterior tibia] tendon transfer in spastic cerebral palsy.' *Journal of Bone and Joint Surgery*, **65A**, 748–754.

Green, W.T., Banks, H.H. (1962) 'Flexor carpi ulnaris transplant and its use in cerebral palsy.' *Journal of Bone and Joint Surgery*, **44A**, 1343–1352.

Greene, W.B. (1987) 'Achilles tendon lengthening in cerebral palsy: comparison of inpatient versus ambulatory surgery.' *Journal of Pediatric Orthopaedics*, 7, 256–258.

Gritzka, T.L., Staheli, L.T., Duncan, W.R. (1972) 'Posterior tibial tendon transfer through interosseus membrane to correct equinovarus deformity in cerebral palsy.' *Clinical Orthopaedics and Related Research*, **89**, 201–206.

Gschwind, C., Tonkin, M. (1992) 'Surgery for cerebral palsy: part 1. Classification and operative procedures for pronation deformity.' *Journal of Hand Surgery*, **17B**, 391–395.

Gwathney, F.W., Fidler, M.O. (1981) 'A dynamic approach to the thumb-in-palm deformity in cerebral palsy.' *Journal of Bone and Joint Surgery*, **63A**, 216-225.

Haddad, R.J. (1977) 'Upper limb surgery in cerebral palsy.' *Regional Course, American Academy for Cerebral Palsy and Developmental Medicine, New Orleans.*

Herring, J.A. (2002a) 'Disorders of the brain, equinovarus deformity.' *In* Tachdjian, M.O. (Ed.) *Pediatric Orthopaedics*. Philadelphia: W.B. Saunders, pp. 1143–1147.

Herring, J.A. (2002b) 'Disorders of the foot, neurogenic abnormalities cavus foot.' *In* Tachdjian, M.O. (Ed.) *Pediatric Orthopaedics*. Philadelphia: W.B. Saunders, pp. 984–1011.

Heyman, C.H. Herndon, C.H., Strong, J.M. (1958) 'Mobilization of the tarso–metatarsal and intermetatarsal joints for the correction of resistant adduction of the forepart of the foot in congenital clubfoot or congenital metatarsus varus.' *Journal of Bone and Joint Surgery*, **40A**, 299–310.

Hirasawa, Y., Katsumi, Y., Tokioka, T. (1985) 'Evaluation of sensibility after sensory reconstruction of the thumb.' *Journal of Bone and Joint Surgery*, **67B**, 814–819.

Hiroshima, K., Hamada, S., Shimizu, N., Ohshita, S., Ono, K. (1988) 'Anterior transfer of the long toe flexors for the treatment of spastic equinovarus and equinus foot in cerebral palsy.' *Journal of Pediatric Orthopaedics*, 8, 164–168.

Hoffer, M.M. (1976) 'Basic considerations and classification of cerebral palsy.' *American Academy of Orthopaedic Surgeons: Instructional Course Lectures*, **25**, 96–106.

—— (1985) 'Tendon transfer to the extensors of the wrists and fingers in cerebral palsy.' *Paper No. 3 presented at the Annual Meeting of the Pediatric Orthopaedic Society of North America, San Antonio, TX.*

—— (1993) 'The use of the pathokinesiology laboratory to select muscles for tendon transfers in the cerebral palsy hand.' *Clinical Orthopedics and Related Research*, **288**, 135–138.

—— Reswig, J.A., Garrett, A.M., Perry, J. (1974) 'The split anterior tibial tendon transfer in treatment of spastic varus of the hindfoot in childhood.' *Orthopedic Clinics of North America*, **5**, 31–38.

—— Perry, J., Melkonian, G.J. (1979) 'Dynamic electromyography and decision-making for surgery in the upper extremity of patients with cerebral palsy.' *Journal of Hand Surgery*, 4, 424–431.

—— Garcia, M., Bullock, D. (1983) 'Adduction contracture of the thumb in cerebral palsy.' *Journal of Bone and Joint Surgery*, **65A**, 755–759.

—— Barakat, G., Koffman, M. (1985) '10-year follow-up of split anterior tibial tendon transfer in cerebral palsied patients with spastic equinovarus deformity.' *Journal of Pediatric Orthopaedics*, 5, 432–434.

—— Lehman, M., Mitani, M. (1986) 'Long term follow-up on tendon transfers to the extensors of the wrist and fingers in patient with cerebral palsy.' *Journal of Hand Surgery*, **11A**, 836–840.

Holstein, A. (1980) 'Hallux valgus—an acquired deformity of the foot in cerebral palsy.' *Foot and Ankle*, 1, 33–38.

Horstmann, H.M., Eilert, R.E. (1977) 'Triple arthrodesis in cerebral palsy.' *Paper presented at annual meeting of the American Academy of Orthopaedic Surgeons, Las Vegas, NV.*

House, J.H. (1975) 'A dynamic approach to the "thumb-in-palm" deformity in cerebral palsy.' *Instructional Course Syllabus, American Academy for Cerebral Palsy.*

—— Gwathmey F.W., Fidler, M.O. (1981) 'A dynamic approach to the thumb-in-palm deformity in cerebral palsy.' *Journal of Bone and Joint Surgery*, **63A**, 216–225.

Huet de la Tour, E., Tardieu, C., Tabary, J.C., Tabary, C. (1979) 'Decrease of muscle extensibility and reduction of sacromere numbers in soleus muscle following local injection of tetanus toxin.' *Journal of the Neurological Sciences*, **40**, 123–131.

Hui, J.H., Goh, J.C., Lee, E.H. (1998) 'Biomechanical study of tibialis anterior tendon transfer.' *Clinical Orthopedics and Related Research*, **349**, 249–255.

Hullin, M.G., Robb, J.E., Loudon, I.R. (1996) 'Gait patterns in children with hemiplegic cerebral palsy.' *Journal of Pediatric Orthopaedics B*, 5, 247–251.

Inglis, A.E., Cooper, W. (1966) 'Release of flexor-pronator origin for flexion deformities of the hand and wrist in spastic paralysis: a study of eighteen cases.' *Journal of Bone and Joint Surgery*, **48A**, 847–857.

Inman, V.T. (1976) *The Joints of the Ankle*. Baltimore: Williams & Wilkins.

—— Mann, R.A. (1978) 'Biomechanics of the foot and ankle.' *In* Mann, R.A. (Ed.) *DuVries Surgery of the Foot, 4th edn*. St Louis: C.V. Mosby.

Ireland, M.L., Hoffer, M.M. (1985) 'Triple arthrodesis for children with spastic cerebral palsy.' *Developmental Medicine and Child Neurology*, **27**, 623–627.

Jahss, M.H. (1980) 'Tarsometatarsal truncated-wedge arthrodesis for pes cavus and equinovarus deformity of the forepart of the foot.' *Journal of Bone and Joint Surgery*, **62A**, 713–722.

Japas, L.M. (1968) 'Surgical treatment of pes cavus by tarsal V-osteotomy.' *Journal of Bone and Joint Surgery*, **50A**, 927–943.

Jebsen, R.H., Taylor, N., Trieschmann, R.B., Trotter, M.J., Howard, L.A. (1969) 'An objective standardized test of hand function.' *Archives of Physical Medicine and Rehabilitation*, **50A**, 331–339.

Jenter, M., Lipton, G.E., Miller, F. (1998) 'Operative treatment for hallux valgus in children with cerebral palsy.' *Foot and Ankle International*, **19**, 830–835.

Johnson, K.A. (1983) 'Tibialis posterior tendon rupture.' *Clinical Orthopaedics and Related Research*, **177**, 140–147.

—— Cofield, R., Morrey, B. (1979) 'Chevron osteotomy for hallux valgus.' *Clinical Orthopaedics and Related Research*, **142**, 44–47.

Jones, M. (1976) 'Differential diagnosis and natural history of the cerebral palsied child.' *In* Samilson, R.L. (Ed.) *Orthopaedic Aspects of Cerebral Palsy. Clinics in Developmental Medicine, Nos 52/53*. London: Spastics International Medical Publications with Heinemann Medical; Philadelphia: J.B. Lippincott.

Kagaya, H., Yamada, S., Nagasawa, T., Ishihara, Y., Kodama, H., Endoh, H. (1996) 'Splint posterior tibial tendon transfer for varus deformity of hindfoot.' *Clinical Orthopedics and Related Research*, **323**, 254–260.

Kalen, V., Brecher, A. (1988) 'Relationship between adolescent bunions and flatfoot.' *Foot and Ankle*, 8, 331–336.

Keats, S. (1965) 'Surgical treatment of the hand in cerebral palsy: correction of the thumb-in-palm and other deformities.' *Journal of Bone and Joint Surgery*, **47A**, 274–284.

—— (1974) 'Congenital bilateral dislocation of the head of the radius in a seven year old child.' *Orthopaedic Review*, **111**, 33–36.

Kettlekamp, D.B., Alexander, H.H. (1969) 'Spontaneous rupture of the posterior tibial tendon.' *Journal of Bone and Joint Surgery*, **51A**, 759–764.

Kitaoka, H.B. (Ed.) (2002) *The Foot and Ankle*. Philadelphia: Lippincott, Williams & Wilkins, pp. 29–45.

Kling, T.F., Kaufer, H., Hensinger, H. (1985) 'Split posterior tibial-tendon transfers in children with cerebral spastic paralysis and equinovarus deformity.' *Journal of Bone and Joint Surgery*, **67A**, 186–194.

Koman, L.A., Gelberman, R.H., Toby, E.B., Poehling, G.G. (1990) 'Cerebral palsy. Management of the upper extremity.' *Clinical Orthopedics and Related Research*, **253**, 62–74.

Kunkel, A., Kopp, B., Muller, R., Villringer, K., Villringer, A., Taub, E., Flor, H. (1999) 'Constraint-induced movement therapy for motor recovery in chronic stroke patients.' *Archives of Physical Medicine and Rehabilitation*, **80**, 624–628.

Lake, D., Moreau, M., Rittenhous, B. (1985) 'Outpatient percutaneous heel cord lengthening for the treatment of equinus contractures in children.' *Paper read at the annual Meeting of American Academy for Cerebral Palsy and Developmental Medicine, Seattle, Washington.*

Lee, C.L., Bleck, E.E. (1980) 'Surgical correction of equinus deformity in cerebral palsy.' *Developmental Medicine and Child Neurology*, **22**, 287–292.

Leggio, F.J., Kruse, R. (2001) 'Split tibialis posterior tendon transfer with concomitant distal tibial rotation osteotomy in children with cerebral palsy.' *Journal of Pediatric Orthopaedics*, **21**, 95–101.

Lesny, I, Stehlik, A., Tomasek, J., Tomankova, A., Havlicek, I. (1993) 'Sensory disorders in cerebral palsy.' *Developmental Medicine and Child Neurology*, **35**, 402–405.

Lester, E.L., Johnson, W.L. (1985) 'Posterior tibial tendon transposition/ rerouting (Baker's slide

procedure).' *Paper read at the Annual Meeting of Shrine Surgeons.*

Liepert, J., Miltner, W.H., Bauder, H., Sommer, M., Dettmers, C., Taub E., Weiller, C. (1998) 'Motor cortex plasticity during constraint-induced movement therapy in stroke patients.' *Neuroscience Letter*, **250**, 5–8.

Lin, J.P., Brown, J.K. (1992) 'Peripheral and central mechanisms of hindfoot equinus in childhood hemiplegia.' *Developmental Medicine and Child Neurology*, **34**, 949–965.

Lipp, E.B., Jones, D.A. (1984) 'Flexor carpi ulnaris transfer in cerebral palsy.' *Orthopaedic Transactions*, **8**, 101.

Mann, R.A., Coughlin, M.J. (1999) *Adult Hallux Valgus in Surgery of the Foot and Ankle*. St Louis: C.V. Mosby, pp. 150–269.

—— Soecht, L.H. (1982) 'Posterior tibial tendon ruptures—analysis of eight cases.' *Foot and Ankle*, **2**, 350. (Abstract.)

—— Rudicel, S., Graves, S.C. (1992) 'Repair of hallux valgus with a distal soft-tissue procedure and proximal metatarsal osteotomy.' *Journal of Bone and Joint Surgery*, **74A**, 124–129.

Manske, P.R. (1984) 'Extensor pollicis longus re-routing for treatment of spastic thumb-in-palm deformity.' *Orthopaedic Transactions*, **8**, 95.

—— (1985) 'Redirection of extensor pollicis longus in the treatment of spastic thumb-in-palm deformity.' *Journal of Hand Surgery*, **10A**, 553–560.

Matev, I. (1963) 'Surgical treatment of spastic "thumb-in-palm" deformity.' *Journal of Bone and Joint Surgery*, **45B**, 703–708.

—— (1991) 'Surgery of the spastic thumb-in-palm deformity.' *Journal of Hand Surgery*, **16B**, 127–132.

Matsuo, T., Lai, T., Tayama, N. (1990) 'Combined flexor and extensor release for activation of voluntary movement of the fingers in patients with cerebral palsy.' *Clinical Orthopedics and Related Research*, **250**, 185–193.

—— (2002) *Cerebral Palsy: Spasticity-control and Orthopaedics—An Introduction to Orthopaedic Selective Spasticity-control Surgery (OSSCS)*. Tokyo: Soufusha. p. 153, 293, 180–181, 213–219.

Mayer, L. (1937) 'The physiological method of tendon transplantation in the treatment of paralytic drop-foot.' *Journal of Bone and Joint Surgery*, **19**, 389–394.

McBride, E.D. (1928) 'A conservative operation for bunions.' *Journal of Bone and Joint Surgery*, **10**, 735–739.

McCall, R.E., Frederick, H.A., McCluskey, G.M., Riordan, D.C. (1991) 'The Bridge procedure: a new treatment for equinus and equinovarus deformities.' *Journal of Pediatric Orthopaedics*, **11**, 83–89.

McKeever, D.C. (1952) 'Arthrodesis of the first metatarsophalangeal joint for hallux va1gus, hallux rigidus, and metatarsus primus varus.' *Journal of Bone and Joint Surgery*, **34A**, 129–134.

Meals, R. A. (1988) 'Denervation for the treatment of acquired spasticity of the brachioradialis.' *Journal of Bone and Joint Surgery*, **70A**, 1081–1084.

Medina, P.A., Karpman R.R., Yeung, A.T. (1989) 'Split posterior tibial tendon transfer for spastic equinovarus foot deformity.' *Foot and Ankle*, **10**, 65–67.

Menelaus, M.B. (1984) 'Open flexor tenotomy for hammer toes and curly toes in childhood.' *Journal of Bone and Joint Surgery*, **66B**, 770–771.

Meyer, R.D., Gould, J.S., Nicholson, B. (1981) 'Revision of the first web space: technics and results.' *Southern Medical Journal*, **74**, 1204–1208.

Miller, G.M., Hsu, J.D., Hoffer, M.M., Rentfro, R. (1982). 'Posterior tibial tendon transfer: a review of the literature and analysis of 74 procedures.' *Journal of Pediatric Orthopedics*, **2**, 363–370.

Mital, M.A. (1979) 'Lengthening of the elbow flexors in cerebral palsy.' *Journal of Bone and Joint Surgery*, **61A**, 515–522.

Mitchell, C.L., Fleming, J.L., Allen, R., Glenney, C., Sanford, G.A. (1958) 'Osteotomy-bunionectomy for hallux valgus.' *Journal of Bone and Joint Surgery*, **40A**, 41–60

Möberg , E. (1962) 'Criticism and study of methods for examining sensibility in the hand.' *Neurology*, **12**, 8–19.

—— (1976) 'Reconstructive hand surgery in tetraplegia, stroke, and cerebral palsy: some basic concepts in physiology and neurology.' *Journal of Hand Surgery*, **1**, 29–34.

—— (1984) *Splinting in Hand Therapy*. New York: Thieme-Stratton; Stuttgart/New York: Georg Thieme, pp. 17–21.

Moreau, M.J., Lake, D.M. (1987) 'Outpatient percutaneous heel cord lengthening in children.' *Journal of Pediatric Orthopedics*, **7**, 253–255.

Mosca, V.S. (1995) 'Calcaneal lengthening for valgus deformity of the hindfoot. Results in children who had severe, symptomatic flatfoot and skewfoot.' *Journal of Bone and Joint Surgery*, **77A**, 500–512.

Mowery, C.A., Gelberman, R.H., Rhoades, C.E. (1985) 'Upper extremity tendon transfers in cerebral palsy: electromyographic and functional analysis.' *Journal of Pediatric Orthopedics*, **5**, 69–72.

Mulier, R., Moens, P., Molenaers, G., Spaepen, D., Dereymaeker, G., Fabry, G. (1995) 'Split posterior tibial tendon transfer through the interosseus membrane in spastic equinovarus deformity.' *Foot and Ankle International*, **16**, 754–759.

Nather, A., Balsubramaniam, P., Bose, K. (1984) 'Tendon lengthening—an experimental study in rabbits.' *Orthopaedic Transactions*, **8**, 109.

Nishioka, E., Yoshida, K., Yamanaka, K., Inoue, A. (2000) 'Radiographic studies of the wrist and elbow in cerebral palsy.' *Journal of Orthopaedic Science*, **5**, 268–274.

Noronha, J., Bundy, A., Groll, J. (1989) 'The effect of positioning on the hand function of boys with cerebral palsy.' *American Journal of Occupational Therapy*, **43**, 507–512.

Olney, B.W., William, P.F., Menelaus, M.B. (1988) 'Treatment of spastic equinus by aponeurosis lengthening.' *Journal of Pediatric Orthopaedics*, **8**, 422–425.

Ōunpuu, S., Gage, J.R., Davis, R.B. (1991) 'Three-dimensional lower extremity joint kinetics in normal pediatric gait.' *Journal of Pediatric Orthopaedics*, **11**, 341–349.

Parsch, K. Rubsaamen, G. (1992) 'Die Behandlung des spastischen Klumpfusses.' *Orthopäde*, **21**, 332–338.

Patella, V., Martucci, G. (1980) 'Transposition of the pronator radio teres muscle to the radial extensors of the wrist, in infantile cerebral paralysis. An improved operative technique.' *Italian Journal of Orthopaedics and Traumatology*, **6**, 61–66.

Paulos, L., Coleman, S.S., Samuelson, K.M. (1980) 'Pes cavovarus.' *Journal of Bone and Joint Surgery*, **62A**, 942–953.

Perlstein, M.A., Hood, P. M. (1956) 'Infantile spastic hemiplegia, intelligence, oral language and motor development.' *Courier*, **6**, 567.

Perry, J. (1977) 'Preoperative and postoperative dynamic electromyography as an aid in planning tendon transfers in children with cerebral palsy.' *Journal of Bone and Joint Surgery*, **59A**, 531–537.

—— Hoffer, M.M., Giovan, P., Antonelli, D., Greenberg, R. (1974) 'Gait analysis of the triceps surae in cerebral palsy. A preoperative clinical and electromyographic study.' *Journal of Bone and Joint Surgery*, **56A**, 511–520.

—— (1992) *Gait Analysis. Normal and Pathological Functions*. Thorofare, NJ: Slack.

Pletcher, D.F.-J., Hoffer, M.M., Koffman, D.M. (1976) 'Non-traumatic dislocation of the radial head in cerebral palsy.' *Journal of Bone and Joint Surgery*, **58A**, 104–105.

Purohit, A.K., Raju, B.S., Kumar, K.S., Mallikarju, K.D. (1998) 'Selective musculocutaneous fasciculotomy for spastic elbow in cerebral palsy: a preliminary study.' *Acta Neurochirugia* (Wein), **140**, 473–478.

Rang, M. (1993) 'Neuromuscular disease.' *In* Wenger, D.R., Rang, M. (Eds) *The Art and Practice of Children's Orthopaedics.* New York: Raven Press, pp. 550, 558.

—— (2000) *The Story of Orthopaedics.* Philadelphia: W.B. Saunders, pp. 101–104.

—— Silver, R., de la Garza, J. (1986) 'Cerebral palsy.' *In* Lovell, W.W., Winter, R.B. (Eds) *Pediatric Orthopaedics, 2nd edn, vol. 1.* Philadelphia: J. B. Lippincott, p. 345.

Rattey, T.E., Leahey, L., Hyndman, J., Brown, D.C., Gross, M. (1993) 'Recurrence after Achilles tendon lengthening in cerebral palsy.' *Journal of Pediatric Orthopaedics*, 13, 184–187.

Rayan, G.M., Young, B.T. (1999) 'Arthrodesis of the spastic wrist.' *Journal of Hand Surgery*, 24A, 944–952.

Reimers, J. (1990) 'Functional changes in the antagonists after lengthening the agonists in cerebral palsy.' *Clinical Orthopedics and Related Research*, 253, 30–34.

Renshaw, T., Sirkin, R., Drennan, J. (1979) 'The management of hallux valgus in cerebral palsy.' *Developmental Medicine and Child Neurology*, 21, 202–208.

Renshaw, T.S., Green, N.E., Griffin, P.P., Root, L. (1996) 'Cerebral palsy: orthopaedic management.' *In* Pritchard, D.J. (Ed.) *Instructional Course Lectures.* Rosemont, IL: American Academy of Orthopaedic Surgeons, 45, 1591–1593.

Rodda, J., Graham, H.K. (2001) 'Classification of gait patterns in spastic hemiplegia and spastic diplegia: a basis for management algorithm.' *European Journal of Neurology*, 8 (Suppl. 5), 98–108.

Root, L., Kirz, P. (1982) 'The result of posterior tibial tendon surgery in 83 patients with cerebral palsy.' *Developmental Medicine and Child Neurology*, 24, 241–242. (Abstract.)

—— Miller, S.R., Kirz, P. (1987) 'Posterior tibial tendon transfer in patients with cerebral palsy.' *Journal of Bone and Joint Surgery*, 69A, 1133–1139.

Rose, S.A., DeLuca, R.A., Davis, R.B. III, Õunpuu, S., Gage, J.R. (1995) 'Kinematic and kinetic evaluation of the ankle after lengthening of the gastrocnemius fascia in children with cerebral palsy.' *Journal of Pediatric Orthopaedics*, 131,727–732.

Rosenthal, R.K., Deutsch, S.D., Miller, W., Schumann, W., Hall, J.E. (1975) 'A fixed ankle below-the-knee orthosis for the management of genu recurvaturn in spastic cerebral palsy.' *Journal of Bone and Joint Surgery*, 57A, 545–547.

—— Simon, S.R. (1992) 'The Vulpius gastrocnemius–soleus lengthening.' *In* Sussman, M.D. (Ed.) *The Diplegic Child*, Rosemont, IL: American Academy of Orthopaedic Surgeons, 355–363.

Ruda, R., Frost, H.M. (1971) 'Cerebral palsy spastic varus and forefoot adductus, treated by intramuscular posterior tibial tendon lengthening.' *Clinical Orthopaedics and Related Research,* 79, 61–70.

Ryan, G.M., Saccone, P.G. (1996) 'Treatment of spastic thumb-in-palm deformity: a modified extensor pollicis longus tendon rerouting.' *Journal of Hand Surgery*, 21B, 834–839.

Sage, F.P. (1992) 'Cerebral palsy.' *In* Crenshaw, A.H. (Ed.) *Campbell's Operative Orthopaedics.* St Louis: C.V. Mosby, p. 2316–2317.

Saji, M.J., Upadhyay, S.S., Hsu, L.C.S., Leong, J.C.Y. (1993) 'Split tibialis posterior transfer for equinovarus deformity in cerebral palsy. Long-term results of a new surgical procedure.' *Journal of Bone and Joint Surgery*, 75B, 498–501.

Sakellarides, H.T., Mital, M.A., Lenzi, M.D. (1981) 'Treatment of pronation contractures of the forearm in cerebral palsy by changing the insertion of the pronator radii teres.' *Journal of Bone and Joint Surgery*, 63A, 645–652.

—— —— Matza, R.A., Dimakopoulos, P. (1995) 'Classification and surgical treatment of the thumb-in-palm deformity in cerebral palsy and spastic paralysis.' *Journal of Hand Surgery*, 20A, 428–431.

Sala, D.A., Grant, A.D., Kummer, F.J. (1997) 'Equinus deformity in cerebral palsy: recurrence after tendo Achilles lengthening.' *Developmental Medicine and Child Neurology*, 39, 45–48.

Salter, R.B. (1993) *Continuous Passive Motion.* Baltimore: Williams & Wilkins.

Saltzman, C.L., Fehrle, M.J., Cooper, R.R., Spencer, E.C., Ponsetti, I.V. (1999) 'Triple arthrodesis: twenty-five and forty-four year average follow-up of the same patients.' *Journal of Bone and Joint Surgery*, 81A, 1391–1402.

Samilson, R.L. (1976) 'Crescentric osteotomy of the os calcis for calcanealcavus feet.' *In* Bateman, J.E. (Ed.) *Foot Science.* Philadelphia: W. B. Saunders, pp. 18–25.

—— Morris, J.M. (1964) 'Surgical improvement of the cerebral palsied upper limb; electromyographic studies and results of 128 operations.' *Journal of Bone and Joint Surgery*, 46A, 1203–1216.

Saraph, V., Zwick, E. B., Uitz, C., Linhart, W., Steinwender, G. (2000) 'The Baumann procedure for fixed contracture of the gastrosoleus in cerebral palsy.' *Journal of Bone and Joint Surgery*, 82B, 535–540.

Schneider, L.H. (1999) 'Flexor tendons—late reconstruction.' *In* Green D.P., Hotchkiss, R.N., Pederen, W.C. (Eds) *Green's Operative Hand Surgery, 4th edn.* New York: Churchill Livingstone, pp. 1906–1908.

Schneider, M., Balon, K. (1977) 'Deformity of the foot following anterior transfer of the posterior tibial tendon and lengthening of the Achilles tendon for spastic equinovarus.' *Clinical Orthopaedics and Related Research*, 125, 112–117.

Schwartz, J.R., Carr, W., Bassett, F.H., Coonrad, R.W. (1977) 'Lessons learned in the treatment of equinus deformity in ambulatory spastic children.' *Orthopaedic Transactions*, 1, 84.

Seelenfreund, M., Fried, A. (1973) 'Correction of hallux valgus deformity by basal phalanx osteotomy of the big toe.' *Journal of Bone and Joint Surgery*, 55A, 1411–1415.

Segal, L.S., Thomas, S.E., Mazur, J.M., Mauterer, M. (1989) 'Calcaneal gait in spastic diplegia after heel cord lengthening: a study with gait analysis.' *Journal of Pediatric Orthopaedics*, 9, 697–701.

Sharrard, W.J.W., Bernstein, S. (1972) 'Equinus deformity in cerebral palsy.' *Journal of Bone and Joint Surgery*, 54B, 272–276.

Silfverskiöld, N. (1923–24) 'Reduction of the uncrossed two-joint muscles of the leg to one-joint muscles in spastic conditions.' *Acta Chirurgica Scandinavica*, 56, 315–330.

Silver, C.M. (1977) *Instructional Course on Management of Spastic Hemiplegia.* Las Vegas: American Academy of Orthopaedic Surgeons.

—— Simon, S.D. (1959) 'Gastrocnemius-muscle recession (Silfverskiöld operation) for spastic equinus deformity in cerebral palsy.' *Journal of Bone and Joint Surgery*, 41A, 1021–1028.

—— Spindell, E., Lichtman, H.M., Scala, M. (1967) 'Calcaneal osteotomy for valgus and varus deformities of the foot in cerebral palsy.' *Journal of Bone and Joint Surgery*, 49A, 232–246.

—— Lichtman, H.M., Motamed, M. (1976) 'Surgical correction of spastic thumb-in-palm deformity.' *Developmental Medicine and Child Neurology*, 18, 632–639.

Simon, S.R., Ryan, A.W. (1992) 'Biomechanical/neurophysiologic factors related to surgical correction of equinus deformity.' *In* Sussman, M.D. (Ed.) *The Diplegic Child.* Rosemont, IL: American Academy of Orthopaedic Surgeons, pp. 365–381.

Sirna, E., Sussman, M.D. (1985) 'Immediate mobilization of patients following tendo Achilles lengthening in short leg casts.' *Paper read at Annual Meeting of American Academy for Cerebral Palsy and Developmental Medicine, Seattle, Washington.*

Smith, R.J. (1982) 'Flexor pollicis longus abductor-plasty for spastic thumb-in-palm deformity.' *Journal of Hand Surgery*, 7, 327–334.

Sorial, R., Tonkin, M.A., Gschwind, C. (1994) 'Wrist arthrodesis using a sliding radial graft and plate fixation.' *Journal of Hand Surgery*, 19B, 217–220.

Strayer, L.M. (1950) 'Recession of the gastrocnemius.' *Journal of Bone and Joint Surgery*, 32A, 671–676.

—— (1958) 'Gastrocnemius recession. Five year report of cases.' *Journal of Bone and Joint Surgery*, 40A, 1019–1030.

Strecker, W.B., Via, M.W., Oliver, S.K., Schoenecker, P.L. (1990) 'Heel cord advancement for the treatment of equinus deformity in cerebral palsy.' *Journal of Pediatric Orthopaedics*, 10, 105–108.

Strickland, J.W. (1999) 'Flexor tendons—acute injuries.' *In* Green, D.P., Hotchkiss, R.N., Pedersen, W.P. (Eds) *Green's Operative Hand Surgery.* New York: Churchill Livingstone, pp. 1680–1861.

Sutherland, D.H., Cooper, L., Daniel, D. (1980) 'The role of the ankle plantar flexors in normal walking.' *Journal of Bone and Joint Surgery*, 62A, 354–363.

Swanson, A.B. (1982) 'Surgery of the hand in cerebral palsy.' *In* Flynn, J.E. (Ed.) *Hand Surgery, 3rd edn.* Baltimore: Williams & Wilkins, pp. 476–488.

—— Browne, H.S., Coleman, J.D. (1960) 'Surgery of the hand in cerebral palsy and the swan-neck deformity.' *Journal of Bone and Joint Surgery*, 42A, 951–964.

—— —— —— (1966) 'The cavus foot-concepts of production and treatment by metatarsal osteotomy.' *Journal of Bone and Joint Surgery*, 48A, 1019. (Abstract.)

Tachdjian, M.O. (1972) *Pediatric Orthopaedics*. Philadelphia: W.B. Saunders.

—— (1994) *Atlas of Pediatric Orthopaedic Surgery*. Philadelphia: W.B. Saunders, pp. 1252–1257.

Tardieu, C., Tabary, J.S., Huet de la Tour, E., Tabary, C., Tardieu, G. (1977) 'The relationship between sarcomere length in the soleus and tibialis anterior and the articular angle of the tibia-calcaneum in cats during growth.' *Journal of Anatomy*, **124**, 581–588.

Taub, E., Parella, P., Barro, G. (1973) 'Behavioral development after forelimb deafferentation on day one of birth in monkey with and without blinding.' *Science*, **181**, 959–960.

—— Uswatte, G., Pidikiti, R. (1999) 'Constraint-induced movement therapy: a new family of techniques with broad application to physical rehabilitation—a clinical review.' *Journal of Rehabilitation Research Development*, **3**, 228–236.

—— —— Elbert, T. (2002) 'New treatments in neurorehabilitation founded on basic research.' *Nature Reviews. Neuroscience*, **3**, 228–236.

Taylor, N., Sand, P.L., Jebsen, R.H. (1973) 'Evaluation of hand functrion in children.' *Archives of Physical Medicine and Rehabilitation*, **54**, 129–135.

Throop, F.B., DeRosa, G.P., Reeck, C., Waterman, S. (1975) 'Correction of equinus in cerebral palsy by the Murphy procedure of tendo calcaneus advancement. A preliminary communication.' *Developmental Medicine and Child Neurology*, **17**, 182–185.

Tonkin, M., Gschwind, D. (1994) 'Surgery for cerebral palsy: part 2, flexion deformity of the wrist and fingers.' *Journal of Hand Surgery*, **17**, 396–400.

Townsend, D.R., Wells, L., Lowenberg, D. (1990) 'The Cincinnati incision for the split posterior tibial tendon transfer: a technical note.' *Journal of Pediatric Orthopaedics*, **10**, 667–669.

Truscelli, D., Lespargot, A., Tardieu, G. (1979) 'Variation in the long-term results of elongation of the tendo achilles in children with cerebral palsy.' *Journal of Bone and Joint Surgery*, **61B**, 466–469.

Turner, J.W., Cooper, R.R. (1972) 'Anterior transfer of the tibialis posterior through the interosseus membrane.' *Clinical Orthopaedics and Related Research*, **83**, 241–244.

Van Heest, A.E., House, J., Putnam, M. (1993) 'Sensibility deficiencies in the hands of children with spastic hemiplegia.' *Journal of Hand Surgery*, **18**, 278–281.

—— —— Cariello, C. (1999) 'Upper extremity surgical treatment of cerebral palsy.' *Journal of Hand Surgery*, **24A**, 323–330.

Vogt, J.C. (1998) 'Split anterior tibial transfer for spastic equinovarus foot deformity: retrospective study of 73 operated feet.' *Journal of Foot and Ankle Surgery*, **37**, 2–7.

Vulpius, O., Stoffel, A. (1913) *Orthopädische Operationslehre*. Stuttgart: Ferdinand Enke.

Waters, P.M., Van Heest, A. (1998) 'Spastic hemiplegia of the upper extremity of children.' *Hand Clinic*, **14**, 119–134.

Watkins, M.B., Jones, J.B., Ryder, G.T., Brown, T.H. (1954) 'Transplantation of the posterior tibial tendon.' *Journal of Bone and Joint Surgery*, **36A**, 1181–1189.

Westin, G.W., Dye, S. (1983) 'Conservative management of cerebral palsy in the growing child.' *Foot and Ankle*, 4, 160–163.

Westwell-O'Connor, M., Delucca, P., ?unpuu, S. (2002) 'Comparison of percutaneous tendo-Achilles lengthenings with gastrocnemius lengthenings to treat equinus in children with cerebral palsy.' *Developmental Medicine and Child Neurology*, 44 (Suppl. 91), 15. (Abstract.)

White, J.W. (1943) 'Torsion of the Achilles tendon.' *Archives of Surgery*, 46, 784–787.

White, W.F. (1972) 'Flexor muscle slide in the spastic hand. The Max Page operation.' *Journal of Bone and Joint Surgery*, 54B, 453–459.

Wilcox, P.G., Weiner, D.S. (1985) 'The Akron midtarsal dome osteotomy in the treatment of rigid pes cavus: a preliminary review.' *Journal of Pediatric Orthopedics*, 5, 333–338.

Williams, P. F. (1976) 'Restoration of muscle balance of the foot by transfer of the tibialis posterior.' *Journal of Bone and Joint Surgery*, 58B, 217–219.

Willis, J.K., Morello, A., Davie, A., Rice, J.C., Bennett, J.T. (2002) 'Forced use treatment of childhood hemiparesis.' *Pediatrics*, 110, 949–956.

Winter, D. (1991) *The Biomechanics and Motor Control of Human Gait: Normal, Elderly and Pathological*. Waterloo, Ontario: University of Waterloo Press.

Winters, T.F., Gage, J.R., Hicks, R. (1987) 'Gait patterns in spastic hemiplegia in children and young adults.' *Journal of Bone and Joint Surgery*, 69A, 437–441.

Wu, K.K. (1986) *Surgery of the Foot*. Philadelphia: Lea & Febiger.

Wynn-Davies, R. (1970) 'Acetabular dysplasia and familial joint laxity: two etiological factors in congenital dislocation of the hip.' *Journal of Bone and Joint Surgery*, 52 B, 704–716.

Yekutiel, M., Jariwala, M., Stretch, P. (1994) 'Sensory deficit in the hands of children with cerebral palsy: a new look at assessment and prevalence.' *Developmental Medicine and Child Neurology*, 36, 619–624.

Yngve, D.A., Chambers, C. (1996) 'Vulpius and Z-lengthening.' *Journal of Pediatric Orthopaedics*, 16, 759–764.

Yude, C., Goodman, R. (1999) 'Peer problems of 9- to 11-year-old children with hemiplegia in mainstream schools. Can these be predicted?' *Developmental Medicine and Child Neurology*, 41, 4–8.

Zancolli, E.A. (1979) *Structural and Dynamic Bases of Hand Surgery, 2nd Edn.* Philadelphia: J.B. Lippincott.

—— Goldner, J.L., Swanson, A.B. (1983) 'Surgery of the spastic hand in cerebral palsy; report of the committee on spastic hand evaluation.' *Journal of Hand Surgery*, 8, 766–772.

—— Zancolli, E.R. (1981) 'Surgical management of the hemiplegic spastic hand in cerebral palsy.' *Surgical Clinics of North America*, 61, 395–406.

Ziv, I., Blackburn, N., Rang, M., Koreska, J. (1984) 'Muscle growth in normal and spastic mice.' *Developmental Medicine and Child Neurology*, 26, 94–99.

8
SPASTIC DIPLEGIA

SNAPSHOT: SPASTIC DIPLEGIA

- *Communication*: practically normal
- *Mobility*: community
- *Activities of daily living*: all
- *Walking*: usually between 24 and 36 months; latest at 48 months (some need external supports, crutches, canes or walker depending on the equilibrium reactions.

SNAPSHOT: MANAGEMENT

- *Orthopaedic problems*:

  upper limbs: in some only fine-motor incoordination
  lower limbs: equinus, pes valgus, spastic hamstrings and quadriceps, hip internal rotation gait, spastic adductors, hip-flexion contracture
- *Physiotherapy*: muscle strengthening exercises, adaptive sports, balance training
- *Orthoses*: AFO for dynamic equinus
- *Neurosurgery*: rhizotomy recommended and done at some centers; need good balance reactions
- *Botlinum toxin*: before age 7 for dynamic equinus; trial in hip-adductors and hamstrings

- *Orthopaedic surgery*:

  fixed equinus: Achilles or gastrocnemius–soleus aponeurotic lengthening

  pes valgus: subtalar stabilization or calcaneal lengthening osteotomy

  flexed-knee gait: fractional hamstring lengthening; distal rectus femoris transfer

  hip adduction: adductor longus myotenotomy

  hip-flexion contracture: psoas tenotomy at the pelvic brim or lengthening of tendon

  hip internal rotation gait: derotation femoral osteotomy

CHARACTERISTICS

Spastic diplegia associated with preterm birth now appears to be less common than previously noted in the developed western nations. The distribution of all cases diagnosed as spastic diplegic cerebral palsy ranged from 18% to 44.9% in a review of multiple studies from northern Europe as well as Western Australia (Stanley *et al.* 2000). Colver (2003) reviewed 18 references and similarly noted an average of 33% with diplegia. The rate of cerebral palsy among neonatal survivors born before 33 weeks' gestation is 30 times higher than among those born at term (Stanley et al. 2000). In Sweden, spastic diplegia accounted for 70% of all patients with cerebral palsy in 1989 (Hagberg *et al.* 1989), but in subsequent studies by the same group, the incidence of spastic diplegia among children with cerebral palsy in Western Sweden decreased to 35% of the total, with hemiplegia becoming more common at 38% and spastic quadriplegia at 6%. They attributed the decreased incidence in spastic diplegia to a decrease in post-hemorrhagic hydrocephalus in very preterm children (Himmelmann et al., 2005). Additionally, 15% had dyskinetic or ataxic cerebral palsy (6%). Similarly the distribution of cerebral palsy noted in a cohort study from Victoria, Australia, showed of 374 children with cerebral palsy that 35% had hemiplegia, 28% had diplegia and 37% had quadriplegia. Adding to the increasing numbers of children with cerebral palsy is the rise in multiple births deemed to be due to the widening use of fertility enhancing drugs and therapies for infertility in developed countries (Stanley *et al.* 2000). In the clinic at Children's Hospital at Stanford in 1979, 66.5% of the children with spastic diplegia had been born preterm. Shevell and coworkers (2003) studied the total group of patients with cerebral palsy in their neurological practice. Of the 217 patients with cerebral palsy, 18% had spastic

TABLE 8.I
Causes of spastic diplegia in 39 patients with cerebral palsy

54%	periventricular leukomalacia
41%	unknown
15%	intracranial hemorrhage
12%	intrapartum asphyxia
8%	toxins

From Shevell *et al.* (2003).

diplegia, compared to 35.5% with spastic quadriplegia, and 31.3% with spastic hemiplegia, with the remainder in other categories. The etiologies of cerebral palsy could be ascertained in 82% of their patients. The causes of cerebral palsy among the spastic diplegic children are noted in Table 8.I. With better diagnostic tools and improved prenatal and prenatal care it is interesting to see the shift in associated risk factors in cerebral palsy as well as the topographical shift in cerebral palsy.

Diplegia is defined as the presence of grossly spastic muscles in the lower limbs, with minor motor deficits in the upper limbs. In contrast, paraplegia involves just the lower limbs, with no deficits in the upper limb. If the latter pattern of paralysis is observed, high spinal-cord lesions should be considered especially if the patient has urinary bladder problems. Hereditary spastic paraplegia must also be included in the differential diagnosis.

The general characteristics in the child with spastic diplegia are as follows:

1. Upper-limb gross-motor function is good, with only minor incoordination of the fingers on fine-motor skill testing (e.g. approximating each fingertip to the thumb in sequence).

2. The lower-limb muscles are definitely spastic; the typical pattern is shown in Figure 8.1. (a) Hip-flexion spasm and contracture; (b) hip internal rotation with excessive femoral anteversion; (c) hip-adduction spasm and contracture; (d) knee-flexor or extensor spasticity predominate or are equal in the degree of spasticity; (e) equinus of the ankle; (f) pes valgus with a plantarflexed talus and hindfoot equinus.

3. Speech and intellect are usually normal or only slightly impaired.

4. Esotropia and perceptual and visual–motor deficits are common.

5. The neurological examination finds hyperactive lower-limb reflexes, positive Babinski sign, increased stretch reflexes in spastic calf, hamstring, and hip-adductor muscles.

Most children can walk independently. Those who have deficient anterior equilibrium reactions need crutches, and a few who are deficient in these reactions in all planes require walkers.

NATURAL HISTORY

Most of these children walk by 48 months. The deficient posterior equilibrium reactions seem to persist throughout life, but independent walking continues. Some children who have deficient equilibrium reactions as noted in Chapter 2 (anterior and posterior, or lateral) seem able to discard crutches and get about the household when puberty begins. Why this occurs is a

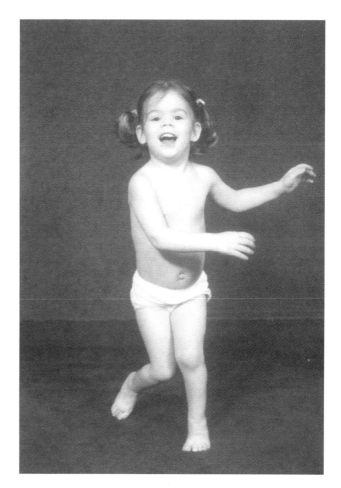

Fig. 8.1. Typical posture lower limbs: spastic diplegia.

matter of speculation, but it may be related to the increased sex-hormone levels and their influence on the neuromuscular system at this time or perhaps better muscular strength.

Almost all can be 'integrated' into regular school by the age of 7 or 8 years. These days, Californian children with spastic diplegia rarely begin in a special school. The usual course is from preschool programs into regular school.

Almost all should be able to lead independent and useful lives provided they have not been conditioned or segregated into the 'disabled' population through well-intentioned 'treatment' of their neurological defect. We can give parents of this group an optimistic prognosis on long-term function, but we must avoid talking about the disease which cannot be cured. Among the adult patients in our study, many diverse occupations were represented: computer programmer, mother and housewife, soap salesman, pizza cook, banker, secretary, teacher of physically disabled children, insurance agent, recreation playground director, librarian, amusement-park worker, and mayor of Antelope Valley, California. Of the 44 who were 18 years or older (37% of the group) only one was unemployed or not in school; only one was in a sheltered workshop.

The following is a vignette of coping and achieving, which should give inspiration to all parents and children with spastic diplegia. Dr Jan Brunstrom, an internationally recognized neurologist, was born 3 months preterm and weighed a little more than 3 lb. Diagnosed with cerebral palsy at the age of 2, she underwent treatments such as submersion in a tub of crushed ice. For years she wore 'really horrible' braces, including hip waders made of metal twister cables. As a teen, Brunstrom defied medical advice and took up swimming. 'I found that I moved better in water,' she said. Three operations at 16, 20 and 27 years freed her from braces. She earned her MD from the Medical College of Virginia, then completed a 5-year residency program in pediatrics and neurology at Washington University School of Medicine in St Louis. She got married and in 1993 gave birth to a son, Ian. Since 1998 she has worked exclusively with children who have cerebral palsy at the St Louis Children's Hospital (Hales 2003).

The one predominant disability in adolescents and adults that blocks development of adult independence has been anxiety neurosis. It may be that parental and professional over-treatment, and excessive striving to remedy deficits rather than compensate for them, is the cause of the mental distress. Examples of such remedial efforts include: (1) nagging to practice walking better; (2) attempts to master abstract subjects that may not be possible, and (3) practice to improve handwriting when typewriting or word-processing with a computer is more efficient.

'Therapeutic choices in the locomotor management of the child with cerebral palsy,' according to Patrick *et al.* (2001), could be due to 'more luck than judgement'. The words are particularly relevant to those with spastic diplegia, our largest group of children with cerebral palsy and for whom we wish to do our best. Orthopaedic surgery has been a treatment of choice for more than half a century. Refinements of patient selection and objective evaluations will undoubtedly continue to enhance judgement for a good functional and safe outcome. Orthopaedic surgery has improved in all areas compared to what was the case 50 or even 20 years ago.

NON-SURGICAL MANAGEMENT

The services available from physical and occupational therapists and orthotists have been discussed in Chapter 6. In this group, as in spastic hemiplegia, physical and occupational therapy services need not be prolonged and should be functionally oriented. We have to temper our zeal to recommend more 'intensive' therapy. A randomized controlled study by Bower and colleagues (2001) compared 'intensive' physical therapy of 56 children aged 3 and 12 years and a Gross Motor Function Measure (GMFM) classification of level III with 'routine' therapy. No statistically significant changes in the scores in the therapy group or in the goal or aim-oriented group could be found. In an editorial commentary, 'Does "therapy" have a future,' Bax (2001) questioned whether the effects of therapy can be fairly measured with the GMFM, and asked whether efficacy should be assessed rather in terms of parental satisfaction and ease in the management of the child. (Perhaps, after the 'age of reason', commonly assumed to be 7 years, the child might be the better judge.)

Children who have spastic diplegia need muscle strengthening and preparation for fun and games in regular school so that they can be properly integrated with their peer groups. Most children with spastic diplegia in regular school make only sporadic visits to a therapist during their academic years. After completing secondary school and college, some seek the help of a private athletic trainer who supervise the exercise and stretching programme that the patient thinks beneficial. In this regard, does a health club for the disabled make sense? It seems so for the unimpaired who have created the boom in 'fitness centers'.

Anecdotes about children who have never had physical therapy are difficult to find. In 35 years of practice Bleck encountered only one adolescent who had escaped the special school and the therapy unit. At age 17 years he had developed contracture of the hamstrings and a flexed-knee gait. Up to this time he had always attended regular school; he was in high school at the time, and a member of basketball team. His parents did not realize he had cerebral palsy and attributed his tight hamstrings to the residuals of poliomyelitis. Apparently his family physician ignored the mild gait abnormality as he matured.

Physical therapy management using active assistive and resistive exercise and joint mobilization is very useful for restoring gait function after orthopaedic surgery, but usually should not last more than 6 months.

SURGICAL MANAGEMENT

Although there seem to be many options for the management of spastic diplegia, e.g. botulinum toxin injections, rhizotomy, intrathecal baclofen and orthotics, this chapter covers only orthopaedic surgery in spastic diplegia. After selective posterior rootlet rhizotomy was introduced in about 1985, neurosurgeons and some orthopaedic surgeons issued a flood of reports on its efficacy in spastic diplegia. Two decades later it is evident that rhizotomy does not preclude orthopaedic surgery; 66%–75% still required orthopaedic surgery particularly for in-toed gait due to fixed femoral torsion and for pes valgus (Thomas *et al.* 1997). Using 3D gait analysis, Thomas and colleagues found that improvements in the gait pattern occurred between the first and second years after surgery, but the changes were not significant. Enthusiasm for rhizotomy seems to be tempered.

Intrathecal baclofen has been tried in patients with spastic diplegia who are able to walk (Albright 1996), but after reviewing options for management of cerebral palsy in general, Patrick and colleagues (2001) did not express much eagerness to try it in their patients.

WHAT IS BEST: ORTHOPAEDIC SURGERY OR RHIZOTOMY?

Gage and Novacheck (2001) attempted to answer the question of best outcomes with orthopaedic surgery or rhizotomy in a study 32 patients who had spastic diplegia or triplegia at their center (Gillette Children's Specialty Heathcare, St Paul, Minnesota). Seventeen had only orthopaedic surgery, seven had only posterior rootlet selective rhizotomy, and eight had both rhizotomy and orthopaedic surgery to correct deformities. The best technical outcomes (decreased oxygen cost and a 'normalcy index' of quantifying walking) were in those who had both the neurosurgery and the orthopaedic surgery. Using a 10-level parent-reported walking scale, four of 17 with orthopaedic surgery only decreased their walking, none of seven who had only rhizotomy decreased walking ability, and none of eight who had both surgeries had decreased function.

There is no established relationship between normalcy of gait pattern and function.

The questionnaire entailed delineation of observed 22 skills, for example: walk carrying an object, walk carrying a fragile object or glass of liquid, walk up and down stairs with or without using a railing, run, jump off single step. In all three groups of surgical experience, all patients and families reported a high level of satisfaction.[1] Gage and Novacheck (2001) added that the series was very small. They thought it would be 'beneficial' to critically study the patients who did not improve and thereby improve the selection of their patients for treatment.

So we still find it impossible to generalize as to what is the best in the long run for the child with spastic diplegia. The study by Gage and Novacheck that gave most approbation to the combined rhizotomy and orthopaedic group, but we do not know the basis of selection of the patient for the rhizotomy or orthopaedic surgery. We do not know if those who improved the most in the two outcome measures used had normal or deficient balance reactions, nor if the orthopaedic surgery group had more severe limb deformities.

OBJECTIVE OF ORTHOPAEDIC SURGERY

In spastic diplegia, the main purpose of orthopaedic surgery is to make the gait pattern more functional and energy-conserving as well as to preserve muscle power (i.e. moments as measured by kinetics). Inadequate or inappropriate ranges of motion, malrotation, and inadequate muscle power are components of abnormal gait. Data on muscle power during gait has been measured and estimated using 3D kinetic data (Winter 1987, Õunpuu *et al.* 1991).

Although instrumented gait analysis is time-consuming, labor-intensive for professionals and costly,[2] it can and does show significant changes in the gait of the child with spastic diplegia.

---

1 One wonders why parents and families expressed a 'high degree of satisfaction' with any one of the three surgical approaches. Is this a psychological phenomenon due to the exemplary interpersonal relationships with the professionals of the treating institution and nor wanting to disappoint? Or as occurs when people see a play at a high-priced theater and then praise it to friends despite a low opinion by a professional critic; could it be that they don't want to say they spent their money for no entertainment?

2 In 2003 the estimate for a complete gait analysis varies among institutions and laboratories; it may range from $1000 to $2000 or higher depending on the location of the laboratory, personnel, etc.

Gait analysis supplements the clinical examination and has enhanced the decision process for orthopaedic surgery. Although direct comparison with the reported preoperative and postoperative gait analyses is not possible with random patient selection and controls, the studies we have done show improvement comparable to the 1- and 2-year results after rhizotomy. Figure 8.2 gives some examples from a very detailed 30-page gait analysis before surgery in a 10-year-old boy with spastic diplegia and the postoperative analysis 13 months after surgery. The analyses entailed both right and left sides, passive ranges of lower-limb joint motion (Table 8.II), kinematic data in the frontal, sagittal and transverse planes, ankle, knee, hip and trunk/pelvis kinetics, electromyographs of selected muscle groups, energy analysis, balance measurements (Table 8.III), video analysis, temporal spatial measurements, and a narrative description and interpretation of the gait analysis data. This is a lot of data to digest. At one time *Acta Scandinavica Orthopaedica* decided to publish all the raw data of clinical research with each paper accepted. It can be easily appreciated that if all the original data of gait analysis of each patient in a study were published, one issue could be the length of a 300–500 page book. The only solution is to trust the authors of the reports to interpret the data correctly and honestly.

So as not to burden the reader unduly we present only the pre- and postoperative graphic and numerical data from the right lower limb and pelvis and the kinetic data of the right ankle. Table 8.III details the energy requirements and balance data of the same patient. Our objective is to inform the reader of the

TABLE 8.II
Passive ranges of motion of lower-limb joints, patient BN, spastic diplegia

	Preoperative (°)	Postoperative (°)
Ankle		
Dorsiflexion (knee flexed)	15	0
Plantarflexion	35	45
Knee		
Flexion	160	150
Extension	−10	0
Popliteal angle	55	55
Hip		
Flexion	135	110
Extension	10 flexion (Thomas test)	0 flexion (Thomas test)
Internal rotation*	70	35
External rotation	20	25
Adduction	40	30
Abduction	35	35
Thigh–foot axis	10 external	15 internal
Rectus test prone lying	+	+

Data for the right lower limb only; both sides had similar ranges of motion. All clinical measurements of ranges of joint motion subject to error of 10°. Decrease in hip flexion postoperatively cannot be explained. *Major change is decreased internal rotation of the hip correlating with the subtrochanteric derotation osteotomy. The increase in the thigh foot axis cannot be explained. This measurement combines both femoral and tibial torsion. Graphic display of hip rotation and foot progression in gait analysis shows improvement toward normal postoperatively.

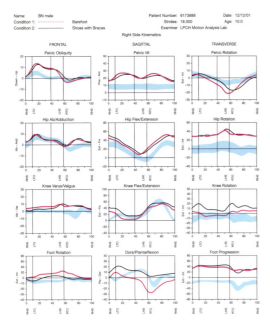

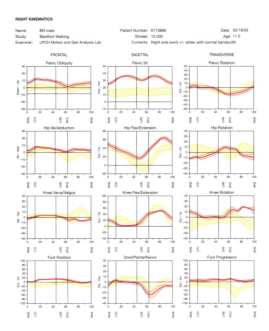

Fig. 8.2. (*a*) Patient BN, spastic diplegia, preoperative right-side kinematics. *Red line*: barefoot; *dark blue line*: shoes and AFO; *light blue shading*: mean normal with SD. Note: anterior pelvic tilt increased at about 30°; increased internal rotation of hip- and foot-progression angle, hip extension limited to about –10°. Abduction/adduction normal. Knee flexion/extension continued flexion beyond terminal swing and at toe-off (stance). Stance begins on bottom line at 0, swing at 60 (%) of cycle. (By courtesy of Jessica Rose Agramonte PhD and Leslie Torburn MS, PT, of the Gait and Motion Analysis Laboratory, Lucile Salter Packard Children's Hospital at Stanford University, and Todd A. Lincoln MD of the Department of Orthopaedic Surgery, Stanford University School of Medicine.)

Fig. 8.2. *contd.* (*b*) Patient BN, spastic diplegia, 13 months postoperative, right-side kinematics. *Red line*: barefoot; *yellow shading paths*: normal and standard deviations. Note: anterior pelvic tilt increased to 40°; hip extension decreased slightly to about –18°; hip internal rotation within normal limits; foot-progression angle near normal. Knee flexion/extension normal. Stance begins at 0 on bottom line, swing begins at 60% of gait cycle. (Equipment by Motion Analysis Corp., Santa Rosa, CA; 8 camera Falcon system. Data collection software by EVaRT 3.2.1; data analysis software by Orthotrak 5.0.4; Motion Lab Systems for MA-200 EMG and footswitch system; Windac Acquisition Pro. 2.04; B & L Engineering, Tustin, CA EMG Analyzer3.54.)

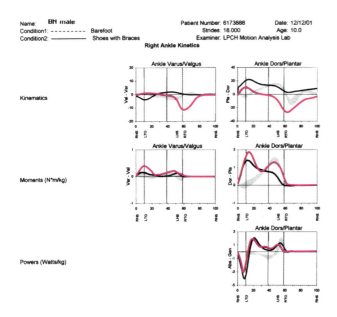

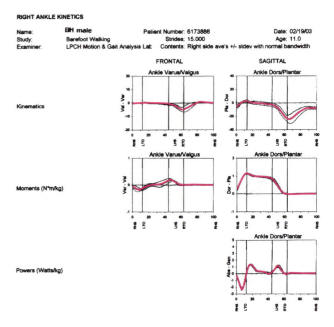

Fig. 8.2. *contd.* (*c*) Patient BN, preoperative, kinetics and kinematics, right ankle. *Red line*: barefoot; *black line*: shoes and AFO. Excessive plantarflexion when barefoot on terminal swing. Ankle plantarflexion moments increased on stance.

Fig. 8.2. *contd.* (*d*) Patient BN, postoperative, kinetics and kinematics right ankle. Improved to near normal in all parameters. No surgery of the foot or ankle. Only derotation femoral osteotomy and medial hamstring lengthening. Moments = force × distance from center of rotation (nm/kg). Joint power = net joint moment × joint angular velocity (watts/kg). Power decreased in early stance, then increases from first 20%–60% of the cycle. RHS, right heel strike; LTO, left toe-off; LHS, left heel strike; RTO, right toe-off. No significant changes with or without shoes and orthosis.

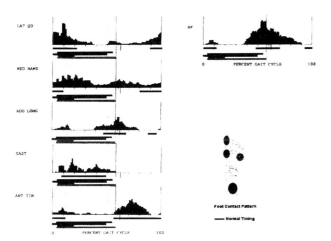

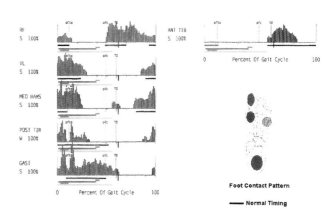

Fig. 8.2, *contd.* (*e*) Patient BN. Preoperative dynamic integrated electromyograms, surface electrodes, barefoot, right lower limb. Color codes foot switch pressure points. Vastus lateralis (LAT QD), medial hamstrings (MED HAMS), adductor longus (ADD LONG), gastrocnemius (GAST), anterior tibial (ANT TIB), rectus femoris (RF). Vastus lateralis: normal timing; hamstrings: continuous activity; adductor longus: out-of-phase in loading response and premature onset in terminal stance; anterior tibial curtailed in terminal swing; rectus femoris: prolonged into mid-swing and absent in terminal swing.

Fig. 8.2, *contd.* (*f*) Patient BN. Postoperative dynamic electromyograms, surface electrodes except posterior tibial recorded with fine wire electrodes, barefoot, right lower limb. Rectus femoris (RF), vastus lateralis (VL), medial hamstrings (MED HAMS), posterior tibial (POST TIB), gastrocnemius (GAST), anterior tibial (ANT TIB). Rectus femoris: prolonged throughout swing; vastus lateralis: normal; medial hamstrings = prolonged to mid-stance and out-of-phase pre-swing; posterior tibial: premature onset in terminal swing and premature cessation in mid-stance; gastrocnemius: onset is premature in terminal swing and somewhat prolonged in pre-swing; anterior tibial: premature cessation in mid-swing. Compared with preoperative analysis medial hamstrings have more phasic activity. Posterior tibial not done preoperatively. In this study the posterior tibial does not appear to be highly abnormal and not likely to be responsible for the mother's perceived turning-in of the right foot; the kinematics depict neutral rotation and neutral foot-progression angle.

Name:	BN male					
Condition1:	Barefoot					
Condition2:	Shoes with Braces					

Patient Number: 6173888 Date: 12/12/1
Strides: 18 000 Age: 10.0
Examiner: LPCH Motion Analysis Lab

Temporal Spatial

		Subject	StDev	Norm	StDev	%Norm
Velocity	(cm/s)	122.1	6.36	119.6	17.83	102%
Cadence	(steps/min)	150.3	4.11	124.6	8.52	121%
Stride Length	(cm)	98.3	4.31	115.2	15.05	85%
Step Width	(cm)	18.2	1.02	12.0	3.32	152%
Pelvic Width	(cm)	-	-	-	-	-
Pelvic to Step Ratio	(cm)	-	-	-	-	-
Velocity	(cm/s)	122.9	7.40	119.6	17.83	103%
Cadence	(steps/min)	142.1	4.11	124.6	8.52	114%
Stride Length	(cm)	104.2	5.89	115.2	15.05	91%
Step Width	(cm)	23.6	0.83	12.0	3.32	197%
Pelvic Width	(cm)	-	-	-	-	-
Pelvic to Step Ratio	(cm)	-	-	-	-	-
Right						
Step Length	(cm)	58.6	5.79	65.2	8.35	90%
Weight Accept	(% cycle)	4.9	1.40	10.2	0.77	48%
Single Support	(% cycle)	40.6	4.59	39.5	0.68	103%
Weight Release	(% cycle)	7.7	2.98	10.2	0.77	75%
Stance	(% cycle)	53.1	2.49	60.5	0.68	88%
Swing	(% cycle)	46.9	2.49	39.5	0.68	119%
Right						
Step Length	(cm)	56.3	9.14	65.2	8.35	86%
Weight Accept	(% cycle)	6.1	0.86	10.2	0.77	60%
Single Support	(% cycle)	42.8	6.71	39.5	0.68	108%
Weight Release	(% cycle)	5.7	1.90	10.2	0.77	55%
Stance	(% cycle)	57.3	4.45	60.5	0.68	95%
Swing	(% cycle)	42.7	4.45	39.5	0.68	108%

Fig. 8.2, *contd.* (*g*) Patient BN. Preoperative. Temporal spatial measurements computer generated. Data in shaded area are walking barefoot. Black-and-white data are with shoes and AFOs. Only pronounced changes from normal values seem to be cadence and step width.

Name:	BN male					
Study:	Barefoot Walking					
Examiner:	LPCH Motion & Gait Analysis Lab					

Patient Number: 6173888 Date: 2/18/63
Strides: 15 000 Age: 11
Contents: Temporal Spatial Data

Temporal Spatial

		Subject	StDev	Norm	StDev	%Norm
Velocity	(cm/s)	117.1	6.15	121.1	22.11	97%
Cadence	(steps/min)	145.8	5.66	121.2	16.22	120%
Stride Length	(cm)	97.3	3.92	119.9	12.44	81%
Step Width	(cm)	15.2	2.60	10.2	2.25	149%
Pelvic Width	(cm)	-	-	-	-	-
Pelvic to Step Ratio	(cm)	-	-	-	-	-
Right						
Step Length	(cm)	50.4	5.76	44.7	6.43	113%
Weight Accept	(% cycle)	7.3	1.93	7.7	1.68	95%
Single Support	(% cycle)	43.3	4.52	42.7	1.85	101%
Weight Release	(% cycle)	7.3	2.17	7.7	1.68	96%
Stance	(% cycle)	57.6	4.49	57.3	1.85	101%
Swing	(% cycle)	42.4	4.49	42.7	1.85	99%

Fig. 8.2, *contd.* (*h*) Patient BN. Postoperative. Temporal spatial measurements, barefoot. Stance and swing phases are nearly normal walking barefoot compared with the preoperative data. Weight release preoperatively barefoot was 75% of the cycle and postoperatively 55%. The preoperative and postoperative data are not dramatic variations from normal values.

TABLE 8.III
Pre- and postoperative energy analysis and balance measurement, patient BN, spastic diplegia, Fig. 8.2 (a-h)

Energy analysis (tested barefoot)

Floor walking speed (m/min); mean (SD) †

	Preoperative		Postoperative 13 months		
Control					
Slow 39 (11)	Comfortable 70 (11)	Fast 105 (12)	Controls same		
Patient			*Patient*		
Slow 60.5	Comfortable 71.6	Fast 66.7	Slow 58.2	Comfortable 66.7	Fast 72.2

Energy Expenditure Index (EEI) (beats/min) ‡

Control					
Slow 0.7 (0.3)	Comfortable 0.5 (0.1)	Fast 0.6 (0.2)	Controls same		
Patient			*Patient*		
Slow 0.99	Comfortable 1.06	Fast 0.72	Slow 0.89	Comfortable 0.96	Fast 1.0

Balance (tested barefoot) *
Parameter mean (SD)

	Eyes open	Eyes open	
	Normal	Patient	Patient
Path length (cm/sec)	1.1 (0.3)	1.1 (0.1)	1.1 (0.24)
Average radial displacement (cm)	0.5 (0.1)	1.4 (0.4)	1.4 (0.21)
	Eyes closed	Eyes closed	
Path length (cm/sec)	1.5 (0.4)	1.4 (0.5)	1.3 (0.12)
Average radial displacement (cm)	0.5 (0.1)	1.0 (0.2)	0.9 (0.26)

† Pre- and postoperative walking speeds are not significantly changed

‡ Pre- and postoperative energy expenditures are slightly less postoperatively on slow and comfortable walking, but somewhat greater on faster pace.

*Center of pressure is the centroid with respect to the feet. Average radial displacement is the radial deviation of the center of pressure centroid relative to the mean centroid location. Path length is the distance traveled by the centroid per second and primarily influenced by way frequency. The radial displacement is influenced by sway amplitude.

The balance data show a postoperative increase in the average radial displacement. This indicates that the center of pressure between feet has moved outside the base of support. The path lengths are unchanged and indicate no increase in body sway frequency.

complexity of gait analysis, the obvious professional time consumed, and to appreciate what goes into 'evidence-based' studies now being demanded. We wonder if a software program could be developed to sort out only the abnormal findings in the massive amount of data. Schutte and colleagues (2000) attempted to do so. Obviously more studies and more techniques and more money would be needed to develop and simplify outcome analysis.

Pediatric orthopaedic surgeons at several centers worldwide have reported the results of surgery in spastic diplegia. A prospective study of 30 patients using gait analysis for kinematic changes in the joints, temporal gait factors (25% increase in velocity and 18% increase in stride length), documented improvements in these parameters that were maintained 2 years after surgery (Abel *et al.* 1999). GMFM scores changed little as might be expected in spastic diplegia in these children with a mean age of 8.7 years. But they did improve significantly in standing, walking, running and jumping.

Zwick and colleagues (2001) from Graz, Austria, have used gait analysis in spastic diplegia before and after surgery. Postoperative improvements in the kinematics of the ankle, hip and knee were noted. Kinetic studies demonstrated that most of the power generation was in the hip muscles while the ankle contributed only a small part. Power generation at the hip in stance and at the ankle during push-off indicated the importance of function of the muscles at these joint levels.

Gait velocity as a temporal measurement in gait analysis was studied in 47 patients by Kay and associates (2001) of Los Angeles to see if gait velocity would predict a surgical outcome. Alas, this simple measurement was not increased reliably in all children with cerebral palsy who had surgery, particularly if they were older than 12 years. Of note is that the diagnosis, type of surgery, number of procedures done or the preoperative ambulation level did not predict postoperative velocity.

Will my child walk faster after surgery?—Not necessarily.
Will he walk better?—We expect so.

Additional outcome measurements for walking, such as the Gillette Functional Assessment Questionnaire (FAQ) (Novacheck *et al.* 2000) and the Pediatric Orthopaedic Society of North America (POSNA) Musculoskeletal Functional Health Questionnaire (Tervo *et al.* 2002), have been found to be useful and valid as clinical measures. Investigators use these questionnaires along with instrumented gait analysis to determine effectiveness of orthopaedic surgery.

EVOLUTION OF GAIT FUNCTION IN SPASTIC DIPLEGIA

Three studies of the natural history of gait in spastic diplegia should provide the justification for orthopaedic surgery. Bell *et al.* (2002) studied with instrumented gait analysis 28 children of whom 19 had diplegia, seven had hemiplegia and two with quadriplegia. None had surgery. Assessments were at least 2 years apart with a mean of 4.4 years (SD 2.2) between the tests. At the time of the first examination the mean age was 7.8 years (SD 2.4) and on the second examination the mean age was 12.2 years (SD 3.8). The results of the detailed assessments demonstrated a decrease in stride and temporal parameters, gait kinematics and passive range of motion over time. Peak hip extension in stance worsened between tests. Hip rotation in stance did not change. The knee range of motion deteriorated in the sagittal plane along with peak knee flexion in swing. Highly significant decreases in motion were at the ankle. The clinical measurement of the ranges of motion revealed a decline in hip abduction and the popliteal angle. Of concern was a lack of correlation of the passive joint range of motion measure and joint function in gait. The concern was in using the passive range of joint motion as the sole tool in surgical decisions.

Complementing the foregoing study, an earlier study of the natural history of gait in spastic diplegia was by Johnson *et al.* (1997) in 18 patients with spastic diplegia age 4–14 years during a time interval of a mean of 32 months. The analysis with 3D gait analysis confirmed deterioration of the gait over the period of time. Loss of excursion of the pelvis, ankle and knee were statistically significant. A cross-sectional study Norlin and Odenrick (1986) reported a decrease in cadence and an increase in stance duration as the age of the patient with spastic cerebral palsy increased.

TIMING OF ORTHOPAEDIC SURGERY

Surgery for improvement of gait cannot be performed until the child has actually developed a gait pattern that can be observed and, if facilities are available, measured in a laboratory. Although the mature gait pattern develops at about the age of 7 years (Sutherland *et al.* 1980), it is reasonably close to the mature pattern before this age. The consensus is that most of the surgical treatment can be accomplished between the ages of 4 and 8 years (Rang *et al.* 1986). In spastic diplegia we strive to finish the more formal and intensive treatment program by this age.

Surgery should only be done earlier than age 4–8 years if there are structural changes such as subluxation of the hip, contracture of the knee joint due to spastic hamstrings and, in rare cases, a contracture of the gastrocnemius–soleus muscles.

Surgery should not be regarded as the last resort or as 'something that can be done when all other methods have failed'. The increased incidence of postoperative psychological problems in adolescents (Williams, 1977), and the sudden disruption of the body-image which appears to reach its peak during adolescence, are probably related to the more frequent emotional upheavals and slow recovery from surgery in this age-group.

In spastic diplegia orthopaedic surgery is confined to the lower limb. Surgery should not be unduly staged so that the phenomenon of marking birthdays with surgery and hospitalization becomes the predominant feature of life for the child with cerebral palsy (Figs 6.23, 8.2). With careful clinical examinations and analysis combined with the information gleaned from gait analysis, multilevel surgery (ankle, knee,

hip) at one stage has been found effective by many orthopaedic surgeons (Hadley *et al.* 1992, Norlin and Tkaczuk 1992, Nene *et al.* 1993, Fabry *et al.* 1999, Patrick *et al.* 2001, Saraph *et al.* 2002). Although simultaneous operations on the ankle, knee and hip are quite feasible, the decision on the right procedure demands exposition of the complex functional and structural deformities and their surgical management. So it is necessary to discuss each as a separate entity even though they almost always coexist. We expect that the surgeon has the ability to synthesize into the whole of the gait pattern with the assistance of instrumented gait analysis if available or at the minimum depend on the published accounts of gait analysis in the normal and in spastic diplegia preoperative and postoperative orthopaedic surgery.

The preoperative assessment and decisions for multilevel surgery will consume more time than the operation.

The task for the surgeon is to carefully examine and reexamine the patient's gait, joints and muscles so that the appropriate surgical procedures can be combined and excessive staging avoided (Fig. 8.3). The preoperative assessment and decisions for multilevel surgery will consume more time that the operation. Even orthopaedic surgeons need 'cognitive skills'—a paradigm enunciated by specialists in internal medicine in the context of better fees. Orthopaedic surgery in the lower limb in spastic diplegia is relatively simple and so allows one stage multilevel surgery to be feasible and not excessively traumatic. Examination techniques have been described in Chapter 2 and measurement methods (gait analysis) in Chapter 3.

POSTURE AND GAIT PATTERNS
IN DIPLEGIA

When we observe the posture and gait of a child with spastic diplegia anywhere in the world it is as though each child came from the same mold. The common pattern in the frontal plane

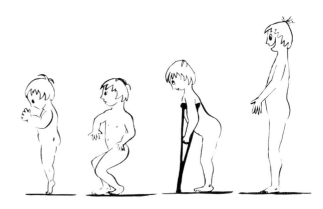

Fig. 8.3. Usual staging of orthopaedic surgery in spastic diplegia to be avoided. *From left to right*: talipes equinus; crouch after Achilles tendon lengthening; crouch corrected by hamstring lengthening; final erect posture after hip-flexion contracture corrected. (Drawing reproduced by courtesy of the artist, Mercer Rang MD, Toronto.)

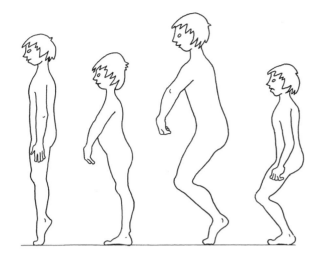

Fig. 8.4. Gait and posture patterns in spastic diplegia (Rodda and Graham 2001). (*A*) True equinus. Ankles in equinus, hip and knee in extension throughout stance. (*B*) True equinus. Can be hidden when patient stands with feet flat; knee bends into recurvatum. (*C*) Jump without stiff knee. Ankle equinus, knee and hip in flexion. Jump with stiff knee is the same posture as in panel A during gait with a spastic quadriceps overpowering the hamstrings. (*D*) Crouch. Excessive ankle dorsiflexion and excessive knee and hip flexion. Most common after too much lengthening of the Achilles tendon.

is flexed, adducted and internally rotated hips. In the sagittal plane we see an increased anterior pelvic tilt, lumbar lordosis, either flexed or hyperextended knees, and equinus.

Rodda and Graham (2001) drew from a variety of sources to publish a classification of posture and gait patterns in spastic diplegia and construct an algorithm of management. Sagittal patterns were as follows:

1. *True equinus.* The ankles are in plantarflexion throughout stance and the hips and knees extended. The equinus can be hidden when the patient stands flat foot; the knee is then in recurvatum. The relationship between the foot–ankle and knee is a plantarflexion–knee extension couple (PF–KE). A strong gastrocnemius–soleus controls forward progression of the tibia during stance. The ground reaction force vector falls anterior the the knee joint to provide an extensor moment to the knee and reduces the demand on the quadriceps. If the gastrocnemius–soleus is overlengthened a crouch gait results.

Botulinum toxin injections into the gastrocnemius in dynamic equinus (4U/kg each side) may be helpful. If a contracture is present, lengthening of the gastrocnemius is the preferred management.

2. *Jump gait—with or without a stiff knee.* The jump is due to spasticity of the hamstrings, hip flexors and calf muscles. The ankle is in equinus, the knee and hip in flexion, and an anterior pelvic tilt with increased lumbar lordosis. The stiff knee gait is due to the spastic quadriceps.

In young children the equinus can be managed short term with botulinum toxin injections of the gastrocnemius and hamstrings and an ankle–foot orthosis (AFO). As the child ages (between the ages of 4 and 8 years), multilevel surgery consisting of gastrocnemius, hamstring (with transfer of the distal rectus

femoris tendon as indicated by limited knee flexion on swing – < 35°) and iliopsoas lengthening.

3. *Crouch gait* is due to excessive ankle dorsiflexion and the ankle with excessive flexion of the hip and knee. The commonest cause is overlengthening of the Achilles tendon. Management requires iliopsoas and hamstring lengthening, a ground-reaction AFO to restrict forward progression of the tibia, osteotomies to correct excessive medial femoral and lateral tibial torsion, as well as correction/stabilization of the pes valgus.

Coronal- and transverse-plane problems are mainly excessive hip adduction and hip internal rotation. Surgical management is adductor longus myotenotomy for the adduction deformity and femoral derotation osteotomy for the internal femoral torsion. The above classification was detailed by Bleck (1987) with reference to the effects of the hip-flexion deformity, but without the concept of Gage's 'lever arm dysfunction'.

O'Byrne and colleagues (1998) of Seattle, Washington, described a technique using quantitative data of the hip, knee, and ankle in the sagittal plane in 55 hemiplegic and 91 diplegic patients. From these studies of kinematics using cluster statistical analysis they derived eight groups of gait patterns, e.g. stiff leg gait, genu recurvatum and crouch gait. They proposed their system to automatically classify the gait patterns in the spastic types of cerebral palsy. Whether this system is helpful in reaching decisions for specific surgery at all levels is not known.

Classification of gait patterns in spastic diplegia has branched out across the Pacific to Taiwan. Here Lin *et al.* of the National Cheng Kung University (2000) categorized the gait patterns in 23 children by the kinetic characteristics that defined internal moments at the knee. The four patterns were jump, crouch, recurvatum and mild cases. By defining the kinetic patterns they hoped this would help in the management of the patient. But they did not report how they applied this knowledge to clinically test the method of classification, except that the 'mild' cases had kinetic data close to that found in unaffected children and therefore needed no treatment. This should be a plus for the children who have the classification of 'mild'—no weekly physical therapy sessions, orthotics or surgery.

LEVER-ARM DYSFUNCTION

As an introduction to elementary physics, Dr Jim Gage (Gage 1991; Gage and Novacheck 2001) introduced the concept of 'lever-arm dysfunction' (also termed 'lever-arm disease' by Rodda and Graham 2001) in the gait of cerebral palsy. A moment is defined as a force acting on a lever creating motion or acceleration around an axis. A lever-arm or moment-arm is the perpendicular distance between a force and the fulcrum. Lever-arms are three-dimensional in the body involving planes in flexion/extension, abduction/adduction, internal/external rotation. The force as measured in Newtons when multiplied by the length of the lever-arm in meters is equal to the moment that acts around the center of rotation (or fulcrum). A moment or the magnitude of a moment is expressed in *Newton-meters* [moment = force (Newtons) × lever-arm (meters)]. In the skeleton the lever acts along the length of the bone and the joint at the end of the bone

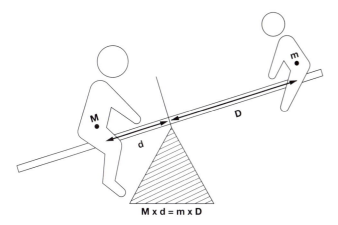

Fig. 8.5 Larger and smaller children can balance each other on a teeter-totter (see-saw) by varying their distance from the fulcrum. In gait the skeleton acts as the lever, the muscle or ground reaction force creates the force perpendicular to the lever, and the joint acts as the fulcrum to create a moment. This is useful for throwing a ball but not for moving a mountain. (Reproduced from Gage 1991, by permission.)

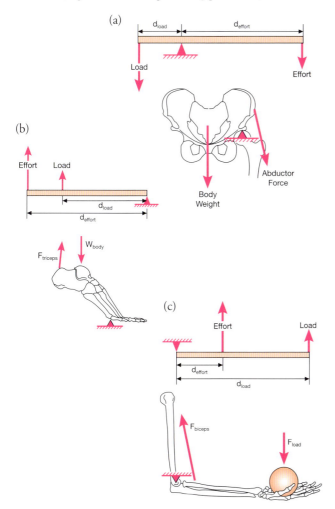

Fig. 8.6 Three classes of levers with musculosketal examples. (*a*) First-class lever with fulcrum in the middle; as in the hip joint during single limb support. (*b*) Second-class lever with the load in the middle; as in the foot during push-off where the heads of the metatarsals serve as the fulcrum. (*c*) Third-class lever with the force in the middle. This is useful for throwing a ball but not to move a mountain. (Reproduced from Gage and Schwartz 2002, by permission.)

is the center of rotation or fulcrum. As an example of moments, the see-saw may help to clarify matters.[3] The physics of muscle forces uses similar principles as see-sawing. Children of unequal weight can balance each other by varying the distance to the fulcrum so that Force × distance equals force × Distance. As the child pushes off the ground he creates a moment (Fig. 8.5). Similarly, in the skeleton, muscles create force through the lever-arm of the bones and motion around the joint which acts as a fulcrum.

There are three classes of levers which are all represented in the musculoskeletal system. These are based on the relative positions of the fulcrum (axis of motion), the load and the force. The see-saw is an example of a first-class lever where the fulcrum is in the middle of the load and the force. Use of a crowbar to lift an object is another example. Use of the principles of first-class levers to allow movement of great forces with a smaller force helped build the Egyptian pyramids and the great cathedrals of Europe. In the body, this type of lever action is used through the pelvis during single limb support. In this case the hip acts as the fulcrum while the hip-abductors are the force countering the load of body weight (Fig. 8.6). In a second-class lever the load is in the middle of the effort and the fulcrum. A common example of this is the wheelbarrow. During gait this principle is noted through the foot–ankle complex at push-off when the metatarsal phalangeal joints of the foot serve as the fulcrum of motion with the load of body weight more central and countered by the force generated by the ankle plantarflexors. Third-class levers have the effort or force in the middle and the fulcrum and load at either end of the lever. In the body this occurs through the elbow and forearm when lifting an object in the hand or throwing a ball (Fig. 8.7).

As can be noted around the ankle, the class of lever varies with the particular phase of the gait cycle. For example, as the foot accepts weight during loading response, the fulcrum is the heel, body weight comes down through the ankle and the force-resisting body weight comes from the ankle dorsiflexors and long toe extensors acting on the forefoot. The foot is thus acting as a second-class lever (similar to a wheelbarrow being pulled). In mid-stance, when the foot is plantargrade, the foot acts as first-class lever with the fulcrum at the ankle. The ground reaction force pushing up on the forefoot is resisted by the force of the soleus acting on the os calcis (lie a teeter-totter). Finally, in terminal stance the foot reverts to the status of a second-class lever with the fulcrum at the metatarsal heads. Now, body weight is coming through the ankle, and muscle force generated by the plantarflex-ors is acting on the os calcis (similar to a wheelbarrow being pushed). Since the heel is off the ground, we essentially have a

---

3 A see-saw (teeter-totter) is common in children's playgrounds. It is a long plank that is balanced on a central fulcrum. When one person is seated at each end, one end goes up while the other goes down. If a boy on one end has a large mass (e.g. weight 200 lb) it is multiplied by his distance from the fulcrum which is equal to the mass of the lighter boy (weight 100 lb) multiplied by his distance from the fulcrum. The further the lightweight boy is from the fulcrum the greater the length of the lever arm needed to counter balance the heavier boy at the other end.

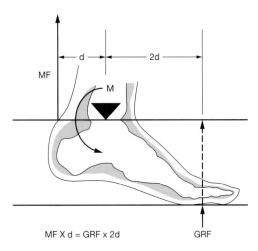

MF X d = GRF x 2d

Fig. 8.7 Ground reaction force acts on the foot during gait and the gastrocsoleus muscles act on the skeletal levers of the forefoot and hindfoot. Since the distance of the forefoot to the ankle fulcrum is twice that of the hindfoot to the ankle fulcrum, the forces posteriorly must be double the GRF to balance. (Reproduced from Gage 2004, Fig. 4.6, p.48, by permission.)

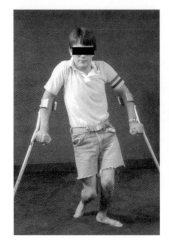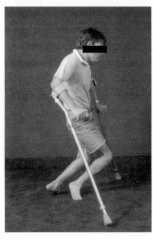

Fig. 8.8. Teenager with spastic diplegia. Knee-flexion contracture, lever-arm dysfunction, external tibial torsion, valgus feet.

wheelbarrow situation, which is what occurs during third rocker. Therefore the muscle force is acting at a distance of 3d from the fulcrum (the metatarsal heads) and the load at a distance of 2d. The mechanical advantage in that situation would be 3/2 = 1.5 (that is, one Newton of force would lift 1½ Newtons of weight). In second rocker during mid-stance, when the foot is flat on the floor and the ankle is the fulcrum, we have a true first-class lever in which case Muscle Force × d = GRF × 2d (Gage 2004) (Fig. 8.7).

The ground reaction force in walking produces external moments; forces due to inertia and the segment weights are resisted by internal moments generated by muscle action, tendons and/or ligaments.[4] Muscles and/or ground reaction forces act most effectively on rigid bony levers which are in the line of progression to produce walking.

Deformities of the lever-arm interfere with walking ability. Gage and co-authors, Novacheck (2001) and Schwartz (2002) identified five types of lever-arm deformity: (1) short lever-arm (coxa valga); (2) flexible lever-arm (pes valgus); (3) malrotated lever-arm (external tibial torsion; femoral torsion); (4) abnormal pivot or action point (hip subluxation /dislocation); (5) positional lever-arm dysfunction (erect versus crouch gait).

As an example of common lever-arm dysfunction in spastic diplegia, Gage *et al.* (2001) explained that in the stance phase of gait, knee stability is maintained without quadriceps muscle contraction. This is due to the 'plantarflexion/knee-extension couple'. The contraction of the soleus muscle restrains the forward progression of the tibia over the foot to keep the ground reaction force anterior to the knee. The ground reaction force acts on the leg lever-arm so that the knee joint is kept in extension without

quadriceps muscle function. If the lever-arm is crooked or twisted as in external tibial torsion (i.e. greater than the normal mean of 20º), the magnitude of the extension moment acting on the knee will be reduced. The clinical message of the concept of lever-arm dysfunction in abnormal gait patterns is to correct the skeletal deformity of the lever-arm (Fig. 8.8).

SURGICAL PROCEDURES

Rather than review the century-long history of orthopaedic surgery in cerebral palsy, Table 8.IV lists past and discarded interventions and current favored operative procedures, i.e. what's in and what's out. Approval of specific surgery is a process of osmosis among the orthopaedic surgical community as it spreads through the voluminous medical literature, seminars, conferences, meetings, instructional courses, and personal informal exchange. Disapproval based on disappointing results is not often expressed in publications even though negative reports capture the interest of surgeons. Generally we pay more attention to reports of negative results probably because part of our human nature is the mood expressed as *Schadenfreude*.[5] Physicians traditionally are skeptics.

Muscle–tendon lengthenings in spastic cerebral palsy do change the gait pattern in some measurable parameters. Other than kinematic and kinetic data, joint angular velocity appears to be an important change. This was measured in 73 age-matched normal controls and spastic gait patterns in 40 patients with a mean age of 8.3 years by Granata *et al.* (2000) of the University of Virginia. Joint angular velocity was measured before and 9 months after surgery. The measurements of the ankle, knee and hip showed only changes in the reduced ankle dorsiflexion velocity at foot strike and improved dorsiflexion velocity through mid-stance. Hip- and knee-joint angular velocities

---

4 Inertia as used in physics is defined as the tendency of a body at rest to resist acceleration, to remain at rest, or to stay in motion in a straight line unless disturbed by an external force.

5 *Schadenfreude* (German): malicious pleasure; connotes joy (*freude*) at another's misfortune (*schaden*: damage, harm). The term is frequently used by contemporary journalists and essayists in current English publications.

TABLE 8.IV
Past history, refinements and simplification of orthopaedic surgery in spastic diplegia

Gait deformity	Current preferred surgery What's in ☺	Past and abandoned surgery What's out ☹
Hip adduction	Adductor longus myotenotomy	Obturator neurectomy Adductor brevis myotenotomy Adductor origin transfer to ischium Gracilis myotomy
Hip-flexion contracture	Iliopsoas tenotomy at or above pelvic brim (lengthening, recession) Z-lengthening iliopsoas tendon	Iliopsoas tenotomy at lesser trochanter Iliopsoas recession Iliopsoas transfer to greater trochanter Ober–Yount fasciotomy Soutter or Campbell muscle-slide Proximal rectus femoris tenotomy Myotomy of anterior gluteus medius
Hip internal rotation	Femoral subtrochanteric derotation osteotomy	Posterior transfer origin tensor fascia femoris Adductor longus myotomy and ant. obturator neurectomy or transfer adductor origins to ischium Neurectomy of superior gluteal nerve Gluteus medius and minimus transfer Transfer of semitendinosus to anterior-lateral femur
Knee flexion	Fractional hamstring lengthening	Transfer of hamstring insertions Proximal hamstring origin release
Knee extension with limited knee flexion on swing	Transfer distal tendon of rectus femoris tendon	Proximal rectus femoris tenotomy Distal rectus femoris tenotomy
Excessive tibial torsion	Tibial derotation osteotomy (proximal or distal)	Ignoring lever-arm dysfunction
Equinus	Gastrocnemius aponeurosis lengthening (modifications)	Tendoachilles lengthening (except rarely) Gastrocnemius or soleus neurectomy Transfer Achilles insertion
Pes valgus	Medial displacement calcaneal osteotomy Subtalar extra-articular arthroreisis STA-peg arthroreisis Lengthening calcaneal osteotomy Triple arthrodesis at maturity as last resort	Calcaneal (posterior open wedge) osteotomy Peroneus brevis tenotomy or transfer

were unchanged. Electromyographic data changed to reduced amplitude of the gastrocnemius–soleus during the loading phase and decreased activation of the hamstrings and quadriceps at toe-off. The data suggested that the underlying neural stimulus of the knee and hip remained unchanged. The most important effect of was an altered response to stretch of the gastrocnemius–soleus muscle. Does this study mean we should do nothing about the hip flexion or adduction contracture and only concentrate on the ankle and foot? We think not. The purpose of the study was to show that joint-angle data offered better discrimination between gait patterns of normal and subjects with cerebral palsy.

HIP

HIP-ADDUCTION DEFORMITY
In the past, surgeons focused almost exclusively on the hip-adductors and the Achilles tendon as the surgery of choice in cerebral palsy. Because of knowledge of muscle function derived from gait analysis and the more critical appraisal of outcomes and many more publications, the consensus among orthopaedic surgeons has reduced the surgery for the hip-adduction deformity to one simple procedure in spastic diplegia.

ANATOMY, PHYSIOLOGY AND BIOMECHANICS
The adductor muscles of the hip originate from the pubis anteriorly and insert on the femur medially. Strange (1965) proposed that anatomically the hip-adductors function as external rotators. They are innervated by the obturator nerve, except for one half of the adductor magnus which is supplied by the tibial division of the sciatic nerve. The anterior branch of the obturator nerve supplies the adductor longus and gracilis and usually the adductor brevis; the posterior branch distributes branches to the adductor magnus and brevis when the brevis does not receive a branch from the anterior division (Gardner *et al.* 1969, Clemente 1985).

Electromyograms of the adductors during level gait in normal persons have demonstrated that they contract at the end of stance phase (Fig. 8.9). Murray and Sepic (1968) showed that the maximum output of the gluteus medius and minimus muscles (hip adductors) occurs when the hip is in 5° of adduction. Matsuo *et al.* (1984, 1986), in a clinical study of the results of adductor myotomy with and without obturator neurectomy, concluded that the adductor brevis is an important antigravity muscle in quadripedal and bipedal locomotion, and essential for a stable erect posture. However, Matsuo (2002) still believes the gracilis is important.

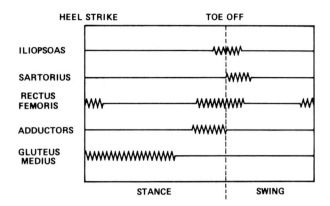

Fig. 8.9. Normal electromyograms of hip muscles in level gait.

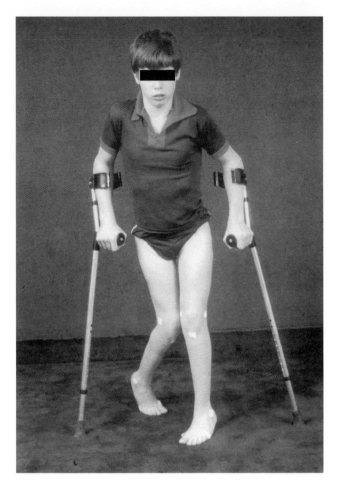

Fig. 8.10. Spastic diplegia, age 14 years. Does he have hip internal rotation or adduction? Ranges of motion each hip: abduction 30°, extension −35°, internal rotation 90°, external rotation 10°. A case of 'pseudo-adduction' (Steinwender *et al.* 2001).

The function of the hip abductors during gait has been well established (Inman 1947, Saunders *et al.* 1953); these muscles are essential for energy conservation because they prevent excessive lateral shift of the trunk during the single-limb phase of stance when their action pulls the pelvis down on the weightbearing limb. Approximately 2 cm of lateral trunk shift occurs quickly from limb to limb during level walking. Without good functioning of abductor muscles, a lurching gait occurs which expends high levels of energy.

The hip-adductor muscles fire during stance phase and keep the femur in approximately 5° adduction during stance. Adduction of the femur is necessary for optimum function of the hip abductors. Abduction of the femur beyond 0° during the stance phase of walking weakens the abductors.

The base of the gait in normal subjects measures 5–10 cm from heel to heel, though in some individuals it may be as narrow as 1 cm (mean in children 7.6 cm, according to Scrutton 1969). These measurements are correlated with the need to keep the femora in slight adduction for efficient gait. Consequently, in children with spastic diplegia and adductor spasticity, the goal of treatment should be to keep the base of the gait within normal limits (5–10 cm) and not 'broad-based'. Standing with feet apart may be more restful when standing to attention, but the benefits do not carry over to walking.

The goal of treatment should be to keep the base of the gait within normal limits (5–10 cm) and not 'broad-based'.

Are the hip-adductors the main cause of the hip internal rotation gait pattern so common in children with spastic diplegia? The theory that the hip-adductor muscles are the culprit responsible for the in-toed gait pattern in these patients has been discarded. The former controversy probably arose because of differences in the perception of what constitutes hip internal rotation during gait—one surgeon's hip adduction may be another's internal rotation (Fig. 8.10). Steinwender and colleagues (2001a) of Graz, Austria, termed this perception 'pseudo-adduction'. They used computerized gait analysis in a study of diplegic children, half of whom had a crouch gait pattern and half did not. Children in both groups showed more internal rotation

in the first half of stance compared with unaffected children, most importantly the degree of hip adduction was the same in both groups.

Furthermore, adduction spasticity usually can be found simultaneously with hip-flexion spasticity and internal rotation during gait. Occasionally, we have observed the gait of children with spastic hemiplegic who internally rotated only the involved limb while walking. In these children no hip-adduction spasticity or contracture or the adductors could be found. As will be discussed in the section on hip internal rotation, the major anatomical pathology is excessive femoral anteversion 2 SD or more beyond the normal mean degree for age (properly termed 'torsion'). The gluteus medius is the major internal rotator muscle of the femur as described by Duchenne (1867). If the surgeon cuts its insertion on the greater trochanter, femoral rotation during gait is eliminated. But the trade-off is a severe gluteus medius limp.

Banks and Green (1960), in their report of 89 patients who had adductor myotomy and anterior branch obturator neurectomy, found that 15 had persistent hip internal rotation gait patterns postoperatively. Bleck (1987) observed the same results even after intrapelvic obturator neurectomy.

270

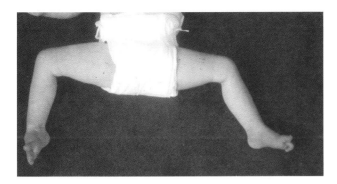

Fig. 8.11. Postoperative hip-abduction posture after adductor myotomy and anterior branch neurectomy, bilateral two months' abduction casting. Two-year-old patient with tension athetosis and dystonia. Lessons: do not mistake dystonia/ athetosis for spasticity. Rare indication for anterior branch neurectomy could be with spastic total body involvement. Use removable hip splint or brace when possible to monitor adductor tightness.

While electrical stimulation of the obturator nerve in surgery appears to cause hip internal rotation, a more careful observation shows that these patients have the knees flexed, so that as the heel rests on the table it acts merely as a pivot point which allows gravity to rotate the limb internally when adduction occurs. This phenomenon can be observed in normal awake children who have femoral torsion and their knees are splinted in flexion. When asked to bring the knees together voluntarily, they internally rotate the limb.

CLINICAL EXAMINATION

When the child walks, adduction spasticity is obvious and characterized by close approximation of the knees and thighs and a short stride-length. More severe adduction spasticity causes 'scissoring'—one limb crosses over the other.

The measurement of hip-adduction contracture is made with the hips in extension, the pelvis level and the child supine. When abducting one limb, the other needs to be held securely to prevent the pelvis from moving. The degree of abduction is determined with one limb of the goniometer placed along the line between the anterior superior iliac spines, and the other along the femur. With the hips flexed 90° the pelvis must be kept level by holding the other limb securely; not to do so allows the pelvis to rotate to the side of the abducted limb and a false measurement of hip abduction.

Athetosis and dystonic posturing must be differentiated from spasticity. With slow passive movements combined with relaxation of the patient, the lack of contracture of the muscle will be evident. In athetosis, particularly dystonic posturing, surgery to relieve the apparent adduction deformity may reverse to an abduction deformity (Fig. 8.11).

As might be expected, the electromyographic examination will show almost continuous activity of the adductor muscles during both phases of the gait (Fig. 8.12).

INDICATIONS FOR SURGERY

In the ambulatory patient, surgery to relieve adduction spasticity is indicated when each hip is limited in abduction to 20° or less with the hip extended, or when there is scissoring (Sharrard 1975). Hoffer's limit (1986) of passive abduction of the hip was 30° or less. Given the errors in accurate clinical measurements, we can compromise and state that the limits are between 20° and 30°.

When in doubt about the need for surgery and what its effects might be, myoneural blocks of the adductor longus with botulinum toxin may help make the decision (see Chapter 3). The belly of the muscle should be injected. An injection deep to the belly of the adductor longus in its proximal portion may block the anterior branch of the obturator nerve. The resulting paralysis of the adductor muscles will last about 3 months, which gives the physician, therapist, parents and patient sufficient time to observe the gait and make a decision for or against surgery. Lidocaine (1%) can also be used in older children and adults. However, Lidocaine may cause light-headedness often enough for a detailed and valid observation of the gait to be compromised; the dose to avoid toxicity needs to be remembered. Botulinum toxin intramuscularly has the advantage of a longer effect of paralyzing the muscle.

TYPES OF ADDUCTOR 'RELEASE'

'Release' appears as a general term for muscle-tendon surgery in cerebral palsy. But it is meaningless when the intended results of surgery demand specificity.

1. *Adductor longus and gracilis myotomy with anterior branch obturator neurectomy* used to be the recommended approach (Keats 1957, Banks and Green 1960, Silver *et al.* 1966, Samilson *et al.* 1967). However, in spastic diplegia a more critical appraisal of results has led to abandonment of the obturator neurectomy, which causes paralysis not only of the adductor longus but also

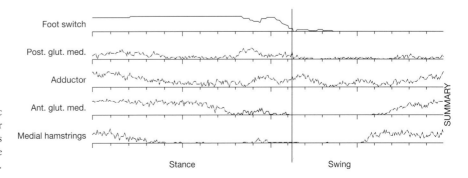

Fig. 8.12. Gait EMG of 8-year-old with spastic diplegia: shows continuous firing of adductor muscles (surface electrodes); gluteus medius appropriate stance-phase activity (fine-wire electrodes). Medial hamstring activity normal.

of the adductor brevis (in the majority of cases where the anterior branch of the nerve supplies the adductor brevis). The results were judged quite adequate, but surgeons did not recognize the effects of widening the base of the gait beyond normal and the need for adduction of the femur for the maximum pelvic stabilization of the hip during the stance phase of gait. Matsuo *et al.* (1984, 1986, Matsuo 2002) made the point that the adductor brevis is the main hip stabilizer, and the loss of its strength results in over-abduction of the hip. In an analysis of their 42 cases, they recommended cutting only the adductor longus to improve gait efficiency and preserve the function of the other adductor muscles, particularly the adductor brevis, which keep the femur slightly adducted during the stance phase of gait. Adduction of the femur during the stance phase maintains tension on the gluteus medius for maximum strength of muscle. Thus, it does not seem logical to cut the anterior branch of the obturator nerve in patients who are ambulatory; to do so risks paralysis of the adductor brevis. (In spastic diplegia anterior or posterior branch obturator neurectomy is not desirable or needed. Those who scissor rarely are independent ambulators who need no external support.)

Posterior and anterior branch obturator neurectomies produce too much weakening of the adductors. The broad-based hip-abducted gait pattern might appear to be 'stable' (like an A-frame), but it is definitely not functional.

2. *Adductor origin transfer to the ischial tuberosity (origin of the hamstrings)* first suggested by Perry in the flaccid paralysis of poliomyelitis to reinforce weakened hip-extensor muscles (Westin 1965, Garrett 1976) (Fig. 8.13).

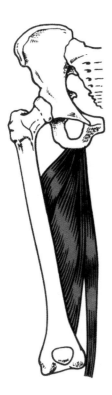

Fig. 8.13. Adductor origin transfer to ischial tuberosity. No longer popular among orthopaedic surgeons. Results no different than adductor longus myotenotomy.

After Stephenson and Donovan (1971) reported their results of transfer of the origins of the adductor longus, brevis and gracilis to the ischium in cerebral palsy, other surgeons also reported their results (Baumann 1972, Couch *et al.* 1977, Griffin *et al.* 1977, Baumann *et al.* 1978, Root and Spero 1981; E.B. Evans and M.M. Hoffer, personal communications).

In the end-result studies of this operation, one criterion of success appeared to be improvement of the hip internal rotation gait in two reports (Krom 1969, Couch *et al.* 1977). Another criterion for success was the measurement of the base of the gait. In the study by Couch *et al.* (1977), the mean preoperative measurement was 13.5 cm and the postoperative mean was 24 cm (range 12–37 cm). If the normal range is 5–10 cm, is the broad-based gait a satisfactory goal for optimum function?

Other studies on the results of adductor transfer have focused on the improvement of hip radiographs which assessed the degree of subluxation and/or acetabular dysplasia, utilizing the center edge (CE) angle method or the migration index of the femoral head (Reimers and Poulsen 1984, Schultz *et al.* 1984). Radiographs were also used to assess the results of adductor tenotomy and anterior branch obturator neurectomy by Wheeler and Weinstein (1984). None of these studies segregated potentially ambulatory patients from those who were ambulatory with or without support or were non-ambulatory. The importance of these functional differences in analyzing the results of surgery in prevention of subluxation and dislocation of the hip will be discussed in Chapter 9. The independently walking child with spastic diplegia rarely dislocates the hip, if ever, and only those who have partial weight bearing with crutches or walkers have subluxation.

Goldner (1981) challenged the need to transfer the origins of the adductor longus, brevis and gracilis to the ischium (1981); his operative question was 'compared to what'? He reported equally satisfactory results by merely recessing the detached muscles distally and anchoring them with a suture to the epimyesium overlying the adductor brevis. The same procedure appears to have been the unintended result by Loder *et al.* (1992) who found that after the adductor longus tendon was marked with a metallic marker at the time of transfer in 33 hips, it had pulled away from the ischium in 11 of 30 hips. Evidence of detachment of the transfer was higher in patients with spastic diplegia.

Scott and colleagues at the Shriners Hospital for Crippled Children in Houston, Texas, studied 33 ambulatory patients with gait analysis an average of 9.6 years after adductor transfer (Scott *et al.* 1996). Although functional improvement was observed, gait analysis documented pelvic obliquity in 85% and unilateral hip subluxation in 36%. Consequently, these surgeons abandoned adductor origin transfer.

Beals and colleagues from Portland, Oregon (1998), did a modified adductor transfer and in an average follow-up of 51 months were satisfied with their results because the passive range of hip abduction was improved 43° and maintained in 141 patients. However, their results need interpretation in the context of spastic diplegia because only nine of the patients were 'free' walkers; eight used walkers. The majority were non-walkers whose ages ranged from 18 months to 15 years (mean 5 years 10 months). Assessment of results was the effect on the migration index of the femoral head, the acetabular index, and the CE angles, and the range of abduction obtained and maintained. The modification was to do the adductor transfer on the most severe side of the adduction contracture if it was asymmetrical and then achieve asymmetry by 'release' on the other side. These surgeons transferred only the anterior half of the gracilis tendon to the ischium and then sutured the origin of the adductor brevis to the remaining posterior half of the gracilis. The adductor longus was sectioned at the origin and sutured with the anterior half of the gracilis to the adductor brevis. Improvement in abduction averaged 43°.

Adductor transfer appears to have no advantages, and in the few in which Bleck (1987) tagged the transferred origin with a metal clip, it was dismaying to see that the clip had moved distally from the ischial tuberosity in a radiograph made 24 hours postoperatively (Fig. 8.14). In effect the spasticity had performed Goldner's adductor origin recession postoperatively.

3. *Adductor longus myotenotomy*, allowing its proximal end to slide distally with a suture to anchor it to the underlying brevis, is simple and the choice for most patients with spastic diplegia. The consensus now seems to be to do only the adductor longus myotomy (Gage *et al.* 1996, Davids *et al.* 2001). According to long-standing recommendations and traditions of most orthopaedic surgeons, we also did a myotomy of the proximal portion of the gracilis in patients who are walking independently.

4. *Gracilis myotomy?* Following the party line and tradition of most orthopaedic surgeons, we also did a myotomy of the

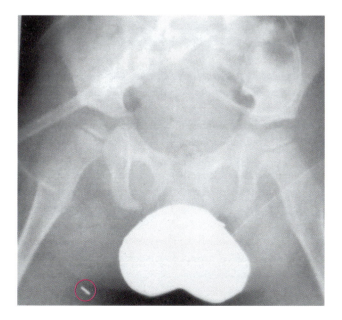

Fig. 8.14. Anterior–posterior radiographs of pelvis and hips made 18 hours postoperative bilateral adductor longus and gracilis transfer to ischium. Michele metallic clips placed at site of transfer; the clip on the left has retracted far distally from the ischium, while the right has remained in place. Results identical on both sides. Lorder *et al.* (1992) tagged the adductor longus tendon after transfer. Radiographs in 11 of 30 hips showed it had pulled away from the ischium.

proximal portion of the gracilis in patients who also had an adductor longus myotenotomy. But the indication for a gracilis myotomy seems to have been more tradition than science. It was initiated by Phelps (1959), who reasoned that because the gracilis originates from the symphysis pubis it exerted a diagonal force directed proximally and medially to cause a dislocation of the hip. Phelps based his decision to cut the gracilis on a test done with the patient supine and the knee flexed 90° with the hips abducted to the maximum. Then, with gradual extension of the knee if the hip adducts, a 'tight' gracilis was deemed responsible for the adduction deformity of the hip, and the muscle should be cut.

The gracilis muscle, along with the iliacus and sartorius, and in contrast to the hip-adductors, acts only in the initial swing phase of gait to advance the thigh. As two joint muscles the gracilis and sartorius also contribute to swing phase flexion of the knee in initial and early swing (65%–75% of the gait cycle) (Perry 1992). In light of the electromyographic studies, cutting the slender gracilis muscle in a dynamic spastic adduction of the hip and sacrificing its function on the knee during gait does not seem rational. Furthermore, no study confirms that a myotomy of the gracilis prevents subluxation of the hip. It seems we can safely eliminate gracilis myotomy. But Matsuo (2002) continues to believe that it is important to section this muscle near its origin.

5. *Intrapelvic obturator neurectomy* may be indicated in those patients in whom an anterior branch obturator neurectomy has failed to relieve a sufficient amount of adductor spasticity, and its only indication may be in the total body involved non-ambulatory patient (Fig. 8.15). It must be combined with adductor tenotomy and myotomy to correct the adduction contracture of the hips (Samilson *et al.* 1967). Certainly, it is never indicated in spastic diplegia.

What to choose for excess adduction of the hip in spastic diplegia? For functional improvement of gait in spastic diplegia, adductor longus myotenotomy seems quite sufficient for the majority. It should not be done just because it's there. The temptation to do the quick and easy subcutaneous adductor longus tenotomy should be resisted. Not only can one inadvertently cut the saphenous vein or one of its branches, one can also risk a recurrence of the adduction contracture in 75% of cases who had subcutaneous adductor myotenotomies (Feyen *et al.* 1984).

For functional improvement of gait in spastic diplegia, adductor longus myotenotomy seems quite sufficient in the majority.

OPERATIVE TECHNIQUE FOR ADDUCTOR LONGUS MYOTENOTOMY

The linear incision begins about 2 cm distal to the origin of the adductor longus and continues along the longus for 4–5 cm. The deep fascia is incised, and with blunt dissection the posterior portion of the muscle is clearly defined and separated from the adductor brevis. A myotenotomy of the adductor longus can be done with remarkably little bleeding. The longus muscle is put under stretch by putting a hemostat under the muscle. The tip of a second hemostat is used closed to bluntly divide the muscle

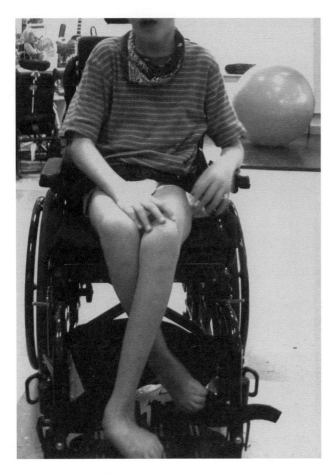

Fig. 8.15. Total body involved adolescent. Crossed lower limbs. Intrapelvic obturator neurectomy may be indicated if spastic paralysis—not athetosis or dystonia.

belly transversely just distal to the musculotendinous junction. The muscle divided this way seldom bleeds much. The anterior branch of the obturator nerve will not be inadvertently cut using this technique. No suturing of the longus is needed. Any small fascia or tendon slips that do not divide bluntly can be divided with a scalpel. The hip is abducted to about 40°.

To prevent the postoperative wound hematoma, all bleeding points are electrocoagulated and large veins ligated or avoided. Wound closure is with absorbable subcutaneous and subcuticular sutures, reinforced with sterile adhesive tapes. In young children, who may urinate uncontrollably after surgery, sealing of the wounds with a collodian dressing prevents infection, maceration and delayed wound healing.

If anterior branch obturator neurectomy is thought necessary in the severe total body involved patient (spastic quadriplegia), the nerve and its branches can be seen within the veil of connective tissue on the surface of the adductor brevis. The branches are stimulated by pinching with the hemostat or by an electric stimulus to make sure these are indeed the nerves. Then with a hemostat the nerves are isolated, picked up and cut distal to the hemostat and dissected proximally for about 2 cm to the point where the main anterior branch is cut.

POSTOPERATIVE CARE

In children, postoperative immobilization with a hip abduction brace or abduction pillow used at night to keep each hip in 30°–40° of abduction for three weeks is sufficient. Forced over-abduction can lead to compression of the articular surfaces of the hip joints and may result in postoperative stiffness. Within a few days, the patients can be mobilized as soon as they are comfortable, with graduation to crutches or a walker, and if they have adequate equilibrium reactions can resume independent walking.

Some surgeons advocated the use of abduction splints at night to maintain the correction. Houkom *et al.* (1986) studied the incidence of hip subluxation with and without nap- and night-bracing after surgery for an average of 10.5 months. They concluded that bracing lowered the incidence of recurrent subluxation of the hip. However, 10 of 21 braced patients developed abduction contractures; two of 36 unbraced children had abduction contractures. Their recommendation was to use a Lorenz-type brace with a thoracic extension for nap- and night-time use for at least 1 year. This brace holds the thighs in 90° flexion and 60° abduction. Perhaps this degree of desired abduction obtained at surgery and the postoperative regimen might apply to non-ambulatory total body involved children with hip subluxation. In their series of 57 patients, only nine were classified as 'assisted ambulators'. Consequently, in spastic diplegic children, postoperative night splinting (especially with the hips flexed 90°) is probably not applicable or necessary. Early mobilization, active hip-abduction exercise (preferably in a swimming pool) and early ambulation seem more physiological in spastic diplegia.

Furthermore, we are not absolutely certain that the braces are really used as specified. Compliance in the Houkom *et al.* study (1986) was assessed by interview with the parents. We presume that the parents were candid. But parents often do not want to disobey the physician and earn his wrath for not complying with directions. Consequently, we remain skeptical of night bracing and its efficacy. We are against night-bracing. The parents have enough do to and enough sleepless nights to impose this ritual without reasonable certainty of its effectiveness.

Early mobilization and ambulation without any postoperative immobilization has been used and found very satisfactory by Sussman (1984). He used Buck's skin traction on the lower limbs for a few days after surgery (to overcome the flexor spasms as the result of the first few days of postoperative pain), and then began an intensive physical therapy program which used passive positioning devices between therapy sessions. This regimen worked for Sussman primarily because his patients were confined to a rehabilitation type hospital for longer than the usual acute hospital stay of 3–5 days. In the United States, long hospitalization during the postoperative days was abandoned as a standard of care 30 or 40 years ago. Home care is possible with minimal disruption to the household.

In young adults who needed only a relief of their adductor spasticity and contracture by adductor tenotomy, cast immobilization postoperatively has not been necessary. A foam or sheepskin padded triangular wedge, the type used for postoperative total hip-joint replacement surgery, was easily tolerated and satisfactory for the first 6 weeks when combined with early resumption of ambulation and active and passive hip abduction exercise.

PROBLEMS WITH ADDUCTOR TENOTOMY WITH OR WITHOUT ANTERIOR BRANCH OBTURATOR NEURECTOMY

1. Failure to prevent continued subluxation and dislocation of the hip with adductor weakening alone. This problem will be discussed fully in Chapter 9.

2. Recurrence of the adduction contracture. Samilson *et al.* (1967) noted reattachment of the adductor tendons in only 23 of 178 adductor tenotomies. Recurrence of the adduction contracture in spastic diplegia after adductor longus myotenotomy has been very rare in our experience over a period of 40 years.

The fear of orthopaedic surgeons of recurrence of the deformity after surgery in cerebral palsy has probably led to too much 'release' of adductor muscles in the failure to appreciate the normal parameters of gait.

3. Failure to correct the hip internal rotation gait. This 'failure' is actually due to mistaking hip internal rotation in stance for adduction. Hip internal rotation during gait depends upon the degree of femoral torsion.

4. A broad-based gait with marked trunk lurch may result from too much adductor weakening. In spastic diplegia there is little or no indication for myotenotomy of the adductor brevis or for obturator neurectomy.

5. A permanent postoperative 'frog leg' or abduction deformity. This might be avoided by immobilization no longer than 3–6 weeks, and by not immobilizing the hips in exaggerated and forced abduction. Forced abduction can cause pressure necrosis of the articular cartilage of the hip joint (Salter and Field 1960). Samilson *et al.* (1967) had 13 total body involved patients whose hips were stiff in the 'frog-leg' position; 10 of these patients had been immobilized in double hip spica plasters for 2.4 months (Fig. 8.9 *b*).

Abduction deformities have been seen in patients who had athetosis and/or dystonic posturing, and adductor 'releases' with obturator neurectomies. Although preoperatively they probably had dynamic excessive adduction of the hips, the contracture was minimal. Before adductor-weakening surgery is performed on this type of patient, it is prudent to use myoneural blocks of the adductor longus and/or the anterior branch of the obturator nerve.

6. Wound infection. Samilson *et al.* (1967) had an increased infection rate with a transverse incision (of the 14 patients who had wound infection in a series of 189 operations, 12 had a transverse incision in the groin). The longitudinal incision is preferred. Also, careful hemostasis by the use of electrocautery and closed suction drainage of the wound for 24–48 hours should help reduce the infection rate.

Adductor myotenotomy, anterior branch obturator neurectomy and other adductor muscle weakening procedures were probably the most overused operations in cerebral palsy. Now,

with a better understanding of the physiology of normal gait and the mechanisms of the various hip deformities, more critical assessments have been done. The result seems to be fewer but more selective operations. As in 20th-century architecture, orthopaedic surgery in spastic diplegia has evolved to 'less is more'.[6]

As in 20th-century architecture, orthopaedic surgery in spastic diplegia has evolved to 'less is more'.

HIP-FLEXION DEFORMITY

Because 60% of the gait cycle is stance, adequate hip extension is necessary for maximum gait efficiency to ensure a good stride length (Fig. 8.16). A spastic hip-flexion contracture that limits extension provides the rationale for correction.

ANATOMY, PHYSIOLOGY AND BIOMECHANICS
Lacking an animal model that is bipedal and has spastic paralysis, we have to rely on anatomical, radiographic, electromyographic,

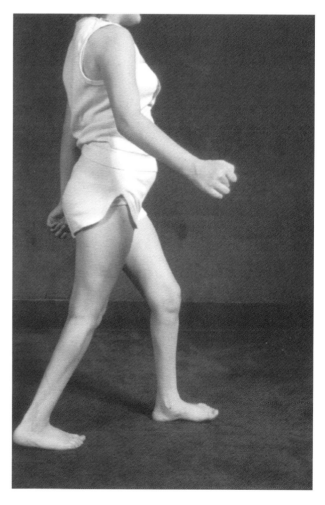

Fig. 8.16. Stance is 60% of the gait cycle so hip normal extension is necessary for optimum function.

6 Ludwig Mies van der Rohe, architect director of Bauhaus style, Berlin, 1930–33.

kinematic and kinetic studies of function of the hip-flexors. From this knowledge and surgical experience a consensus that the iliopsoas is the main cause of the hip-flexion contracture in cerebral palsy has developed.

The sartorius, tensor fascia femoris, rectus femoris, adductors and the iliopsoas are all considered to be flexors of the hip (Duchenne 1867, Brunnstrom 1962). Although these muscles act synergistically and vary with joint position, a consideration of their probable isolated function helps to determine the specific muscle or muscles that might produce flexion deformities in spastic paralysis.

The sartorius and rectus femoris flex the hip up to 90°, but are weak flexors. The rectus femoris is more effective if the knee flexes simultaneously. Our studies have shown that spasticity of the rectus femoris is not an isolated one, and that the vastus medialis and lateralis (and probably the vastus intermedius) share in the spasticity of the entire quadriceps (Csongradi *et al.* 1979).

The pectineus adducts the hip and also flexes it, though not beyond 90°. The adductor longus, brevis and magnus act as hip flexors from the hyperextended position, but not beyond 50°–70°. After these ranges the adductors become extensors. In the erect position, the lower portion of the adductor magnus is an extensor and this function increases as the joint is flexed. In the extended position, the adductor longus is a weak internal rotator. The gracilis acts as a flexor up to 20°–40° of flexion, and then it becomes an extensor.

Pure adductor spasticity in spastic diplegia is rare, and in a practice spanning over 40 years I have only encountered 10 cases of it (E.E.B). In these patients the amount of hip-flexion deformity was no greater than 10°. Furthermore, in three of these patients with a preoperative hip-flexion deformity when measured with the prone hip extension test of Staheli (see Chapter 2), no decrease in the hip-flexion contracture after adductor myotomy and anterior branch of obturator neurectomy resulted. Severe hip-flexion deformities in two total body involved patients who had bilateral intrapelvic obturator neurectomies were unchanged postoperatively using the prone hip-extension test (with the Thomas test in spastic hip flexion contractures you can measure any degree you want, from 0° to 60°) (Bleck 1987).

The *iliopsoas* is the main and powerful flexor of the hip. It is composed of the iliacus muscle, arising from the medial wall of the ilium, and the psoas portion, which originates from the transverse processes and sides of the bodies of all the lumbar vertebrae and the intervertebral disc annular ligaments from the 12th thoracic to the fifth lumbar interspaces. This psoas major muscle ends below the pelvic brim as a broad tendon which inserts into the lesser trochanter of the femur.

The fibers of the iliacus muscle join this tendon at its lateral edge. The psoas tendon is the most medial structure crossing the hip-joint capsule, and is obscured from view laterally by overlapping bulky fibers of the iliacus.

The psoas minor muscle is slender, anterior to the psoas major, and arises from the sides of the bodies of the 12th thoracic and first lumbar vertebra and the intervening intervertebral disc. It inserts into the arcuate (or terminal) line of the iliac fossa

and the iliopectineal eminence of the pelvis and sometimes it extends its lateral border into the iliac fascia. Because of its anatomy, this little muscle would seem unimportant in hip-flexion deformities.

Perry's studies (1992) show that 'the hip flexors advance the limb during swing, but the demand is low'. It is low because of the momentum generated in pre-swing initiated by the gastrocnemius–soleus that provides more than 80% of the acceleration force. This muscle complex provides the power to advance the limb and flex the knee and maintains the steady state for normal walking. But changing the speed of walking is dependent on the iliopsoas (Perry 1992). Although the plantarflexors of the ankle contribute most of the power generation in walking, kinetic studies of gait estimate that the hip-flexors account for 15%–20% (Gage *et al.* 1987, Winter 1987, Õunpuu *et al.* 1991). Because of the lower demand of the hip-flexors in walking, weakening them results in notable gait impairment. Electromyographic analyses of the psoas major while walking have shown that it contracts during heel rise (terminal stance) and the first 40% of the swing phase (Keagy *et al.* 1966, Morinaga 1973). The iliacus has a similar pattern (Hagy *et al.* 1973, Perry 1992) (Fig. 8.9).

The observations of paralysis of the iliopsoas by Brunnstrom (1962) correlates with the biomechanical factors. Walking on a level surface was possible without the muscle; the gait of a patient with a bilateral iliopsoas paralysis resulting from poliomyelitis was characterized by an anterior tilt of the pelvis and lumbar lordosis, and lacked speed and smoothness. But without an iliopsoas to flex the hip, the person cannot lift the foot more than a few inches from the ground, cannot climb stairs and cannot run or jog. Basmajian (1962) recorded continuous slight electrical activity of the iliacus while subjects were standing, and large action potentials in all degrees of hip flexion. The inability of the other hip-flexors to substitute completely for weakening of the iliopsoas should should preclude iliopsoas tenotomy in patients who can walk or who have the potential to do so based upon the prognostic signs for walking as described in Chapters 1 and 5.

In patients who had spastic diplegia and hip-flexion deformities, Perry *et al.* (1976) used gait electromyograms to document abnormal and prolonged electrical activity of the iliacus. In 11 separate gait electromyograms of the iliacus muscle in spastic diplegic patients, we found normal electrical activity in five; in six the activity was prolonged and out of phase (Fig. 8.17). In two patients who had iliopsoas recession the contractions were normal in phase (Bleck 1980) (Fig. 8.18). To

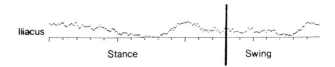

Fig. 8.17. Gait EMG, iliacus, fine-wire electrodes; 10-year-old spastic diplegic with 10° hip-flexion contracture. Iliacus dysphasic, active in stance and swing. Computer plot is summary of seven gait cycles.

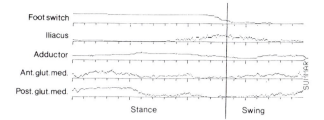

Fig. 8.18. Gait EMG of 20-year-old with spastic diplegia. No previous surgery; 50° hip-flexion contracture and hip internal rotation gait. Adductors continuous activity; anterior and posterior gluteus medius contract in both stance and swing phases, iliacus normal activity. Lesson: the electromyograph alone does not confirm a hip-flexion contracture due to the iliopsoas or the hip adductors or the gluteus medius. It is a bit difficult to insert a fine-wire electrode into the iliacus in a child. Given the contrasting information of the electromyograms this additional study might be eliminated in routine gait analysis. Note: it is muscle shortening that accounts for contracture in cerebral palsy. Delp *et al.* (1996) used gait analysis in showing in 14 subjects with crouch gait that the psoas was shorter more than 1 SD. Hamstring lengths were either normal or longer despite knee flexion instance in 80%.

study the psoas muscle alone would entail insertion of the recording electrodes through the back and localization with imaging—a technical feat that is unattractive to both patient and investigator.

Delp *et al.* (1996) used a graphics-based model with kinematic data derived from three-dimensional gait analysis to estimate the length of the hamstrings and psoas muscle in 14 subjects with crouch gait. 80% had hamstrings that were normal in length or longer despite knee flexion in stance. In all subjects with a crouch gait the psoas was shorter by more than 1 SD while walking. Hip-flexion posture during gait accounts for the flexed knees rather than short hamstrings. This finding provides the rationale for attacking the iliopsoas as the main deforming force.

Delp and his team now at Stanford University (Arnold *et al.* 2000b) constructed models from MR images of three cadaveric models. They compared hip- and knee-flexion moment arms from the three cadaveric models with the calculations derived from the MR images and graphic-based modeling. They found that this method was accurate and efficient to estimate muscle–tendon lengths and moment arms in vivo. Arnold and colleagues (2001) used the MR images to construct deformable computer models to replicate the muscle–tendon structures of four subjects with crouch gait. The differences of normalized hamstring lengths of the deformable models and MRI-based models was less than 5 mm and less than 3 mm for the psoas lengths. This is another tool to provide rapid and accurate estimates of medial hamstring and psoas lengths to assist the surgeon in decisions.

Although we can find no reports on the clinical use of computer modeling in decisions for surgery of spastic gait patterns, the orthopaedic surgeons at the A.I. duPont Institute, Wilmington, Delaware (Miller *et al.* 1999), did use the technique to determine the muscles to be lengthened in spastic dislocations of the hip (to be addressed in a section to follow).

In all individuals with a crouch gait the psoas was shorter than normal by more than 1 cm during walking.

PELVIS AND LUMBAR SPINE ADAPTATION TO HIP-FLEXION CONTRACTURE

Biomechanical adaptation to the hip-flexion deformity occurs in two ways, depending upon the position of the knee, the degree of spasticity of the quadriceps and hamstrings, and the strength of the gastrocnemius–soleus.

1. *Posterior inclination of the pelvis.* When the knees are flexed due to predominant hamstring spasticity and contracture, the pelvis inclines posteriorly and the lumbar spine flattens (Fig. 8.19 *a*, *b*). The patient assumes a sitting posture while trying to stand erect.

2. *Anterior inclination of the pelvis.* When the knees cannot be flexed due to quadriceps spasticity, the pelvis increases its anterior inclination and the lumbar spine becomes more lordotic (Fig. 8.20 *a*, *b*). Anterior pelvic inclination also occurs if the patient has had lengthening or transfer of the hamstrings to the femur and retained the same hip-flexion deformity; the compensating effect of knee flexion is lost. The pelvis then inclines anteriorly and lumbar lordosis increases. Because there are limits to extension of the lumbar spine, the patient may have to lean his trunk forward to bring the trunk's center of gravity anterior to the ankle joint between the base of support (Fig. 8.21).

The correction of these undesirable postural adaptations of the pelvis and lumbar spine is relief of the hip-flexion deformity. Radiographic depiction of the pelvic and spinal compensatory mechanisms can be ascertained with lateral radiographs of the lumbar spine, pelvis and proximal femur with the patient

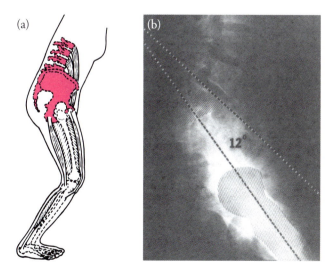

Fig. 8.19. (*a*) Posterior inclination of the pelvis and flattening of the lumbar spine as compensation for flexed hips and flexed knees: sitting down while standing-up ('Jump'; if Achilles overlengthened becomes 'Crouch'). (*b*) Tracing of lateral radiograph of lumbar spine, pelvis and femora with patient standing erect as possible. Femora become more horizontally parallel with the top of the sacrum, posterior inclination of the pelvis with decrease in lumbar lordosis.

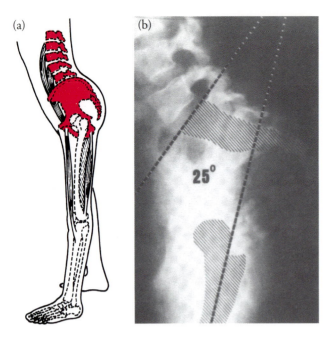

Fig. 8.20. (*a*) Anterior inclination of the pelvis and increased lumbar lordosis as compensation for flexed hips and extended knees due to spastic quadriceps and/or lengthening of hamstrings without correction of the hip-flexion contracture. (*b*) Tracing of lateral radiograph of the lumbar spine, pelvis and femora with patient standing erect. Femora become more vertically parallel with the top of the sacrum, anterior inclination of the pelvis and increased lumbar lordosis.

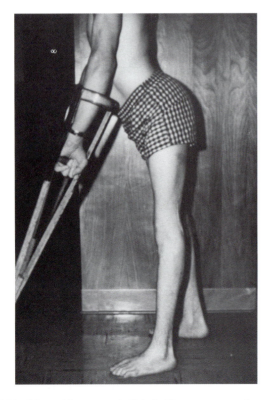

Fig. 8.21. Male, FC, age 34 years, spastic diplegia; 22 years postoperative bilateral total hamstring transfers to femoral condyles. Hip-flexion contracture not corrected. Stiff knee gait. Extreme lumbar lordosis and anterior pelvic inclination. Leans trunk forward on crutches to bring the trunk's center of gravity anterior to the ankle joint between the base of support.

standing as erect as possible (Bleck 1971a, b). On the radiograph a line was drawn along the top of the sacrum to locate the pelvic inclination (for all practical purposes the sacrum moves with the pelvis; its independent motion is no more than 4º). A second line was drawn along the shaft of the femur. The angle formed by the intersection of these two lines was called the *sacrofemoral angle*. In normal children and adolescents this angle measured between 50º and 65º (Fig. 8.22).

In the patient with a hip-flexion deformity and flexed knees, the femora were horizontally parallel with the sacrum and the sacrofemoral angle was less than 50º (Fig. 8.19 *b*).In the patient with a hip-flexion deformity and spastic quadriceps muscles and extended knees with a hip-flexion deformity, the femora were vertically parallel with the sacrum and the sacrofemoral angle was less than 50º (Fig. 8.20 *b*). With acceptable compensation of the hip-flexion deformity, the sacrofemoral angle, although less than normal, was 35º–45º.

Almost all *lordosis* of the lumbar spine was confined to the lumbosacral articulation (L5–S1). When the degree of lordosis between the first and fifth lumbar vertebrae was measured by the Cobb method, the resultant angles were between 45º and 65º and within the limits of normal for children (Propst-Proctor and Bleck 1983). These spinal measurements did not vary either with the degree of the hip-flexion deformity or with the sacrofemoral angle (Bleck 1975).

Although radiographic studies of the compensatory effect of a hip-flexion contracture in an erect patient were useful in depicting the skeletal mechanics, they are *not* necessary in the clinical examination and do not necessarily correlate significantly with the hip-flexion deformity. Bar-on *et al.* (1992) found a poor association between their measurements of the sacral inclination and the estimation of the hip-flexion contracture with either the Thomas or Staheli methods. The radiographs were made with the patient lying prone. The patient then

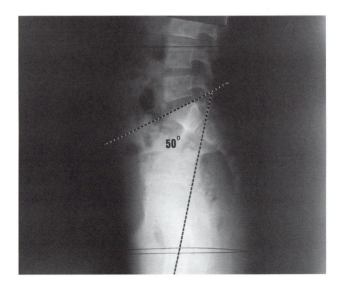

Fig. 8.22. Lateral radiograph of lumbar spine, pelvis and proximal femora; 13-year-old female, normal neurological status, standing erect. Sacrofemoral angle, formed by a line parallel to the top of the sacrum with a line parallel to the femoral shaft is within normal limits (45º–60º).

attempted to attain maximal hip extension. One line was drawn perpendicular to the posterior sacral wall and the other along the femoral shaft.

Although radiographic studies of the compensatory effect of a hip-flexion contracture were useful in depicting the skeletal mechanics, they are not necessary in the clinical examination.

Excessive *anterior bowing of the femoral shaft* does not seem to occur in response to the hip-flexion deformity. In 27 patients who had spastic hip-flexion deformities and sacrofemoral angles that ranged from 15º to 48º, the anterior bow of the femur as measured on the lateral radiographs had a mean of 8º (range 1º–20º). The normal mean femoral shaft anterior bow is considered to be 7º.

CLINICAL MEASUREMENT OF HIP-FLEXION DEFORMITY
The *clinical measurement* of the hip-flexion deformity has been described in Chapter 2. The Staheli prone extension method is most accurate. The Thomas test can be an inaccurate measure-ment of the hip-flexion contracture in spastic paralysis of the

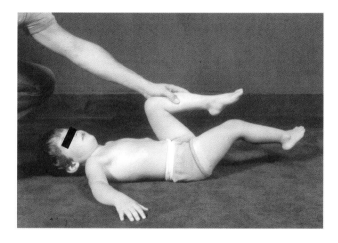

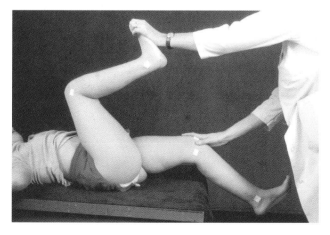

Fig. 8.23. Classic Thomas test for hip-flexion contracture. May be accurate in non-spastic conditions, but very inaccurate in cerebral palsy. How do you discern that the lumbar spine is flat when you flex the opposite hip on the abdomen?

lower limbs (Figs 2.30, 8.23). Stuberg and colleagues (1988) tested the reliability of gonimetric measurements in children with cerbebral palsy and found significant errors. Interrater measurements had a 10º–15º difference between examinations by a single tester. Intrarater measurements were acceptable for hip abduction and knee extension, but not for straight leg-raising or ankle dorsiflexion.

Is there a more accurate way to document a hip-flexion contracture in cerebral palsy? One group used the Thomas test and kinematic gait analysis in 41 patients who had bilateral hip-flexion contractures (Lee *et al.* 1997). Limited hip extension was most closely correlated with anterior pelvic tilting (*p* <0.0001). They found a weak association between the Thomas test and the degree of peak hip extension and anterior pelvic tilt in gait (r=0.41 and 0.36 respectively). So this study confirms that the Thomas test is unreliable in spastic cerebral palsy. The prone hip-extension test of Staheli appears more accurate, but it is neither quick nor easy, and it needs repeating several times on different occasions (Fig. 2.31). Do it slowly and be calm. Anterior pelvic tilt is strongly correlated with reduced dynamic hip extension as measured in the gait laboratory.

Pelvic–femoral fixation is another factor that can account for the gait abnormality. It can be demonstrated by asking the child to stand on one limb and hold onto a table with one hand while swinging the other limb back and forth. The femur moves with the pelvis as a unit. This partial pelvic–femoral fixation is due to spasticity and contracture of the hip musculature. The flexion deformity limits hip extension that is so essential to gait (stance is 60% of the gait cycle). The lumbar spine absorbs this limited hip extension mainly at the lumbosacral articulation. These patients walk with an anterior and posterior pelvic motion as well as an increase in transverse pelvic rotation. Their gait is similar to that of patients who have had an arthrodesis of the hips. Hoffinger *et al.* of Seattle (1992) noted a 'double bump' pelvic motion in the sagittal plane with gait analysis in 36 patients with cerebral palsy (also confirmed by Gage *et al.* 1996). They reasoned that this phenomenon may be due to the lumbar spine compensating for the hip-flexion contracture. As the hip begins to extend when the opposite hip is in extension, pelvic tilt increases. They also thought that hip-flexor weakness might account for the pattern.

Three gait patterns were described in children with spastic diplegia by Bleck (1971a, b). The following are perhaps simplified from the sagittal patterns detailed by Rodda and Graham (2001); the majority have internally rotated hips in stance, and all have equinus. Upper-leg internal rotation during gait may be masked by compensatory external tibial torsion:

1. Flexed internally rotated hips and flexed knees-spastic hamstrings ('crouch').
2. Flexed internally rotated hips and hyperextended knees-spastic quadriceps ('jump' with stiff knees).
3. Flexed internally rotated hips and balanced knee func-tion—neither hamstring nor quadriceps spasticity predominates ('jump' without stiff knees). Their stride length is shorter than normal; knee excursion may be less than normal, and they walk

with an in-toed gait almost identical to that of normal children who have excessive femoral anteversion (Crane 1959).

INDICATIONS FOR SURGERY IN SPASTIC HIP-FLEXION DEFORMITY

When measurements of the hip-flexion deformity were made in children with spastic paralysis (particularly using the prone extension test recommended), neither we nor anyone else ever observed a decrease in the hip-flexion deformity by passive stretching, prone lying, any physical therapeutic methods or orthotics. Instead, compensation with increased pelvic anterior or posterior inclination, knee flexion, or forward lean of the trunk occurs (Fig. 8.24). If this compensation results in a near to normal posture and acceptable gait, there is no need to apply direct surgical treatment. In general, if the hip-flexion deformity is more than 10°–20°, surgical correction is indicated.

It is especially important to reduce the hip-flexion deformity if the flexed knee gait is to be corrected by lengthening of the hamstring muscles. If the hamstrings alone are weakened in such patients, increased anterior inclination and lumbar lordosis can be anticipated as a compensatory mechanism (Fig. 8.21). This postural adaptation does not resolve with time, and low back pain may occur as the patient ages (if you can follow your patients for 15 or more years).

A 10° hip-flexion contracture is the inevitable accompaniment of excessive femoral anteversion (torsion). If Bleck's (1987) observations of decreasing dynamic and passive hip internal rotation following iliopsoas recession (which would be comparable to lengthening) are correct, even a 10° hip-flexion contracture merits correction with surgery along with other multi-level procedures. But it is probable that the iliopsoas lengthening would have to be done between the ages of 4 and 6 years. If so, the patient, parents and surgeon will need patience for the following 3–4 years to see the result. While walking in-toed is considered a subjective disability[7], a torsion either internal of the femur and/or external of the tibia comprise the 'lever-arm dysfunction' affecting efficient gait function.[8]

ABANDONED SURGICAL INTERVENTIONS FOR SPASTIC HIP-FLEXION CONTRACTURE

The following have been tried and found wanting in spastic paralysis.

1. *Ober-Yount fasciotomy* of the tensor fascia femoris and the distal iliotibial band. The operation was used to correct flexion–abduction contractures of the hip due to the flaccid paralysis of poliomyelitis (Yount 1926, Ober 1936, Irwin 1949, Ingram 1987). The contracture in the spastic paralysis of cerebral palsy is not in the fascia on or about the muscles, rather the muscles in spastic paralysis are shortened.

2. *Soutter or Campbell muscle-slide operation* (Campbell 1912, Soutter 1914), which detaches the origins of the sartorius, rectus femoris and tensor fascia femoris muscles and displaces them

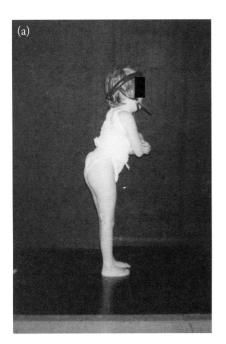 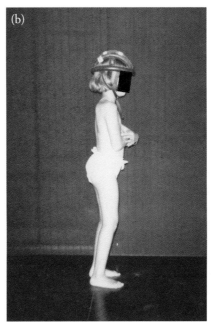 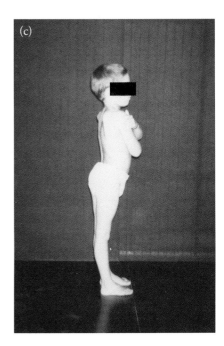

Fig. 8.24. Posture of three 6-year-old children with spastic diplegia, adaptation to hip-flexion deformity: (*a*) knees extended, trunk leans forward; (*b*) flexed knees slightly; compensation for hip-flexion contracture; (*c*) recurvatum of knees, lumbar lordosis.

7 Subjective disability = 'evokes a negative reaction in the observer majority'—Lynn Staheli MD, at International Pediatric Orthopaedic Seminars, circa 1980–85.
8 Rotation terminology: version = twist or rotation of the bone that is within the limits of normal values; torsion implies rotation greater than 2 SD beyond the mean for age, e.g. femoral anteversion is normal; excessive anteversion is torsion. Internal = medial rotation; external = lateral rotation. Medial and lateral are perhaps more accurate terms, e.g. internal connoting something inside as in 'internal medicine'.

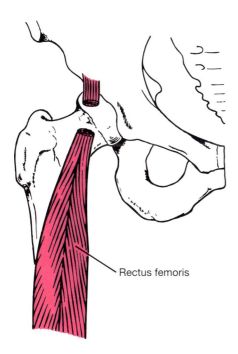

Fig. 8.25. Proximal rectus femoris tenotomy.

distally. The operation was used extensively in hip-flexion contractures due to poliomyelitis. Lamb and Pollock (1962) reported a 66% recurrence rate with this operation.

3. *Proximal rectus femoris tenotomy* (Fig. 8.25). This operation detaches the rectus femoris from its origin on the anterior inferior iliac spine and allows this tendon to retract distally (Fig. 8.25). It should not be done just because the surgeon feels it is 'tight'. Normal rectus femoris tendons are tight. The release of this muscle proximally weakens the quadriceps. If there is minimal co-spasticity of the quadriceps, the hamstrings will overpower the quadriceps so that a flexed knee posture can result within 6 months to 1 year postoperatively.

4. *Myotomy of the anterior fibers of the gluteus medius* as an addition to the release of the sartorius and tensor fascia femoris origins (Roosth 1971). Certainly, as Roosth reported, the procedure diminished the hip internal rotation during gait because the major internal rotator of the hip is the gluteus medius. The trade-off for eliminating the in-toed gait pattern is a bilateral limp due to the weakening of the major hip abductor muscle. Although J. Perry and M.M. Hoffer (personal communication), in their gait electromyograms of the gluteus medius in patients with cerebral palsy and adult stroke, noted no abnormal contractions of the muscle, our EMG studies did show that the anterior fibers had more activity when normal children simulated an in-toed gait by internally rotating their hips—'pigeon-toed' walking. In nine of 11 children with cerebral palsy the muscle had prolonged abnormal contractions (Csongradi *et al.* 1980).

Hip internal rotation in gait does not appear to compromise function significantly. A more important function for energy conservation during gait is the pelvic stabilization by the gluteus medius when weight-shifting from limb to limb during the stance phase of gait. It does not seem worthwhile to use surgery to

compromise this function of the hip-abductor muscles, which would incur excessive lateral displacement of the body for the sake of appearance.

5. *Iliopsoas tenotomy at its insertion* on the lesser trochanter is not advisable in the ambulatory patient. Bleck and Holstein (1963) performed iliopsoas tenotomy in 17 patients with cerebral palsy and spastic paralysis. All had a permanent loss of hip-flexion power that did not return in 13 years of follow-up. Fortunately the patients who were ambulatory and selected for the procedure were dependent on crutches which always can compensate to some degree for deficiencies in hip-muscle function. M.M. Hoffer (personal communication) and Bleck (1987) tagged the end of the iliopsoas tendon with a metallic clip at the time of tenotomy. Postoperative radiographs revealed cephalad retraction of the tendon to unpredictable and varying levels. Some tendons retracted to the level of the femoral head, and others to the mid-ilium (Fig. 8.26). Don't do iliopsoas tenotomy at the lesser trochanter in ambulatory patients.

Don't do iliopsoas tenotomy at the lesser trochanter in ambulatory patients.

In the *non-ambulatory patient*, or in one whose prognosis for walking is poor, and has early or established subluxation of the hip, iliopsoas tenotomy is sufficient together with other muscle-lengthenings or part of the bone procedures. Tenotomy is a far simpler operation than either recession or lengthening. The operative technique is described in Chapter 9. In normal children without spasticity in whom tenotomy of the iliopsoas has been

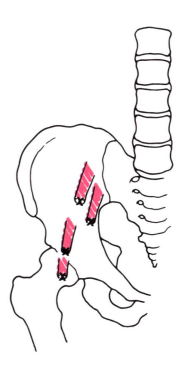

Fig. 8.26. Graphic representation of radiographs of the pelvis and hips after iliopsoas tenotomy with metallic clips placed in the iliopsoas tendon proximal to the cut. Note the variation in the levels to which the tendon retracted.

routinely performed as part of the procedure for open reduction of a congenital dislocation of the hip, no functional loss of hip flexion has been noted. However, in children with cerebral palsy the muscle is spastic and can retract too far superiorly, depending upon the degree of spasticity; in effect the muscle is overlengthened by tenotomy.

6. *Iliopsoas recession.* The objective of iliopsoas recession was to reduce the flexion contracture of the hip, avoid over lengthening of the iliopsoas tendon and preserve the strength of the muscle, and to remove the compression of the tendon on the medial aspect of the hip joint so that reduction of subluxation of the hip would be facilitated. The obstruction to reduction of subluxations and dislocations of the hip by the iliopsoas tendon was a concept in the early treatment of congenital dislocation of the hip (Ferguson 1973, 1975) (Fig. 8.27). The rationale of iliopsoas recession was to reduce the contracture and prevent or reduce the spastic paralytic subluxation of the hip. Accordingly the psoas tendon was recessed to the anterior capsule at the base of the femoral neck, and so remove it from its medial capsular position where it would block reduction of subluxation when the hip was extended and at the same time preserve the strength of

the muscle. It was feared that with z-lengthening and subsequent healing of the tendon by scar additional compression of the medial joint capsule would occur.[9]

Iliopsoas recession detaches the iliopsoas tendon at its insertion on the lesser trochanter, freeing the iliacus fibers from the tendon, and then suturing it to the anterior capsule of the hip joint—a technique inspired as part of cup arthroplasty of the hip for osteoarthritis (Stinchfield and Chamberlain 1966).

Bleck (1971 a, b) reported satisfactory results in 61 patients (55 bilateral iliopsoas recessions and six unilateral). The best results were in children who had the operation between the ages of 5 and 7 years. In a follow-up of a mean of 6.8 years the flexion contractures were reduced from a mean of 30° (15°–60°) to a mean of 0° (0°–30°). Pre-operative subluxation of the hip was reduced completely in six and persisted in 10. Hip-flexion power was reduced in all but three patients to a good to fair strength. In two strength was poor and in one it was zero.

Correction of the hip-flexion deformity failed in some patients older than 11 years. Anterior incision of the joint capsule, while theoretically logical, has not in practice resulted in additional correction. Also, in the few patients in whom Bleck (1987) tried it, he noted limited passive flexion of the hip to 90°— possibly due to the increased anterior cicatrix formation of the joint capsular incision.

Assessment of the pelvic tilt with standing lateral radiographs of the lumbar spine, pelvis and femur to measure the tilt confirmed that the anterior pelvic tilt was reduced from an average of 32° in 21 patients who had the radiographs.

Iliopsoas recession was done as part of a multilevel surgery that usually included fractional medial and lateral hamstring lengthening in 27 patients and adductor longus myotenotomy with anterior branch obturator neurectomy in 11, and Achilles tendon lengthening if a contracture of the gastrocnemius–soleus was evident (Fig. 8.28 *a, b*).

Although patient, family and surgeon were favorably impressed with the result and improvement in the gait and posture, the loss of long-term persistent hip-flexion power of one grade (Normal to Good [5 to 4], or Good to Fair [4 to 3]), and the surgical technique of removing the iliacus attachment to the tendon even though contracture of this muscle was not evident, prompted Bleck to change to z-lengthening of the tendon circa 1980. The electrical activity of the iliacus during level walking has been shown to be similar to that of the psoas major (Close 1964, Perry 1992). In the subsequent years more surgeons became convinced of the importance of the iliopsoas as a deforming force and began to tackle the contracture with more direct and simpler methods that would not compromise the strength of the muscle unduly.

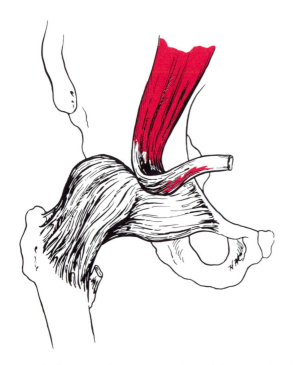

Fig. 8.27. The iliopsoas tendon can compress the medial joint capsule and block the entrance of the femoral head into the acetabulum. (Redrawn from Ferguson 1975, Bleck 1979.)

9 This rationale appeared to be confirmed by Griffith *et al.* (1982) in a review of their original 131 patients who had 255 adductor transfers. After an average of 3 years' follow-up, they found a need for secondary surgery for subluxation in 13%, while 11% required secondary acetabuloplasties. These results caused them to add iliopsoas recession to the adductor transfer surgery in 30 patients (60 hips), with the result that secondary surgery for subluxation dropped to 7% and there was no need for secondary acetabuloplasties

CONTEMPORARY SURGERY FOR SPASTIC HIP-FLEXION CONTRACTURE
Some type of surgical lengthening of the iliopsoas has been accepted to improve hip extension in gait and to preserve the strength of the muscle. Kinematic and biomechanical modeling studies of the psoas and hamstrings lengths in the 14 individuals

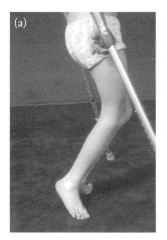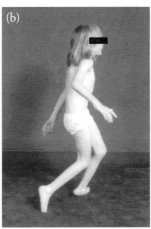

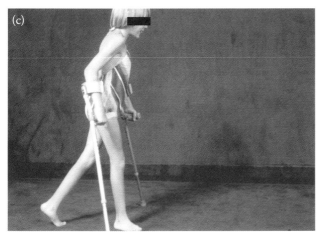

Fig. 8.28. Eight-year-old girl with no previous surgery stood (*a*), and walked (*b*) in a crouched position. Marked improvement in function and position after hamstring lengthenings (*c*). Cerebral palsy is a motion disorder. Still photographs cannot depict the function in gait: only observational gait analysis, videotaping or instrumented gait analysis can document a result fully. However, 'Posture accompanies movement like a shadow; movement begins in posture and ends in posture' (Sherrington, quoted by Rushworth 1964).

who had the crouch gait of cerebral palsy by Delp *et al.* (1996) found that all had maximum psoas lengths shorter than more than 2 SD at approximately 50% of the gait cycle. All individuals had minimum psoas lengths that were shorter than normal by more than 1 SD in approximately 90% of the gait cycle.

Aponeurotic lengthening of the iliopsoas was initiated by Tylkowski and Price (1986), who reported their results in 10 patients with spastic hip-flexion deformities. They described 'aponeurotic lengthening' as an incision the psoas tendon just after it crossed over the brim of the pelvis. The section of the tendon is similar to the procedure described by Salter (1961) for open reduction of the developmental hip subluxation done with innominate osteotomy. This 'aponeurosis' is the broad beginning of the psoas tendon which at this level, by its fusion with the fibers of the iliacus muscle, prevents inordinate retraction of the tendinous portion. Tylkowski's and Price's (1986) preoperative and postoperative careful gait analyses and measurements showed improvement of the flexion contracture (mean 12º) and no loss

of function. Rinsky (1988) reported that he did the same procedure, and finds it easier to do and just as effective as z-lengthening or recession.

Z-lengthening was reported by Anthosen (1966) and Baumann (1970) with apparent good results (Fig. 8.27). Anthosen's postoperative regimen entailed a prolonged hospital stay where the patient was kept prone and the hips maintained in extension.

Z-lengthening seemed satisfactory in ambulatory patients, and it did not appear to bring as much risk of hip-flexion weakness as iliopsoas recession did. Bleck (1987) followed 10 patients who had bilateral iliopsoas tendon z-lengthening for a mean of 4 years. At the time of surgery, nine were between 6 and 14 years (mean 9 years), and one was an adult age 25 years. The mean preoperative flexion contracture measured by the prone extension test of Staheli was 26º (range 15º–45º) and the mean postoperative contracture was 10º (range 0º–30º). The 30º preoperative flexion contracture of one girl at age 6 years was the same postoperatively at age 8 years. None had any evidence preoperatively or postoperatively of subluxation, lateral migration of the femoral head or an abnormal CE angle of the hip.

After z-lengthening of the tendon, healing must be by scar formation. As with all cicatrix formation, contracture of the fibrous tissue occurs. Hence early recurrence of the flexion contracture is a risk with lengthening. The patients must be carefully supervised postoperatively to ensure that they do not sit upright for long periods during the day. In one of my first patients in whom we did a lengthening on one side and a recession on the other, contracture recurred on the side of lengthening within 3 weeks postoperatively. Fortunately aggressive hip extension, passive and active exercise, together with strict prone positioning in bed, overcame this complication in 6 weeks.

The proximal half of the z-lengthened tendon may be inadvertently severed and retract proximally into the pelvis with resultant weakness of hip-flexion power. However, recovery can occur in time. The following anecdote may assuage the anxiety of the surgeon if such occurs. We don't have a 'series' or a controlled study for obvious reasons.

Bleck recommended bilateral iliopsoas tendon lengthenings for a 45º hip-flexion contracture in a 25-year-old man with the objective of relieving constant low back pain. The tendon was inadvertently cut completely on one side at the level of the femoral head. The proximal portion retracted approximately 10 cm into the pelvis. Hip flexion strength was extremely poor for one year after which normal strength returned; on the z-lengthened side there was no weakness. After 5 years the flexion contractures of both hips were 0 as measured by the prone extension method of Staheli and strength was normal. His low back pain was relieved immediately postoperatively and never returned.[10]

---

10 Anecdotes do not qualify for 'evidence-based' studies. But who would want to repeat the surgical experience of the one case of the 25-year-old man 50 times and select patients randomly? 'One case is enough for me' (EEB).

Operative technique for iliopsoas tendon z-lengthening (modified from Baumann 1970). The patient is supine and the lower limbs draped free. Under general anesthesia when the muscles are relaxed a Thomas test measures the hip-flexion contracture and the popliteal angle measures the hamstring contracture. Note that if the hamstrings are contracted beyond the normal of 20° the flexion of the opposite hip in the Thomas test can roll the pelvis posteriorly to give a greater hip-flexion contracture than actually is present. An incision is made beginning about 1.5 cm distal and lateral to the anterior superior iliac spine and continued medially and obliquely parallel with the groin crease. The incision terminates approximately at the junction of the medial one-third and lateral two-thirds of the anterior surface of the thigh. The medial border of the sartorius is identified and retracted laterally with the lateral femoral cutaneous nerve. Deeper in the wound the tendinous origin of the rectus femoris ('the silver fish') is noted. Medial to it and blending with the fascia surrounding the rectus tendon is the iliacus muscle. The femoral nerve is found on the anterior surface of the iliacus, freed up and retracted *gently* medially. The bulky fibers investing the psoas tendon are retracted laterally to expose the tendon. With blunt dissection the tendon is cleared of fatty connective tissue to expose its length.

Kocher clamps placed distally and proximally, with one on the medial half of the tendon and the other on the lateral half, prevent the unwanted retraction of the tendon into the pelvis when it is z-lengthened. The Thomas test can be done to ascertain the correction of the contracture and the amount of lengthening of the tendon (in the fully anesthetized patient the test may be more reliable due to relaxation of the hamstrings). The lengthened ends are sutured together.

How much to lengthen is indicated by the computer model studies of Delp and Zajac (1992). A 1–2 cm increase in the psoas tendon length decreased its hip flexion moment by only 4% and 9% respectively. Identical lengthening of the Achilles tendon

produced dramatically different results: 1 cm increase in length decreased the maximum isometric moment of the soleus by 30% and 85% with a 2 cm increase in length.

Matsuo (1987, 2002) does a sliding lengthening the psoas tendon through a similar approach as described above. He exposes about 5–8 cm of the tendon, isolates it with a blunt dissector or elevator and places a z-sag suture though the area of tendon to be lengthened. Half the tendon is cut medially and proximally, and the other half laterally and distally. Then in a non-described manner he slides the tendon to the desired unspecified length. The z-sag suture is tied to secure the tendon lengthened area. He immobilized the lower limbs in a spica cast to the nipple line for 3 weeks, followed by intensive physiotherapy for 6 months.

In Matsuo's report the average correction of the hip flexion contracture was 18.4°. The gait pattern improved in nine of 13 patients who walked independently. Muscle testing of patients walked had good and fair strength in 89 % and poor in 11 %. About half of the patients had spastic diplegia and the other half spastic quadriplegia, spastic quadriplegia with tension athetosis or triplegia. Of significance is that subluxation of the hip was reduced in about half those who were classified as sitters.

Postoperative care. No hip spica casts are necessary. When the child is comfortable with analgesics, usually by 3 days at the most, gait training should start: first in parallel bars or with a walker, then graduating to crutches as balance improves, and finally leading to independent walking, if this was feasible preoperatively. Usually this process is complete in 6 weeks. Supervised exercise and balance training are continued for an average of 6 months after surgery.

Iliopsoas 'recession', 'intramuscular lengthening', 'release' at or below the pelvic brim: a tenotomy by any other name is still a tenotomy.

ILIOPSOAS RECESSION AT THE PELVIC BRIM
Sutherland and colleagues (1997) at the San Diego Children's Hospital described 'psoas recession' at the pelvic brim in 17 patients followed for an average of 28 months (range, 12–57). All patients had pre- and postoperative gait analysis from which the results were derived and analyzed for statistical significance. Hip flexion and extension were measured with the patient supine according to the standards of clinical measurement of joint motion published by the American Academy of Orthopaedic Surgeons (Greene and Heckman 1994). Postoperatively the passive range of hip extension decreased from 20° to an average of 12° and was statistically significant (p = 0.001). Hip-flexion strength was preserved. According to gait analysis the stride length was increased; maximal hip flexion changed from 56° to 48° in stance. In the representative case the graphic display (Fig. 8B in Sutherland *et al.* 1997) of dynamic hip flexion and extension preoperative extension was 20°; postoperatively hip extension reached 0° comparable to the normal range. Dynamic tilt during stance changed little (26°–23°). The authors attribute this minimal improvement due to the use of assistive devices when walking. After assistive devices were removed from the lower

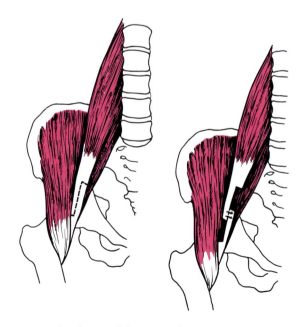

Fig. 8.29. Z-lengthening of the psoas tendon.

284

limbs of five patients, improved pelvic tilt became statistically significant (p = 0.0001). Pelvic tilt improvement declined as age increased at the time of surgery (p = 0.001). At the same operative time, all patients had bilateral distal hamstring lengthenings, and distal rectus femoris to gracilis transfers.

OPERATIVE TECHNIQUE OF PSOAS RECESSION AT THE PELVIC BRIM (Sutherland *et al.* 1997)[11]

The lower limb and lower anterior pelvis and hip are draped free. A vertical mark is made over the femoral artery palpation. The hip-flexion crease is identified by flexing the hip so that the skin incision can be made parallel and slightly distal to the flexion crease. This oblique incision extends from lateral to the femoral artery to the adductor longus if an adductor longus myotenotomy is to be included. The iliac fascia is divided lateral to the femoral artery and exposes the femoral nerve.[12] A rubber drain is passed around the nerve proximal to its branches and then *gently* retracted over a moist laparotomy pad with a smooth retractor toward the femoral sheath medially (no strong armed assistants wanted). The medial border of the iliacus is identified and rolled

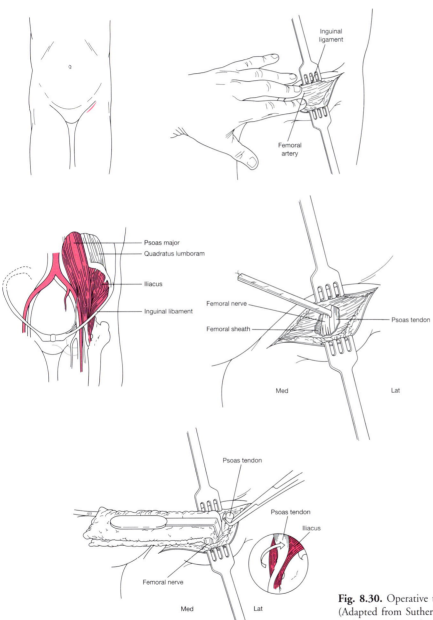

Fig. 8.30. Operative technique for psoas recession at the pelvic brim. (Adapted from Sutherland *et al.* 1997, by permission of the *Journal of Pediatric Orthopaedics* and the Raven Press, New York.)

11 The term has been adopted by pediatric orthopaedic surgeons and begs definition: A brim is the upper edge or rim of a hollow structure. 'The pelvic 'brim' anatomically is the upper pelvic aperture or inlet. This brim is in the plane of the terminal lines. The terminal or arcuate line consists of: (1) pubic crest, (2) pectineal line, (3), medial border of the lower half of the ilium, (4) the ala of the sacrum, (5) sacral promontory. This plane slopes downward and forward as it passes from the sacral promontory to the pubic symphysis. It forms an angle of about 45º with the horizontal' (Gardner *et al.* 1969).

12 Remember the anatomy with NAVY: from lateral to medial the position of important structures below the inguinal ligament is N (femoral nerve), A (femoral artery), V (femoral vein), and Y (empty space).

laterally to expose its surface adjacent to the inner wall of the pelvis using blunt dissecting instruments. The hip is flexed and externally rotated to expose the psoas tendon which is isolated and sectioned at the level of the pelvic brim. It is essential that the inguinal ligament be retracted proximally so that the tendon is *at the pelvic brim and not below it* (Fig. 8.30).

Carroll (Tachdjian 1994) described the same procedure with apparent good results. As pointed out by Sutherland and colleagues (1997), this approach to the psoas tendon entails less risk to the femoral nerve than the intramuscular approach. A femoral nerve injury resulting in paralysis of the quadriceps can be long-term and not very successfully restored by nerve suture to approximate the cut ends. If you are confused as to what is a tendon and what is the nerve, use an electrical nerve stimulator in the operative field.

Intramuscular psoas lengthening over the pelvic brim. The technique of sectioning the psoas tendon within the muscle proximal to the pelvic brim was devised by Skaggs and adopted by Chung *et al.* (1994) and from the same institution, Novacheck and colleagues (2002) at the Gillette Children's Hospital, St Paul, Minnesota. They did the operation along with hamstring lengthening and femoral derotation osteotomy. Results were assessed with pre- and postoperative physical examination and extensive gait analysis, the normalcy index derived from the gait study as well as the 10-point walking scale from the parent FAQ. They compared the results with a group of children who had hamstring lengthening and subtrochanteric osteotomies but no psoas surgery.

In the psoas surgery group the hip-flexion contracture decreased from 10º to 6.1º while there was no change in those who did not have psoas surgery. This negative result was explained because this group had only a 1.74º hip-flexion contracture (in their report the hip-flexion contracture was measured by a 'modified Thomas test' rather than the prone hip-extension test of Staheli). Given the accepted interobserver variation of ±5º in manual measurements of joint ranges of motion, patients in this study could have had a 5º, 10º, a 15º preoperative hip-flexion contracture, or none (Greene and Heckman 1994). The single observer has as much as a 30% difference in the range of motion (Lea and Gerhardt 1995). As measured in the gait analysis maximum hip extension in stance was only 3.56º and postoperatively a minuscule 0.86º in those who had psoas lengthening.

In those who did not have psoas surgery hip extension in stance was –1.84º preoperatively and –1.71º postoperatively. Pelvic tilt improved 5.12º in the psoas surgery group and 2.57º in the no psoas surgery. The normalcy index for both groups improved by 23.4 and 23.8 respectively. Oxygen consumption was unchanged in both groups. Stride length and velocity showed no significant changes. The gait analysis parameters indicated improved hip function for those who had psoas surgery. Walking ability was statistically improved as measured by the FAQ given to parents. No evidence was found that the intramuscular psoas tenotomy caused hip-flexor weakness. Concomitant hamstring lengthenings compounded the postoperative assessment of efficacy. The exquisite outcome data presented strongly suggests

that intramuscular psoas lengthening in the patients of Novacheck and colleagues (2002) had minimum if any significant improvements in the parameters measured. The saving grace was that the surgeons reported no neurovascular complications, e.g. femoral nerve palsy which is the major risk in the procedure.

The exquisite outcome data of Novacheck et al. (2002) of intramuscular over-the-brim iliopsoas lengthening suggest minimum improvement.

McCarthy and Otsuka (2002), in a critique of the paper by Novacheck *et al.* (2002), complimented the authors for their meticulous gathering of a plethora of data even though they reported 'relatively small improvements in overall function'. As admitted by Novacheck *et al.* (2002) their study was not random, and a prospective trial of intramuscular psoas lengthening is indicated. A multicenter trial has been instituted by the Shriners Hospitals for Children, so we may eventually have a more informed opinion on the efficacy of the surgery.[13]

Surgeons other than McCarthy and Otsuka (2002) have doubted the efficacy of iliopsoas 'release'. Feldkamp and Denker (1989) of Munster, Germany, compared two groups of 20 patients. One group had adductor tenotomy and medial hamstring lengthening only, and the other had the same surgery with the addition of 'iliopsoas release'. They found that hip extension did not improve with iliopsoas release (instrumented gait analysis was not reported). However, they did note that hip dislocations and subluxations were positively influenced by iliopsoas release. After adductor transfer, proximal hamstring release and iliopsoas release, Smith and Stevens (1989) found a similar positive effect on the migration percentage, acetabular angle and CE angle in their review of 22 patients who had surgery at an average age of 4 years 9 months. So something may have changed for the better: although some questions remain unanswered. What particular muscle was the main deforming force to cause subluxation when three muscles were included in one surgery?

Another negative view of psoas lengthening with the 'over-the-brim' of the pelvis was expressed by DeLuca *et al.* (1998) from the Connecticut Children's Medical Center. The reported on 73 patients in four groups: medial hamstring lengthening in 37, medial and lateral hamstring lengthening in 12, medial hamstring lengthening with the psoas over-the-brim technique in nine, and medial and lateral hamstring lengthening with the same psoas surgery in 15. Their study entailed the use of gait analysis. They found no significant increase in pelvic tilt (a clinically insignificant 4º) after the medial and lateral hamstrings were lengthened with or without the psoas release.

Although instrumented gait analysis for joint kinematics is considered the *sine quo non* of measurement of lower-limb

---

13 McCarthy and Otsuka (2002) in the context of confusion in results of psoas over-the-brim lengthening in cerebral palsy cite the witty comments of Dr Stephen Skinner about the learning process for the treatment of cerebral palsy as three phases: I. Overwhlemed with information; II finally understanding the diagnostic and treatment protocols; III with fuller knowledge of the literature, one is completely confused.

function in gait, Ramakirishnan and Kadaba (1991) of the Helen Hayes Orthopaedic Engineering Center, New York, studied its accuracy. They used the concepts of Euler and helical (screw) angles to define three-dimensional relative joint angular motion in the lower limbs. To do this they used data from normal subjects and patients with cerebral palsy. Hip- and knee-flexion angles were not changed by perturbing ± 15º in 5º steps from the reference position. Abduction, adduction and rotation angles were significantly affected in the gait cycle. An error of 15º in the flexion–extension angle caused maximum errors of 8º and 12º in the abduction/adduction angle and 10º–15º for rotation angles of the hip and knee. So, in patients who have a flexed-knee gait pattern, there can be a distorted estimation of adduction, abduction and rotation. This study might be recalled when interpreting minimal changes in joint kinematics of patients who have flexed knee gait patterns.

OPERATIVE TECHNIQUE OF INTRAMUSCULAR PSOAS LENGTHENING (Novacheck *et al.* 2002)

A 4 cm oblique incision is made along the inguinal ligament from medial to the anterior superior iliac spine (Fig. 8.31). The external oblique fascia is exposed and incised 3 cm cephalad and parallel to the inguinal ligament. The lateral femoral cutaneous nerve is identified medial to the anterior superior iliac spine and retracted laterally or medially. With extraperiosteal dissection the iliacus muscle fibers are freed of the inner table of the ilium. The muscle mass of the iliacus protects the neurovascular bundle.

With flexion of the hip and the index finger over the superior pubic ramus (the pelvic brim), the finger is placed under the psoas tendon. The iliacus is retracted medially to visualize the tendon which is cut with electrocautery (the authors state that the electrocautery gives confirmation that the tendon seen is not the femoral nerve—a nerve-stimulator might be better and not risk burning the nerve). The index finger palpates the tendon with

the hip in extension to confirm it has been lengthened. No immobilization is necessary and physical therapy to 'promote hip extension' begins on the third day.

Patrick (1996) described the technique of intramuscular 'psoas tenotomy' similar to that of Novacheck *et al.* (2002) with the exception that the skin incision is made on the abdominal wall just medial and anterior to the anterior superior iliac spine. By dissection to the external oblique aponeurosis in the same line of the incision, the outer inguinal ligament as well as the conjoined tendon is identified. The external oblique is opened to expose the internal oblique and transversus abdominis that are freed from the inner edge of the iliac crest with sharp dissection. The inner aspect of the ilium is stripped with blunt dissection to push the iliacus muscle medially and distally and retracted medially. The sacroiliac joint can be palpated at the bottom of the wound. The psoas muscle can be palpated here over the brim of the pelvis. With rotation of the hand into supination the index finger can feel the psoas tendon while an assistant flexes and extends the hip. A Moynihan forceps 'teases' apart the iliacus fibers and the muscle that envelopes the psoas tendon on its medial side. The tendon is isolated and brought laterally with a curved forceps (Fig. 8.29 *b, c*). By flexing the hip slightly the psoas is rolled over on itself. Blunt dissection will reveal the thick tendon with the muscle inserting into it. The psoas tendon is divided with a knife. To avoid mistaking the nerve for the tendon, a nerve stimulator can be used. The Thomas test is repeated to assure that the tendon has been divided. No data on the outcome of the procedure is recorded in Patrick's paper. Before embarking on this procedure in a patient, it might be wise to try it in a cadaver or to assist at surgery with one who is experienced in the approach.

Skaggs *et al.* (1997) were concerned with injury to the neurovascular structures in the process of isolating and cutting the psoas tendon as described above. They did an anatomical study with magnetic resonance imaging of 54 children younger

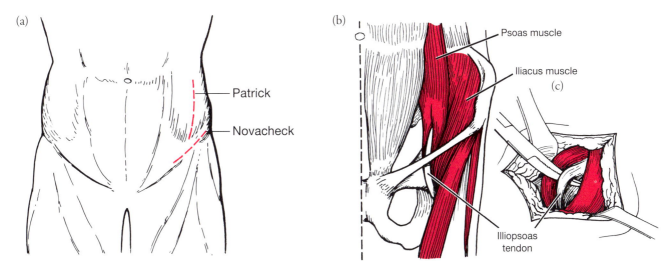

Fig. 8.31. Details of operative technique of intramuscular psoas lengthening over the pelvic brim (see text). (*a*) Skin incision, abdominal wall medial and anterior to anterior superior iliac spine. (*b*) Anatomic relationship of iliopsoas muscle anterior and medial to iliacus. (*c*) Iliacus muscle freed from inner edge of iliac crest and ilium stripped of iliacus which is pushed medially and distally and retracted medially away from the surgeon. Psoas muscle palpated at brim of pelvis. Assistant flexes and extends hip while the surgeon locates the psoas tendon with the index finger. Iliacus teased from the psoas. Tendon brought into wound with a forceps and divided. (Redrawn from Patrick 1996, by permission of the *Journal of Pediatric Orthopaedics* and the Raven Press, New York.)

than age 10 years. The mean distance between the neurovascular structures (femoral nerve) and the psoas tendon in the 'over-the-brim' position was only 1 cm, but might be as close as 4 mm in a child. Caution and careful identification of the psoas tendon deep in the iliacus is particularly important in intramuscular psoas tendon lengthening (it is really a tenotomy). There is no control of the lengthening except that the attachment of the iliacus muscle fibers should restrain excessive proximal retraction of the tendon.

SUMMARY COMMENTARY ON 'PSOAS RELEASE', 'PSOAS RECESSION AT THE PELVIC BRIM', 'INTRAMUSCULAR PSOAS LENGTHENING', 'PSOAS TENOTOMY'

Different terms have been used to title the operative procedure to lengthen and weaken the spastic force and contracture of the iliopsoas muscle and still preserve its strength. Either 'at the brim' or 'over the brim' of the pelvis the tendon is actually cut as in a tenotomy but with the hope that the fibers of the iliacus that blend with an attach to the psoas tendon will prevent undue and unwanted retraction. Such seems to be the case as reported by two experienced surgeons who found no postoperative weakness in hip-flexion strength postoperatively. However, the gains in the method of Sutherland and colleagues (1997) from San Diego, California, were much better than the minimal gains recorded by Novacheck and colleagues (2002) from St Paul, Minnesota. How to explain the differences in the results? Does intramuscular tenotomy of the psoas tendon fail to alter the force of the psoas major muscle as a cause of the hip-flexion contracture? Were the clinical measurements comparable? The degree of contracture preoperatively and lack of dynamic hip extension were minimal in the series of Novacheck *et al.* while these same parameters were greater in the cases of Sutherland *et al.* (1997). Were the patients and/or gait laboratory methods different?

Although the outcomes of iliopsoas tendon z-lengthenings are sparse in the literature and few gait studies have been done pre-and postoperatively, there remains a strong indication that it is the better procedure for a spastic hip-flexion contracture. Finally, does a hip-flexion contracture which by necessity limits hip extension in the stance phase of gait merit surgical treatment and if so, what is the best procedure? The surgeon has to decide to do either something or nothing. For simplicity and less dissection and safety, iliopsoas tenotomy (recession) at the pelvic brim seems the more desirable procedure.

Psoas wars in spastic diplegia: at-the-brim or over-the-brim 'release' vs z-lengthening or nothing?—stay tuned.

HIP INTERNAL-ROTATION DEFORMITY

ANATOMY, PHYSIOLOGY AND MECHANISMS

The internal rotator muscles of the hip are considered to be the gluteus medius and minimus, semitendinosus, adductors and the tensor fascia femoris (Duchenne 1867, Brunnstrom 1962). Anatomists and physiologists have established that the anterior portion of the gluteus medius is the main internal rotator of the

hip (Duchenne 1867, Hollinshead 1951, Brunnstrom 1962, Anderson 1983). Clinical experience confirms these observations; if the tendon is cut or transferred (Steel 1980), the femur no longer internally rotates. Direct measurements of transverse rotations of the segments of the lower limb during level gait show that the pelvis, femur and tibia all internally rotate during swing phase and continue to do so until mid-stance, when abrupt shift to external rotation occurs and continues until toe-off as swing phase begins. The gluteus medius contracts at the beginning of stance and continues to contract until mid-stance (Fig. 8.9). This early stance-phase activity correlates with internal rotation of the entire limb.

In a gait electromyographic telemetry study using fine-wire electrodes in the anterior and posterior portions of the gluteus medius, Csongradi *et al.* (1980) were able to demonstrate biphasic activity of both the anterior and posterior portions, with one phase lasting from late swing to mid-stance and a shorter phase at toe-off in 15 normal children aged 5 and over (Table 8.V). In the normal children who simulated the hip internal rotation gait, the activity of the anterior gluteus medius lasted significantly longer than normal (p<0.001); the posterior part was also of longer duration, but not significantly. In nine children with cerebral palsy and hip internal rotation gaits, the anterior fibers had a longer period of firing than the posterior, and the duration of firing was longer than normal (p<0.05). Surprisingly, in normal children who had femoral antetorsion (anteversion > 2 SD beyond the mean for age), the duration of both anterior and posterior gluteus medius activity was less than the normals and the children with cerebral palsy (p<0.01). The results of this study seem to indicate that overactivity or spasticity of the gluteus medius is not the etiology of excessive femoral anteversion (femoral antetorsion). These data also suggest that the anterior fibers of the gluteus medius in both normal and spastic children account for the hip internal-rotation gait patterns.

The *semitendinosus* internally rotates the thigh medially when the knee is extended, but this rotation diminishes as the knee flexes (Duchenne 1867). The strength of the semitendinosus is much less than the biceps femoris, which is a powerful lateral rotator of the leg. The semimembranosus has no rotator function, but it is the strongest of the hamstring muscles in flexing the knee. Sutherland *et al.* (1969) studied gait electromyograms, and transverse rotation of the lower limbs in seven patients with spastic paralysis and hip internal rotation; all patients consistently

TABLE 8.V
EMG gluteus medius during gait cycles

	Anterior gluteus medius		Posterior gluteus medius	
	% activity	SD	% activity	SD
Normal–normal gait	64	11.3	62	16.2
Normal–internal rotation gait	87	11.6 p<0.001	70	17.4 NS
Spastic cerebral palsy	73	20.6 p<0.05	66	22.4 NS
Increased antetorsion	50	10.9, p<0.01	55	15.0

From Csongradi *et al.* (1980).

had prolonged contraction of the semitendinosus in the stance phase. Chong *et al.* (1978) recorded electromyographic activity in 12 children with cerebral palsy who had lower-limb internal rotation gaits. Spasticity of the medial hamstrings was deemed the most important causative factor. Our own studies of spastic gait patterns that were not confined to only in-toed walking in 32 children demonstrated dysphasic and prolonged activity of the medial hamstrings (Csongradi *et al.* 1979).

These data do not contradict the suggestion that the semitendinosus may contribute to the in-toed gait, but they do indicate that other factors may account for hip internal-rotation gait. Recorded overactivity of a muscle does not necessarily correlate with the abnormal motion observed. Only by removing the muscle function by surgery or isolated paralysis, and then observing the effects, can one be certain it is the prime cause of the gait abnormality: clinical observations still have an important role.

The *adductors* were described as lateral rotators by Duchenne (1867). The lower portion of the adductor magnus is thought to be an internal rotator. Electromyographic studies of the adductors show contraction in late stance (Mann and Hagy 1973); an additional burst of activity in early stance occurs according to Brunnstrom (1962). Most electrical activity occurred after heel contact. These investigators considered the adductors to be weak internal rotators.

In patients with cerebral palsy but with no flexion contracture of the hip (measured with the prone hip-extension method) and only adducted lower limbs during gait, no internal rotation was noted. Conversely, one can find children who have hip internal rotation gaits and no significant limitation of abduction (>40° each hip); these children invariably have clinical evidence of excessive femoral anteversion (range of hip internal rotation >60° and external rotation <30°) and a hip-flexion contracture.

The tensor fascia femoris was noted to be a weak internal rotator by Duchenne (1867). The fact is confirmed by the disappointing results of transfer of its origin posteriorly with the intent of correcting the in-toed gait in spastic paralysis in children (Majestro and Frost 1971).

Bleck (1987) observed four children who had spastic hip-abduction contractures; they had large bulging tensor fascia femoris muscles. These children did not have an internally rotated hip posture, and the passive range of internal rotation and external rotation of their hips was within normal limits.

The rotary function of the *iliopsoas* can be discounted, according to electromyographic evidence in several studies (Basmajian 1962, Close 1964, Guillot *et al.* 1977). In one study of the psoas major during gait (Keagy *et al.* 1966) the contraction of the muscle at the time of heel rise, and continuing through the first 40% of the swing phase, correlated well with Strange's concept (1965) that the psoas major contracts to counteract the lateral rotation of the pelvis. When weight is placed on the hip as the body is propelled forward, the force generated leaves the pelvis behind. The iliopsoas muscle probably prevents excessive lateral pelvic rotation, and even rotates a little medially. Increased transverse rotation of the pelvis has frequently been seen and

photographed in patients with cerebral palsy who have pelvic–femoral fixation due to the marked spasticity of the muscles of the hip and thigh (Bleck 1975).

Tylkowski *et al.* (1982), in a massive and detailed motion-analysis study of hip internal rotation gait patterns in cerebral palsy, depicted the complexity of the problem and delineated three groups of patients who had some distinct gait analysis characteristics to account for the problem. Group I children had the least involvement; internal rotation gait was primarily the result of abnormal muscle activity (gluteus medius, adductors, hamstrings) and pelvic and femoral rotation. In this group, muscle surgery and correction of the coexisting femoral rotation appeared logical to correct the in-toed walking. Group II children were more severely involved, had abnormal muscle activity and dissociated pelvic–femoral motion, and depended on assistive devices; in this group, hip internal rotation was not consistently found and femoral rotation was not an indicator of the hip rotation. In this pattern, soft-tissue surgery would have a limited effect. From this report one might gather that in this group the main problem was pelvic rotation. Group III children had no measurable rotation movements of the femur and pelvis, and the hip appeared fixed in internal rotation position. This group comprised the most severely neurologically involved. Their walking pattern was one of falling and catching oneself—a description of poor equilibrium reactions. In this group there may be no surgical procedure that would significantly improve their gait.

In an attempt to tease apart the problem of which muscle causes the dynamic hip internal rotation during gait bioengineers constructed a three-dimensional model of hip muscles and the effect of hip internal rotation in varying degrees of hip flexion (Delp *et al.* 1999). In the muscles studied (gluteus maximus, medius and mininus, iliopsoas, piriformis, quadratus femoris, obturator internus and externus) they found that hip internal rotation moment arms increased in some muscles with hip flexion but decreased with others, especially the gluteus maximus. The trend toward hip internal rotation with hip flexion occurred in 15 of the 18 muscle compartments. These results suggested that excessive hip flexion might exacerbate the internal rotation of the hip and perhaps somehow activating the gluteus maximus could help correct the excessive hip flexion and internal rotation.

Using gait analysis, Steinwender *et al.* (2001a) of Graz, Austria, described two locomotion patterns in spastic diplegia; one group had a crouch gait and the other did not. In both groups these children had significantly more internal rotation in the first half of the stance phase compared with normal children. An important finding was that the degree of hip adduction was the same in all giving rise to the term 'pseudo-adduction' for limb internal rotation during gait. Subsequently, Steinwender and colleagues (2000) assessed the efficacy of surgical correction of the internal rotation gait of 16 children with spastic diplegia. They concluded that 'multilevel' soft-tissue surgery, particularly medial hamstring lengthening, was effective in correcting the gait pattern *absent fixed bony rotational deformities.*

The same group from Graz, Austria (Saraph *et al.* 2002), resorted to bone surgery for 'fixed internal-rotation deformity of the hip' in eight children with spastic diplegia and 14 with spastic hemiplegia. These patients had multilevel surgery as well as a femoral derotation osteotomy. After surgery, those with hemiplegia had their compensatory external rotation of the pelvis corrected and those with diplegia had significant improvements in hip rotation with no change in pelvic rotation.

In view of the lack of convincing evidence of spastic muscles as the only cause of excessive hip internal rotation gait, some other mechanism must be responsible. This mechanism, which has been studied and verified by several investigators, is excessive femoral anteversion (antetorsion) for the age of the child.

The obverse opinion was rendered by Aktas *et al.* (2000) who found no predictability of hip rotation in gait of children with cerebral palsy with CT measurements for femoral anteversion and the physical examination. But the CT measures of the tibia correlated highly with the physical findings. They concluded that the 'dynamic component' of hip rotation during gait was significant. What specific 'dynamic component' is responsible remains, we suppose, controversial.

The dynamic component of hip internal rotation in children with cerebral palsy was addressed by the bioengineers at Northwestern University, Evanston, Illinois (Arnold *et al.* 2000a). Computer models of three subjects revealed that the medial hamstrings, adductor longus, adductor brevis and gracilis had negligible or small external rotation moment arms through the gait cycle. They suggest these muscles should not be lengthened to correct in-toed gait and that 'other factors' were likely operative. These 'other factors' were probably femoral torsion.

EXCESSIVE FEMORAL ANTEVERSION

A more correct term is antetorsion ('version' is the normal; 'torsion' is abnormal rotation, 2 SD above or below the mean value). However, common usage is anteversion' and we use it here so that the subject will not be even more confusing to the reader. *Clinical and anatomical analyses* support the concept that the one consistent deformity associated with femoral internal rotation in the gait of patients with cerebral palsy is excessive femoral anteversion. The anatomical feature is a twist forward of the head, neck and trochanteric region of the femur with respect to the transcondylar axis of the knee beyond the range expected for normal humans at a given age.

Radiographic measurements using the Magilligan (1956) or the Ryder–Crane technique (Ryder and Crane 1953, Ryder 1972) for determining femoral anteversion in 50 children with spastic diplegia who had hip internal rotation gaits demonstrated femoral anteversion beyond the range of normal for their age. Ten children with cerebral palsy who did not have a hip internal-rotation gait had femoral anteversion within the limits of normal (Bleck 1987) (Fig. 8.32). Lewis *et al.* (1964), Staheli *et al.* (1968), Beals (1969) and Fabry *et al.* (1973) have documented excessive femoral anteversion in ambulatory and non-ambulatory patients with cerebral palsy.

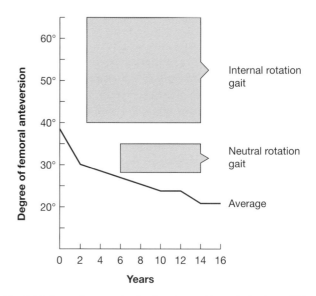

Fig. 8.32. Femoral antetorsion in 50 patients with cerebral palsy and hip internal rotation gait compared with 10 children with cerebral palsy who did not internally rotate with average femoral anteversion values according to age in years.

Coxa valga (a femoral neck-shaft angle >145º) is derived from an anterior–posterior projection of the proximal femur in a radiograph. Because plain radiographs depict images only in two dimensions and are shadows cast on the screen, femoral torsion with the hip in neutral rotation give the perception of coxa valga. Bleck (1987) measured the true angles of inclination of the femoral necks in 60 hips of children with cerebral palsy who had excessive femoral anteversion, and found only three femoral neck-shaft angles above the normal range for age as reported by Shands and Steele (1958). In the study of femoral anteversion in cerebral palsy by Lewis *et al.* (1964), the average anteversion was

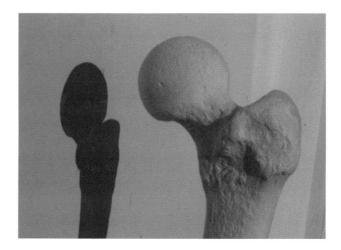

Fig. 8.33. Photograph of anatomical specimen of the proximal femur with simulated 90º femoral anteversion. Spotlight casts a shadow of the proximal femur as in anterior–posterior plain radiographs. The light source was lateral and inferior to the specimen accounting for a near normal femoral neck angle. If the light was directed 90º to the specimen, the extreme femoral anteversion would project as almost a straight head and neck with the shaft, i.e. coxa valga.

54.8° and femoral neck-shaft angle average was 147°; if 145° is accepted as the upper limit of normal, this is not significant coxa valga. Laplaza *et al.* (1993) studied 289 hips in 157 children who had cerebral palsy. They found that the neck-shaft angles were not markedly increased and did not differ substantially from that of the normal population (135°–140°). These radiographic findings of the normal femoral neck-shaft angles in cerebral palsy should alert the surgeon to resist operating on the x-ray to create a varus angle (< 135°) with femoral subtrochanteric osteotomy to reduce a subluxation or dislocation of the hip. Better to realize that we are dealing with excessive femoral anteversion and do derotation osteotomies.

Radiographic findings of the normal femoral neck-shaft angles in cerebral palsy should alert the surgeon to resist operating on the x-ray to create a varus angle (<135 °).

NATURAL HISTORY OF FEMORAL ANTEVERSION

At birth, infants have angles of femoral anteversion from 10° to 60°; the mean is variously given as 31° (Michele 1962) and 38° (Shands and Steele 1958) (Fig. 8.34). During skeletal maturation,

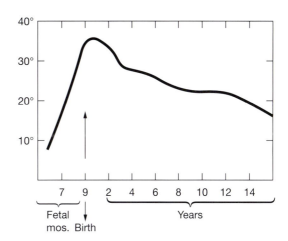

Fig. 8.35. Normal mean values of femoral anteversion from 6th month of fetal life to age 16 years. Note gradual decrease with advancing skeletal maturity (from Shands and Steele 1958; Crane 1959; Fabry *et al.* 1973).

this angle decreases to the adult value of 19° (Shands and Steele 1958, Crane 1959, Fabry *et al.* 1973) (Figs 8.32, 8.35). This spontaneous decrease in most normal children probably has a biomechanical basis.

EXPERIMENTAL DATA ON FEMORAL ANTEVERSION

At birth the proximal end of the femur (head, neck and greater trochanteric region) is entirely cartilaginous and pliable; this proximal segment is fixed to a rigid osseus diaphysis that terminates at the subtrochanteric level (Fig. 8.36). When we manipulated fresh stillborn specimens of the femur, the proximal cartilaginous end could be made to rotate on the rigid osseus diaphysis. Mechanically and mathematically, the point of femoral torsion has been located in the subtrochanteric region of the

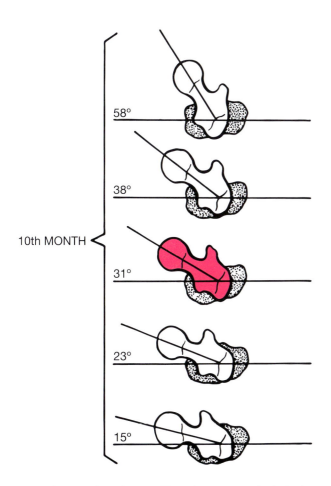

Fig. 8.34. Mean values of ranges of femoral anteversion at birth. (Redrawn from Michele 1962.)

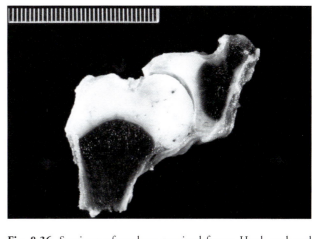

Fig. 8.36. Specimen of newborn proximal femur. Head, neck and trochanter not yet ossified (head ossification begins to show about the fourth postnatal month). Note the osseus diaphysis. The cartilaginous proximal end is attached to the more rigid diaphysis. The point of femoral torsion is considered in the subtrochanteric region (Michele 1962). (Photograph of specimen, by courtesy of John A. Ogden MD.)

femur (Michele 1962). With progressive ossification of the femoral head, neck and greater trochanteric region, the more elastic cartilage is replaced by bone and no further derotation can occur. Fabry *et al.* (1973) documented no further reduction of normal femoral anteversion after the age of 8 years. In Fabry's (1977) study of 180 hips in 91 children with spastic diplegia and hemiplegia, the femoral anteversion did not decrease after the age of 3 years. Laplaza *et al.* (1993) confirmed in cerebral palsy that femoral anteversion at the age of 4 years did not improve with time.

Lee (1977a) studied the possible mechanisms of derotation of the proximal femur in the hips of fresh stillborn specimens. The muscles were dissected from the hips leaving only the capsule intact; the newborn hip-flexion contracture was entirely in the capsule and not in the muscles. He found that a 2º–4º external torque strain was needed to derotate the proximal end of the femur at the cartilaginous–osseous subtrochanteric junction. This derotation occurred as the hips were extended and externally rotated. The torque strains in external rotation were absent when the hips were flexed 90º (Fig. 8.37).

Wilkinson (1962) used skeletally immature rabbits whose hips were immobilized internally rotated for several weeks in plaster to create femoral anteversion; in the same rabbits, retroversion resulted when the hips were immobilized in external rotation. Somerville (1957) discussed 'persistent foetal alignment of the hip' in the context of congenital dislocation. He found that with the hip in full flexion it was possible to rotate the femur 'through nearly 90 degrees, but as the hip extended the femur rotates medially until in full flexion it lies in 20 degrees of medial rotation and cannot be further laterally rotated.' He attributed this lack of hip external rotation because the anterior capsule becomes 'taut' when the hip is extended. 'He also opined that an equal torsional strain must fall on the femoral neck which is partly cartilaginous and malleable. The strain on the proximal femur gradually 'molds the anteversion' until it is reduced to the normal range at skeletal maturity. But if the capsule stretches or is lax, anteversion may not be molded away. Instead persistent fetal femoral anteversion persists.

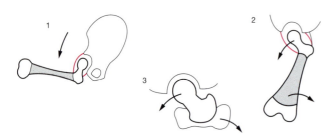

Fig. 8.37. Graphic summary of anatomical experiment with fresh stillborn specimens of the pelvis, hip and femur. All muscles removed; hip capsule left intact. Newborn hip-flexion contracture persisted, indicating that the contracture was in the joint capsule and not the muscle. (1) As the hip was extended pressure from the joint capsule was on the femoral head and proximal femur. (2) A 2º–4º external torque strain was needed to derotate the proximal end of the femur at the cartilage-osseous subtrochanteric junction. (3) As the femoral shaft rotated laterally, the proximal femur as a unit rotated in the opposite direction to reduce the anteversion.

The experiments of Arkin and Katz (1956) on the pressure effects of epiphyseal growth demonstrated that this growth responded to stress on the physis. Torque caused torsional growth. All changes in bone shape were due to new bone laid down by the cartilage cells aligned in the stressed pattern.

These data strongly suggest that in humans the mechanisms necessary for the natural reduction of newborn femoral anteversion are: (1) external rotation of the hip, and (2) hip extension to produce optimal derotation.

Measurements of newborn hip passive extension and internal rotation confirm that all newborn children have a flexion contracture of the hip of 28º (Haas *et al.* 1973). At 6 weeks the flexion contracture decreases to a mean value of 19º, and at 3–6 months it decreases to 7º (Coon *et al.* 1975). Phelps *et al.* (1985) used the prone hip-extension test rather than the Thomas test to measure hip extension at ages 9 and 24 months in unaffected infants: a 10º flexion contracture was present at 9 months and at 24 months it decreased to 3º. Internal rotation of the hip decreased from the age of 6 weeks to 3 months as this hip extended (p=0.005, Coon *et al.* 1975). In the study by Phelps *et al.* (1985), at age 9–24 months hip internal rotation increased from 41º (SD =7.8) to 52º (SD=10.1), and external rotation decreased from 56º (SD =6.6) to 47º (SD =8.5). These serial measurements of the passive range of hip rotation were thought to confirm Pitkow's description (1975) of the spontaneous reduction of the hip external-rotation contracture of the newborn. A hypothesis to explain excessive femoral anteversion in cerebral palsy with spastic paralysis of the lower limbs can be constructed with the experimental and clinical data available. These children are born with spastic paralysis that results in spasticity of the iliopsoas muscle so that the newborn hip-flexion contracture persists. The persistent pull of spastic hip flexor muscle does not permit the pressure of the anterior capsule of the hip on the proximal femur as in normal infants when the hip extends. The lack of hip extension decreases the torque strains on the proximal end of the femur, and derotation cannot occur. We might then deduce that persistent flexion contracture of the hip from birth causes persistence of the infantile femoral anteversion which generally exceeds that of the skeletally mature human. Why the infantile femoral anteversion persists in children with no paralysis leads to speculation. Are they propped in the sitting position as infants too much? Or is it a genetic defect in development of the femur?

Deduction: persistent infantile hip flexion contracture causes persistent infantile femoral anteversion in cerebral palsy.

IN-TOED GAIT AND FEMORAL ANTEVERSION

Why does excessive femoral anteversion cause the in-toed gait seen in some neurologically normal children and some with cerebral palsy? The best explanation was offered by Merchant (1965), who constructed a mechanical model to study the function of the gluteus medius. This muscle is a major stabilizer of the pelvis, and by its contraction during the stance phase of gait allows the shift of the trunk and its center of gravity over the head of the femur. With Merchant's model the hip-abductors exerted optimum force when the insertion of the abductor muscles on the greater trochanter were in a neutral relationship to their origins on the ilium. In femoral antetorsion the greater trochanter is in a posterior position with the femur in neutral rotation; thus, in order to gain optimum strength of the hip abductor during the stance phase of gait, the greater trochanter must shift from its posterior position by internal rotation of the femur. This internal rotation of the femur is necessary to shift the trunk laterally during the stance phase for optimum efficiency and energy conservation during forward progression. Clinical observations seem to confirm this explanation. According to parents interviewed, normal children who in-toe due to excessive femoral anteversion often do so more toward the end of the day when they are fatigued.

The three-dimensional computer model of an adult lower limb that replicated increased femoral anteversion developed by Arnold *et al.* (1997) confirmed the hypothesis that hip internal rotation during gait was a compensatory mechanism to preserve hip-abductor muscle power. When the anteversion angle was increased in the model to 30º–40º there was a 40%–50% decrease in the abduction moment arm of the gluteus medius.

Further fuel was added to the controversy regarding the spastic hip adductors and medial hamstrings by the biomechanical engineers at Stanford University (Arnold and Delp 2001). They used their deformable model of the femur with kinematic data from gait analysis to determine muscle moment arms for various joint angles and femoral anteversion. In marked contrast to opinions of many surgeons in the past they found that with increasing femoral anteversion the adductor muscles shifted toward *external rotation*; the medial hamstrings had negligible or external rotation moment arms with flexed knees or hip internal rotation in gait.

The evidence is strong that the cause of the internal rotation gait in spastic lower limbs is not primarily in a spastic muscle, but due to excessive femoral anteversion. So why continue to attack a muscle? Stay with the bone.

The cause of the internal rotation gait . . . is not primarily in a muscle, but due to excessive femoral anteversion.

Radiographic measurements of the degree of femoral anteversion can be made with a variety of techniques. In the Magilligan technique (1956), an anterior–posterior radiograph of the hips is made with the hips and pelvis in neutral rotation; the femoral neck-shaft angle is measured on the film. Next, a true lateral radiograph is made with the hip in neutral rotation and with the film cassette held on the lateral aspect of the pelvis and femur, and parallel to the neck angle as measured on the first film. The projected angle of anteversion on this second film is obtained by drawing one line along the shaft and another along the center of the neck. Based upon a trigonometric calculation, the angle of rotation of the neck can be worked out. Magilligan constructed a chart so that the true angles of femoral anteversion could be determined without calculations, using the angles of femoral inclination derived from the two films.

In the Ryder–Crane technique (1953), an anterior–posterior radiograph with the hips and pelvis in neutral rotation is made to measure the neck-shaft angle on the film. The second radiograph is an anterior–posterior projection with the hips abducted exactly 30º and flexed 90º; the limb is held on a special frame (MacEwen 1972). The projected angle of femoral neck anteversion is measured by a line through the neck and a second line along the horizontal reference marker of the frame. Trigonometry calculates the true angle of anteversion. Dr C.T. Ryder (personal communication) produced computer-generated tables so that the true angles of anteversion and femoral neck shaft could be easily determined from the two measurements obtained. This method is reasonably accurate, with a reported error of ±10º.

The disadvantage of the Magilligan technique is the demand for a true lateral radiograph of the hip. The disadvantage of the Ryder–Crane technique is the requirement for the hip to be abducted 30º; in cerebral palsy this may not be possible if the child has spastic and contracted hip-adductor muscles.

Other techniques are fluoroscopic (LaGasse and Staheli 1972), axial tomographic (Hubbard and Staheli 1972), computerized axial tomographic (Peterson *et al.* 1981, Horstmann and Mahboubi 1987) and ultrasonographic (Graf 1983, Phillips *et al.* 1985). All methods have been compared for accuracy. Ruby *et al.* (1979) studied the fluoroscopic and biplane methods and concluded that both were comparable in accuracy, but he favoured the Ryder–Crane technique. Computerized axial tomography has the advantage of a more direct visualization, and the radiation can be justified in special problem cases, but its routine use is questionable.[14]

Now that we know excessive femoral anteversion exists and can explain the in-toed gaits of children with spastic diplegia, is radiographic confirmation necessary in every case? It seems unlikely that more studies are needed to prove the point. A more prudent policy would be to rely on the published data and the clinical examination; the radiographic examinations could be reserved for special structural problems in the hip as part of the preoperative planning. Horstmann and Mahboubi (1987) have recommended CT of the hip in planning reconstructive surgery. Computerized axial tomography, as well as magnetic resonance imaging, can be of enormous value in defining the location and integrity of the femoral head in relationship to the acetabulum in the analysis of structural changes in the hip joint when planning surgery.

The clinical examination of hip rotation in children who have a hip internal rotation gait is good enough to assess excessive femoral anteversion. If it is present, the passive range of rotation of the hips, with the hips extended, patient prone and knees flexed

---

14 At the Stanford University Medical Center the mean skin dose from a CT scan was 2.4 rads to the adult pelvic area, 0.6 rads to the male gonads and 2.5 rads to the bladder. Compared with plain radiographs using earthfiltered screens, the active bone marrow does from a radiograph of the pelvis of a 1-year-old child was 3 millrads (millirad=1/1000 of a rad) for the anterior–posterior view, and 2 millirads for the lateral view (Bleck 1984). The ultrasonographic technique studied by Phillips *et al.* (1985) concluded that it was too inaccurate to be useful.

90º, will show internal rotation greater than 60º and external rotation less than 30º. A range of internal rotation of the femur in the 70º–90º range, and external rotation of less than 20º, is good evidence of excessive anteversion. A cautionary note: children who have increased ligamentous laxity may have 80º–90º of rotation in *both directions* not due to excessive femoral anteversion (Wynne-Davies 1970).

Schutte and associates (1997) at the Gillette Children's Hospital used a clinical method to measure the degree of femoral anteversion in a study of its effects on psoas and hamstring muscle lengths during crouch gait. They considered their method to be accurate to within 5º–10º as determined at the time of surgery. The patient lies prone with the knee flexed 90º. The hip is then externally rotated until the greater trochanter is in its most lateral position. The degree that the shin (leg) deviates from the vertical line of zero rotation is the degree of femoral anteversion (e.g. 90º minus 40º = 50º). Six years prior to the preceding study, Ruwe *et al.* (1992) found that the lateral trochanteric prominence method correlated within 4º of the radiographic measurement of femoral anteversion.

The clinical examination of hip rotation in children who have a hip internal rotation gait is good enough to assess excessive femoral anteversion.

ABANDONED SURGICAL PROCEDURES TO CORRECT HIP INTERNAL ROTATION

Various soft tissue procedures have fallen into disuse because critical assessment confirmed their ineffectiveness in correcting the in-toed gait. The following have fallen by the wayside.

(1) Posterior transposition of the origin of the tensor fascia femoris, known as the Durham procedure (Edmonson 1963); Majestro and Frost (1971) reported failure.

(2) Adductor myotomy with anterior branch obturator neurectomy or transfer of the adductor origins to the ischium (Majestro and Frost 1971, Baumann 1972).

(3) Neurectomy of the superior gluteal nerve (Majestro and Frost (1971).

(4) Semitendinosus transfer to the anterior-lateral femur (Baker and Hill 1964, Sutherland *et al.* 1969)—the hamstrings had normal lengths in crouch gait determined by models (Schutte *et al.* 1997).

(5) Gluteus medius and minimus tendon transfer (Steel 1980); the major problem was a severe Trendelenberg gait postoperatively in six of 26 patients (42 hips). Bleck (1987) tried the operation in only three patients; it did correct the in-toed gait, but one patient who walked unassisted at a three year follow-up had a painful subluxation of the hip that was not present preoperatively. Why? Probably because of excessive femoral anteversion and dynamic internal rotation kept the hip located; after gluteus medius transfer, dynamic external rotation caused the proximal femur roll-out of the acetabulum and uncover the femoral head. Independent walkers with spastic diplegia rarely, if ever, develop subluxations of the hip. If it occurs in later childhood, it seems plausible that such cases have an unrecognized developmental subluxation of the hip (incidence estimated as 1 in 1000 live births) that remained silent until symptomatic in later childhood.

Joseph (1998) of Manipal, India, cut only the anterior fibers of the gluteus medius to correct excessive hip and pelvic internal rotation. Joseph's approach to the problem was based on spastic 'overactivity' of the anterior fibers of the gluteus medius and minimus. He did the procedure on 12 hips and stated that the gait improved in all without weakness of the hip-abductor power. No other confirming reports of the efficacy and functional outcomes of this operation have appeared.

(6) Iliopsoas recession (Bleck 1971a, b, 1987). The operation was not intended to correct in-toed gait in spastic diplegia because there is no evidence that the iliopsoas is a hip-rotator muscle. However, in a postoperative follow-up Bleck (1987) noted that in some patients their hip internal rotation in the stance phase of gait had diminished considerably with concomitant decreasing passive hip internal rotation in 3–5 postoperative years so that femoral rotation osteotomy was not necessary. In the follow-up between 7 and 10 years of 21 patients who had iliopsoas recession, seven (33.3 %) had a subsequent derotation subtrochanteric femoral osteotomy (three bilateral and four unilateral) to correct the objectionable in-toeing. The passive range of hip internal rotation had decreased in the others or probably was masked by compensatory external tibial torsion postoperatively. Preoperative radiographic measurements of femoral anteversion were made with the Ryder–Crane technique in only six patients because of the common fear of excessive radiation. The measurements from the radiographs gave equivocal results so no definitive statement to correlate with the anatomical change in rotation of the proximal end of the femur and with the observed decreased internal rotation of the femur throughout the stance phase of gait.

If the surgeon, parents, and the child after iliopsoas lengthening before the age of 7 years can be patient to wait for an expected decrease in femoral anteversion and the in-toed gait, femoral osteotomy can be deferred. After age 8 years femoral torsion does not change in normal children (Fabry *et al.* 1973, Fabry 1977). Our study (Lee 1977a) on the possible mechanism of derotation of the proximal end of the femur on extension and external rotation of the hip indicates that the earlier hip extension is obtained, the more likely correction of the torsion will occur. While the age of the child is important, the chronological age does not always correlate with skeletal age; children who have cerebral palsy may have growth retardation (Horstmann 1986). It might be best to allow the proximal femur to derotate after psoas lengthening, recession, or tenotomy at or above the pelvic brim. Femoral rotation osteotomy can be kept as an arrow in the quiver in case the child older than age 9 years decides to have it. Internal fixation of larger bones can be more secure to ensure a smooth postoperative course without the need for plaster immobilization

DEROTATION FEMORAL OSTEOTOMY

Derotation subtrochanteric femoral osteotomy has produced definite and permanent results (Majestro and Frost 1971, Bost and Bleck 1975, Tylkowski *et al.* 1980, Hoffer *et al.* 1981, Ōunpuu *et al.* 2002). It is indicated in children in whom a marked in-toed gait persists after the age of 8, whose major deformity is femoral rotation and not pelvic rotation, and whose passive range of hip internal rotation is 70°–90°, and whose external rotation is limited to less than 30° with the hip extended. The site of the osteotomy can be any place in the femur, but the supracondylar or subtrochanteric levels are the predominant choices.

Supracondylar derotation femoral osteotomy with pins and plaster. Hoffer *et al.* (1981) prefer the supracondylar level because the femur can be sectioned here through a very small incision, blood loss is minimal and a long-leg cast rather than a hip spica, which could be necessary for osteotomies at the subtrochanteric level. Threaded pins were inserted through the lateral to the medial cortices of the femur above and below the osteotomy site, with the distal pin at an angle to the proximal for the intended correction, so that the foot during gait would not exceed 15°of external rotation from the line of progression. The pins were removed after 4–8 weeks and the long-leg plaster replaced. Early weightbearing was encouraged; the usual time of immobilization was 8 weeks.

Supracondylar osteotomy, especially when pins are used for fixation, does have some complications. In Hoffer *et al.*'s (1981) report of 11 patients, three had pin-tract infections which subsequently healed; two had a 10° limitation of knee extension which resolved in 6 months; one required wedging of the plaster before healing was secure to correct anterior–posterior angulation of the distal fragment.

Thompson *et al.* (1986) made an even smaller incision to derotate the femur at the supracondylar region. The use of intraoperative fluoroscopy with image intensification makes 'peep-hole' surgery feasible. Their operation also used two threaded Steinman pins above and below the osteotomy site. The method was percutaneous in that they drilled the cortices of the supracondylar region of the femur, performed a manual osteoclasis, derotated to the desired degree and immobilized in a long-leg or spica plaster 5–9 weeks. Of their 19 patients, 11 had a 'gait abnormality'; 14 patients had cerebral palsy. They reported good results with only two complications: 5° of varus angulation and one pin breakage. An additional patient required knee manipulation under anesthesia. There can be little argument with these good results of supracondylar osteotomy.

SUPRACONDYLAR DEROTATION FEMORAL OSTEOTOMY WITH SIX-HOLE COMPRESSION PLATE

Cooke *et al.* (1989) used a six-hole compression plate on the lower femoral shaft above the eiphyseal line. After the plate was contoured they fixed it to the proximal portion of the intended osteotomy site with three screws. Then the bone was divided

through 90% of its circumference. After the osteotomy was completed, with osteoclasis and rotation of the distal fragment, three screws were inserted into it and dynamic compression closed the osteotomy site. Weightbearing was not permitted for 3 weeks and then walking aids were used until solid union occurred. Correction occurred in all cases and osteotomies united in 3 months. Walking function improved in all.

DISADVANTAGES OF SUPRACONDYLAR DEROTATION OSTEOTOMY

Bleck (1987) concerns with supracondylar osteotomy were: (1) immobilization of the knee and subsequent stiffness when we know the knee a major determinant of gait; (2) posterior angulation of the distal fragment causing genu recurvatum; (3) pin-tract infection; and (4) a postoperative incision and pin tract scars on the visible lateral distal aspect of the thigh. So many young men and women wear shorts that such scars may be objectionable when showing off their legs. True, there is a postoperative incision scar on the proximal lateral thigh with subtrochanteric osteotomies. It can be hidden with shorts and skirts, though not with a bikini.

Seconding Bleck's opinion against supracondylar derotation osteotomy were Payne and DeLuca (1994) who had a 14.7 % complication rate with supracondylar derotation osteotomies fixed with cross pins in 17 patients (34 osteotomies). This led them to adopt the intertrochanteric osteotomy with the blade-plate fixation in 10 patients with no complications. A slight difference in their approach was to do the operation with the patient prone.

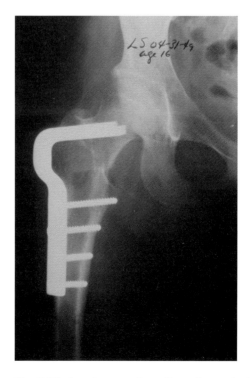

Fig. 8.38. Anterior–posterior radiograph, proximal femur; healed subtrochanteric osteotomy; ASIF hip-compression nail plate.

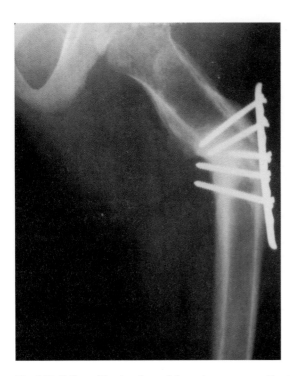

Fig. 8.39. Failure of fixation, femoral derotation osteotomy. Fixation out-moded and inadequate. If you want to use a lateral side plate for fixation, choose a sturdier six-hole plate.

SUBTROCHANTERIC DEROTATION OSTEOTOMY WITH A RIGHT-ANGLE HIP-COMPRESSION NAIL

Since 1967, Bleck (1987) has preferred the subtrochanteric osteotomy with the secure internal fixation of the right-angled hip-compression nail (ASIF) (Fig. 8.38). Staheli *et al.* (1980) reported a 15.5% complication rate in 78 children who had derotation subtrochanteric femoral osteotomy for medial femoral torsion. Among the complications were loss of fixation, errors in the amount of correction, fractures, heel ulcer and infection (Fig. 8.39). Bost and Bleck (1975) reported no infections or failures of fixation using the ASIF hip-compression nail for derotation subtrochanteric osteotomies in 24 patients with spastic diplegia (31 hips).

Brunner and Baumann (1997) of Switzerland also preferred the intertrochanteric femoral osteotomy to correct in-toeing gait. They found the results in 63 hips observed from 11 to 18 years. There was loss of the femoral neck-shaft and anteversion angles in those who had subluxation or dislocation with surgery before the age of 4 years. The osteotomy alone did not result in adequate coverage of the femoral head. Subluxation and dislocation require a different solution and might be prevented as delineated in the section to follow.

It does not make any difference whether you use an ASIF 90° fixed-angle hip-compression blade plate or the Richards intermediate hip screw according to a study of 164 proximal femoral osteotomies by Hau and associates (2000) at the Royal Children's Hospital, Australia. The incidence of complications was 9%.

PROXIMAL FEMORAL ROTATION OSTEOTOMY WITH THE ILIZAROV TECHNIQUE

As might be suspected the wave of enthusiasm for the Ilizarov technique in leg-lengthening and the fixation device modified by Cattoneo and Catagni (cited by Bianchi-Maiocchi and Aronson 1991). The system with the hoops and cross pins through the bone was adopted by Moens *et al.* (1995) of Pellenbereg, Belgium. With this fixation device they were able to cut the cortex of the diaphysis of the femur (corticotomy) between two hoops and externally rotate the distal segment. Walking with partial weight bearing in unilateral cases was allowed on the fifth postoperative day and in bilateral osteotomies in 2 weeks. Healing occurred in 8–10 weeks. Then the fixation was removed under general anesthesia. Physiotherapy to preserve knee flexion was instituted on the first postoperative day and continued after the fixation was removed. Even so the average range of knee flexion was limited to 45°?at this time. Complications were minimal, consisting of slight varus angulation (< 5°) in three and pin-track infections in five. In-toed gait was corrected in all. Objections to the Ilizarov method for derotation osteotomy would be the cumbersome apparatus and most importantly its restrictive postoperative knee flexion.[15]

SUBTROCHANTERIC DEROTATION OSTEOTOMY WITH A FEMORAL INTRAMEDULLARY NAIL

Renshaw and Green (1996) reamed the femoral canal and inserted the proximal and distal locking nail to secure the osteotomy of the shaft to correct femoral torsion. As discovered when this method became popular for femoral fractures in children and adolescents, the risk was avascular necrosis of the femoral head in children due to disruption of its blood supply if the nail were introduced through the fovea. Rather they emphasized that the nail should enter proximally through the tip of the trochanter. And, as with most internal fixation in children, it should be removed when mature bone continuity has been established.

SOME UNINTENDED CONSEQUENCES OF DEROTATION SUBTROCHANTERIC OSTEOTOMY, AND HOW TO AVOID THEM

1. *A postoperative increase in the hip flexion.* The preoperative assessment should include the measurement of the hip-flexion contracture with a clinical measurement (prone hip-extension test) and/or with gait analysis that shows lack of normal hip extension on stance and increased anterior pelvic tilt. The unintended result appears to be due to increased tension on the iliopsoas when the lesser trochanter is rotated in either direction (Fig. 8.40). The calculation of hamstring and psoas lengths in the

15 In France where the Ilizarov method was applied with considerable zeal for leg lengthening, non-union of fractures and deformity the process caused in some patients considerable anxiety with the wires through their thighs and legs surrounded by hoops. The emotional reaction was termed 'St Sebastian syndrome', in memory of the Christian martyr who according to legend and as memorialized in paintings was put to death by multiple arrows through his body (c. 288 AD) (S. Terver, personal communication).

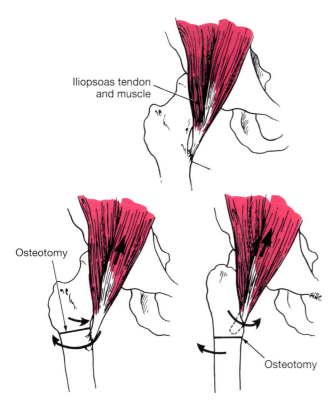

Fig. 8.40. Probable effect of femoral rotation osteotomy below the lesser trochanter and effect on iliopsoas tendon and muscle.

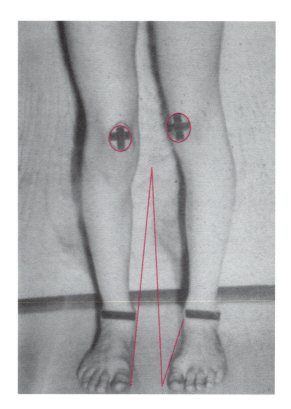

Fig. 8.41. Spastic diplegia; male, age 12 years. Bilateral femoral torsion masked by secondary external tibial torsion beyond normal mean of 22°.

crouch gait of children with cerebral palsy derived from computer generated musculoskeletal models by Schutte *et al.* (1997) showed that rotation of the femur with an average femoral anteversion of 48° affected the muscle lengths. The hamstrings were not significantly short, whereas the psoas lengths were 2 SD below their maximum lengths. Rotation about the axis of the femur at the lesser trochanter caused a substantial movement of the psoas insertion on the lesser trochanter and the shortening of the psoas. Note that the hamstrings were not significantly shortened. Consequently, it appears that the postoperative crouch gait seen in some patients is due almost entirely as a compensation for the worsened hip-flexion contracture.

Another study (Schmidt *et al.* 1999), using three dimensional computer analysis of simulated rotation osteotomies at the intertrochanteric, subtrochanteric or supracondylar levels of the femur, revealed no substantial change in the length of the hamstrings or gracilis. The origin-to-insertion lengths of the adductor longus and brevis decreased to less than 4 mm with sub-trochanteric osteotomies; intertrochanteric osteotomies and 60° of rotation increased adductor brevis lengths 8 mm (6.3%).

The foregoing scientific data explains why a derotation osteotomy of the femur for excessive femoral anteversion can cause an increase in the flexion contracture of the hip. If a preoperative flexion-contracture of the hip is discerned, then a psoas lengthening would be justified at the time of the osteotomy.

Unless it has been done prior to a derotation femoral osteotomy, do a psoas lengthening at the same time of osteotomy.

2. *Excessive out-toeing.* If compensatory external tibial torsion is not recognized preoperatively, femoral derotation osteotomy will result in markedly excessive lateral rotation of the foot from the line of progression (Fig. 8.41). The foot compensates with uncomfortable pes varus. The disability is also subjective; nobody wants to walk like a duck.

External tibial torsion is a normal development from birth as it gradually increases in childhood to the adult value of 22° (Fig. 8.42) If the compensatory external torsion more than the average of 22° and in the range of 30°–40°, an internal rotation osteotomy of the tibia and fibula should be planned at the same time as the femoral osteotomy or at a later date.

It may be that with the prospect of four osteotomies in the lower limbs, the patient and family will elect to do nothing. When standing with the heels together and the lower limbs exposed from above the knees to the feet, the combination of the rotational deformities of the femur and tibia give the appearance of bow legs. The solution to this objectionable cosmetic problem would be to wear either long skirts or trousers.[16] But if you believe in 'lever-arm disease', then imperfect function may be a problem.

3. Persistent anterior rotation of the pelvis evident in unilateral femoral derotation osteotomies and increased pelvic and

---

16 Another solution to mask apparent bow legs when wearing a short skirt or short pants is to pose for photographs as professional models do: don't stand with your feet together, instead stand with one foot and leg in front of the other to create the illusion of normally aligned shapely lower limbs.

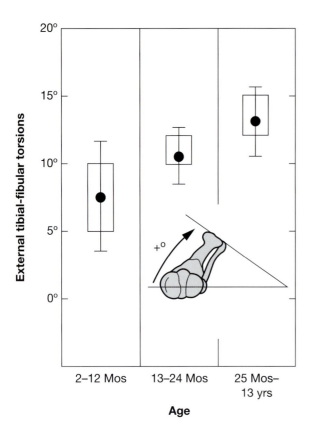

Fig. 8.42. Development of external tibial torsion in normal children from age 2 months to 13 years. (From Bleck and Minaire 1983.)

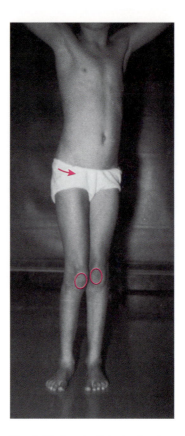

Fig. 8.43. Spastic diplegia, female, age 13 years, postoperative subtrochanteric derotation osteotomy, right side. Persistent anterior rotation of the right side of the pelvis due to overcorrection of internal rotation to zero external rotation. The pelvis cannot rotate externally if the range of internal rotation is so restricted. Lesson: in femoral rotation osteotomy leave 30°–40° of external rotation.

trunk rotation in bilateral osteotomies. The tendency is to overdo corrections for fear of recurrence. The hip needs to have a normal range of internal rotation of 30°–45°. Overcorrection of the internal rotation prevents external rotation of the pelvis on the hip in normal walking (Fig. 8.43). It can also result in posterior subluxation of the hip as the leg seeks to normalize leg rotation. In derotation osteotomies of the femur preserve at least 30°–45° of internal rotation of the hip measured with the limb lying extended on the table and also with limb abducted over the edge of the table with the thigh resting on the table and the knee flexed 90°. The time to check the rotation is in the operating room before wound closure and correct it to the right degree rather than discover the problem 8–12 weeks postoperatively when the patient is fully weightbearing.

Before wound closure and with one or two screws in the fixation nail-plate the degree of internal and external rotation of the hip can be checked.

OPERATIVE TECHNIQUE OF DEROTATION SUBTROCHANTERIC FEMORAL OSTEOTOMY

Because a hip-flexion contracture is inevitably found in spastic diplegic patients who have excessive femoral internal rotation during gait, Bleck (1987) did an iliopsoas recession or lengthening at the time of the osteotomy unless the flexion contracture has been previously corrected (Fig. 8.44).

The subtrochanteric osteotomy is done through the usual lateral approach to the proximal femoral shaft; the incision extends proximally to the tip of the greater trochanter. The origin of the vastus lateralis is detached, and through the posterior portion of this muscle the femur is stripped subperiosteally to expose the entire shaft all around. It is necessary to detach the posterior intramuscular septum from the linea aspera.

With the hip in internal rotation, a guide pin is introduced into the basal region of the femoral neck at a 90° angle to the shaft; this pin is placed slightly more superior to the intended line where the blade of the hip-compression nail is to be inserted. Radiographic control with the image intensifier is used throughout the procedure. The special chisel for the nail is then inserted to create the channel for the blade portion and, if in the correct position on both anterior–posterior and lateral radiographic fluoroscopic projects, the blade of the nail is driven into the bone. The holding device which is used to drive in the blade is kept on it so that the hip can be maintained internally rotated.

To determine the degree of external rotation of the femur distal to the osteotomy, the preoperative passive ranges of motion need to be remembered. There should be 30°–40° of hip external

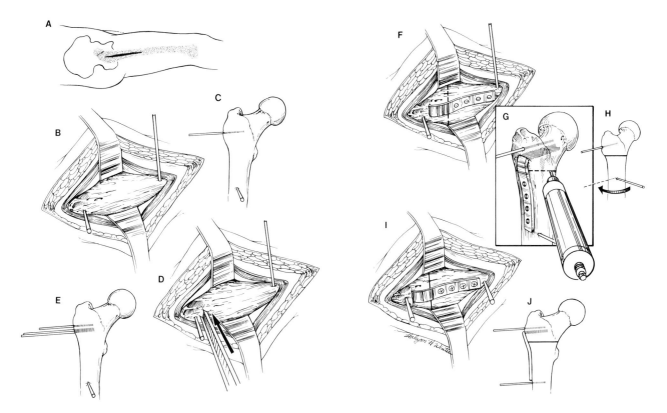

Fig. 8.44. Operative technique of femoral derotation osteotomy. (*A*) Incision lateral thigh over proximal femur. (*B*) Fascia lata split and vastus lateralis fibers separated in posterior portion to expose femoral shaft subperiosteally. (*C*) Two Steinman pins inserted at appropriate angle to derotation desired. (*D, E*) Blade guide inserted distal to guide pin. Localization and blade length of nail determined with fluoroscopy image intensifier. (*F*) Blade and plate portion inserted. (*G*) Osteotomy with a reciprocating saw through subtrochanteric region is made parallel with the blade. (*H*) Proximal fragment held in internal rotation and distal portion of femur externally rotated to point where both pins are parallel. (*I*) Pins parallel and plate fixed to femoral shaft with screws. (*J*) Schematic representation of completed osteotomy. N.B.: blade portion of the device is parallel to the osteotomy to ensure compression forces and secure fixation.

rotation after the osteotomy has been secured. The degree of external rotation can be reasonably estimated by marking the femoral shaft anteriorly with a visible line crossing the proximal and distal portions; an osteotome works best for this. Then, as the femoral shaft is almost a 360° circle, one quarter will represent 90° and one eighth will be 45°. So if the range of hip internal rotation is 80°, derotation of 50° will be about right. Dr L.A. Rinsky (personal communication) has a more elegant and accurate method of determining the exact degree of derotation— a testimony to a superior mathematical mind (Fig. 8.45).

A transverse osteotomy at the subtrochanteric level about l cm from the blade of the nail in the femoral neck is completed with a reciprocating saw. Bone-holding forceps (the c-type seem to work best) grasp the side-plate and femoral shaft, which is then rotated externally the desired degree while an assistant holds the proximal end with the nail-plate driver. The bone-holding forceps are clamped as securely as possible to secure the fixation. At this point the hip can be abducted so that the knee can be flexed over the edge of the table, with the range of internal rotation remaining checked. If satisfactory, the self-compressing plate is fixed to the shaft with the screws using the appropriate and particular technique. After two screws have been placed (out of a usual four to five), the range of hip internal rotation can be checked again. Closed suction drainage is used and wound closure is usual.

Nichols (1980) modified the original Synthes® hip-compression nail by eliminating the lateral offset of the nail to a simple 90° 'L' hip-compression nail (Fig. 8.46). These are manufactured in infant, child, adolescent and adult sizes. The reason for eliminating the lateral protruded part of the original nail was to avoid discomfort over the greater trochanter in patients and tenting of the skin in especially thin children. In this way we are not forced to remove the nail before full recovery has occurred and at a time when schooling would be disrupted. In those patients who are near or beyond skeletal maturity, the need to remove the internal fixation devices is not absolute, unless it is causing discomfort or passing through security checks create undue annoyance as the alarms go off.

Caution: after removal of internal fixation in the femur, protected weightbearing with crutches is advisable for a few weeks. Each hole that was occupied by a screw becomes a 'stress riser' until filled in with bone[17] (Burstein *et al.* 1972). The risk is subtrochanteric fracture. Crutches remind the patient to be careful and guarded in excessive activity.

17 You don't have to wait for the radiograph to show new bone in the drill holes. These holes will be visible in radiographs for longer than 6 months. In 4 weeks, dense-woven bone fills the holes and gradually is incorporated into cortical bone (Burstein *et al.* 1972).

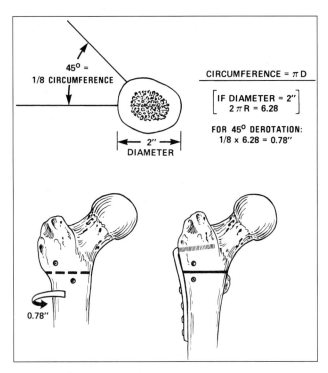

Fig. 8.45. Rinsky (1980) method of determining degree of rotation for derotation osteotomy: measure diameter of femoral shaft with a caliper; calculate circumference = Bd = 2 × 3.14 =6.28 inches; then divide the circumference by the amount of rotation desired, e.g. if 45° = 1/8 of 360° circle of the circumference = 1/8 × 6.28 inches = 0.78 inches. Mark the proximal portion of femur with a drill hole; measure the calculated distance of 0.78 inch and here drill second hole distal to intended site of osteotomy. After osteotomy rotate to that the two drill-holes are in alignment. To speed up the process in the operating room, perhaps the circulating nurse or anesthesiologist ought to be provided with a calculator. Preoperative templating and calculations from the X-ray and the CT scans gives reasonable estimation.

Caution: after removal of internal fixation in the femur, protected weightbearing with crutches is advisable for a few weeks.

The *postoperative care* is non-weightbearing for up to 8 weeks if secure internal fixation has not been achieved. If iliopsoas recession or lengthening has been done, 6–8 hours of hip-extension posture such as with prone lying for up to 3 weeks. Hip-strengthening exercises should be performed. In some patients, even those who have unilateral osteotomies, a bed–wheelchair regime has been required. In bilateral cases this need is greater. In unilateral osteotomies in spastic diplegia, crutch-walking and non-weightbearing on the operated limb increases the risk of falling down in some children because of the commonly associated deficient equilibrium reactions, particularly the posterior ones, which are lacking in almost all.

At the end of 8 weeks, union is secure enough to permit resumption of full weightbearing: beginning in parallel bars, graduating to crutches or walkers within 2–5 days, and without external support (for those who have never needed it) in another month (12 weeks postoperatively). No cast immobilization has been used except for 3 weeks in those who had short- or long-leg casts when foot surgery was also done.

The advantage of this approach to subtrochanteric osteotomy has been the obvious ability to maintain muscle strength and joint range of motion while healing occurs. The disadvantages, in contrast to supracondylar osteotomy, are a longer and more precise operation, more blood loss (usually 350–500 ml), a long lateral scar (10–15 cm) on the proximal thigh, and the need for children to have a second operation a year or two later to remove the internal fixation.

HIP SUBLUXATION AND ACETABULAR DYSPLASIA

Subluxation of the hip occurs in spastic diplegia when the child is only partly weightbearing with the use of crutches or walkers. Dislocation rarely occurs in this kind of patient who at least has independent mobility with assistive devices to compensate for the deficient anterior and posterior equilibrium reactions. Because acetabular dysplasia is secondary to the developmental dislocation at birth, the etiology of the dislocation is probably congenital (changed to 'developmental' in the litigious USA) with super-imposed spastic paralysis in a 2- or 3-year-old child with spastic diplegia. This combination is rare, because the incidence of congenital (developmental) dislocation of the hip is reported to be between eight and 10 per 10,000 births (Coleman 1978).

In spastic diplegia, full weightbearing without support and the usual hip internal rotation gait pattern prevents subluxation. The suggested mechanisms for the development of subluxation and dislocation of the hip are delineated in Chapter 9.

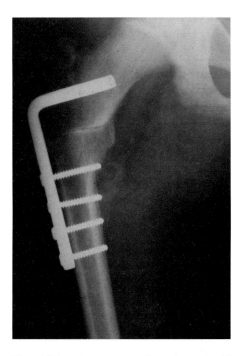

Fig. 8.46. Anterior–posterior radiograph, proximal femur, subtrochanteric derotation osteotomy, fixation with hip compression nail plate without lateral offset (designed by Ted Nichols, MD, Stanford University). The deletion of the lateral offset of the ASIF nail avoids tenting of the skin and bursitis over the lateral projection of the nail in thin patients.

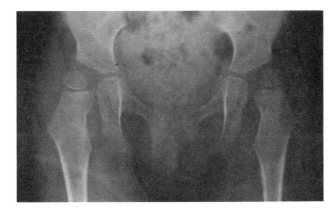

Fig. 8.47. Anterior–posterior radiograph of pelvis and hips, patient HH, female, age 3 years, spastic diplegia, non-ambulatory.

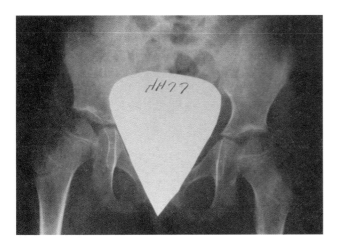

Fig. 8.48. Patient HH, 5 years postoperative, bilateral iliopsoas lengthening only, now independently ambulatory; subluxations reduced.

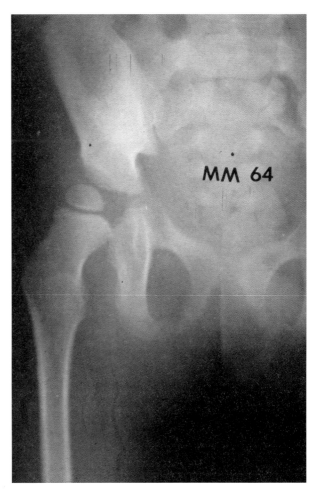

Fig. 8.49. Anterior–posterior radiograph of left hip. Patient MM, male, age 3 years, spastic diplegia, dependent ambulator with triceps crutches, subluxation of left hip.

From our data and experience on the prevention of spastic paralytic subluxation and dislocation of the hip, it seems apparent that reducing the spasticity and contracture of the major deforming muscles before the age of 5 years results in success in the majority of patients (Kalen and Bleck 1985). They found that adductor myotomy with anterior branch obturator neurectomy even before the age of 5 years did not necessarily prevent later subluxation or dislocation. We do have patients who did not have a notable limitation of hip abduction but did have flexion contractures and subluxations of the hip before the age of 5 years; in these children iliopsoas recession resulted in long-lasting reduction of the subluxation and well located hips without acetabular dysplasia on follow-up examination (Figs 8.47–8.50).

Reimers (1980, 1985) disputed that the iliopsoas had any effect, on the basis of his results of iliopsoas lengthening in 11 patients to effect reduction of the subluxation and prevent dislocation of the hip. However, as pointed out in a letter to the editor on the subject (Bleck 1985), no study other than the one by Kalen and Bleck (1985) took into account the ambulatory status of the patient. None of our 99 patients walked independently; 48 walked with crutches, canes or walkers; 51 were non-walkers. Of those who had adductor myotomy and iliopsoas

recession the success rate in preventing further subluxation and additional surgery was 72%, but for those who had only adductor myotomy (with or without anterior branch obturator neurectomy) the success rate was only 36%. In addition there was a 100% success rate after iliopsoas recession and adductor myotomy in those who were ambulatory with assistive devices.

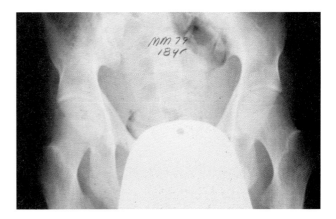

Fig. 8.50. Patient MM, age 18 years, 15 years postoperative bilateral iliopsoas recession. Hips normal. Continued walking with triceps crutches.

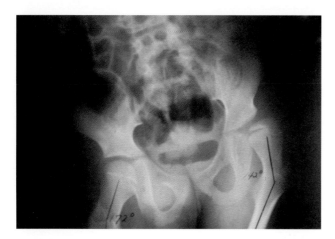

Fig. 8.51. Anterior–posterior radiograph of pelvis and both hips. Patient KK, 7-year-old non-ambulatory boy with spastic diplegia; pelvic obliquity, uncovering of left hip, adduction contracture, left hip; subluxation left hip. Combination of adduction and flexion deformity.

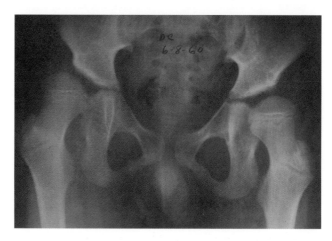

Fig. 8.52. Anterior–posterior radiograph of pelvis and both hips. Patient PC, spastic diplegia, age 9 years, ambulatory with bilateral crutches.

The success of the soft-tissue surgery alone was in children younger than age 5 years. The median age in Reimers' 11 patients was 9.9 years.

In summary, we can recommend lengthening of the psoas *alone* in spastic diplegic children under age 5 who have subluxation of the hip, a flexion contracture of the hip and a range of abduction of each hip more than 30º, and either are ambulatory or have a good prognosis for walking. If this type of child has a range of abduction of the hip less than 30º, adductor longus myotenotomy should be added. If there is no flexion contracture and only an asymmetrical adduction contracture, the hip on the adducted side will *appear* uncovered (Fig. 8.51). In these cases, release of the adduction contracture to correct the resultant pelvic obliquity may reduce this apparent 'subluxation'.

Derotation subtrochanteric osteotomy in addition to psoas lengthening and adductor longus myotenotomy (if the latter is indicated) should be considered for children who have hip subluxation discovered after the age of 5 years (recognizing the differences in skeletal age). Acetabular reconstruction for dysplasia can be added, after age 8–9 years; femoral osteotomy by itself is not likely to result in acetabular remodeling toward normal coverage after this age (Tylkowski *et al.* 1980; Brunner and Baumann 1997) (Figs 8.52–8.54). The exact age after which acetabular remodeling will occur cannot be specifically stated. Skeletal ages vary among children, according to factors such as sex and how much weightbearing they do. If the femoral head is well seated in the acetabulum after the psoas lengthening, you can afford to wait a year or two before attacking the acetabulum surgically. Patience pays.

Recommend . . . lengthening of the psoas alone in spastic diplegic children under age 5 who have a subluxation of the hip.

Derotation subtrochanteric osteotomy in addition to psoas lengthening . . . for hip subluxation discovered after the age of 5 years.

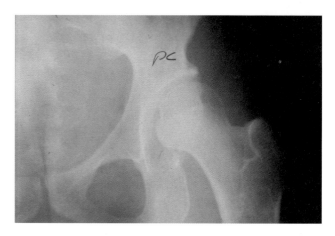

Fig. 8.53. Anterior–posterior radiograph left hip. Patient PC, skeletally mature, age 20 years, 11 years postoperative, bilateral iliopsoas recession and derotation subtrochanteric osteotomies. Approximately 35% of femoral head outside of bony acetabulum which is well formed. Patient asymptomatic, weightbearing with crutches.

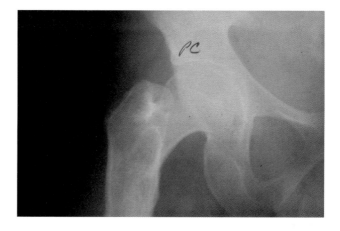

Fig. 8.54. Anterior–posterior radiograph right hip. Patient PC, skeletally mature, age 20 years, 11 years postoperative, bilateral iliopsoas recession and adductor longus myotenotomy. Hip well seated in acetabulum. Asymptomatic, weightbearing with crutches.

Acetabular reconstruction for dysplasia, can be added after age 8–9 years.

KNEE

KNEE-FLEXION DEFORMITY

MUSCLE FUNCTION AND KINEMATICS

The lack of extension of the knee when walking becomes obvious with a flexed knee gait. The hamstring muscles have been the obvious target of surgical attack—their tendons are easily accessible. In the *initial swing* phase of the gait cycle they provide adequate knee flexion of 40º so that the foot can clear the ground as it trails in the plantarflexed position of 20º (Perry 1992). This is why catching your toe on the ground ('stubbing') is not necessarily due to ankle–foot equinus—the surgeon should not jump to gastrocnemius–soleus lengthening.

At *mid-swing* as the gait cycle progresses hamstring action becomes 'intensive' as knee flexion to 60º lifts the foot off the ground and hip flexion primarily through the action of the iliacus advances the thigh. 'The most consistent knee flexor is the short head of the biceps femoris' (Perry 1992). Because the long and short heads of the biceps share the same tendon, the long head acts as a hip-extensor, consequently if the long head is erroneously considered as a knee-flexor, its action on flexion would inhibit hip extension. This is why z-lengthening of the whole biceps tendon should be avoided; instead do fractional lengthening.

In the first half of *terminal swing* all three hamstrings, semitendinosis, semimembranosis and long head of the biceps femoris eccentrically lengthen to inhibit hip extension. At that time the quadriceps begin firing to complete knee extension. The rectus femoris acts as a restraint to excessive knee flexion.

Gait electromyography of the hamstring muscles will demonstrate prolonged and out-of-phase action potentials, often throughout most of the stance phase. Our electromyographic studies have shown concomitant quadriceps prolonged and dysphasic contractions. This has been the case in most ambulatory patients with spastic diplegia. It seems as if the two antagonistic muscle groups frequently balance one another, so that neither excessive knee flexion nor extension dominate (see Figs 3.10, 3.12).

CAUSES AND FUNCTIONAL EFFECTS OF SPASTIC KNEE-FLEXION DEFORMITY

The mechanism of the knee-flexion deformity may be due to spastic and contracted hamstring muscles, secondary to surgically weakened triceps surae muscles, or secondary to a hip-flexion contracture. In crouch gait Hoffinger *et al.* (1993) noted increased anterior pelvic tilt after medial hamstring lengthening. Using three-dimensional gait analysis they found that the medial hamstrings in 12 of 16 patients with spastic diplegia had prolonged electrical activity. In eight of these 12 the hamstrings were contracting concentrically to aid extension of the hip. They concluded that although the hamstrings might be important as hip-extensors, a hip-flexion contracture may contribute to the crouch and should be addressed before the hamstrings are lengthened. As the result of the persistent knee-flexed posture, secondary contractures of the posterior capsule of the knee joint and shortening of the sciatic nerve occur.

The literature is replete with reports year after year for the past 40 years from world orthopaedic community on the management of knee-flexion deformities in cerebral palsy (Keats and Kambin 1962, Hein 1969, Porter 1970, Hyashi 1970, Frost 1971, Banks 1972, Reimers 1974, Feldkamp and Katthagen 1975, Fixsen 1979, Ray and Ehrlich 1979, Baumann *et al.* 1980, Sullivan *et al.* 1984, Simon *et al.* 1986, Hsu 1986, Thometz *et al.* 1989, Reimers 1990, Hsu and Li 1990, Damron *et al.* 1991, Atar *et al.* 1993, DeLuca *et al.* 1998, Damiano *et al.* 1999, Kay *et al.* 2002). Because the knee flexion and extension are more important major determinants of an energy-efficient gait, and because a long 'reach' and stride-length are necessary for this efficiency, it is no wonder that the spastic hamstrings have received so much attention. If you or your therapists doubt that walking with a flexed-knee gait is disabling try walking for an hour or even all day with your knees flexed 30º!

Knee-flexion contracture increases the energy requirements of gait. When the knee-flexion posture is 40º, calculations show an increase in energy requirements from the normal in men of 0. 101 kcal/m to 0.265 kcal/m in cerebral palsy (Sutherland and Cooper 1978, Sutherland 1980). Biomechanical calculations have shown that a 150 lb (68 kg) person who stands with the knee flexed 50º increases the quadriceps femoris tension to 342 lb and the knee joint pressure to 472 lb (Kottke 1966).

ANTERIOR KNEE PAIN

Anterior knee pain can evolve and cause deterioration of gait in children usually age 10–16 years who have been walking with flexed knees. The knee pain can be explained by the lateral radiograph that depicts a patella riding superiorly above the femoral articulation ('patella alta'). Special measurements of 'patella alta' as in otherwise normal persons do not seem necessary in cerebral palsy. The structural change will be obvious. But if you want to measure, the paper by Koshino and Sugimoto (1989) of Yokohama details their method to calculate from the radiograph in children. Lotman (1976) found patella alta in 72% of 100 knees in patients with spastic knee joints compared with only 2% in 25 normal individuals. The inferior pole of the patella will be either fragmented or avulsed fragmentation or avulsion of the distal pole of the patella (Kaye and Freiberger 1971, Rosenthal and Levine 1977, Lloyd-Roberts *et al.* 1985, Feldkamp 1990). The cause is considered to be 'overload of the quadriceps muscle' comparable to 'jumper's knee' (Feldkamp 1990). The cure is correction of the knee-flexion deformity (Fig. 8.55).

When patients who walk with flexion contractures of the knee are seen in the adult years, pain in the knee joint and inability to tolerate walking occurs due to degenerative arthritis of the knee joint. Adult patients with a long-standing knee-flexion contracture can have unremitting knee-joint pain; the initial stage of the degenerative arthritis began with patellar chondromalacia.

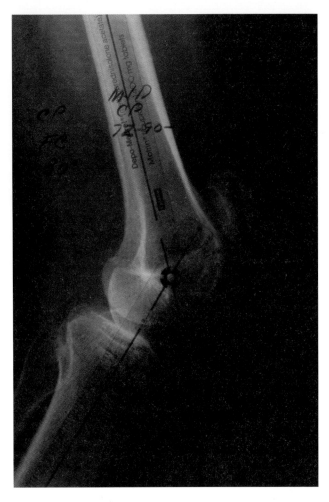

Fig. 8.55. Lateral radiograph of right knee, spastic diplegia, female age 20 years, ambulatory, with severe anterior pain in the right knee, fixed 30° flexion contracture, patella alta, retropatellar crepitus. Pain relieved after bilateral fractional hamstring lengthening and distal rectus femoris transfer to iliotibial band.

CLINICAL EXAMINATION

The clinical examination of the gait, hamstring spasticity and contracture have been described in Chapter 2. Of all the tests for hamstring contracture, the measurement of the popliteal angle with the hip flexed 90° is the best (normal <20°). Contracture of the posterior joint capsule is present if the knee cannot be completely extended when the thigh and leg is extended to rest on the examining tabletop.

How 'tight' hamstrings in normal infants and children are might temper the zeal to lengthen hamstrings based on the limited straight leg-raising or popliteal angles alone without considering the gait pattern and function. In a study by Kuo *et al.* (1997) they assessed the tightness of hamstrings using three tests: straight leg raising, popliteal angle and touching-toes. At birth, straight leg-raising averaged 100°; it increased to 110° at one year, and remained constant at 60° after the age of 5 or 6 years. The popliteal angle was 155° (or 25° from the 0 position) at age 6 years and stayed constant thereafter. An angle of less than 125° (55° lack of extension of the knee) with the hip and knee flexed 90° indicated significant hamstring tightness. Girls were less tight. Tests for ligamentous laxity correlated with the degree of tightness.

The clinical tests for quadriceps spasticity are: (1) to sharply flex the knee when the patient is prone—the increased resistance to knee flexion will be readily appreciated ('pendulum' test); (2) to seat the patient with knees flexed over the table's edge—those with marked quadriceps spasticity will not be able to allow the knees to flex to 90°; passive knee flexion quickly done reveals the resistance of the quadriceps.

Voluntary knee extension from the flexed position indicates that the patient may have a good result from appropriate correction of the knee-flexed posture. In such patients a manual muscle test may possibly indicate the residual strength of the quadriceps. However, a more important concept is that surgery to weaken the hamstrings is essentially a 'balancing act', in which just enough quadriceps spasm will predominate to keep the knee extended at initial stance and to mid-stance and still allow the knee to flex in initial swing (normal 35°–40°) to complete swing (normal 60°–70°). In most patients this ideal result does not occur; but usually there is sufficient quadriceps spasticity to maintain correction so that postoperative orthoses are not required. Knee–ankle–foot orthoses with locked knee joints have only been necessary in older patients who have not only contracted hamstrings but also a joint capsule contracture that required a posterior capsulotomy of the knee joint. The orthosis is used until quadriceps strength is sufficient to ensure complete knee extension at the beginning of stance and to prevent recurrence of the contracture.

Patients who have had weakening of the gastrocnemius–soleus muscle, following lengthenings or neurectomies, will have a 'crouch' position of knee flexion and ankle dorsiflexion. The function of the gastrocnemius–soleus is to prevent forward acceleration of the tibia in the stance phase of gait. When these muscles are too weak, ankle dorsiflexion increases and the strength and/or spasticity of the quadriceps is insufficient to maintain knee extension. To assess the effect of this weakness on knee flexion, the wearing of short-leg walking casts, braces or CAM walkers with the ankle in neutral dorsiflexion can be helpful.

INDICATIONS FOR HAMSTRING LENGTHENING

Surgical weakening of the hamstring muscles is indicated if the knee-flexion deformity is more than 15° during the stance phase of gait. Why 15°? This recommendation is based not only on clinical observations but on experimental studies as well. Patients who can tolerate more than 15° of knee flexion are those who have good hip extension that locks the knee and brings the trunk forward anterior to the knee. In addition, the ankle-plantarflexors serve to overcome the flexed knee at midstance and beyond (Perry *et al.* 1975).

Perry and associates (1975) in their study of knee-flexion posture during gait, measured the quadriceps force needed to stabilize the knee: in 15° of flexion, 75% of the load on the femoral head was taken up by the knee; at 30° of flexion, 210%; at 60°, 400%. The quadriceps muscle force exerted at 15° of flexion was equivalent to 20% of the maximal quadriceps strength; at 30° of flexion, this equivalent force was 30% of the quadriceps strength. The quadriceps force needed when the knee is flexed beyond 15° is greatly increased because the weightbearing surfaces of the femoral condyles are relatively flat in the first 15° of flexion; beyond this point the condyles are rounder and thus more muscle strength is required to maintain extension.

Because flexed knees are so obvious, the surgeon might be tempted to treat this deformity without considering the associated hip-flexion and equinus deformities. If there are structural deformities at the hip and ankle, these should be corrected at the same time as the knee-flexion deformity. The research of Delp *et al.* (1996) using computer modeling techniques during normal and crouch gait should dissuade the surgeon from overlengthening the hamstrings of which 80% were normal or longer. The psoas was shorter by 1 SD while walking. This data is the clue to psoas lengthening along with the hamstring lengthening.

If the hamstrings are weakened and a hip-flexion deformity of any degree exists, increased lumbar lordosis due to increased anterior inclination of the pelvis can be anticipated. If the hip-flexion contracture is over 15°, unacceptable pelvic and spinal compensation may be expected (Fig. 8.56). Studies of the sacrofemoral angle measured on the standing radiographs after

hamstring lengthening have shown a decrease in this angle which indicated correction of the pelvic and lumbar spine adaptations to the hip-flexion deformity (Bleck 1966).

PASSIVE STRETCHING OF HAMSTRINGS?

Passive stretching of the hamstring muscles was a long-standing practice that we intuitively knew more as a tradition than as an effective treatment. Halbertsma and Goeken (1994) did a study of 14 volunteers, age 20–38 years, who had straight leg-raising limited to about 80°. Half the group were 'treated' for 4 weeks with daily stretching exercises at home; the other half as controls had no exercise regimen. Data was obtained with instrumented straight leg-raising. They concluded that exercises did not make short hamstrings any longer or less stiff, but had some influence on tolerance to stretching that was accompanied by an increase of the stretching moment.[18] This should be good news for parents and children. We need not burden parents of children with cerebral palsy to add intensive hamstring stretching exercises as one more daily task.

Exercises did not make hamstrings any longer or less stiff. . . . We need not burden parents and children with hamstring stretching exercises.

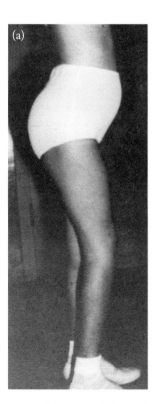 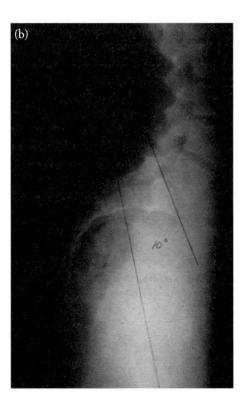 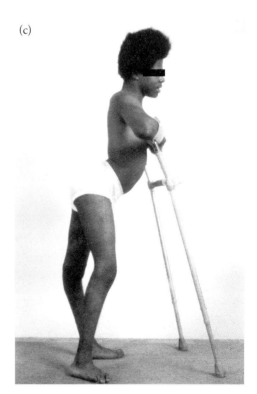

Fig. 8.56. (*a*) Patient NC, Spastic diplegia, posture, age 13 years, female, spastic quadriceps with hip-flexion contracture and severe compensatory lumbar lordosis. (*b*) Lateral radiograph of lumbar spine and pelvis standing erect. Patient NC, spastic diplegia, age 13 years, female. Sacrum is almost horizontal with the floor indicating that most of the lordosis occurs at the lumbosacral articulation. (*c*) Skeletally mature male with severe hip-flexion contracture, recurvatum of knees following hamstring lengthening, hip derotation osteotomies. Compensatory lumbar lordosis.

18 Increased tolerance for hamstring stretching is a probability in persons with a normal neuromuscular system. Anyone who has observed the high kicks by ballerinas and dancers must appreciate that their joint capsules and muscles have been subjected to systematic, daily and rigorous stretching exercises.

BOTULINUM TOXIN INTRAMUSCULAR INJECTION

The pelvic adaptation to the hamstring spasticity was noted by Corry and colleagues of Belfast (1999). After injection of the hamstrings with botulinum-A toxin in 10 children who had cerebral palsy and a flexed knee gait, the mean pelvic tilt increased after the injections. They suggested that isolated hamstring weakening be approached with 'caution'. Although the energy cost of walking was not significantly changed in six of 10 patients, a small increase in knee extension in stance was appreciated by the patients.

Thompson *et al.* (1998) studied the effect of botulinum-A toxin injections in 10 children who had a crouch gait using kinematics derived from gait analysis and calculations of maximum hamstring lengths and excursions from computer modeling. Gait analysis before injection was compared with that 2 weeks after injections. The lengths of the semimembranosus and semitendinosus increased significantly after injection. None of the subjects had short lateral hamstrings. Pelvic tilt and hip flexion increased non-significantly. The study concluded with 'short hamstrings are over-diagnosed in crouch gait'.

SURGICAL PROCEDURES

HAMSTRING TENOTOMY, TRANSFER OR LENGTHENING?
Tenotomy of the hamstrings in spastic diplegia is almost certain to risk overcorrection in knee extension and a loss of knee flexion. The disability will be worse than with knee flexion.

Transfer of the hamstring tendon insertion to the femoral condyles has not fulfilled the promise that these muscles would then act as hip-extensors (Eggers 1952). The procedure was progressively modified from transferring all the hamstrings to just transferring two and finally one medial hamstring. The total transfer often resulted in a straight knee which could not flex. The partial transfers of two hamstrings (usually the medial only) preserved more function, but knee flexion during gait was limited due to the unopposed action of the spastic quadriceps. The transfer of the semitendinosus only improved the results when the semimembranosus was lengthened. The only advantage gained with this latter procedure was perhaps that the semi-tendinosus could not retract proximally into the middle third of the femur, as occurred with tenotomy or if the z-lengthened tendon suture was too weak (Evans 1975). Because of the risk of knee hyperextension due to too much hamstring weakness, surgeons appear to have abandoned all hamstring transfers and the z-lengthening of the semimembranosus. The loss of the semimembranosus tendon strength probably accounts for the loss of its 'check rein' function and the resultant recurvatum of the joint (Fig. 8.57).

FRACTIONAL LENGTHENING OF HAMSTRINGS

This is the technique that most surgeons now employ (Green and McDermott 1942). It allows some control over the degree of lengthening, and although the muscles are weakened, some flexion power is preserved to begin initial swing during gait. Gage *et al.* (1987) quoted Perry's studies (1985) that initial swing is provided

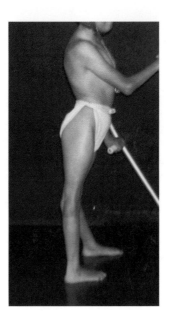

Fig. 8.57. Posture of patient JR. Postoperative medial hamstring transfer. Severe recurvatum of both knees. Such results have been far and few between. One does not need 100 cases to prove an untenable operation for an 'evidenced-based study'; an analysis of one case should be enough.

by the gracilis, short head of the biceps and sartorius. The usual hamstring lengthening does not include the short head of the biceps or sartorius, but very often the gracilis tendon is cut. Perhaps we should leave the gracilis intact in less severe cases.

Generally the results of fractional hamstring lengthening have been satisfactory. However, we know that the total excursion of the knee joint from flexion to extension does not improve in the majority of cases (Rab 1985, Simon *et al.* 1986, Thometz *et al.* 1989, Abel *et al.* 1999). Maximum knee flexion during swing during gait analysis showed no significant effect after multiple soft-tissue releases in patients with cerebral palsy, but the total range of motion and minimum knee flexion in stance improved significantly (Hadley *et al.* 1992).

Do not expect total knee joint excursion to improve significantly after hamstring lengthening.

Surgeons fear recurrence of the contracture, and their fear is well grounded. Dhawlikar *et al.* (1992), at the Hospital for Special Surgery, New York, did a retrospective study of their 126 patients who had distal lengthenings of the hamstrings. In a long follow-up of 3–14 years, 22 patients required reoperation because of recurrence; only 10 had a mild recurvatum of the knee. Only limitation of preoperative straight leg-raising predicted recurrence.

Reimers (1990) studied 38 patients who had distal hamstring lengthenings at a mean age of 5.6 years. He found on follow-up that the strength of the quadriceps was reduced 70%. Seven months after surgery the strength of the muscle had been regained strength by a median value of 22%. Reimers concluded that quadriceps function is strengthened when the hamstrings are weakened and that 6 months elapses before gait improves and the rectus femoris spasticity increases. Damiano *et al.* (1999) confirmed Reimers' conclusions. After hamstring lengthening quadriceps strength improved significantly and hamstring strength regained their preoperative strength in 9 months.

Hsu and Li of the Duchess of Kent Hospital, Hong Kong (1990), did z-lengthenings of the semitendinosus and gracilis and aponeurotic lengthenings of the semimembranosus and biceps femoris in 49 patients, 40 of whom improved their crouch position, while nine recurred and one developed recurvatum.

Hsu's method of hamstring lengthening is practically the same as Bleck's (1987) has been for the past 9 years. In Bleck's series of 33 patients who had a mean age of 7 years (range 3–13 years), and were followed an average of 4½ years (range 3–11 years), had good results in correcting the flexed knee posture during stance phase; three had a recurrence of the knee flexion; two had slight hyperextension of the knee. Most of the patients who had lengthened hamstrings for a flexed knee gait gained extension on stance phase but usually had only the minimum knee flexion on initial swing phase (20º–30º). Rectus femoris distal tendon transfer promises to improve the degree of knee flexion on swing.

MEDIAL HAMSTRING LENGTHENING ONLY OR BOTH MEDIAL AND LATERAL?

Sullivan *et al.* (1984) also had success with medial hamstring lengthening in 39 children: 28% were excellent, 68% good and 4% were unchanged. On follow-up from 1 to 5 years they noted a disturbing degree of out-toeing during gait which ranged from 15º to greater than 30º and noted the development of hindfoot valgus. These results may be due to the unopposed action of the biceps femoris, which is known to be a strong lateral rotator of the tibia (Duchenne 1867). Bleck (1987) noted the postoperative lateral rotation of the tibia in his patients in whom he did only medial hamstring lengthening prior to 1977. Bassett *et al.* (1976), in a long follow-up study on patients who had a medial hamstring transfer, found external tibial torsion in 79%. Because of development of external tibial–fibular torsion beyond the normal, fractional lengthening of the distal biceps aponeurosis as well as fractional lengthening of the semimembranosus should be done.

Kay and colleagues from Los Angeles (2002) compared outcomes of medial with combined medial and lateral hamstring lengthenings in two almost equally divided groups. Follow-up gait analysis was done in a mean of 17 months (SD 8) after surgery. Improvements in kinetic and static measurements improved in both groups and a suggestion that the combined lengthenings had a better range of hamstrings and knee extension. But there was a greater risk of knee hyperextension after the combined operation particularly those who had significant calf spasticity. Hamstring weakness persisted during the follow-up. Damiano *et al.* (1999) found that initial hamstring weakness after lengthening increased to preoperative values 9 months later.

A study of the effects of medial and lateral hamstring lengthening combined with psoas recessions (i.e. tenotomy) at the pelvic brim showed that there was minimal effect on pelvic tilt during gait with or without the psoas recession (DeLuca *et al.* 1998). Medial and lateral hamstring lengthening and the psoas recession reduced preoperative pelvic tilt only a clinically insignificant 4º. If the pelvic tilt during gait was normal or posterior preoperatively, the medial and lateral hamstring lengthening with or without the psoas recession increased anterior pelvic tilt during gait significantly.

Combined medial and lateral hamstring lengthening does not compromise function, slightly risks postoperative recurvatum, and should prevent late external tibial torsion.

OPERATIVE TECHNIQUE FOR FRACTIONAL HAMSTRING LENGTHENING

Dr G.W. Westin (personal communication) introduced the incision and the supine position to Bleck that he has used since (Fig. 8.58). The biceps femoris aponeurosis and not the tendon is lengthened as well as the medial hamstrings (this seems to have avoided the late development of excessive lateral rotation). With the patient supine, an assistant flexes the hip 90º and extends the knee to its limit but not beyond and without force. A straight

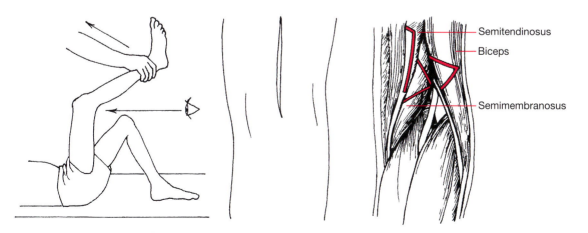

Fig. 8.58. Operative technique for fractional hamstring lengthening. Surgeon seated while assistant extends leg gently to visualize the distal posterior thigh. Straight incision made in distal thigh between hamstring tendons. Semitendinosus z-lengthened. Delta cuts in aponeuroses overlying semimembranosus and biceps femoris. Leg is slowly extended to separate cuts in the aponeuroses to a popliteal angle of 20º from the vertical (160º flexion). Pay attention to the tension on the sciatic nerve especially in older patients who have had long-standing knee-flexion deformities.

incision is made in the midline to the distal one third of the thigh, ending at the popliteal crease (Fig. 8.58). We try to z-lengthen the semitendinosus. In little children with small tendons this is often not possible and a tenotomy results (by design or inadvertently). On follow-up evaluations it is not possible to ascertain the difference between those who had tenotomies or lengthenings of the semitendinosus. Others have made the same observation (L. Diamond, personal communication). The lateral aspect of the semimembranosus distally is freed of fat and connective tissue to expose the whole of its aponeurosis which is incised in a V or delta. As the knee is extended, the ends of the aponeurosis pull apart and the muscle fibers also glide apart; some may tear but continuity is maintained. The aponeurosis on the lateral aspect of the biceps femoris is exposed and similarly incised as the knee is extended. In severe contractures the gracilis tendon is also cut. However, Perry (1985) recommended saving it, because of the role it plays in initiating the swing phase of gait (together with the sartorius and short head of the biceps).

Horstmann prefers to lengthen hamstrings with the patient supine. She makes a midline incision of about 3 cm, ending about 10 cm proximal to the popliteal crease. At this level fractional lengthenings through the aponeurosis overlying the muscle bellies of the biceps, semitendinosis and the underlying semimembranosis can be readily accomplished with excellent visualization. The semitendinosis continuity is maintained. The gracilis is deep in the wound and its bowstringing makes it more easiliy palpated. The tendinous portion of the gracilis is tenotomized at several levels at 1–2 cm intervals through its bipennate muscle insertion, allowing lengthening rather than release. Mindful of Perry's recommendation, only in older children with need for repeat lengthenings and marked contractures is this released.

With the hips flexed 90° extreme force in extending the knee should not be exerted to avoid stretching the sciatic nerve—note that a 20° popliteal angle is within the limits of normal. The sciatic nerve is also shortened in relatively long-standing knee-flexion contractures (children over the age of 12 years may be at particular risk). A sciatic stretch neuropathy causes continuing distressing paresthesias, dysesthesias and loss of sensation of the leg and foot with paralysis of the ankle and foot controlling muscles. The neuropathy lasts a long time. Aspden and Porter (1994) had this complication in one patient with spastic diplegia. They devised a method of calculating the extra strain on the sciatic nerve when the knee is straightened after surgery.[19] However, they pointed out that combined with clinical judgement their method should be a guideline for safe corrective surgery. They surmised that reduction of a hip-flexion deformity by 20° should allow an extra 20° extension at the knee.

Try to avoid postoperative sciatic neuropathy when doing corrective surgery for knee flexion deformities. Do not force the knee into overextension in testing the popliteal angle.

If the knee cannot be completely extended with the limb flat on the table and only 5°–10° of knee-flexion contracture remains, it is safer to apply a cast to be wedged or a long leg adjustable off-the-shelf brace. These can then be gradually extended to reduce or eliminate the knee-flexion contracture. Sudden forced extension risks a sciatic neuropathy or posterior tibial subluxation. Pain in the foot and/or paresthesias are a warning to stop forcing knee extension and to revert to knee flexion.

The postoperative immobilization is a knee immobilizer or adjustable off-the-shelf long brace. The patient is permitted to stand and walk beginning on the first postoperative day. The immobilization is removed in 3 weeks; walking is resumed as the best therapy.

Postoperative knee–ankle–foot orthoses with a drop lock at the knee are rarely necessary in children under age 12 after hamstring lengthening. Orthoses to prevent knee flexion while quadriceps strength is restored seem essential in older children and adolescents who have long-standing hamstring and posterior capsular contractures corrected by surgery.

ABOUT WEDGING CASTS IN KNEE-FLEXION CONTRACTURE

Long-leg casts are occasionally useful to improve residual knee-flexion contracture. An open wedging of a long-leg plaster cast in the supracondylar area is effective in gradually correcting a residual contracture of the posterior capsule (Fig. 8.59). The supracondylar section is chosen to avoid posterior subluxation of the tibia. A residual contracture of 5°–20° may correct with gradual wedging of the cast. Lateral projection radiographs of the knee centered on a film large enough to see the alignment of the femur and tibia is a good practice to discern posterior subluxation of the tibia. If it is occurring, wedging should stop. Posterior subluxation of the tibia is very difficult (or perhaps impossible) to correct. The specific number of degrees beyond which wedging is not advised is unknown. Generally for residual contracture more than 20° a supracondylar extension osteotomy may be best. The general rule for the knee is that extension should be complete at heel contact.

PROXIMAL HAMSTRING MYOTOMY

Proximal myotomy of the hamstring origins was proposed by Seymour and Sharrard (1968). Their indications were a strong quadriceps, 'tightness' of the hamstrings which limited flexion of the hip, a short stride-length, straight leg-raising limited to 30° or less and inability to sit upright with the knees extended. In nine children the results were satisfactory. However, these English surgeons saw no advantage to this procedure over distal elongation of the hamstrings if there was a knee-flexion

---

19 For details of an outline of the mathematical model derived from measurements of the femur and tibia lengths, consult the paper by Aspden, R.M. and Porter, R.W. (1994) 'Nerve traction during correction of knee flexion deformity. A case report and calculation.' *Journal of Bone and Joint Surgery*, **76B**, 471–473. The authors suggest that they can be contacted for further information at the University of Aberdeen, Scotland.

20 W.J.W. Sharrard said the procedure was 'messy', in a 1970 lecture recalled by Bleck.

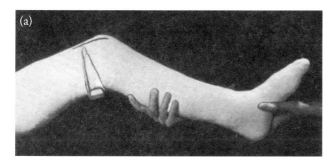

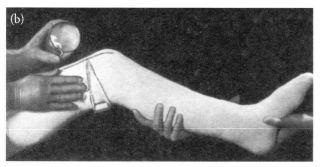

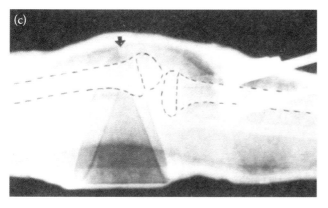

Fig. 8.59. Postoperative wedging cast for residual knee flexion contracture. Anterior hinge and cast cut at the supracondylar level. Knee slowly extended and gap held open with a wood block. (*b*) Apply a petrolatum ointment to area proximal and distal to wedging cut in cast and replaster. The ointment prevents adherence of the plaster and facilitates removal of the plaster wrap around the wedged area so continued opening of the wedge can be done. (*c*) Lateral radiograph of knee in wedging cast. Despite the supracondylar hinge site, posterior subluxation of the tibia has occurred. No further wedging should be done. Kirschner wire traction pin holder and wire incorporated into the plaster to transfer to force on the foot and heel during wedging of the cast.

deformity.[20] Drummond *et al.* (1974) thought the procedure quite satisfactory in 14 patients who had a 'tight hamstring gait' manifested by a short stride-length and who accomplished 'swing-through' by pelvic motion. Fixsen (1979) thought the procedure very effective. Reimers (1974) also seemed to prefer proximal myotomies, even though he had success with the distal lengthenings of the hamstrings. M.M. Hoffer (personal comunication) had two patients whose knee-flexion contracture was not corrected after proximal hamstring release.

Sharps and colleagues (1984) of Philadelphia did a long-term follow-up of 32 of 78 patients who had a proximal hamstring 'release'. They reported generally good results in an average

follow-up of 9 years 5 months. They noted, however, that knee-flexion contractures greater than 10° were not permanently corrected. Only four of 64 knees had mild recurvatum. This led to the conclusion that proximal hamstring 'release' can be used 'without severe lumbar lordosis or devastating genu recurvatum'. Of some significance is that only 40% of the patients returned for follow-up.

Rang *et al.* (1986) recommends this procedure mainly in the total body involved patient when adductor myotenotomy and iliopsoas tenotomy is done; the proximal origins can be sectioned through the same medial incision over the proximal femur.

The procedure seems to have fallen out of favor; there are no reports of its efficacy for the past 20 years.[21] There may be a rare patient with spastic diplegia who would benefit from proximal myotomy of the hamstrings. This is the patient who does not have a hip-flexion deformity but does have both spastic hamstrings and a strong quadriceps that does not allow knee flexion, so that the hamstrings extend the pelvis posteriorly with a secondary kyphosis of the thoracolumbar spine. A myoneural block of the hamstring muscles with 0.5% lidocaine or botulinum toxin may help in evaluating the potential effects of the proximal myotomy. If the pelvis inclines anterior after the temporary paralysis of the hamstring muscles, a proximal myotomy may help to restore pelvic balance and decrease the compensatory and flexible kyphosis.

POSTERIOR CAPSULOTOMY OF THE KNEE JOINT
In a knee-flexion deformity due to spastic and contracted hamstrings, the knee should completely extend when the limb is brought into extension and rests on the tabletop. If the knee joint will not go into complete extension in this position, a contracture of the posterior capsule is present. With this finding the surgeon should be prepared to do a posterior capsulotomy of the knee joint in addition to the hamstring lengthenings. In this case the hamstring lengthenings and posterior capsulotomy can be done through medial and lateral incisions over the distal femur and knee joint. Reliance on wedging casts to correct a residual knee-flexion contracture probably greater than 20° after hamstring lengthening risks posterior subluxation of the tibia, continued knee-flexed posture and recurrence of the flexion posture. When the knee is absolutely in complete extension, no quadriceps force is required to stand erect.

OPERATIVE TECHNIQUE OF POSTERIOR CAPSULOTOMY OF THE KNEE JOINT
If a flexion contracture of the posterior capsule of the knee joint is discerned preoperatively (as determined by the examination described previously in this section), then the midline posterior distal thigh incision to lengthen the hamstrings cannot be used. The patient is prone on the operating table. The hamstrings are

---

21 Proximal hamstring myotomy may have been discarded because of 'heard in the hallways' at meetings anecdotes by orthopaedic surgeons who tried it and found that it caused severe anterior pelvic tilt referred to as 'jack-knife' posture.

fractionally lengthened through posterior medial and lateral longitudinal incisions over the hamstring tendons in the distal thigh and knee joint. The approach to the capsule is from the lateral incision (Wilson 1929, cited by Crenshaw 1963); the iliotibial band can be divided and the biceps aponeurosis incised as previously described. Through the medial incision, the semitendinosus tendon is z-lengthened and the semimembranosus aponeurosis is incised with V or delta cuts. The hip is then flexed 90º and the knee gradually extended but not forced (this is no place for a 'macho' surgeon demonstration). The residual knee-flexion contracture will be apparent as the limb rests on the operating table.

The lengthened hamstring tendons are reflected posteriorly together with the neurovascutar bundle. The heads of the gastrocnemius muscle origins are detached from the femur and stripped distally to expose the joint capsule which is completely incised to obtain additional knee extension. Again do not use undue force—remember, the sciatic nerve is contracted as well.

Cutting the insertion of the anterior cruciate ligament (L.A. Rinsky, personal communication) helps to prevent posterior subluxation of the tibia as the knee is extended. Somerville (1960) maintained that in long-standing flexion contractures of the knee, such as occur in rheumatoid arthritis, the anterior cruciate ligament shortens and prevents the last few degrees of extension. Rinsky observed no instability of the knees post-operatively as a result of sectioning the anterior cruciate ligament in the intercondylar notch posteriorly.

Postoperative care entails a long-leg cast with ample soft padding over the anterior and posterior aspects of the knee and dorsum of the foot in order to bring the knee gradually into complete extension by progressive wedging of the plaster (Fig. 8.59). This is accomplished by making a linear anterior hinge 7.5 cm long in the plaster over the knee and the supracondylar region of the femur, where a circular cut is made in the plaster from medial to lateral. Usually on the third day postoperatively the plaster is cut for wedging, the patient placed prone and the knee extended to the point of pain tolerance and absence of paresthesias in the foot. A block of plastic or wood holds the wedge open; a single roll of cast padding around the area followed by plaster or fiberglass secures the position. It is simple then to remove this cast, extend the knee again and hold the wedge open in the same manner. A lateral radiograph, using a large film with the knee joint in the center, permits more accurate measurement of the degree of extension of the tibia on the femur.

In all cases of posterior capsulotomy with hamstring lengthening, plan to use a knee–ankle–foot orthosis (KAFO) with a drop-lock at the knee joint in 6 weeks postoperatively when the plaster is removed. It is important for the orthosis to be ready as soon as the cast is removed. To delay application of the orthosis risks recurrence. In 3–4 weeks postoperatively, when the knee is straight, we remove the cast and ask the orthotist to make the negative plaster mold of the limb. From this mold a positive plaster is made, from which the orthosis can be constructed. The long-leg cast is reapplied while the orthosis is being made

in the two additional weeks of immobilization. As long as the knee is in extension, weightbearing in the cast can be encouraged.

After the orthosis is applied, active and active assisted knee-flexion and extension exercises can be done by unlocking the knee joint of the orthosis at least three times a day. The patient walks with the knee joints locked until the knee maintains extension at heel contact and throughout mid-stance of gait. Once this occurs, there will be no further need for the orthosis.

If the knee-flexion posture has been aggravated by weakening of the gastrocnemius–soleus muscles and excessive dorsiflexion of the ankle, the knee–ankle–foot orthosis can be converted to an AFO which will block the dorsiflexion of the ankle.

ANTERIOR FEMORAL PHYSEAL STAPLING

A unique and original method to correct a flexion contracture of the knee is to retard the growth of the distal femoral epiphysis anteriorly with staples has as its basis epiphyseal stapling by Blount for genu varum and valgum and linear growth retardation (Blount and Clark 1949). Kramer and Stevens (2001) did anterior stapling of the distal femoral physis for fixed flexion deformities of the knee due to a variety of conditions among which was cerebral palsy in 11 of their 28 patients. Except for two patients who had a congenital knee-flexion deformity at ages 5 and 6 years, all others were between the ages of 11 and 16 years. The flexion deformity varied from 10º–25º and a maximum of 45º.

The operative procedure is simple and entails a supine position on a radiolucent table so that fluoroscopic imaging can be used. Two incisions are made on the anterior medial and anterior lateral aspects of the knee medial and lateral to the patellar sulcus of the femur and centered over the physis. The medial and lateral retinaculum and synovium are incised longitudinally to expose the distal femur. As with all epiphyseal staplings a Keith needle inserted into the physis identifies the physis with image intensification fluoroscopy. *The periosteum is not stripped.* A single 5/8 inch Blount staple is inserted on either side to bridge the physis adjacent to the patellar sulcus. The position is checked by the radiograph. Then the staple is driven home in the anterior–posterior direction. If there is a concomitant valgus of the knee a single staple is inserted anterior and medial. Postoperatively, no immobilization is necessary. As soon as able the patient can resume ambulation and range of motion exercises. The staple is removed when growth has ceased, or when correction has been obtained. If skeletal maturity has not been achieved, the staple can be removed and growth will resume.

Kramer and Stevens (2001) report excellent corrections of the knee-flexion deformity. To be effective at least 12 months of growth should remain at the time of stapling. This decision at to age of stapling will vary; determination of the skeletal age from X-rays of the hand and wrist may be helpful. The margin of safety in not overcorrecting the deformity is that stapling is reversible. No patient in the series developed recurvatum. The only complication reported was wound dehiscence and staple extrusion in one patient. The correction rate is slow and unpredictable. Stapling was done with tendon lengthenings, transfers and foot surgery. This seems to be a good way to avoid the more extensive surgery of capsulotomy of the knee or supracondylar extension osteotomy. But be prepared to lose an amount of knee flexion equal to the extension of the distal femur as is the case with supracondylar osteotomy.

RESULTS AND PROBLEMS

1. *Recurrence of the knee-flexion contracture* has been the dominant concern of surgeons. Lotman (1976) examined 152 patients 3 years after hamstring surgery, and found a 32% recurrence rate, but this high a relapse rate is not the usual experience. Hsu (1986) reported 18% recurred. Bleck (1987) had a 9% recurrence in a 4.5 year follow-up. In the first nine patients (18 knees) with cerebral palsy who had the additional posterior capsulotomies and anterior cruciate ligament insertion incisions for a flexion deformity of the knee, none recurred and there were no posterior subluxations of the tibia or anterior instability of the knee in a mean follow-up of 2 years (Page 1982). Problems other than recurrence have been more prominent and disabling:

2. To avoid *increased postoperative lumbar lordosis and anterior pelvic tilt* (Bleck 1975), the hip-flexion deformity should be corrected either before or during hamstring lengthening. Perhaps a hip-flexion contracture of less than 15º–20º might be tolerated, but not 45º (Fig. 8.56).

3. *Hyperextended knee gait.* When the hamstrings are weakened the quadriceps spasticity becomes evident and can help maintain correction of the flexion contracture of the knees. However, too much quadriceps spasticity and overweakening of the hamstrings will lead to postoperative limited knee flexion on swing phase and genu recurvatum (Fig. 8.57). This straight knee gait will be more disabling than a knee-flexion contracture of 15º. Solution: distal rectus femoris tendon transfer.

4. *Failure to correct the knee-flexion deformity.* This discouraging result is more common when the deformity has been allowed to persist in children older than 10 years. Possible reasons for this failure are: (1) inability to achieve complete extension of the knee due to secondary contracture of the posterior capsule; capsulotomy is required; and (2) quadriceps weakness with lack of terminal extension and insufficient quadriceps spasticity to take up the slack in the stretched-out muscle. This is a rare result and confined mostly to older children who have walked with knees flexed more than 30º. Solution: quadriceps resistance exercise.

5. *Crouch position due to weakness and increased length of the triceps surae.* It is better to underlengthen an Achilles tendon and have a bit of residual equinus or recurrence. Solution: rigid plastic floor-reaction AFO.

6. *Sciatic neuropathy.* A postoperative sciatic stretch paralysis may occur in patients with severe and long-standing knee-flexion contractures if too much force is exerted in extending the knee at the time of surgery. It may not be entirely avoidable, because how far to stretch the hamstrings is a matter of judgement. It could also occur by zealous passive straight leg-raising exercises postoperatively. If in doubt as to how much to extend the knee for residual contracture after hamstring lengthening, with or without posterior capsulotomy, it is probably better to plan on wedging casts (or braces with dial-in-motion limits) postoperatively to extend the knee gradually. Family involvement in this postoperative management requires significant education efforts by the health team. The symptoms of sciatic neuropathy include pain in the plantar aspect of the foot, paresthesias and hyperesthesia of the toes. A stretch paralysis usually recovers, but this may take 6 months to a year.

PATELLAR TENDON ADVANCEMENT

This operation (Chandler 1933, Roberts and Adams 1953, Baker 1956, Keats and Kambin 1962) is no longer used. The decline in interest possibly stems from the lack of need to restore the tension in the quadriceps muscle when hamstring lengthening is done early enough to avoid years and years of a persistent flexed knee gait. Furthermore, the operation of transfer of the patellar tendon distally, in children with open epiphyses, risks premature closure of the proximal anterior portion of the tibial physis when the patellar tendon is detached from its insertion. It has occurred even with the Baker modification (1956), in which the tendon was skived off its insertion rather than removed with block of bone.

Another possible problem with patellar advancement is the aggravation of chondromalacia patellae and accompanying knee pain. When the patella has been chronically displaced proximally and is out of contact with its opposite femoral area, degeneration of its articular cartilage occurs. Radiographs may reveal spur formation at the poles of the patella, fragmentation of its lower pole and elongation of the distal end (Kaye and Freiberger 1971, Rosenthal and Levine 1977). In children with spastic diplegia who have both flexed knees and a spastic quadriceps, patellar pain can be constant.

SUPRACONDYLAR CLOSED WEDGE EXTENSION OSTEOTOMY OF THE FEMUR

An osteotomy of the femur in the supracondylar region is an effective and safe correction for a flexion deformity of the knees in adults with spastic diplegia. The hamstrings are lengthened as usual. A wedge of bone with its base anterior is removed from the supracondylar region of the femur. The amount of bone to be removed is calculated preoperatively. The wedge is closed, and secure internal fixation can be obtained with a contoured lateral plate and screws (the two cancellous bone screws are best in the condylar area distal to the osteotomy) or an external fixator can be applied with appropriate fixation pins.

A closed-wedge extension supracondylar osteotomy will result in a loss of knee flexion equal to the amount of correction. The advantage of the osteotomy is that it shortens the thigh and relaxes the neurovascular structures. Sciatic stretch paralysis and vascular insufficiency are minimized.

A closed-wedge extension supracondylar osteotomy will result in a loss of knee flexion equal to the amount of correction.

SPASTIC HYPEREXTENSION DEFORMITY OF THE KNEE

Two explanations for the hyperextended knee gait have been offered: (1) a spastic quadriceps (Csongradi *et al.* 1979), and (2) poor regulation of ankle plantarflexion power (Simon *et al.* 1978).

Although the spastic rectus femoris muscle was once thought to be an isolated entity (Duncan 1955, Sutherland *et al.* 1975) it is now clear that all segments of the quadriceps muscle can be spastic (Gage *et al.* 1987). In normal subjects, all four portions of the quadriceps contribute to knee extension; the vastus intermedius is a strong extensor (Perry and Lieb 1967).

CO-SPASTICITY OF THE HAMSTRINGS AND QUADRICEPS

Csongradi and colleagues (1979), at the Children's Hospital at Stanford, demonstrated co-spasticity of the quadriceps and hamstring muscles in spastic diplegia. Gage *et al.* (1987) recognized the 'stiff-legged' gait after hamstring lengthening and documented with gait analysis the co-spasticity of the quadriceps and hamstrings. The effect of the spastic quadriceps is limited peak knee flexion in swing. From Perry's (1987) observations that inadequate initial knee flexion is due to the spastic quadriceps and inadequate function of the sartorius, gracilis and short head of the biceps Gage and colleagues (1987) devised transfer of the distal rectus femoris tendon.

In normal gait the knee should fully extend in stance and flex approximately 60° in swing or at least sufficient flexion to allow foot clearance (Gage 1990). Limitation of knee flexion when walking compromises function and a stiff-legged gait is not only ungainly but energy-consuming. It results in vaulting from one foot to the due to other inability of the knee-flexion function that maintains the center of gravity on its low sinusoidal path during forward progression.

The sophisticated study of genu recurvatum in spastic paralysis by Simon *et al.* (1978) pointed to a number of factors responsible. The most important factor was poor ankle plantarflexion; this caused an abrupt halt in tibial motion in early stance if the calf muscles were weak due to overlengthening of the gastrocnemius–soleus with Achilles tendon lengthening and knee hyperextension in late stance if plantarflexor muscles were too strong. From this study Simon *et al.* recommended a rigid plastic ankle–foot orthosis to overcome the genu recurvatum.

INDICATIONS FOR SURGERY OF KNEE HYPEREXTENSION

If the patient has hyperextension of the knee during the stance phase of gait, and the knee does not flex sufficiently in swing phase to allow the foot to clear the floor, the gait is functionally disabling. Confirmation of the spasticity of the quadriceps is obtained by the clinical tests described in Chapter 2 and in this chapter. Electromyography will demonstrate the continuous and out-of-phase activity of the various parts of the quadriceps during level walking. But the clinical tests for quadriceps spasticity and the gait electromyograms have been shown to be of no predictive value. Consequently, reliance has to be on observational gait and instrumented gait analysis for kinematics. Kinematics will show less than 35°–40° of initial flexion during the swing phase and limited complete flexion.

PROXIMAL TENOTOMY OF THE RECTUS FEMORIS ORIGIN

Duncan (1955) proposed tenotomy of the rectus femoris origin to correct knee hyperextension and lack of sufficient knee flexion in swing. The results were not dramatic (Sutherland *et al.* 1975). Sutherland *et al.* (1990) compared the proximal rectus tenotomy with the distal rectus femoris transfer in cerebral palsy. The proximal tenotomy increased peak knee flexion by only 9.1° whereas the distal transfer increased it 16.2°. The proximal tenotomy of the rectus femoris has given way to the distal transfer of its tendon (Waters *et al.* 1979, Gage *et al.* 1987).

The operative technique for rectus femoris origin tenotomy is simple. The tendon can be approached through an oblique incision in the groin region about 1.5 cm between the anterior superior iliac spine. The sartorius is retracted laterally. After removing the investing iliacus fascia from the medial border of the tendon and clearing the tendon of the overlying fatty connective tissue, the direct head of the tendon can be picked up and cut near its origin and allowed to retract distally.

The results of rectus femoris tenotomy, although not extraordinary, have improved gait by allowing a bit more knee flexion on initial swing (Sutherland *et al.* 1975). The operation is no longer popular with surgeons.

DISTAL RECTUS FEMORIS RECESSION

The surgical principle of reducing quadriceps spasticity was derived from the experience of Waters *et al.* (1979) in their management of the 'stiff-legged' gait of adult hemiplegic patients. The technique of distal rectus femoris recession was to expose the distal quadriceps tendon above the superior pole of the patella through a 4–5 cm transverse incision. The thin flat rectus tendon is freed from the underlying quadriceps tendon. The insertion of the tendon on the patella was cut and the tendon cut away proximally from the adjoining fibers of the vastus medialis and lateralis so that when the knee is flexed 90° the rectus tendon slid proximally for an estimated 2–3 cm. A few sutures anchored it in this position.

Although recession of the distal rectus tendon ('release') would seem to accomplish the reduction of quadriceps spasticity more simply, the transfer of the distal tendon to the sartorius as described by Gage *et al.* (1987) gave better results in improving dynamic knee flexion in a study that compared distal 'release' with transfer (Chambers *et al.* 1998).

DISTAL RECTUS FEMORIS TENDON TRANSFER

Gage *et al.* (1987) transferred the distal end of the rectus femoris tendon to the sartorius. The results have been quite satisfactory in most, although the transfer to the sartorius did not change the foot-progression angle to external rotation. In some patients more success in correcting the externally rotated limb was obtained by transfer of this distal rectus tendon to the iliotibial band. Since this first description of the operation the rectus tendon has been transferred to the semitendinosus and gracilis. Transfer to the semitendinosus in biomechanical studies had the largest knee-flexion moment. None of the transfers to the medial tendons had any effect on hip rotation; transfer to the iliotibial band increased the hip internal rotation moment, but only when the hip was externally rotated (Delp *et al.* 1994). Gage *et al.* (1987) did state that transfer of the rectus tendon to the sartorius was difficult because this soft and pliable muscle precluded a secure anchoring suture.

Since the publication of the results of distal rectus femoris transfer the operation was widely adopted and reported by various surgeons (Hsu and Li 1990, Sutherland *et al.* 1990, Õunpuu *et al.* 1993 a, b, Miller *et al.* 1997, Chambers *et al.* 1998, Campos da Paz Jr *et al.* 1998). The results appear to be quite satisfactory in restoring additional knee flexion during the swing phase.

Bioengineering simulations of the swing phase of gait confirmed that the rectus femoris muscle actuator of the model was important (Piazza and Delp 1996). When the actuator was removed from the model, hyperflexion of the knee occurred and when it was excited, reduced knee flexion resulted. Bioengineers Riewald and Delp (1997) threw cold water on the supposition that with a rectus femoris transfer the muscle converts from the knee-extensor to a flexor. They used intramuscular electrodes to stimulate the rectus femoris in four subjects two of whom had transfers to the semitendinosus and two to the iliotibial band. They measured knee moments and obtained electromyograms of the quadriceps, hamstrings and gastrocnemius muscles. The data obtained showed that the rectus femoris generated knee-extension moment in all subjects and suggested that the rectus femoris does not convert to the knee-flexor. So what does it do when transferred as described? Riewald and Delp thought that there was a mechanism which transmitted the force generated by the rectus to a locus anterior to the knee-joint center.

INDICATIONS FOR DISTAL RECTUS FEMORIS TRANSFER

One indication that all agree on is a 'stiff-legged' gait after hamstring lengthening or in cases without prior hamstring lengthening. This gait is characterized by inadequate initial and further knee flexion in the swing phase of gait. Gait analysis and kinematics assist in making the decision. Chambers and colleagues (1998) of San Diego, California, used pre- and post-operative gait analysis to predict the outcomes in either the distal rectus femoris transfer to the sartorius or the distal recession. Peak knee flexion was improved in the transfer group of patients, and deteriorated slightly in the recession group. Abnormal swing phase contractions of the rectus alone as depicted in the electromyograms or combined with the vastus lateralis did not influence the results with either surgery. Neither the preoperative range of knee motion or the Ely test had predictive value in determining efficacy of the operation.

Should the distal rectus femoris tendon transfer be done in most cases of knee-flexed gait in spastic diplegia? It seems as if this is the case with many surgeons and was with the original report of Gage and colleagues (1987). The indication then would be a preoperative decrease of knee flexion on swing phase less than needed for the foot to clear the ground (normal 35º–40º). Gage *et al.* decided on the rectus femoris transfer if sagittal-plane motion was reduced by at least 20% (less than 45º flexion and extension total motion compared to the normal value of 56º). Others working with Gage in analyzing results of rectus femoris transfer (Õunpuu *et al.* 1993b) noted that when the preoperative range of knee motion was greater than 80º preoperatively there were no significant changes postoperatively. But if knee motion totaled more than 80º, knee flexion was maintained in swing. By comparison the patients who had either no transfer of the rectus or a distal rectus femoris release decreased their range of motion 6º and 10º respectively. The results of hamstring lengthening show that although knee extension is usually completely restored on stance, the preoperative restriction of knee flexion is the same postoperatively. Therefore this would be the rationale for combining hamstring lengthening with distal rectus femoris tendon transfer.

'*[Do] rectus femoris transfer if sagittal-plane motion is reduced by at least 20% (less than 45º flexion and extension total motion compared to the normal value of 56º).*'

(Gage *et al.* 1987)

'*Rectus femoris transfer is not indicated if the range of knee motion is greater than 80º.*'

(Õunpuu *et al.* 1993b)

OPERATIVE TECHNIQUE DISTAL RECTUS FEMORIS TENDON TRANSFER

(Gage *et al.* 1987)

A short, transverse anterior–lateral or medial incision is made in the distal thigh at the supracondylar level (depending on the site of transfer). The rectus femoris tendon is isolated at its insertion in the quadriceps. It might be easier to dissect free the rectus femoris muscle proximally from this adherence to the vastus medialis and lateralis and free it distally to isolated the thin flat tendon of the rectus. The rectus femoris is then mobilized with blunt dissection from the underlying vasti muscles. A Bunnell-type suture is placed through the distal part of the tendon. It is then displaced medially or laterally to the intended transfer site. If it is to be medial, the medial intermuscular septum is opened for about 10 cm. The sartorius is palpated through this septal opening and brought up into the anterior wound. With the knee flexed approximately 20º, the rectus tendon is passed through the sartorius and sutured back on itself with strong non-absorbable suture. Additional sutures are placed to secure the tendon (Fig. 8.60).

If the tendon is to be transferred to the iliotibial band it is sutured to the posterior aspect of the band. Transfer to the gracilis tendon was rejected because complete tenotomy of the gracilis

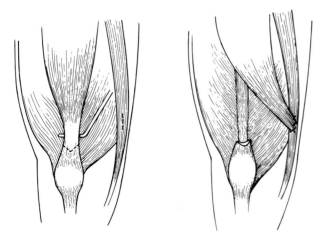

Fig. 8.60. Operative technique of distal rectus femoris transfer to the sartorius muscle. There appears to be no difference in the results of transfer to the semitendinosus or the iliotibial band.

would be needed with the fear that initial knee flexion by the muscle would be eliminated. Some have transferred the rectus tendon to the distal stump of the semitendinosis after tenotomy along with the fractional lengthening of the semimembranosus and biceps aponeurosis. In an analysis of 78 children (105 sides) of the effects of the transfer to the sartorius, semitendinosus, gracilis or the iliotibial band Ōunpuu and colleagues (1993a) found no significant difference between the four transfer sites. Furthermore, they found no consistent changes in transverse plane motion. So you can use whatever seems easiest for you—probably transfer to the semitendinosus or iliotibial band.

Postoperative immobilization in plaster is not necessary. Available knee immobilizers (foam-padded canvas aluminum-stave reinforced circular splints) support the knee in extension. On the third postoperative day the physical therapist can remove the immobilizer for graduated knee flexion exercises. Walking and weightbearing can begin in 1 or 2 days postoperatively. Support may be needed for as much as 3 weeks. As a precaution against falling, the patient might use crutches for another 3 weeks while strength and knee mobility are regained. If the patient used crutches preoperatively, the operation will not eliminate their need postoperatively.

Quadriceps tendon lengthening has been performed in four patients (Bleck 1987) who had no knee flexion during gait due to severe quadriceps spasticity after total hamstring release by other surgeons not aware of co-spasticity of the quadriceps. When seated these patients could barely bend their knees.

The operation was quite direct. Through a transverse incision the quadriceps tendon was z-lengthened and sutured with the knee flexed 45º. Cast immobilization was for 6 weeks with the knees in 30º of flexion.

The results have been satisfactory in permitting the knee to flex 75º–90º when the patient was seated; their gaits, while not normal, were improved with enough flexion on swing phase. A flexed knee posture did not result. They could sit comfortably without their legs stuck out straight from the chair. But quadri-

ceps weakness was sufficient to cause difficulty arising from a low chair or toilet seat. This result may not occur very often since tenotomy of all hamstrings or transfer of all has been put in the waste basket of operations in cerebral palsy.

FOOT AND ANKLE

EQUINUS DEFORMITY

In spastic diplegia equinus is usually bilateral and almost always dynamic when the child begins to walk. Surgical lengthening at this age when no contracture of the triceps surae can be demonstrated is to be resisted (Fig. 8.61). The risk is of weakening the calf muscle and a crouch posture for the physiological and mechanical reasons already given in the preceding section and in Chapter 7.

Dynamic equinus in some young children with spastic diplegia appears related to defective posterior equilibrium reaction. These children appear to need the equinus to bring the center of gravity of their trunks anterior to the ankles and through the base of support between the feet. Their equilibrium reactions are deficient, especially posteriorly. If they try to put their feet flat on the ground, they fall backward. Backward falling places the center of gravity of the trunk (just anterior to the 10th thoracic vertebra) posterior to the base of support creating instability. They can move the center of gravity anterior by rising on tiptoe (Fig. 8.62).

Whether the spastic hamstrings with co-spasticity of the quadriceps are responsible for the posterior displacement has not been studied with measuring techniques for balance combined with electromyography of the hamstrings. In children who are starting to walk and persist with dynamic equinus for 1–3 years can gradually lose the equinus as the central nervous system progressively matures and balance reactions improve generally until the age of 4 years. Nervous system development may explain the success with botulinum toxin injections for dynamic equinus in children under the age of 5 years.

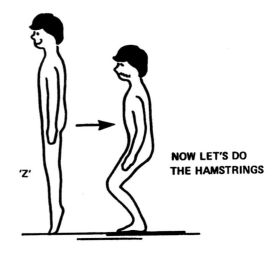

Fig. 8.61. From jump with a z-lengthening of Achilles to crouch.

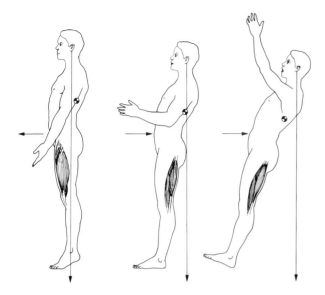

Fig. 8.62. Dynamic equinus compensates for deficient posterior equilibrium reactions. *From left to right*: on tiptoe to keep line of weightbearing just anterior to center of gravity at level of 10th thoracic vertebra and anterior to ankle joints and center of the base of support. Posterior risks displacement posterior to the line of weightbearing falls posterior to base of support. Perturbation of the posture posteriorly causes falling backward.

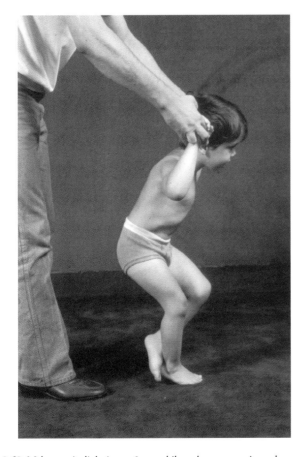

Fig. 8.63. Male, spastic diplegia, age 3 years, bilateral gastrocnemius–soleus spasticity; to keep feet flat on floor he has to sit down when trying to stand erect. Hamstring spasticity and contracture. Line of weightbearing falls posterior to base of support. To avoid falling backward he needs external support.

Some children who have equinus attempt to achieve stability with neutral dorsiflexion of the ankles by flexing the hips and knees so the feet are flat on the ground; they have a sitting posture while trying to stand-up erect (Fig. 8.63).

It may be that in these cases of equinus the 'inhibitive casts' and their companion plastic ankle–foot orthoses can buy time until the equilibrium reactions are more developed, and thus overcome the equinus contracture. Are the hamstrings responsible for persistent equinus? If in doubt about the mechanisms, one can use short-leg walking casts to inhibit the equinus and then observe the knee posture and balance. Additionally, doubts on the efficacy of proposed gastrocnemius lengthening can be resolved by myoneural blocks of the muscle using botulinum toxin injections into four quadrants of the gastrocnemius.

KINEMATIC CHARACTERISTICS OF NORMAL AND EQUINUS GAIT

Baddar and colleagues (2002) of the Motion Analysis Laboratory at the University of Virginia produced a highly detailed study of the characteristics of equinus gait in spastic diplegia compared with normal controls. Of the 34 subjects studied, 11 (22 limbs) had mid-calf recessions of the gastrocnemius-soleus tendon unit. In equinus foot contact is initiated by landing on the forefoot. Mean peak dorsiflexion occurs at 15% of the gait cycle in spastic diplegia compared with 42% in the normal. Dorsiflexion reached only 5.6º in spastic diplegia and 13º in the normal. In those with equinus gait the cycle began at foot contact with five times more knee flexion than normal (40º vs 8º). The ankle–knee couple during single-limb stance was knee extension while the ankle dorsiflexed. With equinus gait the opposite occurred: the knee extended while the ankle plantarflexed. Length curves of the calf muscle showed that the gastrocnemius–soleus was shortened throughout the gait cycle in the normal subjects. In those with equinus gait the mean maximum length of the calf muscle group at the end of single limb stance reached only 121% mean length of the muscle–tendon unit at 22% of the gait cycle compared with 125% at 44% of the gait cycle in the normal subjects.

After gastrocnemius–soleus recession in the mid-calf, mean peak ankle dorsiflexion increased from 7.1º to 15º. Dorsiflexion occurred closer to push-off and close to the normal gait pattern. Knee extension improved at foot contact while midswing knee flexion was reduced. Postoperatively the maximum length of the gastrocnemius–soleus increased from 121% preoperatively to 124% (similar to normal). The timing of maximum lengths improved from 20% of the gait cycle to 33%, but this time was still earlier than in the normal subjects. Ankle plantarflexion moments during loading was reduced, but moment at push-off was increased. The data indicated that adding length with surgery to the gastrocnemius–soleus unit created greater power generation in late stance when the center of the body is in front of the stance limb. The gastrocnemius–soleus mid-calf recessions affected primarily ankle kinematics and not muscle strength. Because the study showed that when the muscle–tendon unit operates in a shortened position as it does in equinus gait, lengthening of the unit can enhance function.

Baddar *et al.* (2002) also noted that they found persistent increased knee flexion to initiate stance and thought this might be due to overactivity or contracture (shortening) of the hamstring muscles. As might be surmised given that spastic paralysis in cerebral palsy is due to a brain dysfunction, the electromyographic patterns of the muscle did not change significantly with surgery.

The results of the surgery were deemed superior to those of 'z-lengthening' of the Achilles tendon which according to the computer modeling study of Delp and Zajac (1992) would reduce the total force-generating capacity of the gastrocnemius–soleus muscle unit.

SURGERY FOR EQUINUS DEFORMITY–CONTRACTURE OF THE GASTROCNEMIUS–SOLEUS

There are two basic surgical procedures that attack equinus gait in cerebral palsy.

1. GASTROCNEMIUS–SOLEUS LENGTHENING (RECESSION)

Gastrocnemius–soleus aponeurotic lengthening intended to preserve more function of the muscle in gait and avoid the risk of a postoperative calcaneus gait was begun by Vulpius and Stoffel (1913), reported in an American journal by Stoffel (1913), described again by Vulpius and Stoffel (1920), adopted in principle by Strayer (1950, 1958), modified by Baker (1954, 1956), by Rosenthal and Simon (1992), modified by Baumann as reported by Saraph *et al.* (2000), and preferred by Matsuo (2002) who 'abandoned' Achilles tendon lengthening. (Details of the operative techniques of Achilles tendon and gastrocnemius–soleus lengthening other than the Baumann technique are in Chapter 7.)

The Baumann procedure has been favored by Saraph and colleagues (2000) in Graz, Austria.[22] The Baumann modification lengthens the gastrocnemius–soleus complex through a medial mid-leg incision. While the ankle is dorsiflexed to the limit, the plantaris tendon is resected and the aponeurosis over the gastrocnemius is divided by two or three parallel cuts. The septum between the medial and lateral gastrocnemius heads is cut. The aponeurosis over the soleus is sectioned. The foot is dorsiflexed to the neutral position and either a short- or long-leg cast applied depending on additional surgery. Four to seven days after surgery the patient stands in a frame and gait training begun. After 3 weeks the cast is removed and a KAFO applied for night-time use and an AFO for daytime walking.

They reported no overcorrections or recurrence in a mean follow-up of 2.2 years (range 2.1– 4.0). Kinetic and kinematic studies of the ankle showed a change toward normal. The authors thought the Baumann procedure was superior to other gastrocnemius–soleus lengthenings since it avoided the musculotendinous junction of a presumed muscle 'growth plate' as

proposed by Ziv *et al.* (1984) in an experimental study using the spastic mouse.

In a letter to the editor, H.K. Graham (2000) of Melbourne, Australia, questioned the validity of the muscle 'growth plate' theory. He noted that there have been no randomized clinical trials comparing lengthening of the Achilles tendon with the various gastrocnemius–soleus lengthenings. He also pointed out that the type of cerebral palsy is more important than the type of surgery, i.e. children with hemiplegia are more likely to have a recurrence of equinus and those with diplegia to have calcaneus.

The same authors from Graz, Austria, reported on multilevel surgery for gait improvement in 29 children with spastic diplegia (Steinwender *et al.* 2001b). The focus was on fixed equinus deformities in 17 patients. Twelve patients had dynamic equinus and did not have surgery. Ankle function was assessed with gait analysis pre and postoperatively for a minimum of 3 years after surgery. They concluded that intramuscular lengthening of the gastrocnemius–soleus muscles improved function and did not cause weakening of the muscle.

2. ACHILLES TENDON LENGTHENING

Z-lengthening of the Achilles tendon has a historic beginning with Stromeyer and Little in 1837 when Little had a tenotomy of his Achilles for an equinus deformity of his foot (Rang 1993), but its reputation has waned (Borton *et al.* 2001, Matsuo 2002). All too often the z-method overlengthens the muscle–tendon unit; it is difficult to maintain the normal tension in the calf muscle group by suturing the split ends of the lengthened tendon. Restoration of adequate tension in the muscle–tendon unit depends on the judgement and proprioception of the surgeon. The justified fear of overlengthening of the Achilles is conversion from a 'jump' posture and gait to a 'crouch'. We recognize now the sensitivity of the soleus to surgical lengthening. Delp *et al.* (1995) through computer modeling demonstrated that a 1 cm lengthening of the soleus results in a 50% loss in force-generating capacity of the soleus. The soleus is rarely contracted in ambulatory diplegic children while it is possible to be contracted in hemiplegia or quadriplegia. Thus we conclude that there is almost no indication for the standard Z-tendo-achilles lengthening in a diplegic. Failures in the past may be more related to the wrong choice of operation than to technique.

Caveat emptor: '*There have been no randomized clinical trials comparing lengthening of the Achilles tendon with the various gastrocnemius-soleus lengthenings.*'

(Graham 2000)

POSTOPERATIVE IMMOBILIZATION, NIGHT SPLINTS AND ORTHOSES?

In contrast to the elaborate postoperative regimen with orthotics as described by Saraph *et al.* was that described by Lee and Bleck (1980). Walking was permitted on the first postoperative day in a long-leg cast for 3 weeks and converted to a short-leg cast for an additional 3 weeks. After cast removal the patients wore

---

22 Saraph *et al.* (2000) cite Baumann, J.U. and Koch, H.G. (1989) 'Ventrale aponeurotische, Verlänge des Musculus gastrocnemius.' *Operat Orthop. Traumatol.* **1**, 254–258.

flexible athletic shoes. All of 71 lengthenings were unbraced, unsplinted at night and unstretched. The minimum follow-up was 2 years. The recurrence rate was 9%; all recurrences occurred in those children who had surgery before age 7 years; five of six recurrences were in patients who had surgery at ages 2 and 4 years. Only two patients (3%) developed a postoperative calcaneus deformity. We do not know if the calcaneus deformity after the Hoke sliding lengthening was due to lack of attention to the ankle position after the cuts in the tendon were made or when the postoperative cast was applied—such is the variability of human perceptions and endeavours. All Achilles lengthenings were bilateral. In the same study 51 bilateral Strayer-Baker lengthenings had a recurrence rate of 29%. Note that this study was done in 1980 before the current sophisticated gait analysis laboratories were established.

Sharrard and Bernstein (1972) of England, Ratty *et al.* (1993) of Nova Scotia, Canada, and Katz *et al.* (2000) of Israel in their study of recurrences after Achilles tendon lengthening also concluded that postoperative night splinting and daytime orthoses did not alter the published and accepted recurrence rates. It was the patient's 'own muscle activity' that maintained the correction (Sharrard and Bernstein 1971). All found that the recurrences of equinus were more frequent when the Achilles lengthenings were done before the age of 4 or 5 years.

If you want simplicity, reproducibility, and predictability it seems as if the *sliding* Hoke Achilles tendon lengthening without postoperative night splints or orthoses should be considered. We will have to wait for a sufficiently large randomized clinical trial comparing the gastrocnemius–soleus recession techniques with sliding Achilles tendon lengthening in spastic diplegia. It is rather doubtful that the trial would want include the z-lengthenings so often referred to in the reports given the variations in controlling the tension of the muscle–tendon unit when suturing the cut tendon ends.

TENOTOMY OF THE GASTROCNEMIUS–SOLEUS MUSCLE–TENDON JUNCTION

A unique method of Achilles lengthening that would be feared by most orthopaedic surgeons was presented by Weigl *et al.* (2001) of Zerifin, Israel. They found that the Achilles tendon could be lengthened with a simple transverse cut at the muscle–tendon junction. They followed the healing of the gap in the tendon in 12 patients (21 Achilles tendons) with sonography. The gap in the tendon healed in six distinct stages. These surgeons concluded that their method was safe and without risk of overlengthening.

Gastrocnemius neurectomy and anterior translocation of the Achilles tendon insertion appear to have been relegated by the majority of orthopaedic surgeons to orthopaedic history (see Chapter 7 for details).

PES VALGUS

Pes valgus is more common in spastic diplegia than pes varus. In one study of 230 patients, 94% of hemiplegic children had pes varus; 64% of the spastic diplegics and quadriplegics had pes

valgus (Bennet *et al.* 1982). Children with spastic diplegia can have varus deformities of the foot; the management of these is discussed in Chapter 7.

PATHOLOGICAL ANATOMY

The spastic pes valgus foot has an eversion and equinus inclination of the calcaneus and abduction of the midfoot which results in a prominence of the head of the talus medially (Fig. 8.64). It is a flexible deformity until adolescence. Until that age the foot can be passively manipulated into the corrected position by plantarflexion of the ankle and inversion of the foot.

Lateral radiographs of the foot when the patient is standing show greater than normal plantarflexion of the talus and varying degrees of loss of dorsiflexion of the calcaneus (Fig. 8.65). According to our studies, the normal plantarflexion of the talus is 26.5º (SD 3º). In children younger than 5 years, the normal plantarflexion of the talus can be as much as 35º so that a line through the center of the talar neck and body falls just inferior to the first metatarsal shaft. The normal calcaneal

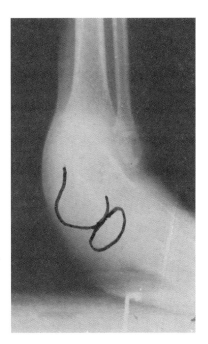

Fig. 8.64. Anterior–posterior radiograph of ankle, talus and navicular. Head of talus prominent medially and navicular displaced laterally on the head of the talus.

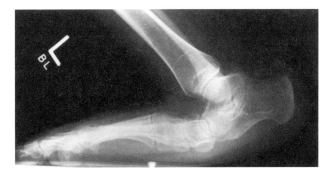

Fig. 8.65. Lateral radiograph of left foot, spastic diplegia, skeletally mature, severe pes valgus. Talus plantarflexed and hindfoot in equinus. Tibia angled far anteriorly secondary to Achilles tendon lengthening.

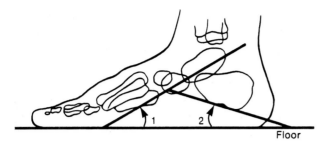

Fig. 8.66. Tracing of weightbearing lateral radiograph of normal foot. Two angles to measure: 1. Plantarflexion of talus (normal mean 26.5°, SD 5.3); 2. Calcaneal dorsiflexion (normal mean 16.8°, SD 5.6).

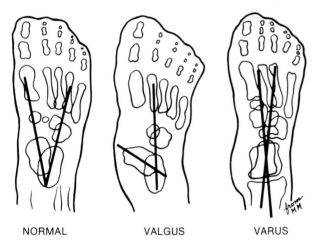

NORMAL   VALGUS   VARUS

Fig. 8.67. Tracings of weightbearing anterior–posterior radiographs of normal, valgus, and varus deformities of the foot. Normal talar–calcaneal divergence angle: mean 15°; valgus more than 25°; varus less than 15°.

dorsiflexion angle is 16.8° (SD 5.6°) (Bleck and Berzins 1977) (Fig. 8.66).

On the anterior–posterior radiograph of the foot with the patient weightbearing, the normal angle formed by a line bisecting the talar neck and another line parallel to the lateral border of the calcaneus is a mean of 18° (SD 5°). If this angle is greater than 25°, valgus is present; if less than 15° the heel is in varus (Fig. 8.67).

MECHANISMS OF SPASTIC PES VALGUS

The axis of rotation of the subtalar joint has been compared to a mitered hinge; its axis is more horizontal than oblique, accounting for the greater degree of eversion than inversion of this joint. The mean angle of inclination of this joint projected on the sagittal plane when measured on anatomical specimens was 42°, with a great variation ranging from 20.5° to 68.5° (Inman 1976).

Spastic peroneal muscles abduct the mid- and forefoot excessively and continuously; this abnormal movement pulls the navicular laterally and with it the supporting plantar ligaments for the talar head. The result is plantarflexion of the talus. Skinner

and Lester (1985) analyzed the dynamic electromyograms in 13 children with spastic diplegia to observe their hindfoot valgus deformities. They described three different patterns of muscle activity to account for the valgus: (1) hyperactive peroneal muscles with a strong posterior tibial muscle; (2) hyperactive peroneals with a weak posterior tibial; and (3) hyperactive extensor digitorum longus muscles (Fig. 8.68).

Orthopaedic surgeons have recognized the spastic peroneals as the major deforming force, and have lengthened the peroneus brevis in an attempt to prevent further deformity in young children (Nather *et al.* 1984). An electromyographic study of the posterior tibial muscle in spastic pes valgus came to the opposite conclusion: in five of six spastic diplegic children, the posterior tibial muscle was electrically silent. This led to the conclusion that without the counterbalancing effect of the posterior tibial muscle, valgus occurred (Bennet *et al.* 1982). Accordingly, transfer of the peroneus brevis to the posterior tibial tendon was proposed.

Calcaneal plantarflexion due to gastrocnemius–soleus contracture contributes to the deformity but unfortunately cannot be the sole cause. If it were, Achilles tendon lengthening would not only prevent but also correct the flexible pes valgus. This we know does not occur. Equinus deformity is seen without valgus and also with varus deformities.

Variations in *ligamentous laxity* among children may account for the early development of severe pes valgus in some and not in others (Wynne-Davies 1970). This variation in laxity of connective tissues among individuals has been ascribed to defects in the cross-linking of collagen (Eyre 1984).

Persistent fetal medial deviation of the talar neck is an anatomical departure from the norm and may account for the internal axial rotation of the foot that is sometimes observed after arthrodesis of the talonavicular joint when the navicular is placed in its anatomical alignment on the talar head. The newborn talus has a greater degree of medial deviation of its neck at birth than in the adult form (Lisowski 1974) (Fig. 8.69). Attenborough (1966) first called our attention to the 'persistent fetal medial deviation of the talar neck' in the 'easy' type of club feet that corrected well with casts, taping or splinting. Although not confirmed by subsequent reports (Bleck and Minaire 1983), persistence of the newborn talar neck angle is one cause of in-toeing in children. Some normal children who at first merely have

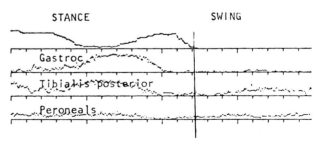

Fig. 8.68. Electromyographs, integrated signals, spastic diplegia, walking, pes valgus. Gastrocnemius normal firing; tibialis posterior firing strongly and normally in stance, and weakly in swing; peroneals firing in swing and stance. Meaning: underneath every valgus is a potential varus and vice versa.

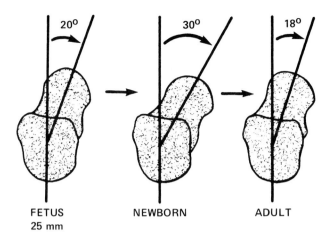

Fig. 8.69. Talar neck angles increasing from fetal life to newborn and normally decreasing at maturity.

in-toeing may develop pes valgus with a prominent head of the talus on the medial aspect of the foot.

ASSESSMENT

In addition to the examination of the deformity, the surgeon must confirm the flexibility and correctibility of the foot by passive manipulation. The foot will have to be brought into varying degrees of equinus before it can be placed in the corrected position. If in doubt about the mobility of the talus, a lateral radiograph of the foot held in equinus and inversion resolves the question and differentiates a fixed from a flexible deformity.

It is essential to obtain anterior–posterior and lateral radiographs of the foot with the patient weightbearing[23] and, most importantly, an anterior–posterior radiograph of the ankle when weightbearing. The ankle radiographs are necessary to determine any valgus tilt of the talus in the ankle mortise (Fig. 8.70). If so, reconstructive surgery of the foot only will be insufficient to correct all of the valgus deformity.

In pes valgus before embarking on surgery to correct the foot deformity, obtain an anterior–posterior radiograph of the ankle with the patient weightbearing to determine valgus tilt of the talus in the ankle mortise—avoid a disappointing result.

Another assessment instrumented tested by Chang *et al.* (2002) of the duPont Hospital for Children is the *dynamic pedobarograph.*[24] This is a pressure sensitive floor-mat that contains a grid of 87 rows by 96 columns of pressure sensing cells. The patient walks on the mat and the resulting signals from the mat are converted to a graphic outline of the plantar aspect of the foot to depict pressures in five sections of the foot. As might be expected varus feet exhibited higher impulses over the lateral aspect and valgus feet over the medial aspect. The heel area had low impulses due to the dynamic equinus.

INDICATIONS AND TIMING OF SURGERY

An obvious and severe pes valgus in spastic diplegia can be corrected only with surgery. One possible classification of severity is the degree of valgus of the heel in relation to the longitudinal alignment of the tibia: less than 10º is mild; 10º–15º is moderate, and greater than 15º is severe (Fig. 8.71).

The measurement of the degree of plantarflexion of the talus on the lateral radiograph, made when weightbearing, may be an additional way to assess severity: 35º–40º is mild; 40º–50º is moderate, and greater than 50º is severe. The lateral radiograph of the foot may also show a decrease in the calcaneal dorsiflexion angle of less than 10º and is an indicator of additional severity.

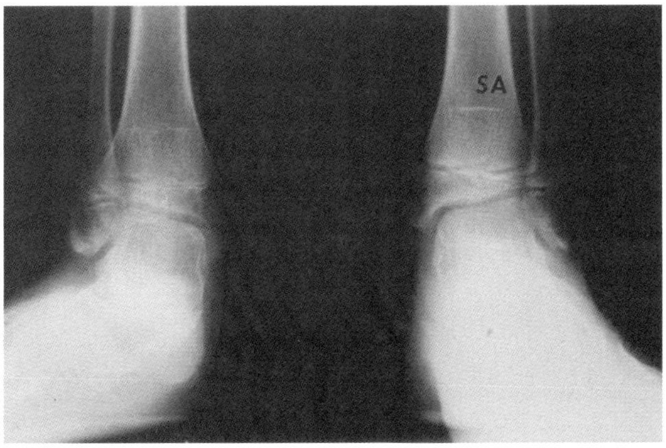

Fig. 8.70. Anterior–posterior radiographs of both ankles in weightbearing, spastic diplegia, bilateral pes valgus, secondary valgus tilt of distal tibial articular surface.

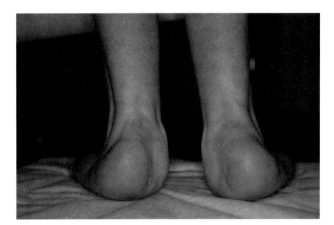

Fig. 8.71. Photograph of hindfeet, spastic diplegia, pes valgus. Clinical estimate of severity according to degree of heel eversion measured with a line bisecting the calf and another bisecting the heel.

23 In making the anterior–posterior projection of the foot with the patient in full weight bearing, it is important to be certain that the patient does not shift to a slight varus position voluntarily. The resultant radiograph will give an erroneous depiction of the skeletal alignment.

24 Tekscan High Resolution Pressure Assessment System (Tekscan, Inc., South Boston, Massachusetts, USA).

A slightly more complicated method of determining the alignment of the talus and calcaneus is the lateral talo–calcaneal angle by measure of the weightbearing lateral radiograph of the foot. A line drawn through the long axis of the calcaneus forms an acute angle with a line through the mid-axis of the talus. Normally this angle varies between 25° and 50°. Another line can be drawn through the inferior cortex of the calcaneus that intersects with a line through the inferior cortex of the 5th metatarsal. The normal obtuse angle is 150° with a slight variation from 133.5° to 149.5° and does not vary with the age of the child (Hensinger 1986). It is a way to make an objective evaluation of a high or low arch.

Anterior–posterior radiographic projections of the foot when weightbearing can define the varus or valgus deformity. Lines are drawn through the long axis of the talus and calcaneus. A normal variation of the angle is found up to the age of five years from about 20°–50°. After age 5 years the normal mean angle with a neutral heel position is 15°. A lesser angle than in the normal range indicates varus and an angle greater than 25°, valgus (Fig. 8.67).

Pes valgus thought to be 'severe' in children under age 4 years may not be as severe at 6–7 years of age. This decrease in severity seems to occur as the foot equilibrium reactions reverse from the primitive infantile eversion reaction to the more mature inversion foot reaction (Gunsolus *et al.* 1975). Another natural phenomenon to account for a decrease in pes valgus may be decreasing ligamentous laxity with age, presumably due to more cross-linking of the collagen.

> *Pes valgus thought to be 'severe' in children under age 4 years may not be as severe at age 6–7 years. . . . Surgery can wait—the foot won't run away.*

Because of these observations, one should be reluctant to advise early surgical treatment of pes valgus (generally younger than age 5 years). We know that the mature gait parameters emerge at about the age of 7 years (Sutherland *et al.* 1980). Parents and grandparents often focus on the feet. They need to know that the foot won't run away. The foot is not the seat of the soul. Children without feet or uncorrected talipes equinovarus can walk. There is more to walking than the feet. Bleck (1987) preferred to delay surgery until about 7 years. Occasionally corrective surgery may be done for a severe deformity of a more skeletally mature foot in children between the ages of 5.5 and 6.5 years. However, early surgery seems to bring a risk of late pes varus. Lee (1977b) found failures in 11 of 13 of Bleck's patients who had extra-articular subtalar arthrodesis under the age of 7 years. This type of arthrodesis is difficult to achieve in young children, owing to the smallness and cartilaginous bulk of their tarsal bones.

Though premature surgery seems to create problems, delaying surgery until adolescence is not wise either. The moderate and severe pes valgus seen in cerebral palsy eventually becomes rigid and impossible to correct with passive manipulation. At this time a triple arthrodesis is the procedure of last resort. At this later age, however, correction is not so satisfactory.

Because bone and articular cartilage must be removed from the subtalar joint, the height of the foot is decreased. This results in uncomfortable impingement of the malleoli on the top edge of the lower quarter shoe (Banks 1977).

Special shoes, sole and/or heel wedges, arch supports and orthotics have not been successful in prevention of spastic pes valgus or in treatment. These might be a type of long-acting placebo for the physician, therapist and parents.

> *Special shoes, sole and/or heel wedges, arch supports and orthotics . . . a type of long-acting placebo for the physician, therapist and parents.*

Correction by extra-articular subtalar arthrodesis or lateral border calcaneal osteotomy is indicated by the incipient development of hallux valgus, which indicates excessive pressure on the medial aspect of the foot on weightbearing. Hallux valgus will often get worse and become painful due to callosities on the medial border of the great toe and the first metatarsal head (Fig. 8.72).

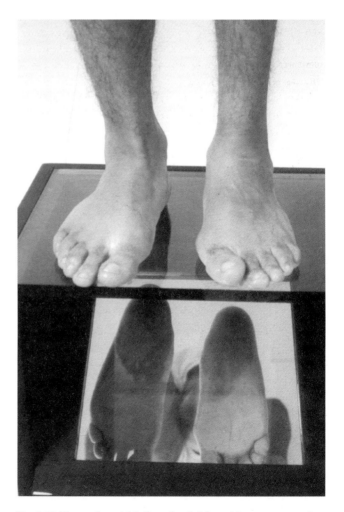

Fig. 8.72. Teenage boy with hallux valgus left foot with great toe pronation, mild midfoot and hindfoot valgus. Correct only if symptomatic.

SURGICAL PROCEDURES: SPASTIC PES VALGUS

There are several choices for correction of pes valgus in cerebral palsy. Only three are effective: two for correction before adolescence and one for adolescents and adults. But first a full review of the choices and a critique seems appropriate.

1. *Peroneal tendon transfer* seems logical. Unfortunately, pes varus has been the frequent result and explains why so little has been written about peroneal tendon transfer in spastic pes valgus. Bennet *et al.* (1982) found no electromyographic activity in five of six posterior tibial muscles in spastic pes valgus. This evidence encouraged them to try transfer of the peroneus brevis to the posterior tibial tendon, with good preliminary results. Time will tell. Late varus could be expected. The electromyograph is not so much quantitative as qualitative. Low-voltage output may be the result of fewer motor units in the area of muscle sampled, and electrical silence can be due to technical adjustments in an attempt to eliminate background noise so that only the strongest signals are recorded. Lengthening of the peroneus brevis at the time of extra-articular subtalar arthrodesis caused a reversal to varus deformities in five of seven feet (Lee 1977b).

2. *Peroneus brevis intramuscular tenotomy* was reported in 30 cases of spastic pes valgus by Nather *et al.* (1984) of Singapore. The mean age of 20 patients was 6 years (range 2–14 years). Severity was graded by the eversion angle of the heel: mild, less than 10° (N=14); moderate, 10° (N=12); severe, greater than 10° (N=4). Using these criteria, the postoperative results on hindfoot valgus were: 14 decreased, 12 were unchanged and four increased. Mild cases showed the most improvement. Experimental lengthenings of leg tendons in rabbits and the effects of immobilization did demonstrate that intramuscular tenotomy did not require immobilization to maintain the separation of tendons ends while healing occurred (Nather *et al.* 1986).

Perhaps intramuscular tenotomy of the peroneus brevis could be considered in children under age 7 years with mild spastic pes valgus. Is mild pes valgus is any more disabling in a child with cerebral palsy than it is in normal children who seem to tolerate and often 'outgrow' mild hindfoot valgus? With moderate deformities will reversal to varus occur in time when the peroneus brevis spasticity has been reduced with lengthening? In more severe cases this simple operation is not likely to work.

3. *Extra-articular subtalar arthrodesis* has been the standard operation to correct spastic pes va1gus in children since Grice (1952) originated this operation for va1gus foot deformities in the residuals of poliomyelitis. The objective was to prevent eversion of the hind-foot by permanently eliminating subtalar joint motion with an arthrodesis exterior to the articular surfaces (Fig. 8.73 *a, b*). Thus children under age 13 years would have preservation of the tarsal bone growth; growth arrest of the tarsal bones would occur with intra-articular arthrodesis—each articular surface is comparable to a growth plate in a long bone.

After Grice published his technique and results (1952), some surgeons saw the operation as a solution to correct pes valgus in children with cerebral palsy and avoid the very severe valgus feet seen in adults (Baker and Dodelin 1958, Baker and Hill 1964). Since that time there have been many reports on the efficacy of

the procedure, not only in poliomyelitis but also in cerebral palsy and myelomeningocele (Pollock and Carrell 1964, Banks 1977, Moreland and Westin 1977, 1986, Ross and Lyne 1980, Aronson *et al.* 1983, Mohaghegh and Stryker 1983, McCall *et al.* 1985, Alman *et al.* 1993).

Banks (1977) had the best results: 86% were described as 'successful', and 63% as 'excellent'. Other surgeons have not had as much success in cerebral palsy: Pollock and Carrell (1964) reported a 31% failure rate (15% had graft failure); Ross and Lyne reported 64% failure and 28% complications. Moreland and Westin (1977) had satisfactory results in 73%, but in 1986 they had unpredictable results with pes valgus except in cases due to poliomyelitis. 21% were fused in an unacceptable position; in cerebral palsy the non-union rate was 31%. McCall *et al.* (1985) had unsatisfactory results in 46%; 25 of 75 feet in cerebral palsy had bone-graft failure.

In contrast to these pessimistic results, Alman and colleagues (1993)—from the city of origin of the Grice procedure, Boston, Massachusetts—had no recurrence of the valgus deformity in 17 patients in an average follow-up of 8.9 years. These were less severely involved patients with cerebral palsy. Five patients who had spastic quadriplegia had recurrences.

Bleck's results were studied by Lee (1977b). Of 44 Grice procedures in cerebral palsy, only 50% had good corrections. Eventually, with secondary procedures, the poor results were converted to satisfactory results in 85%. The procedures used for postoperative varus were posterior tibial tendon transfer or

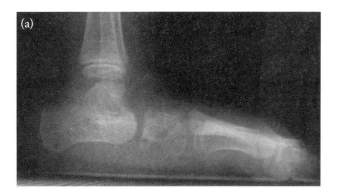

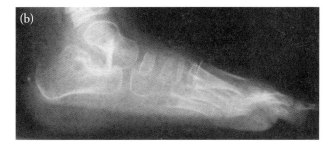

Fig. 8.73. (*a*) Radiograph, lateral projection, foot weightbearing, spastic diplegia, patient TM, age 4 years, pes valgus. Typical plantarflexed talus. (*b*) Radiograph, lateral projection, foot weightbearing, spastic diplegia, patient TM, 1 year postoperative, classic Grice subtalar extra-articular arthrodesis; tibial bone graft in perfect position, but difficult to maintain while consolidating in young children accounting for a high failure rate.

lengthening or anterior tibial tendon transfer in dynamic varus deformities; if the varus was fixed, a closed wedge lateral calcaneal osteotomy sufficed. For dynamic forefoot valgus, peroneus brevis tendon lengthening alleviated this problem which occurred in only two feet.

4. *Modifications of extra-articular subtalar arthrodesis.* We orthopaedic surgeons are like composers of orchestral music: we create variations of operations with the same theme. L.D. Baker (personal communication) used rib homografts and not the original tibial cortical bone grafts. Baker and Hill (1964) did laterally based open wedge osteotomies of the posterior calcaneal facet, holding the wedge open with a cortical bone graft, to block eversion of the subtalar joint. When Bleck used Baker's modification in conjunction with the Grice procedure as originally described, and his results improved dramatically (Bleck 1987). With the tibial cortical grafts alone in the sinus tarsi the failure was 83%, but with the Grice and Baker combined procedures only 25% failed. The rationale for combining the two was that if the tibial bone graft in the sinus tarsi failed to unite or was resorbed, the calcaneal facet osteotomy would hold the correction.

Brown (1968) and Seymour and Evans (1968) used a fibular bone graft in a method Brown learned from Mr J.S. Batchelor at Guy's Hospital in London (unpublished). The fibular shaft bone graft was driven through a hole in the neck of the talus and into the calcaneus to maintain the correction of the pes valgus. Graft failure and breakage occurs with this method because the graft is inserted almost exactly parallel with the axis of rotation of the subtalar joint. Ideally, all grafts should be placed perpendicular to this axis (Fig. 8.74); they will then be under compression and rotation will be minimal.

Hsu *et al.* (1986) used the fibular graft method devised by Batchelor, but added another fibular graft parallel to the tibial shaft as originally recommended by Grice. The risk of fibular shaft removal for a bone graft is failure of reformation of the fibula, which results in valgus of the ankle joint (Wiltse *et al.* 1972, Hsu *et al.* 1974). Bhan and Malhotra (1998) of New Delhi, India, used both a fibular dowel graft and the screw with the bone graft in the sinus tarsi as described by Dennyson and Fulford (1976). Pirani *et al.* (1990) had generally good results with the dowel graft method and learned that one of the major sources of unsat-

isfactory results was simultaneous lengthening of the peroneal tendons.

Mohaghegh and Stryker (1983), applying the principle of stopping eversion by extra-articular arthrodesis, used a dowel graft from the calcaneus in the sinus tarsi. Jeray *et al.* (1998) had success with a bone graft from the calcaneus combined with internal fixation. Guttmann (1990) had success in correction with an iliac bone plug in the sinus tarsi.

Hamel *et al.* (1994) of Wetter, Germany, wrote a candid report on modification of the Grice subtalar arthrodesis for which surgeons should be grateful as it might stem them from embellishment of the procedure—27.9% had poor results. The German surgeons operated on 43 valgus feet of 28 children with cerebral palsy and a mean follow-up of 6.7 years. To the classic Grice bone graft in the sinus tarsi, they added the Schede modification which was to 'roughen' the cartilage surfaces of the talonavicular joint. (They state that they now omit this procedure.)[25] And they added a lot more: an Achilles tendon lengthening leaving the medial part of the tendon attached to the calcaneal insertion; transferred the distal half of the anterior tibial tendon to the plantar calcaneonavicular ligament, and advanced the navicular insertion to the posterior tibial tendon to the first tarsometatarsal joint. Despite this more extensive surgery only 58.1% were judged to have excellent results and 27.9% had poor results. They concluded that their operation could be recommended for patients with spastic hemiplegia and diplegia, but not those who had total body involvement.

According to the 27.9% poor results of modifications of the classic Grice subtalar extraarticular arthrodesis by Hamel et al. (1994), surgeons might resist embellishments of the procedure.

To simplify the technique of extra-articular arthrodesis, Cahuzac (1977) and the orthopaedic surgeons of Montpelier, France, used the technique of Cavalier and Judet (cited by Trouillas 1978). After the valgus foot was manipulated into the correct position, a single screw was inserted from the superior surface of the talar neck obliquely into the calcaneus. Only 10% bad results were reported in 50 feet. The presumption apparently was that the corrections will be sustained, either because of arthrofibrosis of the subtalar joint secondary to immobilization, or because of a possible redirection of the tarsal bone growth. Since this screw is in the axis of rotation of the subtalar joint, the risk of failure in time seems likely. During gait the subtalar joint does rotate in order to absorb the torques generated between the foot and the floor. It seems more logical to add a bone graft to assure solid extra-articular fusion while the screw holds the correction. This is one reason why we should be very selective in recommending subtalar arthrodesis in children with spastic diplegia and pes valgus. 'Mild' valgus needs no correction and 'moderate' may need correction if hallux valgus and medial

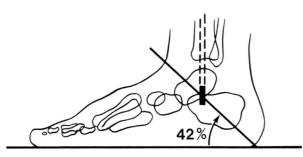

Fig. 8.74. Tracing of weightbearing radiograph of the foot depicting normal mean axis of rotation of subtalar joint (wide variations), and position of bone tibial bone graft, dowel fibular graft, or other fixation that should cross the axis of rotation parallel with the tibial shaft and not be in alignment with it.

25 Hamel *et al.* (1994) cite Schede, F. (1929) 'Die operation der Plattfussbis', *Zeitschrift Orthop. Chir.* **50**, 528–538.

callouses on the head of the first metatarsal and great toe are developing.

Dennyson and Fulford (1976) used the same screw fixation but added an iliac bone graft to the sinus tarsi. They had good results, with a 93.7% fusion rate. An additional advantage of the procedure is that it allows a shorter period of plaster immobilization and earlier weightbearing than the classic Grice procedure. Dr J. Cary (personal communication) introduced the operation to Bleck at the Newington Children's Hospital, Newington, Connecticut, and Bleck used it since. Barrasso and surgeons (1984) of this hospital have reported results that paralleled Bleck's (1987): in 40 feet (26 patients), 95% were rated good or excellent with no poor results. Union of the iliac bone graft with the talus and calcaneus was reported to occur within a mean time of 10 weeks. In 25 feet Bleck (1987) had one failure of correction, and had to remove only one screw (Fig. 8.75 *a*, *b*).

Typical of orthopaedic surgeons who always find a way to modify and original operation were Rang *et al.* (1986) and L.A. Rinsky (personal communication). Rang also used internal fixation and a dowel graft from the calcaneus, rather than an iliac graft. He drove the screw upward from the lateral aspect of the calcaneus into the talus. Rinsky used a Steinman pin from the lateral aspect of the calcaneus to the talus; the pin held the correction until fusion with the iliac bone graft occurs; then the pin was extracted.

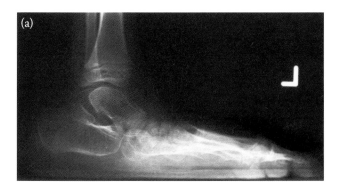

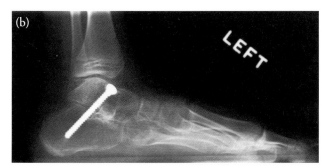

Fig. 8.75. (*a*) Lateral radiograph, left foot, weightbearing, spastic diplegia, patient AB, age 7 years, typical pes valgus with plantarflexed talus and calcaneal dorsiflexion angle at 0. (*b*) Lateral radiograph, left foot, weightbearing, spastic diplegia, patient AB, 2 years postoperative correction with screw through neck of talus to calcaneus and iliac bone graft in sinus tarsi. Calcaneal dorsiflexion same as preoperatively.

5. *Extra-articular subtalar stabilization with staples (arthroereisis)* was introduced by Crawford and associates (1986). In this operation the spastic valgus foot is placed into the corrected position which is secured by a laterally placed staple across the subtalar joint in the body of the talus and the calcaneus. Of the 20 patients 18 patients had cerebral palsy (28 feet), followed for an average of 4.1 years. The results were satisfactory in 84% and unsatisfactory in 16% based on the radiograph of the foot to measure the lateral talocalcaneal angle.

Crawford's original intention was to use the staple as a temporary correction until the child was old enough to have an extra-articular arthrodesis with a bone graft. Crawford and colleagues (1990) from Cincinnati published the results of the subtalar joint stabilization with a staple in 31 procedures (termed 'arthroereisis')[26] in 20 patients with a follow-up of 2–7 years (mean 4.1 years). The age of surgery ranged from 2 years to 10 years 10 months. The surgical incision is the lateral half of the circumferential Cincinnati incision devised originally for club-foot reconstruction. A complete release of the anterior, lateral and posterior articulations of the subtalar joint is done. The calcaneus is reduced and held in position by the blade of an osteotome directed vertically in the subtalar joint. A 1.6 cm (5/8 inch); 1.9 cm if the foot is more than 13 cm long. Vitallium staple is aligned parallel with the tibia and driven across the joint to engage the talus and the calcaneus). But first, a notch to receive the staple flush with the talus is cut in the lateral margin of the calcaneus (Fig. 8.76). An above-knee cast is worn for 6 weeks after which a polypropylene AFO is used for 6 months.

Complications were minor and only one staple extruded. In all cases radiographs suggested some continued subtalar motion manifested by resorption of bone adjacent to the staple's prongs. The original intention of the operation was to stabilize the joint temporarily until the child was old enough for stabilization with bone. Because the follow-up indicated maintenance of the correction with the staple, removal of it and addition of bone was not thought necessary. Whether bone bridges developed around to staple to cross the joint or whether the immobilization caused arthrofibrosis and cartilage degeneration as occurs in other immobilized joint over a period of time cannot be ascertained (Fig. 8.77).

It was Crawford's concept to do the operation at a very young age to prevent more severe and fixed deformity at the child matured. One might be reluctant to recommend surgical correction of pes valgus under the age of 6–7 years particularly at age 2–3 years (in Crawford's series the age at the time of surgery was less than 6 years in 15 of the 20 patients) because mild and moderate pes valgus (less than 15° of heel eversion) may not be any more significant in spastic diplegia than it is in non-

26 Arthroereisis or arthroresis stems for the Greek ᾽αρθρο (joint) and ᾽ερεισις (a propping up). Presumably this Greek term was chosen instead of 'arthrodesis' (δησις = a binding together) which connotes fusion of the joint to differentiate the staple fixation of the joint from the extraarticular arthrodesis, although the staple does secure the joint comparable to arthrodesis. Arthroereisis does sound rather grand. The same term is used for the plastic plug implant in the sinus tarsi.

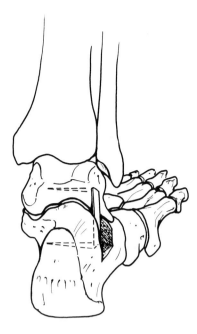

Fig. 8.76. Drawing of placement of staple between corrected alignment of talus and calcaneus for correction of pes valgus. Note the trough cut into the lateral aspect of the calcaneus to counter-sink the staple so it remains flush with the lateral aspect of the talus.

paralytic flexible pes valgus. Also 2- to 3-year-old children with spastic diplegia whose foot appeared to be in severe valgus have been observed to gradually correct as the child's central nervous system develops and matures—in general to the age of 7 years. Bleck has attributed the early pes valgus to equilibrium reactions of the feet with eversion when the child first begins to stand and walk and reversal to the normal inversion reactions at about the age of 4 years (Gunsolus *et al.* 1975)

Not ones to have a closed mind, the pediatric orthopaedic surgeons at the Children's Hospital, San Diego, California (Sanchez *et al.* 1999), did the subtalar joint stapling in flexible, severe planovalgus feet due to neuromuscular conditions. They did the operation in 34 feet at an average age of 5 years (range 2.5–9 years). Of the 34 feet an alarming 16 feet required revision

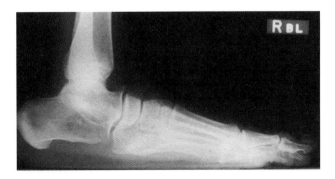

Fig. 8.77. Radiograph, right foot, spastic diplegia, patient BB, age 22 years, with spastic diplegia and bilateral subtalar extra-articular arthrodesis, 15 years postoperative. Subtalar joint fused. Bone spur on dorsal articular surface of talar neck at the talonavicular joint. Asymptomatic.

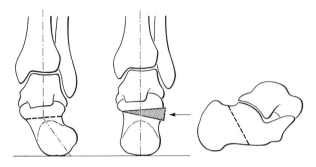

Fig. 8.78. Drawing, open wedge osteotomy of calcaneus with insertion of tibial allograft for valgus of the hindfoot in spastic diplegia. No longer recommended (Sage 1987).

at an average of 39 months after surgery in a range of 9–63 months. Revisions consisted of staple removal, repeat subtalar stapling in one case, triple arthrodesis in two, and calcaneal, cuboid and cuneiform osteotomies in nine feet. Their conclusion was that the long-term results of the staple arthroereisis were unpredictable and no longer recommended it for the correction of pes valgus due to neuromuscular conditions. A close to 50% failure rate is too much to accept for any operation.[27]

Pes valgus in toddlers may be the primitive foot equilibrium reactions that begin in eversion and reverse to inversion with maturation of the nervous system.

6. *Open wedge calcaneal osteotomy* (Silver *et al.* 1967, 1974, Silver 1977) was proposed to preserve the mobility of the subtalar joint and correct the valgus by shifting the weight-bearing area of the calcaneus from an everted to an inverted position. A sterile slice of cadaver cortical bone kept the laterally based osteotomy open while healing occurred (Fig. 8.78). Silver had success with this procedure. From a study of the radiographs in Silver's publications, it appeared that this osteotomy will realign the valgus foot if the talus has moderate plantar flexion of 45°–55°. If plantarflexion of the talus is greater than this (60°–80°), calcaneal osteotomy may not suffice for an adequate correction (R.L. Samilson, F. Sage, personal communications).

The late Fred Sage of the Campbell Clinic, Memphis, Tennessee, came to a firm conclusion: after an experience with calcaneal osteotomies: 'We do not recommend opening wedge osteotomies of the calcaneus' (Sage 1987). The reason is the skin overlying the calcaneus laterally and medially is not very mobile so that open wedge osteotomy puts too much tension on the suture line increasing the risk of necrosis and slough of the incision. In addition, the medial calcaneal nerves are stretched with an open wedge osteotomy resulting in painful neuromas.

'We do not recommend opening wedge osteotomies of the calcaneus.'

(Sage 1987)

27 Crawford's ingenious subtalar stapling, in the parlance of medical etiquette, remains 'controversial'—a useful euphemism.

7. *Medial displacement osteotomy of the calcaneus* was mentioned by Coleman (1983) as yet another way to overcome pes valgus. This oblique osteotomy in the coronal plane of the calcaneus made through a lateral approach can shift the heel directly medially. It brings the heel into direct alignment with the tibia. Correction of the valgus of the hindfoot can occur. It is not likely to correct the mid- and forefoot pathological anatomy characteristic of pes valgus in spastic diplegic children. Gleich (1893) of Germany is credited by Koutsoviannis (1971) of Larrisa, Greece, reporting from Bristol, England, and Silver *et al.* (1967) with the original concept as a treatment for flat foot.[28]

The technique and follow-up results of the medial displacement osteotomy for pes valgus was detailed by Koman *et al.* (1993). Ten patients (18 feet) had the following procedure: a lateral incision inferior to the peroneal tendons; identification and preservation of the sural nerve; incision and elevation of the periosteum over the lateral aspect of the calcaneus; a transverse osteotomy parallel to the subtalar joint confirmed by a fluoroscopic image; the medial periosteum must be incised through the osteotomy to ensure displacement (caution: avoid injury to the flexor hallucis longus); the distal fragment of the calcaneus is displaced up to 50% and maintained without tilting of the fragment. The osteotomy is secured with pins inserted from the anterior aspect of the talus and directed obliquely and posteriorly to the plantar cortex of the calcaneus, but *not penetrating it* (Fig. 8.79).

A short-leg non-weightbearing cast is worn for 3–4 weeks. The pins are then removed and a short-leg walking cast applied and used for 2–3 weeks. The average age at the time of surgery was 9 years, 4 months and had a follow-up of a mean 42 months. Percutaneous Achilles lengthenings had been done at the time of surgery in five of the nine patients. A functional evaluation showed good or excellent results in 17 of 18 feet. One patient required reoperation because of overcorrection and a varus tilt of the displaced calcaneal fragment. Most of the patients continued to have a 'mild' valgus but did not require further surgery. Radiographic improvement of the weightbearing lateral projections was measured in all patients. The objective of the surgery is to correct the valgus deformity and preserve subtalar joint motion. Whether this motion was preserved or not is not mentioned in the paper: it is a very difficult range of motion to measure. Horstmann has used this procedure for the past 20 years and has noted similar results with good preservation of subtalar motion.

8. *Calcaneal lengthening.* Mosca (1995) of Seattle drew on the concept of the structural abnormality of a calcaneal–valgus deformity proposed by Dillwyn Evans (1975) of Wales. Pes valgus consists of a short lateral column and a long medial column of the bones. It seems as if the valgus foot is a box like a trapezoid

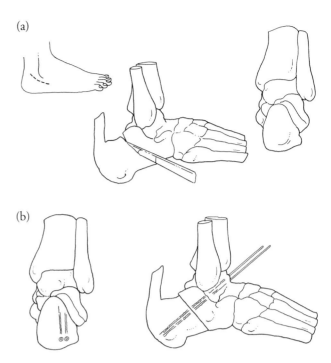

Fig. 8.79. (*a*) Schematic drawing of technique of medial displacement osteotomy of calcaneus for pes valgus. Lateral curvilinear incision over calcaneus, osteotome transects calcaneus parallel to the subtalar joint. (*b*) Calcaneus displaced 50% medially and fixation with two pins from talar neck into calcaneus stopping in the cortex, but not through it. (Redrawn from Koman *et al.* 1993, Figs 1 and 2.)

with a short and long side enclosed at either end. Depending on the lengths of the columns, pes valgus and varus are mirror images. The theory is that the normal foot has equal medial and lateral lengths. Whether this is actual or perceptual cannot be ascertained in the absence of actual linear measurements. Evans used the concept to correct the valgus deformity with an open wedge osteotomy of the calcaneus just posterior to the cuboid bone.

Mosca took the concept further to an open wedge osteotomy of the calcaneus between the anterior and middle facets (sustenaculum tali) of the subtalar joint. It is a distraction-wedge osteotomy held apart by a trapezoidal tricortical iliac bone graft (either an allograft or autogenous graft). After an incision over the sinus tarsus is made, and soft tissue retracted, the site of the osteotomy is delineated about 1.5 cm proximal to the calcaneal-cuboid joint. Elevator retractors are placed between the middle and anterior facets (Fig. 8.80 *a*). The position should be corroborated with fluoroscopy. Then mark the position with Steinman pins proximal and distal to the osteotomy site. The osteotomy will advance obliquely from proximal laterally to more distal medially. The tricortical bone graft can be from the child or allograft. It is trapezoidal (Fig. 8.80 *c*), with the lateral border twice the width of the medial and of sufficient depth to fill the os calcis osteotomy from lateral to medial, usually 2–2.5 cm. Preoperative templating is helpful to optimize surgical outcome. Distract the osteotomy site with a laminar spreader and stack the grafts horizontally with the tricortical position lateral. Make sure

28 Gleich's paper is in German with the onomatopoetic title Plattfussbehandlung that needs no English translation. The date 1893 reminds one of the advice of the late Robert Jameson MD, Stanford University faculty: 'If you think you have something new, always search the German literature.'

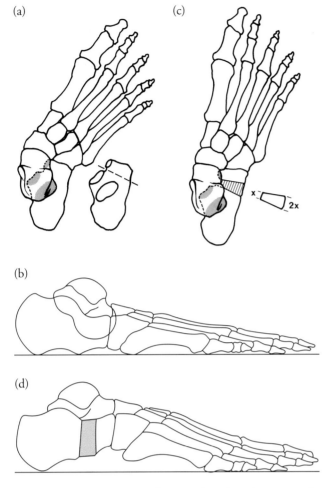

(a)

(c)

(b)

(d)

Fig. 8.80. Schematic drawing of open wedge calcaneal osteotomy for lengthening lateral border of the foot in pes valgus; allograft inserted to keep wedge open. (*a*) Osteotomy through os calcis is oblique and exits medially between the anterior and middle facet. (*b*) Lateral sag of midfoot associated with valgus plantarflexed hindfoot. (*c*) Tricortical wedges are put into the distracted osteotomy site in the os calcis. (*d*) Lateral shows optimal graft position. Two or three grafts are stacked on each other. Graft size is typically 10–12 mm at the tricortical side and 4–6 mm medially. (Redrawn from Mosca 1995, Fig. 2A–D, by permission.)

the calcanealcuboid joint does not sublux. If not stable, fix with percutaneous Steinman pins. The operative technique described in great detail by Mosca (1995) should be consulted.

Mosca did the operation in eight patients with cerebral palsy, out of the 20 who had a variety of etiologies for the deformity. The age at time of surgery ranged from four years to 16 years, seven months. At the time of average follow-up of 2 years 7 months, all except two had satisfactory results assessed by clinical examination and radiographic studies. The main objective of the osteotomy, preservation of subtalar joint motion could not be measured, but seemed to be the same as it was preoperatively with the arc of motion having shifted from valgus to neutral. Whether subtalar motion will be preserved over the years given that the osteotomy enters the subtalar joint area is not known. If there is late subtalar joint pain due to degenerative arthritis, Mosca rightly opines that arthrodesis of the joint would be easy to do because of no deformity to correct.

The mechanism of correction 'is unknown'. Mosca thought that correction occurred because of the 'windlass' effect of the osteotomy on the plantar fascia to elevate the longitudinal arch. This effect appears comparable to the Jack toe raising test' (Jack 1953) in which the great toe of the fully weightbearing foot is passively dorsiflexed to its maximum range. If the sag in the flat foot is at the naviculocuneiform joint, the arch will raise providing a justification for naviculo-cuneiform fusion to correct flexible ('relaxed') flat foot.

Another mechanism to explain correction may be a shift of the sustentaculum tali under the head of the talus where it belongs and realignment of the navicular bone to the center of the head of the talus. But this is only a speculation that could be probably worked on in anatomic modelling techniques.

As might be expected the effectiveness of Mosca's operation was investigated by Andreacchio and colleagues (2000) at the A.I. duPont Hospital for Children. They selected 12 children with spastic diplegia, two with hemiplegia and one with triplegia for the lateral column lengthening at a mean age of 7.3 years. They had a comparison group of seven feet in four children with an average age of 10.8 years in whom they did an open wedge osteotomy–arthrodesis of the calcaneal–cuboid joint. Only feet that could be passively manipulated into the corrected position were accepted for the surgery. The surgical technique for calcaneal lengthening was the same as described by Mosca with the exception that fixation of the osteotomy and bone graft was with a semitubular plate and two screws in eight feet. Peroneus brevis and or longus tendon lengthenings were done according to the 'tightness' judged by the surgeon. In addition, when indicated, Achilles tendon or gastrocnemius lengthenings were included.

Four patients whose calcaneal articular surface appeared severely rounded instead of the normal flat calcaneal–cuboid joint surface had an open wedge resection of the calcaneal–cuboid joint with a tricortical bank bone rather than osteotomy between the anterior and middle calcaneal facets. Internal fixation with a semitubular plate and screws was used to secure this joint.

Andreacchio *et al.* (2000) had poor results in 25% of the feet that had lengthenings through the calcaneus; all needed a surgical revision. In this group one foot developed subtalar fusion although the result was judged 'good'. In the cases that had a calcaneal–cuboid joint resection and an open wedge osteotomy–arthrodesis, three failed to unite, but were asymptomatic with maintenance of the correction. The duPont group concludes that Mosca's calcaneal lengthening is a good operation to correct the valgus deformity and preserve subtalar motion. But as in Mosca's study subtalar joint motion is impossible to measure with usual goniometric techniques and no measurements are given to certify that the goal of preserving subtalar joint motion has been met. As in Mosca's experience radiographic measurements pre- and postoperatively did not correlate well with the clinical result even though 'changes' were found. Finally, one patient also had a peroneus longus tendon lengthening and postoperative forefoot supination with recurrence of the planovalgus deformity. Thus lengthening of the peroneal longus tendon with calcaneal lengthening is not recommended. Despite the duPont group's poor results in one-fourth of their patients these orthopaedic surgeons wrote that it is good operation primarily, it appears, because of the promise of preservation of subtalar joint motion. It may be that their technique was faulty but this was not detailed.

9. *Calcaneal–cuboid–cuneiform osteotomy*. Rathjen and Mubarak (1998) detailed a calcaneal–cuboid–cuneiform osteotomy to combine the features of some of the preceding operations while avoiding violation of the subtalar joint for correction of the valgus foot. Initially any necessary soft-tissue lengthenings are done such as gastrocnemius lengthening or peroneus brevis lengthening. Their procedure calls for a medial displacement osteotomy of the calcaneus in a manner similar to that previously described under medial displacement of the calcaneus. This is performed through a lateral longitudinal incision starting just distal to the tip of the lateral malleolus and continuing to the distal edge of the cuneiform. The sural nerve is noted and retracted dorsally. Curved retractors are used protectively as the osteotomy is made. The osteotomy line is about 1cm proximal to the posterior facet joint, extends obliquely to 1cm short of the calcaneal–cuboid joint at an angle of about 40° from the bottom of the foot. This is done very carefully to avoid plunging through to the medial structures. Additionally, a medially based wedge of the calcaneus can be removed as is clinically indicated. This is facilitated by initially shifting the posterior portion of the os calcis laterally then spreading the osteotomy site open laterally. Then the posterior position of the os calcis is slid medially and the wedge is closed. Double pin fixation is added after the cuboid and cuneiform osteotomies are done. While retracting the peroneal tendon inferiorly, a laterally based cuboid osteotomy is performed with an osteotome through the middle of the bone with care to avoid the calcaneal–cuboid joints and the cuboid–metatarsal joint. To correct the valgus subluxation of the midfoot, a plantar-based closing wedge osteotomy of the medial cuneiform is done removing a pie-shaped wedge of the middle ⅔ of the cuneiform bone. This is approached with a u-shaped capsular incision over the navicular with the base proximally for later reefing. This closing wedge osteotomy helps reconstruct the sagging medial longitudinal arch and corrects the lateral talo–horizontal angle. The wedge taken from mid-third of the base of the medial cuneiform is inserted into the cuboid to lengthen the lateral column of the foot (Fig. 8.81). If necessary, additional bone graft from the os calcis can be used. When optimal positioning has been achieved, the osteotomy sites are secured with smooth 0.62-inch K wires through each of these osteotomy sites beginning with two pins through the medially shifted calcaneal osteotomy. The talonavicular joint can be medially reefed advancing the flap of capsule overlying the navicular. Pins are left protruding through the skin and bent at 90°. The foot is splinted initially then casted when the swelling subsides. The foot is non-weight-bearing until pin removal and recasting.

Rathjen and Mubarak (1998) reported on the results of correction of valgus feet using this technique in 24 feet in 17 patients with a variety of diagnosis in addition to severe valgus

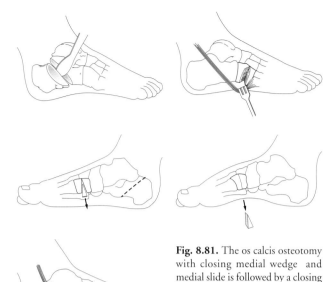

Fig. 8.81. The os calcis osteotomy with closing medial wedge and medial slide is followed by a closing medial cuneiform osteotomy. The wedge of bone from the base of the medial cuneiform is rotated and used to create a laterally based opening wedge at the cuboid osteotomy site. (Modified from Rathjen and Mubarak 1998, by permission.)

deformities (8 cerebral palsy) were reviewed in follow-up on average of 17 months. On average lateral talo–horizontal angle improved from a sagging 43° to a respectable 29° while the AP talo–navicular coverage angle (the AP edges of the navicular to the AP perpendicular line of the talar shaft) in standing x-rays went from 32° to 18°. Clinically, these feet had 7 excellent results, 16 good and 1 fair result. The fair result was due to overcorrection into varus causing lateral foot pain.

Addressing foot deformities while not violating the subtalar joint seems in these authors' opinion most optimal. It is important to preoperatively plan by making templates from the standing x-rays of the foot prior to surgery to anticipate the effect of the anticipated osteotomies. Additionally, fluoroscopy is used throughout the above procedures to ensure optimal placement of the osteotomies.

Wait—wait—there's more surgery for pes valgus.

10. *Subtalar arthroereisis*. The principle of this operation is to block eversion of the subtalar joint with a polyethelene Stapeg implant inserted laterally into the subtalar joint (Fig. 8.82). The principle is a throwback to that designed by Chambers (1946) when he published his operation of elevating the floor of the sinus tarsi to block eversion at the subtalar joint in flexible pes valgus. The same principle of blocking eversion to correct paralytic pes valgus was introduced by Grice (1952). Apparently with the intention of avoiding subtalar joint fusion and restriction of its motion, Smith and Millar (1983) designed a polymethyl-methacrylate ultra-high molecular weight polyethylene peg that was implanted on the dorsal surface of the calcaneus just anterior to the posterior facet of the subtalar joint to correct valgus and

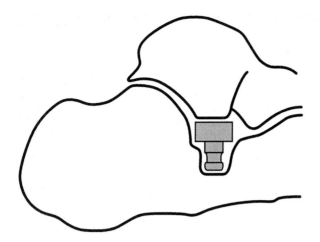

Fig. 8.82. Drawing of STA-peg in sinus tarsi to block subtalar joint eversion and correct pes valgus. (Redrawn from Vedantam et al. 1998, Fig. 3, by permission.)

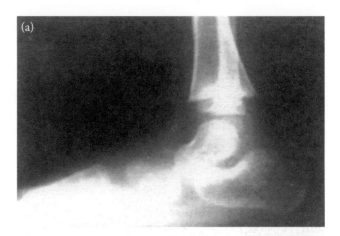

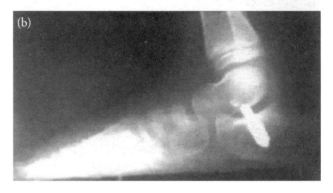

Fig. 8.83. (*a*) Lateral radiograph of foot, weightbearing, pes valgus, spastic diplegia, patient RPS, age 4 years 9 months. (*b*) Lateral radiograph of foot, weightbearing, patient RPS, with screw and cap of polyethylene in sinus tarsi to block eversion of subtalar joint (arthroereisis), 3 years postoperative. (Radiographs reproduced by permission of Dr Patricia Fucs, São Paulo, Brazil and *Revista de Orthopedia*.)

to increase the medial longitudinal arch in the growing child. In subsequent years the subtalar joint peg has been used with claimed extraordinary success primarily by podiatrists for correction of flexible flat feet and valgus feet in cerebral palsy (Lepow and Smith 1989, Tompkins *et al.* 1993, Smith and Ocampo 1997, Bruyn *et al.* 1999, Dockery and Crawford 1999, Grady and Dinnon 2000, Forg *et al.* 2001, Giannini *et al.* 2003).

The operation found its way into the orthopaedic departments of the Shriners Hospitals in Chicago and St Louis (Vedantam *et al.* 1998, Smith *et al.* 2000). The orthopaedic surgeons at the St Louis unit did the procedure in 78 children who had valgus deformities of the foot secondary to neuromuscular diseases. Surgery was done at a mean age of 7 years 9 months. At an average follow-up of 4 years 6 months, satisfactory results were obtained in 96.4% of the 135 feet. In only five cases was the implant removed. Triceps surae fractional lengthening, transfer of the triceps surae, fractional lengthening of the peroneal tendons, posterior tibial tendon transfers, and reefing of the medial soft tissue and talonavicular capsule was done in conjunction with the implant insertion. A short leg cast was worn for 4 weeks and then an ankle–foot orthosis for 6 months or more.

Most of the published results of the use in flexible pes planus ('flexible pes valgo planus', 'hypermobile flat foot', 'flexible flat foot') give enthusiastic approbation to the operation with few and minimal complications. Smith and colleagues (2000) of the Shriners Hospital in Chicago reporting on its use and results in cerebral palsy issue a disclaimer: 'The procedure is rarely needed in the flexible flatfoot of a normal child.'

Fucs *et al.* (1997) of the Department of Orthopaedic Surgery, Santa Casa School of Medicine, São Paulo, Brazil, published their results of the insertion of a plastic cap with a screw in the sinus tarsi for the pes valgus in 18 patients (36 feet) 15 of whom had spastic diplegia and three with tetraplegia[29] (Fig. 8.77). The

age of surgery ranged from 3 years 10 months to 9 years (mean 6.1). The screw and plastic cap allowed the foot to grow and correct the deformity (Fig. 8.83 *a, b*). The average follow-up was 2 years 9 months. They reported good results and maintenance of the correction in 29 feet and unsatisfactory in seven (20%). Dr Fucs and her group considered this a temporary measure to correct the deformity; accordingly, in most cases they removed the plastic cap and screw. After the second operation the patients are said to be 'doing well'. These 'Paulista' orthopaedic surgeons like the procedure (P.M. Fucs, personal communication).

The plastic peg in the sinus tarsi blocks eversion of the hindfoot and so corrects the valgus deformity. Does it preserve subtalar joint motion as intended? Husain and Fallat (2002) did a biomechanical analysis of the Maxwell–Brancheu arthroereisis implants[30] by testing five different sizes (6, 8, 9, 10 and 12 mm diameters) in fresh frozen cadaver limbs. They found that restrictions of subtalar joint motion ranged from 32% to 76.8% restrictions (SD 5.4%–7.6%). Therefore, there is restriction of eversion of the subtalar joint motion with the implant in place.

---

29 Design of the plastic capped screw attributed to Pisani cited in a reference: Milano, L. and Scala, A. (1985), 'La risi extraarticuolare della sottoastraglalica con endortesi calcaneale nel tratamento chirurgico delle deformità in valgo del calcagno.' *Chir del Piede*, **9**, 303–308.

30 Maxwell–Brancheau implant (MBA) is titanium alloy button 15 mm in length and available in 6, 8, 10 and 12 mm diameters. It is screwed into the floor of the sinus tarsi to abut the lateral talus to restrict eversion.

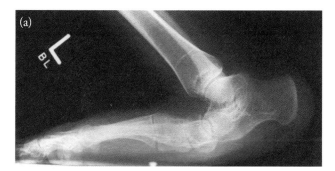

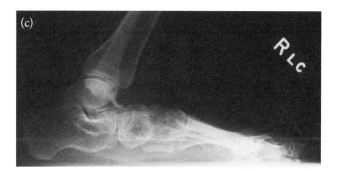

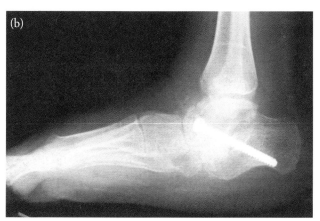

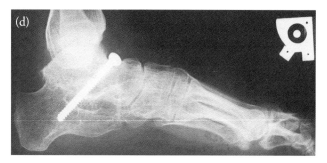

Fig. 8.84. Radiographs, lateral projections, weightbearing of feet of two patients, skeletally mature, spastic diplegia, pes valgus, correction with triple arthrodesis and screw from talus to calcaneus. (*a*) Left foot, severe pes valgus, almost rigid, patient KS, spastic diplegia, age 15 years. (*b*) Left foot, patient KS, 1 year postoperative triple arthrodesis with screw fixation; correction maintained. Solid arthrodesis of the three joints. Given severe preoperative fixed deformity the result is 'as good as it gets'. As in almost all valgus foot corrections in cerebral palsy, calcaneal dorsiflexion angle not restored. Functional result: good. (*c*) Right foot, patient MH, age 18 years, with pes valgus, partially flexible and manipulable. (*d*) Right foot, patient MH, age 20 years, excellent restoration of normal anatomy. Solid fusion of talonavicular, calcaneal–cuboid and subtalar joints.

One wonders if this restriction of joint motion will lead to cartilage degeneration, arthrofibrosis and eventual fusion (articular cartilage gets its nutrition only from the synovial fluid; motion of the joint is necessary for diffusion of the fluid into the cartilage cells). The subtalar joint has an important function. As a mitered hinge joint it permits transverse rotation of the leg without slippage of the foot on the ground. It absorbs the rotation of the leg in the stance phase of gait (Inman *et al.* 1994). So restriction of motion of the subtalar joint should not be taken lightly although it is practically impossible to measure clinically.

Sta-peg polyethylene arthroereisis (Smith *et al.* 2000): '*The procedure is rarely needed in the flexible flatfoot of a normal child.*'

11. Although *triple arthrodesis* has been the standard operation for severe pes valgus in adolescents and adults it should be used as a last-resort procedure when none of the foregoing procedures can result in a painless foot with corrected position. If performed before adolescence when skeletal maturity begins (age 13 years and older), foot growth will not be significantly stunted by removal of the articular surfaces of the talus, calcaneus, navicular and cuboid bones. Although triple arthrodesis offers good correction of the varus deformities, the results have not been as pleasing for valgus deformities (Duckworth 1977, Horstmann and Eilert 1977). All too often the postoperative foot still has the appearance of pes valgus. The talus usually returned to its plantarflexed position and the calcaneus remained in relative equinus (less than 10° of dorsiflexion). To improve these results, Bleck (1987) added Grice's principle as modified by Dennyson

and Fulford (1976) to the procedure; the talus is brought out of its plantarflexed position and secured with a screw from the talar neck to the calcaneus while healing with solid arthrodesis occurs (Fig. 8.84 *a, b*). Correction of the calcaneal equinus has not been attempted. Some non-paralytic 'flat feet' have relative equinus of the calcaneus and function very well. There is a notion that this position of the calcaneus provides a longer lever arm for the gastrocnemius–soleus to increase plantarflexion muscle power needed in competitive running and jumping. Achilles or gastrocnemius–soleus lengthening will not restore the normal dorsiflexed angle of the calcaneus. Other than possibly a posterior ankle joint capsulotomy, zealous attempts to restore the dorsiflexed angle of the calcaneus by calf and/or flexor tendon lengthenings will result in a calcaneus deformity.

Tenuta *et al.* (1993) reported a mean follow-up of 17.8 years (range 11–45 years) of triple arthrodesis for equinovarus deformities in 12 feet and in 23 valgus deformities of patients who had cerebral palsy. Although 43% had degenerative changes in the ankle joint depicted in the radiographs as well as some loss of motion, it did not cause a problem in function or pain for this group of patients. The most important observation was the failure to correct the valgus deformity in 12 of the 23 feet in contrast to the good corrections of equinovarus deformities. The persistent valgus deformity was related to the poor subjective outcome.

In contrast to triple arthrodesis of equinovarus deformity, failure to correct a valgus deformity of the foot with triple arthrodesis is common.

Experienced surgeons have noticed that the result of triple arthrodesis in the valgus foot is to have a foot that appears the same as it did preoperatively. The addition of screw fixation of the talus to the calcaneus with triple arthrodesis as described by Bleck (1987) has improved the results of triple arthrodesis of the valgus foot. The numbers of patients who have had this procedure are too small to have significance primarily because most severe valgus feet in cerebral palsy have been corrected with subtalar extraarticular arthrodesis in childhood; severe deformity meriting triple arthrodesis in adolescence or adulthood in developed countries is uncommon.

For very long-term follow-up of triple arthrodesis, as usual, we have to rely on the orthopaedic surgery department of the University of Iowa (Saltzman *et al.* 1999). They were able to do a 25- and 44-year average follow-up of 67 feet in the same 57 patients who had triple arthrodeses for a foot deformities due to a variety of causes among which was cerebral palsy in three (4 %). At the time of the first follow-up (25 years), good results obtained in 75%, and fair in 25%. In the 44 year follow-up good results decreased to 28%, fair increased to 69%, and two became poor (3%). Results were judged mainly on the basis of pain, residual deformity, callosities, pseudoarthrosis and ankle-joint deterioration. Pseudoarthrosis was found in 19% particularly of the talonavicular joint in 16%. The ankle had no degenerative changes in 31%, mild in 64%, moderate in 3%, and severe in 1% at the 25-year follow-up. At the second follow-up all ankles had degenerative changes; 9% were severe.

The Iowa study documents that the results of triple arthrodesis deteriorate with aging of the patient, but 95% were very satisfied with the result. The authors note that the study lacked a control group or how much of the deterioration was due to such factors as the underlying disease process or aging. At the first follow-up 37 ankles or feet were not painful; by the second follow-up 14 of these became painful. The anticipated result of progressive degeneration of the ankle joint articular cartilage due to restriction of the motion of the subtalar joint and transfer of rotation of the foot during gait to the anklet was confirmed, but not disabling for the major portion of the patients' lives (Fig. 8.85). The operation 'was a satisfactory solution for imbalance of the hindfoot in this group of patients' (p.1391). Other authors of long-term follow-ups of triple arthrodesis were cited by the Iowa orthopaedic surgeons. Radiographs depicted osteoarthritis of the ankle, naviculocuneiform and tarsometatarsal joints in varying percentages but without a clear relationship to pain on relatively long-term follow-up (Fig. 8.78). Improved operative techniques that include internal and external fixation are expected to reduce the incidence of pseudoarthrosis particularly of the talonavicular joint.

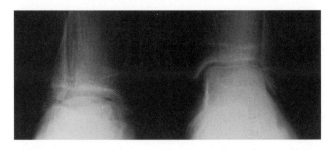

Fig. 8.85. Anterior–posterior radiograph of ankles, bilateral, weightbearing, spastic diplegia, age 18 years, 5 years postoperative triple arthrodesis, left foot. Ball and socket left ankle joint due to dome-shaped talar articular surface; symptoms tolerable and not disabling.

OPERATIVE TECHNIQUES

Two operations which have been reliable in a reasonable restoration of the normal anatomy and configuration of the foot. Given the obvious discrepancies between chronological and skeletal age, a general policy is to recommend the extra-articular arthrodesis before age 13 years in boys and 11 years in girls (with variations in skeletal age) and the intra-articular arthrodesis after that age.

Extra-articular subtalar arthrodesis with internal fixation (Dennyson and Fulford 1976, Barrasso *et al.* 1984). With the patient anesthetized, the foot is inverted and dorsiflexed. If the heel remains in equinus, a sliding Achilles tendon lengthening (Hoke or White) is first performed. The foot is dorsiflexed with the foot held in varus just to the neutral position where the plantar surface of the heel is in 90º relationship to the tibia. Zealous dorsiflexion beyond this point should be avoided. The superior surface of the talar neck and sinus tarsi are exposed through an oblique posteriorly directed incision beginning at the talar head to bisect the heel and ending at the peroneal tendon sheaths. The inferior aspect of the talar neck, sinus tarsi and superior surface of the calcaneus are denuded of all fat and fibrous tissue. It is desirable to preserve a thick posterior flap of skin and subcutaneous tissue. The bone surfaces are cleanly exposed and gently roughened with a curette and small osteotome.

The foot is then manipulated into the corrected anatomical position, which is confirmed by a lateral fluoroscopic view with the image intensifier. The foot is held securely and steadily in this position by the surgeon as the assistant inserts the screw. Monitoring with intraoperative fluoroscopy assures accuracy of screw placement and position of the tarsal bones.

The spot for screw insertion on the superior aspect of the talar neck is found by blunt dissection of the soft tissue between the extensor digitorum longus tendons and the neurovascular bundle. A small dissecting elevator can be placed on either side of the talar neck. The space created should be just large enough to accommodate the cancellous bone screw. The screw length and direction can be estimated by overlaying a depth gauge on the lateral aspect of the foot, checking the position with the image intensifier fluoroscope, and marking the skin for the direction.

Others (Barrasso *et al.* 1984) introduce a Kirschner wire as a guide pin driven posterior to the intended site of the screw. With the proper size drill to match the screw, and through a drill sleeve to protect the adjacent tissues, a hole is drilled from the center of the talar neck and through to the body of the calcaneus. Use of AO cannulated large screw (7.3 mm) system improves the precision of screw placement. The screw is then inserted to maintain the new position of the talus securely. The screw can end near the plantar surface of the calcaneus but not through it. A cortical cancellous bone graft and chips are removed from the outer wall of the ilium and packed into the sinus tarsi.

A short-leg cast, with the foot well padded, immobilizes the foot and ankle. At 4 weeks postoperative this plaster is changed for wound inspection and a walking boot added. Weightbearing to tolerance is permitted for the next 4 weeks. After cast removal, supportive elastic bandages or elastic stockingette with temporary felt arch supports usually give more comfort to the patient for the next week or two while walking in ordinary sports shoes. Although some surgeons (Barrasso *et al.* 1984) have prescribed plastic ankle–foot orthoses as additional protection postoperatively, it is recommended that these custom-molded orthotics are prescribed only in large and heavy children.

Foot-skin and soft-tissue tenderness persists for several weeks in children who have had overprotection of their feet preoperatively. The only way the skin and fat on the plantar aspect of the foot can hypertrophy enough to diminish this hypersensitivity is through consistent and persistent weightbearing. Walking barefoot on grass, sand or carpets seems to help.

Triple arthrodesis. If the hindfoot is in equinus when the foot is inverted and dorsiflexed, a sliding Achilles tendon lengthening to allow dorsiflexion just to the neutral position is necessary. The incision for the arthrodesis of the three joints is the same as described in the preceding section for extra-articular arthrodesis: oblique beginning at the head of the talus, crossing the sinus tarsi and continued posteriorly to the peroneal tendons. The fibrous tissue and fat should be removed from the sinus tarsi in almost one piece and remain attached as a flap of the posterior skin of the incision to facilitate wound closure after the foot has been corrected. At time of wound closure this thick flap will aid in suturing the skin without tension.

The three joints (calcanealcuboid, talonavicular and subtalar) are denuded of articular cartilage to expose the subchondral bone (the details of the technique have been described for varus feet in Chapter 7). Medially based wedges of bone are cautiously removed only if necessary to obtain good contact of the raw and roughened subchondral surfaces when the foot is manipulated into the corrected position in which the talus is brought out of its plantarflexion. The entire head of the talus is not removed as described in the Hoke method. Rather the talar articular surface should be removed leaving the round contour of the head to match the concave surface of the navicular that is removed with a curette. For better visualization of the navicular, a second incision over the medial aspect of the joint is recommended (Coleman 1983). The foot is firmly held in its corrected position by the surgeon while the assistant introduces the fixation screw

from the talar neck into the calcaneus, as described for extra-articular arthrodesis (Fig. 8.84 *a*, *b*). The plantarflexion of the talus should be corrected and maintained with the screw.

Triple arthrodesis for pes valgus: 'Medially based wedged of bone are cautiously removed only if necessary.'

A Steinman pin from the plantar surface of the heel is inserted anterior to its weight-bearing area into the calcaneus and talus. A second pin can be driven from the first metatarsal shaft to cross the talonavicular joint.[31] Internal fixation can be performed with solid or cannulated screws instead of the pins. This avoids potential pin breakage or pin track infection. The technique ensures good fixation at the time of surgery but does not allow further manipulation of the position later. With this combination of internal and external fixation, a bulky padding comprised of dorsal and plantar pads secured with several layers of rolled padding prevents constriction by the plaster or fiberglass. The cast should extend from the toes to below the knee. The postoperative cast and dressings can be removed for wound inspection in 2–3 weeks and the position of the foot changed with pin removal and manipulation under anesthesia if thought desirable.

The pins and cast are removed in 4–6 weeks and replaced with a short-leg walking cast. Weightbearing to tolerance is permitted for the next 4–6 weeks. When the cast is removed, elastic bandages or elastic support-hose control postoperative edema which can last for a month or more. Ordinary sturdy sports shoes are adequate.

Because fusion of the joints will not be evident radiographically from 6 months to 1 year postoperatively both patient and surgeon can be relieved of anxiety if solid union is not seen at the time of final plaster removal.

Williams and Menelaus (1977) described an inlay bone graft for correction and arthrodesis of pes valgus. A vertical trough was created in the sinus tarsi to include the talonavicular and calcanealcuboid joints. A slightly oversized tibial bone graft was then hammered into this trough. Subtalar joint cartilage was removed with a gouge, and the cavity packed with bone chips (Fig. 8.86). This modification has merit because the bone graft would act as a prop for the repositioned talus.

PROBLEMS WITH SUBTALAR EXTRA-ARTICULAR OR TRIPLE ARTHRODESIS IN PES VALGUS
The main problems are as follows.

1. Failure to recognize concomitant valgus of the ankle joint. If subtalar correction is done and valgus of the ankle is present, the foot will still be in valgus. A preoperative weightbearing anterior–posterior radiograph of the ankle joints forewarns and allows additional operative planning. In young children who

---

31 Bleck does not recommend staples or plate fixation of the subtalar or midtarsal joints in triple arthrodesis. The reason is that if the surgeon finds that on cast change in 2–3 weeks he or she is not happy with the position of the foot, pins can be removed and the foot can be manipulated to the desired position without reopening the operative wound.

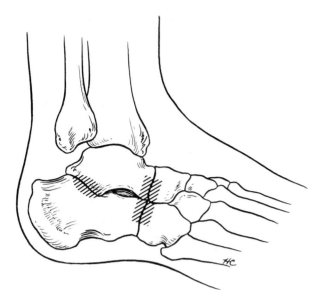

Fig. 8.86. Schematic drawing of Williams and Menelaus technique (1977) for triple arthrodesis in pes valgus. A trough is excised from the sinus tarsi to include the talonavicular and calcanealcuboid joints. A tibial bone graft slightly larger than the trough is hammered in for a snug fit. Subtalar joint cartilage removed with gouge and packed with bone chips.

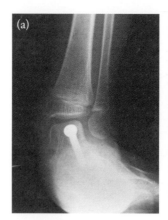

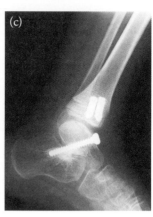

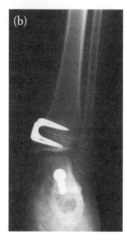

Fig. 8.87. (*a*) Anterior–posterior radiograph of right ankle postoperative subtalar arthrodesis with screw fixation, bilateral pes valgus, spastic diplegia, age 7 years, with valgus tilt of talus in ankle mortice. (*b*) Anterior–posterior radiograph of right ankle 1 year postoperative stapling of medial distal physis showing correction of valgus of the distal tibial plafond. (*c*) Lateral radiograph of right ankle, postoperative subtalar arthrodesis with screw and iliac bone graft in sinus tarsi showing fusion and two staples in the medial distal tibial physis.

have valgus of the ankle, stapling of the distal medial tibial physis; may gradually restore a horizontal ankle joint parallel with the floor and eliminate a supramalleolar osteotomy (Butkus *et al.* 1983) (Fig. 8.87 *a–c*). In adolescents there may be insufficient growth potential for staples to be effective. Supramalleolar closed wedge tibial and fibular osteotomies will be required.

2. Overcorrection into varus with the extra-articular arthrodesis occurs most often in young children. This can be partly avoided by observing the position of the heel at the time of surgery when the foot is manipulated into the correct position before fixation. After fixation, the heel position can be checked in an anterior-posterior radiograph of the foot made in the operating room. The measured angle between the talus and calcaneus indicates heel position. A neutrally aligned heel will have an angle of approximately 15º. If varus of the heel is observed after the joints are fused, the problem can be corrected by a laterally based closed wedge osteotomy of the calcaneus (Figs 8.88, 8.89). Slight valgus is residually is much better than varus. Remember the old adage: 'Thou shalt not varus.'

3. Undercorrection and valgus of the hind-foot can be due in a triple arthrodesis to recurrence of plantarflexion of the talus. This return of the talus to its plantarflexed position can be minimized with screw fixation of the talus and calcaneus as described. Even with this extra fixation, the configuration of the foot may not appear as entirely normal after triple arthrodesis for severe spastic pes valgus.

What seems evident in these flat-looking feet after surgery is a calcaneal equinus which is not corrected by Achilles tendon lengthening. Posterior capsulotomy of the ankle might allow dorsiflexion of the calcaneus; however, in severe pes valgus of adolescents and adults, the tibial articular surface of the talus

becomes limited in area anteriorly due to the deformity of the talus. Perhaps a crescentric osteotomy of the posterior portion of the calcaneus to simulate its dorsiflexed position might improve the result (Wu 1986). This osteotomy is the reverse of that described by Samilson (1976) for pes calcaneal cavus. Because Bleck has not performed this additional procedure, it is only a suggestion and not based on results.

4. Varus of the mid-foot is a problem due to lengthening of one or both peroneal tendons. In this instance, lengthening or a split transfer of the posterior tibial tendon should resolve the

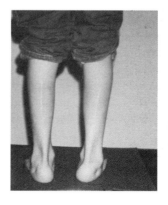

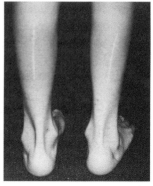

Fig. 8.88. (*a*) Both legs and hindfeet, postoperative varus deformity of right foot after subtalar extraarticular arthrodesis. (*b*) Both legs and hind feet, 1 year postoperative, closed wedge osteotomy of calcaneus to correct varus of the hindfoot.

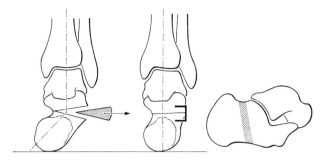

Fig. 8.89. Schematic drawing of closed wedge osteotomy of calcaneus with staple fixation for correction of fixed varus of hindfoot.

problem. In some cases of forefoot varus, a split anterior tibial tendon transfer may be the solution. The decisions should be based on the clinical examination and confirmed with dynamic electromyography if available.

5. Valgus deformity of the ankle postoperatively may result from removal of a segment of the fibular shaft to be used as a bone graft and reossification does not occur (Wiltse 1972, Hsu *et al.* 1974).

6. Postoperative in-toe gait can be confused with a dynamic varus. The gait problem is due to internal axial rotation of the entire foot. Preoperatively, either internal tibial–fibular torsion or persistent excessive medial deviation of the talar neck is not recognized as associated with the spastic pes valgus. The in-toeing becomes evident after surgical correction when the navicular bone is aligned in its normal position on the head of the talus. In spastic valgus feet the navicular bone is displaced laterally on the talar head (Fig. 8.90).

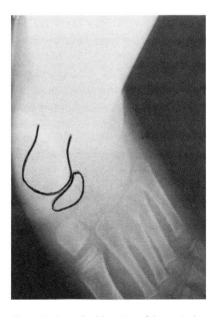

Fig. 8.90. Lateral subluxation of the navicular on the talus noted with pes valgus. Corrective surgery for valgus midfoot deformity restores the navicular to its normal position on the articular surface of the talus with resultant medial alignment of the foot compared to preop. If the talar neck deviation exceeds the adult norm of 18º consider the possible result of excess medial rotation of the limb from the line of progression.

This result might be avoided by careful preoperative evaluation. When the foot is passively manipulated with the knee flexed 90º into the desired corrected position, the internal rotation of the foot will be appreciated. When this is observed, a derotation osteotomy of the tibia and fibula at the time of subtalar arthrodesis can be planned and accomplished at the same operation or at a second stage.

TIBIAL–FIBULAR TORSION, INTERNAL OR EXTERNAL

Excessive external tibial–fibular torsion is more common than internal in cerebral palsy as a compensation for femoral torsion or as the result of medial hamstring tendon lengthening (Bassett *et al.* 1976).

Internal tibial–fibular torsion is probably the congenital type superimposed on spastic diplegia. Spontaneous correction is dubious. It can be masked by spastic pes valgus. We have no evidence that orthotics correct the torsion in either direction.

Surgical correction of excessive external tibial torsion (greater than 30º) is indicated: (1) if it causes symptoms in the foot or ankle as the result of excessive stress on the medial side of these joints; (2) if the foot assumes a varus position in the attempt to rectify the abnormal position; or (3) if a knee–ankle–foot orthosis cannot accommodate the degree of torsion either at the knee or ankle joints.

The indications for correction of internal tibial torsion in spastic diplegia are present when the patient walks in-toed so badly as to create a subjective disability. Usually the request for surgery comes from an emerging adolescent who has a fairly good gait pattern and is independent. The other indication has been mentioned in the previous section on in-toeing after extra-articular subtalar arthrodesis for spastic pes valgus.

Operative technique for derotation osteotomy of the tibia and fibula. The choice is either a proximal or distal osteotomy. Bleck (1987) has preferred the transverse osteotomy of the proximal tibia just below the tibial tubercle and a fibular osteotomy 1–2 cm distal to the tibial site. The fibular osteotomy is done through a small lateral incision with an osteotome. The exact desired area of the tibia is located with the fluoroscope; the skin is marked and a straight 3 cm incision is made on the center of the medial cortex of the tibia. The incision can be slightly oblique if one wants it to be straight after the rotation (oblique from lateral to medial for an external rotation osteotomy, and the opposite for the internal). To control the proximal tibial fragment and to enable wedging of the plaster to correct malalignment postoperatively, a Steinman pin is inserted medially to engage both cortices of the proximal tibia and parallel to the knee joint. It is not necessary to penetrate the lateral muscular compartment or the skin. The tibia is exposed subperiosteally distal to the pin; retractors are inserted around the entire bone to protect the posterior neurovascular structures. A power oscillating saw cuts the bone transversely. *Be sure to continuously irrigate the saw with cool saline solution to avoid killing the bone cells and delaying union.*

With the hip in neutral position (patella facing forward) and the knee extended, the correct degree of rotation can be determined by 10° of external axial rotation of the foot when the ankle is dorsiflexed to the neutral position.

The fascia of the anterior compartment is easily reached and routinely slit proximally and distally.[32]

Continuous suction drainage of the wound for 24–48 hours obviates a hematoma. After wound closure and dressing, the osteotomy site is dressed anteriorly and posteriorly with ABD pads secured with rolled cotton as usual. The first section of the plaster incorporates the thigh, knee, pin and the leg to its distal third. The knee is kept in almost complete extension, taking care not to overextend the leg and cause a posterior angulation at the osteotomy site. The pin is prevented from sliding with a slotted metal dial and screw-holding device, which is also incorporated in the plaster. When this section of the plaster has 'set', then rotation is manually checked and the foot and ankle are joined with plaster to the proximal portion. We then check the position of the osteotomy in the operating room with fluoroscopy. If unacceptable angulation is noted, the plaster can be cut at the osteotomy site, manipulated appropriately and replastered. Obviously a major portion of the operation depends upon who holds the limb while plaster is applied. The surgeon holds and the assistant wraps.

On the second or third day postoperatively, anterior–posterior and lateral radiographs are made of the limb with the knee centered on a large film (35 × 45 cm). The alignment of the bones can be measured and the plaster cut if realignment is required.

The patient is non-weightbearing for 4–5 weeks, after which the pin and plaster are removed and replaced with a long-leg walking plaster. Standing and walking to tolerance are encouraged in plaster for an additional 4–5 weeks. At 8–10 weeks postoperatively, radiographs usually show sufficient union to allow weightbearing without plaster. Knee-flexion and extension exercises are necessary to restore function.

Osteotomy of the distal tibia and fibula has been heralded as a more satisfactory and cosmetic procedure (Bennett *et al.* 1985). A 1 cm horizontal incision was made anteriorly over the distal tibia. With the aid of fluoroscopy and 'tactile sensation' of the surgeon's hands, multiple drill holes were made through a single hole in the anterior cortex. The osteotomy was completed with a small osteotome. The fibular osteotomy is similarly made through a 1 cm incision, 2 cm proximal to the tibial site. With the knee flexed 90° the foot was rotated to the desired position with reference to the knee axis. A long-leg plaster was applied with the knee flexed 60°–90°.

Postoperatively additional correction was obtained by circumferentially cutting the plaster at the osteotomy sites. After 4–6 weeks, a short-leg walking cast was applied until there was radiographic evidence of union (usually in 4–6 weeks).

Distal tibial osteotomies can be slow to heal and without fixation as in the technique of Bennett *et al.* (1985) it is not easy to match and hold rotation of both legs reliably. The only modification of the foregoing procedure was by Stefko *et al.* (1998) of the San Diego Children's Hospital. They used percutaneous crossed Kirschner wires to secure the osteotomy. From the same institution Dodgin *et al.* (1998) documented with gait analysis correction of the medial rotation of the tibia and the foot progression angle. If postoperatively you have second thoughts on the amount of correction, it would be necessary to extract the wires before cutting the cast circumferentially and rotating the distal leg and foot to the desired rotation. It is doubtful that one would want to reinsert the fixation wires without thorough preparation of the skin which would necessitate removal of the cast, preparation of the skin, manipulation, and reapplication of the plaster. But apparently this was never necessary in the hands of the pediatric orthopaedic surgeons of San Diego.

Bennett *et al.* (1985) stated that the major reason to perform the distal osteotomies was to avoid the cosmetically objectionable scar of the proximal sites. Inasmuch as abnormal foot rotation is a subjective disability, they have a point. Their other reasons included a high complication rate reported with proximal tibial osteotomies (Steel *et al.* 1971). Steel *et al.* reported that of 46 proximal tibial osteotomies in children for genu varum or valgum, nine had a serious complication which they attributed to compression or stretching of the anterior tibial artery. In studying this paper it now appears that these were all instances of anterior compartment syndromes due to a rise in compartment pressures—an entity that has been defined and become common knowledge in the past 30 years. The complications reported with the distal osteotomies in 19 patients (32 rotation osteotomies) were remanipulation (9%), posterior bowing in six (19%), transient 'numbness' in three patients, delayed healing, tendinitis and a cast sore in one patient (Bennett *et al.* 1985). Their mean healing-time necessitating plaster immobilization was 14.5 weeks (range 10–24 weeks). Most of their postoperative casts required splitting to accommodate apparent swelling (70%). These surgeons also believe that derotation of the tibia could be best accomplished with the knee flexed 90° rather than with the knee extended.

Although the distal osteotomy of tibia seems to have gained favor with many orthopaedic surgeons, the proximal osteotomy of the tibia has some advantages: healing is rapid within a range of 8–10 weeks; rotation of the tibia with the knee extended at the time of surgery is the position of the knee at heel contact to mid-stance when excessive external rotation of the foot is obvious and the effects of the foot lever arm decreases the plantarflexion–knee extension couple as well as ankle power generation just before push-off; coexistent genu valgum or varum of the tibia cannot be corrected with a distal tibial osteotomy. While posterior bowing of the tibia in six distal osteotomies reported by Bennett *et al.* (1985) did not adversely affect the result, it does not seem desirable unless the bowing corrects ankle equinus, but proximal osteotomies can bow posteriorly to create genu recurvatum.

---

32 Keep the Metzenbaum scissor blades closely adjacent to the fascia—going too deep risks cutting the nerve to the extensor hallucis longus muscle. It has happened.

OPERATIVE TECHNIQUE DISTAL TIBIAL AND FIBULA ROTATION OSTEOTOMY (MORRISSY AND WEINSTEIN 2001)

The fibula is divided first through a 3 cm incision over the subcutaneous border of the fibula, just above the flare. Drill holes are placed at the intended osteotomy site and an osteotome completes it. The osteotomy should be *transverse. Warning:* stay beneath the periosteum to avoid cutting a small vein close to the medial border of the fibula. If cut there will be 'considerable bleeding'.

The 4 cm incision for the tibial osteotomy is just lateral to the anterior border of the bone to extend just above the ankle crease proximally. The incision can be oblique to result in a straight scar line depending on the intended rotation. If it is to be external the incision angles from proximal–lateral to distal–medial. If it is to be internal, the opposite incision is made.

The exposure of the distal tibia is limited and medial to the anterior tibial tendon. The physis should be identified. Crego and small chandler elevators around the tibia give all the exposure needed. Multiple drill holes are made 1 cm above the physis and kept in line so that the osteotomy to be completed with an osteotome between the drill holes is *transverse—not oblique.* If you want to use a small blade power saw, be sure to use a lot of irrigation with cool saline solution to avoid heating the bone which delays healing. Frequent lifting of the saw from the edge to be cut also helps to reduce heat build-up of the blade and results in a clean osteotomy.

The knee is flexed 90º and the tibia is rotated to the desired correction. A smooth Steinman pin is inserted from the medial malleolus across the osteotomy site and through the lateral cortex of the tibia. If desired, but not essential a second pin can be inserted from the lateral side. Intraoperative fluoroscopy adds more precision.

Rotation of long bones is tricky and does not resolve with growth. . . . Normal external rotation of the foot is between 7º and 10º from the line of progression in walking.

Before wound closure and the fixation pin in place Bleck would bring the knee into complete extension resting on the table with the patella pointing straight-up to keep the hip in neutral rotation. Then the foot is dorsiflexed to neutral making sure it is in neither varus nor valgus. The angle of the medial border of the foot with the vertical plane will give a good estimate of the amount of rotation obtained (the normal external rotation of the foot is between 7º and 10º from the line of progression in walking—a line bisecting the body in the frontal plane) (Fig. 8.91) (Elftman 1969). Sutherland *et al.* (1994) measured normal foot rotation with respect to the line of progression in children. At heel rise the foot is in 5º–7º external rotation and then internally rotates on swing. If the osteotomy is of only one tibia, then preoperatively measure the external rotation of the opposite foot with the knee extended and the hip in neutral and a line through bisecting the body in the frontal plane.[33] If you are not satisfied with the rotation obtained, you can remove the pin while the wound is open and rotate the tibia again to the desired position and reinsert the pin.

After wound closure a long leg cast with the knee flexed 90º is applied. Morrissy and Weinstein (2001) advised that the pin should be 'well-padded so that it does not move with the cast and cause wound problems.' After 6 weeks and depending on the status of healing in radiographs, the pin can be extracted with pliers. The authors state this is not painful, but may cause anxiety.

Although pin fixation works surprisingly well, Horstmann has changed to internal fixation with a six-hole plate and a short leg cast. This prevents pin-track infections and reduces worries about alignment, movement within the cast and loss of precise correction.

ANTERIOR COMPARTMENT SYNDROME

The most serious complication after a proximal tibial osteotomy is an anterior compartment syndrome which also occurs with a proximal tibial tuberosity transfer, a proximal tibial epiphyseal arrest or fracture. It does not seem to have occurred in any of the distal tibial rotation osteotomies. Bleck (1987) avoided this problem by doing a routine lateral and anterior compartment fasciotomy at the time of the proximal tibial and fibular osteotomies through the same operative incision. But do not let this prophylactic measure give you total security and a good night's sleep.

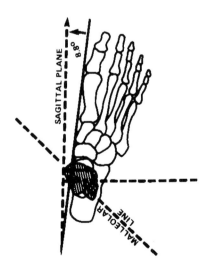

Fig. 8.91. The 'bottom-line' of rotation of the tibia: medial rotation of the foot from the line of progression, average 8.8º (range 7º–10º). Measure with the knee extended and the hip in neutral rotation. Measure the angle between the medial border of the foot with the foot in neutral dorsiflexion and the line of progression, i.e. the mid-sagittal plane or bisection of the frontal plane of the head, neck, trunk and pelvis.

33 Rotation of lone bones is tricky and does not resolve with growth. A sterile goniometer in the operating room may allow the surgeon to do it right the first time. Malrotation may be a perceptual problem. You can measure foot rotation with the knee extended on the table and also with the knee flexed 90º over the table edge, assuming you do not rotate the tibia at the knee joint.

The most serious complication after a proximal tibial osteotomy is an anterior compartment syndrome.

Continuous monitoring of compartment pressures with a slit catheter in the compartment and connected to a pressure/monitor display will remove worry of missing an elevated compartment pressure after an osteotomy or other surgery about the proximal tibia. Pressures above 30 mmHg should be taken seriously and fasciotomy considered after judging the clinical status (Mubarak and Hargens 1981). Monitoring compartment pressures with the transducer and a monitor screen for digital read-out is more reliable than instructing the nurse to 'check the circulation of the feet' or the skin color of the toes (especially difficult at night in a darkened room). Increasing pain in the limb is a sign of an impending compartment syndrome. But with children who have spastic muscles and are apt to be given muscle relaxants and narcotics that suppress anxiety and cerebral function, increasing pain as a sign is probably not entirely reliable as an indication of the compartment syndrome. Because of the potential for compartment syndrome or numbness associated with the proximal osteotomy, Horstmann prefers the distal tibial and fibular osteotomy.

PHILOSOPHY

Children with spastic diplegia are subjected to these myriad surgical procedures and therapies. By reviewing the past we hope to help out the young professional in his or her quest for optimal treatment. Our philosophy includes these tenets of care: keep realistic goals in mind, use gait analysis to plan surgical intervention and measure results, study past experiences to avoid some of the pitfalls of treatment, maximize therapeutic time and use health-care expenditure wisely. At the end of the day the child with cerebral palsy is most of all a child.

FURTHER READING

Canale, S.T., Ed. (2003) *Campbell's Operative Orthopaedics, 10th edn.* Philadelphia: Mosby.

Morrissy, R.T., Weinstein, S.L., Eds (2001) *Lovell and Winters Pediatric Orthopaedics, 5th edn.* Philadelphia: Lippincott Williams & Wilkins.

Robb, J.E. (1994) 'Orthopaedic management of cerebral palsy.' *In* Benson, M.K.D., Fixsen, J.A., Macnicol, M.F. (Eds) Edinburgh: Churchill Livingstone, pp. 255–275.

REFERENCES

Abel, M.F., Damiano, D.L., Pannunzio, M., Bush, J. (1999) 'Muscle–tendon surgery in diplegic cerebral palsy: functional and mechanical changes.' *Journal of Pediatric Orthopaedics*, 19, 366–375.

Aktas, S., Aiona, M.D., Orendurff, M. (2000) 'Evaluation of rotational gait abnormality in the patients with cerebral palsy.' *Journal of Pediatric Orthopaedics*, 20, 217–220.

Albright, A.L. (1996) 'Intrathecal baclofen in cerebral palsy movement disorders.' *Journal of Child Neurology*, 11 (Suppl.1), S29–S35.

Alman, B.A., Craig, C.L., Zimbler, S. (1993) 'Subtalar arthrodesis for stabilization of valgus hindfoot in patients with cerebral palsy.' *Journal of Pediatric Orthopaedics*, 13, 634–641.

Anderson, J. (1983) *Grant's Atlas of Anatomy, 8th edn.* Baltimore: Williams & Wilkins, pp. 4–29.

Andreacchio, A., Orellana, C.A., Miller, F., Bowen, T.R. (2000) 'Lateral column lengthening as treatment for planovalgus foot deformity in ambulatory children with spastic cerebral palsy.' *Journal of Pediatric Orthopaedics*, 20, 501–505.

Anthosen, W. (1966) 'Treatment of hip flexion contracture in cerebral palsy patients.' *Acta Orthopaedica Scandinavica*, 37, 387–393.

Arkin, A.M., Katz, J.F. (1956) 'The effects of pressure on epiphyseal growth.' *Journal of Bone and Joint Surgery*, 38A, 1056–1076.

Arnold, A.S., Komattu, A.V., Delp, S.L. (1997) 'Internal rotation gait: a compensatory mechanism to restore abduction capacity decreased by bone deformity.' *Developmental Medicine and Child Neurology*, 39, 40–44.

—— Asakawa, D.J., Delp, S.L. (2000a) 'Do the hamstrings and adductors contribute to excessive internal rotation of the hip in persons with cerebral palsy?' *Gait and Posture*, 12, 181–190.

—— Salinas, S., Asakawa, D.J., Delp, S.L. (2000b) 'Accuracy of muscle moment arms estimated from MRI-based musculoskeletal models of the lower extremity.' *Computer Aided Surgery*, 5, 108–119.

—— Blemker, S.S., Delp, S.L. (2001) 'Evaluation of a deformable musculoskeletal model for estimating muscle–tendon lengths during crouch gait.' *Annals of Biomedical Engineering*, 29, 263–274.

—— Delp, S.L. (2001) 'Rotational moment arms of the medial hamstrings and adductors vary with femoral geometry and limb position: implications for the treatment of internally rotated gait.' *Journal of Biomechanics*, 34, 437–447.

Aronson, J., Nunley, J., Frankovitch, K. (1983) 'Lateral talocalcaneal angle in assessment of subtalar valgus: follow-up of seventy Grice-Green arthrodeses.' *Foot and Ankle*, 4, 56–63.

Aspden, R.M., Porter, R.W. (1994) 'Nerve traction during correction of knee flexion deformity. A case report and calculation.' *Journal of Bone and Joint Surgery*, 76B, 471–473.

Atar, D., Zilberger, L., Votemberg, M., Norsy, M., Galil, A. (1993) 'Effect of distal hamstring release on cerebral palsy patients.' *Bulletin of the Hospital for Joint Disease*, 53, 34–36.

Attenborough, D.G. (1966) 'Severe congenital talipes equinovarus.' *Journal of Bone and Joint Surgery*, 48B, 31–39.

Baddar, A., Granata, K., Damiano, D.L., Carmines, D.V., Blanco, J.S., Abel, M.F. (2002) 'Ankle and knee coupling in patients with spastic diplegia: effects of gastrocnemius–soleus lengthening.' *Journal of Bone and Joint Surgery*, 84A, 736–744,

Baker, L.D. (1954) 'Triceps surae syndrome in cerebral palsy.' *Archives of Surgery*, 68A, 216–221,

—— (1956) 'A rational approach to the surgery needs of the cerebral palsy patient.' *Journal of Bone and Joint Surgery*, 38A, 313–323.

—— Dodelin, R.A. (1958) 'Extra-articular arthrodesis of the subtalar joint (Grice procedure).' *Journal of the American Medical Association*, 168, 1005–1008.

—— Hill, L.M. (1964) 'Foot alignment in the cerebral palsy patient.' *Journal of Bone and Joint Surgery*, 46A, 1–15.

Banks, H.H., Green, W.T. (1960) 'Adductor myotomy and obturator neurectomy for correction of adduction contracture of the hip in cerebral palsy.' *Journal of Bone and Joint Surgery*, 42A, 111–126.

—— (1972) 'The knee and cerebral palsy.' *Orthopaedic Clinics of North America*, 3, 113-129.

—— (1977) 'Management of spastic deformities of the foot and ankle.' *Clinical Orthopedics and Related Research*, 122, 70–76.

Bar-on, E., Malkin, C., Eilert, R.E., Luckey, D. (1992) 'Hip flexion contracture in cerebral palsy. The association between clinical and radiologic measurement methods.' *Clinical Orthopedics and Related Research*, 281, 97–100.

Barrasso, J.A., Wile, P.B., Gage, J.R. (1984) 'Extra-articular subtalar arthrodesis with internal fixation.' *Journal of Pediatric Orthopedics*, 4, 455–459.

Basmajian, J.V. (1962) *Muscles Alive.* Baltimore: Williams & Wilkins.

Bassett, F.H., Poehling, G.G., Moorefield, W.G., Riley, K., Minnich, J. (1976) 'Hamstring procedures in cerebral palsy. A: sequelae after long follow-up. B: recommendations for current practice.' *Journal of Bone and Joint Surgery*, 58A, 725. (Abstract.)

Baumann, J.V. (1970) *Operative Behandlung der Infantilen Zerebralparesen.* Stuttgart: Georg Thieme.

—— (1972) 'Hip operations in children with cerebral palsy.' *Reconstructive Surgery and Traurnatology*, 13, 68–82.

—— Meyer, E., Schurmann, K. (1978) 'Hip adductor transfer to the ischial tuberosity in spastic and paralytic hip disorders.' *Archives of Orthopaedic and Traumatic Surgery*, 92, 107–112. (German.)

—— Ruetsch, H., Schurmann, K. (1980) 'Distal hamstring lengthening in cerebral palsy. An evaluation by gait analysis.' *International Orthopaedics*, **3**, 305–309.

—— Koch, H.G. (1989) 'Ventrale aponeurotische Verlängerung des Musscullus gastrocnemius.' *Operat Orthop Traumatol*, **1**, 254–258.

Bax, M. (2001) 'Does "therapy" have a future?' *Developmental Medicine and Child Neurology*, **45**, 3.

Beals, R.K. (1969) 'Developmental changes in the femur and acetabulum in spastic paraplegia and diplegia.' *Developmental Medicine and Child Neurology*, **11**, 303–313.

Beals, T.C., Thompson, N.E., Beals, R.K. (1998) Modified adductor transfer in cerebral palsy.' *Journal of Pediatric Orthopaedics*, **18**, 522–527.

Bell, K.J., Õunpuu, S., DeLuca, P.A., Romness, M.J. (2002) 'Natural progression of gait in children with cerebral palsy.' *Journal of Pediatric Orthopaedics*, **22**, 677–682.

Bennet, G., Rang, M., Jones, D. (1982) 'Valgus and varus deformities of the foot in cerebral palsy.' *Developmental Medicine and Child Neurology*, **24**, 499–503.

Bennett, J.T., Bunnell, W.P., MacEwen, G.D. (1985) 'Rotational osteotomy of the distal tibia and Fibula.' *Journal of Pediatric Orthopedics*, **5**, 294–298.

Bhan, S., Malhotra, R. (1998) 'Subtalar arthrodesis for flexible hindfoot deformities in children.' *Archives Orthopaedic and Trauma Surgery*, **117**, 312–315.

Bleck, E.E. (1966) 'Management of hip deformities in cerebral palsy.' *In* Adams, J.P. (Ed.) *Current Practice in Orthopaedic Surgery*. St Louis: C.V. Mosby.

—— (1971a) 'Postural and gait abnormalities caused by hip flexion deformity in spastic cerebral palsy.' *Journal of Bone and Joint Surgery*, **53A**, 1468–1488.

—— (1971b) 'The hip in cerebral palsy.' *In: Instructional Course Lectures, American Academy of Orthopaedic Surgeons*. St Louis: C.V. Mosby.

—— (1975) 'Spinal and pelvic deformities in cerebral palsy.' *In* Samilson, R.L. (Ed.) *Orthopaedic Aspects of Cerebral Palsy. Clinics in Developmental Medicine, Nos 52/53*. London: Spastics International Medical Publications with Heinemann Medical; Philadelphia: J.B. Lippincott.

—— (1980) 'The hip in cerebral palsy.' *Orthopedic Clinics of North America*, **11**, 79–104.

—— (1984) 'Computerized axial tomography for developmental problems of the hip.' *Developmental Medicine and Child Neurology*, **26**, 231–235. (Annotation.)

—— (1985) 'Spastic paralytic dislocation of the hip.' *Developmental Medicine and Child Neurology*, **27**, 401–403. (Letter.)

—— (1987) *Orthopaedic Management in Cerebral Palsy*. London: Mac Keith Press with Blackwell Scientific; Philadelphia: J.B. Lippincott.

—— Holstein, A. (1963) 'Iliopsoas tenotomy for spastic hip flexion deformities in cerebral palsy.' *Paper presented at the Annual Meeting American Academy of Orthopaedic Surgeons, Chicago.*

—— Berzins, U.J. (1977) 'Conservative management of pes valgus with plantar flexed talus flexible.' *Clinical Orthopaedics and Related Research*, **122**, 85–94.

—— Terver, S., Wheeler, R., Csongradi, J., Rinsky, L.A. (1981) 'Joint laxity in children: statistical correlations with scoliosis, congenital dislocations of the hip and talipes equinovarus.' *Orthopaedic Transactions*, **5**, 5–6.

—— Minaire, P. (1983) 'Persistent medial deviation of the neck of the talus: a common cause of in-toeing in children.' *Journal of Pediatric Orthopaedics*, **3**, 149–159.

Bianchi-Maiocchi, A., Aronson, J. (Eds) (1991) *Operative Principles of Ilizarov*. Milan: ASAMI.

Borton, D., Walker, K., Pirpiris, M., Nattrass, G., Graham, H.K. (2001) 'Isolated calf lengthening in cerebral palsy: outcome analysis of risk factors.' *Journal of Bone and Joint Surgery*, **83B**, 364–370.

Blount, W.P., Clark, G.R. (1949) 'Control of bone growth by epiphyseal stapling, preliminary report.' *Journal of Bone and Joint Surgery*, **31A**, 464–478.

Bost, F.W., Bleck, E.E. (1975) 'Rotation osteotomies for spastic paralytic internal rotation deformities of the femur.' *Paper read at the Annual Meeting American Academy for Cerebral Palsy, New Orleans.*

Bower, E., Michell, D., Burnett, M., Campbell, M.J., McLellan, D.L. (2001) 'Randomized controlled trial of physiotherapy in 56 children with cerebral palsy followed 18 months.' *Developmental Medicine and Child Neurology*, **43**, 4–15.

Brown, A. (1968) 'A simple method of fusion of the subtalar joint in children.' *Journal of Bone and Joint Surgery*, **50B**, 369–371.

Brunner, R., Baumann, J.V. (1997) 'Long-term effects of intertrochanteric varus-derotation osteotomy on femur and acetabulum in spastic cerebral palsy: an 11- to 18-year follow-up study.' *Journal of Pediatric Orthopaedics*, **17**, 585–591.

Brunnstrom, S. (1962) *Clinical Kinesiology*. Philadelphia: F.A. Davies.

Burstein, A.H., Currey, J., Frankel, V.H., Heiple, K.G., Lunseth, P., Vessely, J.C. (1972) 'Bone strength. The effect of screw holes.' *Journal of Bone and Joint Surgery*, **54A**, 1143–1156.

Buryn, J.M., Cerniglia, M.S., Chaney, D.M. (1999) 'Combination of Evans calcaneal osteotomy and STA-Peg arthroreisis for correction of the severe pes valgo planus deformity.' *Journal of Foot and Ankle Surgery*, **38**, 339–346.

Butkus, J.K., Moore, D.W., Raycroft, J.F. (1983) 'Valgus deformity of the ankle in myelodysplastic patients. Correction by stapling of the medial part of the distal tibial physis.' *Journal of Bone and Joint Surgery*, **65A**, 1157–1162.

Cahuzac, M. (1977) *L'Enfant Infirme Moteur d'Origine Cérébrale*. Paris: Masson.

Campbell, W.C. (1912) 'Transference of the crest of the ilium for flexion contracture of the hip.' *Southern Medical Journal*, **166**, 235.

Campos da Paz Jr, A., Nomura, Á. M., Burnett, S.M., Dennuci, S.M. (1998) 'Rectus femoris surgery in children with spastic cerebral palsy; does it improve function?' *Unpublished study SARAH/Rede Nacional de Hospitais da Aprelho Locomotor, Brasilia, Brasil.*

Chambers, E.F.S. (1946) 'An operation for the correction of flexible flat feet of adolescents.' *Western Journal of Surgery, Obstetrics, and Gynecology*, **54**, 77–86.

Chambers, H., Lauer, A., Kaufman, K., Cardelia, J.M.., Sutherland, D. (1998) 'Prediction of outcome after rectus femoris surgery in cerebral palsy: the role of cocontraction of the rectus femoris and vastus lateralis.' *Journal of Pediatric Orthopaedics*, **18**, 703–711.

Chandler, F. A. (1933) 'Re-establishment of normal leverage of patella in knee flexion deformity in spastic paralysis.' *Surgery, Gynecology and Obstetrics*, **57**, 523–527.

Chang, C.H., Miller, F., Schuyler, J. (2002) 'Dynamic pedobarograph in evaluation of varus and valgus foot deformities.' *Journal of Pediatric Orthopaedics*, **22**, 813–818.

Chong, K.C., Vojnic, C.D., Quanbury, A.O., Eng, P., Letts, R.M. (1978) 'The assessment of the internal rotation gait in cerebral palsy: an electromyographic gait analysis.' *Clinical Orthopaedics and Research*, **132**, 145–150.

Chung, C.Y., Novacheck, T.F., Gage, J.R. (1994) 'Hip function in cerebral palsy: the kinematic and kinetic effects of psoas surgery.' *Gait and Posture*, **2**, 61. (Abstract.)

Clemente, C. (1985) *Gray's Anatomy of the Human Body, 13th US edn*. Philadelphia: Lea & Febiger, p. 397.

Close, J. R. (1964) *Motor Function in the Lower Extremity: Analysis by Electronic Instrumentation*. Springfield, IL: C.C. Thomas.

Coleman, S. S. (1978) *Congenital Dysplasia and Dislocation of the Hip*. St Louis: C.V. Mosby.

—— (1983) *Complex Foot Deformities in Children*. Philadelphia: Lea & Febiger.

Colver, A.F., Sethumadhavan, T. (2003) 'The term diplegia should be abandoned.' *Archives of Disease in Childhood*, **88**, 286–290.

Cooke, P.H., Carey, R.P.L., Williams, P.F. (1989) 'Lower femoral osteotomy in cerebral palsy: a brief report.' *Journal of Bone and Joint Surgery*, **71B**, 146–147.

Coon, V., Donato, G., Houser, C., Bleck, E.E. (1975) 'Normal ranges of motion of the hip in infants six weeks, three months and six months of age.' *Clinical Orthopaedics and Related Research*, **110**, 256–260.

Corry, I.S., Cosgrove, A.P., Duffy, C.M., Taylor, T.C., Graham, H.K. (1999) 'Botulinum toxin A in hamstring spasticity.' *Gait and Posture*, **10**, 206–210.

Couch, W.H., Jr De Rosa, G.P., Throop, F.B. (1977) 'Thigh adductor transfer for spastic cerebral palsy.' *Developmental Medicine and Child Neurology*, **19**, 343–349.

Crane, A. (1959) 'Femoral torsion and its relation to toeing-in and toeing-out.' *Journal of Bone and Joint Surgery*, **41A**, 421–428.

Crawford, A.H., Bilbo, J.T., Schniegenberg, G. (1986) 'Subtalar stabilization by staple arthrodesis in the young child.' *Orthopaedic Transactions*, **10**, 152.

—— Kuchrzyk, D., Roy, D.R., Bilbo, J. (1990) 'Subtalar stabilization of the planovalgus foot by staple arthroereisis in young children who have neuromuscular problems.' *Journal of Bone and Joint Surgery*, **72A**, 840–845,

Crenshaw, A.H. (1963) *Campbell's Operative Orthopaedics, vol. 2, 4th edn*. St Louis: C.V. Mosby, pp. 1061–1062.

Csongradi, J., Bleck, E.E., Ford, W.F. (1979) 'Gait electromyography in normal and spastic children with special reference to the quadriceps femoris and hamstring muscles.' *Developmental Medicine and Child Neurology*, **21**, 738–748.

—— Terver, S., Mederios, J., Bleck, E.E. (1980) 'Electromyographic study of the gluteus medius during the gait of normal children and cerebral palsy children.' *Orthopaedic Transactions*, 4, 72.

Damiano, D.L., Abel, M.F., Pannunzio, M., Romano, J.P. (1999) 'Interrelationships of strength and gait before and after hamstring lengthening.' *Journal of Pediatric Orthopaedics*, 19, 352–358.

Damron, T., Breed, A.L., Roecker, E. (1991) 'Hamstring tenotomies in cerebral palsy: long-term retrospective analysis.' *Journal of Pediatric Orthopaedics*, 11, 514–519.

Davids, J.R., DeLuca, P.A., Mencio, G.A., Novacheck, T.F., Waters, P.M. (2001) 'Cerebral palsy: current concepts in orthopaedic management.' *Instructional Course Lectures, American Academy of Orthopaedic Surgeons, 68th Annual Meeting, San Francisco, CA.*

Delp, S.L., Zajac, F.E. (1992) 'Force- and moment-generating capacity of lower-extremity muscles before and after tendon lengthening.' *Clinical Orthopedics and Related Research*. 284, 247–259.

—— Ringwelski, D.A., Carroll, N.C. (1994) 'Transfer of the rectus femoris: effects of transfer site on moment arms about the knee and hip.' *Journal of Biomechanics*, 27, 1201–1211.

—— Statler, K., Carroll, N.C. (1995) 'Preserving plantar flexion strength after surgical treatment for contracture of the triceps Surae: a computer simulation study.' *Journal of Orthopaedic Research*, 13, 96–104.

—— Arnold A.S., Speers, R.A., Moore, C.A. (1996) 'Hamstrings and psoas lengths during normal and crouch gait: implications for muscle–tendon surgery.' *Journal of Orthopaedic Research*, 14, 144–151.

—— Hess, W.E., Hungerford, D.S., Jones, L.C. (1999) 'Variation in moment arms with hip flexion.' *Journal of Biomechanics*, 32, 493–501.

DeLuca, P.A., Õunpuu, S., Davis, R.B., Walsh, J.H. (1998) 'Effect of hamstring and psoas lengthening on pelvic tilt in patients with spastic diplegic cerebral palsy.' *Journal of Pediatric Orthopaedics*, 18, 712–718.

Dennyson, W.G., Fulford, R. (1976) 'Subtalar arthrodesis by cancellous grafts and metallic fixation.' *Journal of Bone and Joint Surgery*, 58B, 507–510.

Dhawlikar, S.H., Root, L., Mann, R.L. (1992) 'Distal lengthening of the hamstrings in patients who have cerebral palsy. Long-term retrospective analysis.' *Journal of Bone and Joint Surgery*, 74A, 1385–1391.

Dockery, G.L., Crawford, M.E. (1999) 'The Maxwell–Brancheau arthroereisis (MBA) implant in pediatric and adult flexible flatfoot conditions.' *Foot and Ankle Quarterly*, 12, 107–120.

Dodgin, D.A., De Swart, R.J., Stefko, R.M., Wenger, D.R., Ko, J.Y. (1998) 'Distal tibial/fibular derotation osteotomy for correction of tibial torsion: a review of technique and results in 63 cases.' *Journal of Pediatric Orthopaedics*, 18, 95–101.

Drummond, D.S., Rogala, E., Templeton, J., Cruess, R. (1974) 'Proximal hamstring release for knee flexion and crouched posture in cerebral palsy.' *Journal of Bone and Joint Surgery*, 56A, 1598–1602.

Duchenne, G.B. (1867) *Physiologie des Mouvements*. Paris: J.-B. Baillière et Fils, pp. 328–341.

Duckworth, T. (1977) 'The surgical management of cerebral palsy.' *Prosthetics and Orthotics International*, 1, 96–104.

Duncan, W.R. (1955) 'Release of rectus femoris in spastic children.' *Journal of Bone and Joint Surgery*, 37A, 634.

Edmonson, A.S. (1963) *Campbell's Operative Orthopaedics*. St Louis: C.V. Mosby.

Eggers, G.W.N. (1952) 'Transplantation of hamstring tendons to femoral condyles in order to improve hip extension and to decrease knee flexion in cerebral spastic paralysis.' *Journal of Bone and Joint Surgery*, 34A, 827–830.

Elftman, H. (1969) 'Dynamic structure of the human foot.' *Artificial Limbs*, 13, 49–58.

Evans, D. (1975) 'Calcaneal-valgus deformity.' *Journal of Bone and Joint Surgery*, 57B, 270–278.

Evans, E.B. (1975) 'The knee in cerebral palsy.' *In* Samilson, R.L. (Ed.) *Orthopaedic Aspects of Cerebral Palsy. Clinics in Developmental Medicine, Nos 52/53.* London: Spastics International Medical Publications with Heinemann Medical; Philadelphia: J.B. Lippincott.

Eyre, D.R. (1984) 'Collagen cross-linking in normal and diseased skeletal connective tissues.' *In* Jacobs, R.R. (Ed.) *Pathogenesis of Idiopathic Scoliosis.* Chicago: Scoliosis Research Society. pp. 107–118.

Fabry, G. (1977) 'Torsion of the femur.' *Acta Orthopaedica Belgica*, 43, 454–459.

—— MacEwen, G.D., Shands, A.R. (1973) 'Torsion of the femur. A study in normal and abnormal conditions.' *Journal of Bone and Joint Surgery*, 55A, 1726–1739.

—— Liu, X.C., Molenaers, G. (1999) 'Gait pattern in patients with spastic diplegic cerebral palsy who underwent staged operations.' *Journal of Pediatric Orthopaedics B*, 8, 33–38.

Feldkamp, M., Katthagen, E.W. (1975) 'Results of surgical correction of flexion contractures of the knee joint in cerebral palsy children.' *Zeitschrift für Orthopädie und ihre Grenzgebiete*, 113, 181–188.

—— Denker, P. (1989) 'Importance of the iliopsoas muscle in soft-tissue surgery of hip deformities in cerebral palsy children.' *Archives of Orthopaedic and Trauma Surgery*, 108, 225–230.

—— (1990) 'Patella fragmentation bei Zerebralparese.' *Zeitschrift für Orthopädie und ihre Grenzgebiete*, 128, 160–164. (German.)

Ferguson, A.B. (1973) 'Primary open reduction of congenital dislocation of the hip using a median adductor approach.' *Journal of Bone and Joint Surgery*, 55A, 671–689.

—— (1975) *Orthopaedic Surgery in Infancy and Childhood.* Baltimore: Williams & Wilkins.

Feyen, J., Libricht, P., Fabry, G. (1984) 'Adductor myotorny, hamstring lengthening and Achilles tendon lengthening in cerebral palsy.' *Acta Orthopaedica Belgica*, 50, 180–189.

Fixsen, J.A. (1979) 'Surgical treatment of the lower limbs in cerebral palsy: a review.' *Journal of the Royal Society of Medicine*, 72, 761–765.

Forg, P., Feldman, K., Flake, E., Green, D.R. (2001) 'Flake-Austin modification of the STA–Peg arthroereisis: a retrospective study.' *Journal of the American Podiatric Medical Association*, 91, 394–405.

Frost, H.M. (1971) 'Cerebral palsy, the spastic crouch.' *Clinical Orthopaedics and Related Research*, 80, 2–8.

Fucs, P.M. de Moraes Barros, Svartman, C., Kertzman, P.F., Kusabara, A., Bussolaro, F.A., Rossetti, F.T.R. (1997) 'Tratmento do pé plano-valgo espástico pela artrorrise de Pisani.' *Revista de Ortopedia*, 32, 145–152. (Portuguese.) Website: http://www.sbot.org (Sociedade Brasileira de Orthopedia e Traumatologia).

Gage, J.R., Perry, J., Hicks, R.R., Koop, S., Wrentz, J.R. (1987) 'Rectus femoris transfer as a means of improving knee function in cerebral palsy.' *Developmental Medicine and Child Neurology*, 29, 159–166.

—— (1990) 'Surgical treatment of knee dysfunction in cerebral palsy.' *Clinical Orthopedics and Related Research*, 253, 45–54.

—— (1991) *Gait Analysis in Cerebral Palsy.* London: Mac Keith Press with Blackwell Scientific; Philadelphia: J.B. Lippincott.

—— (1995) 'Gait analysis: principles and applications.' *Journal of Bone and Joint Surgery*, 77A, 1607–1623.

—— Ed. (2004) *The Treatment of Gait Problems in Cerebral Palsy.* London: Mac Keith Press with Cambridge University Press.

—— Stout, J.L., Novacheck, T.F. (1996) 'A Rational Approach to the Surgical Treatment of Gait Problems in Spastic Diplegia.' *Instructional Course Lecture, American Academy of Cerebral Palsy and Developmental Medicine, 50th Annual Meeting, Minneapolis, MN.*

—— Novacheck, T.F. (2001) 'An update on the treatment of gait problems in cerebral palsy.' *Journal of Pediatric Orthopaedics Part B*, 10, 265–274.

—— Schwartz, M.H. (2002) 'Dynamic deformities and lever-arm considerations.' *In* Paley, D. (ed.) *Principles of Deformity Correction.* Berlin: Springer, pp. 761–775.

Gardner, E., Gray, D.J., O'Rahilly, R. (1969) *Anatomy—A Regional Study of Human Structure.* Philadelphia: W.B. Saunders, p. 457.

Garrett, A.L. (1976) 'Discussion of papers by Couch *et al.* and Griffin *et al.* on adductor transfer.' *Paper presented at the Annual Meeting of the American Academy for Cerebral Palsy, Los Angeles.*

Giannini, S., Ceccarelli, F., Vannini, F., Baldi, E. (2003) 'Operative treatment of flatfoot with talocalcaneal coalition.' *Clinical Orthopedics and Related Research*, 411, 178–187.

Gleich, A. (1893) 'Beitrag zur operativen Plattfussbehandlung.' *Archiv für Klinische Chiurgie*, 46, 358–362.

Goldner, J.L. (1981) 'Hip adductor transfer compared with adductor tenotomy in cerebral palsy.' *Journal of Bone and Joint Surgery*, 63A, 1498. (Letter.)

Grady, J.F., Dinnon, M.W. (2000) 'Subtalar arthroereisis in the neurologically normal child.' *Clinics in Podiatric Medicine and Surgery*, 17, 443–457.

Graf, R. (1983) 'New possibilities for the diagnosis of congenital hip joint dislocation by ultrasonography.' *Journal of Pediatric Orthopedics*, 3, 354–359.

Graham, H.K. (2000) Correspondence re 'The Baumann procedure for fixed contracture of the gastrosoleus in cerebral palsy' (Saraph *et al.* 2000). *Journal of Bone and Joint Surgery*, 82B, 1084–1085, and author's reply.

Granata, K.P., Abel, M.F., Damiano, D. L. (2000) 'Joint angular velocity in spastic gait and the influence of muscle-tendon lengthening.' *Journal of Bone and Joint Surgery*, **82A**, 174–186.

Green, W.T., McDermott, L.J. (1942) 'Operative treatment of cerebral palsy of the spastic type.' *Journal of the American Medical Association*, **118**, 434–440.

Greene, W.B., Heckman, J.D. (1994) *The Clinical Measurement of Joint Motion.* Rosemont, IL: American Academy of Orthopaedic Surgeons.

Grice, D.S. (1952) 'Extra-articular arthrodesis of the subastragalar joint for correction of paralytic flat feet in children.' *Journal of Bone and Joint Surgery*, **43A**, 927–940.

Griffin, P.P., Wheelhouse, W.W., Shiavi, R. (1977) 'Adductor transfer for adductor spasticity: clinical and electromyographic gait analysis.' *Developmental Medicine and Child Neurology*, **19**, 783–789.

Griffith, B., Donavan, M.M., Stephenson, C.T., Franklin, T. (1982) 'The adductor transfer and iliopsoas recession in the cerebral palsy hip.' *Orthopaedic Transactions*, **6**, 94–95.

Guillot, M., Terver, S., Betrand, A., Vanneuville, G. (1977) 'Radiographie, electromyographie et approche fonctionnelle du muscle psoas-iliaque.' *Acta Anatomica*, **99**, 274.

Gunsolus, P., Welsh, C., Houser, C.E. (1975) 'Equilibrium reactions in the feet of children with spastic cerebral palsy and of normal children.' *Developmental Medicine and Child Neurology*, **17**, 580–591.

Guttmann, G.G., (1990) 'Subtalar arthrodesis in children with cerebral palsy: results using iliac bone plug.' *Foot and Ankle*, **10**, 206–210.

Haas, S.S., Epps, C.H., Adams, J.P. (1973) 'Normal ranges of hip motion in the newborn.' *Clinical Orthopaedics and Related Research*, **91**, 114–118.

Hadley, N., Chambers, C., Scarborough, N., Cain, T., Rossi, D. (1992) 'Knee motion following multiple soft-tissue releases in ambulatory patients with cerebral palsy.' *Journal of Pediatric Orthopaedics*, **12**, 324–328.

Hagberg, B., Hagberg, G., Olow, I., von Wendt, L. (1989) 'The changing panorama of cerebral palsy in Sweden. V. The birth period 1979–1982. *Acta Pediatrica Scandavica*, **78**, 283–290.

Hagy, J.L., Mann, R.A., Keller, C. (1973) *Normal Gait Electromyograms and Lower Limb Ranges of Motion.* San Francisco: Shriner's Hospital for Crippled Children.

Halbertsma, J.P., Goeken, L.N. (1994) 'Stretching exercises: effective on passive extensibility and stiffness in short hamstrings of healthy subjects.' *Archives of Physical Medicine and Rehabilitation*, **75**, 976–981.

Hales, D. (2003) 'Who says I can't?' *Parade*, July 27.

Hamel, J., Kissling, C., Heimkes, B., Stotz, S. (1994) 'A combined bony and soft-tissue tarsal stabilization procedure (Grice-Schede) for hindfoot valgus in children with cerebral palsy.' *Archives of Orthopaedic and Trauma Surgery*, **113**, 237–243.

Hau, R., Dickens, D.R., Nattrass, G.R., O'Sullivan, M., Torode, I.P., Graham, H.K. (2000) 'Which implant for proximal femoral osteotomy in children? A comparison of the AO (ASIF) 90 degree fixed-angle blade plate and the Richards intermediate hip screw.' *Journal of Pediatric Orthopaedics*, **20**, 336–343.

Hein, W. (1969) 'Surgical therapy of the knee contracture in cerebral paresis.' *Zeitschrift für Orthopädie und ihre Grenzgebiete*, **106**, 755–759. (German.)

Hensinger, R.N. (1986) *Standards in Pediatric Orthopedics.* New York: Raven Press, pp. 266–269.

Heydarian, K., Akabarnia, B.A., Jabalameli, M., Tabador, K. (1984) 'Posterior capsulotomy for the treatment of severe flexion contractures of the knee.' *Journal of Pediatric Orthopaedics*, **4**, 700–704.

Himmelmann, K., Hagberg, G., Beckung, E., Hagberg, B., Uvebrant, P. (2005) 'The changing panorama of cerebral palsy in Sweden. IX. Prevalence and origin in the birth-year period 1995–1998.' *Acta Paediatrica*, **93**, 287–294.

Hoffer, M.M. (1986) 'Management of the hip in cerebral palsy.' *Journal of Bone and Joint Surgery*, **68A**, 629–631.

—— Prietto, C., Koffman, M. (1981) 'Supracondylar derotational osteotomy of the femur for internal rotation of the thigh in the cerebral palsied child.' *Journal of Bone and Joint Surgery*, **63A**, 389–393.

Hoffinger, S.A., Augsburger, S., Graubert, C. (1992) 'The "double bump" pattern of sagittal plane pelvic motion in cerebral palsy gait.' *Abstract, Program American Academy for Cerebral Palsy and Development Medicine*, September 30–October 3, 1992, p.15.

—— Rab, G.T., Abou-Ghaida, H. (1993) 'Hamstrings in cerebral palsy crouch gait.' *Journal of Pediatric Orthopaedics*, **13**, 722–726.

Hollinshead, W.H. (1951) *Functional Anatomy of the Limbs and Back.* Philadelphia: W.B. Saunders.

Horstmann, H. (1986) 'Skeletal maturation in cerebral palsy.' *Orthopaedic Transactions*, **10**, 152.

—— Eilert, R.E. (1977) 'Triple arthrodesis in cerebral palsy.' *Paper presented at annual meeting of the American Academy of Orthopaedic Surgeons, Las Vegas.*

—— Mahboubi, S. (1986) 'Use of CT scan in cerebral palsy hip reconstruction.' *Paper No. 20, Annual meeting of the Pediatric Orthopaedic Society of North America, Boston.*

Houkom, J.A., Roach, J.W., Wenger, D.R., Speck, G., Herring, J.A., Norris, R.N. (1986) 'Treatment of acquired hip subluxation in cerebral palsy.' *Journal of Pediatric Orthopedics*, **6**, 285–290.

Hsu, L.C. (1986) 'Results of hamstring lengthening at the Duchess of Kent Hospital, Hong Kong.' *Paper presented at Second Symposium on Cerebral Palsy, Singapore.*

—— O'Brien, J.D., Yau, A.C.M.C., Hodgson, A.R. (1974) 'Valgus deformities of the ankle in children with fibular pseudoarthrosis.' *Journal of Bone and Joint Surgery*, **56A**, 503–510.

—— Jaffray, D., Leong, J.C.Y. (1986) 'The Batchelor–Grice extra-articular subtalar arthrodesis.' *Journal of Bone and Joint Surgery*, **68B**, 125–127.

—— Li, H.S. (1990) 'Distal hamstring elongation in the management of spastic cerebral palsy.' *Journal of Pediatric Orthopaedics*, **10**, 378–381.

Hubbard, D.D., Staheli, L.T. (1972) 'The direct radiographic measurement of femur torsion using axial tomography.' *Clinical Orthopaedics and Related Research*, **86**, 16–20.

Husain, Z.S., Fallat, L.M. (2002) 'Biomechanical analysis of Maxwell–Brancheau arthroereisis implants.' *Journal of Foot and Ankle Surgery*, **41**, 352–358.

Hyashi, Y. (1970) 'The surgery of hamstring tendons for knee flexion contracture in cerebral palsy.' *Journal of the Kumamoto Medical Society*, **44**, 144–149.

Ingram, A.J. (1987) 'Paralytic disorders.' *In* Crenshaw, A.H. (Ed.) *Campbell's Operative Orthopaedics, 7th edn.* St Louis: C.V. Mosby, pp. 2985–2990.

Inman, V.T. (1947) 'The functional aspects of the abductor muscles of the hip.' *Journal of Bone and Joint Surgery*, **29A**, 607–619.

—— (1976) *The Joints of the Ankle.* Baltimore: Williams & Wilkins.

—— Ralston, H.J., Todd, F. (1994) Human locomotion.' *In* Rose, J., Gamble, J.G. (Eds) *Human Walking.* Baltimore: Williams & Wilkins, pp.16–21.

Irwin, C.E. (1949) 'The iliotibial band. Its role in producing deformity in poliomyelitis.' *Journal of Bone and Joint Surgery*, **31A**, 141–146.

Jack, E.A. (1953) 'Naviculo-cuneiform fusion in the treatment of flat foot.' *Journal of Bone and Joint Surgery*, **35B**, 75–82,

Jeray, K.J., Rentz, J., Ferguson, R.L. (1998) 'Local bone-graft technique for subtalar extraarticular arthrodesis in cerebral palsy.' *Journal of Pediatric Orthopaedics*, **18**, 75–80.

Johnson, D.C., Damiano, D.L., Abel, M.F. (1997) 'The evolution of gait in childhood and adolescent cerebral palsy.' *Journal of Pediatric Orthopaedics*, **17**, 392–396.

Joseph, B. (1998) 'Treatment of internal rotation gait due to gluteus medius and minimus overactivity in cerebral palsy: anatomical rationale of a new surgical procedure and preliminary results in twelve hips.' *Clinical Anatomy*, **11**, 22–28.

Kalen, V., Bleck, E.E. (1985) 'Prevention of spastic paralytic dislocation of the hip.' *Developmental Medicine and Child Neurology*, **27**, 17–24.

Katz, K., Arbel, N., Aper, N., Soudry, N. (2000) 'Early mobilization after sliding achilles tendon lengthening in children with spastic cerebral palsy.' *Foot and Ankle International*, **21**, 1011–1014.

Kay, R.M., Rethlefsen, S.A., Dennis, S.W., Skaggs, D.L. (2001) 'Prediction of postoperative gait velocity in cerebral palsy.' *Journal of Pediatric Orthopaedics B*, **10**, 275–280.

—— —— Skaggs, D., Leet, A. (2002) 'Outcome of medial versus combined medial and lateral hamstring lengthening in surgery in cerebral palsy.' *Journal of Pediatric Orthopaedics*, **22**, 169–172.

Kaye, J.J., Freiberger, R.H. (1971) 'Fragmentation of the lower pole of the patella in spastic lower extremities.' *Radiology*, **101**, 97–100.

Keagy, R.D., Brurnlik, J., Bergin, J.L. (1966) 'Direct electromyography of the psoas major muscle in man.' *Journal of Bone and Joint Surgery*, **48A**, 1377–1382.

Keats, S. (1957) 'Combined adductor-gracilis tenotomy and selected obturator nerve resection for the correction of adduction deformity of the hip in children with cerebral palsy.' *Journal of Bone and Joint Surgery*, **39A**, 1087–1090.

—— Kambin, P. (1962) 'An evaluation of surgery for the correction of knee-flexion contracture in children with cerebral spastic paralysis.' *Journal of Bone and Joint Surgery*, **44A**, 1146–1154.

Koman, L.A., Mooney, J.F., Goodman, A. (1993) 'Management of valgus hindfoot deformity in pediatric cerebral palsy patients by medial displacement osteotomy.' *Journal of Pediatric Orthopaedics*, **13**, 180–183.

Koshino, T., Sugimoto, K. (1989) 'New measurement of patellar height in the knees of children using the epiphyseal line midpoint.' *Journal of Pediatric Orthopaedics*, **9**, 216–218.

Kottke, F.J. (1966) 'The effects of limitation of activity upon the human body.' *Journal of the American Medical Association*, **196**, 825–830.

Koutsoviannis, E. (1971) 'Treatment of mobile flat foot by displacement osteotomy of the calcaneus.' *Journal of Bone and Joint Surgery*, **53B**, 96–100.

Kramer, A., Stevens, P. M. (2001) 'Anterior femoral stapling.' *Journal of Pediatric Orthopaedics*, **21**, 804–807.

Krom, W. (1969) 'An evaluation of the posterior transfer of the adductor muscles of the hip in the ambulatory patient with cerebral palsy.' *Resident conference paper, unpublished. Downey, CA: Rancho Los Amigos Hospital.*

Kuo, L., Chung, W., Bates, E., Stephen, J. (1997) 'The hamstring index.' *Journal of Pediatric Orthopaedics*, **17**, 18–88.

LaGasse, D.J., Staheli, L.T. (1972) 'The measurement of femoral anteversion. A comparison of the fluoroscopic and biplane roentgenographic methods of measurement.' *Clinical Orthopedics and Related Research*, **86**, 13–15.

Lamb, D.W., Pollock. G.A. (1962) 'Hip deformities in cerebral palsy and their treatment.' *Developmental Medicine and Child Neurology*, **4**, 488–497.

Laplaza, F.J., Root, L., Tassanawipas, A., Glasser, D.B. (1993) 'Femoral torsion and neck-shaft angles in cerebral palsy.' *Journal of Pediatric Orthopaedics*, **13**, 192–199.

Lea, R.D., Gerhardt, J.J. (1994) 'Current concept review: range of motion measurements.' *Journal of Bone and Joint Surgery*, **77A**, 784–789.

Lee, C.L. (1977a) 'Forces acting to derotate exaggerated femoral anteversion of the newborn hip.' *Unpublished thesis as part of a fellowship from the United Cerebral Palsy Research and Education Foundation, New York and the Children's Hospital at Stanford.*

—— (1977b) 'The Grice subtalar extra-articular arthrodesis.' *Unpublished thesis of fellowship from the United Cerebral Palsy Research and Education Foundation. Palo Alto, CA: Children's Hospital at Stanford, Pediatric Orthopaedic–Rehabilitation Service.*

—— Bleck, E.E. (1980) 'Surgical correction of equinus deformity in cerebral palsy.' *Developmental Medicine and Child Neurology*, **22**, 287–292.

Lee, L.W., Kerrigan, D.C., Della Croce, U. (1997) 'Dynamic implications of hip flexion contracture.' *American Journal of Physical Medicine and Rehabilitation*, **76**, 502–508.

Lepow, G.M., Smith, S.D. (1989) 'A modified subtalar arthroereisis implant for the correction of flexible flatfoot in children. The STA peg procedure.' *Clinics in Podiatric Medicine and Surgery*, **6**, 585–590.

Lewis, F.R., Samilson, R.L., Lucas, D.B. (1964) 'Femoral torsion and coxa valga in cerebral palsy–a preliminary report.' *Developmental Medicine and Child Neurology*, **6**, 591–597.

Lin, C.J., Guo, L.Y., Su, F.C., Chou, Y.L., Cherug, R.J. (2000) 'Common abnormal kinetic patterns of the knee in gait in spastic diplegia of cerebral palsy.' *Gait and Posture*, **11**, 224–232.

Lisowski, F. P. (1974) 'Angular growth changes and comparisons in the primate talus.' *Folia Primatologia (Basel)*, **7**, 81–97.

Lloyd-Roberts, G.E., Jackson, A.M., Albert, J.S. (1985) 'Avulsion of the distal pole of the patella in cerebral palsy. A cause of deterioration of gait.' *Journal of Bone and Joint Surgery*, **67B**, 252–254,

Loder, R.T., Harbuz, A., Aronson, D.D., Lee, C.L. (1992) 'Postoperative migration of the adductor tendon after posterior adductor transfer in children with cerebral palsy.' *Developmental Medicine and Child Neurology*, **34**, 49–54.

Lotman, D.B. (1976) 'Knee flexion deformity and patella alta in spastic cerebral palsy.' *Developmental Medicine and Child Neurology*, **18**, 315–319.

MacEwen, G.D. (1972) *Adjustable Frame for the Lower Limb for Radiographs by the Ryder-Crane Technique.* Washington, DE: A.I. Dupont Institute.

Magilligan, D.J. (1956) 'Calculation of the angle of anteversion by means of horizontal lateral roentgenography.' *Journal of Bone and Joint Surgery*, **38A**, 1231–1246.

Majestro, T.C., Frost, H.M. (1971) 'Cerebral palsy: spastic internal femoral torsion.' *Clinical Orthopaedics and Related Research*, **79**, 44–56.

Mann, R., Hagy, J. (1973) *Normal Electromyographic Data.* San Francisco: Shriner's Hospital for Crippled Children.

—— (1983) 'Biomechanics in cerebral palsy.' *Foot and Ankle*, **4**, 114–118.

Matsuo, T., Hajime, T., Tada, S., Fujii, T., Hara, H. (1984) 'The role of hip adductors. for adduction contracture of the hip in cerebral palsy.' *Seikeigeka (Orthopedic Surgery)*, **35**, 1265–1272. (Japanese.)

—— Tada. S., Hajime., T. (1986) 'Insufficiency of the hip-adductor after anterior obturator neurectomy in forty-two children with cerebral palsy.' *Journal of Pediatric Orthopedics*, **6**, 686–692.

—— Hara, H., Tada. S. (1987) 'Selective lengthening of the psoas and rectus femoris and preservation of the iliacus for flexion deformity of the hip in cerebral palsy patients.' *Journal of Pediatric Orthopedics*, **7**, 690–698.

—— (2002) *Cerebral Palsy: Spasticity-control and Orthopaedics.* Tokyo: Soufusha, 285.

McCall, R.E., Lillich, J.S., Harris, J.R., Johnston, F.A. (1985) 'The Grice extra-articular subtalar arthrodesis: a clinical review.' *Journal of Pediatric Orthopedics*, **5**, 442–445.

McCarthy, J., Otsuka, N.Y. (2002) 'Letter to the Editor.' *Journal of Pediatric Orthopaedics*, **22**, 827.

Merchant, A.C. (1965) 'Hip abductor muscle force.' *Journal of Bone and Joint Surgery*, **47A**, 462–475.

Michele, A.A. (1962) *Iliopsoas.* Springfield, IL.: C.C. Thomas.

Miller, F., Cardoso Dias R., Lipton, G.E., Albarracin, J.P., Dabney, K.W., Castagno, P. (1997) 'The effect of rectus EMG patterns on the outcome of rectus femoris transfers.' *Journal of Pediatric Orthopaedics*, **17**, 603–607.

—— Slomczykowski, M., Cope, R., Lipton, G.E. (1999) 'Computer modeling of the pathomechanics of spastic hip dislocation in children.' *Journal of Pediatric Orthopaedics*, **19**, 486–492.

Moe, J.H., Winter, R.B., Bradford, D.S., Lonstein, J.E. (1978) *Scoliosis and Other Spinal Deformities.* Philadelphia: W.B. Saunders, p. 538.

Moens, P., Lammens, J., Molenaers, G., Fabry, G. (1995) 'Femoral derotation osteotomy for increased hip anteversion. A new surgical technique with a modified Ilizarov frame.' *Journal of Bone and Joint Surgery*, **77B**, 107–109.

Mohaghegh, H.A., Stryker, W. (1983) 'Grice procedure using dowel iliac graft.' *Orthopaedic Transactions*, **7**, 166.

Moreland, J.R., Westin, G.W. (1977) 'Further experience with Grice subtalar arthrodesis.' *Orthopaedic Transactions*, **1**, 109.

—— (1986) 'Further experience with Grice subtalar arthrodesis.' *Clinical Orthopaedics and Related Research*, **207**, 113–121.

Morinaga, H. (1973) 'An electromyographic study on the function of the psoas major muscle.' *Journal of Japanese Orthopaedic Association*, **47**, 47. (English abstract.)

Morrissy, R.T., Weinstein, S.L. (2001) *Atlas of Pediatric Orthopaedic Surgery.* Philadelphia: Lippincott Williams & Wilkins, pp. 687–692.

Mosca, V.S. (1995) 'Calcaneal lengthening for valgus deformity of the hindfoot. Results in children who had severe symptomatic flatfoot and skewfoot.' *Journal of Bone and Joint Surgery*, **77A**, 500–512.

Mubarak, S.J., Hargens, A.R. (1981) *Compartment Syndromes and Volkmann's Contracture.* Philadelphia: W.B. Saunders.

Murray, M.P., Sepic, S.B. (1968) 'Maximum isometric torque of hip abductor and adductor muscles.' *Physical Therapy*, **43**, 1327–1335.

Nather, A., Fulford, G.E., Stewart, K. (1984) 'Treatment of valgus hindfoot in cerebral palsy by peroneus brevis lengthening.' *Developmental Medicine and Child Neurology*, **26**, 335–340.

—— Balasubramaniam, P., Bose, K. (1986) 'A comparative study of different methods of tendon lengthening: an experimental study in rabbits.' *Journal of Pediatric Orthopedics*, **6**, 456–459.

Nene, A.V., Evans, G.A., Patrick, J.H. (1993) 'Simultaneous multiple operations for spastic diplegia. Outcome and functional assessment of walking in 18 patients.' *Journal of Bone and Joint Surgery*, **75B**, 488–494.

Nichols, T. (1980) 'Modified hip compression nail-plate.' *Postdoctoral student project, orthopaedic surgery, Stanford University School of Medicine.*

Novacheck, T.F., Stout, J.L., Tervo, R. (2000) 'Reliability and validity of the Gillette Functional Assessment Questionnaire as an outcome measure in children with walking disabilities.' *Journal of Pediatric Orthopaedics*, **20**, 75–81.

—— Trost, J.P., Schwartz, M.H. (2002) 'Intramuscular psoas lengthening improves dynamic hip function in children with cerebral palsy.' *Journal of Pediatric Orthopaedic Surgery*, **22**, 158–164.

Norlin, R., Odenrick, P. (1986) 'Development of gait in spastic children with cerebral palsy.' *Journal of Pediatric Orthopedics*, **6**, 674–680.

—— Tkaczuk, H. (1992) 'One session surgery on the lower limb in children with cerebral palsy. A five year follow-up.' *International Orthopaedics*, **16**, 291–293.

Ober, F.R. (1936) 'The role of the iliotibial band and fascia lata as a factor in the causation of low-back disabilities and sciatica.' *Journal of Bone and Joint Surgery*, 18, 105–110.

O'Byrne, J.M., Jenkinson, A., O'Brien, T.M. (1998) 'Quantitative analysis and classification of gait patterns in cerebral palsy using a three-dimensional motion analyzer.' *Journal of Child Neurology*, 13, 101–108.

Odding, E., Roebroeck, M.E., Stam, H.J. (2006) 'The epidemiology of cerebral palsy: incidence, impairments and risk factors.' *Disability and Rehabilitation*, 28, 183–191.

Õunpuu, S., Gage, J.R., Davis, R.B. (1991) 'Three-dimensional lower extremity joint kinetics in normal pediatric gait.' *Journal of Pediatric Orthopaedics*, 11, 341–349.

—— Muik, E., Davis, R.B. 3rd, Gage, J.R., DeLuca, P.A. (1993a) 'Rectus femoris surgery in children with cerebral palsy. Part I: The effect of rectus femoris transfer location on knee motion.' *Journal of Pediatric Orthopaedics*, 13, 325–330.

—— —— —— —— —— (1993b) 'Rectus femoris surgery in children with cerebral palsy. Part II: A comparison between the effect of transfer and release of the distal rectus femoris on knee motion.' *Journal of Pediatric Orthopaedics*, 13, 331–335.

—— DeLuca, P., Davis, R., Romness, M. (2002) 'Long-term effects of femoral derotation osteotomies: an evaluation using three-dimensional gait analysis.' *Journal of Pediatric Orthopaedics*, 22, 139–145.

Page, J. (1982) 'Results of posterior capsulotomy of the knee with section of the anterior cruciate ligament insertion.' *Thesis for orthopaedic graduate education program in orthopaedic surgery, Stanford, CA: Stanford University School of Medicine.*

Patrick, J.H. (1996) 'Techniques of psoas tenotomy and rectus femoris transfer: "new" operations for cerebral palsy diplegia—a description.' *Journal of Pediatric Orthopaedics Part B*, 5, 242–246.

—— Roberts, A.P., Cole, G.F. (2001) 'Therapeutic choices in the locomotor management of the child with cerebral palsy—more luck than judgement?' *Archives of Disease in Childhood*, 85, 275–279.

Perry, J., Lieb, F.J. (1967) 'A study of the quadriceps extension mechanism at the knee.' *Final Project Report, Downey, CA: Rancho Los Amigos Hospital.*

—— Antonelli, D., Ford, W. (1975) 'Analysis of knee joint forces during flexed-knee stance.' *Journal of Bone and Joint Surgery*, 57A, 961–967.

—— Hoffer, M.M., Antonelli, D., Plut, J., Lewis, G., Greenberg, R. (1976) 'Electromyography before and after surgery for hip deformity in children with cerebral palsy.' *Journal of Bone and Joint Surgery*, 58A, 201–208.

—— (1985) 'Normal and pathological gait.' *In: Atlas of Orthotics: Biomechanical Principles and Application.* St Louis: C.V. Mosby.

—— (1987) 'Distal rectus femoris transfer.' *Developmental Medicine and Child Neurology*, 29, 153–158.

—— (1992) *Gait Analysis.* Thorofare, NJ: Slack; New York: McGraw Hill, pp. 97, 120, 155–157, 163.

Payne, L.A., DeLuca, P.A. (1994) 'Intertrochanteric versus supracondylar osteotomy for severe femoral anteversion.' *Journal of Pediatric Orthopaedics*, 14, 39–44.

Peterson, H., Klassen, R., McLeod, R., Hoffman, A. (1981) 'The use of computerized tomography in dislocation of the hip and femoral neck anteversion in children.' *Journal of Bone and Joint Surgery*, 63B, 198–208.

Phelps, E., Smith, L.J., Hallum, A. (1985) 'Normal ranges of hip motion of infants between nine and 24 months of age.' *Developmental Medicine and Child Neurology*, 27, 785–792.

Phelps, W.M. (1959) 'Prevention of acquired dislocation of the hip in cerebral palsy.' *Journal of Bone and Joint Surgery*, 41A, 440–448.

Phillips, H.O., Greene, W., Guilford, W.B., Mittelstaedt, C.A., Gaisie, G., Vincent, L.M., Durell, C. (1985) 'Measurement of femoral torsion: comparison of standard roentogenographic techniques with ultrasound.' *Journal of Pediatric Orthopaedics*, 5, 546–549.

Piazza, S.J., Delp, S.L. (1996) 'The influence of muscles on knee flexion during the swing phase of gait.' *Journal of Biomechanics*, 29, 723–733.

Pirani, S.P., Tredwell, S.J., Beauchamp, R.D. (1990) 'Extraarticular subtalar arthrodesis: the dowel method.' *Journal of Pediatric Orthopaedics*, 10, 244–247.

Pitkow, R.B. (1975) 'External rotation contracture of the extended hip: a common phenomenon of infancy obscuring femoral neck anteversion and the most frequent cause of out-toeing, gait in children.' *Clinical Orthopaedics and Related Research*, 110, 139–145.

Pollock, J.H., Carrell, B. (1964) 'Subtalar extra-articular arthrodesis in the treatment of paralytic valgus deformities.' *Journal of Bone and Joint Surgery*, 46A, 533–541.

Porter, R.E. (1970) 'Hamstring transfers in cerebral palsy.' *New York State Journal of Medicine*, 70, 1866–1867.

Propst-Proctor, S.L., Bleck, E.E. (1983) 'Radiographic determination of lordosis and kyphosis in normal and scoliotic children.' *Journal of Pediatric Orthopedics*, 3, 344–346.

Rab, G.T. (1985) 'Static and dynamic muscle length model use in cerebral palsy.' *Paper no. 34, Annual Meeting of Pediatric Orthopaedic Society of North America, San Antonio, TX.*

Ramakrishnan, H.K., Kadaba, M.P. (1991) 'On the estimation of joint kinematics during gait.' *Journal of Biomechanics*, 24, 969–977.

Rang, M., Silver, R., de la Garza, J. (1986) 'Cerebral palsy.' *In* Lovell, W.W., Winter, R.B. (Eds) *Pediatric Orthopedics, vol. 1, 2nd edn.* Philadelphia: J.B. Lippincott.

—— (1993) 'Neuromuscular disease.' *In* Wenger, D.R., Rang, M. (Eds) *The Art and Practice of Children's Orthopaedics.* New York: Raven Press, p.534–587.

Rathjen, K.E., Mubarak, S.J. (1998) 'Calcaneal–cuboid–cuneiform osteotomy for the correction of valgus foot deformation in children.' *Journal of Pediatric Orthopaedics*, 18, 775–782.

Ratty, T.E., Leahey, L., Hyndman, J., Brown, D.C.S., Gross, M. (1993) 'Recurrence after Achilles tendon lengthening in cerebral palsy.' *Journal of Pediatric Orthopaedics*, 13, 184–187.

Ray, R.L., Ehrlich, M.G. (1979) 'Lateral hamstring transfer and gait improvement in the cerebral palsy patient.' *Journal of Bone and Joint Surgery*, 61A, 719–723.

Reimers, J. (1974) 'Contracture of the hamstrings in spastic cerebral palsy.' *Journal of Bone and Joint Surgery*, 65B, 102–109.

—— (1980) 'The stability of the hip in children. A radiological study of the results of muscle surgery in cerebral palsy.' *Acta Orthopaedica Scandinavica* (Suppl.), 184, 1–97.

—— Poulsen, S. (1984) 'Adductor transfer versus tenotomy for stability of the hip in spastic cerebral palsy.' *Journal of Pediatric Orthopedics*, 4, 52–54.

—— (1985) 'Spastic paralytic dislocation of the hip.' *Developmental Medicine and Child Neurology*, 27, 401. (Letter).

—— (1990) 'Functional changes in the antagonists after lengthening the agonists in cerebral palsy. II. Quadriceps strength before and after distal hamstring lengthening.' *Clinical Orthopedics and Related Research*, 253, 35–37.

Renshaw, T.S., Green, N.E., Griffin, P.P., Root, L. (1996) 'Cerebral palsy: orthopaedic management.' *In* Pritchard, D. J. (Ed.) *Instructional Course Lectures*, Rosemont, IL: American Academy of Orthopaedic Surgeons, 45, 1591–1593.

Riewald, S.A., Delp, S.L. (1997) 'The action of the rectus femoris muscle following distal tendon transfer: does it generate knee flexion moment?' *Developmental Medicine and Child Neurology*, 39, 99–105.

Rinsky, L.A. (1988) 'Surgery for the upper and lower extremity deformities in cerebral palsy.' *In* Chapman, M.N., Madison, M. (Eds) *Operative Orthopaedics.* Philadelphia: J.B. Lippincott.

Roberts, W.M., Adams, J.P. (1953) 'The patellar-advancement operation in cerebral palsy.' *Journal of Bone and Joint Surgery*, 35A, 958–966.

Rodda, J., Graham, H.K. (2001) 'Classification of gait patterns in spastic hemiplegia and spastic diplegia: a basis for management algorithm.' *European Journal of Neurology*, 8, 98–111.

Roosth, H.P. (1971) 'Flexion deformity of the hip and knee in spastic cerebral palsy: treatment by early release of spastic hip-flexor muscles.' *Journal of Bone and Joint Surgery*, 53A, 1489–1510.

Root, L., Spero, C.R. (1981) 'Hip adductor transfer compared with adductor tenotomy in cerebral palsy.' *Journal of Bone and Joint Surgery*, 63A, 767–772.

Rosenthal, R.K., Levine, D.B. (1977) 'Fragmentation of the distal pole of the patella in spastic cerebral palsy.' *Journal of Bone and Joint Surgery*, 59A, 934–939.

—— Simon, S.R. (1992) 'The Vulpius gastrocnemius–soleus lengthening.' *In* Sussman, M.D. (Ed.) *The Diplegic Child.* Rosemont, IL: American Academy of Orthopaedic Surgeons, pp. 355–363.

Ross, P.M., Lyne, D. (1980) 'The Grice procedure: indicators and evaluation of long term results.' *Clinical Orthopaedics and Related Research*, 153, 195–200.

Ruby, L., Mital, M., O'Conner, J., Patel, U. (1979) 'Anteversion of the femoral neck. A comparison of methods of measurements in patients.' *Journal of Bone and Joint Surgery*, 61, 46–51.

Ruwe, P.A., Gage, J.R., Ozonoff, M.B., DeLuca, P.A. (1992) 'Clinical determination of femoral anteversion. A comparison with established techniques.' *Journal of Bone and Joint Surgery*, 74A, 820–830.

Ryder, C.T., Crane, L. (1953) 'Measuring femoral anteversion: the problem and the method.' *Journal of Bone and Joint Surgery*, 35A, 321–328.

Sage, F. (1987) 'Cerebral palsy.' *In* Crenshaw, A.H. (Ed.) *Campbell's Operative Orthopaedics*. St Louis: C.V. Mosby, p. 2870.

Salter, R.B. (1961) 'Innominate osteotomy in the treatment of congenital dislocation and subluxation of the hip.' *Journal of Bone and Joint Surgery*, 43B, 518–539, p.528.

—— Field, P. (1960) 'The effects of continuous compression in living articular cartilage: an experimental investigation.' *Journal of Bone and Joint Surgery*, 42A, 31–49.

Saltzman, C.L, Fehrle, M.A., Cooper, R.R., Spencer, E., Ponseti, I. (1999) 'Triple arthrodesis: twenty-five and forty-four-year average follow-up of the same patients.' *Journal of Bone and Joint Surgery*, 81A, 1391–1402.

Samilson, R.L., Carson, J.J., James, P., Raney, F.L. (1967) 'Results and complications of adductor tenotomy and obturator neurectomy in cerebral palsy.' *Clinical Orthopaedics and Related Research*, 54, 61–73.

—— (1976) 'Crescentric osteotomy of the os calcis for calcanealcavus feet.' *In* Bateman, J.E. (Ed.) *Foot Science*. Philadelphia: W.B. Saunders, pp. 18–25.

Sanchez, A.A., Rathjen, K.E., Mubarak, S.J. (1999) 'Subtalar staple arthroereisis for planovalgus foot deformity in children with neuromuscular disease.' *Journal of Pediatric Orthopaedics*, 19, 34–38.

Sandrow, R.E., Sullivan, P.D. (1971) 'Complications of tibial osteotomy in children for genu varum or valgum.' *Journal of Bone and Joint Surgery*, 53A, 1629–1635.

Saraph, V., Zwick, E.G., Uitz, D., Linhart, W., Steinwender, G. (2000) 'The Bauman procedure for fixed contracture of the gastrosoleus in cerebral palsy.' *Journal of Bone and Joint Surgery*, 82B, 535–540.

—— —— Zwick, G., Dreier, M., Steinwender, G., Linhart, W. (2002) 'Effect of derotation osteotomy of the femur on hip and pelvis rotations in hemiplegic and diplegic children.' *Journal of Pediatric Orthopaedics B*, 11, 159–166.

—— —— —— Steinwender, C., Steinwender, G., Linhart, W. (2002) 'Multilevel surgery in spastic diplegia: evaluation by physical examination and gait analysis in 25 children.' *Journal of Pediatric Orthopaedics*, 22, 150–157.

Saunders, J.B., Inman, V.T., Eberhart, H.D. (1953) 'The major determinants in normal and pathological gait.' *Journal of Bone and Joint Surgery*, 35A, 543–558.

Schultz, R.S., Chamberlain, S.E., Stevens, P.M. (1984) 'Radiographic comparison of adductor procedures in cerebral palsied hips.' *Journal of Pediatric Orthopedics*, 4, 741–744.

Schmidt, D.J., Arnold, A.S., Carroll, N.C., Delp, S.L. (1999) 'Length changes of the hamstrings and adductors resulting from derotational osteotomies of the femur.' *Journal of Orthopaedic Research*, 17, 279–285.

Schutte, L.M., Hayden, S.W., Gage, J.R. (1997) 'Lengths of hamstrings and psoas muscles during crouch gait: effects of femoral anteversion.' *Journal of Orthopaedic Research*, 15, 615–621.

—— Narayanan, U., Stout, J.L., Selber, P., Gage, J.R., Schwartz, M.H. (2000) 'An index for quantifying deviations from normal gait.' *Gait and Posture*, 11, 25–31.

Scott, A.C., Chambers, C., Cain, T.E. (1996) 'Adductor transfers in cerebral palsy: long-term results studied by gait analysis.' *Journal of Pediatric Orthopaedics*, 16, 741–746.

Scrutton, D.R. (1969) 'Foot sequences of normal children under five years old.' *Developmental Medicine and Child Neurology*, 11, 44–53.

Seymour, N., Evans, D.K. (1968) 'A modification of the Grice subtalar arthrodesis.' *Journal of Bone and Joint Surgery*, 50B, 372–375.

—— Sharrard, W.J.W. (1968) 'Bilateral proximal release of the hamstrings in cerebral palsy.' *Journal of Bone and Joint Surgery*, 58B, 274–277.

Shands, A.R., Steele, M.K. (1958) 'Torsion of the femur.' *Journal of Bone and Joint Surgery*, 40A, 803–816.

Sharps, C.H., Clancy, M., Steel, H.H. (1984) 'A long-term retrospective study of proximal hamstring release for hamstring contracture in cerebral palsy.' *Journal of Pediatric Orthopedics*, 4, 443–447.

Sharrard, W.J.W. (1975) 'The hip in cerebral palsy.' *In* Samilson, R. L. (Ed.) *Orthopaedic Aspects of Cerebral Palsy. Clinics in Developmental Medicine, Nos 52/53.* London: Spastics International Medical Publications with Heinemann Medical; Philadelphia: J.B. Lippincott.

—— Bernstein, S. (1972) 'Equinus deformity in cerebral palsy.' *Journal of Bone and Joint Surgery*, 54B, 272–276.

Shevell, M.I., Majnemer, A., Morin, I. (2003) 'Etiologic yields of cerebral palsy.' *Pediatric Neurology*, 28, 352–359.

Silver, C.M., Simon, S.D., Lichtman, H.M. (1966) 'The use and abuse of obturator neurectomy.' *Developmental Medicine and Child Neurology*, 8, 203–205.

—— —— Spindell, E., Lichtman, H.M., Scala, M. (1967) 'Calcaneal osteotomy for valgus and varus deformities of the foot in cerebral palsy.' *Journal of Bone and Joint Surgery*, 49A, 232–246.

—— —— Lichtman, H.M. (1974) 'Long term follow-up observations on calcaneal osteotomy.' *Clinical Orthopedics and Related Research*, 99, 181–187.

—— (1977) 'Calcaneal osteotomy results in 100 operations and 64 feet followed longer than 5 years.' *In: Instructional Course Lectures, American Academy of Orthopaedic Surgeons.* St Louis: C.V. Mosby.

Simon, S.D., Lichtman, H.M. (1966) 'The use and abuse of obturator neurectomy.' *Developmental Medicine and Child Neurology*, 8, 203–205.

—— Spindell, E., Lichtman, H.M., Scala, M. (1967) 'Calcaneal osteotomy for valgus and varus deformities of the foot in cerebral palsy.' *Journal of Bone and Joint Surgery*, 49A, 232–246.

—— Lichtman, H.M. (1974) 'Long term followup observations on calcaneal osteotomy.' *Clinical Orthopedics and Related Research*, 99, 181–187.

Simon, S.R., Deutsch, S.D., Nuzzo, R.M., Mansour, M.J., Jackson, J.L.F., Koskinen, M., Rosenthal, R.K. (1978) 'Genu recurvaturn in spastic cerebral palsy.' *Journal of Bone and Joint Surgery*, 60A, 882–894.

—— Thometz, J., Rosenthal, R.K., Griffin, P. (1986) 'The effect of medial hamstring lengthening on the gait of patients with cerebral palsy.' *Orthopaedic Transactions*, 10, 152.

Skaggs, D.L., Kaminsky, C.K., Eskander-Richards, E., Reynolds, R.A., Tolo, V.T., Bassett, G.S. (1997) 'Psoas over the brim lengthenings. Anatomic investigation and surgical technique.' *Clinical Orthopedics and Related Research*, 339, 174–179.

Skinner, S.R., Lester, D.K. (1985) 'Dynamic EMG findings in valgus hindfoot deformity in spastic cerebral palsy.' *Orthopaedic Transactions*, 9, 91.

Smith, J.T., Stevens, P.M. (1989) 'Combined adductor transfer, iliopsoas release, and proximal hamstring release in cerebral palsy.' *Journal of Pediatric Orthopaedics*, 9, 1–5.

Smith, P.A., Millar, E.A., Sullivan, R.C. (2000) 'Sta-Peg arthroereisis for treatment of the planovalgus foot in cerebral palsy.' *Clinics in Podiatric Medicine and Surgery*, 17, 459–469.

Smith, S.D., Millar, E.A. (1983) 'Arthrorisis by means of a subtalar polyethylene peg implant for correction of hindfoot pronations in children.' *Clinical Orthopedics*, 181, 15–23.

—— Ocampo, R.F. (1997) 'Subtalar arthrorisis and associated procedures.' *Clinics in Podiatric Medicine and Surgery*, 14, 87–98.

Somerville, E.W. (1957) 'Persistent foetal alignment of the hip.' *Journal of Bone and Joint Surgery*, 39B, 106–113.

—— (1960) 'Flexion contractures of the knee.' *Journal of Bone and Joint Surgery*, 42B, 730–735.

Soutter, R. (1914) 'A new operation for hip contractures in poliomyelitis.' *Boston Medical and Surgical Journal*, 170, 380–381.

Staheli, L.T., Duncan, W.R., Schaefer, R. (1968) 'Growth alterations in the hemiplegic child.' *Clinical Orthopaedics and Related Research*, 60, 205–212.

—— Clawson, D.K., Hubbard, D.D. (1980) 'Medial femoral torsion: experience with operative treatment.' *Clinical Orthopaedics and Related Research*, 146, 222–225.

Stanley, F., Blair, E., Alberman, E. (2000) *Cerebral Palsies: Epidemiology & Causal Pathways*. London: Mac Keith Press with Cambridge University Press, p. 15.

Steel, H.H., Sandrow, R.E., Sullivan, P.D. (1971) 'Complications of tibial osteotomy for children for genu varum or valgum,' *Journal of Bone and Joint Surgery*, 53A, 1629–1635.

—— (1980) 'Gluteus medius and minimus insertion advancement for correction of internal rotation gait in spastic cerebral palsy.' *Journal of Bone and Joint Surgery*, 62A, 919–927.

Stefko, R.M., de Swart, R.J., Dodgin, D.A., Wyatt, M.P., Kaufman, K.R., Sutherland, D.H., Chambers, H.G. (1998) 'Kinematic and kinetic analysis of distal derotational osteotomy of the leg in children with cerebral palsy.' *Journal of Pediatric Orthopaedics*, 18, 81–87.

Steinwender, G., Saraph, V., Zwick, E.B., Uitz, C., Linhart, W. (2000) 'Assessment of hip rotation after gait improvement surgery in cerebral palsy.' *Acta Orthopaedica Belgica*, 66, 259–264.

—— —— —— Steinwender, C., Linhart, W. (2001a) 'Hip locomotion mechanisms in cerebral palsy crouch gait.' *Gait & Posture*, **13**, 78–85.

—— —— —— —— —— (2001b) 'Fixed and dynamic equinus in cerebral palsy: evaluation of ankle function after multilevel surgery.' *Journal of Pediatric Orthopaedics*, **21**, 102–107.

Stephenson, C.T., Donovan, M.M. (1971) 'Transfer of hip adductor origins to the ischium in spastic cerebral palsy.' *Developmental Medicine and Child Neurology*, **13**, 247. (Abstract.)

Stinchfield, F.E., Chamberlain, A.C. (1966) 'Arthroplasty of the hip.' *Journal of Bone and Joint Surgery*, **48A**, 564–581.

Stoffel, A. (1913) 'The treatment of spastic contractures.' *American Journal of Orthopaedic Surgery*, **10**, 611–644.

Strange, F.G. St C. (1965) *The Hip*. Baltimore: Williams & Wilkins.

Strayer, L.M. (1950) 'Recession of the gastrocnemius.' *Journal of Bone and Joint Surgery*, **32A**, 671–676.

—— (1958) 'Gastrocnemius recession. Five year report of cases.' *Journal of Bone and Joint Surgery*, **40A**, 1019–1030.

Stuberg, W.A., Fuchs, R.H., Miedaner, J.A. (1988) 'Reliability of goniometric measurements of children with cerebral palsy.' *Developmental Medicine and Child Neurology*, **30**, 657–666.

Sullivan, R.C., Gehringer, K.M., Harris, G.F. (1984) 'A computer assisted survey of the results of medial hamstring surgery in children with cerebral palsy.' *Orthopaedic Transactions*, **8**, 109.

Sussman, M. (1984) 'Adductor and iliopsoas releases: results after early mobilization.' *Orthopaedic Transactions*, **8**, 112.

—— (Ed.) (1992) *The Diplegic Child*. Rosemont, IL: American Academy of Orthopaedic Surgeons.

Sutherland, D.H. (1980) *Lecture, International Pediatric Orthopaedic Seminar, San Francisco*.

—— Schottstaedt, E.R., Larsen, L.I., Ashley, R.K., Callander, J.N., James, P.M. (1969) 'Clinical and electromyographic study of seven spastic children with internal rotation gait.' *Journal of Bone and Joint Surgery*, **51A**, 1070–1082.

—— Larsen, L.I., Mann, R. (1975) 'Rectus femoris release in selected patients with cerebral palsy: a preliminary report.' *Developmental Medicine and Child Neurology*, **17**, 26–34.

—— Cooper, L. (1978) 'The pathomechanics of progressive crouch gait in spastic diplegia.' *Orthopaedic Clinics of North America*, **9**, 142–154.

—— Olshen, R., Cooper, L., Woo, S.K. (1980) 'The development of mature gait.' *Journal of Bone and Joint Surgery*, **62A**, 336–353.

—— Santi, M., Abel, M.F. (1990) 'Treatment of stiff-knee gait in cerebral palsy: a comparison by gait analysis of distal rectus femoris transfer versus proximal rectus release.' *Journal of Pediatric Orthopaedics*, **10**, 433–441.

—— Kaufman, K.R., Moitoza, J.R. (1994) 'Kinematics of normal human walking.' *In* Rose, J., Gamble, J.G. (Eds) *Human Walking, 2nd edn.* Baltimore: Williams & Wilkins, pp. 34–35.

—— Zilberfarb, J.L., Kaufman, K.R., Wyatt, M.P., Chambers, M.D. (1997) 'Psoas release at the pelvic brim in ambulatory patients with cerebral palsy: operative technique and functional outcome.' *Journal of Pediatric Orthopaedics*, **17**, 563–570.

Tachdjian, M. (1994) *Atlas of Pediatric Orthopaedic Surgery*. Philadelphia: W.B. Saunders, pp. 570–572.

Tenuta, J., Shelton, Y.A., Miller, F. (1993) 'Long-term follow-up of triple arthrodesis inpatients with cerebral palsy.' *Journal of Pediatric Orthopaedics*, **13**, 713–716.

Tervo, R.C., Azuma, S., Stout, J., Novacheck, T. (2002) 'Correlation between physical functioning and gait measures in children with cerebral palsy.' *Developmental Medicine and Child Neurology*, **44**, 185–190.

Thomas, S.S., Aiona, M.D., Burckon, C.E., Piatt, J.H. Jr (1997) 'Does gait continue to improve 2 years after selective dorsal rhizotomy?' *Journal of Pediatric Orthopaedics*, **17**, 387–391.

Thometz, J., Simon, S., Rosenthal, R. (1989) 'The effect on gait of lengthening of the medial hamstrings in cerebral palsy.' *Journal of Bone and Joint Surgery*, **71A**, 345–353.

Thompson, G.H., Shaffer, J.W., Zdeblich, T. (1986) 'Percutaneous distal femoral derotation osteotomy.' *Paper No. 19, Annual Meeting, Pediatric Orthopaedic Society of North America*, Boston.

Thompson, N.S., Baker, R.J., Cosgrove, A.P., Corry, I.S., Graham, H.K. (1998) 'Musculoskeletal modelling in determining the effect of botulinum toxin on the hamstrings of patients with crouch gait.' *Developmental Medicine and Child Neurology*, **40**, 622–625.

Tompkins, M.H., Nigro, J.S., Mendicino, S. (1993) 'The Smith STA-peg: a 7 year retrospective study.' *Journal of Foot and Ankle Surgery*, **32**, 456–457.

Trouillas, J. (1978) 'La chirurgie des membres inferieurs chez l'infirme moteur cérébrale spastique.' *Thesis for the Faculty of Medicine, Montpellier, France.*

Tylkowski, C.M., Rosenthal, R.K., Simon, S.R. (1980) 'Proximal femoral osteotomy in cerebral palsy.' *Clinical Orthopedics and Related Research*, **151**, 183–192.

—— Simon, S.R., Mansour, J.M. (1982) 'Internal rotation gait in spastic cerebral palsy.' *Hip*, 89–125.

—— Price, C.T. (1986) 'Aponeurotic lengthening of the iliopsoas muscle for spastic hip flexion deformities–assessment by gait analysis.' *Paper No. 25, Pediatric Orthopaedic Society of North America Annual Meeting, Boston.*

Vedantam, R., Capelli, A.M., Schoenecker, P.L. (1998) 'Subtalar arthroereisis for the correction of planovalgus foot in children.' *Journal of Pediatric Orthopaedics*, **18**, 294–298.

Vulpius, O., Stoffel, A. (1913) *Orthopädische Operationslehre.* Stuttgart: Ferdinand Enke, pp. 29–31.

—— (1920) *Orthopädische Operationslehre, 2nd edn.* Stuttgart: Ferdinand Enke.

Waters, R.L., Garland, D.E., Perry, J., Habig, T., Slabaugh, P. (1979) 'Stiff-legged gait in hemiplegia: surgical correction.' *Journal of Bone and Joint Surgery*, **61A**, 927–933.

Weigl, D., Copeliovitch, L., Itzchak, Y., Strauss, S. (2001) 'Sonographic healing stages of Achilles tendon after tenomuscular lengthening in children with cerebral palsy.' *Journal of Pediatric Orthopaedics*, **21**, 778–783.

Westin, G.W. (1965) 'Tendon transfers about the foot, ankle, and hip in the paralyzed lower extremity.' *Journal of Bone and Joint Surgery*, **47A**, 1430–1443.

Wheeler, M.E., Weinstein, S.L. (1984) 'Adductor tenotomy–obturator neurectomy.' *Journal of Pediatric Orthopedics*, **4**, 48–51.

Wilkinson, I. (1962) 'Femoral anteversion in the rabbit.' *Journal of Bone and Joint Surgery*, **44B**, 386–397.

Williams, I. (1977) 'The consequences of orthopaedic surgery to the adolescent cerebral palsied: medical, educational and parental attitudes.' *Paper presented at the Study Group on Integrating the Care of Multiply Handicapped Children, St. Mary's College, Durham, England.* London: Spastics Society Medical Education and Information Unit.

Williams, P.F., Menelaus, M.B. (1977) 'Triple arthrodesis by inlay grafting— a method suitable for undeformed or valgus foot.' *Journal of Bone and Joint Surgery*, **59B**, 333–336.

Wilson, P.D. (1929) 'Posterior capsuloplasty in certain flexion contractures of the knee.' *Journal of Bone and Joint Surgery*, **11**, 40–58.

Wiltse, L.L. (1972) 'Valgus deformity of the ankle. A sequel to acquired or congenital abnormalities of the fibula.' *Journal of Bone and Joint Surgery*, **54A**, 595–606.

Winter, D.A. (1987) *The Biomechanics and Motor Control of Human Gait.* Waterloo, Ontario: University of Waterloo Press.

Winter, S., Autry, A., Boyle, C., Yeargin-Allsopp, M. (2002) 'Trends in the prevalence of cerebral palsy in a population-based study.' *Pediatrics*, **110**, 1220–1225.

Wu, K.K. (1986) *Surgery of the Foot.* Philadelphia: Lea & Febiger.

Wynne-Davies, R. (1970) 'Acetabular dysplasia and familial joint laxity: two etiological factors in congenital dislocation of the hip.' *Journal of Bone and Joint Surgery*, **52B**, 704–716.

Yount, C.C. (1926) 'The rôle of the tensor fasciae femoris in certain deformities of the lower extremities.' *Journal of Bone and Joint Surgery*, **8**, 171–193.

Ziv, I., Blackburn, N., Rang, M., Koreska, J. (1984) 'Muscle growth in normal and spastic mice.' *Developmental Medicine and Child Neurology*, **26**, 94–96.

Zwick, E.B., Seraph, V., Linhart, W.E., Steinwender, G. (2001) 'Propulsive function during gait in diplegic children: evaluation after surgery for gait improvement.' *Journal of Pediatric Orthopaedics B*, **10**, 226–233.

9
TOTAL BODY INVOLVEMENT

SNAPSHOT: TOTAL BODY INVOLVED

- *Communication*: vocal may be absent or not intelligible. Non-verbal methods feasible in most
- *Activities of daily living*: limited
- *Mobility*: feasible with assistive devices
- *Walking*: very limited if at all possible
- *Major orthopaedic problems*: Scoliosis; hip dislocation
- *Intellect*: varying mental retardation; athetosis often has normal intellectual function.

CHARACTERISTICS

'Total body involved' is the term now generally used to describe cerebral palsy in persons who have quadriplegia spastic or athetosis, trunk, head and neck dysequilibrium, speech and hearing deficits and a variety of intellectual dysfunctions (e.g. mental retardation, perceptual and visual defects). The most serious defect in many is an inability to orally communicate needs, thoughts and feelings. The overall incidence of communication disorders in this group was estimated as 40% unable to write, 10% non-verbal and 20% non-vocal (Bureau of Education for the Handicapped 1976).[1] In one study of drooling prevalence in cerebral palsy, 45% had quadriplegia (Tahmassebi and Curzon 2003). The number of total body involved children appears to vary among countries. In North India, spastic quadriplegia accounted for 61% of 1000 children identified with cerebral palsy. Dyskinetic cerebral palsy was found in 7.8% (Singhi *et al.* 2002).

Deafness is common in those whose cerebral dysfunction was due to maternal rubella or erythroblastosis fetalis. Deafness with cerebral palsy is now rare due to prevention of both these etiologies. Blindness due to retrolental fibroplasia, associated with the neonatal respiratory distress syndrome, has fortunately disappeared due to the discovery of the effects of hyperoxygenation. Convulsive disorders are common and add to the turmoil of existence and care.

Mental retardation is not inevitable, even though first impressions can lead to rash judgements. Non-verbal persons who were taught to communicate with alternative methods were found to have normal intelligence (McNaughton 1975). Root (1977a) reported that 55% of his total body involved patients had IQs over 80; normal intelligence was documented in 36% of those who had spastic paralysis and in 68% involved with athetosis.

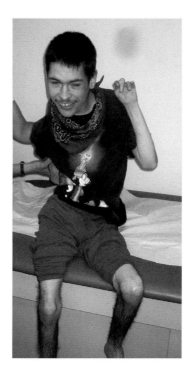

Fig. 9.1. Patient with spastic quadriplegia. He lacks trunk control, balance and speed. He mobilizes with a motorized wheelchair and communicates through a computer.

---

1 No additional data on the incidence of communication disorders in the total body involved child have been found to date. However, we suspect from our own observations of this group of children that the incidence is approximately the same in 2006.

Head and trunk control are often deficient. Standing equilibrium reactions are usually nil. Total extensor patterns of the trunk and limbs predominate in some, while others have a mixture of flexor (usually in the upper limbs) and extensor (in the lower limbs) involuntary or spastic muscle activity. The upper limbs may be more involved in athetosis, and there are patients who have better foot and toe control than in their hands and fingers. Often one upper limb is not as involved as the other, which will have better voluntary control of some sort. We have patients whose only voluntary control is with their head and neck and/or eyes.

The most common skeletal problems are subluxation and dislocation of the hip and scoliosis.

The most common skeletal problems are subluxation and dislocation of the hip and scoliosis. Knee-flexion contractures and ankle equinus are frequent, but in the patient who does not walk are not particularly disabling. If hip subluxation leading to dislocation is not prevented and/or corrected, degenerative joint disease results to cause pain and added disability as the person ages (see Chapter 5). Those who have athetosis seem especially prone to pain in the spine and limb joints due to the effects of continuous contorted motion as they grow older (Bleck 1975, Hirose and Kadoya 1984). Recurrent dislocation of the shoulder in athetosis has been observed occasionally.

PROGNOSIS

Prognosis for function in communication, activities of daily living, mobility and walking have been discussed in Chapter 3. Walking is almost always impossible or not functional. The level of wheelchair mobility can be categorized according to ability to transfer in and out of the chair: (1) able to transfer independently, (2) able to transfer with assistance, and (3) totally dependent.

Mobility in the wheelchair is subdivided according to those who are able to use a manual chair efficiently or a motorized wheelchair effectively. Some can do neither and are dependent on another person to push them about. Most total body involved children and adults need motorized wheelchairs and can use them effectively with appropriate interfaces and control mechanisms.

Because most of these patients lack trunk balance, supportive sitting has become recognized as most important. Rang *et al.* (1981) classified sitting as follows: (1) by ability—hands-free, hand-dependent, or propped; (2) by pattern of deformity—asymmetrical slouch or windswept hips and pelvis; and (3) by severity of deformity—none, amenable to surgery, or beyond surgery. Do we remake the child to fit the seat or do we design the seat to fit the child (Rang 1986)? Interest in seating is reflected in publications on seating analysis and construction (Ring *et al.* 1978, Trefler *et al.* 1978, Paul *et al.* 1980, Rang *et al.* 1981, Fulford *et al.* 1982, Holte and Siekman 1983). Seating clinics have been established in some centers (Rang *et al.* 1986).

ASSESSMENT, MANAGEMENT AND GOALS

These patients require all the clinical orthopaedic and neurological assessments delineated in Chapter 2, with added special assessments according to need (Chapter 3). Assessments for the senses and intellect will be required, depending upon the individual's deficits in function and physiology.

Management is based upon the goal-oriented approach according to the priorities for optimum independent living as described in Chapter 6. Because these persons present an almost overwhelming number of problems, efforts toward rehabilitation are apt to be truncated, the individuals relegated to the waste-basket category of medical care, and their potential as persons neglected.

The late Dr Samilson noted, with reference to orthopaedic surgery as part of the treatment of the total body involved and mentally retarded person: 'I have found that the physicians most adamant about strict non-operative management of the retarded cerebral-palsied patients are precisely the same physicians who rarely, if ever, see such patients' (Samilson 1981, p.89). But times and attitudes have changed as reflected in a review of the medical literature in the quarter century since Samilson's criticism. There are abundant clinical reports on the need and efficacy of preventing and treating the dislocation of the hips and progressive scoliosis in the total body involved patient (also termed 'quadriplegia' or 'double hemiplegia' by some authors).

Goals need to be established and changed if repeated evaluations require reorientation of recommended management. To rely on one's own values and culture to judge the 'quality of life' of disabled persons would be highly subjective and prejudicial. Because of increasing life-expectancy due to advances in medicine and sanitation, we have a constant outpouring of rhetoric concerning cost-benefit ratios. Samilson added this perspective: 'The interpretation of what is cost and what is benefit varies from person to person and is dependent on individual interests and biases' (Samilson 1981, p.89). The only rational approach in this group of severely disabled persons is to focus on them as individuals who will need the resources to achieve optimum independence in function consistent with the limitations imposed by the neurological and orthopaedic condition.

A happy and comfortable life exclusive of gainful employment can be a reasonable goal.

A happy and comfortable life exclusive of gainful employment can also be a reasonable goal. Achievement of optimum independence should be 'cost-effective' in the long run.

ORTHOPAEDIC PROBLEMS

The major orthopaedic problems which require orthopaedic surgery for prevention and reconstruction in the total body involved patient are dislocation of the hip and scoliosis. Structural deformities of other joints in the upper and lower limbs can be surgically treated depending upon the feasibility for improving function. An occasional patient may have hand function improved with surgery, as outlined in Chapter 7. Correction of knee-flexion contractures and severe foot deformities can be justified in wheelchair users if assistive or independent transfers will be facilitated. Reconstructive surgery for the lower-limb deformities are the same as described for spastic hemiplegia and diplegia (Chapters 7 and 8).

The most common problem in limb surgery in the total body involved is the preoperative differentiation of spasticity from tension athetosis and/or dystonia. Tenotomies or lengthenings in the athetoid patient can result in the opposite and more disabling deformity (known as 'athetoid shift').

The most common problem in limb surgery in the total body involved is the preoperative differentiation of spasticity from tension athetosis and/or dystonia.

Hospitalization for orthopaedic surgery in this group has been two to four times longer than the average length of stay for spastic diplegia and hemiplegia (Hoffer and Bullock 1981). However, surgery for hip and knee deformities did produce gains, primarily in hygiene and sitting tolerance. Surgery can be complicated by compromised pulmonary function, urinary-tract infections and decubitus ulcers, especially in patients who require postoperative plasters. Inpatient preoperative preparation, pulmonary function assessment and treatment can decrease postoperative complications. Discharge planning, to facilitate home nursing care, must be more detailed than with other types of patients. Since not all patients will be from traditional nuclear families with the space for bed care and energetic caregiving family members, some sort of continuous inpatient care facility will be required during the time for healing of skeletal structures. In all patients who have hip and/or spine surgery, the skills of the rehabilitation engineering team will be needed for assessment and fabrication of seating and mobility equipment.

FRACTURES OF LONG BONES

Fractures in the severely total body involved patient are another complication of management and seem to occur more commonly in those in long-term care institutions. McIvor and Samilson (1966) had 92 patients who had 134 fractures in a 10-year period. The mechanism of fracture in 70 was undetermined. In others it was from falling, catching a limb in the railing of a bed, turning in bed or in a radiology department, or during a bath. Closed treatment was preferred: the healing time with closed treatment was 3.5 months, and with surgery 5.3 months. Cast and splint application was adapted to the patient's particular limb deformity. Of 69 fractured femora, 45 had malunion but function was not compromised.

Pritchett (1990) evaluated total body involved 100 patients with unstable hips, half of which were treated surgically. Sixteen untreated patients had 16 closed fractures and nine surgically treated had 11 fractures. Tibial fractures had closed treatment. Three of seven femoral fractures had an open reduction with internal fixation. Femoral fractures occurred below a retained fixation device from previous surgery.

Supracondylar fractures of the femur occurred often, and always with osteopenia. Over-zealous and vigorous passive exercise of the knee by the physical therapist can cause the supracondylar fracture (sometimes called the 'oops' fracture when the physical therapist or caregiver hears a crack in the knee region); the complication is not entirely avoidable nor should it be overdrawn as a catastrophic event.

In one series the most important cause of the fracture was physical therapy; Brunner and Doderlein (1996) reviewed 37 patients, with a total of 54 fractures without significant trauma, and found that physical therapy was the cause in 50% of cases. The risk of fracture was estimated to be 0.065% per year. All fractures healed mainly with conservative care primarily plaster casting. For proximal femoral fractures internal fixation was chosen. Twenty-two of these fractures occurred within a year of reconstructive surgery primarily of the hip, thus implicating immobilization in plaster which advances osteopenia as a major risk factor. Therefore immobilization should be kept as short as possible. Rehabilitation should be 'carried out extremely carefully'.

Osteopenia always occurs in the absence of gravity and the forces of weightbearing. It is one of the physiological changes in space travel. Calcium and vitamin D intake alone will not prevent it. All these fractures heal with simple immobilization. If there is a flexion contracture of the knee, extension of the distal femoral fragment will correct the contracture; or if there is an internal rotation deformity of the femur, external rotation of the distal fragment will be corrective. Paradoxically, one can use an opportunity to turn what seems bad into some good.

HIP AND PELVIC DEFORMITIES

HIP-ADDUCTION CONTRACTURES

Adduction contractures in the total body involved patient are usually with a subluxation or dislocation of the hip (Fig. 9.2). If asymmetrical, a pelvic obliquity results. If there is no evidence of subluxation or dislocation by radiographs, adduction contractures that interfere with perineal hygiene and sitting can be corrected with adductor myotenotomies and, in this group, anterior branch obturator neurectomy. The operative techniques are described in Chapter 8. If there is the rare recurrence of scissoring after these procedures when one leg crosses over the other, intrapelvic obturator neurectomy can alleviate the severe adductor spasticity.

Intrapelvic obturator neurectomy is a rarely needed operation. In recurrences of severe adduction spasticity it has the advantage of not dissecting through postoperative scar as the result of prior adductor myotenotomy and anterior branch obturator neurectomy in a search for the posterior branch of the obturator nerve. However, Sage (1987) advised against it because after intrapelvic neurectomy some adductor power remains due to the femoral nerve supplying the pectineus muscle and the sciatic nerve supplies a portion of the adductor magnus. Nevertheless,

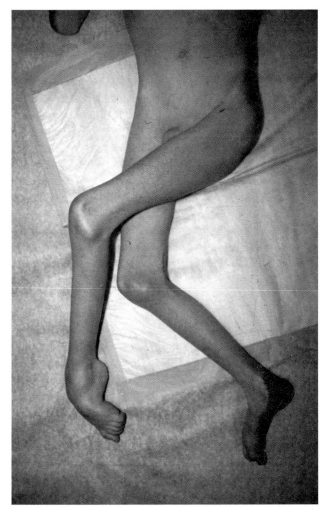

Fig. 9.2. Total body involved; severe adductor muscle spasticity.

intrapelvic obturator neurectomy may have a place in recurrence of severe adductor spasticity after adductor longus myotenotomy and anterior branch obturator neurectomy. The intrapelvic neurectomy was used for sensory denervation of the arthritic hip before the advent of total hip replacements and the sometimes effective femoral osteotomies (Chandler and Seidler 1939, Obletz *et al.* 1949). It may be only of historical interest, and a bit of embellishment to this text, but we include it because a very occasional patient with recurrence of severe hip adduction might benefit.[2]

The *operative approach* is extraperitoneal through slightly curved transverse incision just above the symphysis pubis and ending at the linea semmilunaris that borders the rectus abdominis sheath (Pfannenstiel incision). The patient is placed in the Trendelenberg position for ease of exposure. The rectus sheath is split transversely across the rectus muscles. Using finger dissection, the distal portion of the rectus is separated from the

anterior sheath. The lateral border of the rectus is exposed. Staying extraperitoneal the finger dissection reflects the bladder and peritoneum medially and then sweeps over the obturator foramen until the nerve is palpated. A Mixter forceps or aneurysm hook carefully dissects the nerve and when isolated pinches it with the forceps to observe the contraction of the adductor muscles. Ligation of the nerve proximally and distally before removing 2–3 cm of it ensures prevention of difficult to control bleeding. Wound closure in layers is routine.

HIP-FLEXION CONTRACTURES

Hip-flexion contractures alone, without subluxation or dislocation in the total body involved patient, rarely need correction. After all, these patients are sitters. One can imagine surgical correction of hip-flexion contractures in wheelchair-bound patients if they stand for assistive transfers and have hamstring lengthenings to correct untenable knee-flexion contractures (more than 20º). Iliopsoas tenotomy to prevent severe and possible painful lumbar lordosis due to adaptive increased anterior inclination of the pelvis might then be a necessary accompaniment to the correction of the knee-flexion posture with these limited goals.

HIP-EXTENSION AND ABDUCTION CONTRACTURES

Hip-extension and abduction contractures have been observed in total body involved patients who have a dyskinetic motor disorder (athetosis and dystonia) rather than spasticity. In such patients an iliopsoas tenotomy may result in the shift of the dystonic pattern from flexion to extension. In these patients, alternating flexion and extension posturing without a hip-flexion contracture can be observed. But preoperatively you have to determine if there is a true hip-flexion contracture which is difficult. When the hamstrings are contracted, the Thomas test will be misleading. The repeated, careful and tedious examination with the prone hip-extension test may change the decision to perform an iliopsoas tenotomy at the lesser trochanter. A calm, unhurried and repetitive examination of the patient should assist in the diagnosis of athetosis and dystonia. In this case, if there is a hip-flexion contracture and a hip subluxation, iliopsoas tenotomy (also termed 'recession') at the pelvic brim or an iliopsoas lengthening may be the more prudent procedure rather than tenotomy at the lesser trochanteric insertion.

Extension deformity of the hips with anterior dislocation has been reported (Copeliovitch *et al.* 1983), but we have never seen it. The functional problem was the inability to sit in a wheelchair. Treatment was surgical, with release of the proximal hamstring muscle origins, gluteus maximus, hip external rotator muscles and, if necessary to gain flexion of the hip to 90º for sitting, incision of the posterior capsule of the hip joint (Bowen *et al.* 1981, Szalay *et al.* 1986a). Selva *et al.* (1998) reported 27 anterior hip dislocations in 17 patients that were treated with acetabular reconstruction, femoral shortening or proximal femoral head and neck resection. Perhaps intrathecal baclofen could be considered in such cases.

2 In my experience, this is a 'fun' operation. It worries the general surgeon who pokes his head into the room noticing the preparation of the abdominal wall and asks what we are doing. I like to respond: 'I thought today we'd do an end-to-end' (EEB).

The 'frog-leg' abduction deformity of the hips following adductor myotomy and anterior branch obturator neurectomy in a total body involved patient can be usually attributed to athetosis and dystonic posturing mistaken for spasticity (Fig. 9.3). Another cause of this unintended result may be due to forced compression of the femoral head in the acetabulum with immobilization in excessive hip abduction and for too long (longer than 6 weeks). This can result in cartilage degeneration, arthrofibrosis of the joint, and stiff hips.

PELVIC OBLIQUITY (PELVIC 'TILT')

SAGITTAL PLANE

Pelvic obliquity in the sagittal plane in the total body involved patient who sits is rarely as much of a problem as it is in spastic diplegia. Excessive posterior tilt of the pelvis can occur with spinal fusion and instrumentation for correction of scoliosis if the lumbar lordosis is not preserved. Posterior inclination of the pelvis and the absence of lordosis shifts the weight to the trunk when sitting to the distal sacrum and coccyx rather than to the posterior thighs. The resultant excessive pressure on the tail of the spine can cause painful sitting and skin breakdown over the sacrococcygeal area. When fusion is into the sacrum, the spinal fixation rods need to be bent to accommodate some lordosis (Figs 9.4, 9.5).

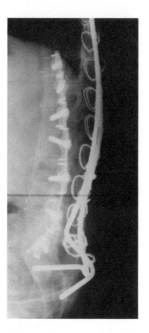

Fig. 9.4. Anterior spine fusion with Dwyer fixation and posterior Luque–Galveston fixation and spinal fusion. Lordosis eliminated by anterior instrumentation; sacrum is vertical; when sitting pressure is concentrated on the tip of the sacrum and coccyx.

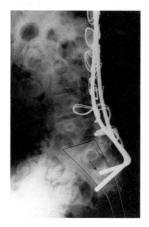

Fig. 9.5. Luque–Galveston fixation and posterior spine fusion. Rods bent to create lordosis. Sacrum becomes more horizontal in a more normal position.

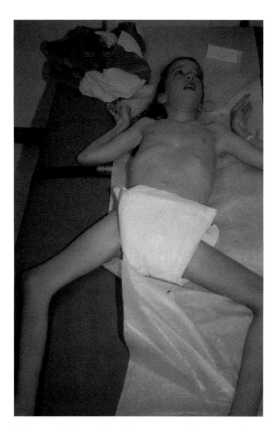

Fig. 9.3. Postoperative adductor myotenotomy and anterior branch obturator neurectomy; wide abduction posture of the hips ('frog-leg'). Occurs in tension athetosis and dystonia, not spasticity.

CORONAL PLANE

Pelvic obliquity in the coronal plane is frequent in the total body involved. In the coronal plane, pelvic obliquity can be due to contractures above and/or below the iliac crest. The most common cause is an adduction contracture of the hip (see above). Asymmetrical adduction contractures cause pelvic obliquity and appear as acetabular 'uncovering' of the femoral head of the most adducted hip (Fig. 9.6). The 'uncovered' femoral head on the high side can be interpreted on radiographic examination as 'subluxation'. This may explain the reports of success of preventing and/or reducing subluxation of the hip with adductor myotenotomies. If there is no flexion contracture or hip subluxation or scoliosis, adductor myotorny and anterior branch obturator neurectomy alone will correct the pelvic obliquity. But if there is scoliosis in which the pelvis is part of the spinal curvature as in effect, the terminal vertebra (Dubousset 1985), adductor myotenotomy or iliopsoas tenotomy will not correct the deformity. To level the pelvis correction of the scoliosis is essential.

(a)

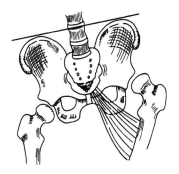

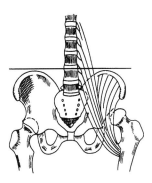

Fig. 9.7. Pelvis can be level with hip dislocation due primarily to the spastic iliopsoas.

(b)

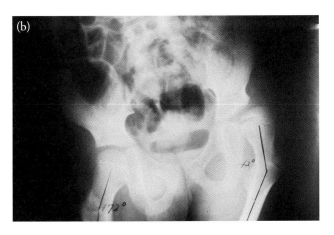

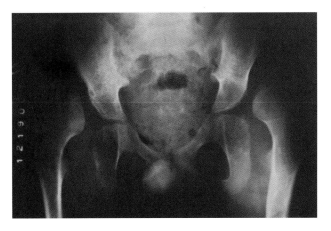

Fig. 9.6. (*a*) Asymmetrical adduction contracture with pelvic obliquity and apparent hip subluxation. (*b*) Radiograph pelvis and both hips, pelvic obliquity due to hip adduction contracture with apparent 'uncovering' of the femoral head. The coxa valgum is due to femoral torsion and is only a projection of it.

Fig. 9.8. Radiograph. Total body involved. Level pelvis. Bilateral hip dislocation.

TRANSVERSE PLANE

Pelvic obliquity in the transverse plane (rotation) also accompanies scoliosis when the curvature includes the pelvis (Dubousset 1985). Fixed rotation of the pelvis is usually first observed after scoliosis correction by spinal instrumentation and arthrodesis. It can be difficult to derotate the pelvis completely by rotation of the end lumbar vertebra in the correction of spinal curvature.

PELVIC OBLIQUITY, SCOLIOSIS, AND SUBLUXATION OR DISLOCATION OF THE HIP

Lonstein and Beck (1986), Cristofaro *et al.* (1985) and Hodgkinson *et al.* (2002) found no association between hip subluxation and dislocation and pelvic obliquity (Fig. 9.7). Black and Griffin (1997) studied 80 patients who had 86 subluxated or dislocated hips. Eight patients had no pelvic obliquity with bilateral subluxations or dislocations (Fig. 9.8). Seventy patients had subluxation or dislocation on the high side of the pelvic obliquity. The contralateral hip was contained. The authors conclude that infrapelvic obliquity (muscle spasticity and contracture below the iliac crest) usually precedes suprapelvic obliquity (scoliosis).

Hip instability and scoliosis are separate entities, each with its own etiology in muscle imbalance. Prevention or correction of hip dislocation has no effect on scoliosis prevention, although the two often coexist.

Prevention or correction of hip dislocation has no effect on scoliosis prevention, although the two often coexist.

CLASSIFICATION OF PELVIC OBLIQUITY ('TILT')

Surgeons have a penchant in reviewing their surgical experience to classify the deformities in retrospective studies and thus provide guidelines for appropriate prevention and treatment. Frischhut and colleagues (2000) of Innsbruck, Austria, studied pelvic tilt in the neuromuscular disorders of Duchenne muscular dystrophy, spinal muscular atrophy, spina bifida and cerebral palsy. They detailed four types of pelvic tilt. All had scoliosis. They concluded that only correction of the scoliosis and fusion to the sacrum can correct the pelvic obliquity, and that hip surgery had no effect on pelvic tilt.

Another classification of pelvic obliquity in cerebral palsy was developed by Black and Griffin (1997). They described five classes of body alignment in 80 patients who had subluxation or dislocation of the hip with pelvic obliquity. Hip dysplasia was found in all.

The term 'wind-blown' was introduced by Letts *et al.* (1984). The type III pelvic 'tilt' described by Frischhut *et al.* (2000) was termed the 'windblown' or 'windswept'. The configuration of the trunk and pelvis is due to a combination of an adduction contracture of one hip and displacement of the other hip in

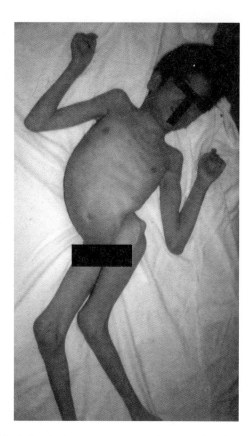

Fig. 9.9. Total body involved, age 12 years. Wind-swept pelvis, hip dislocation and scoliosis.

abduction and pelvic obliquity secondary to scoliosis (Figs 9.9, 9.10). Unilateral dislocation is often present. The abducted hip may have a contracture of the iliotibial band. Letts *et al.* (1984) described the typical deformity as a scoliosis convex on the side away from the side in which the hip was dislocated and the pelvis tilted superiorly on the side of the dislocation. In 22 teenage children who had radiographs from the time of infancy

to the ages of 13–19 years, they noted that the hip pathology appeared first, followed by pelvic obliquity and then scoliosis. By age 12 years all had a subluxation of the hip on the high side of the pelvis. The acetabular index (average 27° at age 3 years) was not affected until the hip had been subluxated or dislocated for several years. To prevent this ugly deformity they recommended bilateral adductor 'release' as soon as Shenton's line is broken (i.e. early subluxation) and iliopsoas 'release' if there is a hip flexion contracture.[3] The role of the iliopsoas as the cause of the deformity was deemed 'very significant'. Abduction seating postoperatively was strongly emphasized.

Abel *et al.* (1999) analyzed surgical treatment in 37 cerebral palsy patients to evaluate the development of the 'wind-blown' deformity over a period of 73 months. Infrapelvic obliquity appeared first but at the end of the 73-month observation period all obliquities encompassed both infrapelvic and suprapelvic factors. The final pattern of infrapelvic obliquity and the hip with the most subluxation could not be predicted from the initial radiographs or the pattern of scoliosis. Scoliosis increased during the 73-month observation time. The range of hip adduction strongly correlated with subluxation; suprapelvic obliquity due to scoliosis had a weak correlation. Severe hip abduction deformities usually followed unilateral adductor 'releases'. Soft-tissue surgery did not have an effect on the final migration index of the hip, but initially the migration index improved in 33% of the hips with the greater subluxation.

The final pattern of infrapelvic obliquity and the hip with the most subluxation could not be predicted from the initial radiographs or the pattern of scoliosis.

INCIDENCE OF HIP DISLOCATION IN CEREBRAL PALSY

Orthopaedic surgeons have discerned for at least 30 years that dislocation of the hip occurs almost exclusively in the total body involved non-ambulatory patient (Hoffer *et al.* 1972, Samilson *et al.* 1972, Le Foll 1980, Le Foll *et al.* 1981, Vidal 1982, Howard *et al.* 1985, Kalen and Bleck 1985). In these series subluxation was also found but subluxation in this group of patients leads to dislocation (Fig. 9.11). Of the 29 children with hemiplegia in the report by Howard *et al.* (1985), only two had abnormal hip architecture; one had a bilateral dislocation. This one case probably represents a developmental dislocation of the hip occurring at the time of birth. In Miranda's 1979 study of 119 children spastic diplegia, none had hip dislocations at follow-up (S. Miranda, personal communication). In another review of 694 patients with cerebral palsy followed from 1957 to 1980 by Bleck (unpublished personal observations), only the total body involved had dislocations.

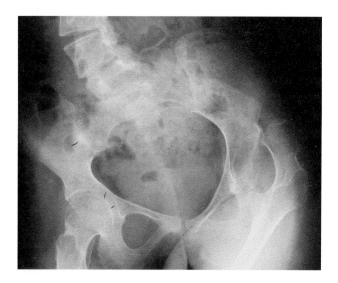

Fig. 9.10. Radiograph. Total body involved, age 16 years. Marked pelvic obliquity, hip dislocation on the left, and scoliosis.

3 The discontinuity of Shenton's line in radiographs to discern early subluxation of the hip is no longer used. Rather, the migration percentage is acknowledged as the best early sign of subluxation of the hip.

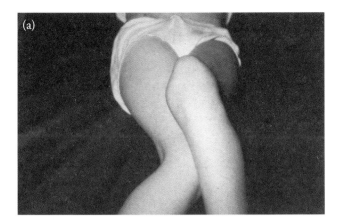

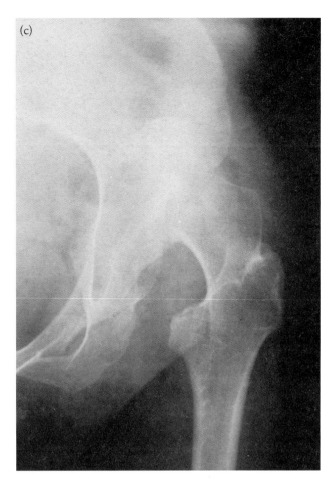

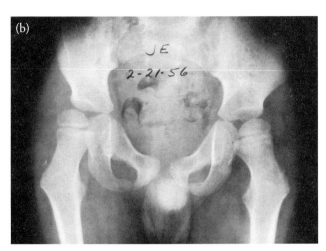

Fig. 9.11. (*a*) Total body involved lower-limb posture: left hip flexed and dislocated; right hip internally rotated and located. (*b*) Radiograph. Patient JE, age 4, subluxation of right hip. Bilateral adductor longus myotenotomy and anterior branch obturator neurectomy. (*c*) Radiograph, Patient JE returned for follow-up at age 20 years. Left hip dislocated and painful.

Dislocation of the hip occurs almost exclusively in the total body involved non-ambulatory patient.

It is possible to have a congenital dislocation of the hip and cerebral palsy. This combination is rare, but may be seen in spastic hemiplegia or diplegia. In western nations, the incidence of congenital dislocation is thought to be between 0.2 and 2.2 children per 1000 livebirths. Ethnic and racial differences have been recognized (Coleman 1978). The major radiological change, in distinguishing between a congenital and an acquired spastic paralytic dislocation, is the absence of any acetabular dysplasia in the infant and young child with cerebral palsy and subluxation of the hip. In contrast, congenital dislocations of the hip (currently termed 'developmental' dislocations in the United States) will develop very early acetabular dysplasia, manifested in the radiograph by increased acetabular angles (Fig. 9.12). Cooke *et al.* (1989) found nine dislocated hips in the perinatal period out of 683 in patients with cerebral palsy. All of these had 'pronounced' acetabular dysplasia which indicates that the hip was dislocated at or around the time of birth.

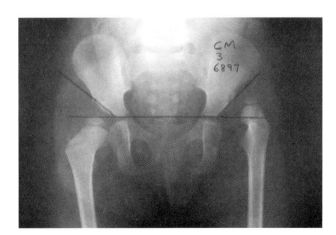

Fig. 9.12. Radiograph. Three-year-old child without any neurological impairments. Left hip dislocation and severe acetabular dysplasia. Developmental dislocation of the hip. The marked acetabular dysplasia is not seen at age three years in cerebral palsy with spasticity.

NATURAL HISTORY OF HIP DISLOCATION IN CEREBRAL PALSY

In the total body involved baby, the radiographs of the hips at first appear normal, then lateral subluxation without acetabular dysplasia occurs, followed by acetabular dysplasia, and finally dislocation (Fig. 9.13). The acetabular shallowing occurs as a response to the lack of contact of the femoral head in the acetabulum. Concentrically located femoral heads will have normal acetabular development up to the age of 4 years (Harris *et al.* 1975).

The ability to walk independently or with external supports by age 4 or 5 years profoundly influences the outcome. Those who are household and neighborhood walkers, and use crutches or walkers retain the subluxation and acetabular dysplasia but do not dislocate. Those who never walk dislocate. The mean age of dislocation was thought to be approximately 7 years (Samilson *et al.* 1972). In the series reported by Kalen and Bleck (1985) the average age of detection by any medical authority was 11.5 years.[4]

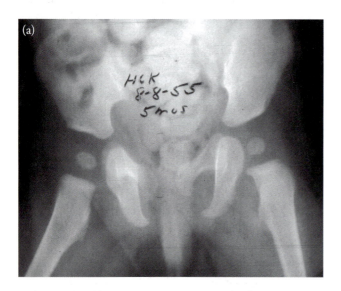

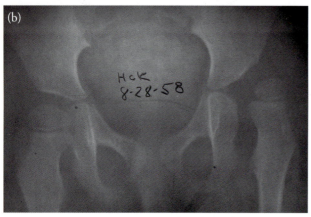

Fig. 9.13. (*a*) Radiograph. Patient HCK. Total body involved. Age 5 months. Hips normal. (*b*) Radiograph. Patient HCK. Age 41 months. Subluxation of left hip.

4 The late age of discovery of dislocation of the hip in these patients indicates a lack of radiographic surveillance from age 30 months to 5 years.

The ability to walk independently or with using external supports by age 4 or 5 years profoundly influences the outcome.

PATHOMECHANICS OF HIP DISLOCATION IN CEREBRAL PALSY

Two structural changes appear to be the major factors in spastic paralytic dislocation of the hip: persistence of the infantile hip-flexion contracture, and infantile excessive femoral anteversion. The femoral anteversion's radiographic shadow interpreted as 'coxa valga' has been discussed in Chapter 8.

ILIOPSOAS, ADDUCTORS, HAMSTRINGS

The continuous spasticity of the iliopsoas muscle leads to its shortening and contracture, because it fails to have appositional growth as suggested by the experimental data reviewed by Rang *et al.* (1986, see pp. 110, 248). The spastic adductor muscles have long been implicated as the major deforming force (Fig. 9.14). Asymmetrical adduction contracture and pelvic obliquity does compound the problem, but the evidence does not point exclusively to these factors. The contracture of the medial hamstrings also contributes to the dislocation when the knee extends with hip adduction and the femoral head drifts out of the acetabulum (Hiroshima and Ono 1979). The iliopsoas during gait acts at the very end of the stance phase and in the first 40% of the swing phase (Fig. 9.15). It appears to act to bring the trunk over the advancing femoral head during level walking.

Computer modeling of spastic hip dislocations showed that the hip has a hip-force magnitude of three times that of a child with a normal hip (Miller *et al.* 1999). The mathematical model demonstrated that to normalize the hip-joint reaction force the psoas, iliacus, gracilis, adductor longus and brevis muscle should be lengthened.

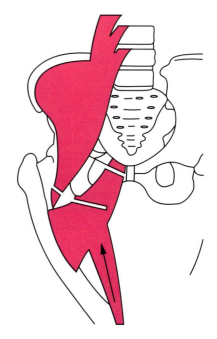

Fig. 9.14. Three major spastic muscles act to cause hip subluxation–dislocation: iliopsoas, adductors and hamstrings.

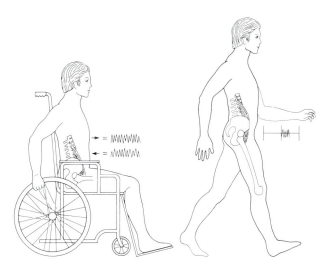

Fig. 9.15. Pictorial representation of an electromyographic study of the psoas major muscle when sitting and walking (from Morigana 1975).

ILIOPSOAS ELECTRICAL ACTIVITY ON SITTING AND STANDING

The iliopsoas can be active when sitting or standing as recorded with wire electrodes in non-weightbearing and sitting postures by Guillot *et al.* (1977). Flexion of the hip more than 110° against resistance elicited the greatest activity of the psoas major. Adduction of the hip or external rotation in flexion beyond 90° produced moderate contractions. When the subjects stood, elevation of the pelvis on the same side resulted in moderate to strong action potentials. The muscle also contracted as the trunk was brought up into extension (with a *redressement du tronc*, or straightening up) when hip flexion and extension were resisted, as occurs when you adjust your slumped posture in a chair to 'sit up straight'.

Morigana (1973) also studied the function of the iliopsoas with needle electrodes inserted to a depth of 7 cm from the back at the level of the third lumbar vertebra together with electrodes in the rectus abdominis and sacrospinalis muscles. In easy standing and sitting upright, slight to moderate activity of the psoas was found in most of the 10 subjects. When leaning forward or backward as well as with flexion of the opposite hip, large amplitude action potentials from the psoas were always evident (Fig. 9.15). In summary, these two electromyographic studies indicate that the iliopsoas contracts with trunk and opposite hip motions in the non-ambulatory total body involved patient when sitting or lying down.

Electromyographic studies indicate that the iliopsoas contracts with trunk and opposite hip motions in the non-ambulatory total body involved patient when sitting or lying down.

HIP SUBLUXATION PROGRESSION TO ACETABULAR DYSPLASIA AND DISLOCATION

As depicted by Ferguson (1973, 1975) in his studies of congenital dislocation of the hip, the iliopsoas tendon as it crosses the medial capsule of the hip pushes the femoral head laterally when the muscle is contracted (Fig. 9.16). In the non-weightbearing patient with femoral excessive anteversion as hip flexion and external rotation the subluxation increases, and the lesser trochanter becomes the center of rotation (Somerville 1959, Sharrard *et al.* 1975). Because of the lack of pressure by the femoral head, the acetabulum fails to deepen and dysplasia occurs (Smith *et al.* 1958, Salter 1966, Beals 1969). Finally, hip flexion and adduction pushes the head posteriorly to complete the dislocation. Eventually the femoral head comes to rest on the lateral superior and posterior aspect of the ilium.

Usually, by the age of 13 years, the femoral head becomes flattened laterally due to the pressure of the overlying abductor muscles,[5] and a deep groove appears on the center of the femoral head due to the pressure of the ligamentum teres (Samilson *et al.* 1972) (Fig. 9.17). A study of 12 dislocated proximal femora by Lundy *et al.* (1998) described a wedge shaped deformation of the femoral head and furrow across the superior lateral head due the pressure of the superior rim of the acetabulum. The furrow creates a fulcrum upon which the hip progressively subluxates and then dislocates. In the specimens the degree of valgus of the femoral neck was insignificant.[6] The lesser trochanter was hypertrophic and angulated anteriorly and superiorly due to the

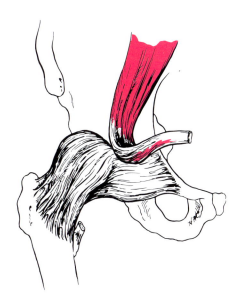

Fig. 9.16. The spastic iliopsoas and tendon compress the hip-joint capsule medially with resultant lateral displacement of the femoral head. (Redrawn from Ferguson 1975; Bleck 1979.)

---

5 An anatomic study of femoral head deformation in dysplasia of the hip by Beck *et al.* (2001) found lateral notching in all cases of dysplasias due cerebral palsy. The notching was attributed to the pressure of the gluteus minimus thought to be hypertonic, but no electromyographic studied was reported to confirm this speculation.

6 The absence of significant coxa valga in the anatomical specimens of the 12 dislocated proximal femora in children with cerebral palsy is important in subtrochanteric femoral osteotomies. These are frequently done as 'varus osteotomies' for presumed coxa valga as visualized on plain anterior–posterior radiographs. Subtrochanteric derotation osteotomy to correct the pathology of excessive femoral anteversion should be the correct procedure.

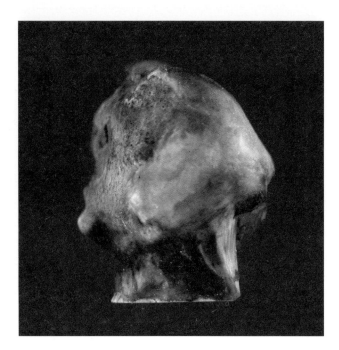

Fig. 9.17. Specimen of femoral head of dislocated hip in total body involved patient. Lateral aspect of the head is flattened and the articular cartilage destroyed.

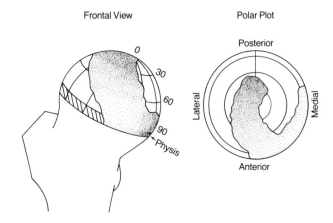

Fig. 9.18. Result of study of containment area of the femoral head in a normal male seated; hip flexed 105º, abducted 20º, externally rotated 5º (Rab 1981a). Dark areas represent contact of the femoral head with the acetabulum. Very little 'containment' of the posterior and lateral surfaces of the femoral head. (By courtesy of George Rab MD. Redrawn from computer-generated diagrams.)

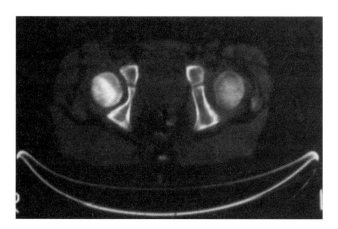

Fig. 9.19. CT scan of hips, subluxation of the right hip, total body involved. Acetabular development on the right is deficient compared with the left.

pull of the spastic iliopsoas. In the end, cartilage of the femoral head out of contact with the acetabular cartilage degenerates completely.

One might imagine and presume that sitting would 'contain' the hip. Such is not the case based on mathematical models of the hip and computerized simulations of the hip orientation and mobility. Rab (1981b) constructed a model of femoral head containment with the subject seated. The contact areas of the femoral head with the acetabulum were small, and less so on its posterior portions (Fig. 9.18). These findings correlate with transverse plane computerized axial tomograms of acetabula in spastic paralytic dislocations of the hip; the posterior acetabulum appeared deficient (Fig. 9.19). Coleman (1983) and Lau *et al.* (1986) described similar acetabular changes in paralytic dislocations.

Computed axial tomography showed that the acetabuli in patients with cerebral palsy had significant posterior deficiency compared with those who had spina bifida and developmental (congenital) hip dysplasia (Buckley *et al.* 1991). However, another study using three-dimensional computer tomography depicted that the acetabular defect was not always posterior-superior in cerebral palsy (Kim and Wenger 1997).

Unilateral subluxation of the hip in spastic diplegic patients can be explained as due to only partial weightbearing when full weight is not borne on the supporting limb so the full force of the hip abductor muscles does not occur. In particular, the internal rotation function of the gluteus medius during the stance phase of gait is diminished. Consequently, the femoral head is not repetitively contained in the acetabulum with hip internal rotation in stance to counteract the excessive femoral anteversion that is persistent from infancy. Absent the pressure of the femoral

head in the acetabulum, dysplasia of it occurs and subluxation results.

Independent functional neighborhood and community walking have a hip internal rotation gait and located hips—typical of spastic diplegia. Full weightbearing without external support in gait analysis demonstrates contraction of the gluteus medius in the stance phase. As the gluteus medius is a powerful internal rotator of the hip the femoral head is driven into the acetabulum and 'contained'.

HIP PAIN—IS IT A PROBLEM?

O'Brien and Sirkin (1977) described a patient with dislocated hips, and wrote that pain, perineal care and loss of functional status were not major problems, but the majority of experienced orthopaedic surgeons considered pain of major importance in adolescent and adult patients (Hoffer *et al.* 1972, Samilson *et al.* 1972, Sharrard *et al.* 1975, Cooperman *et al.* 1987). In a study of 99 patients, 75 were seen for subluxation of the hip and 24 for dislocation; 8% of those with subluxation and 24% of those with dislocation had pain at a mean age of 18 years with a range of 9.8–24.8 years (Kalen and Bleck 1985). In one detailed study by Pritchett (1990), pain in the dislocated hip was absent in 29 of 50 untreated patients and in 31 of 50 treated patients; pain was minor in 19 untreated and 16 treated; it was moderate (requiring only analgesics such as acetaminophen) in only two untreated hips and in three treated. The author admitted that pain levels were difficult to ascertain because most patients were incoherent so that assessment had to be based on posturing, groaning, grimacing and crying as well as attendant's assessment.

Hodgkinson and colleagues (2000) of Lyon, France, did an extensive review of the literature confined to 'excentration' of the hip in cerebral palsy.[7] They found no known marker that could distinguish dislocated or subluxated hips that would be become painful. They did note that irreversible cartilage degeneration can cause pain. The same group of Lyonnaise physicians conducted a multicenter study of 234 non-ambulatory patients over age 15 years (Hodgkinson *et al.* 2001). The mean age was 27 years, 10 months. Hip pain was present in 47.2% and tolerable in 35.6%. Because the pain was provoked, linked to position or spontaneous, these French physicians advised medical treatment, i.e. drugs, before embarking on surgery.

Of 234 non-ambulatory patients over age 15 years (Hodgkinson et al. 2001) hip pain was present in 47.2% and tolerable in 35.6%.

Knapp and Cortes (2002) looked at pain in adults in an age range of 21 to 52 years with dislocated hips. Of 38 dislocated hips, 71% were not painful. Yet Cooperman *et al.* (1987) stated that of 38 non-institutionalized patients with spastic quadriplegia half of the 51 dislocated hips were painful.

American orthopaedic surgeons appear reluctant to 'wait and see' before attempting to restore the anatomy of the dislocated hip in the child and adolescent with cerebral palsy. This attitude may be inherent in the American character—the penchant for decision and action, as a nation of 'Godsakers'.[8] It takes long and consistent follow-up to make a judgement on pain incidence, and there is no way to predict which patients will have pain and when it will occur. So, why wait until the hip joint has degenerated so much that reconstructive surgery to preserve the hip joint integrity will not be feasible? Should we launch a preemptive strike on the hip?

PREVENTION OF HIP DISLOCATION UNDER AGE 5 YEARS
Orthotics and physical therapy methods have not been demonstrated to have any effect on prevention of subluxation or dislocation of the hip. Unfortunately the late Dr Ronald Mac Keith's hope expressed many years ago that keeping the infant prone most of the time on a 'shallow inclined plane' when lying down would prevent hip dislocation has not been fulfilled (Mac Keith 1966). He based his recommendation on the observation that 'excessive extensor tone is an overactive response of the tonic labyrinth reflex evoked in the supine position'.

Efforts continue to prevent progression of hip subluxation and dislocation with devices. Hankinson and Morton (2002) of Derbyshire, UK, tried a lying hip abduction system (Jenx Dreama, Jenx Limited, Sheffield, UK) in seven children with hip subluxation due to cerebral palsy. The hip migration percentage changed from 7% to 4%. Sleeping and seating improved and pain was less. The authors cautioned that this was a pilot study. Also from the UK, Pountney *et al.* (2002) of East Sussex tried the Chailey Adjustable Postural Support systems in lying, standing or sitting in 59 children with bilateral cerebral palsy. They found that those hips that had a subluxation were stabilized, i.e. maintained their 'integrity.' As in the case of failure of adductor myotomy and anterior branch obturator neurectomy to prevent dislocation, a long follow-up (5 years or longer) depending on the age when management was instituted is essential to determine the hoped-for result. The physician and/or therapist might not implement an orthotic system that has undetermined long term results. Such devices entail more struggle for the parents so that the treatment can become more burdensome than the disease (Fig. 9.20).

Houkom *et al.* (1986) had good results with prolonged postoperative bracing. They used a Lorenz type orthosis at nap and night-time for one year postoperatively in 27 patients with severe involvement; the hip subluxation improved 69% in those braced and showed no improvement in those who were not braced. Bracing caused a hip-abduction contracture in 21%.

We have been reluctant to impose additional burdens on the family by insisting on postoperative bracing after adductor and psoas surgery of these total body involved children. It would mean application and removal of the device twice each during the 24 hours. Many of these children awaken frequently during the

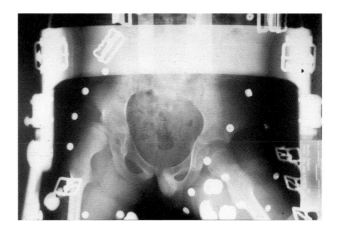

Fig. 9.20. Radiograph. Total body involved in hip orthosis and subluxation of right hip.

7 'Excentration' is a favored term for hip subluxation and dislocation in Europe, as is 'luxation' for dislocation.
8 'This means that Americans tend to feel it is better to do something rather than not do anything. I call them a nation of Godsakers, said the Englishman Dr Fry. For God's sake do something.' (Payer 1988, p. 131.)

night even without bracing. The compliance of night-bracing is doubtful. Parents need sleep to face the next day.

We have been reluctant to impose additional burdens on the family by insisting on postoperative bracing for these total body involved children.

Kalen and Bleck had an 83% success rate in psoas and adductor lengthenings without bracing in those who did not have a pelvic obliquity and scoliosis, and with these additional deformities a 60% success—almost comparable to Houkom *et al.*'s results with bracing.

Selective posterior rootlet rhizotomy has not been effective in reduction of a hip subluxation in 25% of cases (Carroll *et al.* 1998). Orthopaedic surgery was required.

Adductor myotenotomy alone or with anterior branch obturator neurectomy has a long history as the treatment of choice to prevent evolution of hip dislocation in cerebral palsy (Tachdjian and Minear 1956, Phelps 1959, Sharrard *et al.* 1975, Reimers 1980, Reimers and Poulsen 1984, Schultz *et al.* 1984, Wheeler and Weinstein 1984, Parsch 1985, James 1986). In these studies reported since 1980, the migration percentage and index devised by Reimers (1980) and/or the center edge angles of Wiberg (1939) were the radiographic criteria used to judge the efficacy of adductor tenomyotomy with or without anterior branch obturator neurectomy or adductor origin transfer.

Success with adductor myotomy, with or without anterior branch obturator neurectomy or adductor origin transfer, is limited if the ambulatory status of the patients is carefully defined. When all cases regardless of geographic involvement of the spastic paralysis and walking ability are grouped together, adductor tenomyotomy failed to prevent progressive subluxation and dislocation in ranges from 25% to 75% (Table 9.I).

ILIOPSOAS TENOTOMY, RECESSION, 'RELEASE'
The failures of adductor myotenotomy were due to the lack of appreciation of the important role of the iliopsoas as a major force

in causing subluxation progressing to dislocation in the total body involved patient. Since the mid-1980s many orthopaedic surgeons have come to recognize the need for weakening of the spastic iliopsoas by tenotomy at the lesser trochanter or below or above the pelvic brim.

The radiographic successes of adductor myotomy with or without anterior branch obturator neurectomy in improving or stopping progression of subluxation of the hip can be related to the ambulatory status of the child. There is 100% success when the child is a fully independent walker. In those who must use crutches or walkers (in effect partial or non-weightbearing), the successes of adductor weakening may appear only if there is an asymmetrical adduction with pelvic obliquity, no flexion contracture, and an 'uncovered' hip on the adducted side that appears as but not an actual subluxation (Fig. 9.21). It is rare not to find a hip-flexion contracture due to the iliopsoas spasticity in spastic diplegia and the total body involved (if you use the prone-lying hip-extension test).

With confidence in preventing progressive subluxation to dislocation of the hip in total body involved patients less than 5 years of age and a poor prognosis for walking, the surgeon can recommend iliopsoas tenotomy at the lesser trochanter along with adductor longus myotenotomy and anterior branch obturator neurectomy. If the prognosis for walking is guarded, the iliopsoas tenotomy below or above the pelvic brim may preserve hip-flexion power when they do begin to walk (in the spastic diplegic child the mean age of walking is 36 months).

With confidence in preventing progressive subluxation to dislocation of the hip in total body involved patients less than 5 years of age and a poor prognosis for walking, the surgeon can recommend iliopsoas tenotomy at the lesser trochanter.

TABLE 9.1
Reported failures to prevent or reduce subluxation/dislocation of the hip in cerebral palsy with adductor myotenotomy or adductor transfer

Author	%
Banks and Green (1960)	30
Sharrard *et al.* (1975)	25 (48 % independent walkers)
Samilson *et al.* (1972)	25
Reimers (1980)	43
Griffith *et al.* (1982)	'Disappointing high percentage later subluxation after adductor transfer' (Stephenson and Donavan 1971)
Kalen and Bleck (1985)	75 (crutches or walkers); 59 (non-walkers)
Cobeljic *et al.* (1994)	100
Scott *et al.* (1996)	36 (unilateral subluxation; adductor transfers)
Cornell *et al.* (1997)	17–77 (dependent on migration percentage) 45 (of all 56 hips)
Beals *et al.* (1998)	38 (worse head coverage and acetabular index)
Cottalorda *et al.* (1998)	8–65 (dependent on migration percentage) 33 (of all 57 hips)
Turker and Lee (2000)	58

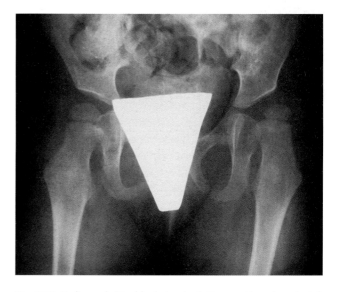

Fig. 9.21. Radiograph. Total body involved. Femur adducted on the left with 'uncovering' of approximately half the femoral head. This may be the case when only adductor longus myotenotomy will level the pelvis and 'cover' the femoral head.

In the late 1970s and early 1980s the role of the iliopsoas in subluxation and dislocation of the hip was recognized by a few surgeons (Sharrard *et al.* 1975, Fettweis 1979, Letts *et al.* 1984, Kalen and Bleck 1985). Kalen and Bleck (1985), in their review of the effects of adductor surgery alone compared with adductor surgery and iliopsoas tenotomy or recession, reported a 100% radiographic success rate in reduction of subluxation those who had an iliopsoas recession and needed crutches or walkers. The clinical success rate was 84% (meaning that no further surgery was necessary). In contrast, the clinical failure rate in these walkers with adductor surgery alone was 59%. In the non-walkers the clinical success rate in the iliopsoas group fell to 58% and the radiographic result to 67%; however, in those who had no pelvic obliquity, clinical success rose to 83% and radiographic success to 95% (Fig. 9.22). The mean age of surgery with success in both groups was 4.4–4.9 years, and the failures had a mean age range of 5.3–6.0 years. Radiographic success was determined by the migration percentage devised by Reimers (1980) (Fig. 9.23). If the last follow-up radiographs showed a more than 10% increase in the migration percentage, progressive subluxation occurred and result was called a failure. The center edge angles of Wiburg were not used because of their unreliability under the age of 5 years (Coleman 1978, Kalen and Bleck 1985).

More reports have come from various Western nations in the 1990s on the efficacy of adductor and iliopsoas 'releases' in reduction of subluxation and prevention dislocation (France: Onimus *et al.* 1991; Yugoslavia, Cobeljic *et al.* 1994; Canada, Moreau *et al.* 1995; USA, Miller *et al.* 1997; Czech Republic, Sindelarova and Poul 2001). Onimus *et al.* (1991) found 90% successful results in prevention of dislocation of the hip with iliopsoas and adductor tenotomies in total body involved children if the surgery was done under age 4 years and a migration percentage less than 33%. These orthopaedic surgeons from Besançon, France, opined that preventive surgery should be done before 2–3 years of age.

ILIOPSOAS INSERTION TRANSFER TO GREATER TROCHANTER

The late John Sharrard of Sheffield, UK, devised the successful transfer of the iliopsoas tendon to the great trochanter to stabilize the hip in spina bifida and applied the same operation to hip subluxations and dislocations in cerebral palsy (Sharrard and Burke 1982). They combined the procedure with adductor 'release' and open reduction of the hip when deemed necessary. Of 23 patients' hips, all become stable and pain-free.

In Johannesburg, South Africa, the iliopsoas transfer of Sharrard was successful in reducing the dislocation of the hip, but 45 of 47 patients with total body involved cerebral palsy had unintended results (Erken and Bischof 1994). Twenty of 28 patients who had a posterolateral iliopsoas transfer developed

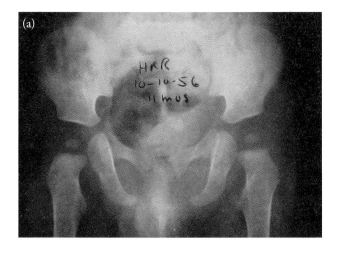

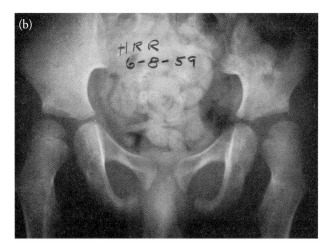

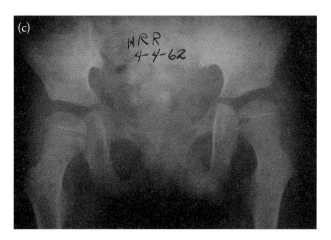

Fig. 9.22. (*a*) Radiograph. Patient HHR, total body involved, age 11 months. Hips normal. (*b*) Radiograph. Patient HHR, age 44 months. Early subluxation of both hips. (*c*) Radiograph. Patient HHR, age 7 years 5 months, 3 years postoperative bilateral iliopsoas tenotomy and adductor longus myotenotomy and anterior branch obturator neurectomy.

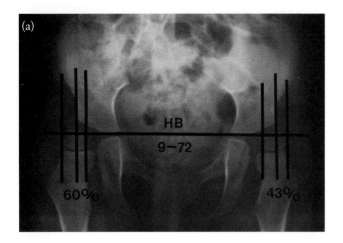

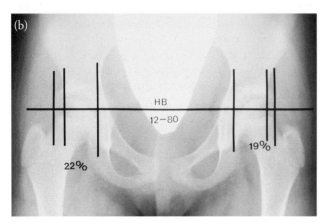

Fig. 9.23. (*a*) Radiograph. Patient HB, spastic diplegia, age 3 years, bilateral hip subluxation. (*b*) Radiograph. Patient HB. 8 years postoperative bilateral iliopsoas recession. Reduction of subluxation maintained in both hips. (From Kalen and Bleck 1985; reproduced by permission of the Mac Keith Press.)

scoliosis and became so severe in 10 patients that it caused impingement of the ribs on the pelvis. More disabling was deterioration of postoperative sitting. Seven could not be in a sitting position; six had extension contractures of the hip and 72% had a range of flexion of only 0°–60°. Because sitting was so compromised in these patients who had to sit, Erken and Bischof (1994) recommended iliopsoas transfer not to be used in cerebral palsy.

> *Erken and Bischof (1994) recommended iliopsoas transfer not to be used in cerebral palsy.*

PREDICTABILITY OF SUBLUXATION AND DISLOCATION

The following are risk factors for development of subluxation leading to dislocation of the hip in cerebral palsy.

1. ABILITY TO WALK AND WALKING PROGNOSIS
(a) Total body involved (spastic quadriplegia), poor prognosis, non-walking = dislocation (59%) (Howard *et al.* 1985).

(b) Spastic diplegia, good prognosis, walk with crutches, canes or walkers = subluxation (6.5%); spastic hemiplegia, good

prognosis, independent = 0 subluxation or dislocation (Howard *et al.* 1985).

2. RADIOGRAPHIC RISK FACTORS AT 30 MONTHS AND EVERY 6 MONTHS TO AGE 5 YEARS
(a) *Migration percentage* greater than 15% increasing to 40% indicates surgery.[9]

   Various authors recommend surgery at varying migration percentages: Miller and Bragg (1995) and Flynn and Miller (2002) advised surgery at 25% or more; 60% progressed to 90% (Fig. 9.24); Cornell *et al.* (1997) had 83% good results with muscle lengthenings if the percentage was less than 40%. If more than 40%, only 23% had good results. All hips with a percentage greater than 60% failed. Cornell (2001) commented: 'Although we agree that there is no absolute cut-off value for the migration percentage for the production of a good result, we found 40% to be a good guide in most cases.'

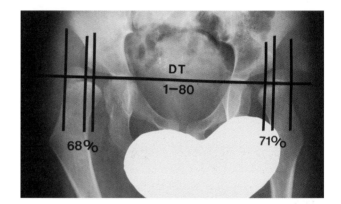

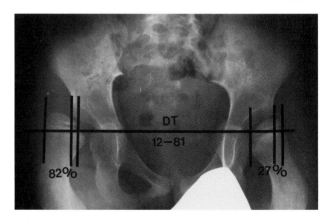

Fig. 9.24. (*a*) Radiograph. Patient DT. Spastic diplegia, age 36 months, dependent walker, subluxation of both hips. Migration index right 68% and left 71%. (*b*) Radiograph. Patient DT. One year postoperative bilateral adductor myotenotomies and anterior branch obturator neurectomies. Reduction of subluxation failed. Migration index right 82%. Left improved to 27%. A migration index of 60% or greater will fail to have a reduction of the subluxation. (From Kalen and Bleck 1985; reproduced by permission of the Mac Keith Press.)

---

9 Migration percentage, Reimer (1980): 10% by age 4 years in normal children. See Chapter 2, p.12. The anterior–posterior radiographic projection must be made with the pelvis level, the legs together and the patellae pointing straight-up (neutral rotation).

Brunner and Robb (1996) pointed out that the migration percentage can be inaccurate in depicting the displacement of the femoral head in the sagittal plane. In four patients with total body involved cerebral palsy the femoral head was dislocated anteriorly. This is not surprising given that the migration index is measured on the anterior–posterior view. Three-dimensional computer axial tomograms accurately reflected that pathology as did *faux profil* projections (lateral projection of the pelvis and hips). But, this report does not diminish the value of plain anterior–posterior radiographs on the pelvis and hips to determine the risk of subluxation in the 1- to 5-year age-group.

Arthrographic radiographs of 51 hips in 31 children with cerebral palsy defined five levels of hip instability by the migration index in one study (Heinrich *et al.* 1991). Deformation of the femoral head increased with an increase in the migration index. Their measurement was an angle constructed by line defined by the intersection of Hilgenreiner's horizontal line with a tangent drawn from the most lateral point of contact between the cartilaginous capital femoral epiphysis and the lateral acetabular cartilaginous anlage.[10] The angle so constructed decreased with the increase in the migration index. This finding was considered as evidence that the progressive deformation of the femoral head and acetabulum occurs during and sometimes before the hip becomes unstable. The authors believed that it should be done in all cases. Although arthrograms can further define the pathological anatomy, the professional time and radiographic exposure in doing arthrograms of the hips does not seem worthwhile especially the need to repeat the procedure every 6 months in a surveillance protocol from age 18–48 months. It may be valuable to some surgeons when planning reconstruction of established subluxations of the hip in children beyond the age of 5 years if three-dimensional computerized axial tomography (3D CT) scans are not available.

(b) *Acetabular index* (Cooke *et al.* 1989) more than 30°. The anterior–posterior radiograph should be made without pelvic rotation; the width of the right and left obturator foramina should be 1:1.[11] The consensus is that the acetabular index is not the best measurement as a risk factor for subluxation. Acetabular dysplasia becomes evident too late for good results with only iliopsoas and adductor myotenotomy.

The two major risk factors for progressive subluxation of the hip are the walking ability of the child and the hip migration percentage.

PREDICTABILITY OF OUTCOME OF ADDUCTOR AND ILIOPSOAS SURGERY

The following factors are important in predicting a good outcome of adductor and iliopsoas weakening to prevent progressive subluxation and eventual dislocation of the hip.

1. AGE OF ILIOPSOAS TENOTOMY/LENGTHENING AND ADDUCTOR MYOTENOTOMY

The data indicate that in children under the age of 5 years iliopsoas recession/tenotomy at or above the pelvic brim will have the best results (Kalen and Bleck 1985). The results are apt to be better if the decision for surgery is made at the ages less than 3–4 years (Onimus *et al.* 1991).

If the range of abduction of either hip in extension with the pelvis leveled while under anesthesia, is less than 40°–45°, adductor myotenotomy is indicated. Because anterior branch obturator neurectomy improved the results from 56% to 69% in one study (Kalen and Bleck 1985), the neurectomy appears indicated at the time of surgery in the total body involved child. The exception to performing the iliopsoas recession or tenotomy would be the rare case if no flexion contracture is demonstrated with the prone extension test (see Chapter 2).

2. WALKING ABILITY

If the child under the age of 5 years has a good prognosis for walking (see Chapter 1 for locomotor prognostic signs), the result will be good. If the prognosis for walking is poor and/or the child is not walking, the prognosis for prevention of subluxation and dislocation with iliopsoas tenotomy will be good. But with only adductor myotenotomy and/or anterior branch obturator neurectomy the result will be poor in preventing progressive subluxation to dislocation.

3. MIGRATION PERCENTAGE

Good results occur in 90% if the migration percentage is 33% or less when done under age 5 years (Onimus *et al.* 1991). The consensus is that surgical lengthening of the iliopsoas and adductors is indicated in a child younger thatn 8 years if the migration percentage is 25%–60%, if greater than 60% bony surgery is indicated (Flynn and Miller 2002); 8 years old and even 7 years appears to be too late (Fig. 9.25).

There is no absolute cut-off value for the migration percentage; for the production of a good result, we found 40% to be a good guide in most cases.

Pelvic obliquity due to scoliosis was present in 66% of the patients in the study by Kalen and Bleck (1985) and was prevented by iliopsoas tenotomy or adductor tenomyotomy. Prevention of the subluxation and dislocation of the hip with muscle-lengthening occurs independently of the scoliosis.

---

10 Hilgenreiner's horizontal line is drawn through the triradiate cartilages on the anterior-posterior radiograph of the hips and pelvis.

11 Normal mean acetabular angles at age 18 months to 2 years: 25° (range 20°–30°) (Tonis 1976, Hensinger 1986). If there is a flexion contracture of the hip, holding one in maximum flexion or both hips flexed on a pad or pillow to flatten the lumbar spine and pelvis will produce a more accurate image of the pelvis for measurement of the acetabular angles (Cornell *et al.* 1994, Scrutton *et al.* 2001).

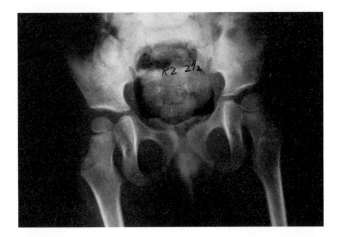

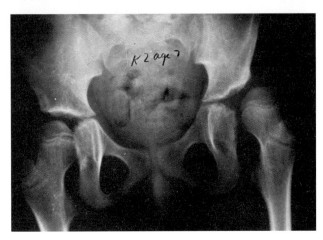

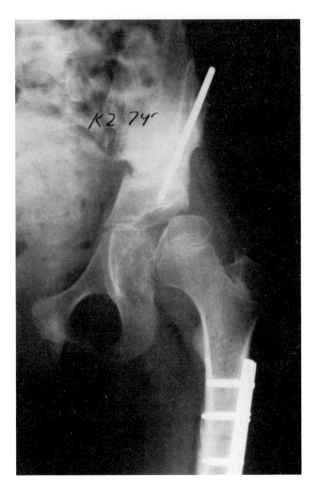

Fig. 9.25. (*a*) Radiograph. Patient KZ. total body involved, age 30 months. Normal appearing hips. (*b*) Radiograph. Patient KZ, age 7 years. Left hip subluxation and acetabular dysplasia. Too old for a good result with iliopsoas tenotomy and adductor myotenotomy and anterior branch obturator neurectomy. Bone surgery required. (*c*) Radiograph. Patient KZ, postoperative innominate osteotomy and derotation femoral osteotomy. Reduction of subluxation failed. The innominate osteotomy of Salter uncovers the hip posteriorly. Iliopsoas tenotomy at the pelvic brim is always done with the innominate osteotomy.

ILIOPSOAS TENOTOMY AT THE LESSER TROCHANTER

Iliopsoas tenotomy for spastic hip-flexion contractures was first described in the American literature by Peterson (1950) in the surgical treatment of spastic paraplegia resulting from spinal-cord injury. Bleck and Holstein (1963) reported its use in cerebral palsy. The medial approach to the proximal femur was devised by Ludloff (Crenshaw 1963), and brought to Bleck's attention by Dr C. Young (personal communication) as a way to expose the lesser trochanteric region of the femur. Keats and Morgese (1967) published a description of the operation.

Iliopsoas tenotomy should be performed bilaterally when both hips have spasticity and contracture, even though only one has a subluxation. In unilateral procedures, the opposite untreated hip is apt to dislocate postoperatively (R.L. Samilson, personal communication). The same case against unilateral hip surgery in severe cerebral palsy was made by Noonan *et al.* (2000). In 35 patients 10 of the non-operated hips dislocated and 16 subluxated.

Uematsu *et al.* (1977) performed, in effect, iliopsoas tenotomies when they did posterior iliopsoas transfers for hip instability in cerebral palsy. In the 30 hips in which this transfer

was performed, they noted a marked tendency to convert unilateral to bilateral deformities.

In addition to iliopsoas tenotomy, adductor longus myotenotomy with anterior branch obturator neurectomy is usually necessary in most cases of early subluxation of the hip in the total body involved child. If the hamstrings are spastic and contracted (popliteal angle greater than 20°), lengthening of the hamstrings either by proximal origin myotomy or distal fractional lengthening may achieve a higher percentage of good results (Hiroshima and Ono 1979, Rang *et al.* 1986).

OPERATIVE TECHNIQUE—ILIOPSOAS TENOTOMY AT THE LESSER TROCHANTER[12]

With the hip flexed, abducted and externally rotated an incision is begun 1–1.5 cm distal to the origin of the adductor longus and extended directly over the adductor longus distally for 5 cm

---

12 The operative technique for iliopsoas tenotomy above or below the pelvic brim is described in Chapter 8. In the total body involved non-walking patient, iliopsoas tenotomy at the lesser trochanter is easier. It can be combined through the same incision with adductor longus tenomyotomy and anterior branch obturator neurectomy.

(Fig. 9.26). If required, the adductor myotomy and anterior branch obturator neurectomy are then performed. With finger dissection the interval between the pectineus and adductor brevis muscles is developed to palpate the lesser trochanter. A spade-type retractor (Chandler retractor) is placed medially around the lesser trochanter to retract the adductor magnus medially, and a similar retractor laterally retracts the pectineus. The veil of connective tissue and fat is swept off the psoas tendon under which is passed a 90°-angled forceps (Mixter type) and the tendon is cut as well as some of the fibers of the iliacus which accompany it a bit distal to the tendon. The tendon is freed by blunt dissection proximally; it then retracts.

The proximal hamstring origin myotomy can be done through the same incision (Gurd 1984, Rang *et al.* 1986). The gracilis origin is sectioned; then the blunt dissection is carried medially around the adductor magnus to the origins of the medial hamstring muscles on the ischium. The semitendinosus origin is partly tendinous and can be easily mistaken for the sciatic nerve or vice versa. When one is certain of the location of the sciatic nerve, then the semitendinosus is sectioned. The semimembranosus origin is cut. Use of the electrocautery lessens the bleeding and risk of a hematoma. Continuous suction of the wound is essential for 24–48 hours.

POSTOPERATIVE CARE

Hip spica plasters have not been used for postoperative immobilization. Instead bilateral long-leg plasters connected with a stick, to abduct each hip 40°–45° has been sufficient for 3 weeks. Alternatively, hip-abduction braces with adjustable hinges allow for titration of abduction to an appropriate comfort level for the child. After plaster or brace removal, an abduction pillow splint or a triangular abduction wedge splint can be used for 10–12 weeks at night while the postoperative scar matures (although night splinting has not been routine). In small children (age 18 months to 3 years) who did not have hamstring spasticity or contracture the pillow hip-abduction splint seemed quite adequate. But the number of cases who qualified for this sort of postoperative management is too small to give a data-based result. Hip-abduction wedges in the wheelchair seat are routine. Early mobilization of the hip and knee joints with gentle and regular passive exercise allows an early return to comfortable sitting and resumption of functional goals. The hot-tub whirlpool at home (comparable to those used in many health clubs and modern hotels for the 'tired executive') has been the single most valuable relaxation and mobility device for these total body involved children.

SUBLUXATION OF THE HIP AND ACETABULAR DYSPLASIA OVER AGE 5 YEARS

GENERAL CONSIDERATIONS

Barrie and Galasko (1996) of Manchester, UK, found that in 67 total body involved patients with 86 hips that 'soft-tissue release alone led to recurrence of dislocation or subluxation in many

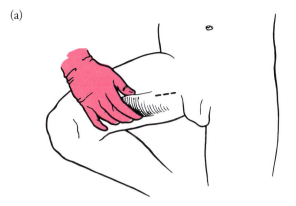

(a)

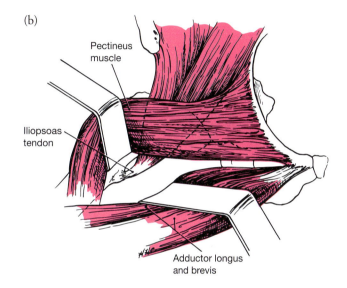

(b)

Pectineus muscle

Iliopsoas tendon

Adductor longus and brevis

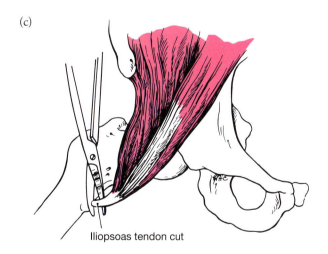

(c)

Iliopsoas tendon cut

Fig. 9.26. (*a*) Medial proximal thigh approach for iliopsoas tenotomy. Incision over the adductor longus. (*b*) Adductor longus, brevis and pectineus muscle retracted to expose the iliopsoas tendon insertion on the lesser trochanter. (*c*) Iliopsoas tendon isolated, cut and allowed to retract proximally.

patients and has been abandoned.' In their description, it appears that the 16 'releases' were of the adductor muscles and of these eight also had anterior branch obturator neurectomies. Only one had an iliopsoas transfer. The mean age of surgery was 6.3

years. The failure of the 'soft-tissue' surgery convinced them that the combined pelvic and femoral osteotomies with 'soft-tissue release' corrected the migration percentage better than with femoral osteotomy and soft-tissue release alone.

The indications for a femoral osteotomy and acetabular reconstruction in addition to the adductor tenomyotomies and iliopsoas tenotomy are age-related. Our data (Kalen and Bleck 1985) suggest that iliopsoas tenotomy to prevent dislocation is less successful after age 5 years. Remember, however, that skeletal and developmental ages may lag a year or two behind normal children (Horstmann 1986). In all children under age 6 or 7 years' skeletal age, the surgeon might wait for a year or two after tenotomies and myotomies to determine whether or not additional bone surgery will be required. Reimers (1992) documented improved acetabular angles in 21 of 31 hips that had femoral osteotomies after the age of 4 years. Surprising improvement in the acetabular angle was recorded in a follow-up of 4–7 years in three who had the operation at age less than 10 years and even in three older than 10 years. Reimers's message was that in his 28 quadriplegic patients hip stability was achieved with femoral osteotomy alone. Acetabuloplasty was not needed.

In all children under age 6 or 7 years' skeletal age, the surgeon can wait for a year or two after tenotomies and myotomies to determine whether or not additional bone surgery will be required.

FEMORAL OSTEOTOMY

The femoral varus-derotation osteotomy is primarily correction of excessive femoral anteversion (torsion), although the common operation continues to include with the title, 'varus'. The procedure has been used by many surgeons (Eilert and MacEwen 1977, Tylkowski *et al.* 1980, Steeger and Wunderlich 1982, Horstmann and Rosabal 1984, Vanderbrink *et al.* 1984, Bunnell 1985, Roye *et al.* 1990, Herndon *et al.* 1992, Reimers 1992, Bagg *et al.* 1993, Parent *et al.* 1994, Brunner and Baumann 1997, Hau *et al.* 2000, Settecerri and Karol 2000, Noonan *et al.* 2001).

An exception to the enthusiasm for varus-derotation femoral osteotomy was expressed by Brunner and Baumann (1997) in their review of 63 hips in 45 patients followed for 11–18 years. Patients younger than age 4 years had a 96% loss of correction of the neck-shaft angle and a 42% loss of the anteversion angle. The result was insufficient coverage of the femoral head in subluxation and dislocation as measured by the center-edge angles. Additional surgery was adductor 'elongation' or 'transfer'. *The iliopsoas was not addressed.* They concluded that because 'osseus correction on the femur in cerebral palsy deteriorates more rapidly the younger the patient and the more severe spasticity at the time of surgery, corrective operations should be postponed until the age of 8–10 years'. An important conclusion was that hip-adductor weakening had no effect as an adjunct to derotation-varus osteotomy on the neck-shaft angle or the femoral anteversion angle or centralizing the femoral head in the acetabulum. The oversight of not lengthening the iliopsoas at the time of the osteotomy and the effect on preventing further

subluxation and dislocation is significant in the report of these Swiss orthopaedic surgeons. Only eight of their 45 patients were younger than 4 years. A year later, Brunner (1998), had much better results with 'iliopsoas' transfer together with the femoral and pelvic osteotomies.

Varus derotation femoral osteotomy has not always been successful in correcting subluxation or preventing dislocation of the hip. Noonan *et al.* (2001) reported that in 65 patients who had 79 femoral osteotomies in an average follow-up of 5.2 years, three were dislocated, 19 had subluxation and 57% were stable (Fig. 9.27).

Although the varus component of the osteotomy seems important to many surgeons, coxa valga is a radiographic artifact, a shadow on the anterior–posterior radiograph, due to the one-dimensional projection of antetorsion of the head and neck rather than actual valgus of the femoral neck.[13] The major correction is derotation of the femur. The osteotomy should restore the femoral neck angle to about 135° and femoral anteversion to 15°–30°. Too much varus in the femoral neck will create an adduction deformity of the hip.

That coxa valga is not a major component of the spastic paralytic hip is the detailed radiographic study of 215 patients with cerebral palsy by Laplaza and Root (1994). Femoral anteversion angles in independent and non-walkers were beyond the normal in both groups (42°–43°, SD 9.7°–11.7°); the neck-shaft angles were within a normal range of 139°–143° (SD 6.5°–7.6°). Additional analysis of these angles according to the center-edge angle and the migration index do not appear significant. The message of the study is that excessive femoral anteversion as 'persistence of the femoral fetal geometry' is the major deformity rather than the radiographic appearance of coxa valga.

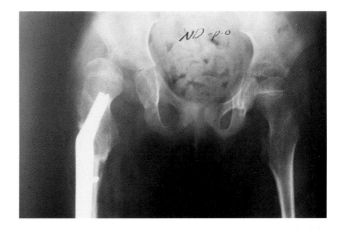

Fig. 9.27. Radiograph. Subtrochanteric femoral osteotomy failed to reduce subluxation of the hip. Iliopsoas tenotomy/recession must always be included with the femoral osteotomy.

13 One way to appreciate the true neck shaft angle is to make the anterior–posterior radiograph with the hip in maximum internal rotation. Internal rotation of the femur will allow a measurement of the neck-shaft angle within 10° (Kay *et al.* 2000).

Coxa valga is a radiographic artifact, a shadow on the anterior–posterior radiograph, due to the one-dimension projection of antetorsion of the head and neck rather than actual valgus of the femoral neck.

Surgeons of the Hôpital St Vincent de Paul, Paris (Parent *et al.* 1994), modified the varus osteotomy by medial displacement of the distal fragment and fixation with a 100° Synthes blade plate. They created extreme varus with a mean neck-shaft angle of 104.5°, i.e. coxa vara. At follow-up two hips of 39 redislocated in the postoperative period and one hip dislocated on the longer follow-up despite a Chiari pelvic osteotomy. In their description of the operative procedure no mention was made of iliopsoas or adductor tenotomy. The message is that a varus osteotomy, even extreme, to 'cover' the hip on the one-dimensional anterior–posterior radiograph as imagined is not successful.

As with derotation osteotomy for hip-internal rotation gait, the derotation must not be overdone; a residual passive range of 20°–30° of internal rotation is more functional even when sitting. A contemporary adage might apply here: 'Nothing exceeds like excess.' For normal external rotation of the pelvis, a range of internal rotation of the femur is necessary. With secure internal fixation the range of passive hip rotation in flexion and extension can be assessed before wound closure. Radiographic measurements of the degree of femoral anterversion are not necessary.

Various internal fixation devices for the osteotomy have been recommended (Bleck 1979, Greene 1985, Alonso *et al.* 1986). A more recent innovation was the modified Richards' intermediate hip screw to improve the stability of the fixation (Wilkinson *et al.* 2001). With this screw only 16% of the patients who had a femoral osteotomy required plaster casts. However, orthopaedic surgeons from Wilkinson's institution in Victoria, Australia, found little difference in complications between the Synthes 90° fixed-angle blade plate and the Richards intermediate hip screw (Hau *et al.* 2000) Both devices were effective.

Increasingly, femoral osteotomy has been combined with pelvic osteotomies and iliopsoas and adductor lengthening as a single stage procedure in patients who had either subluxation or dislocation (Mubarak *et al.* 1992, Onimus *et al.* 1992, Brunner and Baumann 1994, Atar *et al.* 1995, Jerosch *et al.* 1995, Root *et al.* 1995, Barrie and Galasko 1996, Gordon *et al.* 1996, Miller *et al.* 1997, Brunner 1998, Song and Carroll 1998, Knelles *et al.* 1999, McNerney *et al.* 2000, Wu *et al.* 2001).

COMPLICATIONS OF FEMORAL OSTEOTOMY
Complications of femoral osteotomy in 79 children with cerebral palsy included 16 who had 25 fractures, decubitus ulcers in five (Stasikelis *et al.* 1999). All fractures healed uneventfully with casts or splints. More complications occurred in non-ambulatory patients (66 %) compared with only one of 13 ambulatory patients.

Epiphyseal changes in postoperative radiographic examinations 'suggestive' of avascular necrosis were found in 10% of the hips that had only a femoral osteotomy and in 46% of the hips that had a pelvic osteotomy at the same time (Stasikelis *et al.* 2001). The radiographic findings of avascular necrosis were a subchondral radiolucency (fracture) of the femoral head, a change in shape of the head, an increased radiodensity, or coxa magna. As devastating as this complication seems, it was 'of little clinical consequence' according to the investigators. No surgical techniques or patient characteristics could be ascertained as causative factors of the suggestive radiographic findings of avascular necrosis after femoral or pelvic osteotomies. This interesting study should alleviate the anxiety of surgeons who have enough to worry about when doing surgery of the hip in patients with cerebral palsy.

Heterotopic ossification about the hip after femoral osteotomy was diagnosed in four of eight patients with spastic quadriplegia and a prior selective posterior rhizotomy (Payne and DeLuca 1993). No heterotopic ossification occurred in 118 hips of 69 patients who did not have a selective posterior rhizotomy or in seven patients with spastic diplegia who did have a selective posterior rhizotomy. In another study of postoperative heterotopic ossification, 21 had mild degrees of it, but in two or five patients who had both hip and spine surgery it was severe.

Lee *et al.* (1992) documented heterotopic ossification around the hip in two patients after bilateral adductor 'releases' and one after spinal fusion but at a site unrelated to the surgery. Krum and Miller (1993) documented mild to moderate heterotopic ossification in 21 of 61 children who hip adductor lengthening. In two of five patients who had concomitant spinal fusions, heterotopic ossification was so severe that hip fusion occurred. An unusual occurrence of heterotopic ossification caused ankylosis of the non-operated hip in a 15-year-old male with spastic quadriplegia after a unilateral adductor tenotomy (Ushmann and Bennett 1999). McHale (1991) had one case of bilateral spontaneous arthrodesis of the hips in a child after bilateral shelf augmentations and femoral varus osteotomies (Fig. 9.28). Kalen and Gamble (1984) reported a very high incidence of heterotopic ossification in 89% and ankylosis in 28% of proximal femoral resections for a chronic painful dislocated hip (Fig. 9.29).

Heterotopic ossification was found to be a common occurrence after total hip replacements in adults without cerebral palsy. In 100 consecutive patients it occurred in 21% (Brooker *et al.* 1973). From this experience a classification of the ectopic bone was formulated (Table 9.II). Unless ankylosis of the hip resulted, there was no compromise of the functional result. The four classes of ossification might lend some precision in describing the degree of postoperative new bone formation about the hip.

There are two choices for prevention of heterotopic ossification postoperatively in orthopaedic surgery: oral non-steroidal anti-inflammatory agents or single dose radiation.

Indomethacin. The medical literature supports the oral administration of indomethacin for prevention of heterotopic ossification in total hip arthroplasty (Dorn *et al.* 1998, Hofmann *et al.* 1999, Burd *et al.* 2001, D'Lima *et al.* 2001). It is also effective in decreasing the incidence of heterotopic ossification in spinal cord injuries (Banovac *et al.* 2001). Most physicians

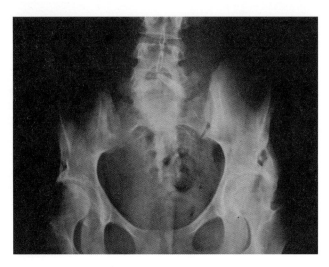

Fig. 9.28. Ankylosis of the left hip due to heterotopic ossification after an acetabular 'shelf' procedure.

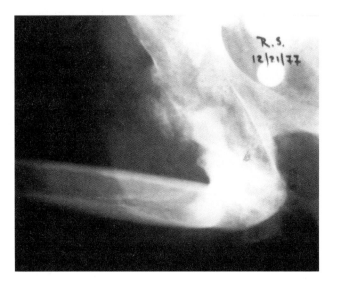

Fig. 9.29. Heterotopic ossification and hip fusion after proximal femoral head and neck resection of dislocated hip in a total body involved patient.

continue its use for 8–14 days; a 3-day administration was ineffective (van der Heide *et al.* 1999).

Among the ineffective non-steroidal anti-inflammatory agents are ibuprofen (Koorevaar *et al.* 1999), and acetylsalicylic acid (Knelles *et al.* 1997). Alternatives to indomethacin reported as effective are celecoxib (Romano *et al.* 2004), and meloxicam

TABLE 9.II
Classification of postoperative heterotopic ossification about the hip
(Brooker *et al.* 1973)

Class I. Islands of bone within the soft tissues.

Class II. Bone spurs from the pelvis or proximal end of the femur with a least 1 cm between the opposing bone surfaces.

Class III. Bone spurs from the pelvis or proximal end of the femur with less than 1 cm between the opposing bone surfaces.

Class IV. Apparent bony ankylosis.

(Legenstein *et al.* 2003). But Bathel and colleagues (2002) of Wurzburg, Germany, found that meloxicam was no more effective than indomethacin (which was 'almost half the price of meloxicam therapy'). Celecoxib as a selective cyclo-oxygenase (COX-2) inhibitor was found to have the same efficacy as indomethacin (Romano *et al.* 2004). Salmon calcitonin was stated by Turkish orthopaedic surgeons to be more effective than indomethacin in 60 adults without cerebral palsy after total hip replacements (Gunal *et al.* 2001). Although both drugs were more effective than the placebo, Naproxen (750 mg/day) was shown to be significantly more effective in preventing heterotopic ossification than indomethacin (75 mg/day) in a French stody of at-risk men undergoing total hip replacement (Vielpeau *et al.* 1999).

Indomethacin or its alternatives appear to be an effective preventative of heterotopic ossification. We wonder why it has not been reported in proximal femoral resections for the salvage of a dislocated painful hip with the very high incidence of heterotopic ossification. Risk factors such as prior heterotopic ossification or hypertrophic arthritis are not usual in the age group of patients with total body involvement who are candidates for salvage surgery of the painful dislocated hip.

Indomethacin or its alternatives appear to be an effective preventative of heterotopic ossification.

The risk of indomethacin and other like non-steroidal anti-inflammatory agents is primarily gastrointestinal bleeding. Other adverse effects are listed among which are central nervous system symptoms so that patients who have epilepsy should not be given the drug. An alarming side-effect was psychosis in one patient and three others reported in the pharmacologic literature (Nassif and Ritter 1999).

Radiation. Radiotherapy postoperatively has been known for a long time as a preventative for heterotopic ossification. Ashton *et al.* (2000) of Concord, Australia, had 20 patients who had a single fraction radiotherapy after total hip-replacements. They selected patients on the basis of risk factors: previous heterotopic ossification and bilateral hypertrophic arthritis. 60% also were given a 13-day course of indomethacin.

A comparative study of radiation or indomethacin following total hip replacement by orthopaedic surgeons of the Scripps Clinic (La Jolla, California) found that indomethacin was equal in effectiveness to radiation in low to moderate risk for heterotopic ossification. They made the point of cost effectiveness, i.e. the patient-billed cost of radiation was $1400 versus approximately $100 for the course of indomethacin (D'Lima *et al.* 2001). Another study compared localized irradiation with indomethacin following surgery of acetabular fractures (Burd *et al.* 2001). They found no significant difference in Brooker grade III or IV ossification (7% in the treated group and 38% in those not receiving prophylaxis). Radiotherapy is an alternative measure for patients who cannot tolerate indomethacin or similar compounds.

BLADDER INFECTION AND HETEROTOPIC OSSIFICATION—A THEORY

Based on the experimental transplantation of bladder epithelium to the anterior rectus sheath of dogs with the induction of ossification and bone formation by Huggins (1931). Bleck (1962) in an experimental tissue culture protocol hypothesized that when bladder epithelium was actively growing as replacement due to infection some molecular compound might be released to the circulation to induce heterotopic ossification. Bleck speculated that the coincidence of a high rate of heterotopic ossification in spinal cord injury paraplegia, spina bifida (21.6%) and in cerebral palsy (8.6%) (Bouchard and D'Astous 1991) could be associated with chronic bladder infections known to occur frequently in such patients.

Bladder infections are more common in cerebral palsy than we usually suppose (6.9%, Drigo *et al.* 1988, Moulin *et al.* 1998). Incontinence occurs in an estimated one-third of patients with cerebral palsy (Decter *et al.* 1987, Borzyskowski 1989). Accordingly, to prevent heterotopic ossification after limb surgery in paralytic patients, it might be reasonable to sterilize the urine with an injectable gram negative sensitive antibiotic just prior to the operation. Gram-negative bacterial infections are common: E. coli, Pseudomonas and Enterococcus (Moulin *et al.* 1998). Certainly urine cultures in would be in order. Further research in the induction of the heterotopic ossification is needed.

ACETABULAR DYSPLASIA

Acetabular dysplasia in children older than the skeletal age of 4 years is not likely to self-correct with growth as in congenital dislocation of this hip after femoral osteotomy (Harris *et al.* 1975). However, in spastic paralytic dislocations one could wait a year or two after femoral osteotomies with iliopsoas and adductor tenomyotomies have been performed between the ages of 5 and 7 years. Tylkowski *et al.* (1980) found no acetabular remodeling after femoral osteotomies in children older than 8 years. The mean age of the combined iliopsoas and adductor tenotomies, femoral and pelvic osteotomies in the series reported ranged from 5 to 12 years.

RADIOGRAPHIC MEASUREMENTS

Radiographic assessment using the plain anterior–posterior view of the pelvis and hips and a *faux profil* ('false view') of the hips, as well as anterior–posterior views with the hips in abduction and internal rotation have been advised (Gillingham *et al.* 1999). The frog-leg lateral projection would be difficult in cerebral palsy due to the usual contracture of the adductor muscles. 3D CT will give a more comprehensive view of the abnormal skeletal anatomy.

Shenton's line can be assessed but not measured. The acetabular sourcil (from the French for 'eyebrow') is a smooth curvature of dense subchondral bone in the lateral acetabulum indicative of asymmetric loading of the hip joint (Gillingham *et al.* 1999). The most useful measurements are the acetabular index in children and the acetabular angle in adults. In infants

and children the index is the angle formed by the intersection of a line (Helgenreiner's horiztonal line) through the triradiate cartilage and the edge of the acetabulum (Hensinger 1986, Scoles *et al.* 1987); in adults the angle is that formed by the horizontal line is through the tips of the obturator tear shadows (the U) and the line drawn from the obturator tear-drop to the edge of the acetabulum (Sharp 1961). The normal acetabular angle ('index') in children after 24 months is less than 24º and in adults the angle is less than 43º. Although the radiograph may be made to distort the true angle, bad positioning will account to no more than 4º in variation (Sharp 1961). But to be reasonably accurate the anterior–posterior projection should be made with minimal rotation of the pelvis so that the width of the obturator foramina are in a ratio of 1:1 (Fig. 9.30).

SALTER INNOMINATE OSTEOTOMIES: SINGLE, DOUBLE, TRIPLE

Inasmuch as the posterior acetabulum is most often deficient in paralytic dislocations (Coleman 1983, Lau *et al.* 1986), innominate osteotomies that rotate the pelvis anteriorly and laterally do not seem logical. These are the single innominate osteotomy of Salter (1961), the double one of Sutherland and Greenfield (1977), and the triple type of Steel (1977). Molloy (1986) had good results in both flaccid and spastic paralytic subluxation or dislocation of the hip with the Salter innominate osteotomy combined with a femoral osteotomy and transiliac transfer of the iliopsoas posteriorly. Eight patients had cerebral palsy and 10 myelomeningocele. She found no differences in the results between these two groups.

The Salter innominate osteotomy has some biomechanical limits. Whether if will be sufficient to contain the femoral head in the acetabulum can be determined with preoperative radiographic examination. The hip is held in 25º of flexion, neutral rotation, 10º abduction and the x-ray beam directed 25º posteriorly and caudally to the coronal plane (Rab 1978, 1981b).

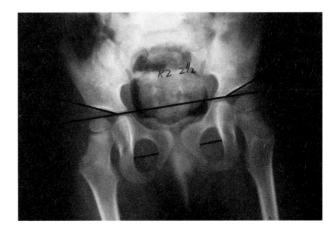

Fig. 9.30. Anterior–posterior radiograph of the hips and pelvis. To measure acetabular angles with reasonable accuracy there should be no pelvic rotation. The widths of the obturator foramina should be equal.

PEMBERTON ILIAC OSTEOTOMY

The Pemberton iliac osteotomy in paralytic subluxation of the hip and acetabular dysplasia has had favorable results by some surgeons (Coleman 1983, Barry and Staheli 1986, Hoffer 1986). In a follow-up study of 30 subluxated hips in children, age 23 months to 12 years, with either cerebral palsy or myelomeningocele, Barry and Staheli (1986) had satisfactory results at the time of evaluation at an average of 4 years (range 2–9 years) postoperatively.

Because the Pemberton iliac osteotomy depends upon the flexibility of the triradiate cartilage when prying down the roof of the acetabulum, the operation is most satisfactory in children at or under age 7 years (Pemberton 1965, Eyre-Brook *et al.* 1978) (Fig. 9.31). However, age 8–9 years is probably not too old. Again age is relative and depends upon the skeletal maturity of the child.

PERICAPSULAR ACETABULOPLASTY

The pericapsular acetabuloplasty devised by Dega (1974) is preferred by Mubarak and colleagues (1992) and modified as part of the combined procedure to reduce the dislocated hip. It includes femoral shortening at the subtrochanteric level as well as the varus-derotation osteotomy at the same site (Figs 9.32, 9.33).

CHIARI ILIAC OSTEOTOMY

In more skeletally mature children over age 10 years and certainly in adolescents, the Chiari iliac osteotomy seems the easiest and most effective operation (Chiari 1974, Bailey and Hall 1985). The Chiari osteotomy was abandoned by Mubarak *et al.* (1992) in younger patients who had a bone age of less than 12 years. Their reason was that the acetabular cartilage at these younger ages can be saved by hinging at the triradiate cartilage. Bleck (1987) preferred the Chiari osteotomy in the combined procedures in the skeletally mature patient who had a dislocated hip. In 31 established dislocations followed from 2 to 14 years, 26 hips remained reduced and only one that had the Chiari osteotomy redislocated, and one that had a Salter innominate osteotomy redislocated (Gamble *et al.* 1990). The other three patients did not have a pelvic osteotomy to correct the acetabular dysplasia.

PERIACETABULAR OSTEOTOMY
(GANZ *ET AL.* 1988)

The Ganz (1988) osteotomy from Berne, Switzerland, can be done only after skeletal maturity because it crosses the triradiate cartilage. It is indicated primarily for older adolescent or young adult patients who have dysplastic hips (Trousdale *et al.* 1995, Gillingham *et al.* 1999). Its use in cerebral palsy has not been established and is unlikely to be used for dislocation or subluxation in the total body involved patient. For a non-walking or limited walking patient it seems a bit much to do the extensive reorientation of the acetabulum with osteotomies through the pubis, ilium and ischium. It is mentioned here for completeness. It might be considered the ambulatory adult with spastic diplegia

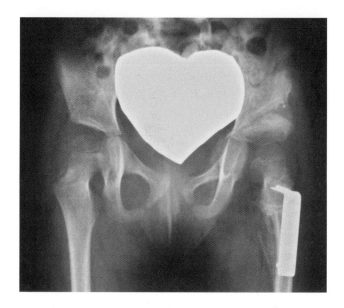

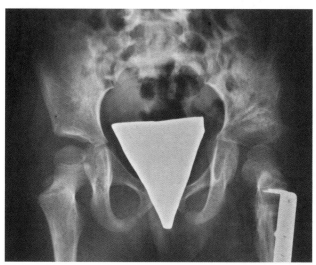

Fig. 9.31. Radiograph. Correction of acetabular dysplasia in total body involved with Pemberton pelvic osteotomy and derotation subtrochanteric femoral osteotomy.

who has a painful early degenerative joint disease due to long standing subluxation. Of course, it would need to be accompanied by partial release or lengthening of the deforming forces—the iliopsoas and the adductor muscles.

ACETABULAR COVERAGE: WHICH PROCEDURE GIVES THE BEST RESULTS?

The reports in the literature do not unequivocally support any particular operation to ensure acetabular coverage of the femoral head. Pope *et al.* (1994) reviewed three types of pelvic osteotomies, the Salter, the Steel and the Chiari, in 21 patients that included 12 with total body involvement. The mean age at the time of surgery was 10.6 years. Generally all improved in the center-edge angles, neck-shaft angles, and the migration percentage. Resubluxation occurred in four patients: three had Chiari osteotomies and one had bilateral Salter osteotomies. Two patients had advanced degenerative joint changes with pain. The

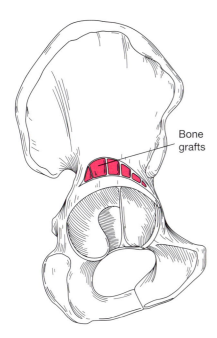

Bone grafts

Fig. 9.32. Dega pericapsular pelvic osteotomy. Bone grafts from the iliac crest keep the osteotomy open to correct the shallow acetabular roof. (Redrawn from Flynn and Miller 2002, by permission.)

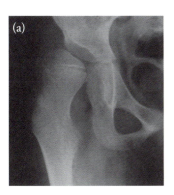 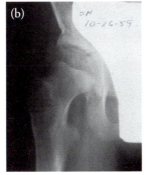

Fig. 9.33. (*a*) Radiograph. Patient SH. Spastic diplegia. Crutch dependent. Age 8 years. Subluxation of right hip. (*b*) Radiograph, Patient SH. Age 11 years, 6 months, 3.5 years postoperative iliopsoas recession, adductor longus myotenotomy, anterior branch obturator neurectomy, varus derotation subtrochanteric femoral osteotomy and Dega acetabuloplasty.

number of patients is so small that no definite conclusion can be made as to the efficacy of one procedure over the other.

Dietz and Knutson (1995) evaluated their results of Chiari osteotomies in patients with cerebral palsy who had subluxation or dislocation. They did the operation without femoral osteotomies. In a follow-up of more than 7 years, 79% were painless. A migration index equal to or greater than 30% was found in 29%. The authors suggested that their results would be better if they had done femoral osteotomies or 'alternative acetabular procedures'. Their conclusion leads to the need for a combined operative approach to spastic paralytic subluxation or dislocation of the hip.

It seems reasonable to state that for children under the age of 12 years, or with an open triradiate cartilage, the modified

Dega is apt to give the best results. When the triradiate cartilage is closed, the Chiari iliac osteotomy in the total body involved patient seems satisfactory *but only when femoral osteotomies, iliopsoas and adductor tenotomy are included in a one stage operation.*

For children under the age of 12 years, the modified Dega procedure is apt to give the best results. When the triradiate cartilage is closed, the Chiari iliac osteotomy in the total body involved patient seems satisfactory.

OPERATIVE TECHNIQUE OF VARUS DEROTATION SUBTROCHANTERIC OSTEOTOMY (FIG. 9.34)

Preoperative templating of hip x-rays with the true neck-shaft angle is imperative. The neck-shaft angle is usually around 140º but appears higher due to rotation. The true neck-shaft angle can be determined under image intensification by rotating the hip internally to compensate for the anteversion. Appropriately sized instrumentation for internal fixation is chosen based on these measurements. The proper level for the osteotomy is critical to the proper use of the instrumentation. Confirmation of these measurements and the surgical plan can be done by fluoroscopic examination of the hips just prior to surgical incision. Surgery can be done with the patient either prone or supine. Each has its benefits, especially regarding what other surgery needs to be done.

Surgery starts with adductor tenotomies and, if needed, anterior branch obturator neurectomy and iliopsoas tenotomy. When indicated, a proximal hamstring myotomy through the medial groin approach (as previously described) is done. Alternatively an over-the-pelvic-brim intramuscular lengthening of the psoas can be utilized if retention of optimal hip-flexor power is of concern, particularly in ambulators (Novacheck *et al.* 2002)

Varus osteotomy is then done, starting with a longitudinal incision along the lateral aspect of the proximal femur distal to the flare of the greater trochanter. Its length should be about the same as the blade plate being used.

Next, under radiographic fluoroscopic control, a guide pin is introduced from below the greater trochanter into the head and neck of the femur and checked for position in both planes. If a Synthes cannulated 90º angle blade plate is used to obtain a desired 120º end neck-shaft angle, the pin is inserted on the AP image to allow the axis of the head and neck to be 30º over the pin placement (Fig. 9.34 *a*). This should be inferior in the neck but above the calcar. On the lateral X-ray the guide pin should be placed centrally (Fig. 9.34 *b*).

The cannulated chisel is put in over the guide wire in neutral, i.e. perpendicular to the femoral shaft, taking care to monitor rotation to avoid unwanted flexion or extension. Appropriate depth can be gauged from the guide pin and the optimally sized plate chosen from this measurement. The amount of derotation can be monitored by scoring the femoral shaft longitudinally prior to osteotomy or derotation pins can be put in above and below the osteotomy site. The proximal osteotomy using a power saw is done first, parallel to the osteotomy plate just distal to

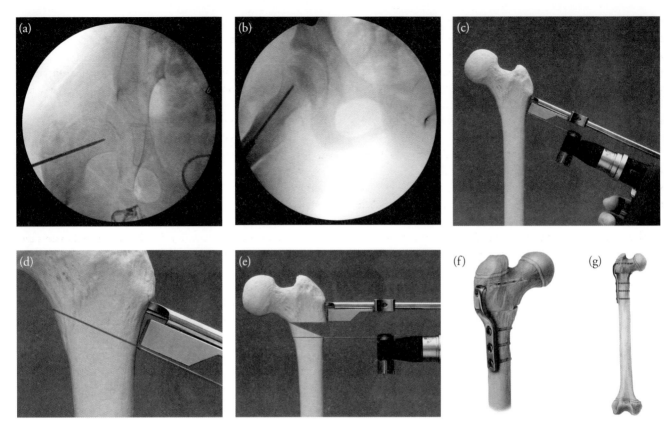

Fig. 9.34. Varus osteotomy for Synthes cannulated pediatric osteotomy system. (*a*) Image intensification view of pin placement in AP, inferior in the neck and above the calcar. (*b*) In the lateral view pin should appear central in the neck. (*c*) The cannulated chisel is inserted over the guide pin with the chisel guide aligned with the femoral shaft so as not to create flexion or extension. (*d*) The first osteotomy cut is parallel to the saw guide to end just below the femoral neck. (*e*) The second cut is perpendicular to the femoral shaft. The distal femur should be derotated or shortened as indicated prior to plate fixation. (*f*) The plate is inserted in the track of the chisel and held in desired position with a clamp with the osteotomy site coapted. Oblique of plate with dynamic compression screws in place after the osteotomy. (*g*) AP of femur with Synthes Cannulated Pediatric Osteotomy Plate in place. Reproduced from Synthes 2003, by permission.)

the saw guide, below the femoral neck and perpendicular to the longitudinal axis of the femoral shaft (Fig. 9.34 *c*, *d*). The cannulated chisel is then levered into varus and the distal osteotomy is made perpendicular to the femoral shaft to remove a medially based wedge of bone (Fig. 9.34 *e*). If femoral shortening is desirable, it should be done at this time. In a subluxated or dislocated hip this may be 1–2 cm. If the osteotomy is being done only to correct rotational malalignment, no shortening may be needed. The end result of derotation should allow both internal and external passive rotation but normalize previous pathology.

Most modern hip-compression plates have offset holes to allow compression without the use of a special compression device. After removal of the guide pin and chisel, the blade is gently pushed down the track made by the chisel and the plate is fixed to the femoral shaft with a bone clamp. Then cortical dynamic compression screws are used to fix the plate to the femoral shaft (Fig 9.34 *f*, *g*). Instrumentation continues to improve so it is important to consult the manufacturer's technical guides for exact details and recommendations prior to surgery. The Synthes Cannulated Pediatric Osteotomy System screw medializes the femoral shaft slightly, resulting in better biomechanical configuration and preventing a wide gap at

the perineal level. With the surfaces coapted by the plate and compression screws there should be adequate stability. Casting or postoperative bracing may be useful to maintain hip reduction or decrease pain from movement. When hip reduction is not an issue, weightbearing can be started as long as fixation is stable.

Iliac osteotomies can be done at the same time. A separate oblique incision beginning 1–2 cm medial and 1.5 cm distal to the anterior superior iliac spine and continued laterally 1 cm distal to the mid-portion of the iliac crest usually affords sufficient exposure for these osteotomies. (In complete dislocation of the hip one single incision for both the femoral and iliac osteotomies as described in the next section is used.)

PERICAPSULAR ILIAC OSTEOTOMY OPERATIVE TECHNIQUE (PEMBERTON)

As in the Salter osteotomy, a transverse incision beginning medial to the anterior superior iliac spine and carried laterally over the anterior two-thirds of the ilium gives adequate exposure (Pemberton 1965, Coleman 1978). The usual anterior iliofemoral exposure of the lateral aspect of the ilium is then made after subcutaneous reflection of the skin. The sartorius is sectioned at its origin and retracted distally. With a sharp elevator or an osteotome, the cartilaginous apophysis of the ilium is peeled off the crest and reflected medially. The iliacus muscle is easily dissected subperiosteally to expose the inner wall of the ilium. The gluteus medius is similarly stripped from the outer wall. Blunt retractors are placed on both sides of the ilium against the bone circumscribing the sciatic notch. The anterior aspect of the ilium is stripped to the origin of the rectus femoris muscle. The attachment of the capsule of the hip joint is exposed anteriorly and laterally.

The osteotomy of the outer wall of the ilium is curvilinear and parallels the capsule; it begins at the anterior inferior iliac spine just above the reflected head of the rectus femoris. The bone is cut posteriorly and inferiorly toward (but not into) the triradiate cartilage. The posterior cut is directed anterior to the sciatic notch and posterior to the hip-joint edge. The inner wall cut is made in the same line, and usually inferior to the outer wall cut, in order to provide more lateral coverage in the case of the paralytic dysplastic acetabulum.

The two cuts in the ilium are joined with a curved osteotome as far as the triradiate cartilage. The inferior portion of the cut ilium is then rotated laterally with a lamina spreader between the two osteotomized segments. With a small gouge, grooves are made in the opposing two slabs of the ilium. These help stabilize the bone graft, which is cut from the anterior–superior aspect of the ilium above the anterior–inferior iliac spine. The graft is wedged into place to hold the osteotomy open. No internal fixation is necessary. The image intensifier fluoroscope throughout the procedure with a radiopaque dye in the joint (30% Renografin) can give the surgeon more assurance that the operation has accomplished the correction as intended.

Muscles are reapproximated as usual and the skin closed. Suction drainage should prevent hematoma formation. A ½ spica plaster for 6 weeks is sufficient for bone healing so that early mobilization is possible.

PERICAPSULAR ILIAC OSTEOTOMY–DEGA (1974) MODIFIED, OPERATIVE TECHNIQUE (MUBARAK ET AL. 1992)

After an adductor tenotomy and psoas tenotomy through a medial approach the acetabuloplasty is begun. A modified Smith-Peterson anterior curvilinear longitudinal incision is made parallel to the iliac crest and avoiding the injury to the lateral femoral cutaneous nerve. The iliac apophysis is elevated from the crest of the iliac wing. The muscles are bluntly stripped subperiosteally from the iliac wing. The hip joint capsule is swept clean and the reflected and direct heads of the rectus femoris are cut and reflected distally. The capsule is opened with a T-shape incision with the bottom of the T going down the femoral neck. The capsular edges are secured with non-absorbable number 1 sutures for use in closure later. The ligamentum teres is resected and the transverse acetabular ligament divided. The joint is cleared of the fibrofatty tissue. The femoral head is inspected for the integrity of the articular cartilage in cases of dislocation to ascertain whether or not to reduce the hip. If more than 50% of the articular cartilage is damaged, resection of the femoral head or valgus osteotomy should be done instead of a reduction.

At this point a varus shortening derotation osteotomy can be done as described earlier to allow reduction of the femoral head.

The pelvic osteotomy is done under image intensification. A straight osteotome, about 1.5 cm wide, is used to start the osteotomy at 0.5–1 cm above the acetabular edge.

A straight osteotome, 1.3–1.9 cm wide makes a cut 0.5–1.0 cm above the acetabulum in a line from the anterior inferior iliac spine to the sciatic notch. The osteotomy is completed from the lateral cortex but *not through* the medial wall of the pelvis. Both cortices (the corners) should be cut at the anterior inferior iliac spine and the sciatic notch with a large Kerrison rongeur (Fig. 9.35).

The next cut is made with a 1.9–2.5 cm curved osteotome guided by the image-intensifier fluoroscope. This osteotome cuts halfway between the articular surface and the inner pelvic cortex. Only the outer cortex is cut medially and distally to the triradiate cartilage. Gentle downward pressure with the osteotome or a smooth laminar spreader opens the osteotomy 1.0–1.5 cm (Fig. 9.36).

Next a bicortical bone graft is obtained from the anterior superior iliac crest and shaped into three or four small triangles. These triangular grafts are placed in the pelvic osteotomy site. The

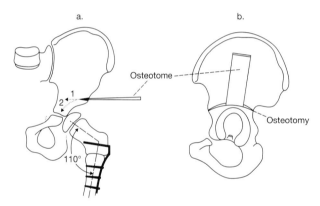

Fig. 9.35. Modified Dega. Direction of the osteotomy cuts. Note the elliptical shape of the dysplastic acetabulum in (*b*). (Redrawn from Mubarak *et al.* 1992, by permission of the *Journal of Bone and Joint Surgery.*)

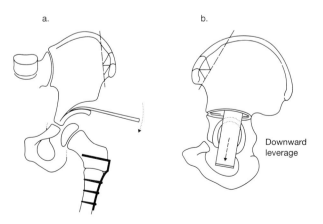

Fig. 9.36. Downward leverage to open the osteotomy without violating the triradiate cartilage. (Redrawn from Mubarak *et al.* 1992, by permission of the *Journal of Bone and Joint Surgery.*)

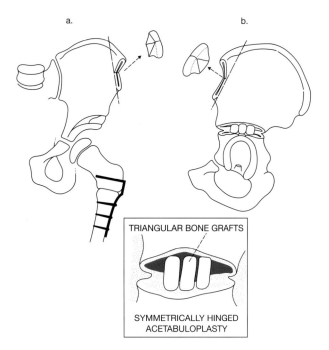

Fig. 9.37. Triangular bone grafts from the iliac crest complete the acetaboplasty. (Redrawn from Mubarak *et al.* 1992, by permission of the *Journal of Bone and Joint Surgery.*)

largest graft is placed where maximum coverage of the head is wanted (usually superiorly). Equal-size grafts anteriorly to posteriorly allow symmetrical hinging of the acetabulum at the triradiate cartilage so that posterior coverage of the femoral head is assured. The wedges of graft are close to each other to prevent collapse, rotation or displacement. Thus no fixation pins are necessary (Fig. 9.37).

The capsule is closed and skin closure is usual. Intraoperative radiographs document the correction of the acetabular angle usually from a preoperative mean of 30° to a postoperative mean of 14°. A high spica cast is applied. In planned sequentially staged bilateral procedures, the cast is removed 2 weeks after the first operation. After the second hip surgery the cast is left on for 6 weeks, changed under anesthesia and an above-the-knee hip-spica cast applied and used for another 4 weeks. The position of the hip in the cast is 45° of flexion and 30° of abduction to allow sitting.

PROBLEMS WITH PERICAPSULAR PELVIC OSTEOTOMIES

TECHNICAL DEMANDS

The Pemberton and modified Dega procedures are more technically demanding than the Chiari iliac osteotomy, acetabular augmentation, or the method of Albee (1915). In Albee's operation the acetabulum was deepened with a semicircular osteotomy of the ilium just above the joint capsule, bent down and secured with tibial bone grafts. Before doing the Pemberton or modified Dega procedure for the first time, the surgeon might practice the operation on a cadaver pelvis or plastic model. But specimens or models that have the triradiate cartilage are rare. No

videotape demonstrations on these pelvic osteotomies are available through the usual resource of the American Academy of Orthopaedic Surgeons (www.aaos.org). Perhaps the best way is the traditional way of 'see one, do one, teach one'.

AGE AND FLEXIBILITY OF THE TRIRADIATE CARTILAGE

As pointed out by Coleman (1978), one disadvantage of the Pemberton osteotomy is that it is dependent upon the flexibility of the triradiate cartilage which is the hinge on which all the correction depends. The same is true with the Dega modification. Thus it works best in children with a skeletal age of 7 years or younger, and is progressively more difficult to do until it becomes impossible by 10 or 12 years. In the series reported by Mubarak and colleagues (1992), the age range was 5½–13 years (one patient only).

PREMATURE CLOSURE OF TRIRADIATE CARTILAGE

A major pitfall of the Pemberton or Dega osteotomy would be growth arrest of the triradiate cartilage; this would result in a small acetabulum and a larger femoral head, which obviously would not be contained. This problem can be minimized by avoiding entrance into the triradiate cartilage during the procedure. Mubarak *et al.* (1992) had no cases of premature closure of the triradiate cartilage.

EXCESSIVE ANTERIOR DISPLACEMENT OF THE DISTAL SEGMENT

Too much anterior displacement of the distal segment will block hip flexion and uncover the posterior portion of the femoral head in paralytic subluxations. Therefore the displacement of this distal segment should be lateral and equal in both anterior and posterior segments.

POSTOPERATIVE STIFFNESS OF THE HIP

In contrast to the Salter osteotomy, pericapsular pelvic osteotomies can have postoperative stiffness which can persist for several weeks (Bleck 1987). Avoiding more correction than necessary, and restoring the acetabular roof to the more normal angle (15°–20° acetabular angle) may prevent compression of the articular cartilage and resultant limited motion of the hip.

AVASCULAR NECROSIS OF THE FEMORAL HEAD

Avascular necrosis of the femoral heads with subsequent recovery occurred in two cases reported by Mubarak *et al.* (1992). This late complication may be the result of increased pressure on the femoral head, or due to disruption of the medial femoral circumflex artery in the course of iliopsoas tenotomy reported by Manjarris and Mubarak (1984). It might be avoided by confining the exposure of the iliopsoas tendon to its distal 2–3 cm. The artery winds around the medial aspect of the femur between the iliopsoas the pectineus muscles.

This postoperative fracture occurs occasionally. Osteopenia is usual in the total body involved non-walking patient. Other than awareness of the fragility of the bones in these patients, it is not absolutely preventable. Caregivers can inadvertently lift the patient by the legs a patient in a pantaloon spica or after the spica has been removed.[14] Fortunately, these fractures heal with conservative care and without compromising function.

Acetabular augmentation ('shelf procedure') was resurrected and greatly improved in technique by Staheli (1981) for congenital acetabular dysplasia. Zuckerman *et al.* (1984) reported good results from this procedure in subluxation of the hip in cerebral palsy in 17 patients. These orthopaedic surgeons combined acetabular augmentation with additional procedures on 14 hips, including six varus derotation femoral osteotomies and, significantly, one Pemberton iliac osteotomy. No subsequent reports on the efficacy of acetabular augmentation in cerebral palsy can be found. Their institution also had good results with Pemberton iliac osteotomies in paralytic subluxations (Barry and Staheli 1986). Pous (1985) described an ingenious new method of acetabular augmentation by using a vascularized graft of the iliac crest which resulted in immediate stability of the hip in three children with cerebral palsy and subluxation. So there are choices. Most surgeons have reserved acetabular augmentation for congenital acetabular dysplasias, where the round uncovered portion of the femoral head matches that equally round contour of the acetabulum. This is hardly ever the case in cerebral palsy.

HIP DISLOCATION MANAGEMENT

Although it is true that not all dislocated hips in total body involved adolescents are painful (as discovered in an analysis of 3922 patients with cerebral palsy by Gandy and Meyer 1983), we cannot predict which ones will become painful. We can agree that the painless dislocated hip in the skeletally mature patient can be left alone (Fig. 9.38). There is no point in using surgery to produce a painful located hip.

The painless dislocated hip in the skeletally mature patient can be left alone. There is no point in using surgery to produce a painful located hip.

The mean age of dislocation of the hip is about 7 years. Secondary changes occur as the dislocation persists, not only as acetabular development lags but also in the femoral head. The head becomes deformed and the cartilage degenerates as described in Chapter 5 (see Figs 5.11, 5.13). It should be obvious that placing this deformed and degenerated femoral head in the acetabulum would be unwise. If the dislocation is painless in these older mature patients, there is no need for salvage operations, unless performed to enhance sitting and perineal hygiene.

---

14 Caregivers should be instructed to lift the patient with the hands under the buttocks and trunk.

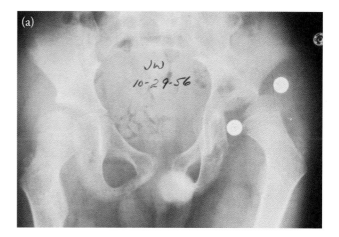

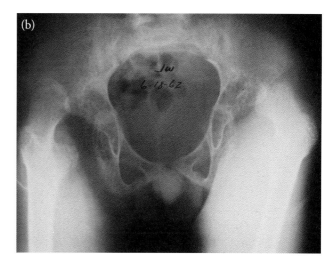

Fig. 9.38. (*a*) Radiograph. Patient JW. Total body involved. Age 12 years. Subluxation of both hips, 50% on right. Bilateral adductor myotenotomies and anterior branch obturator neurectomies done. (*b*) Radiograph. Patient JW. Age 22 years. Both hips dislocated and painless. 10 years postoperative adductor myotenotomies and anterior branch obturator neurectomies.

Given these perspectives and the inability to predict the painful adolescent or adult dislocated hip, then it seems logical to relocate these hips in children before skeletal maturity, preferably under age 12 years. There is no better substitute for a located and stable femoral head in a reconstructed acetabulum. Nor are 'simple' solutions, such as femoral head and neck resection, entirely satisfactory for pain relief (Cristofaro *et al.* 1977, Root 1977a).

In older children with hip dislocation and deformation of the femoral head (flattening of its lateral surface) seen on the radiographic examination, the femoral head is exposed first and inspected. If the articular cartilage is intact then proceed with the entire reconstructive operation (Fig. 9.39). If the cartilage has degenerated, then proceed with a salvage procedure and make no attempt to do an elaborate reconstruction to relocate the femoral head.

The indications to relocate the dislocated hip in children and adolescents before skeletal maturity can be summarized as follows:

1. To prevent a painful hip in adult life; a painful hip can compromise their mobility and render their care more difficult.

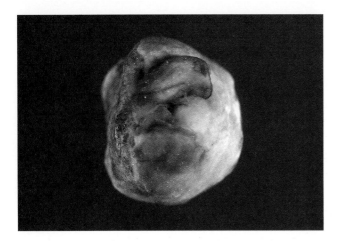

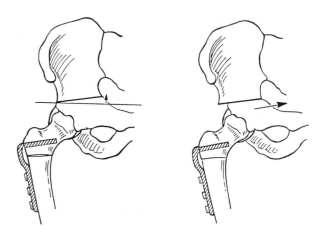

Fig. 9.39. Specimen of femoral head, dislocated hip, total body involved. Articular surface extensively degenerated and destroyed. Before proceeding with operative reduction of the dislocated hip with a femoral shortening and derotation osteotomy, open the joint capsule to inspect the articular surface of the femoral head. If cartilage damage is obvious, do not proceed with the reconstruction. A painful located hip is not a desired result.

Fig. 9.40. One-stage reconstruction for dislocated hip. Note that the inclination of the pelvic osteotomy is no more than 10° superiorly.

2. To prevent and correct severe pelvic obliquity which interferes with sitting balance. However, if the pelvic obliquity is due to concomitant scoliosis, relocating the hip will not correct the pelvic obliquity.

3. To prevent painful bursal formation over the greater trochanter on the dislocated side and over the ischial tuberosity due to pelvic obliquity as the result of the dislocation only (*i.e.* no scoliosis).

4. To prevent and correct severe adduction of the femur that makes perineal hygiene difficult.

DISLOCATED HIP AND SCOLIOSIS
With this combination, the scoliosis should be corrected first, and then followed (if the femoral articular surface is intact) by surgical reconstruction to reduce the dislocation. If the hip is painful in the adolescent and the femoral head obviously deformed, the surgeon can do a resection interposition capsular arthroplasty first and use the femoral head as part of the bone graft in the spinal fusion.

**OPERATIVE PLAN OF
ONE-STAGE RECONSTRUCTION:
HIP DISLOCATION** (Fig. 9.40)

Surgeons from both hemispheres have reported satisfactory long-term results in spastic paralytic dislocations of the hip with several operations done at one stage (Samilson *et al.* 1972, Sherk *et al.* 1983, Gross *et al.* 1984, Root and Brourman 1985, Ibrahim *et al.* 1986, Gamble *et al.* 1990, Mubarak *et al.* 1992, Onimus *et al.* 1992, Atar *et al.* 1995, Jerosch *et al.* 1995, Barrie and Galasko 1996, Gordon *et al.* 1996, Brunner 1998, Jozwiak *et al.* 2000, McNerney *et al.* 2000, Wu *et al.* 2001, de Moraes Barros Fucs *et al.* 2002) as follows:

1. Adductor longus, gracilis myotomy, anterior branch obturator neurectomy and iliopsoas tenotomy.[15] If the hamstring

muscles are contracted, add proximal hamstring myotomy, all this can be done through the medial thigh incision previously described.

2. Capsulotomy to inspect the femoral head before proceeding. As mentioned previously, if the articular cartilage is degenerated, proceed no further and perform a salvage operation.

3. Femoral shortening with a varus derotation subtrochanteric femoral osteotomy and internal fixation (90° hip osteotomy compression nail-plate). Klisiç and Janovic (1976) introduced femoral shortening that greatly facilitated reduction of congenital dislocations of the hip. Femoral shortening alone will not necessarily reduce a dislocated hip as reported by Terjesen and Hellum (1998) of Oslo. Of 16 hips, 11 remained subluxated or dislocated. These Norwegian surgeons opined that the aim of surgery was not reduction of the dislocation, but rather to relief of pain and the improvement of perineal hygiene and sitting function. Most of us now believe it is better to do femoral shortening as a combined procedure to reduce the dislocated hip if the femoral head articular surface is reasonably preserved.

4. Pemberton or modified Dega iliac osteotomy in patients 5–16 years with open triradiate cartilage. Chiari (1974) iliac osteotomy over bone age 13 years with closed triradiate cartilage.

5. Capsulorrhaphy of the hip.

Surgeons from both hemispheres have reported satisfactory long-term results in spastic paralytic dislocations of the hip with several operations done at one stage.

CHIARI ILIAC OSTEOTOMY: OPERATIVE TECHNIQUE

The Chiari iliac osteotomy (1974) alone has been used for painful subluxation and dislocation of the hip in cerebral palsy (Bailey

---

15 I am not certain that a gracilis myotomy is necessary, but it is tradition since it was advocated by Phelps (1959) to prevent spastic subluxation/dislocation of the hip.

and Hall 1985, Grogan *et al.* 1986) but in only three of the five patients was pain relieved and secondary intertrochanteric osteotomies required. Since Chiari of Vienna first described his innovative operation for congenital subluxation of the hip in 1955, a plethora of papers have reported successes, complications, modifications of the technique and biomechanical analyses (Colton 1972, Hoffman *et al.* 1974, Mitchell 1974, Salvati and Wilson 1974, Canale *et al.* 1975, Benson and Evans 1976, Drummond *et al.* 1979, Herold and Daniel 1979, Onimus and Vergnat 1980, Malefijt *et al.* 1982, Betz *et al.* 1988, Delp *et al.* 1990, Dietz and Knutson 1995). In general the results have been good when assessed by the relief of pain. In ambulatory patients with congenital subluxation, a postoperative limp is usual. One issue has been the amount of medial displacement of the distal portion of the osteotomy. Colton (1972) recommended that it be no more than 55%. Salvati and Wilson (1974) contended it should be enough to cover the femoral head completely with the proximal ilium, and Bailey and Hall (1985) would do even a 100% displacement and used a cortical–cancellous bone graft between the two segments in order to achieve anterior femoral head coverage when necessary.

Onimus and Vergnat (1980) said that the iliac osteotomy did not hinge solely on the symphysis pubis, but that both sacroiliac joints moved to cause upward and lateral displacement of the iliac crest; the opposite acetabulum was displaced laterally, while that on the osteotomized side slid medially.

Benson and Evans (1976) used cadaver specimens and found that the sciatic nerve was stretched over the brim of the sciatic notch when displacement occurred. They surmised that when unwanted posterior drift of the distal segment of the osteotomy occurred, it prevented sciatic neuropathy. They also believed that splintering of the bone in the sciatic notch puts the nerve in jeopardy. Their radiographic study suggested that some poor results might be explained by a tendency for the iliac osteotomy to hinge posteriorly at the sciatic notch and open anteriorly like a book. Radiographs may give the illusion that the femoral head is covered.

The important points of the technique of Chiari's osteotomy are: (1) the osteotomy must begin at the margin of the acetabulum—not too far above it or in it; (2) the osteotomy must be ascending and directed no more than 10° cephalad to end in the sciatic notch and not in the sacroiliac joint. A biomechanical analysis of the effects of the Chiari osteotomy showed cephalad inclinations greater than 10° reduced the gluteus medius muscle length and abductor torque; (3) if possible, the osteotomy should be curved slightly posteriorly in order to prevent posterior slippage of the distal segment. Bleck (1987), after observing long follow-ups, found that it did not seem to make much difference in the contour of the acetabulum if the osteotomy was almost straight and not curved (Fig. 9.38). With bone remodeling the curved shape of the shifted ilium becomes curved to cover the head. In postoperative computerized axial tomographs the proximal ilium overlies the femoral head 'like an umbrella' (S. Terver, personal communication), or perhaps more appropriately 'like a plank' (J.E. Hall, personal communication) (Fig. 9.39).

Important points . . . of Chiari's osteotomy . . .: (1) the osteotomy must begin at the margin of the acetabulum—not too far above it or in it; (2) the osteotomy must be ascending and directed no more than 10° cephalad to end in the sciatic notch and not in the sacroiliac joint.

OPERATIVE TECHNIQUE OF ONE-STAGE RECONSTRUCTION FOR SPASTIC DISLOCATION OF THE HIP

1. The patient is supine. No towels or sandbags are used under the hip to rotate the pelvis. This position will distort the radiographic image. Fluoroscopy with image intensification and a video monitor help to achieve optimum accuracy in the techniques.

2. An anterior–medial groin incision and approach (as described above) is used for the myotomies of the adductors, anterior branch obturator neurectomy, iliopsoas tenotomy, and when indicated, proximal hamstring myotomy.

3. The anterior iliofemoral approach to the hip is made through an incision that begins at the mid-crest of the ilium and continues just below the crest to the anterior superior iliac spine, where it curves medially and then laterally toward the greater trochanter. There it turns distally over the lateral aspect of the proximal femoral shaft. The incision has the configuration of a question mark.

The proximal dissection is first done by detaching the origins of the sartorius and rectus femoris and the tensor fascia femoris and gluteus medius muscles. The latter is stripped off the outer wall of the ilium, and its fibers are separated from the joint capsule over the dislocated femoral head. The capsule is opened with a 'T' incision paralleling the acetabular edge with a perpendicular cut in line with the femoral neck. The articular cartilage is inspected. If it is in reasonably normal condition, we proceed with the operation of relocation. If it is degenerated, a salvage procedure such as femoral head and neck resection with capsular interposition is carried out.

4. With the capsule open, the ligamentum teres is excised and the acetabulum visualized. In contrast to congenital dislocations, it is rarely necessary to remove fat and fibrous tissue from the acetabulum. The lateral aspect of the femur and subtrochanteric region is exposed by detaching the origin of the vastus lateralis and stripping the muscle subperiosteally from the femur, as well as stripping the periosteum circumferentially and including the insertion of the posterior-lateral intermuscular septum.

Varus osteotomy is then done starting with a longitudinal incision along the lateral aspect of the proximal femur starting at the flare of the greater trochanter.

The varus osteotomy is performed with the appropriate compression blade plate as noted previously. Usually, 1–2 cm femoral shortening is needed to reduce the hip without pressure on the femoral head. The anteversion is corrected to about 20° and the hip is set in varus of 110°–120°. Care should be taken to retain at least 20°–30° of internal rotation and 10°–20° of anteversion to avoid posterior subluxation of the femoral head

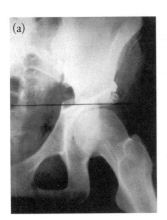
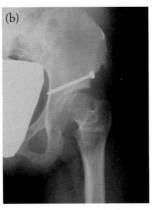

Fig. 9.41. (*a*) Radiograph. Chiari osteotomy for subluxation of the hip and acetabular dysplasia. Skeletally mature patient. (*b*) Radiograph. Follow-up of Chiari osteotomy in panel (*a*). The osteotomy was straight. Bone remodeling created a cup shaped roof over the femoral head. Mother Nature can be wondrous.

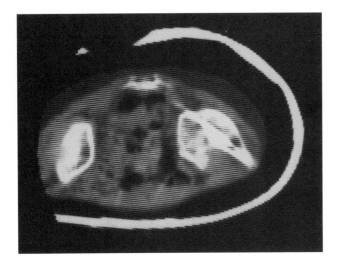

Fig. 9.42. CT scan. Postoperative Chiari osteotomy, right. The ilium puts a 'plank' over the femoral head.

or an externally rotated femoral shaft. The wound is packed but left open while returning to the pelvic wound to do the pelvic osteotomy.

5. The pelvic osteotomy can be the modified Dega with an open triradiate cartilage or a Chiari osteomy after skeletal maturity. To perform the Chiari iliac osteotomy, a guide pin is placed just at the edge of the acetabular margin below the anterior inferior iliac spine but above the site of intended osteotomy. To ensure that the osteotomy is neither too high nor too low, visualization of the articular cartilage of the joint through a tiny incision in the capsular attachment is very helpful. The guide pin is inserted under radiographic control and directed 5°–10° cephalad to end in the greater sciatic notch. Blunt retractors must be inserted on both sides of the ilium in the sciatic notch.

The osteotomy cut is made with a narrow osteotome in the lateral wall of the ilium, and must always ascend slightly toward the inner wall (Fig. 9.40). The cut can curve slightly posteriorly

to follow the margins of the capsular attachment. 'Repeated checking of the osteotome position by X-ray is very helpful' (Chiari 1974, p. 58). When the osteotomy is completed, displacement can be attempted by holding the proximal ilium with a forceps while abducting and internally rotating the hip. Because of the previous femoral osteotomy and the relaxed abductor muscles, it is usually necessary and safer to push the femoral head medially by applying lateral pressure on the greater trochanter. At times the insertion of a dull spade elevator to act as a lever between the osteotomy surfaces is helpful to initiate the displacement.

If more displacement is needed than is possible, iliac bone grafts can be added, similar to the technique used for acetabular augmentation described by Zuckerman *et al.* (1984). The main cause of inability to displace the distal segment medially is allowing the osteotomy to drift inferiorly during the procedure. Then the only remedial measure will be to recut the osteotomy surfaces so gliding can occur. This may produce a little gap in the site, but in growing children it will eventually fill in with new bone. The osteotomy is secured with oblique threaded Steinman pins or bone screws. The long cortical cancellous type are ideal, but only if the ilium is wide enough to accommodate. The screw direction needs checking with the fluoroscope to ensure that the fixation screw or pin in the proximal ilium enters the distal segment superiorly and medially to the acetabulum and not in it. Suction drainage is used in all cases, and wound closure is in the routine manner (Figs 9.43, 9.44).

6. A 1½ spica plaster with the hip in slight flexion, unstressed abduction and neutral rotation is applied and removed 6–8 weeks postoperatively. Because we use internal fixation, we extend the spica to below the rib margins so that the patient can be semi-reclining in a wheelchair with an adjustable back-rest rather than be forced to remain flat in bed for weeks. Alternatively, an adjustable hip brace made preoperatively can also accomplish appropriate immobilization. After plaster removal, passive range of motion of the joints and pool therapy, if available, speeds

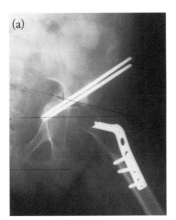
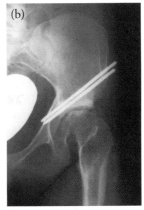

Fig. 9.43. (*a*) Radiograph. Immediately postoperative reduction of dislocated hip, varus-derotation femoral osteotomy, and Chiari pelvic osteotomy. Straight cut across ilium; inclination of the iliac osteotomy 11°. (*b*) Radiograph one year postoperative. Remodeling of the overlying ilium to conform to the femoral head contour.

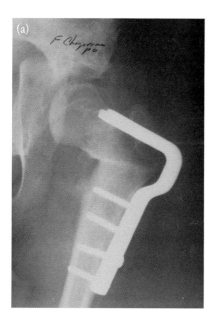

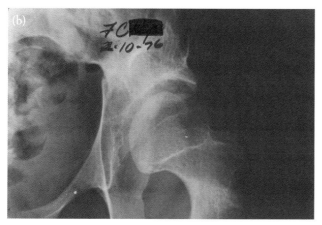

Fig. 9.44. (*a*) Radiograph. Patient FC. Operative reduction of dislocated hip with femoral shortening, derotation femoral osteotomy, Chiari pelvic osteotomy. Total body involved, age 17 years, 3 months postoperative. (*b*) Radiograph. Patient FC. Two years postoperative. Extensive remodeling of the ilium covers the hip.

up the restoration of comfortable sitting. Wheelchair seating modifications may be required.

COMPLICATIONS OF THE CHIARI OSTEOTOMY

The only significant complication was sciatic neuropathy in two patients (Bleck 1987). In one it gradually disappeared; in the other, exposure of the greater sciatic notch revealed that the nerve was stretched tightly over the bone of the notch. Removal of the underlying bone and wrapping the nerve in a cellulose foam sponge relieved the symptoms of pain in the calf and foot. Chiari (1974) also reported a sciatic neuropathy, and presumed it was from stretching of the nerve; the femoral nerve was involved in one case, and six cases had peroneal neuropathies. Malefijt *et al.* (1982) had one case of postoperative sciatic neuropathy in 27 patients.

Benson and Evans (1976), in an anatomical study using human cadavers, concluded that the sciatic nerve was angulated at the osteotomy site; bone splintering at the sciatic notch was also thought to be a contributing factor in the complication of postoperative neuropathies. They reasoned that the nerve was sometimes protected from overstretching when the distal segment of the osteotomy slipped posteriorly.

Non-union of the osteotomy is a possibility. A 100% displacement of the distal pelvic segment led to delayed union of 4 months in one adult patient with congenital dysplasia (Bleck 1987). One case reported by Betz *et al.* (1988) had a delayed union of 8 months.

SALVAGE PROCEDURES FOR PAINFUL DEGENERATED
DISLOCATED HIPS

When the head of the femur is deformed and the cartilage degenerated as usually occurs in the total body involved adolescent and adult who has a painful dislocated hip, four salvage procedures have been proposed: (1) subtrochanteric abduction osteotomy; (2) femoral head and neck resection; (3) hip arthrodesis; and (4) total hip-replacement arthroplasty. Which to choose?

We hope that early preventative surgery or reduction of the dislocated or subluxated hip in childhood before severe degenerative change occur will eliminate the need for these salvage operations.

SUBTROCHANTERIC VALGUS OSTEOTOMY

The authors have had no experience with this procedure in which the femoral head is left dislocated and the femur abducted at the osteotomy distal to the lesser trochanter. It is an old operation for longstanding irreducible congenital dislocations of the hip dating from Kirmisson (1894), modified by Lorenz (1918), Schanz (1922) and finally Hass (1943) (all cited by Crenshaw 1963, p. 1738). Weinert and Ireland (1985) made a further modification, in that they used rigid fixation with the compression hip-screw system. They performed the operation in four total body involved patients who had severe contractures and hip dislocations, apparently with satisfactory results. Other surgeons seem to have tried this procedure in cerebral palsy, but have not published the results. There is no journal of negative results.

FEMORAL HEAD AND NECK RESECTION

Resection of the femoral head and neck has been the most commonly used operation to relieve the pain of a dislocated hip in a skeletally mature total body involved patient. Castle and Schneider (1978) introduced the operation. They were specific in their directions; they resected not just the head and neck of the femur but the entire proximal end to below the lesser trochanter. In three patients who had only femoral head and neck resection, pain and deformity recurred. In 11 who had the entire proximal end of the femur removed and the interposition arthroplasty, pain and deformity were relieved (Fig. 9.45).

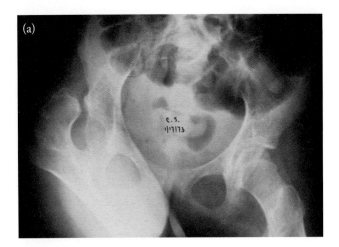

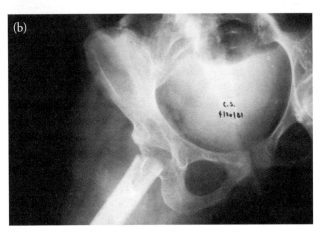

Fig. 9.45. (*a*) Radiograph. Patient CS, Painful dislocated right hip, total body involved, age 20 years. (*b*) Radiograph. Patient CS. Postoperative proximal femur resection. Pain relieved.

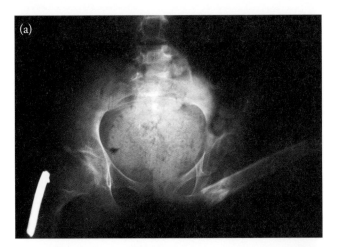

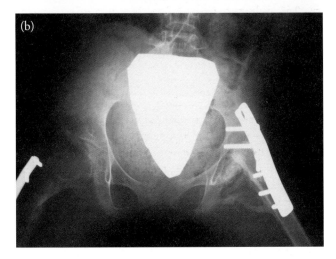

Fig. 9.46. (*a*) Radiograph. Patient MR. Total body involved, age 19 years. Postoperative femoral osteotomy for subluxation of right hip and proximal femur resection for painful dislocation of right hip. Left hip ankylosed in abduction of 120° due to heterotopic ossification. Unable to sit in wheelchair or pass through standard doorways in the chair. (*b*) Radiograph. Patient MR. Wide abduction left hip corrected to 105° flexion, 20° abduction and neutral rotation with arthrodesis and contoured plate fixation. (Radiographs by courtesy of James G. Gamble, MD, PhD.)

An interposition arthroplasty was created by detachment of the hip-joint capsule from the femur and suturing it across the acetabulum. The gluteus medius and minimus muscle insertion was sutured into the space between the proximal femur and the acetabulum and the quadriceps origin was sutured over the resected femoral shaft; iliopsoas tenotomy was always performed. Their patients (14 hips) were placed in Russell's traction postoperatively for an unspecified duration.

Castle and Schneider (1978) 'resected not just the head and neck of the femur but the entire proximal end to below the lesser trochanter.'

The results seemed to have been equivocal for some surgeons who wondered if there is any good salvage procedure for this distressing condition (Koffman 1981). Since 1981 more surgeons have given approbation to the operation to relieve pain. Kalen and Gamble (1984) re-examined the 18 hips in 15 patients in whom the operation was done at an average age of 17.5 years. They found pain was relieved in two-thirds; 89% had heterotopic ossification and 28% were ankylosed (Fig. 9.46).[16] Even though the radiographs were 'not pretty', the goals of pain relief, improved

sitting ability and facilitation of nursing care were accomplished in the majority (Fig. 9.47). Subsequently, other surgeons have found resection-arthroplasty quite effective for pain relief (Raih *et al.* 1985, Baxter and D'Astous 1986, McCarthy *et al.* 1988a, Widmann *et al.* 1999).

McHale and colleagues (1990) resected the proximal femur, placed the lesser trochanter in the acetabulum, did a capsuloplasty and added a subtrochanteric valgus osteotomy. The results were thought to be more sustained if the femur is kept in skeletal traction, using a Kirschner wire through the distal femur or proximal tibia, and balanced suspension with the limb resting on a posterior Thomas splint for 2–3 weeks. During this time,

16 Postoperative heterotopic ossification after myotomies and tenotomies is less common in cerebral palsy than in spina bifida. Bouchard and D'Astous (1991) found it in 8.6% of children with cerebral palsy compared to 21% of those who had spina bifida.

376

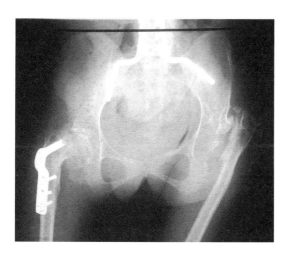

Fig. 9.47. Radiograph. Patient MP, age 24 years, postoperative spinal fusion with Luque–Galveston system, subtrochanteric osteotomy of right femur, and resection of the right proximal femur for painful dislocation. Irregular overgrowth of the proximal femur and shortening did not create a beautiful radiograph, but pain relieved. (Courtesy of James G. Gamble, MD, PhD.)

frequent passive range of motion of the hip would be indicated. This is the regime used by Murray *et al.* (1964) when they had very successful results of femoral head and neck resection as a salvage procedure for arthritis of the hip. But Widmann *et al.* (1999) found that skeletal traction was no better than skin traction in preventing proximal migration of the femur.

As after femoral subtrochanteric osteotomies postoperative heterotopic ossification about the hip varies from 89% (Kalen and Gamble 1984) to 18% (Raih *et al.* 1985). Widmann *et al.* (1999) prescribed single dose radiation postoperatively for five hips. Their incidence of heterotopic ossification was 11% of 18 hips.

HIP ARTHRODESIS

Both arthrodesis of the hip and total hip replacement arthroplasty in cerebral palsy were introduced by Root and colleagues (Root 1977a, b, 1982, Root *et al.* 1986). Arthrodesis is not an attractive option for either patient or physician, but within limitations it can be a useful salvage operation to relieve intractable pain. It is not an option in children. Even though very long follow-up studies of children who had hip arthrodeses (usually for tuberculosis) revealed very satisfactory results, with sustained function for employment and almost all activities of living, we would not recommend arthrodesis of the hip in children who have cerebral palsy (Sponseller *et al.* 1984). The spasticity, and lack of normal patterns of control of knee-flexor and extensor muscles, would inevitably make walking less efficient. The knee is a more important determinant of gait than the hip. The reason why otherwise normal persons have good results with hip arthrodesis is preservation of knee function. Arthrodesis should be reserved for the skeletally mature patients.

Since the report of Root *et al.* (1986) only one paper on the efficacy of arthrodesis for the painful subluxated or dislocated hip in cerebral palsy has been forthcoming (de Moraes Barros Fucs

et al. 2003). These orthopaedic surgeons of São Paulo, Brazil, did arthrodesis of the hip in 14 dislocated hips in patients with cerebral palsy. Of these, eight had quadriplegia; two had a mixed pattern and four were diplegic. Three were sitters, while seven were bedridden. The mean age of surgery was 15 years, 5 months (range 10 years 11 months to 29 years 11 months; Fig. 9.48).

The São Paulo series is instructive for the failure of previous surgery to relieve pain: two had adductor and psoas releases; one with unilateral dislocation had a triple innominate osteotomy; two had a valgus osteotomy of the proximal femur; two had a proximal femoral resection with a valgus subtrochanteric osteotomy (McHale *et al.* 1990). All were relieved of pain after arthrodesis and improved their function. Of the seven bedridden patients, five were able to sit comfortably. Of the three sitters, two became community walkers, and the one household walker was able to be a community walker.

Arthrodesis seems best performed both intra- and extra-articular. The Davis (1954) method of the muscle pedicle inlay

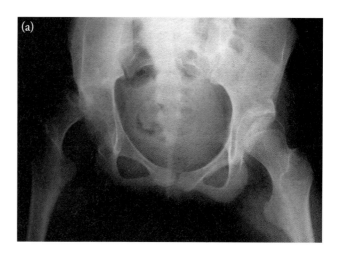

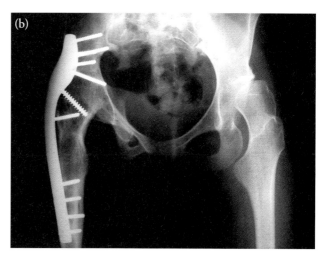

Fig. 9.48. (*a*) Radiograph. Patient SP1. Total body involved female age 13 years, painful dislocation, right hip. Normal left hip, level pelvis, no scoliosis. (*b*) Radiograph. Patient SP1, age 18 years, postoperative arthrodesis with Cobra plate fixation. Courtesy of Celso Svartman MD and Patricia Fucs MD, Santa Casa School of Medicine, São Paulo, Brazil (Ciências Médicas da Santa Casa de São Paulo, Brasil).

graft from the iliac crest has assisted in obtaining better and more rapid fusion, plus some sort of internal fixation. The simple method of cancellous screws inserted from inside the pelvis into the femoral head seems to be a good method for intra-articular fixation (Mowery *et al.* 1986). If necessary, the position of the hip can be set at the site of a subtrochanteric osteotomy performed at the same time. The osteotomy should be secured with a nail plate. The position of arthrodesis for these sitting patients is neutral rotation, 40°–50° of flexion and 10° of abduction (Root *et al.* 1986).

In the São Paulo techniques, intra-articular fusion was secured either with an AO-DCP 4.5 mm large plate or an AO-Cobra plate. All had adductor and psoas tenotomies. A spica cast was used postoperatively for an average of 2 months in eight patients. Six patients had no cast. The AO-Cobra plate provides secure fixation so that the patient can be free of the constraints and discomforts of a cast—a great advantage for the patient with cerebral palsy.

Arthrodesis to relieve a painful hip in cerebral palsy will be rarely indicated. The criteria for selection strictly limit this choice. These are (1) unilateral dislocation, (2) contralateral hip not at risk, (3) skeletal growth completed, and (4) no spinal deformity (Fig. 9.49). Accordingly, anecdotes on its efficacy as a permanent solution for the relief of pain may serve to help a surgeon select this surgical approach. Bleck had occasion to perform arthrodesis of the hip in only two patients with cerebral palsy. One young woman had a severe abduction deformity of the hip with pain after a proximal femoral resection for a dislocated hip. Her hip was so abducted that she could no longer sit in her wheelchair and pass through a doorway. Arthrodesis was accomplished with internal fixation; the hip was moved to a position of 45° flexion, 30° abduction and neutral rotation. Pain was relieved and her sitting became comfortable. Fortunately, she had no scoliosis with a pelvic obliquity that would demand correction with spinal instrumentation, and fusion into the sacrum which would effectively remove the required mobility of the pelvis via the lumbosacral joint after hip arthrodesis.

Bleck's other patient was an adult confined to a wheelchair due to total body involvement with athetosis and spasticity. He had a subluxation of his right hip and degenerative arthritis, and in pain almost continuously. Arthrodesis with the hip in 45° flexion, 10° abduction and neutral rotation using a cobra plate and screws and no spica plaster immobilization completely relieved his pain. He has remained in his wheelchair fully employed in the Department of Rehabilitation of the State of California.

The criteria for selection strictly limit the choice for arthrodesis of the hip: (1) unilateral dislocation, (2) contralateral hip not at risk, (3) skeletal growth completed, and (4) no spinal deformity.

TOTAL JOINT ARTHROPLASTY

Prosthetic replacement of the painful degenerated hip in cerebral palsy has steadily gained acceptance with good results (Skoff and Keggi 1986, Root *et al.* 1986, Buly *et al.* 1993, Weber and Cabanela 1999, Wicart *et al.* 1999). Obviously it is better to have a movable hip rather than a stiff one. It is indicated in patients who have painful hips, usually due to chronic subluxation, and are ambulatory to some degree although Wicart *et al.* (1999) of Paris reported its use in three sitting patients. None of their 14 patients were bedridden.

Unlike arthrodesis of the hip, arthroplasty is the solution for patients who have scoliosis (assuming that the curvature and the pelvic obliquity will be corrected first). The usual total body involved adult patient whose hip is chronically dislocated is probably not a candidate for a total hip-replacement arthroplasty given the complications of infection, dislocation of the femoral component, deep venous thrombosis, and loosening of the femoral or acetabular component.

Total hip arthroplasty in 15 patients relieved the painful hip in 14 (Root *et al.* 1986). Preoperatively 12 of the patients had some ability to walk, most with external support. All were able

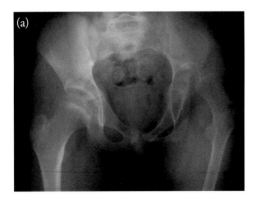 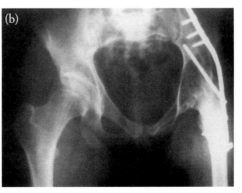 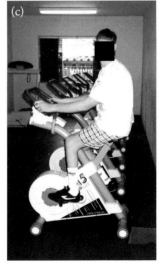

Fig. 9.49. (*a*) Radiograph. Patient SP2. Total body involved male, age 13 years, painful dislocation, left hip. Normal right hip. No pelvic obliquity and no scoliosis. (*b*) Radiograph. Patient SP2. Age 15 years, 6 months. Postoperative intra and extra-articular arthrodesis with long screw and contoured plate fixation. Pain free. (*c*) Patient SP2, Postoperative arthrodesis, right hip. Able to sit comfortably and pedal the exercise bicycle. (By courtesy of Celso Svartman MD and Patricia Fucs MD, Santa Casa School of Medicine, São Paulo, Brazil.)

to resume some functional walking after the arthroplasty. Four had spastic diplegia or paraplegia; three were listed as triplegic and the remaining eight were called quadriplegic. The postoperative complications were probably usual for total hip replacements, but more frequent: bending of the femoral component; dislocation 12 days after surgery, then again at 4 months and 10 months; loosening of the femoral component after 7 years but with mild symptoms; recurrent subluxation of the femoral component requiring its replacement 6 years postoperatively. 53% had heterotopic ossification, but with no obvious clinical significance. Buly and Root's colleagues (1993) of New York did a longer follow-up of a mean of 10 years (range 3–17 years) of their total hip arthroplasties in cerebral palsy. Pain relief was sustained in 94% and function improved. Only one femoral stem and one acetabular component had loosened. Survivorship analysis at 10 years was 95% for loosening and 86% for removal of components (Fig. 9.50).

The results detailed by Buly *et al.* (1993), Wicart *et al.* (1999) and Weber and Cabanela (1999) are comparable to those of Root *et al.* (1986). As might be expected, surgeons selected different prostheses and variations of uncemented or cemented acetabular or femoral components. Certainly if the forces deforming spastic muscles have not been previously released, iliopsoas lengthening/tenotomy at or above the pelvic brim and adductor longus tenomyotomy should be done at the time of the arthroplasty.

Gabos *et al.* (1999) of the Alfred I. duPont Institute of Delaware did an innovative 'prosthetic interposition arthroplasty' in 11 non-ambulatory patients with spastic quadriplegia and severe degenerative hip disease due to chronic dislocation or subluxation. In all but one patient they used a non-cemented shoulder prosthesis in the femoral canal. In seven they used a glenoid component in the false acetabulum. Four hips dislocated within 4 months postoperative, but 10 maintained their stability. As so common in cerebral palsy, five developed heterotopic ossification. Ten patients had complete relief of pain. Sitting tolerance improved in every patient. Three patients had a prior resection of the proximal femur and persistent pain. While this high dislocation rate seems to negate its use in hips, this interposition arthroplasty relieved pain in all. Would this procedure be preferable to the usual salvage operation of resection of the proximal femur?

WHAT IS TO BE DONE, ARTHRODESIS OR ARTHROPLASTY?

We have to answer a question with a question. Is this patient with cerebral palsy specifically total body involved? If so, sitting and standing equilibrium reactions will be deficient. If they are not absent, and the lateral equilibrium reactions are or have been fairly normal when standing, the patient is not total body involved and has the ability to be at least a household walker.

In conclusion, the case can be made for total hip replacement for painful subluxation of the hip in the adult with spastic diplegia or triplegia who has lost the ability for household walking with

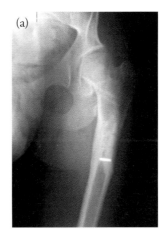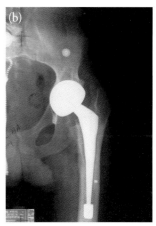

Fig. 9.50. (*a*) Radiograph. Patient MG, total body involved with athetosis and dystonia, ambulatory, male, age 15 years. Age 11 bilateral derotation femoral osteotomies for hip internally rotated gait pattern. Age 13 years pain left hip; total hip replacement; pain relieved. (*b*) Radiograph. Patient MG, age 15 years, loose femoral stem of prosthesis and pain. Total hip replacement revision, left hip. Age 33 occasional pain. (By courtesy of Gene Bruce MD, San Mateo, CA.)

crutches. A patient with spastic diplegia or triplegia who was more than a household walker and never used crutches and had a subluxation of the hip would be rare indeed. If total hip replacement is performed, the patient should be told that revision and replacement of the arthroplasty may be necessary several years later.

One can imagine few indications for complete hip replacement in the non-ambulatory total body involved person.

One can imagine few indications for complete hip replacement in the non-ambulatory total body involved person. Consider carefully the magnitude of the operation and its complications, versus the possible benefits of more comfortable sitting and sleeping. We can hope that early surgery to prevent and correct subluxation and dislocation of the hip will continue to keep the numbers of cases in follow-up studies of salvage surgery very low.

KNEE, FOOT AND ANKLE DEFORMITIES

Knee-flexion contractures in the total body involved patient need correction only if the flexed knee interferes with assistive transfers from the wheelchair, or if positioning in bed becomes uncomfortable. A knee-flexion contracture combined with the osteopenia due to non-weightbearing in these patients makes them prone to supracondylar fractures of the femur (Samilson *et al.* 1972). If the patient has transfer ability from the chair, a knee-flexion contracture beyond 15º–20º is an indication for correction.

Fractional and prudent lengthening of the hamstring tendons, rather than tenotomy or transfer of all, should prevent the conversion of a flexed knee to a constantly extended posture. An underlying quadriceps spasticity is present in most of these patients. If the hamstring muscles are excessively weakened, the predominant extensor pattern which follows would make sitting in a chair more untenable than if the knees were left flexed. If knee flexion is severely limited after hamstring lengthening, quadriceps tendon recession or lengthening should restore knee flexion.

Proximal hamstring lengthening improved hip and spine positioning in 62 non-walking children with spastic quadriplegia, only 35 had 2 or more years of follow-up (Elmer *et al.* 1992). The hamstring contracture was accompanied by difficulty in sitting due to a hip-extensor thrust and increased kyphosis. The 'lengthening' described was a myotomy of the origins of the hamstrings through a transverse anterior–medial incision; the posterior one-fourth to one-third of the adductor magnus origin was sectioned to gain exposure of the hamstring origins.[17] Sitting balance as assessed on a clinical modified scale of Reimers (1972) improved significantly. Apparently conversion to a spastic extended knee position did not occur postoperatively.

Very often these are long-standing contractures which involve the posterior capsule of the knee joint. If so, posterior capsulotomy and section of the anterior cruciate ligament insertion will be indicated. Sudden and forced extension of the knee under anesthesia may be inadvert and cause a temporary sciatic neuropathy. In adolescents and young adults, soft-tissue surgery alone may not be feasible due to the shortening of the neurovascular structures. A closed wedged femoral condylar osteotomy with internal fixation and hamstring lengthening would be the preferred surgical treatment. Knee flexion will be limited depending on the degree of extension of the supra-condylar osteotomy.

Foot and ankle deformities in this group of patients need correction only if they interfere with sitting posture or the mobility of the patient who is capable of transfers, either assistive or independent.

Given the stipulations for surgery with regard to functional potential, equinus, valgus and varus deformities of the foot and ankle can be corrected. Severe equinus, even if the person has no transfer abilities, can be disabling; shoeing is impossible and the foot cannot rest comfortably on the foot-rest of the wheelchair. Without the foot-rests, the equinus foot hangs down so that the toes drag on the floor or else the wheelchair seat has to be raised to a position beyond the usual table or desk height.

The surgical techniques for corrections of these deformities are identical to those described in Chapters 7 and 8.

UPPER-LIMB DEFORMITIES

Upper-limb deformities that are amenable to surgical correction for improved function are rare in the total body involved. As discussed in Chapter 7, hand or elbow surgery has been performed in very few patients with quadriplegia. Before surgery of the upper limb is considered in these patients, it is essential to obtain a detailed and repeated analysis of the potential for function,

especially voluntary control. An occupational therapist can assess the patient's limited function before decisions for surgery are made. As noted in Chapter 7, elbow-flexion contracture correction has been done to allow elbow extension and the use of crutches for at least household walking. The potential for walking can be determined largely based upon testing for infantile automatisms and the development of the normal parachute reactions. To use crutches or canes effectively, there must be good side-to-side equilibrium reactions. In the most severely affected total body involved patients we have only found a few who benefited from correction of upper-limb deformities. These related to problems with hand hygiene because of severe finger flexion contractures or development of severe wrist contractures precluding effective use of motorized wheelchair control or impeding activities of daily living such as dressing. The more intelligent totally involved patient will likely have strong opinions regarding the benefits of surgical intervention. The key is to be both realistic in the potential outcome and selective regarding patient. Electromyographic and video analysis coupled with trial injections with botulinum toxin or use of selective splinting is helpful to optimize a surgical plan. The principles are the same as outlined in Chapter 7.

SPINAL DEFORMITIES

In the total body involved patient, the two spinal problems are scoliosis and cervical spine degenerative changes which cause spinal-cord or nerve-root compression and superimpose a spinal cord paralysis on the motion disorder due to the brain malfunction.

KYPHOSIS AND LORDOSIS

Kyphosis of the thoracic spine is seen in many children with cerebral palsy when first sitting erect. This early kyphosis usually is not structural or fixed. Bobath (1966) explained it as a compensatory mechanism in bringing the trunk over the pelvis in the child who has an extensor pattern of spasticity with resultant insufficient hip flexion.

Fixed kyphosis can be associated with long-standing hamstring spasticity and contracture which is counterbalanced by quadriceps muscle spasticity, so that the pelvis is in constant posterior inclination when the child stands (Fig. 9.51). Ambulatory patients with excessive lumbar lordosis may have a compensatory thoracic kyphosis.

Treatment of the thoracic kyphosis with the usual Milwaukee brace (the cervical–thoracolumbar–spinal orthosis, or CTLSO) has not been successful in the few patients for whom it was prescribed. The addition of a brace adds another restriction to the already seriously disabled person. Furthermore, there is no functional disability from kyphosis in the total body involved. The problem seems to alarm the physical therapist and family more than the patient.

In the sitting patient, lordosis is rarely a problem; in fact if it is eliminated by spinal fusion with straight rods, or anterior Dwyer instrumentation and fusion, sitting becomes a greater

---

17 The procedure is commonly termed a proximal hamstring origin 'release'.

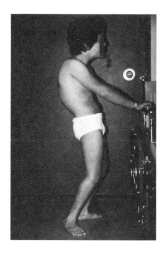

Fig. 9.51. Photograph. Spastic diplegia, male, age 12 years, ambulatory. Spastic hamstrings and quadriceps with posterior inclination of the pelvis and secondary kyphosis. Cosmetically objectionable to some, but no pain and no functional loss.

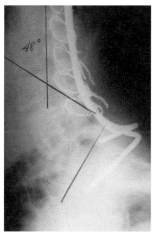

Fig. 9.52. Radiograph. Lateral projection, lumbar spine and sacrum. Luque rods bent to preserve lordosis.

problem. The problem is that without lumbar lordosis, the weight of the head, trunk and upper limbs when sitting is concentrated on the small surface area of the coccyx and end of the sacrum (Fig. 9.52). The surface area for sitting becomes much greater with lordosis, as weight is then on the posterior aspect of the thighs. Hyperlordosis has been reported after selective posterior rootlet rhizotomy (Fig. 9.53.) (Crawford *et al.* 1996, Johnson *et al.* 2000, Turi and Kalen 2000).

Measurement of the thoracic kyphosis and lumbar lordosis on lateral radiographs of the spine with the patient seated or standing is sometimes useful in the assessment of the presumed spinal problem. Measurements of what is considered to be normal have been published (Propst-Proctor and Black 1983). The Cobb method of measurement has been used on the lateral radiographs; for the thoracic kyphosis we used the angle between the top of the 5th and 12th thoracic vertebrae and for lumbar lordosis between the 1st and 5th lumbar vertebrae (Table 9.II).

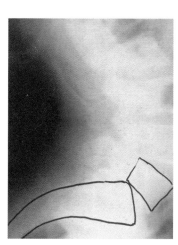

Fig. 9.53. Radiograph. Lateral projection, lumbar spine and sacrum. Severe hyperlordosis. Sacrum horizontal.

Although thoracic kyphosis of 40° is considered normal, 60° seems compatible with a long and useful life. One orthopaedic surgeon recognized that 60° of thoracic kyphosis does not preclude Olympic championship (Nachemson 1980). Kyphosis of 80° and beyond does seem disabling but never encountered in cerebral palsy by the authors. If it ever occurred in an adolescent with a fixed structural deformity, the recommendation would probably be for anterior disc excision and fusion, and second stage posterior fusion and corrective instrumentation (Moe *et al.* 1978).

SCOLIOSIS

PREVALENCE

Scoliosis is more prevalent in the non-ambulatory total body involved patient and in the ambulatory child who has hemiplegia, diplegia or ataxia than idiopathic scoliosis in the general population (Robson 1968, Balmer and MacEwen 1970, Samilson and Bechard 1973, Rosenthal *et al.* 1974, Madigan and Wallace 1981). In the ambulatory patient with cerebral palsy the incidence varies with the particular clinic population and years studied. A clinic in St Louis, Missouri, had a 5% incidence in the years 1950–59 and 3% in 1970–79. Bleck (1987) noted that in ambulatory patients with cerebral palsy the incidence was three times that expected in the normal child and adolescent population (6.0 per 100 versus 2.0 per 100). In the total body involved the prevalence of structural scoliosis greater than 10° varies from 25% (Samilson and Bechard 1973, Moe *et al.* 1978) to 64% (Madigan and Wallace 1981). The only significance and value of the above data is to make the physician aware that scoliosis in cerebral palsy is common, and children should be regularly examined for signs of spinal curvature. When clinical evidence is found, a radiographic examination confirms and measures the degree of scoliosis so that progression can be ascertained and intervention instituted.

Although cerebral palsy has been with us for ages, scoliosis in cerebral palsy was generally ignored prior to 1970 (James 1967, Keats 1970). Awareness of it in cerebral palsy as a serious and treatable problem seems to have arisen with the innovation of effective correction of scoliosis with instrumentation and fusion first with Harrington (1962) and followed by several fixation systems.

ETIOLOGICAL FACTORS

We have not unraveled the puzzle of the cause of idiopathic scoliosis or the scoliosis of cerebral palsy. But we may draw inferences from clinical observations. Factors that may be operative are equilibrium reactions (balance), muscle asymmetry, persistent Galant's reflex, biochemical factors, abnormal endochondral ossification. Of these, deficient equilibrium reactions due to some dysfunction of the central nervous system seem the most important.

Deficient equilibrium reactions. In patients with cerebral palsy who walk the development of the spinal curve during growth, the curve pattern and the prognosis for progression appear no different from idiopathic scoliosis. In one study of 315 children with cerebral palsy (Bleck 1975), the incidence of scoliosis in the ataxic type was three times high than in spastic hemiplegia or diplegia. The curve patterns in the ataxic type were identical to those of idiopathic scoliosis, primarily right thoracic curves. Horstmann and Boyer (1983), in a review of 530 patients with cerebral palsy seen as outpatients at the Alfred I. duPont Institute, noted similar findings with an incidence of scoliosis of 47.6% in athetoid patients, 42% in patients with spastic quadriplegia, 23.8% in those with spastic diplegia, 15.5% in those with spastic paraplegia, and 15% in those with spastic hemiplegia. Friedreich's ataxia is known to have an 80%–100% occurrence of scoliosis (Farmer 1964, Cady and Bobechko 1984). Aronsson *et al.* (1994), in a comparison study of scoliosis, concluded that the curves in Friedreich's ataxia were similar to those in idiopathic scoliosis.

That a sensory defect may be an etiological factor was suggested by the experimental sectioning of dorsal spinal roots in animals with resultant scoliosis (Liszka 1961, MacEwen 1968). The possible role of the central nerve system was Suzuki *et al.*'s (1964) finding of electroencephalographic abnormalities and enlargement of the third ventricle in patients with idiopathic scoliosis. Further implicating the central, nervous system's role in idiopathic scoliosis was the experimental spinal curvature in dogs after unilateral lesions of the caudate nucleus and reversal of the curves by destruction of the opposite caudate nucleus (Martin 1965).

One constant observation in the total body involved patients is the absence of truncal equilibrium reactions. Despite the circumstantial and experimental evidence of a possible defect in the postural equilibrium mechanisms as causative of scoliosis research, along these lines has not confirmed a definitive lesion in the central nervous system (Yamada *et al.* 1969, Sahlstrand *et al.* 1978, Sahlstrand and Lidstrom 1980, Gregoric *et al.* 1981, Driscoll *et al.* 1984, Adler *et al.* 1986).

Sitting balance has been measured with a computerized pressure plate system in 100 individuals with normal and abnormal spines (Smith and Emans 1992). Abnormal patterns of pressure distribution were seen in lumbar curves of idiopathic scoliosis, in severe scoliosis of myelodysplasia and cerebral palsy, and in kyphosis and hyperlordosis. Most interesting and probably dismaying is that after spinal fusion poor sitting balance persisted.

MUSCLE

The spinal curve patterns in the non-walking total body involved patient are similar to those due to poliomyelitis, myelomeningocele and muscular dystrophy. Asymmetrical spasticity/and or dystonia may be operative in cerebral palsy. Biopsies of the paravertebral muscles in scoliosis of patients with cerebral palsy and idiopathic scoliosis compared with normal non-scoliotic individuals showed that fiber-type distribution was different in the scoliosis patients from the normal controls. However, these changes were on *both sides* of the curve (Bleck *et al.* 1976). These findings do not suggest that unilateral muscle weakness in cerebral palsy or idiopathic scoliosis is an etiological factor. Experimental paravertebral muscle contracture in rabbits produced scoliosis (Langeskiöld 1971) but spinal-muscle contracture has not been demonstrated in cerebral palsy.

GALANT'S REFLEX

Samilson and Bechard (1973) opined that scoliosis in their institutionalized patients with total body involvement had persistence of the infantile incurvatum reflex (Galant's). To elicit this reflex the skin alongside the vertebral column is stroked; the trunk bends into the concavity of the stimulated side (Beintema 1968). Only one of Bleck's 16 patients with total body involvement had this reflex.

BIOCHEMICAL FACTORS

Increased ligamentous laxity as a defect in the cross-linking of collagen in idiopathic scoliosis can be discounted as causative (Bleck *et al.* 1981, Mattson *et al.* 1983).

The proteoglycan content of the intervertebral discs in cerebral palsy and idiopathic scoliosis were analyzed and found to be negative (Oegema *et al.* 1983). Any changes from normal were deemed to be secondary to the curvature.

Proton magnetic imaging of human muscle abstracts in idiopathic and cerebral palsy scoliosis showed slight decreases in creatine and lactic acid in idiopathic scoliosis and a significant decrease in cerebral palsy (Arus *et al.* 1984). These changes may indicate that the muscle is more involved in the spinal curvatures of cerebral palsy.

The fascinating studies of Machida *et al.* (1993, 1995, 1994, 2001), in which the pineal gland was removed from chickens to produce scoliosis, suggested that the altered postural and equilibrium mechanisms were associated with melatonin synthesis and a deficiency of it resulted in experimental scoliosis.[18] Pineal gland removal in rats also created scoliosis with decreasing plasma melatonin (Machida *et al.* 1999). The implication was that neurotransmitters or neurohormonal systems in the pineal body are major contributing factors in the experimental scoliosis of chickens. Whether pineal body dysfunction is an etiological factor affecting equilibrium and posture in the total body involved patient with cerebral palsy is a question not yet answered.

---

18 Melantonin is a hormone secreted by the pineal gland. Its synthesis arises from serotonin and has a marked circadian rhythm (Shepherd 1994).

ABNORMAL ENCHONDRAL OSSIFICATION

Histological studies (Enneking and Harrington 1969) revealed more cartilage derangement and retarded enchondral growth on the convex side of idiopathic curves with no increased osteoplastic or osteoblastic activity. With this data it seems evident that extraosseous causes are operative in idiopathic scoliosis and the same conclusion is likely in cerebral palsy. The structural changes in the spine are secondary beginning in the intervertebral discs and then in the vertebra and facet joints.

SCOLIOSIS SECONDARY TO PRIMARY PELVIC OBLIQUITY WITH HIP SUBLUXATION OR DISLOCATION

Because hip dislocation and subluxation with pelvic obliquity often coexist with scoliosis, it was assumed that correction of the hip problem will prevent the pelvic obliquity and the scoliosis. Muscle-release operations below the iliac crest have not prevented or altered the scoliosis. James (1956) made this observation long ago in his paper on paralytic scoliosis. Lonstein and Beck (1986) presented their data in which they could find no association between hip dislocation, pelvic obliquity and scoliosis in cerebral palsy. Scoliosis develops regardless of the hip and pelvic positions.

This review of some of the possible mechanisms of scoliosis, and the lack of a definite etiological factor to explain why some patients develop curvatures and others do not, indicates why the prevention and conservative management of scoliosis in general (and specifically in cerebral palsy) is empirical and not very effective.

CHARACTERISTICS

In the total body involved patient the majority of curves are thoracolumbar. When the pelvis becomes part of the cure, pelvic obliquity results (Samilson and Bechard 1973). Patients who walk usually have double major curves without pelvic obliquity. In some the thoracic curve predominates with a poorly compensated lumbar curve (Lonstein and Beck 1986).

Because the curves begin early in the total body involved child these curves, in contrast to the later onset of idiopathic scoliosis, become more rigid at an earlier age. Severe rotation and wedging of the vertebral bodies as well as distortion of the articular facets is usual.

PROGNOSIS

Despite early diagnosis and attempted conservative treatment the prognosis is for increasing curvature in the total body involved child (Fig. 9.54). Progressive of the scoliosis is also correlated with the velocity of trunk growth (Duval-Beaupère and Grossiord 1967a, b; Duval-Beaupère 1970, 1971; Duval-Beaupère and Combes 1971; Terver *et al.* 1980). Spinal growth ceases when the iliac apophyses are full ossified and fused to the ilium (Risser sign 5) (Risser and Ferguson 1936, Zaoussis and James 1958). In idiopathic scoliosis if the curve is less than 50° progression due to growth usually ceases.

However, scoliosis in the total body involved patient is progressive even after skeletal maturation (Madigan and Wallace

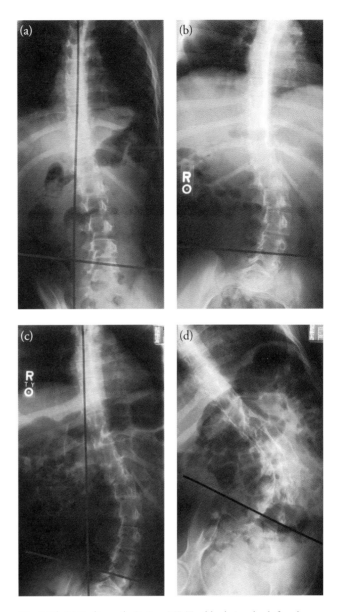

Fig. 9.54. (*a*) Radiograph. Patient MP. Total body involved, female, age 13 years. Slight lumbar scoliosis. (*b*) Radiograph, Patient MP, age 16 years. Scoliosis has progressed. (*c*) Radiograph. Patient MP, age 19 years. Scoliosis progressed. (*d*) Radiograph, Patient MP, age 23 years. Severe curvature. Surgery scheduled.

1986). These authors used the following nomogram to determine progression: Cobb angle minus three times the Risser sign divided by the chronological age (Lonstein and Carlson 1984). If for example, the child is 10 years old and the curve measures 30° with a Risser sign of zero, the chance of progression without treatment is 100%. Untreated scoliosis, in general, has a poor prognosis (Nachemson 1968). Idiopathic curves over 50° progress throughout life at 1° per year (Weinstein *et al.* 1981). Restriction of pulmonary function occurs in all, but is not life-threatening until the thoracic curves were beyond 100°–120°. Horstmann and Boyer (1984) found the greatest progression of scoliosis in quadriplegic cerebral palsy after skeletal maturity particularly in curves over 60°.

Progression of scoliosis in institutionalized adults with cerebral palsy and scoliosis was found after skeletal maturity by Thometz and Simon (1988). If the curve was less than 50° at maturity progression was 0.8 each year; if more than 50° the rate of progression was 1.4° per year. Others have confirmed progression of curves in adults with cerebral palsy (Majd *et al.* 1997). Initial curves of 33.9° progressed to 56.5°. Three curves progressed to 106° and a pelvic obliquity of 45°. Functional decline and decubiti correlated with the rate of progression.

Progression of scoliosis in adults: curves <50° = 0.8°/year; >50° = 1.4°/year

ORTHOTIC MANAGEMENT

In the ambulatory patient with cerebral palsy, scoliosis that does not have a sacral or pelvic component, orthoses of various types used in idiopathic scoliosis are probably just as effective in cerebral palsy. The overall rate of stemming progression is likely to be between 17% and 30%. The Milwaukee brace (or CTLSO) is unsuitable for most patients with cerebral palsy due to their dysequilibrium which made the wearing of the brace most difficult.

Plastic body jackets were reported as successful in arresting the progression of scoliosis in 42 patients with cerebral palsy, most of whom had quadriplegia (Bunnell and MacEwen 1977). In this series the average age of diagnosis of the spinal curve was 9 years; the follow-up ranged from 9 to 60 months (mean 26.4 months). The authors admitted that the follow-up was too short to reach a definite conclusion on the efficacy of the orthosis. If the mean age of application of the orthosis was 9 years, then the mean age at follow-up was only 11 years—almost exactly the time when the velocity of spinal growth accelerates and curves increase dramatically.

Plastic orthoses (the thoracolumbar spinal orthosis, or TLSO) may hold some curves in the total body involved child, but generally they only delay the decision for definitive spinal instrumentation and fusion until the child is old enough for fusion (Moe *et al.* 1978). Zimbler *et al.* (1985) confirmed orthotic failure to stop progression when the curves were more than 40° and the child over age 10 years.

Wilmington custom-made plastic orthoses used for 23 hours a day for 67 months in another study found that 'spinal orthotics had no impact on scoliosis curve, shape, or rate of progression in spastic quadriplegic patients' (Miller *et al.* 1996). In a critique of the study cited, Galasko (1997) opined that the study was flawed because failure of the orthosis was defined as the patient who came to spinal fusion. In response, Miller (1997), one of the co-authors, replied that while their paper did not test the 'supposition that spinal bracing in these children' can prevent development of scoliosis, it did test that there was no effect on progression. Further, there are no data to show that bracing can prevent the development of scoliosis in the patient with total body involvement (Fig. 9.55).

Spinal orthotics had no impact on scoliosis curve, shape, or rate of progression in spastic quadriplegic patients.

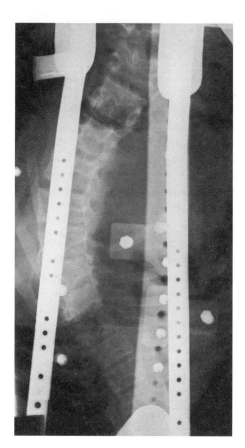

Fig. 9.55. Radiograph in TLSO. Scoliosis is neither corrected nor progression arrested.

The obverse of the negative reports on orthotic efficacy of scoliosis in quadriplegic cerebral palsy was the report of Terjesen *et al.* (2000) of Oslo, Norway. They studied retrospectively 86 patients with spastic quadriplegia who were treated with custom-molded polypropylene thoracolumbar-sacral orthoses. The mean Cobb angle at the beginning of orthotic application in patients at a mean age of 13.8 years was 68.4° (range of 25°–131°). The mean correction in the orthosis was 25°. On a follow-up of a mean of 6.3 years after initiating treatment the mean Cobb angle without the orthosis was 93° (range of 40°–145°) and a mean progression of 4.2° per year. At the conclusion of the study there were 57 patients who did not have a spine fusion were still alive and 72% used their orthoses at a mean age of 22 years. Parents and caregivers were said to be satisfied with the use of the orthosis because it improved sitting stability and better overall function.

Comment: Because the foregoing study in a peer reviewed medical journal appears to give approbation to encasing a patient in a plastic body jacket as management of a progressive paralytic scoliosis, the details in the report have been highlighted. That the curves without the pressure of the orthosis were a mean of 93° and as high as 145° would not seem to be a desirable end result. Progression was not stopped. Furthermore, of the 86 patients, 29 either had died or had a spinal fusion. It may be that North American, British and continental European orthopaedic surgeons are enthusiastic about scoliosis correction and fusion because the tools and techniques have made surgery effective, feasible and safe as well as eliminating the need for orthoses or elaborate wheelchair seating.

The Soft Boston Orthosis (SBO) is a thoracolumbar spinal orthosis that has been used to stabilize scoliosis in total body involved patients. It fits snugly on the trunk. The perception that this encasement of the orthosis around the chest cage would further restrict pulmonary function was shown not to be the case in a study by Leopando *et al.* (1999). They measured pulmonary mechanics and gas exchange in 12 children and young adults with severe cerebral palsy and compared patients with and without the orthosis. The results showed no negative impacts on pulmonary function as measured. Rather the work of breathing was the greatest in the sitting position without the orthosis.

Encasing the trunk in a rigid shell can be compared to a glass of jelly in which a straight straw is inserted. If you push on the straw, it bends despite the outer shell of glass. Gravity and with weight of the head, neck, shoulder girdles and upper limbs exert the downward pressure on the spine.

Winter (1986) had some success in slowing the progression of the curve in the total body involved patient with the use of a polypropylene sitting orthosis. Lonstein (2001) recommends the Gillette seating support orthosis as a holding device with some success. These hard plastic seats can be hard to tolerate for 6–8 hours. Custom made upholstered contour seats with lateral support systems have been used to accommodate the trunk of the total body involved child.

Special seating was studied in non-walking patients with cerebral palsy in an assessment chair with a clear backrest (Holmes *et al.* 2003). Measurements of the spinal curve were recorded as the 'spinous process angle' to approximate the Cobb angle of radiographic studies. Forces on the patient were measured with electrical resistance strain gauge transducers on the lateral support pads and seat base. Significant static correction of the spinal curve was with a 3-point force system to the sides of the trunk. This method of analysis of seating and lateral pads was thought to have a potential in the special seating for patients with scoliosis.

The question raised about seating systems is: do you fit the seat to the child or the child to the seat? With the advance in surgical correction most contemporary orthopaedic surgeons will fit the child to the seat by corrective spinal surgery.

Do you fit the seat to the child or the child to the seat?

ELECTRICAL STIMULATION
Lateral electrical spinal stimulation (LESS) was introduced by Bobechko and Herbert (1986). Intermittent pulsed implantable electrical stimulators were applied to the paravertebral muscles during recumbency at night-time rest. They reported success in stopping curve progression in cerebral palsy in 89% of those treated. A wave of enthusiasm for this appealing method in idiopathic scoliosis was rather short-lived as reports poured in discounting its efficacy, i.e. LESS was less, not more. Curiously, Cady and Bobechko (1984) stated it was useless in the scoliosis of Friedreich's ataxia. Surgical treatment was advised for all cases.

SURGICAL MANAGEMENT

HISTORY AND PROGRESS
Unfortunately for the patient with total body involvement there is no effective treatment for scoliosis other than correction by instrumentation and spinal fusion. The success of spinal instrumentation in scoliosis surgery introduced by Harrington (1962) generated interest in the scoliosis of cerebral palsy. Spinal fusion by posterior element arthrodesis in scoliosis has developed greatly since it was first established by Hibbs (1924) (Cobb 1952, Risser and Nordquist 1958, Goldstein 1959). Prior to effective instrumentation a variety of plaster body casts were used for preoperative correction and postoperative stabilization to hold the correction obtained while fusion occurred. Failure of fusion at one or more levels (pseudoarthrosis) was discouragingly common— as high as 68% (Ponsetti and Friedman 1950). Goldstein's (1959) addition of autogenous iliac bone grafts to the fusion site reduced his pseudoarthrosis rate to 12.9%. But failure of fusion was difficult to determine radiographically so that 'second look' surgery was advised to ascertain the failure of fusion sites and repair them.

The high failure rate of fusion let alone modest corrections and relapses of correction and the chore of plaster cast application discouraged orthopaedic surgeons from tackling scoliosis in cerebral palsy. Since the early 1960s surgical treatment of the curvatures in the total body involved patient has evolved from Harrington's instrumentation and postoperative casting to preoperative halo-femoral traction and Harrington instrumentation with posterior fusion (Bonnett *et al.* 1973) to anterior fusion with Dwyer instrumentation (Dwyer *et al.* 1969), to a two-stage anterior fusion with Dwyer instrumentation and Harrington instrumentation and posterior fusion (Bonnett *et al.* 1975), to anterior discectomy and fusion without instrumentation and posterior fusion with interlaminar wiring of Luque rods or other types of posterior segmental instrumentation system using hooks and screws (Rinsky 1990). Postoperative casting was eliminated. Progress has been rapid so that halo–femoral traction or halo–pelvic traction is no longer used.

Progress in anesthesia, monitoring of neurological function during surgery of the spine, intensive care, autologous blood transfusion, red cell saving devices, availability of supplemental allograft bone, and an array of antibiotics all conspired to encourage the surgery for correction and fusion of the scoliosis in general, and in particular, for the high risk surgery in the total body involved patient with cerebral palsy. Despite the tremendous biotechnical progress Dubousset (2003) sees the need for more to be done such as preoperative simulation of surgery and perioperative control with computer software.

DOES CORRECTION OF SCOLIOSIS AND FUSION MAKE ANY DIFFERENCE?
There are always skeptics who doubt the value of extensive surgery for scoliosis in this group of patients. One study from New Mexico compared 14 adult residents with quadriplegic cerebral palsy, who had untreated scoliosis, with 45 similar adults

who had mild or no curves (Kalen *et al.* 1992). No differences were found in pain levels, incidence of decubiti, pulse rate, oxygen saturation, need for pulmonary therapy, use of pulmonary medication, cardiopulmonary function or time given for daily care. But those with scoliosis greater than 45° had more pelvic and hip deformities and needed modified wheelchairs. Another study from New England compared 17 patients with severe cerebral palsy and scoliosis who had spine fusions with 20 non-fused patient's spines with an average curve of 76° (Cassidy *et al.* 1994). No clinically significant differences were noted in pain levels, pulmonary medication utilization or pulmonary therapy, decubiti, function, or time for daily care. However, the majority of healthcare workers believed that the fused patients were more comfortable.

Do the studies of Kalen *et al.* (1992) and Cassidy *et al.* (1994) throw cold water on the zeal of orthopaedic surgeons to prevent progression or correct severe scoliosis in the total body involved patient? Not necessarily. Those of us who have seen large numbers of such patients brought to us by parents who want 'something done' may advise surgery. These are usually adolescents or young adults deformed as a pretzel, propped in a seating contraption, and in desperate pulmonary straights with recurrent pneumonia (Fig. 9.56). We wish they had been brought to use sooner when correction and fusion would be feasible with acceptable risks and not a last desperate attempt.

A personal interview of caregivers after posterior instrumentation and fusion with and without anterior fusion of total body involved patients conducted by Comstock *et al.* (1998) concluded that 85% were 'very satisfied' with the results of surgery. In particular they noted the benefit of improved sitting, appearance, ease of care and comfort.

Jones *et al.* (2003) used the Pediatric Orthopaedic Society of America outcomes questionnaire in the assessment of spinal fusion of total body involved patients. Of 20 patients, 10 parents completed the questionnaire in 6 months and 1 year postoperatively. Although there were no significant changes in function, health, pain, or happiness, parental satisfaction improved significantly after 1 year. Complications did not significantly alter the questionnaire results (Fig. 9.57).

A questionnaire study of 190 children and 122 educators and therapist determined satisfaction with the outcome of spinal fusion in children with cerebral palsy (Tsirikos *et al.* 2004). Data from the questionnaire revealed a 'positive impact of the surgery on the patients' overall function, quality of life, and ease of care'. The vast majority of parents (95.8 %) and caregivers (83.4 %) would recommend spine fusion.

The vast majority of parents (95.8 %) and caregivers (83.4 %) would recommend spine fusion.

Spinal fusion for scoliosis in patients with total body involvement decreased life-expectancy as described in a study involving patients at the Alfred I. du Pont Hospital, Delaware (Tsirikos *et al.* 2003a). Of 288 patients with cerebral palsy and neuromuscular scoliosis who had spinal fusions at a mean age of 13 years 11 months (SD 3 years 4 months), 12.5% or 36 of 288 patients died within the follow-up period of 2–14 years (1988–2000). The number of days in the intensive care unit after surgery and severe preoperative thoracic kyphosis were the only statistically significant predictive factors for decreased life-expectancy following spinal fusion.

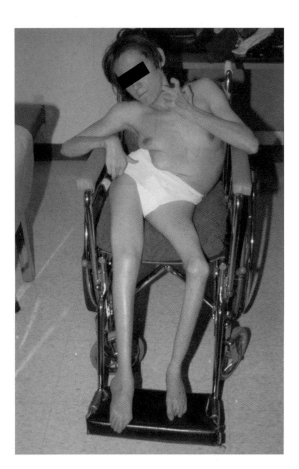

Fig. 9.56. Photograph. Total body involved, 18 year old, female. Untreated severe structural deformities of the spine, pelvis and hips.

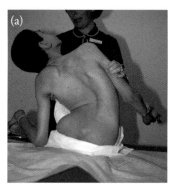
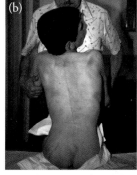

Fig. 9.57. (*a*) Photograph, patient FG. Total body involved male, age 16 years, severe scoliosis, loss of sitting balance. (*B*) Photograph, patient FG. Scoliosis corrected with posterior Luque–Galveston system, and posterior spinal fusion. Sitting balance improved but equilibrium reactions still deficient.

INDICATIONS

A curve over 40º with or without pelvic obliquity in the patient with total body involvement is an indication for surgical correction and fusion. Risk factors for severe scoliosis in cerebral palsy include: curve over 40º before the age of 15 years, bedridden status, total body involvement, and thoracolumbar curve pattern.

A curve over 40º with or without pelvic obliquity in the patient with total body involvement is an indication for surgical correction and fusion.

A decision on when the curve is most easily corrected needs to be made while weighing the immediate gains against the future risks. Surgery of this magnitude may be fatal if the decision has been delayed too long when the curve is very severe (120º or more), if the adolescent's nutritional status is poor, and if respiratory and cardiac function are compromised. Patients with total body involvement cannot cooperate in preoperative respiratory studies. If the patient has a history of recurrent pneumonia, and/ or respiratory arrests, surgery may not be the prudent course. Blood gas determination may help in the preoperative assessment. A major postoperative complication is carbon dioxide retention necessitating artificial respiration with intubation for weeks or months.

In discussion with parents or other caregivers about the risks of surgery in scoliosis, the numerical scoring system of Nachemson (1980) is helpful and understandable even though we have no objective data to arrive at a score. People relate to numbers and our *gestalt* based upon our knowledge and experience can be expressed as follows: if the removal of a wart is one point and a heart transplant is 100 points, an instrumentation and fusion in idiopathic scoliosis is 74. In paralytic scoliosis the risk might be 90.

If the removal of a wart is one point and a heart transplant is 100 points, an instrumentation and fusion in idiopathic scoliosis is 74. In paralytic scoliosis the risk might be 90.

The major complaint of the wheelchair-bound person who has severe scoliosis and pelvic obliquity is marked discomfort when seated due to the descent of the lower ribs into the pelvic brim (Fig. 9.59). Neither seat inserts, lateral pressure pads or thoracic suspension jackets have been satisfactory solutions. Furthermore, plastic or leather body jackets constrict the already restricted respiration. Philosophic deliberations and 'cost-benefit' calculations might be focused on the 'person behind the disability' (N. Clyde, personal communication), the family who provides care, and the costs of continuing nursing care that becomes necessary as the years of the patient and parents advance. The media age engenders focus on the immediate (McLuhan 1964). We need to have a longer and broader view.

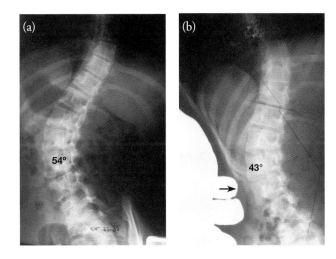

Fig. 9.58. (*a*) Radiograph. Thoracolumbar curve of 54º. (*b*) Radiograph. Patient prone. Manual lateral pressure over the curve with pelvis manually stabilized on the right side. Curve is still flexible with passive correction of 11º. Only posterior instrumentation and fusion are probably required.

SPINAL GROWTH

Spinal growth ceases with spinal fusion (Johnson and Southwick 1960, Moe *et al.* 1964, Letts and Bobechko 1974). After fusion the amount of spinal growth remaining is small and the degree of correction will often make up for the slight loss of trunk height. Each vertebra grows in height approximately 0.07 cm per year. If 12 vertebra are fused at age 12 years, the loss of height at skeletal maturity (age 16 years) will be 3.36 cm (Moe *et al.* 1978).

SPINAL FLEXIBILITY

Spinal flexibility can be assessed preoperatively with radiographic examinations. Anterior–posterior or posterior–anterior projec-

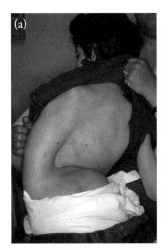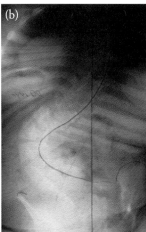

Fig. 9.59. (*a*) Patient GG. Photograph posterior view, patient sitting, total body involved, mentally retarded and non verbal, age 17 years. Very severe deformity. What looks like an arm on the left side of the trunk is the spinal curvature with rotation. (*b*) Radiograph. Patient GG. Curve measures approximately 120º. Surgery not advised because of extreme risk with this severe curve.

tions are made with the patient lying supine or prone on the radiographic table. Passive bending to the right and left (active bending is usually not possible in the total body involved patients) assists in estimated flexibility of the vertebral column. Direct manual pressure over the apex of the curve and countervailing manual pressure on the opposite side of the pelvis can give an estimate of flexibility of the curve. The radiograph will have to be made with the examiner wearing lead gloves and a lead apron to give protection from radiation. Push films simulate what we do and see at the time of posterior instrumentation and fusion (Kleinman *et al.* 1982).

PREOPERATIVE TRACTION

Preoperative traction with pelvic and cervical traction (Cotrel 1975), halo-cervical traction while seated in a wheelchair (Stagnara 1971) or halo femoral traction (Nickel *et al.* 1968), or halo-pelvic hoop traction (DeWald and Ray 1970, O'Brien *et al.* 1971, O'Brien 1977) have been abandoned as attempts to mobilize the rigid scoliotic spine. Anterior intervertebral disc excision and fusion greatly mobilizes the lumbar and thoracic spines effectively.

ANTERIOR SPINAL FUSION AND INSTRUMENTATION

Hodgson (1968) pioneered anterior spinal fusion in tuberculosis of the spine, while Dwyer (Dwyer *et al.* 1969, Dwyer 1973) was a pioneer of anterior instrumentation. Hall (1972) developed the anterior thoracoabdominal approach to the spine. Dwyer's instrumentation of staples and a cable corrected the lumbar curvature with good early results and rapid recovery without the need for a plaster jacket (Bonnett *et al.* 1973). By 1977 enthu-

siasm for Dwyer's instrumentation and fusion had waned because of unacceptably high failure rates of fusion—29% in neuromuscular scoliosis (Hall *et al.* 1977).

Dwyer instrumentation was abandoned because it eliminated lumbar lordosis so essential for sitting with weight distributed on the posterior thighs rather than on the coccygeal region. Also the rigidity of anterior fixation precluded further correction with a second stage posterior instrumentation and fusion. Hopf *et al.* (1997) designed a new anterior spinal device that not only provided firm stabilization for fusion but also derotation, and most importantly, restoration of lordosis. They reported results in 50 patients, three of whom had neuromuscular scoliosis.

Bleck (1987) discovered that excision of the intervertebral discs in two patients with severe rigid curves was useless and that vertebral body excision would be required to mobilize some of these spines (Fig. 9.60 *a, b*) (Leatherman 1969, Heinig 1984).

Zielke (1982) with his rigid anterior fixation of staples, screws and a rod effectively corrected the lateral curvature in a short segment fusion of thoracolumbar curves. Zielke claimed that his effective instrumentation that derotated a short segment of the curve made Dwyer's instrumentation obsolete.

The Texas Scottish Rite Hospital (TSRH) spinal fixation is applied to the anterior spine. Its use by orthopaedic surgeons in Beijing, China was found to be effective in idiopathic scoliosis and one case of neuromuscular scoliosis (Shen *et al.* 2003).

Rather than fuse to the pelvis in neuromuscular scoliosis, Basobas *et al.* (2003) analyzed the results in selected patients who had only an anterior fusion and instrumentation. They found that excellent corrections including pelvic obliquity were obtained and maintained. The system was used in 21 patients, most of whom

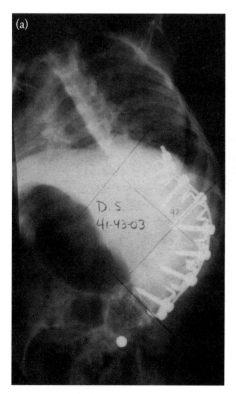

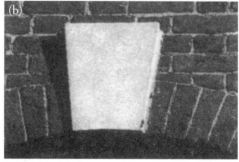

Fig. 9.60. Severe rigid lumbar curve. (*a*) Radiograph. Anterior disc excision and Dwyer instrumentation failed to correct the severe curve. Repeat surgery done with excision of apical vertebra. (*b*) The keystone of an arch of a bridge. The apical vertebra in this case is comparable to the keystone which if removed would collapse the arch of the bridge.

had myelomeningocele. The instrumentation was a single rod fixed with screws to the thoracic vertebral bodies of a correctable thoracic curve as described by Lowe *et al.* (2003) for thoracic hypokyphosis in idiopathic scoliosis.

VIDEO-ASSISTED THORACOSCOPIC SURGERY

Arthroscopy of the knee led the way to endoscopic removal of the gall bladder and has now found its way to the thoracic spine and scoliosis. Papin *et al.* (1998) did anterior spinal releases and arthrodeses using endoscopic video-assistance in adolescent scoliosis with a resultant 63% reduction in the Cobb angle after the second-stage posterior instrumentation. The cosmetic advantage was obvious, but the 'initial enthusiasm' for the procedure waned because the radiologic evidence of fusion seemed less than with an open thoracotomy. The authors concluded that the video-assisted thoracoscopic anterior fusion was reserved only for patients at risk of the 'crankshaft' of the spine as late complication.

Anand and Regan (2002) did video-assisted endoscopic removal of 117 herniated thoracic discs in 100 patients. Clinical improvement occurred in 73% of the patients at a 2-year follow-up. No neurological complications were encountered.

Newton *et al.* (2003) compared anterior fusion and instrumentation with video-assisted thoracoscopic surgery to the open operation in idiopathic scoliosis. The radiographic outcomes in both groups were the similar, but in the open operation group there was significant reduction in forced vital capacity compared to the endoscopic group. Chest wall morbidity was reduced with endoscopic surgery.

Lenke (2003) described his experience using the anterior thoracic endoscopic release and fusion followed by posterior instrumentation and fusion in 21 patients who had idiopathic scoliosis. One patient had a conversion to the open procedure because of bleeding and one developed a pseudoarthrosis necessitating revision surgery.

Thoracoscopic anterior disc excision and fusion has not been reported as an adjunct for surgery in scoliosis of patients with cerebral palsy. But it is possible that it has been tried in the process of evolution of surgical techniques of spine surgery.

POSTERIOR INSTRUMENTATION AND FUSION

Harrington instrumentation. MacEwen (1969) was one of the pioneers in using Harrington instrumentation in scoliosis in the patient with total body involvement. By 1972, MacEwen had discovered that Harrington instrumentation was not the final answer as many had hoped (MacEwen 1972).

Cotrel-Dubousset. Posterior instrumentation has been modified many times since its introduction by Harrington in 1962 (Akeson and Bobechko 1986). The principle was distraction of the curve on the concave side and compression on the convex side. Cotrel-Dubousset of France designed the same distraction-compression system with a twist (Dubousset *et al.* 1986, Johnson *et al.* 1986). They used a rough rod secured with pedicle hooks and screws to derotate the vertebra in addition to the lateral correction. Its use was first confined to idiopathic thoracic and

thoracolumbar curves and was expanded to include paralytic scoliosis (Dubousset *et al.* 1987, M'Rabet and Dubousset 1988). The latter used various instrumentations for correction and fusion of scoliosis in non-walking patients with cerebral palsy: Harrington, Luque or Cotrel-Dubousset systems. Twenty-one had a combined anterior and posterior fusion. About half had some sort of complication, but the results between 2 and 13 years follow-up were 'very encouraging'. French surgeons of Besançon (Onimus *et al.* 1992) also used a variety of spinal fusion techniques in 32 bedridden children with total body involvement. Although the complication rate was high (including three deaths and major complications including sepsis and cutaneous problems in 10 others), sitting was acquired in all cases, pain was relieved in two-thirds, and respiratory problems in two-thirds of cases were diminished postoperatively.

Luque (Cardoso *et al.* 1976, Luque and Cardoso 1977) introduced a new method of spinal fixation fixed with interlaminar wires at each spinal segment fixed to semirigid rods on both sides of the curve. The fixation was sufficiently rigid to eliminate postoperative plaster casts or orthoses while fusion occurred (Fig. 9.61). The elimination of encasing plaster casts made the Luque system very appealing for correction of scoliosis in the total body involved patient. This system was found to be effective in neuromuscular scoliosis and its use was rapidly adopted (Herndon *et al.* 1987, Broom *et al.* 1989)

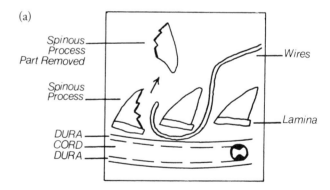

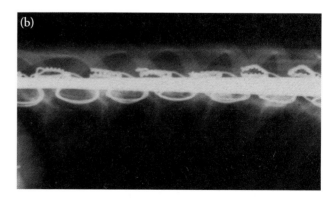

Fig. 9.61. (*a*) Diagrammatic representation of sagittal section of the midline structures of the vertebral column. The interlaminar wires in the Luque system and proximate to the dura and spinal cord. (*b*) Radiograph. Lateral projection of mid-thoracic spine depicting interlaminar wires for Luque rod fixation.

Drummond (1984), as usual in orthopaedic instrumentation, devised a modification. Wires were passed through the spinous processes at each level, and fixed to a Harrington rod on the convex side and a Luque rod on the concave side. Sponseller *et al.* (1986) gave approbation to this combination of systems in a report of a mean correction of 50.5% and a mean loss of correction of only 5% in a 22-month follow-up.

Other adaptation of the Luque principle of segmental wire fixation were combinations with the Harrington distraction rod ('Harri-Luke', 'Lukington', 'Luque-Harrington').

Galveston, Texas orthopaedic surgeons introduced fixation of the distal ends of bent Luque rods into the ilium that facilitated correction of the pelvic obliquity and fusion to include the sacrum (Allen and Ferguson 1981, 1982, Allen 1983). The Galveston fixation with the Luque rods and wires was widely adopted for neuromuscular scoliosis in general and specifically for the scoliosis of the total body involved (Brown *et al.* 1982, Metz and Zielke 1982, Stanitski *et al.* 1982, Cardoso 1984, Kalen *et al.* 1985, Thompson *et al.* 1985, Herndon *et al.* 1987, Gersoff and Renshaw 1988, Boachie-Adjei *et al.* 1989, Gau *et al.* 1991, Benson *et al.* 1998, Thomson and Banta 2001, Kaczmarczyk *et al.* 2003). Kalen and colleagues of Stanford University had encouraging results in 28 patients with neuromuscular scoliosis (Kalen and Bleck 1985, Kalen *et al.* 1985). The corrections of curves from 35° to 100° (mean 69°) was 70%. Blood loss was considerable (average case 5500 ml) and the operations were long, averaging 7 hours (Fig. 9.62 *a*, *b*).

Luque Unit Rod. The loss of correction due to rotation of the Luque rods led McCarthy and McCullough (1985) to add a locking collar to the proximal ends of the two rods. Moseley *et al.* (1986) went a step further to design a closed loop of the proximal end of the two Luque rods with retention of the distal bend of the rods for insertion into the ilium. This addition greatly improved correction of the curve and pelvic obliquity

without a significant loss of correction (Bell *et al.* 1989, Maloney *et al.* 1990) (Fig. 9.63 *a*, *b*). Other orthopaedic surgeons have documented the effectiveness of the unit rod in correcting pelvic obliquity and the spinal curvature better than with the two-rod Luque system (McCarthy *et al.* 1988b, Bulman *et al.* 1996, Dias *et al.* 1996, Lipton *et al.* 2003) (Fig. 9.64). The unit rod without fusion to the sacrum has also been used with good results in ambulatory patients with cerebral palsy (Tsirikos *et al.* 2003b).

Other modifications of posterior instrumentation have evolved since Harrington, Luque and Dubousset. San Julian *et al.* (1995) of Pamplona, Spain, used two short rods at the lumbar curve-one in distraction and the other in compression, and two long rods in distraction to the sacrum, with pedicle screw fixation up to the thoracic spine, pedicular hooks, and fixation of all four rods with sublaminar and basispinous wires; Marchesi and colleagues (1997) of Montreal, Canada, modified the Luque-Galveston technique with sacral screws in the 1st sacral pedicles and a transverse traction device between the distal right-angle bends of the rods (Danek System M-8) (Fig. 9.65); the ISOLA-Galveston system uses integration of hooks, wires, screws and post anchors (Whitaker *et al.* 2000, Yazici *et al.* 2000) reported from Kansas City, USA.

The *Cantilever Bending Technique* was an innovation by Chang (2003) of Taiwan for rigid curves that included neuromuscular causes. The technique entails the insertion of six pedicle screws on the upper, apical and lower segments on both the concave and convex sides. A convex rod is locked to the pedicle screws. *In situ* benders are secured to the convex side above and below the apical pedicle screw. The free ends of the benders, the lever arms, are brought closer to each other to effect a powerful force to correct the curve in the coronal plane. A prebent rod to conform to the corrected curve is secured to the screws on the concave side. Both rods are connected with transverse links. Intraoperative radiographs are used to determine the need for adjustment. The benders are removed when all is secure. No neurological complications occurred. Chang stated that this method obviated the need for anterior release to correct large and rigid curves.

From Freiburg, Germany came a system that consisted of dorsal semi rigid instrumentation with pedicle screws in the lumbosacral spine and sublaminar wiring of rods in the thoracic spine to correct paralytic scoliosis (Knoeller and Stuecker 2002). Corrections were 66.4%.

The *Isola-Galveston* instrumentation is a further evolution for spinal correction and fusion with reported efficacy in a variety of neuromuscular scoliosis patients that included cerebral palsy (Yazici *et al.* 2000). The ISOLA segmental spinal system in scoliosis has had success in idiopathic and neuromuscular scoliosis as delineated in a study from orthopaedic surgeons of Hong Kong (Leung *et al.* 2002).

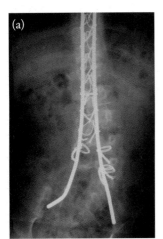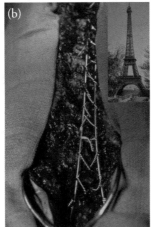

Fig. 9.62. (*a*) Radiograph. Postoperative Luque–Galveston method of posterior instrumentation and fixation to the pelvis. (*b*) Intraoperative photograph of the posterior wound for spinal fusion and Luque–Galveston fixation. Although the photograph reminds us of Paris, the operation was devised in Mexico by the late Eduardo Luque MD.

ANTERIOR DISC EXCISION AND FUSION AND POSTERIOR INSTRUMENTATION AND FUSION

Combined anterior and posterior fusion was described by Floman *et al.* (1982) in 35 patients who had a variety of severe deformities

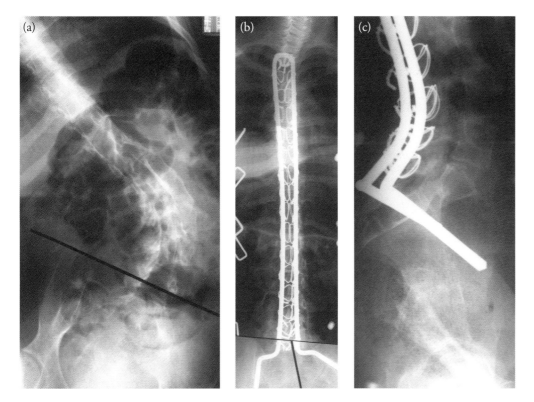

Fig. 9.63 (*a*) Radiograph. Patient MP, age 16 years, severe progressive scoliosis. (*b*) Radiograph. Patient MP, age 23 years. Scoliosis and pelvic obliquity corrected with anterior disc excision and apical vertebrectomy followed by Luque type unit rod and interlaminar wires. (*c*) Radiograph. Lateral projection lumbar spine and sacrum. Distal rods bent to preserve normal lordosis. No instrumentation used anteriorly which would preclude persevation of lumbar lordosis with posterior instrumentation. (By courtesy of L.A. Rinsky MD, Stanford University.)

such as severe kyphosis and major thoracolumbar curves with pelvic obliquity. Optimal corrections were obtained, but the complication rate was high (32/73 patients) leading the authors to caution that the combined anterior and posterior approach should not be undertaken lightly and by inexperienced surgeons. Lonstein and Akabarnia (1983) stated in a long term follow-up study of 107 patients who had scoliosis with cerebral palsy or mental retardation that in those who had pelvic obliquity it was *always* necessary to do the anterior and posterior surgery; fusion to the sacrum was essential. Hopf and Eysel (2000) of Kiel, Germany, recognized that the combined anterior and posterior approach was necessary in most cases of cerebral palsy.

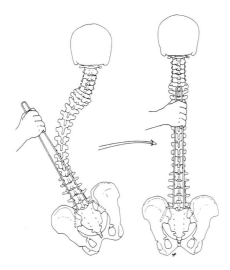

Fig. 9.64. Correction of pelvic obliquity and scoliosis with the unit rod. The pelvic fixation insert first so the rods can act as a 'rudder' to level the pelvis and the unit is brought to the midline of the spine and secured with interlaminar wires (from Maloney *et al.* 1990), by permission.

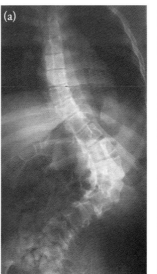
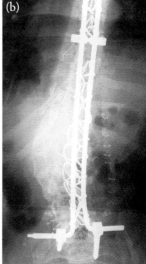

Fig. 9.65. (*a*) Radiograph. Patient AK. Total body involved, male. (*b*) Postoperative segmental spinal fixation with sacral screws for pelvic fixation and traction bar lower thoracic level (Danek System M-8).

The combined anterior and posterior approach should not be undertaken lightly.

Anterior disc excision and fusion without instrumentation and posterior instrumentation and fusion in pelvic obliquity and scoliosis in cerebral palsy have given better correction than with posterior instrumentation and fusion alone (O'Brien 1972, Boachie-Adjei *et al.* 1989, Maloney *et al.* 1990, Rinsky 1990, Dias *et al.* 1996, Thacker *et al.* 2002, Tsirikos *et al.* 2003c).

The decision to do either a one-stage posterior fusion or a two-stage anterior and posterior fusion was based on traction radiographs by Boachie-Adjei *et al.* (1989). If the pelvis was not level or if the torso was not balanced over the pelvis, and the curve was rigid, the two-stage procedure was done.

A same-day two-stage anterior and posterior fusion using the Galveston rods to the pelvis was done with the patient in halo–femoral traction during the operation. The scoliosis and severe pelvic obliquity were corrected and maintained in a 2-year follow-up (Huang and Lenke 2001). The addition of the traction on the spine during surgery might be a solution to correct a very severe curve and severe pelvic obliquity. Although the authors reported no complications, there is one that could occur with halo-traction, i.e. 6th cranial nerve palsy which is most frequent, but also 9th, 10th and 12th traction palsy can occur (Wilkins and MacEwen 1977). Much of the traction is exerted on the upper cervical spine with the result of stretch paralysis of the cranial nerves as they exit the skull. Patients in skeletal cervical traction should be monitored regularly particularly for lack of lateral gaze (Abducens nerve, 6th cranial nerve), swallowing (9th) and voice (10th) changes, and tongue (12th) movement abnormalities. Lateral radiographic projections from the occiput to the third cervical vertebra when traction is applied might alert the surgeon to excessive traction in the upper cervical spine. A maximum weight of 12 kg on the halo and 12 kg divided between the two lower limbs was advised by Moe *et al.* (1978).

OPERATIVE TECHNIQUES FOR ANTERIOR AND POSTERIOR SPINE FUSION AND INSTRUMENTATION

Rather than consume more paper and ink, the reader is referred to several excellent texts on operative techniques listed as 'Further reading' preceding the references. It is probably necessary to see the operations, preferably as a first or second assistant to the experienced surgeon.

CORRECTION WITHOUT SPINAL FUSION

Correction of progressive scoliosis in children too young for fusion with resultant loss of growth has been an attractive option because of orthotic failure. Luque instrumentation without fusion failed to prevent progression of spinal curves (three cases of cerebral palsy) and some rods broke (Fig. 9.66) (Rinsky *et al.* 1985, Eberle *et al.* 1986).

Harrington rod distraction every 6 months without fusion has had more success (Moe *et al.* 1984). Dr E. Ascani of Italy (personal communication) modified the distracting rod with

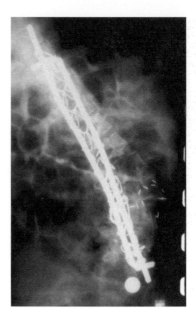

Fig. 9.66. Radiograph. Failure of Luque rods and segmental fixation to restrain progression of scoliosis without fusion in a growing boy. The method is no longer recommended.

two hooks on either side of the distal and proximal ends. They made a small incision to distract the rod at regular intervals for sequential correction without fusion.

SPINAL MUSCLE MYOTOMY

Myotomy of the paravertebral muscles in cerebral palsy to decrease progression of scoliosis has a superficial appeal. Terazawa *et al.* (1980) reported one case of a 21-year-old Japanese male who had a 'remarkable' improvement of scoliosis after 'soft tissue releases' and a transfer to the ipsilateral tendon fasciae lata to the rib cage. One wonders if this young man had pure athetosis with dystonia and not a structural scoliosis.

Matsuo (2002) does selective spinal and abdominal myotomies to relieve 'hypertonicity' of trunk muscles in his general scheme termed Orthopaedic Selective Spasticity-Control Surgery (OSSCS). He proposes the muscle weakening for early intervention of and as a preventative of scoliosis in cerebral palsy, and as an adjunct to spinal fusion. However, no data are provided on the preoperative and postoperative spinal deformities treated. The publication of a study justifying spinal myotomies as referenced in Matsuo's text is in Japanese (Goto *et al.* 1987).

PRINCIPLES OF SURGERY FOR PARALYTIC SCOLIOSIS

The elements or principles to be included in surgery for paralytic scoliosis remain unchanged:

- Spinal fusion is essential. Instrumentation systems are only temporary sutures to maintain the correction while new bone formation creates a permanent strong support.
- Arthrodesis should extend as far lateral as the transverse processes.
- Fusion should extend from the sacrum to the 1st, 2nd or 3rd thoracic vertebra (Fig. 9.67). One surgeon and his colleagues extended the fusion only to the 5th lumbar vertebra thus

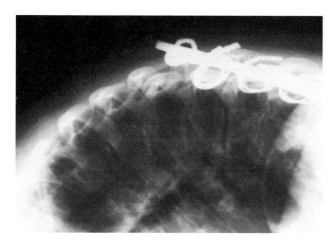

Fig. 9.67. Kyphosis of the upper thoracic spine above the fixation rods. The rods should extend to the 1st, 2nd or 3rd thoracic vertebra. Lower than this, the spine bends anteriorly with growth and gravity.

preserving mobility of the lumbosacral joint (Sussman *et al.* 1996). In their cases, most of whom had muscular dystrophy, pelvic obliquity was improved 50% and only two increased their pelvic obliquity.

Despite not including the sacrum in the fusion, pelvic obliquity was partially corrected due to the strong iliolumbar ligaments that run from the transverse processes of the 5th lumbar vertebra to the iliac crest (Luk *et al.* 1986). These ligaments maintain the vertebra in a 'fairly constant relationship with the sacrum'. This is why the correction of the scoliosis with anterior instrumentation to the fifth lumbar vertebra can partially correct the pelvic obliquity (O'Brien *et al.* 1975, Leong *et al.* 1981).

Most surgeons include the sacrum in spinal fusions for scoliosis in the total body involved with cerebral palsy. An exception was made by Drummond (1996) who fuses the spine only to the 4th lumbar vertebra in scoliosis of ambulatory patients with cerebral palsy and occasionally a short fusion in Duchenne's muscular dystrophy if the pelvic obliquity is 'moderate', flexible, and when the 5th lumbar vertebra is horizontal.

Fusion should extend from the sacrum to the 1st, 2nd or 3rd thoracic vertebra.

- The facet should be excised, although B.L. Allen Jr (personal communication) doubted this was necessary because fixation was so rigid. Bleck (1987) found that facet joints were still open 8 years postoperatively in an area that had an anterior fusion.
- Autogenous iliac bone grafts should be added to the fusion area (Goldstein 1969), but supplemental allografts are necessary and effective (McCarthy *et al.* 1986, Montgomery *et al.* 1990, Bridwell *et al.* 1994). Rib resections on the convex side can provide additional grafts (Hoppenfeld and Gross 1986; L.A. Rinsky, personal communication). Zeller *et al.* (1994) of Paris, France had success results using a tibial bone graft for 72 patients who had posterior fusions for neuromuscular scoliosis. The only complication was a leg length discrepancy of less than 2 cm in four patients related to tibial overgrowth. They believed their results of fusion were superior to those that used 'bank bone'.

- Both anterior discectomy and fusion without instrumentation and posterior fusion with instrumentation are best in the rigid curves of cerebral palsy.
- If the surgeon and anesthesiologist judge that the patient can tolerate the posterior surgery immediately after the anterior first stage, the patient is turned prone for the second posterior stage. If not, the second-stage posterior surgery can be scheduled 7–10 days after the anterior surgery has been done barring complications from the first stage. The patient remains in bed during the interval.
- The anterior thoracoabdominal approach entails removal of the intervertebral discs and cartilagenous end-plates to subchondral bone, and excision of vertebral bodies when the apical vertebrae remain immovable (Heinig 1984). When vertebrae are excised, the anterior longitudinal ligament is preserved. Heinig preserved the cortex and scooped out the cancellous bone to create an 'eggshell'. The shell is crushed and the vertebral fragments are replaced in the sleeve of the ligaments, as in making a sausage.

  Vertebral body excision was rarely done in the past (Compère 1932, VonLackum and Smith 1933, Wiles 1951). Although anesthesia techniques and blood-replacement with transfusion and with washed cells from the 'cell saver' have made vertebral body excision somewhat safer, it is still a formidable procedure. Extreme caution to diminish injury to the spinal cord is obvious. It is not certain that continuous cold saline lavage of the exposed dura mater or intravenous corticosteroids will protect the spinal cord.
- Pelvic obliquity should be corrected as much as possible. Contractures below the iliac crest, i.e. flexion and adduction should be corrected first.
- Correction should aim for compensation so that the occiput remains directly over the sacrum (Fig. 9.68).
- In the non-walking patient with total body involvement the goal is comfortable sitting. In fusion to the sacrum the lumbar lordosis should be preserved. Rods have to be bent to accommodate a lordosis between 20° and 30° (measured on the lateral radiograph of the lumbar spine from the top of first lumbar vertebra to the bottom of the 5th lumbar vertebra; normal median 40°—Table 9.III). Most of the lordosis occurs at the lumbosacral level (normal median 12°—Table 9.III) Lumbar lordosis ensures that the body weight when sitting will be on the posterior thighs which can accept 100 mm mercury per square inch (4.4 cm) before skin ischemia occurs. In contrast, the coccygeal area can tolerate only about 15 mm per square inch. Coccygeal pressure in sitting is the result of elimination of lumbar lordosis (Motloch 1978).
- Correction should not be forced beyond the limits of mobility of the spine.
- Neurological complications are the most feared and may be minimized with spinal cord monitoring using somatosen-

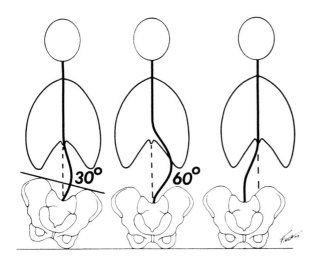

Fig. 9.68. Importance of obtaining alignment of head and trunk over center of sacrum. *Left:* minimal curve but unsatisfactory pelvic obliquity; *center:* the curve is larger but well balanced with head and trunk over the sacrum; *right:* small curve, pelvis level, trunk vertical but shifted out of balance to the left. (Reprinted by permission, from Moe *et al.* 1978.)

sory-evoked cortical potentials (Bunch *et al.* 1983, Brown *et al.* 1984, Williamson and Galasko 1992, DiCindio *et al.* 2003), and the Stagnara wake-up test (Vauzelle *et al.* 1973, Hall *et al.* 1978). Although the patient with cerebral palsy, particularly the total body involved, it may be thought that a disruption of spinal cord function would make little difference in the motor function of the limbs, the interruption of the nerve supply to the bladder or a major sensory deficit in the lower limbs would add another disability.

Minimize neurological complications in scoliosis surgery with somatosensory-evoked potentials during surgery and the wake-up test.

The patient with total body involvement may not have voluntary control or their feet. Stimulation of the plantar aspect of the foot with a small tooth forceps is sufficient stimulus to cause withdrawal of the foot and limb. The wake-up test is facilitated if the inhalation anesthetic is fluothane that can be rapidly reversed to awaken the patient. It ensures continuity of the anterior columns of the spinal cord. *Somatosensory evoked potentials are not perfect* to monitor the integrity of the spinal cord tracts (Ginsberg *et al.* 1985, Szalay *et al.* 1986b) because somatosensory evoked potentials do not monitor the anterior

columns of the spinal cord. Transcranial electric motor-evoked potentials could be monitored in only 39% of cerebral palsy patients who had severe involvement (DiCindio *et al.* 2003) in contrast to 82% success in monitoring somatosensory evoked potentials with stimulation of the posterior tibial nerve.

Spinal-cord dysfunction can occur due to interruption of the blood supply. This may be caused by excessive distraction of the spine. In the anterior approach, electrocoagulation of bleeding vessels in the intervertebral foramina should be avoided. Packing off the bleeder and adding hemostatic agents or gelfoam should be sufficient to control bleeding. The main blood supply of the spinal cord in the mid thoracic region arises from the arteria radiculomedullaris magna (ARM or the artery of Adamkiewicz; Fujisawa *et al.* 2006) to supply the anterior spinal artery in the mid-thoracic region. The origin of the arteria radicullomedullaris is from one of the intercostal arteries from the sixth thoracic distally or an upper lumbar segmental arteries at the first, second or third lumbar levels near the intervertebral foramen. This arises on the left side in 66% of patients. As it passes through the intervertebral foramen with the anterior nerve root, it courses proximally initially then takes a hairpin turn to join into and become the anterior spinal artery coursing distally (Doppman and DiChiro 1968, Keim and Hilal 1971). Electrocoagulation in the intervertebral foramina risks coagulation of an intercostal artery that feeds the major blood supply of the spinal cord.

Closed suction drainage of the wound greatly assists wound healing and complications. Wound dressing changes are usually unnecessary. It does not increase blood loss significantly and the need for blood transfusion (Blank *et al.* 2003). Its use is practically universal among spine surgeons for the past 40 years. Subcutaneous perforated plastic tubes can be placed throughout the entire wound, connected to a suction device and left in situ as long as 72 hours.

PREOPERATIVE PREPARATION

Autologous blood for transfusion can be conserved 1 month in advance of the operation. One unit per week is drawn from the patient and stored for use in the operating room. Correction and spinal fusion in neuromuscular scoliosis risks extensive blood loss (>50% total blood volume). The more vertebral segments are fused, the greater the loss (Edler *et al.* 2003). The risk of more than 50% blood volume in neuromuscular scoliosis surgery was estimated as seven times higher than in idiopathic scoliosis.

The greater loss of blood in neuromuscular scoliosis surgery compared with idiopathic scoliosis was documented and studied

TABLE 9.III
Summary of distribution of lordosis, kyphosis, and L5–S1 angle. (Patients: 104 normal, 114 scoliosis; 2 to > 20 years)

	Lordosis		Kyphosis		L5-Sl angle	
	Normal	*Scoliotic*	*Normal*	*Scoliotic*	*Normal*	*Scoliotic*
Median (°)	40	48.5	27	28	12	*10.5*
20%–75% (°)	31–49	40–55	21–33	16.5–36	9–16	6–14.5
10%–90% (°)	22.5–54	33.5–61.5	11.5–39.5	9–53	5–21	4–18

From Propst-Proctor and Bleck (1983).

by Kannan *et al.* (2002). Prothrombin time was longer over time in the neuromuscular scoliosis patients and Factor VII activity was decreased. These depletions of the clotting factor suggested activation of the extrinsic coagulation pathway.

Small patients who have a neuromuscular disease and have extensive spinal surgery may not be able to donate their blood (autologous) before surgery. Allogeneic red cell transfusions are often required.[19]

Amicar (episolon aminocaproic acid) is an antifibrinolytic agent, administered intraoperatively to reduce blood loss during scoliosis surgery. In a blindly randomized study of 36 patients with idiopathic scoliosis who had posterior spine fusions with segmental spinal instrumentation, postoperative blood loss measured by the amount of suction drainage was decreased in the Amicar group compared to controls. Perioperative blood loss was less, and there was also less need for autologous blood transfusions (Florentino-Pineda *et al.* 2004). Kuklo *et al.* (2003) did a review of data on blood management studies to reduce the need for autologous blood transfusion in spinal surgery. They concluded that the 'judicious' use of thrombotic agents and antifibrinolytics and techniques such as autologous blood donation and red cell augmentation can be effective in reducing the need for blood transfusions in spinal surgery.

Chest physical and respiratory therapy should be done at least 1 day preoperatively.

Assessment of the nutritional status of the patient may be important for optimum results and fewer complications. Serum albumin should be at least 35 g/liter and the total blood lymphocyte count of at least 1.5 giga per liter (1500 cells/mm^3) (Jevsevar and Karlin 1993). If these nutritional indicators are below the stated levels, a nutritional program should be instituted.

A poor nutritional status in the patient with total body involvement who has scoliosis surgery has been associated with more complications that include infections and delayed wound healing. In the study cited, three of four patients who had a feeding tube had normal nutritional parameters. This would be one of the 'aggressive measures' recommended by the investigators to bring the nutritional status to normal.

Enteric supplementation via nasal of gastric tubes between the anterior and posterior stages of spinal fusion may be in order as reflected in low albumin and total protein levels (Mooney 2000). This method for an average of 9.1 days was reported as safe, and less costly than total parental nutrition in the patient with cerebral palsy who had extensive spinal surgery. Supplemental vitamins and iron are presumed.

The nutritional status of these particular patients can be assessed with serum albumin and total protein levels and a lymphocyte count.

An alternative assessment for nutritional status was the measurement of resting energy expenditure and body cell mass

in children with spastic quadriplegia (Azcue *et al.* 1996). Resting energy expenditure was poorly correlated with body cell mass. But in nine of 13 children with spastic quadriplegia had reduced resting energy expenditure per unit of lean tissue or extracelluar water. Consequently, the authors proposed measurement of individual energy expenditure with bioelectrical impedance analysis.

Bone allografts should be on hand to be added to the fusion site.

POSTOPERATIVE CARE
After the posterior instrumentation, sitting can resume in 5–7 days postoperatively in a contoured upholstered seat insert to support the trunk and compensate for the deficient equilibrium reactions. Postoperatively molded plastic shells can be worn for security while the fusion is consolidating. Bleck (1987) used removable anterior and posterior shells postoperatively in only two of 55 cases.

COMPLICATIONS
Spine surgery is big surgery and complications are inevitable. The only point in listing some of the complications is to expect them, watch for them, and deal with them promptly when they arise.

The only point in listing some of the complications is to expect them, watch for them, and deal with them promptly when they arise.

Anterior spine surgery in neuromuscular scoliosis of 111 patients had a complication rate of 44.1%, of which 26.1% were major (Sarwahi *et al.* 2001). Pulmonary complications were the most common major complications and urinary tract infections the most common minor complications. The rate of complications was greater in cerebral palsy scoliosis surgery. Factors affecting complications were thoracoabdominal or transthoracic approaches, operative blood loss more than one liter, previous spine surgery, and a curve greater than 100°.

A larger study of 599 patients who had pediatric anterior spine fusions between the years 1967 and 1991 revealed major complications in 7.5% and minor ones in 33% (Grossfeld *et al.* 1997). Most of the major complications were respiratory (e.g. pneumonia, pneumothorax, respiratory distress syndrome). Atelectasis was frequent as might be expected, but considered a 'minor complication'. One distressing complication was lymph effusion due to a tear in the thoracic duct that required chest tube drainage and exploration to repair the rent in the duct (Fig. 9.69) (Propst-Proctor *et al.* 1983).

In another similar study of risk factors for complications in spinal fusions of 107 patients with cerebral palsy the significant risk factors were a curve greater than 70°, the severity of the neurological involvement, and severity of the history of medical problems (Lipton *et al.* 1999). The weight of the child for height and age or a deficient total lymphocyte count made no statistically significant effect on outcome.

---

19 Allogeneic: different gene constitutions in the same species; antigentically distinct.

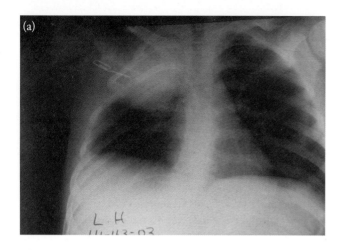

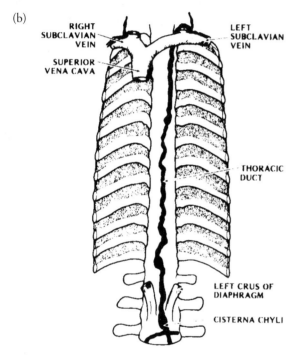

Fig. 9.69. (*a*) Radiograph. Left lung effusion; chyle thorax. (*b*) Drawing of anatomy of the thoracic duct as a reminder to try to avoid injury to it during the thoracoabdominal exposures for scoliosis correction and fusion (from anterior–posterior radiograph of pelvis and hips). Pelvic obliquity due to persistent adduction contracture of right hip—'wind-swept pelvis'. Hip 'uncovered' on adducted side. Age 9 years, female, total body involved. (From Propst-Proctor *et al.* 1983, by permission.)

Deep wound infections occur at a rather high rate in spinal instrumentation and fusion in patients with cerebral palsy with considerable variation among institutions: 8.7% (Szoke *et al.* 1998); 20% (Malamo-Lada *et al.* 1999); 4.3% (Sponseller *et al.* 2000).[20] The infection rate depends on the number of cases and the differing risk factors among a series of patients. The major infecting organisms were coagulase-negative Staphylococcus, Enterobacter, Enterococcus and Escherichia coli. In both studies wound debridement, secondary closure and prolonged antimi-

crobial therapy was necessary for healing. Serial debridement was not always successful; a few healed by allowing the wound to granulate over the rods, or by rod removal. The only significant risk factors determined were the degree of mental retardation and the use of allografts (Sponseller *et al.* 2000).[21]

Pulmonary complications need no special discussion on management. Ample help in managing these is usually available with consulting pediatricians, anesthesiologist, and pulmonologists.

Neurological complications of major proportions such as paraplegia can occur, but minimized with SEP monitoring and the wake-up test during surgery. If the monitoring indicates lack of transmission of conduction in the spinal cord or the wake-up test fails, the advice is to cut the distraction rod in two or remove the instrumentation without undue delay. Prior to cutting or removing the instrumentation it is wise to check the blood pressure. Hypotension can affect spinal cord circulation and should be immediately corrected by the anesthesiologist. Major spinal-cord lesions occurred in 87 of 7885 cases of scoliosis surgery between 1965 and 1971. Complete recovery occurred in 22, partial recovery in 28, and none in 24. Not all were associated with Harrington instrumentation; six patients became paraplegic with skeletal traction only (MacEwen *et al.* 1975). Segmental instrumentation has been accompanied with neurological complications and minor sensory changes that were transient (Wilber *et al.* 1984). Of 507 cases of segmental spinal instrumentation with Luque rods, there were two partial spinal cord syndromes (0.4 %), 13 cases of truncal and limb hyperesthesia (2.6 %) and one femoral neuropathy from a protruding pelvic rod (Allen and Ferguson 1985).

The hyperesthesia following Luque segmental instrumentation is characterized by extreme tenderness of the skin over the anterior trunk and thighs. All Bleck's patients recovered within 2 weeks (Bleck 1987). The cause seems to be a lesion of the posterior spinal cord due to hemorrhage and edema that can be caused the sublaminar wires (Biemond 1964, Braakman and Penning 1971, Liepones *et al.* 1984). Caution and care are necessary when passing the wires under the lamina (Yngve *et al.* 1986). If bleeding occurs on removal of the ligamentum flavum, electrocoagulation or hemostats should not be used to control bleeding. Packing of the bleeding with hemostatic sponges should be used.

Instrumentation breakage or failure is bound to occur, but apparently rarely given the paucity of reports of such and probably because of the superiority of the metallurgy by the manufacturers. Luque rods have snapped, but rarely if quarter-inch rods are used rather than 3/16 inch other than in small and slightly built children. Hooks and screws can inadvertently be dislodged. Magnissalis *et al.* (2003) report a fracture of a quarter-inch ISOLA rod which on testing failed due to loosening of a two-set tandem

---

20 Deep wound infections with anterior spinal surgery in a large series of 599 procedures was only 1.17% (Grossfeld *et al.* 1997).

21 Why the degree of mental retardation was a significant risk factor is difficult to understand, unless these patients had a poor nutritional and immune status due to their need to be fed or had a problem with chewing, swallowing or regurgitation.

connecter and subsequent overloading of the contralateral bar. The system was replaced 22 months later.

Penetration of the pelvic rod portion of the Luque unit rod is not surprising and probably happens occasionally. Salvation was obtained in one case report in which one limb of the distal rod protruded into the hip. The solution was through an anterolateral approach to the hip and shortening the protruded rod with a burr so the hardware could be retained and no loss of correction occurred (Givon and Miller 1999).

Loss of correction or proximal instrument failure in the Luque–Galveston technique occurred in 13 of 41 patients (Sink *et al.* 2003). In four of these a kyphosis developed at the cephalad portion of the instrumentation and in nine the proximal hardware pulled out. Posterior migration of the distal end of the rods occurred in five. Hyerkyphosis preoperatively was considered responsible for loss of proximal instrument failure. Anterior lumbar discectomy and fusion without instrumentation in the thoracolumbar or lumbar spine with kyphosis was deemed the risk factor for instrumentation failure. Presumably one might conclude that if thoracolumbar or lumbar kyphosis is present, anterior instrumentation would be in order to prevent failure.

PERICARDIAL TAMPONADE

Pericardial tamponade is a complication not of the surgery itself, but of anesthesia monitoring of the central venous pressure. The catheter used for this purpose should be only in the superior vena cava. If inadvertently advanced into the right atrium, the pumping of the heart can cause the tip of the catheter to erode through the pericardium with resultant tamponade and heart failure. Kalen *et al.* (1992) reported three patients who had this complication. It can be prevented with a chest radiograph after the catheter has been inserted to make certain it is in the superior vena cava.

CRANKSHAFT PHENOMENON[22]

The crankshaft phenomenon refers to postoperative curve progression with angulation and rotation of the spine after posterior fusion with instrumentation (Dubousset *et al.* 1989). It occurs when fusion is done prior to the Risser I stage as an indicator of spinal growth. The progressive angulation and rotation is due to continued growth of the anterior spinal structures. At risk are patients who are in Tanner I stage of maturation and who have open triradiate cartilages. The prevention of this late structural complication is anterior vertebral body fusion as well as posterior fusion. Several authors have reported on its occurrence and suggested prevention (Dubousset *et al.* 1989, Shufflebarger and Clark 1991, Dohin and Dubousset 1994, Lapinsky and Richards 1995, Sanders *et al.* 1995, 1997, Hamill *et al.* 1997, Lee and Nachemson 1997, Roberto *et al.* 1997,

---

22 *Crankshaft* = a shaft turned by a crank. *Crank* = a device for transmitting rotary motion which consists of a handle or arm attached at right angles to the shaft. The original Model-T Ford was started by turning a crank in the front end of the automobile.

Kesling *et al.* 2003). The scoliosis treated was primarily idiopathic and in one report, congenital (Kesling *et al.* 2003), although Dubousset *et al.* (1989) included paralytic scoliosis as well as idiopathic.

Hamill and colleagues of St Louis, Missouri (1997), in an analysis of 33 skeletally immature patients younger than 12 years and who had posterior spine fusions with instrumentation, found the triradiate cartilage open in 24 patients at the time of surgery. But of those 29 only 9 (37.5%) developed the crankshaft phenomenon. So the open triradiate cartilage was not the only prognostic indicator of late crankshaft phenomena.

Smucker and Miller (2001), of the Alfred I. duPont Hospital for Children, reviewed their 50 patients with cerebral palsy who had posterior only fusion with unit rod instrumentation. All had open triradiate cartilage at the time of fusion. Follow-up of more than 2 years and with closed triradiate cartilages found no clinically significant radiographic changes in the curve patterns. Does this mean that the unit rod to correct and stabilize the spine in children who have spinal growth velocity remaining at the time of fusion is effective in preventing the 'crankshaft' phenomenon?

CERVICAL SPONDYLOSIS AND MYELOPATHIES

Severe athetosis with constant movement of the neck or severe dystonic posturing does play havoc with the cervical vertebrae and the intervertebral discs eventually leading to foraminal occlusion and/or compression of the spinal cord. Bleck (1987) reported only two cases. One was a 34-year-old female with severe athetosis who became suddenly quadriplegic due to a subluxation of the 5th on the 6th cervical vertebra. A computerized axial tomogram with nitrizamide dye in the canal depicted severe atrophy of the spinal cord. The other patient was a 31-year-old man with severe athetosis and constant turning of his head to the left. He had the slow onset of flaccid paralysis of his shoulder girdle musculature. Radiographs of the cervical spine showed extensive degenerative changes and almost complete occlusion of the intervertebral foramina.

Other case reports were by McCluer (1982) of four patients with athetosis. Two of these had almost complete quadriplegia at the 5th cervical spinal cord level. All had cervical spondylosis and a myelopathy. Three of the four patients had surgical decompression of the spinal cord with poor results. Angelini *et al.* (1982) had one case of cervical myelopathy in a child with torsion dystonia. Reese *et al.* (1991), of Buffalo, New York, reported three patients with spastic cerebral palsy without a movement disorder who had a cervical myelopathy that caused a functional loss. The diagnosis was delayed until the clinical manifestations of cervical cord compression were discovered. The authors plead that if functional deterioration is noted in such adults with cerebral palsy, awareness of possible cervical-cord pathology should prompt diagnostic measures such as an MRI study and surgical treatment.

From London comes a case report of a boy with dystonic quadriplegia. An MRI study showed a cervical cord lesion and an os ondontoideum (Amess *et al.* 1998). The cause was ascribed to the cervical spinal-cord trauma due to the excessive movements of the neck. Again the plea was to 'pay careful attention' to changes in the neurological status of children with athetosis so early diagnosis of cervical cord pathology and treatment can be instituted before it is too late.

Pay careful attention to changes in the neurological status of children and adults with athetosis.

Japanese orthopaedic and neurosurgery physicians seem to have the largest experience with cervical cord lesions in athetoid cerebral palsy (Fuji *et al.* 1987, Harada *et al.* 1996, Mikawa *et al.* 1997, Onari *et al.* 2002). This may be due to a higher incidence of cerebral palsy with athetosis in Japan than in North America, the UK or mainland Europe: or perhaps our Japanese colleagues may be more aware than we are. The paper by Onari and colleagues (2002) is particularly instructive and comprises the experience of cervical myelopathy in 23 adult patients who had athetosis. Their patients improved neurologically with a combined anterior–posterior fusion using anterior wave-shaped rods for stabilization. Rigid external fixation was not required.

The intramuscular injection of botulinum-A toxin into dystonic neck muscles may be a very useful adjunct in the process of cervical spine fusion for arresting the progression of cervical myelopathy. The botulinum toxin injections eliminated involuntary neck movements so that halo fixation could be tolerated (Racette *et al.* 1998).

FURTHER READING

Bleck, E.E. (1980) 'The hip in cerebral palsy.' *Orthopaedic Clinics of North America*, 11, 79–104.

Bradford, D.S., Zdeblick, T.A. (2004) *Master Techniques in Orthopaedic Surgery: The Spine*, 2nd edn. Philadelphia: Lippincott Williams & Wilkins.

Canale, S.T. (Ed.) (2003) *Campbell's Operative Orthopaedics*, 10th edn. Philadelphia: Mosby.

Lenke, J.G., Orchowski, J. (2004) 'Segmental posterior spinal instrumentation—thoracic spine to sacrum.' *In* Frymoyer, J.W., Wiesel, S.N. (Eds) *The Adult and Pediatric Spine*, 3rd edn. Philadelphia: Lippincott Williams & Wilkins.

Morrissy, R.T., Weinstein, S.L. (Eds) (2001) *Atlas of Pediatric Orthopaedic Surgery*. Philadelphia: Lippincott Williams and Wilkins.

Vaccaro, A.R., Betz, R.R., Zeidman, S.M. (Eds) (2003) *Principles and Practices of Spine Surgery*. Philadelphia: Mosby.

Lonstein, J.E. (2001) 'Neuromuscular spinal deformities' *In* Weinstein, S.L. (Ed) *The Pediatric Spine*, 2nd edn. Philadelphia: Lippincott Williams & Wilkins.

Watkins, R.G. (2003) *Surgical Approaches to the Spine*, 2nd edn. New York: Springer.

REFERENCES

Abel, M.F., Blanco, J.S., Pavlovich, L., Damiano, D.L. (1999) 'Asymmetric hip deformity and subluxation in cerebral palsy: an analysis of surgical treatment.' *Journal of Pediatric Orthopaedics*, 19, 479–485.

Adler, N., Bleck, E.E., Rinsky, L.A., Young, W. (1986) 'Balance reactions and eye–hand coordination in idiopathic scoliosis.' *Journal of Orthopaedic Research*, 4, 102–107.

Akeson, J., Bobechko, W.P. (1986) 'Treatment of scoliosis by instrumentation with double hook and posterior fusion.' *Orthopaedic Transactions*, 10, 35.

Albee, F.H. (1915) 'The bone graft wedge. Its use in the treatment of relapsing, acquired, and congenital dislocation of the hip. *New York Medical Journal*, 102, 433–435.

Allen, B.L. Jr (1983) 'Spinal instrumentation, Part II. Segmental spinal instrumentation with L-rods.' *In Instruction Course Lectures, American Academy of Orthopaedic Surgeons, Vol. 32*. St Louis: C.V. Mosby.

—— (1985) 'The Galveston technique of L-rod instrumentation—a second generation survey.' *Paper No. 13, read at Annual Meeting of the Pediatric Orthopaedic Society of North America, Boston*.

—— Ferguson, R.L. (1981) 'The Galveston technique for L-rod instrumentation of the scoliotic spine.' *Spine*, 7, 276–284.

—— —— (1982) 'L-rod instrumentation for scoliosis in cerebral palsy.' *Journal of Pediatric Orthopedics*, 2, 87–96.

—— —— (1983) 'Staged correction of neuromuscular scoliosis.' *Journal of Pediatric Orthopedics*, 3, 555–562.

Alonso, J.E., Lovell, W.W., Lovejoy, J.F. (1986) 'The Altdorf hip clamp.' *Journal of Pediatric Orthopedics*, 6, 339–402.

Amess, P., Chong, W.K., Kirkham, F.J. (1998) 'Acquired spinal cord lesion associated with os odontoideum causing deterioration in dystonic cerebral palsy: case report and review of the literature.' *Developmental Medicine and Child Neurology*, 40, 195–198.

Anand, N., Regan, J.J. (2002) 'Video-assisted thoracoscopic surgery for thoracic disc disease; Classification and outcome study of 100 consecutive cases with a 2-year minimum follow-up period.' *Spine*, 27, 871–879.

Angelini, L., Broggi, G., Nardocci, N., Savoiardo, M. (1982) 'Subacute cervical myelopathy in a child with cerebral palsy. Secondary to torsion dystonia?' *Child's Brain*, 9, 354–357.

Aronsson, D.D., Stokes, I.A., Ronchetti, P.J., Labelle, H.B. (1994) 'Comparison of curve shape between children with cerebral palsy, Friedreich's ataxia, and adolescent scoliosis.' *Developmental Medicine and Child Neurology*, 36, 412–418.

Arus, C., Barany, M., Westler, W.M., Markley, J.L. (1984) 'Proton nuclear magnetic resonance of human muscle extracts.' *Clinical Physiology and Biochemistry*, 2, 49–55.

Ashton, L.A., Bruce, W., Goldberg, J., Walsh, W. (2000) 'Prevention of heterotopic bone formation in high risk patients post-total hip arthroplasty.' *Journal of Orthopaedic Surgery (Hong Kong)*, 8, 53–57.

Atar, D., Grant, A.D., Bash, J., Lehman, W.B. (1995) 'Combined hip surgery in cerebral palsy patients.' *American Journal of Orthopedics*, 24, 52–55.

Azcue, M.P., Zello, G.A., Levy, L.D., Pencharz, P.B. (1996) 'Energy expenditure and body composition in children with spastic quadriplegic cerebral palsy.' *Journal of Pediatrics*, 129, 870–876.

Bagg, M.R., Farber, J., Miller, F. (1993) 'Long-term follow-up of hip subluxation in cerebral palsy patients.' *Journal of Pediatric Orthopaedics*, 13, 32–36.

Bailey, T.E., Hall, J.E. (1985) 'Chiari medial displacement osteotomy.' *Journal of Pediatric Orthopedics*, 5, 635–641.

Balmer, G.A., MacEwen, G.D. (1970) 'The incidence of scoliosis in cerebral palsy.' *Journal of Bone and Joint Surgery*, 52B, 134–136.

Banks, H.H., Green, W.T. (1960) 'Adductor myotomy and obturator neurectomy for correction of adduction of the hip in cerebral palsy.' *Journal of Bone and Joint Surgery*, 42A, 111–126.

Banovac, K., Williams, J.M., Patrick, L. D., Haniff, Y.M. (2001) 'Prevention of heterotopic ossification after spinal cord injury with indomethacin.' *Spinal Cord*, 39, 370–374.

Barrie, J.L., Galasko, C.S. (1996) 'Surgery for unstable hips in cerebral palsy.' *Journal of Pediatric Orthopaedics B*, 5, 225–231.

Barry, R.J., Staheli, L.T. (1986) 'Management of neuromuscular hip dysplasia by pericapsular osteotomy.' *Orthopaedic Transactions*, 10, 149.

Basobas, L., Mardjetko, S., Hammerberg, K., Lubicky, J. (2003) 'Selective anterior fusion and instrumentation for the treatment of neuromuscular scoliosis.' *Spine*, 28, S245–248.

Bathel, T., Baumann, B., Noth, U., Eulert, J. (2002) 'Prophylaxis of heterotopic ossification after total hip arthroplasty: a prospective randomized study comparing indomethacin and meloxicam.' *Acta Orthopaedica Scandinavica*, 73, 611–614.

Baxter, M.P. (1986) 'Proximal femoral resection–interposition arthroplasty: salvage hip surgery for the severely disabled child with cerebral palsy.' *Journal of Pediatric Orthopaedics*, 6, 681–685.

—— D'Astous, J. (1986) 'Proximal femoral resection-interposition arthroplasty: salvage hip surgery for the severely disabled child with cerebral palsy.' *Journal of Pediatric Orthopedics*, 6, 681–685.

Beals, R.K. (1969) 'Developmental changes in the femur and acetabulum in spastic paraplegia and diplegia.' *Developmental Medicine and Child Neurology*, **11**, 303–313.

Beals, T.C., Thompson, N.E., Beals, R.K. (1998) 'Modified adductor muscle transfer in cerebral palsy.' *Journal of Pediatric Orthopaedics*, **18**, 522–527.

Beck, M., Woo, A., Leunig, M., Ganz, R. (2001) 'Gluteus minimus-induced femoral head deformities in dysplasia of the hip.' *Acta Orthopaedica Scandinavica*, **72**, 13–17.

Beintema, D.J. (1968) *A Neurological Study of Newborn Infants. Clinics in Developmental Medicine, No. 28*. London: Spastics International Medical Publications with Heinemann Medical.

Bell, D.F., Moseley, C.F., Koreska, J. (1989) 'Unit rod of segmental spinal instrumentation in the management of patients with progressive neuromuscular spinal deformity.' *Spine*, **14**, 1301–1307.

Benson, E.R., Thomson, J.D., Banta, J.V. (1998) 'Results and morbidity in a consecutive series of patients undergoing spinal fusion for neuromuscular scoliosis.' *Spine*, **23**, 2308–2317.

Benson, M.K.D., Evans, D.C.J. (1976) 'The pelvic osteotomy of Chiari: an anatomical study of the hazards and misleading radiographic appearances.' *Journal of Bone and Joint Surgery*, **58B**, 164–168.

Betz, R.R., Kumar, S.J., Palmer, C.T., MacEwen, G.D. (1988) 'Chiari pelvic osteotomy in children and young adults.' *Journal of Bone and Joint Surgery*, **70A**, 182–191.

Biemond, A. (1964) 'Contusio cervicalis posterior.' *Nederlands Tijdschrift voor Geneeskunde*, **108**, 1333–1335.

Black, B.E., Griffin, P.P. (1997) 'The cerebral palsied hip.' *Clinical Orthopaedics and Related Research*, **338**, 42–51.

Blank, J., Flynn, J.M., Bronson, W., Ellman, P., Pill, S.G., Lou, J.E., Dormans, J.P., Drummond, D.S., Ecker, M.L. (2003) 'The use of postoperative subcutaneous closed suction drainage after posterior spinal fusion in adolescents with idiopathic scoliosis.' *Journal of Spinal Disorders and Techniques*, **16**, 508–512,

Bleck, E.E. (1962) 'Heterotopic ossification in tissue culture.' *Thesis submitted to the American Orthopaedic Association.*

—— (1975) 'Deformities of the spine and pelvis in cerebral palsy.' *In* Samilson, R.L. (Ed.) *Orthopaedic Aspects of Cerebral Palsy. Clinics in Developmental Medicine, Nos 52/53*. London: Spastics International Medical Publications with Heinemann Medical; Philadelphia: J.B. Lippincott.

—— (1979) '*Orthopaedic Management in Cerebral Palsy*. Philadelphia: W.B. Saunders.

—— (1987) *Orthopaedic Management in Cerebral Palsy. Clinics in Developmental Medicine, Nos. 99/100*. London: Mac Keith Press with Cambridge University Press; Philadelphia: J.B. Lippincott.

—— Holstein, A. (1963) 'Iliopsoas tenotomy for spastic hip flexion deformities in cerebral palsy.' *Paper presented at Annual Meeting American Academy of Orthopaedic Surgeons, Chicago.*

—— Koehler, J.P., Dillingham, M., Trimble, S. (1976) 'Histochemical studies of thoracis spinalis and sacrospinalis muscles in scoliosis.' *American Academy of Neurology, Program Abstract.*

—— Terver, S., Wheeler, R., Csongradi, J., Rinsky, L.A. (1981) 'Joint laxity in children: statistical correlations with scoliosis, congenital dislocation of the hip and talipes equinovarus.' *Orthopaedic Transactions*, 5, 5–6.

Boachie-Adjei, O., Lonstein, J.E., Winter, R.B., Koop, S., Vanden Brink, K., Denis, F. (1989) 'Management of neuromuscular spinal deformities with Luque segmental instrumentation.' *Journal of Bone and Joint Surgery*, **71A**, 548–562.

Bobechko, W.P., Herbert, M.A. (1986) 'Totally implantable stimulators for treatment of scoliosis in children with C.P.' *Orthopaedic Transactions*, **10**, 156.

Bonnett, C., Brown, J.C., Brooks, H.L. (1973) 'Anterior spine fusion with Dwyer instrumentation for lumbar scoliosis in cerebral palsy.' *Journal of Bone and Joint Surgery*, **55A**, 425. (Abstract.)

—— Perry, J., Nickel, V., Walinski, T., Brooks, H.L., Hoffer, M., Stiles, C., Brooks, R. (1975) 'The evolution of treatment of paralytic scoliosis at Rancho Los Amigos Hospital.' *Journal of Bone and Joint Surgery*, **57A**, 206–215.

—— Grow, T. (1976) 'Thoracolumbar scoliosis in cerebral palsy. Results of surgical treatment.'
Journal of Bone and Joint Surgery, **58A**, 328–336.

Borzyskowski, M. (1989) 'Cerebral palsy and the bladder.' *Developmental Medicine and Child Neurology*, **31**, 693–696.

Bouchard, J., D'Astous, J. (1991) 'Postoperative heterotopic ossification in children: a comparison of children with spina bifida and with cerebral palsy.' *Canadian Journal of Surgery*, **34**, 454–456.

Bowen, J.R., MacEwen, G.D., Mathews, P.A. (1981) 'Treatment of extension contracture of the hip in cerebral palsy.' *Developmental Medicine and Child Neurology*, **23**, 23–29.

Braakman, R., Penning, L. (1971) *Injuries of the Cervical Spine*. Amsterdam: Excerpta Medica, pp. 82–83.

Bridwell, K.H., O'Brien, M.F., Lenke, L.G., Baldus, C., Blanke, K. (1994) 'Posterior spinal fusion supplemented with only allograft bone in paralytic scoliosis. Does it work?' *Spine*, **19**, 2658–2666.

Brooker, A. F., Bowerman, J. W., Robinson, R. A., Riley, L. H. (1973) 'Ectopic ossification following total hip replacement.' *Journal of Bone and Joint Surgery*, **55A**, 1629–1632.

Broom, M.J., Banta, J.V., Renshaw, T.S. (1989) 'Spinal fusion augmented by Luque-rod segmental instrumentation for neuromuscular scoliosis.' *Journal of Bone and Joint Surgery*, **71A**, 32–44.

Brown, J.S., Swank, S., Specht, L. (1982) 'Combined anterior and posterior spine fusion in cerebral palsy.' *Spine*, 7, 570–573.

Brown, R.H., Nash, C.L. Jr, Berilla, J.A., Amaddio, M.D. (1984) 'Cortical evoked potential monitoring. A system for intraoperative monitoring of spinal cord function.' *Spine*, 9, 256–261.

Brunner, R., Baumann, J.U. (1994) 'Clinical benefit of reconstruction of dislocated or subluxated hip joints in patients with spastic cerebral palsy.' *Journal of Pediatric Orthopaedics*, **14**, 290–294.

—— Doderlein, L. (1996) 'Pathological fractures in patients with cerebral palsy.' *Journal of Pediatric Orthopaedics*, **5**, 232–228.

—— Robb, J.E. (1996) 'Inaccuracy of migration percentage and center-edge angle in predicting femoral head displacement in cerebral palsy.' *Journal of Pediatric Orthopaedics*, **5**, 239–241.

—— Baumann, J.U. (1997) 'Long-term effects of intertrochanteric varus-derotation osteotomy on femur and acetabulum in spastic cerebral palsy: an 11- to 18-year follow-up study.' *Journal of Pediatric Orthopaedics*, **17**, 585–591.

—— (1998) 'Which procedure gives the best results in reconstructing dislocated hips in cerebral palsy?' *Acta Orthopedica Belgica*, **64**, 7–16.

Buckley, S.L., Sponseller, P.D., Magid, D. (1991) 'The acetabulum in congenital and neuromuscular hip instability.' *Journal of Pediatric Orthopaedics*, **11**, 498–501.

Buly, R.L., Huo, M., Root, L., Binzer, T., Wilson, P.D. Jr (1993) 'Total hip arthroplasty in cerebral palsy. Long term follow-up results.' *Clinical Orthopaedics and Related Research*, **296**, 148–153.

Bulman, W.A., Dormans, J.P., Ecker, M.L., Drummond, D.S. (1996) 'Posterior spinal fusion for scoliosis in patients with cerebral palsy: a comparison of the Luque rod and unit rod instrumentation.' *Journal of Pediatric Orthopaedics*, **16**, 314–323.

Bunch, W.H., Scarff, T.B., Trimble, J. (1983) 'Spinal cord monitoring.' *Journal of Bone and Joint Surgery*, **65**, 707–710. SPECIFY A OR B

Bunnell, W.P. (1985) 'Varus derotational osteotomy of the hip in cerebral palsy.' *Orthopaedic Transactions*, **9**, 88.

—— MacEwen, G.D. (1977) 'Non-operative treatment of scoliosis in cerebral palsy: preliminary report on the use of a plastic jacket.' *Developmental Medicine and Child Neurology*, **19**, 45–49.

Burd, T.A., Lowry, K.J., Anglen, J.O. (2001) 'Indomethacin compared with localized irradiation for the prevention of heterotopic ossification following surgical treatment of acetabular fractures.' *Journal of Bone and Joint Surgery*, **83A**, 1783–1788.

Bureau of Education for the Handicapped (1976) *Conference on Communication Aids for the Non- Vocal; Severely Physically Handicapped Person, Alexandria, VA.*

Cady, R.B., Bobechko, W.P. (1984) 'Incidence, natural history and treatment of scoliosis in Friedreich's ataxia.' *Journal of Pediatric Orthopedics*, 4, 673–676.

Canale, S.T., Hammond, N.L., Cotler, J.M., Sneddlen, H.E. (1975) 'Pelvic displacement osteotomy for chronic hip dislocation in myelodysplasia.' *Journal of Bone and Joint Surgery*, **57A**, 177–183.

Cannulated Pediatric Osteotomy System/CAPOS (2003) *Technique Guide*. Paoli, PA: Synthes.

Cardoso, A. (1984) 'Paralytic scoliosis.' *In* Luque, E.R. (Ed.) *Segmental Spinal Instrumentation*. Thorofare, NJ: Slack, pp. 119–146.

—— Tajonas, F.A., Luque, E.R. (1976) 'Osteotomias de columna, neuvos conceptos.' *Annals of Orthopaedic Trauma*, **12**, 105–113.

Carroll, K.L., Moore, K.R., Stevens, P.M. (1998) 'Orthopedic procedures after rhizotomy.' *Journal of Pediatric Orthopaedics*, **18**, 69–74.

Cassidy, C., Craig, C.L., Perry, A., Karlin, L.I., Goldberg, M.J. (1994) 'A reassessment of spinal stabilization in severe cerebral palsy.' *Journal of Pediatric Orthopaedics*, **14**, 731–739.

Castle, M.E., Schneider, C. (1978) 'Proximal femoral resection–interposition arthroplasty.' *Journal of Bone and Joint Surgery*, **60A**, 1051–1054.

Chandler, F.A., Seidler, F. (1939) 'Intrapelvic extraperitoneal resection of the obturator nerve.' *Surgery, Gynecology, and Obstetrics*, **69**, 101–102.

Chang, K.W. (2003) 'Cantilever bending technique for treatment of large and rigid scoliosis.' *Spine*, **28**, 2452–2458.

Chiari, K. (1955) 'Ergebnisse mit der Beckenosteotomie als Pfannendachplastik.' *Zeitschrift fïir Orthopädie und ihre Grenzgebiete*, **87**, 14–26.

—— (1974) 'Medial displacement osteotomy of the pelvis.' *Clinical Orthopaedics and Related Research*, **98**, 55–71.

Cobb, J.R. (1952) 'Technique, after-treatment, and results of spine fusion in scoliosis.' *Instructional Course Lectures, vol. 9*. Ann Arbor: J.W. Edwards, pp. 65–70.

Cobeljic, G., Vukasinovic, Z., Djoric, I. (1994) 'Surgical prevention of paralytic dislocation of the hip in cerebral palsy.' *International Orthopaedics*, **18**, 313–316.

Coleman, S.S. (1978) *Congenital Dysplasia and Dislocation of the Hip*. St Louis: C.V. Mosby.

—— (1983) 'Reconstructive procedures in congenital dislocation of the hip.' *In* McKibbin, B. (Ed.) *Recent Advances in Orthopaedics, No. 4*. Edinburgh: Churchill Livingstone, pp. 23–44.

Colton, C.L. (1972) 'Chiari osteotomy for acetabular dysplasia in young adults.' *Journal of Bone and Joint Surgery*, **54B**, 578–589.

Compère, E.L. (1932) 'Excision of hemivertebrae for correction of congenital scoliosis. Report of two cases.' *Journal of Bone and Joint Surgery*, **14**, 555–562.

Comstock, C.P., Leach, J., Wenger, D.R. (1998) 'Scoliosis in total-body-involvement cerebral palsy. Analysis of surgical treatment and patient and caregiver satisfaction.' *Spine*, **23**, 1412–1424.

Cooke, P.H., Cole, W.G., Carey, R.P.L. (1989) 'Dislocation of the hip in cerebral palsy. Natural history and predictability.' *Journal of Bone and Joint Surgery*, **71B**, 441–446.

Cooperman, D.R., Bartucci, E., Dietrick, E., Millar, E. A. (1987) 'Hip dislocation in spastic cerebral palsy: long-term consequences.' *Journal of Pediatric Orthopaedics*, **7**, 268–267.

Copeliovitch, Y., Mirovsky, N., Halperin, D., Hendel, D. (1983) 'Extension deformity of the hips with anterior subluxation of the head of the femur in cerebral palsy.' *Orthopaedic Transactions*, **7**, 557.

Cornell, M.S. (2001) 'Adductor tenotomies in children with quadriplegic cerebral palsy: longer term follow-up.' *Journal of Pediatric Orthopedics*, **21**, 136–137.

—— Boyd, R., Baird, G., Spencer, J.D. (1994) 'Brief reports: imaging the acetabulum in children with cerebral palsy.' *Journal of Bone and Joint Surgery*, **76B**, 982–983.

—— Hatrick, N.C., Boyd, R., Baird, G., Spencer, J.D. (1997) 'The hip in children with cerebral palsy. Predicting the outcome of soft tissue surgery.' *Clinical Orthopaedics and Related Research*, **340**, 165–171.

Cotrel, Y. (1975) 'Traction in the treatment of vertebral deformity.' *Journal of Bone and Joint Surgery*, **57B**, 260. (Abstract.)

Cottalorda, J., Gautheron, V., Metton, G., Charmet, E., Maatougui, K., Chavrier, Y. (1998) 'Predicting the outcome of adductor tenotomy.' *International Orthopaedics*, **22**, 374–379.

Crenshaw, A.H. (1963) *Campbell's Operative Orthopaedics*. St Louis: C.V. Mosby.

Cristofaro, R., Koffman, M., Woodward, R., Baxter, S. (1977) 'Treatment of the totally involved cerebral palsy problem sitter.' *Paper read at the Annual Meeting of the American Academy for Cerebral Palsy and Developmental Medicine, Atlanta.*

—— Taddonio, R.F., Gelb, R. (1985) 'The effect of correction of spinal deformity and pelvic obliquity on hip stability in neuromuscular disease.' *Orthopaedic Transactions*, **9**, 88.

D'Astous, J.L., Baxter, M.E. (1986) 'Proximal femoral resection–interposition arthroplasty—salvage hip surgery for the severely disabled child with cerebral palsy.' *Paper read at the Annual Meeting Pediatric Orthopedic Society of North America, Boston.*

Davis, J.B. (1954) 'The muscle–pedicle bone graft in hip fusion.' *Journal of Bone and Joint Surgery*, **33A**, 790–799.

Decter, R.M., Bauer, S.B., Khoshbin, S., Dyro, F.M., Krarup, C., Colodny, A.H., Retick, A.B. (1987) 'Urodynamic assessment of children with cerebral palsy.' *Journal of Urology*, **138**, 1110–1112.

Dega, W. (1974) 'Osteotomia trans-iliakalna w leczeniu wrodzonej dysplazji biodra.' *Chirurgia Narzadpm Richu i Ortopedia. Polska*, **39**, 601–613.

de Gauzy, J.S., Roux, F.E., Henry, P., Cahuzac, J.P. (1999) 'Somatosensory evoked potentials during surgery of scoliosis: significance of epidural recording.' *Revue de Chirurgie Orthopédique et Réparatrice de l'Appareil Locomoteur*, **85**, 387–392. (French.)

Delp, S.L., Bleck, E.E., Zajac, F.E., Bollini, G. (1990) 'Biomechanical analysis of the Chiari hip osteotomy. Preserving hip muscle strength.' *Clinical Orthopaedic and Related Research*, **254**, 189–198.

de Moraes Barros Fucs, P.M., Svartman, C., de Assumpção, R.M.C., Virgulino, C.C., Gomi, F.H., Silber, M.F. (2002) 'Resultados da reconstrução do quadril subluxado e luxado da paralisia cerebral.' *Revista Brasileira de Ortopedia Pediátrica*, **3**, 9–17.

—— —— —— Kertzman, P. F. (2003) 'Treatment of painful chronically dislocated and subluxated hip in cerebral palsy with hip arthrodesis.' *Journal of Pediatric Orthopaedics*, **23**, 529–534.

DeWald, R.L., Ray, R.D. (1970) 'Skeletal traction for the treatment of scoliosis.' *Journal of Bone and Joint Surgery*, **52A**, 233–238.

Dias, R.C., Miller, F., Dabney, K., Lipton, G., Temple, T. (1996) 'Surgical correction of spinal deformity using a unit rod in children with cerebral palsy.' *Journal of Pediatric Orthopaedics*, **16**, 734–740.

DiCindio, S, Theroux, M., Shah, S., Miller, F., Dabney, K., Brislin, R.P., Schwartz, D. (2003) 'Multimodality monitoring of transcranial electric motor and somatosensory-evoked potentials during surgical correction of spine deformity in patients with cerebral palsy and other neuromuscular disorders.' *Spine*, **28**, 1851–1855.

Dietz, F.R., Knutson, L.M. (1995) 'Chiari pelvic osteotomy in cerebral palsy.' *Journal of Pediatric Orthopaedics*, **15**, 372–380.

D'Lima, D.D., Venn-Watson, E.J., Tripuraneni, P., Colwell, C.W. (2001) 'Prevention of heterotopic bone formation in high risk patients post-total hip arthroplasty.' *Orthopedics*, **24**, 1139–1143.

Dohin, B., Dubousset, J.F. (1994) 'Prevention of the crankshaft phenomenon with anterior spinal epiphysiodesis in the surgical treatment of severe scoliosis in the younger patients.' *European Spine Journal*, **3**, 165–168.

Doppman, J., DiChiro, G. (1968) 'The arteria radicularis magna: radiographic anatomy in the adult.' *British Journal of Radiology*, **41**, 40–45.

Dorn, U., Grethen, C., Effenberger, H., Berka, H., Ramsauer, T., Drekonja, T. (1998) 'Indomethacin for prevention of heterotopic ossification after hip arthroplasty. A randomized comparison between 4 and 8 days of treatment.' *Acta Orthopaedica Scandanavica*, **69**, 107–110.

Drigo, P., Seren, F., Artibani, W., Laverda, A.M., Battistella, P.A., Zacchello, G. (1988) 'Neurogenic vesico-urethral dysfunction in children with cerebral palsy.' *Italian Journal of Neurological Science*, **9**, 151–154.

Driscoll, D.M., Newton, R.A., Lamb, R.L., Nogi, J. (1984) 'A study of postural equilibrium in idiopathic scoliosis.' *Journal of Pediatric Orthopedics*, **4**, 677–681.

Drummond, D.S. (1984) 'The Wisconsin system: a technique of interspinous segmental spinal instrumentation.' *Contemporary Orthopaedics*, **8**, 29–37.

—— Rogala, E.J., Cruess, R., Moreau, J. (1979) 'The paralytic hip and pelvic obliquity in cerebral palsy and myelomeningocele.' *American Academy of Orthopaedic Surgeons; Instructional Course Lectures*, **28**, 7–36.

—— (1996) 'Neuromuscular scoliosis.' *Journal of Pediatric Orthopaedics*, **16**, 281–283. (Editorial.)

Dubousset, J. (1985) 'Scolioses paralytiques et bassin oblique.' *In* Dimeglio, A., Auriach, A., Simon, L. (Eds) *L'Enfant Paralysé*. Paris: Masson, pp. 90–97.

—— Graf, H., Miladi, L., Cotrel, Y. (1986) 'Spinal and thoracic derotation with CD instrumentation.' *Orthopaedic Transactions*, **10**, 36.

—— Guillaumat, M., Miladi, L., Beurier, J., Tassin, J.L., Cotrel, Y. (1987) 'Correction and fusion to the sacrum of the oblique pelvis using CD instrumentation in children and adults.' *Revue de Chirurgie Orthopédique et Réparatrice de l'Appareil Locomoteur*, **73** (Suppl. 2), 164–167.

—— Herring, J.A., Shufflebarger, H. (1989) 'The crankshaft phenomenon.' *Journal of Pediatric Orthopaedics*, **9**, 541–550.

—— Machida, M. (2001) 'Possible role of the pineal gland in the pathogenesis of idiopathic scoliosis. Experimental and clinical studies.' *Bulletin de l'Académie Nationale de Médecine*, **185**, 593–602.

—— (2003) 'Spinal instrumentation, source of progress, but also revealing pitfalls.' *Bulletin de l'Académie Nationale de Médecine*, **187**, 523–533.

Duval-Beaupère, G. (1970) 'Les repères de maturation dans la surveillance des scolioses.' *Revue de Chirurgie Orthopédique et Réparatrice de l'Appareil Locomoteur*, 56, 59–76.

—— (1971) 'Pathogenic relationship between scoliosis and growth.' *In* Zorab, P.A. (Ed.) *Scoliosis and Growth*. London: Churchill Livingstone.

—— Grossiord, A. (1967a) 'Les caractères evolutifs des scolioses polymyeliques; 207 cas de type espiriltoire.' *Presse Médicale*, 75, 2375–2380.

—— (1967b) 'Apport des scolioses polymyetiliques à l'étude des scolioses idiopathiques.' *Acta Orthopedica Belgica*, 33, 575–586.

—— Dubousset, J., Queneau, P., Grossiord, A. (1970) 'Pour une théorie unique de l'évolution des scolioses.' *Presse Médicale*, 78, 1141–1146.

—— Combes, J. (1971) 'Segments supérieur et inférieur au cours de la croissance physiologique des filles.' *Archives Françaises de Pédiatrie*, 28, 1057–1070.

Dwyer, A.F., Newton, C., Sherwood, A.A. (1969) 'An anterior approach in scoliosis: a preliminary report.' *Clinical Orthopaedics and Related Research*, 62, 192–202.

—— (1973) 'Experience of anterior correction of scoliosis.' *Clinical Orthopaedics and Related Research*, 93, 191–206.

Eberle, D.F., Al-Saati, F., Al-Saudairy, M. (1986) 'Complications following segmental spinal instrumentation without fusion in management of paralytic scoliosis.' *Orthopaedic Transactions*, 10, 17.

Ecker, M.L., Dormans, J.P., Schwartz, D.M., Drummond, D.S. (1996) 'Efficacy of spinal cord monitoring in scoliosis surgery in patients with cerebral palsy.' *Journal of Spinal Disorders*, 9, 159–164.

Edler, A., Murray, D.J., Forbes, B.S. (2003) 'Blood loss during posterior spinal fusion surgery in patients with neuromuscular disease: is there an increased risk?' *Paediatric Anaesthesia*, 13, 818–822.

Eilert, R.E., MacEwen, G.D. (1977) 'Varus derotational osteotomy of the femur in cerebral palsy.' *Clinical Orthopaedics and Related Research*, 125, 168–172.

Elmer, E.B., Wenger, D.R., Mubarak, S.J., Sutherland, D.H. (1992) 'Proximal hamstring lengthening in the sitting cerebral palsy patient.' *Journal of Pediatric Orthopaedics*, 12, 329–336.

Enneking, W.F., Harrington, P. (1969) 'Pathological changes in scoliosis.' *Journal of Bone and Joint Surgery*, 51A, 165–184.

Erken, E. H., Bischof, F. M. (1994) 'Iliopsoas transfer in cerebral palsy: the long term outcome.' *Journal of Pediatric Orthopaedics*, 14, 295–298.

Eyre-Brook, A.L., Jones, D.A., Harris, F.C. (1978) 'Pemberton's iliac acetabuloplasty for congenital dislocation or subluxation of the hip.' *Journal of Bone and Joint Surgery*, 60B, 18–24.

Farmer, T.W. (1964) *Pediatric Neurology*. New York: Hoeber.

Ferguson, A.B. (1973) 'Primary open reduction of congenital dislocation of the hip using a median adductor approach.' *Journal of Bone and Joint Surgery*, 55A, 671–689.

—— (1975) *Orthopaedic Surgery in Infancy and Childhood*. Baltimore: Williams & Wilkins.

Fettweis, E. (1979) 'Addukotrenspasmus, Praluxationen und Luxationen und den Huftgelenken bei spastisch geliihmten Kindem und Jugendlichen, klinische Beobachtungen zur Atiologie, Pathogenese, Therapie und Rehabilitation. Part I.' *Zeitschrift für Orthopädie*, 117, 39–49.

Floman, Y., Micheli, L.J., Penny, J.N., Riseborough, E.J., Hall, J.E. (1982) 'Combined anterior and posterior fusion in seventy-three spinally deformed patients: indications, results and complications.' *Clinical Orthopaedics and Related Research*, 164, 110–122.

Florentino-Pineda, I., Thompson, G.H., Poe-Kochert, C., Huang, R.P., Haber, L.L., Blakemore, L.C. (2004) 'The effect of amicar on perioperative blood loss in idiopathic scoliosis; the results of a prospective randomized double-blind study.' *Spine*, 29, 233–238.

Flynn, J. M., Miller, F. (2002) 'Management of hip disorders in patients with cerebral palsy.' *Journal of the American Academy of Orthopaedic Surgeons*, 10, 198–209.

Frischhut, B., Krismer, M., Stoeckl, B., Landauer, F., Auckenthaler, Th. (2000) 'Pelvic tilt in neuromuscular disease.' *Journal of Pediatric Orthopaedics B*, 9, 221–228.

Fuji, T., Yonenobu, K., Fujiwara, K., Yamashita, K., Ebara, S., Onon, K., Okada, K. (1987) 'Cervical radiculopathy or myelopathy secondary to athetoid cerebral palsy.' *Journal of Bone and Joint Surgery*, 69A, 815–821.

Fujisawa, Y., Morishita, K., Murakami, G., Abe, T. (2006) 'Histological and morphometric study of the arterial route from the intercostals/lumbar artery via the Adamkiewicz artery to the anterior spinal artery using elderly

cadavers with or without aortic aneurysms.' *Annals of Vascular Surgery*, 20, 9–16.

Fulford, G.E., Cairns, T.P., Sloan, Y. (1982) 'Sitting problems of children with cerebral palsy.' *Developmental Medicine and Child Neurology*, 24, 48–53.

Gabos, P.G., Miller, F., Galban, M.A., Gupta, G.G., Dabney, K. (1999) 'Prosthetic interposition arthroplasty for the palliative treatment of end-stage spastic hip disease in non-ambulatory patients with cerebral palsy.' *Journal of Pediatric Orthopaedics*, 19, 796–804.

Galasko, C.S.B. (1997) Letter to the editor. *Journal of Pediatric Orthopaedics*, 17, 407.

Gamble, J.G. (1984) 'Resection arthroplasty of the hip in paralytic dislocations.' *Developmental Medicine and Child Neurology*, 26, 341–346.

—— Bleck, E.E. (1985) 'Prevention of spastic paralytic dislocation of the hip.' *Developmental Medicine and Child Neurology*, 27, 17–24.

—— Rinsky, L.A. (1985) 'Preliminary results of Luque instrumentation in neuromuscular scoliosis.' *Orthopaedic Transactions*, 9, 94–95.

—— Bleck, E. (1990) 'Established hip dislocations in children with cerebral palsy.' *Clinical Orthopaedics and Related Research*, 253, 90–99.

Gandy, D.J., Meyer, L.C. (1983) 'Long-term study of the dislocating hip in cerebral palsy.' *Orthopaedic Transactions*, 7, 387.

Ganz, R., Klaue, K., Vinh, T.S., Mast, J.W. (1988) 'A new periacetabular osteotomy for the treatment of hip dysplasias: technique and preliminary results.' *Clinical Orthopaedics and Related Research*, 232, 26–36.

Gau, Y.L, Lonstein, J.E., Winter, R.B., Koop, S., Denis, F. (1991) 'Luque-Galveston procedure for correction and stabilization of neuromuscular scoliosis and pelvic obliquity: a review of 68 patients.' *Journal of Spinal Disorders*, 4, 339–410.

Gersoff, W.K., Renshaw, T.S. (1988) 'The treatment of scoliosis in cerebral palsy by posterior spinal fusion with Luque-rod instrumentation.' *Journal of Bone and Joint Surgery*, 70A, 41–44.

Gillingham, B.L., Sanchez, A.A., Wenger, D.R. (1999) 'Pelvic osteotomies for the treatment of hip dysplasia in children and young adults.' *Journal of the American Academy of Orthopaedic Surgeons*, 7, 325–337.

Ginsberg, H.H., Shetter, A.G., Raudzens, P.A. (1985) 'Postoperative paraplegia with preserved intraoperative somatosensory evoked potentials.' *Journal of Neurosurgery*, 63, 296–300.

Givon, U., Miller, F. (1999) 'Shortening of the unit rod protruding into the hip joint: case report and description of the surgical procedure.' *Journal of Spinal Disorders*, 12, 74–76.

Goldstein, L.A. (1959) 'Results in the treatment of scoliosis with turnbuckle plaster cast correction and fusion.' *Journal of Bone and Joint Surgery*, 41A, 321–335.

—— (1969) 'Treatment of idiopathic scoliosis by Harrington instrumentation and fusion with fresh autogenous iliac bone grafts.' *Journal of Bone and Joint Surgery*, 51A, 209–222.

Gordon, J.E., Capelli, A.M., Strecker, W.B., Delgardo, E.D., Shoenecker, P.L. (1996) 'Pemberton pelvic osteotomy and varus derotational osteotomy in the treatment of acetabular dysplasia in patients who have static encephalopathy.' *Journal of Bone and Joint Surgery*, 78A, 1863–1871.

Goto, K., Matsuo, T., Kasaba, K. (1987) 'Muscle release operation for scoliosis in cerebral palsy.' *Seikei geka to saigai geka (Orthopaedics and Traumatology)*, 36, 171–173. (Japanese.)

Greene, W. (1985) 'Cary plate fixation for varus derotation femoral osteotomy in cerebral palsy.' *Paper read at Annual Meeting of American Academy for Cerebral Palsy and Developmental Medicine, Seattle*.

Gregoric, M., Petak, F., Trontelj, J.V., Dimitrijevic, M.R. (1981) 'Postural control in scoliosis.' *Acta Orthopaedica Scandinavica*, 52, 59–63.

Griffith, B., Donavan, M.M., Stephenson, C.T., Franklin, T. (1982) 'The adductor transfer and iliopsoas recession in the cerebral palsy hip.' *Orthopaedic Transactions*, 6, 94–95.

Grogan, T.J., Krom, W., Oppenheim, W.L. (1986) 'The Chiari osteotomy for hip containment in cerebral palsy.' *Orthopaedic Transactions*, 10, 143.

Gross, M.S., Ibrahim, K., Wehner, J., Dvonch, V. (1984) 'Combined surgical procedure for treatment of hip dislocation in cerebral palsy.' *Orthopaedic Transactions*, 8, 113.

Grossfeld, S., Winter, R.B., Lonstein, J.E., Denis, F., Leonard, A., Johnson, L. (1997) 'Complications of anterior spinal surgery in children.' *Journal of Pediatric Orthopaedics*, 17, 89–95.

Guillot, M., Terver, S., Betrand, A., Vanneuville, G. (1977) 'Radiographie, electromyographie et approche functionnelle du muscle psoas-iliaque.' *Acta Anatomica*, 99, 274. (Abstract.)

Gunal, I., Hazer, B., Seber, S., Gokturk, E., Turgut, A., Kose, N. (2001) 'Prevention of heterotopic ossification after total hip replacement: a prospective comparison of indomethacin and salmon calcitonin in 60 patients.' *Acta Orthopaedica Scandinavica*, 72, 467–479.

Gurd, A.R. (1984) 'Surgical correction of myodesis of the hip in CP.' *Orthopaedic Transactions*, 8, 112.

Hall, J.E. (1972) 'The anterior approach to spinal deformities.' *Orthopedic Clinics of North America*, 3, 81–93.

—— Gray, J., Allen, M. (1977) 'Dwyer instrumentation and spinal fusion: a follow-up study.' *Journal of Bone and Joint Surgery*, 39B, 117. (Abstract.)

—— Levine, C.R., Sudhir, K.G. (1978) 'Intraoperative awakening to monitor spinal cord function during Harrington instrumentation and spine fusion. Description of procedure and report of three cases.' *Journal of Bone and Joint Surgery*, 60A, 553–536.

Hamill, C.L., Bridwell, K.H., Lenke, L.G., Chapman, M.P., Baldus, C., Blanke, K. (1997) 'Posterior arthrodesis in the skeletally immature patient. Assessing the risk for crankshaft: is an open triradiate cartilage the answer?' *Spine*, 22, 1343–1351,

Hankinson, J., Morton, R.E. (2002) 'Use of a lying abduction system in children with bilateral cerebral palsy.' *Developmental Medicine and Child Neurology*, 44, 177–180.

Harada, T., Ebara, S., Anwar, M. M., Okawa, A., Kajiura, I., Hiroshima, K., Ono, K. (1996) 'The cervical spine in athetoid cerebral palsy. A radiological study of 180 patients.' *Journal of Bone and Joint Surgery*, 78B, 613–619.

Harrington, P. (1962) 'Treatment of scoliosis. Correction and internal fixation by spinal instrumentation.' *Journal of Bone and Joint Surgery*, 44A, 591–610.

Harris, N.H., Lloyd-Robert, G.C., Gallien, R. (1975) 'Acetabular development in congenital dislocation of the hip.' *Journal of Bone and Joint Surgery*, 57B, 46–52.

Hau, R., Dickens, D.R., Nattrass, G.R., O'Sullivan, M., Torode, I.P., Graham, H.K. (2000) 'Which implant for proximal femoral osteotomy in children? A comparison of the AO (ASIF) 90 degree fixed-angle blade plate and the Richards intermediate hip screw.' *Journal of Pediatric Orthopaedics*, 20, 336–343.

Heinig, J. (1984) 'Eggshell procedure.' *In* Luque, E.R. (Ed.) *Segmental Spinal Instrumentation*. Thorofare, NJ: Slack, pp. 221–234.

Heinrich, S.D., MacEwen, G.D., Zembo, M.M. (1991) 'Hip dysplasia, subluxation and dislocation in cerebral palsy: an arthrographic analysis.' *Journal of Pediatric Orthopaedics*, 11, 488–493.

Hensinger, R.N. (1986) *Standards in Pediatric Orthopedics*. New York: Raven Press, p. 68.

Herndon, W.A., Sullivan, J.A., Yngve, D.A., Gross, R.H., Dreher, G. (1987) 'Segmental spinal instrumentation with sublaminar wires. A critical appraisal.' *Journal of Bone and Joint Surgery*, 69A, 851–859.

—— Bolano, L., Sullivan, J.A. (1992) 'Hip stabilization in the severely involved cerebral palsy patients.' *Journal of Pediatric Orthopaedics*, 12, 68–73.

Herold, H.H., Daniel, D. (1979) 'Reduction of neglected congenital dislocation of the hip in children over the age of six years.' *Journal of Bone and Joint Surgery*, 61B, 1–6.

Hibbs, R.A. (1924) 'A report of fifty-nine cases of scoliosis treated by the fusion operation.' *Journal of Bone and Joint Surgery*, 6, 3–37.

Hirose, G., Kadoya, S. (1984) 'Cervical spondylotic radiculo-myelopathy in patients with athetoid–dystonic cerebral palsy: clinical evaluation and surgical treatment.' *Journal of Neurology, Neurosurgery, Psychiatry*, 47, 775–780.

Hiroshima, K., Ono, K. (1979) 'Correlation between muscle shortening and derangement of hip joint in spastic cerebral palsy.' *Clinical Orthopaedics and Related Research*, 144, 186–193.

Hodgkinson, I., Vadot, J.P., Metton, G., Berard, C., Berard, J. (2000) 'Prevalence and morbidity of hip excentration in cerebral palsy.' *Revue de Chirurgie Orthopédique et Réparatrice de l'Appareil Locomoteur*, 86, 158–161.

—— Jindrich, M.L., Duhaut, P., Vadot, J.P., Metton, G., Berard, C. (2001) 'Hip pain in 234 non-ambulatory adolescents and young adults with cerebral palsy: a cross-sectional multicentre study.' *Developmental Medicine and Child Neurology*, 43, 806–808.

—— Berard, C., Chotel, F., Berard, J. (2002) 'Pelvic obliquity and scoliosis in non-ambulatory patients with cerebral palsy: a descriptive study of 234 patients over 15 years of age.' *Revue de Chirurgie Orthopédique et Réparatrice de l'Appareil Locomoteur*, 88, 337–341,

Hodgson, A.R. (1968) 'Correction of fixed spinal curves.' *Journal of Bone and Joint Surgery*, 47A, 1222–1227.

Hoffer, M.M. (1986) 'Management of the hip in cerebral palsy.' *Journal of Bone and Joint Surgery*, 68A, 629–631.

—— Abraham, E., Nickel, V. (1972) 'Salvage surgery at the hip to improve sitting posture of mentally retarded, severely disabled children with cerebral palsy.' *Developmental Medicine and Child Neurology*, 14, 51–55.

—— Bullock, M. (1981) 'The functional and social significance of orthopaedic rehabilitation of mentally retarded patients with cerebral palsy.' *Orthopedic Clinics of North America*, 12, 185–191.

Hoffman, D.V., Simmons, E.H., Barrington, T.W. (1974) 'The results of the Chiari osteotomy.' *Clinical Orthopaedics and Related Research*, 98, 162–170.

Hofmann, S., Trnka, H.J., Metzenroth, H., Frank, E., Ritschl, P., Salzer, M. (1999) 'General short-term indomethacin prophylaxis to prevent heterotopic ossification in total hip arthroplasty.' *Orthopedics*, 22, 207–211.

Holmes, K.J., Michael, S.M., Thorpe, S.I., Solomonidis, S.E. (2003) 'Management of scoliosis with special seating for the non-ambulant spastic cerebral palsy population—a biomechanical study.' *Clinical Biomechanics (Bristol, Avon)*, 18, 480–487.

Holte, R., Siekman, A. (1983) *Fundamentals of Postural Seating. Special Bulletin of Rehabilitation Engineering Center*. Palo Alto, CA: Children's Hospital at Stanford.

Hopf, C.G., Eysel, P., Dubousset, J. (1997) 'Operative treatment of scoliosis with Cotrel-Dubousset-Hopf instrumentation. New anterior spinal device.' *Spine*, 22, 618–627.

—— —— (2000) 'One-stage versus two-stage spinal fusion in neuromuscular scoliosis.' *Journal of Pediatric Orthopaedics B*, 9, 234–243.

Hoppenfeld, S., Gross, A.M. (1986) 'Posterior rib resection in scoliosis surgery.' *Orthopaedic Transactions*, 10, 27.

Horstmann, H.M. (1986) 'Skeletal maturation in cerebral palsy.' *Orthopaedic Transactions*, 10, 152.

—— Boyer, B. (1984) 'Progression of scoliosis in cerebral palsy patients after skeletal maturity.' *Orthopaedic Transactions*, 8, 116.

—— Rosabal, D.G. (1984) 'Varus derotation osteotomy.' *Orthopaedic Transactions*, 9, 192.

Hosada, G. (1982) 'Push-film device.' *Special Project: Rehabilitation Engineering Intern*. Palo Alto, CA: Children's Hospital at Stanford.

Houkom, J.A., Roach, J.W., Wenger, D.R., Speck, G., Herring, J.A., Norris, R.N. (1986) 'Treatment of acquired hip subluxation in cerebral palsy.' *Journal of Pediatric Orthopedics*, 6, 285–290.

Howard, D.B., McKibbin, B., Williams, L.A., Mackie, I. (1985) 'Factors affecting the incidence of hip dislocation in cerebral palsy.' *Journal of Bone and Joint Surgery*, 67B, 530–532.

Huang, M.J., Lenke, L.G. (2001) 'Scoliosis and severe pelvic obliquity in a patient with cerebral palsy: surgical treatment utilizing halo-femoral traction.' *Spine*, 26, 2168–2170.

Huggins, E.B. (1931) 'The formation of bone under the influence of epithelium of the urinary tract.' *Archives of Surgery*, 22, 377–408.

Ibrahim, K., Gross, M., Wehner, J. (1986) 'Combined procedure helps relieve pain in cerebral palsy patients.' *Orthopedics Today*, Sept. 4.

James, J.I.P. (1956) 'Paralytic scoliosis.' *Journal of Bone and Joint Surgery*, 38B, 660–685.

—— (1967) *Scoliosis*. Edinburgh: E. & S. Livingstone, p. 145.

Jerosch, J., Senst, S., Hoffstetter, I. (1995) 'Combined realignment procedure (femoral and acetabular) of the hip joint in ambulator patients with cerebral palsy and secondary hip dislocation.' *Acta Orthopedica Belgica*, 61, 92–99.

Jevsevar, D.S., Karlin, L.I. (1993) 'The relationship between preoperative nutritional status and complications after an operation for scoliosis in cerebral palsy.' *Journal of Bone and Joint Surgery*, 75A, 880–884.

Johnson, J.R., Wingo, C.F., Holt, R.T., Leatherman, K.D. (1986) 'A preliminary report of 36 patients treated with the Cotrel–Dubousset procedure.' *Orthopaedic Transactions*, 10, 36.

Johnson, J.T.H., Southwick, W.O. (1960) 'Bone growth after spine fusion.' *Journal of Bone and Joint Surgery*, 42A, 1396–1412.

Jones, K.B., Spoonseller, P.D., Shindle, M.K., McCarthy, M.L. (2003) 'Longitudinal parental perceptions of spinal fusion for neuromuscular spine deformity in patients with totally involved cerebral palsy.' *Journal of Pediatric Orthopaedics*, 23, 143–149.

Jozwiak, M., Marciniak, W., Piontek, T., Pietrzak, S. (2000) 'Dega's transiliac osteotomy in the treatment of spastic hip subluxation and dislocation.' *Journal of Pediatric Orthopaedics B*, 9, 257–264.

Kaczmarczyk, J., Nowakowski, A., Balcerkiewicz, K., Szulc, P. (2003) 'Galveston technique in treatment of paralytic spine deformities.' *Chirurgia Narzadow Ruchu i Ortopedia Polska*, 68, 121–124. (Polish.)

Kalen, V., Gamble, J.G. (1984) 'Resection arthroplasty of the hip in paralytic dislocations.' *Developmental Medicine and Child Neurology*, **26**, 341–346.

—— Bleck, E.E. (1985) 'Prevention of spastic paralytic dislocation of the hip.' *Developmental Medicine and Child Neurology*, **27**, 17–24.

—— —— Rinsky, L.A. (1985) Preliminary results of Luque instrumentation in neuromuscular disorders.' *Orthopaedic Transactions*, **9**, 94–95.

—— Medige, T.A., Rinsky, L.A. (1992) 'Pericardial tamponade secondary to perforation by central catheters in orthopaedic patients.' *Journal of Bone and Joint Surgery*, **74A**, 1110–1101.

Kannan, S., Meert, K.L., Mooney, J.F., Hillman-Wiseman, C., Warrier, I. (2002) 'Bleeding and coagulation changes during spinal fusion surgery: a comparison of neuromuscular and idiopathic scoliosis patients.' *Pediatric Critical Care Medicine*, **3**, 364–369.

Kay, R.M., Jaki, K.A., Skaggs, D.L. (2000) 'The effect of femoral rotation on the projected femoral neck-shaft angle.' *Journal of Pediatric Orthopaedics*, **20**, 736–739.

Keats, S. (1970) *Operative Orthopaedics in Cerebral Palsy.* Springfield, IL: C.C. Thomas, p. 225.

—— Morgese, A.N. (1967) 'A simple anteromedial approach to the lesser trochanter of the femur for the release of the iliopsoas tendon.' *Journal of Bone and Joint Surgery*, **49A**, 632–636.

Keim, H.A., Hilal, S.K. (1971) 'Spinal angiography in scoliosis patients.' *Journal of Bone and Joint Surgery*, **53A**, 904–912.

Kesling, K.L., Lonstein, J.E., Denis, F., Perra, J.H., Schwender, J.D., Transfeldt, E.E., Winter, R.B. (2003) 'The crankshaft phenomenon after posterior spinal arthrodesis for congenital scoliosis: a review of 54 patients.' *Spine*, **28**, 267–271.

Kim, H.T., Wenger, D.R. (1997) 'Location of acetabular deficiency and associated hip dislocation in neuromuscular hip dysplasia: three-dimensional computed tomographic analysis.' *Journal of Pediatric Orthopaedics*, **17**, 143–151.

Kleinman, R.G., Csongradi, J.J., Rinsky, L.A., Bleck, E.E. (1982) 'The radiographic assessment of spinal flexibility in scoliosis.' *Clinical Orthopaedics and Related Research*, **162**, 47–53.

Klisic, P.C., Jankovic, L. (1976) 'Combined procedure of open reduction and shortening of the femur in treatment of congenital dislocation of the hip in older children.' *Clinical Orthopaedics and Related Research*, **119**, 60–69.

Knapp, D.R. Jr, Cortes, H. (2002) 'Untreated hip dislocation in cerebral palsy.' *Journal of Pediatric Orthopaedics*, **22**, 668–671.

Knelles, D., Barthel, T., Karrer, A., Kraus, U., Eulert, J., Kolbl, O. (1997) 'Prevention of heterotopic ossification after total hip replacement. A prospective, randomized study using acetylsalicylic acid, indomethacin and fractional or single-dose radiation.' *Journal of Bone and Joint Surgery*, **79B**, 596–602.

—— Raab, P., Wild, A., Muller, T., Krauspe, R. (1999) 'Complex reconstruction of dislocated hip joints in spastic handicapped children.' *Zeitschrift für Orthopädie und ihre Grenzgebiete*, **137**, 409–413.

Knoeller, S.M., Stuecker, R.D. (2002) 'Impact of early surgical correction of curves in paralytic scoliosis.' *Saudi Medical Journal*, **23**, 1181–1186.

Koffman, M. (1981) 'Proximal femoral resection or total joint replacement in severe disabled cerebral palsy spastic patients.' *Orthopedic Clinics of North America*, **12**, 91–100.

Koorevaar, C.T., Hu, H.P., Lemmens, A., van Kampen, A. (1999) 'No effective prophylaxis of heterotopic ossification with short term ibuprofen.' *Archives of Orthopaedic and Trauma Surgery*, **119**, 183–185.

Krum, S.D., Miller, F. (1993) 'Heterotopic ossification after hip and spine surgery in children with cerebral palsy.' *Journal of Pediatric Orthopaedics*, **13**, 739–743.

Kuklo, T.R., Owens, B.D., Polly, D.W. Jr (2003) 'Perioperative blood and blood product management for spinal deformity surgery.' *Spine Journal*, **3**, 388–393.

Langenskiöld, A. (1971) 'Growth disturbance of muscle: a possible factor in the pathogenesis of scoliosis.' *In* Zorab, P.A. (Ed.) *Scoliosis and Growth.* London: Churchill Livingstone, p. 85.

Lapinsky, A.S., Richards, B.S. (1995) 'Preventing the crankshaft phenomenon by combining anterior fusion with posterior instrumentation. Does it work?' *Spine*, **20**, 1392–1398.

Laplaza, F.J., Root, L. (1994) 'Femoral anteversion and neck-shaft angles in hip instability in cerebral palsy.' *Journal of Pediatric Orthopaedics*, **14**, 719–723.

Lau, J. H. K., Parker, J. C., Hsu, L. C. S., Leong, J. C. Y. (1986) 'Paralytic hip instability in poliomyelitis.' *Journal of Bone and Joint Surgery*, **68B**, 528–533.

Leatherman, K. C. (1969) 'Resection of vertebral bodies.' *Journal of Bone and Joint Surgery*, **51A**, 206. (Abstract.)

Lee, C.S., Nachemson, A.L. (1997) 'The crankshaft phenomenon after posterior Harrington fusion in skeletally immature patients with thoracic or thoracolumbar idiopathic scoliosis followed to maturity.' *Spine*, **22**, 58–67.

Lee, M., Alexander, M.A., Miller, F.A., Steg, N.L., McHugh, B.A. (1992) 'Postoperative heterotopic ossification in the child with cerebral palsy: three case reports.' *Archives of Physical Medicine and Rehabilitation*, **73**, 289–292.

Le Foll, D. (1980) 'Contribution à l'étude de la luxation de la hanche chez l'infirme moteur d'origine cérébrale.' *Thèse pour le Doctorat en Médecine, Académie de Paris, Université René Descartes, Faculté de Médecine Chochin Port, France.*

—— Dubousset, J., Queneau, P. (1981) 'Les defauts de centrage de la tête fémorale chez l'infirme moteur d'origine cérébrale.' *Revue de Chirurgie Orthopedique*, **67**, 121–131.

Legenstein, R., Bosch, P., Ungersbock, A. (2003) 'Indomethacin versus meloxicam for prevention of heterotopic ossification after total hip arthroplasty.' *Archives of Orthopaedic and Trauma Surgery*, **123**, 91–94.

Lenke, L.G. (2003) 'Anterior endoscopic discectomy and fusion for adolescent idiopathic scoliosis.' *Spine*, **28**, S36–43.

Leong, J.C.Y., Wilding, K., Mok, C.K., Ma, A., Chow, S.P., Yau, A.C.M.C. (1981) 'Surgical treatment of scoliosis following poliomyelitis: a review of one hundred and ten cases.' *Journal of Bone and Joint Surgery*, **63A**, 726–740.

Leopando, M.E., Moussavi, Z., Holbrow, J., Chernick, V., Pasterkamp, H, Rempel, G. (1999) 'Effect of a Soft Boston Orthosis on pulmonary mechanics in severe cerebral palsy.' *Pediatric Pulmonlology*, **28**, 53–58.

Letts, R.M., Bobechko, W.P. (1974) 'Fusion of the scoliotic spine in young children.' *Clinical Orthopaedics and Related Research*, **101**, 136–145.

—— Shapiro, L., Mulder, K., Klasen, O. (1984) 'The windblown hip syndrome in total body cerebral palsy.' *Journal of Pediatric Orthopedics*, **4**, 55–62.

Leung, J.P., Lam, T.P., Ng, B.K., Cheng, J.C. (2002) 'Posterior ISOLA segmental spinal system in the treatment of scoliosis.' *Journal of Pediatric Orthopaedics*, **22**, 296–301.

Liepones, J.V., Bunch, W.H., Lonser, R.E., Daley, R.L., Gogan, W.J. (1984) 'Spinal cord injury during segmental sublaminar spinal instrumentation: an animal model.' *Orthopaedic Transactions*, **8**, 173.

Lipton, G.E., Miller, F., Dabney, K.W., Altiok, H., Bachrach, S.J. (1999) 'Factors predicting postoperative complications following spinal fusions in children with cerebral palsy.' *Journal of Spinal Disorders*, **12**, 197–205.

—— Letonoff, E.J., Dabney, K.W., Miller, F., McCarthy, H.C. (2003) 'Correction of sagittal plane spine deformities with unit rod instrumentation in children with cerebral palsy.' *Journal of Bone and Joint Surgery*, **85A**, 2349–2357.

Liszka, O. (1961) 'Spinal cord mechanisms leading to scoliosis in animal experiments.' *Acta Medica Polonia*, **2**, 45–63.

Lonstein, J.E., Akbamia, A. (1983) 'Operative treatment of spinal deformities in patients with cerebral palsy or mental retardation. An analysis of one hundred and seven cases.' *Journal of Bone and Joint Surgery*, **65A**, 43–55.

—— Carlson, J.M. (1984) 'The prediction of curve progression in untreated idiopathic scoliosis during growth.' *Journal of Bone and Joint Surgery*, **66A**, 1061–1071.

—— Beck, K. (1986) 'Hip dislocation and subluxation in cerebral palsy.' *Journal of Pediatric Orthopedics*, **6**, 521–526.

—— (2001) 'Neuromuscular spinal deformities.' *In* Weinstein, S.L. (Ed.) *The Pediatric Spine, 2nd edn.* Philadelphia: Lippincott Williams & Wilkins, pp. 791–792.

Lowe, T.G., Betz, R., Lenke, L., Clements, D., Harms, J., Newton, P., Haher, T., Merola, A., Wenger, D. (2003) 'Anterior single-rod instrumentation of the thoracic and lumbar spine: saving levels.' *Spine*, **28** (Suppl. 20S), S208–216.

Luk, K.D.K., Ho, H.C., Leong, J.C.Y. (1986) 'The iliolumbar ligament. A study of its anatomy, development and clinical significance.' *Journal of Bone and Joint Surgery*, **68B**, 197–200.

Lundy, D.W., Ganey, T.M., Odgen, J.A., Guidera, K.J. (1998) 'Pathologic morphology of the dislocated proximal femur in children with cerebral palsy.' *Journal of Pediatric Orthopaedics*, **18**, 528–534.

Luque, E.R. (1982) 'Segmental spinal instrumentation for correction of scoliosis.' *Clinical or Orthopaedics and Related Research*, **163**, 192–198.

—— Cardoso, A. (1977) 'Segmental correction of scoliosis with rigid fixation. Preliminary report.' *Orthopaedic Transactions*, **1**, 136–137.

MacEwen, G.D. (1968) 'Experimental scoliosis.' *In* Zorab, P.A. (Ed.) *Proceedings of a Second Symposium on Scoliosis: Causation.* Edinburgh: Churchill Livingstone, p. 18.

—— (1969) 'The incidence and treatment of scoliosis in cerebral palsy.' *Paper Presented at Annual Meeting of American Academy for Cerebral Palsy, Miami Beach, FL.*

—— (1972) 'Operative treatment of scoliosis in cerebral palsy.' *Reconstructive Surgery and Traumatology,* **13,** 58–67.

—— Bunnell, W.P., Sriram, M. (1975) 'Acute neurological complications in the treatment of scoliosis. A report of the Scoliosis Research Society.' *Journal of Bone and Joint Surgery,* **57A,** 404–408.

Machida, M., Dubousset, J., Imamura, Y., Iwaya, T., Yamada, T, Kimura, J., Toriyama, S. (1993) 'An experimental study in chickens for the pathogenesis of idiopathic scoliosis.' *Spine,* **18,** 1609–1615.

—— —— —— —— —— —— —— —— (1994) 'Pathogenesis of idiopathic scoliosis: SEPs in chicken with experimentally induced scoliosis and in patient with idiopathic scoliosis.' *Journal of Pediatric Orthopaedics,* **14,** 329–335.

—— —— —— —— —— —— (1995) 'Role of melatonin deficiency in the development of scoliosis in pinealectomized chickens.' *Journal of Bone and Joint Surgery,* **77B,** 134–138.

—— Murai, I., Miyashita, Y.U., Dubousset, J., Tamada, T., Kimura, J. (1999) 'Pathogenesis of idiopathic scoliosis. Experimental study in rats.' *Spine,* **24,** 1985–1999.

—— —— Satoh, T., Murai, I., Wood, K.B., Yamada, T., Ryu, J. (2001) 'Pathologic mechanism of experimental scoliosis in pinealectomized chickens.' *Spine,* **26,** E385–E391.

Mac Keith, R. (1966) 'Prevention is better than cure.' *Developmental Medicine and Child Neurology,* **8,** 379. (Editorial.)

Madigan, R.R., Wallace, S.L. (1981) 'Scoliosis in the institutionalized cerebral palsy population.' *Spine,* **6,** 583–590.

—— (1986) 'Scoliosis in cerebral palsy: short term follow-up and prognosis in untreated institutionalized patients.' *Orthopaedic Transactions,* **10,** 17.

Magnissalis, E.A., Zinelis, S., Demetriades, D., Hager, J. (2003) 'Analysis of a retrieved Isola spinal system fractured in service.' *Journal of Biomedical Materials Research,* **64B,** 6–12.

Majd, M.E., Muldowny, D.S., Holt, R.T. (1997) 'Natural history of scoliosis in the institutionalized adult cerebral palsy population.' *Spine,* **22,** 1461–1466.

Malamo-Lada, H., Zarkotou, O, Nikolaides, N., Kanellopoulou, M., Demetriades, D. (1999) 'Wound infections following posterior spinal instrumentation for paralytic scoliosis.' *Clinical Microbiology and Infection,* **5,** 135–139.

Malefijt, M.C., Dew, W., Hoogland, T., Nielsen, H.K.L. (1982) 'Chiari osteotomy in the treatment of congenital dislocation and subluxation of the hip.' *Journal of Bone and Joint Surgery,* **64A,** 996–1004.

Maloney, W.J., Rinsky, L.A., Gamble, J.G. (1990) 'Simultaneous correction of pelvic obliquity, frontal plane, and sagittal plane deformities in neuromuscular scoliosis using a unit rod with segmental sublaminar wires.' *Journal of Pediatric Orthopaedics,* **10,** 742–749.

Manjarris, J.F., Mubarak, S. (1984) 'Avascular necrosis of the femoral heads following bilateral iliopsoas and adductor releases via the medial approach to the hip.' *Journal of Pediatric Orthopaedics,* **4,** 109–110.

Marchesi, D., Arlet, V., Strickler, V., Achi, M. (1997) 'Modification of the original Luque technique in the treatment of Duchenne's neuromuscular scoliosis.' *Journal of Pediatric Orthopaedics,* **17,** 743–749.

Martin, J.P. (1965) 'Curvature of the spine in post-encephalitic Parkinsonism.' *Journal of Neurology, Neurosurgery and Psychiatry,* **28,** 395–400.

Matsuo, T. (2002) *Cerebral Palsy. Spasticity-control and Orthopaedics—An Introduction to Orthopaedic Selective Spasticity-Control Surgery (OSSCS).* Tokyo: Soufusha.

Mattson, G., Haderspeck-Grib, K., Schultz, A., Nachemson, A. (1983) 'Joint flexibilities in structurally normal girls and girls with idiopathic scoliosis.' *Journal of Orthopaedic Research,* **1,** 57–62.

McCarthy, R.E, McCullough, F.L. (1985) 'Experience with a locking collar for Luque rods.' *Paper read at the Annual Meeting of the Scoliosis Research Society, Coronado, CA.*

—— Peek, R.D., Morrissy, R.T., Hough, A.J. Jr (1986) 'Allograft bone in spinal fusion for paralytic scoliosis.' *Journal of Bone and Joint Surgery,* **68A,** 370–375.

—— Simon, S., Doughlas, B., Zawacki, R., Reese, N. (1988a) 'Proximal femoral resection to allow adults who have severe cerebral palsy to sit.' *Journal of Bone and Joint Surgery,* **70A,** 1011–1016.

—— McCullough, F.L., Peek, R.D., Harrsion, B.H. (1988b) 'A locking collar for Luque rods.' *Orthopaedics,* **11,** 921–926.

McCluer, S. (1982) 'Cervical spondylosis with myelopathy as a complication of cerebral palsy.' *Paraplegia,* **20,** 308–312.

McHale, K.A., Bagg, M., Nason, S.S. (1990) 'Treatment of the chronically dislocated hip in adolescents with cerebral palsy with femoral head resection and subtrochanteric valgus osteotomy.' *Journal of Pediatric Orthopaedics,* **10,** 504–509.

—— (1991) 'Bilateral spontaneous arthrodesis of the hip after combined shelf acetabular augmentation and femoral varus osteotomies.' *Journal of Pediatric Orthopaedics,* **11,** 108–111.

McIvor, W.C., Samilson, R.L. (1966) 'Fractures in patients with cerebral palsy.' *Journal of Bone and Joint Surgery,* **48A,** 858–866.

McLuhan, M. (1964) *Understanding the Media: Extension of Man.* New York: McGraw.

McNaughton, S. (1975) 'Visual symbols: a system of communication for the nonverbal physically handicapped child.' *Regional Course, American Academy for Cerebral Palsy, Palo Alto, CA.*

McNerney, N.P., Mubarak, S.J., Wenger, D.R. (2000) 'One-stage correction of the dysplastic hip in cerebral palsy with the San Diego acetabuloplasty: results and complications in 104 hips.' *Journal of Pediatric Orthopaedics,* **20,** 93–103.

Meert, K.L., Kannan, S., Mooney, J.F. (2002) 'Predictors of red cell transfusion in children and adolescents undergoing spinal fusion surgery.' *Spine,* **27,** 2137–2142.

Metz, P., Zielke, K. (1982) 'Erste Ergebnisse der Operation nach Luque. Voraufiger Bericht über 12 Falle.' *Zeitschrift für Orthopädie,* **120,** 337–338.

Mikawa, Y., Watanabe, R., Shikata, J. (1997) 'Cervical myelo-radiculopathy in cerebral palsy.' *Archives of Orthopaedic and Trauma Surgery,* **116,** 116–118.

Miller, A., Temple, T., Miller, F. (1996) 'Impact of orthoses on the rate or scoliosis progression in children with cerebral palsy.' *Journal of Pediatric Orthopaedics,* **16,** 332–335,

Miller, F., Bagg, M. R. (1995) 'Age and migration percentage as risk factors for progression in spastic hip disease.' *Developmental Medicine and Child Neurology,* **37,** 449–455.

—— Cardoso Dias, R., Dabney, K.W., Lipton, G.E., Triana, M. (1997) 'Soft-tissue release for spastic hip subluxation in cerebral palsy.' *Journal of Pediatric Orthopaedics,* **17,** 571–584.

—— (1997) 'Letter to the editor.' *Journal of Pediatric Orthopaedics,* **17,** 407.

—— Giradi, H., Lipton, G., Ponzio, R., Klaumann, M., Dabney, K.W. (1997) 'Reconstruction of the dysplastic spastic hip with peri-ilial pelvic and femoral osteotomy followed by immediate immobilization.' *Journal of Pediatric Orthopaedics,* **17,** 592–602.

—— Slomczykowski, M., Cope, R., Lipton, G.E. (1999) 'Computer modeling of the pathomechanics of spastic hip dislocation in children.' *Journal of Pediatric Orthopaedics,* **19,** 486–492.

Mitchell, G.P. (1974) 'Chiari medial displacement osteotomy.' *Clinical Orthopaedics and Related Research,* **98,** 146–150.

Moe, J.H. (1958) 'A critical analysis of methods of fusion for scoliosis. An evaluation in two hundred and sixty-six patients.' *Journal of Bone and Joint Surgery,* **40A,** 529–554.

—— Sundberg, A.B., Gustilo, R. (1964) 'A clinical study of spine fusion in the growing child.' *Journal of Bone and Joint Surgery,* **46B,** 784–785. (Abstract.)

—— Winter, R.B., Bradford, D.S., Lonstein, J.E. (1978) *Scoliosis and Other Spinal Deformities.* Philadelphia: W.B. Saunders.

—— Kharrat, K., Winter, R.B., Cummine, J.L. (1984) 'Harrington instrumentation without fusion plus external orthotic support for treatment of difficult curvature problems in young children' *Clinical Orthopaedics and Related Research,* **185,** 35–45.

Molloy, M.K. (1986) 'The unstable paralytic hip: treatment by combined pelvic and femoral osteotomy and transiliac psoas transfer.' *Journal of Pediatric Orthopedics,* **6,** 533–538.

Montgomery, D.M., Aronson, D.D., Lee, C.L., LaMont, R.L. (1990) 'Posterior spinal fusion: allograft versus autograft bone.' *Journal of Spinal Disorders,* **3,** 370–375.

Mooney, J.F. 3rd (2000) 'Perioperative enteric nutritional supplementation in pediatric patients with neuromuscular scoliosis.' *Journal of the Southern Orthopaedic Association,* **9,** 202–206.

Moreau, M., Cook, P.C., Ashton, B. (1995) 'Adductor and psoas release for subluxation of the hip in children with spastic cerebral palsy.' *Journal of Pediatric Orthopaedics*, **15**, 672–676

Morigana, H. (1973) 'An electromyographic study on the function of the psoas major muscle.' *Journal of the Japanese Orthopaedic Association*, **47**, 351–365.

Moseley, C., Mosca, V., Lawton, L., Koreska, J. (1986) 'Improved stability in segmental instrumentation in neuromuscular scoliosis.' *Orthopaedic Transactions*, **10**, 5.

Motloch, W. (1978) 'Analysis of medical costs associated with healing of pressure sores in adolescent paraplegics.' *Thesis for Bachelor of Science Degree in Business Administration, University of San Francisco.*

Moulin, F., Quintart, A., Sauvestre, C., Mensah, K., Bergeret, M., Raymond, J. (1998) 'Nosocomial urinary tract infections: retrospective study in a pediatric hospital.' *Archives de Pédiatrie: Organe Officiel de la Société Française de Pédiatrie*, **5** (Suppl. 3), 274S–278S.

Mowery, C.A., Houkom, J.A., Roach, J.W., Sutherland, D.H. (1986) 'A simple method of hip arthrodesis.' *Journal of Pediatric Orthopedics*, **6**, 7–10.

M'Rabet, A., Dubousset, J. (1988) 'Treatment of spinal deformities in patients with cerebral palsy.' *Revue de Chirurgie Orthopédique et Réparatrice de l'Appareil Locomoteur*, **74**, 647–648. (French.)

Mubarak S.J., Mortensen, W., Katz, W. (1986) 'Combined pelvic (Dega) and femoral osteotomies in the treatment of paralytic hip dislocation.' *Developmental Medicine and Child Neurology*, **28** (Suppl. 53), 33–34. (Abstract.)

—— Valencia, F.G., Wenger, D.R. (1992) 'One-stage correction of the spastic dislocated hip. Use of pericapsular acetabuloplasty to improve coverage.' *Journal of Bone and Joint Surgery*, **74A**, 1347–1357.

Murray, W.R., Lucas, D.B., Inman, V.T. (1964) 'Femoral head and neck resection.' *Journal of Bone and Joint Surgery*, **46A**, 1184–1197.

Nachemson, A. (1968) 'A long-term follow-up study of non-treated scoliosis.' *Acta Orthopaedica Scandinavica*, 39, 466–476.

—— (1980) *Lectures, International Pediatric Orthopaedic Seminar, Chicago.*

Nassif, J.M., Ritter, M.A. (1999) 'Indomethacin-induced postoperative psychosis.' *Journal of Arthroplasty*, **14**, 769–770.

Newton, P.O., Michelle, M.S., Faro, F., Frances, Betz, R., Clements, D., Haher, T., Lenke, L., Lower, T., Merola, A, Wenger, D. (2003) 'Use of video-assisted thoracoscopic surgery to reduce perioperative morbidity in scoliosis surgery.' *Spine*, **28**, S249–S254.

Nickel, V.L., Perry, J., Garrett, A., Heppenstall, M. (1968) 'The halo, a spinal skeletal traction fixation device.' *Journal of Bone and Joint Surgery*, **50A**, 1400–1409.

Noonan, K.J., Walker, T.L., Kayes, K.J., Feinberg, J. (2000) 'Effect of surgery on the non-treated hip in severe cerebral palsy.' *Journal of Pediatric Orthopaedics*, **20**, 771–775.

—— —— —— —— (2001) 'Varus derotation osteotomy for the treatment of hip subluxation and dislocation in cerebral palsy: statistical analysis in 73 hips.' *Journal of Pediatric Orthopaedics B*, **10**, 279–286.

Novacheck, T.F., Trost, J.P., Schwartz, M.H. (2002) 'Intramuscular psoas lengthening improves dynamic hip function in children with cerebral palsy.' *Journal of Pediatric Orthopaedics*, **22**, 158–164.

Obletz, B.E., Lockie, L.M., Milch, E., Hyman, I. (1949) 'Early effects of partial sensory denervation of the hip for relief of pain in chronic arthritis.' *Journal of Bone and Joint Surgery*, **31A**, 805–814.

O'Brien, J.J., Sirkin, R.B. (1977) 'The natural history of the dislocated hip in cerebral palsy.' *Paper presented to the Annual Meeting of the American Academy for Cerebral Palsy and Developmental Medicine, Atlanta.*

O'Brien, J.P. (1977) 'The management of severe spinal deformities with the halo-pelvic apparatus; pitfalls and guidelines in its use.' *Journal of Bone and Joint Surgery*, **59B**, 117–118. (Abstract.)

—— Yau, A.C.M.C., Smith, T., Hodgson, A.R. (1971) 'Halo-pelvic traction.' *Journal of Bone and Joint Surgery*, **53B**, 217–229.

—— (1972) 'Anterior and posterior correction and fusion for paralytic scoliosis.' *Clinical Orthopaedics and Related Research*, **86**, 151–153.

—— Dwyer, A.P., Hodgson, A.R. (1975) 'Paralytic pelvic obliquity: its prognosis and management and the development of a technique for full correction of the deformity.' *Journal of Bone and Joint Surgery*, **57A**, 626–631.

Oegema, T.R., Bradford, D.S., Cooper, K.M., Hunter, R.E. (1983) 'Comparison of the biochemistry of proteoglycans isolated from normal, idiopathic scoliotic and cerebral palsy spines.' *Spine*, **8**, 378–384.

Onari, K. Kondo, S., Mihara, H., Iwamura, Y. (2002) 'Combined anterior–posterior fusion for cervical spondylotic myelopathy in patients with athetoid cerebral palsy.' *Journal of Neurosurgery*, **97** (1 Suppl.), 13–9.

Onimus, M., Vergnat, L. (1980) 'La médialisation du cotyle et les déplacements parasites dans l'ostéotomie pelvienne de Chiari.' *Revue de Chirurgie Orthopédique*, **66**, 299–309.

—— Allamel, G., Manzone, P., Laurain, J.M. (1991) 'Prevention of hip dislocation in cerebral palsy by early psoas and adductor tenotomies.' *Journal of Pediatric Orthopaedics*, **11**, 432–435.

—— Manzone, P., Cahuzac, J.P., Laurain, J.M., Lebarbier, P. (1992) 'Surgical treatment of dislocations and subdislocations of the hip in patients with cerebral palsy by femoral and pelvic osteotomy.' *Revue de Chirurgie Orthopédique et Réparatrice de l'Appareil Locomoteur*, **78**, 74–81.

—— —— Lornet, J.M., Laurain, J.M. (1992) 'Surgical management of scoliosis in bed-ridden patients with cerebral palsy.' *Revue de Chirurgie Orthopédique et Réparatrice de l'Appareil Locomoteur*, **78**, 312–318. (French.)

Papin, P., Arlet, V., Marchesi, D., Laberge, J. M., Aebi, M. (1998) 'Treatment of scoliosis in the adolescent by anterior release and vertebral thoracoscopy. Preliminary results.' *Revue de Chirurgie Orthopedique et Réparatrice de l'Appareil Locomoteur*, **84**, 231–238. (French.)

Parent, H.F., Zeller, R.D., Mascard, E., Miladi, L., Seringe, R. (1994) 'Modified femoral varization osteotomy for the unstable hip in cerebral palsy.' *Journal of Pediatric Orthopaedics B*, **3**, 18–21.

Parsch, V.K. (1985) 'Hanche et infirmite motrice cerebrale.' *In* Dimeglio, A., Auriach, A., Simon, L. (Eds) *L'Enfant Paralysé*. Paris: Masson.

Paul, I.T., Holte, R.N., VonKampen, E. (1980) 'Factors influencing design of modular inserts for disabled children.' *Proceedings of International Conference on Rehabilitation Engineering*, 161–162.

Payer, L. (1988) *Medicine and Culture. Varieties of Treatment in the United States, England, West Germany and France.* New York: Penguin.

Payne, L.A., DeLuca, P.A. (1993) 'Heterotopic ossification after rhizotomy and femoral osteotomy.' *Journal of Pediatric Orthopaedics*, **13**, 733–738.

Pemberton, P.A. (1965) 'Pericapsular osteotomy of the ilium for treatment of congenital subluxation and dislocation of the hip.' *Journal of Bone and Joint Surgery*, **47A**, 65–86.

Peterson, L.T. (1950) 'Tenotomy in the treatment of spastic paraplegia with special reference to tenotomy of the iliopsoas.' *Journal of Bone and Joint Surgery*, **32A**, 875–885.

Phelps, W.M. (1959) 'Prevention of acquired dislocation of the hip in cerebral palsy.' *Journal of Bone and Joint Surgery*, **41A**, 440–448.

Ponsetti, I.V., Friedman, B. (1950) 'Changes in the scoliotic spine after fusion.' *Journal of Bone and Joint Surgery*, **32A**, 381–395.

Pope, D.F., Bieff, H.U., DeLuca, P.A. (1994) 'Pelvic osteotomies for subluxation of the hip in cerebral palsy.' *Journal of Pediatric Orthopaedics*, **14**, 724–730.

Pountney, T., Mandy, A., Green, E., Gard, P. (2002) 'Management of hip dislocation with postural management.' *Child: Care, Health, Development*, **28**, 179–185.

Pous, J.G. (1985) 'Cartilagenous iliac crest transfer to stabilize neurologic hip.' *Orthopaedic Transactions*, **9**, 192.

Pritchett, J.W. (1990) 'Treated and untreated unstable hips in severe cerebral palsy.' *Developmental Medicine and Child Neurology*, **32**, 3–6.

Propst-Proctor, S.L. (1981a) 'Containment of the hip: a theoretical comparison of osteotomies.' *Clinical Orthopaedics and Related Research*, **154**, 191–196.

—— (1981b) 'Preoperative roentgenographic evaluation for osteotomies about the hip in children.' *Journal of Bone and Joint Surgery*, **63A**, 305–309.

—— Bleck, E.E. (1983) 'Radiographic determination of lordosis and kyphosis in normal and scoliotic children.' *Journal of Pediatric Orthopedics*, **3**, 344–346.

—— Rinsky, L.A., Bleck, E.E. (1983) 'The cisterna chyli in orthopaedic surgery.' *Spine*, **8**, 787–792.

Rab, G.T. (1978) 'Biomechanical aspects of Salter osteotomy.' *Clinical Orthopaedics and Related Research*, **132**, 82–87.

Racette, B.A. Lauryssen, C., Perlmutter, J.S. (1998) 'Preoperative treatment with botulinum toxin to facilitate cervical fusion in dystonic cerebral palsy. A report of two cases.' *Journal of Neurosurgery*, **88**, 328–330.

Raih, T.J., Comfort, T.H., Beck, K.O., Vanden Brink, K.D. (1985) 'Proximal femoral resections in severe cerebral palsy.' *Orthopaedic Transactions*, **9**, 492.

Rang, M. (1986) *Course on Cerebral Palsy, Scottish Rite Children's Hospital, Atlanta, Georgia.*

—— Douglas, G., Bennet, G.D., Koreska, J. (1981) 'Seating for children with cerebral palsy.' *Journal of Pediatric Orthopedics*, **1**, 279–287.

—— Silver, R., de la Garza, J. (1986) 'Cerebral palsy.' *In* Lovell, W.W., Winter, R.B. (Eds) *Pediatric Orthopaedics, 2nd edn.* Philadelphia: J.B. Lippincott.

Reese, M.E., Msall, M.E., Owen, S., Pictor, S.P., Paroski, M.W. (1991) 'Acquired cervical spine impairment in young adults with cerebral palsy.' *Developmental Medicine and Child Neurology*, **33**, 153–158.

Reimers, J. (1972) 'A scoring system for the evaluation of ambulation in cerebral palsied patients.' *Developmental Medicine and Child Neurology*, **14**, 332–335.

—— (1980) 'The stability of the hip in children. A radiological study of the results of muscle surgery in cerebral palsy.' *Acta Orthopaedica Scandinavica*, **184** (Suppl.), 1–97.

—— Poulsen, S. (1984) 'Adductor transfer versus tenotomy for stability of the hip in spastic cerebral palsy.' *Journal of Pediatric Orthopedics*, **4**, 52–54.

—— (1992) 'Acetabular development after femoral osteotomy in cerebral palsy after age four years. *Journal of Pediatric Orthopaedics B*, **1**, 35–37.

Ring, N.O., Nelhman, L., Pearson, D.A. (1978) 'Molded supportive seating for the disabled.' *Prosthetics and Orthotics International*, **2**, 30–34.

Rinsky, L.A., Gamble, J.G., Bleck, E.E. (1985) 'Segmental instrumentation without fusion in children with progressive scoliosis.' *Journal of Pediatric Orthopedics*, **5**, 687–690.

—— (1990) 'Surgery of spinal deformity in cerebral palsy. Twelve years in the evolution of scoliosis management.' *Clinical Orthopaedics and Related Research*, **253**, 100–109.

Risser, J.C., Ferguson, A.B. (1936) 'Scoliosis: its prognosis.' *Journal of Bone and Joint Surgery*, **18**, 667–670.

—— Nordquist, D.M. (1958) 'A follow-up study of the treatment of scoliosis.' *Journal of Bone and Joint Surgery*, **40A**, 555–569.

Roberto, R.F., Lonstein, J.E., Winter, R.B., Denis, F. (1997) 'Curve progression in Risser stage 0 or 1 patients after posterior spinal fusion for idiopathic scoliosis.' *Journal of Pediatric Orthopaedics*, **17**, 718–725.

Robson, P. (1968) 'The prevalence of scoliosis in adolescents and young adults with cerebral palsy.' *Developmental Medicine and Child Neurology*, **10**, 447–452.

Romano, C.L., Duci, D., Romano, D., Mazza, M., Meani, E. (2004) 'Celecoxib versus indomethacin in the prevention of heterotopic ossification after total hip arthroplasty.' *Journal of Arthroplasty*, **19**, 14–18.

Root, L. (1977a) 'The totally involved cerebral palsy patient.' *Instructional Course Lectures, Annual Meeting American Academy of Orthopaedic Surgeons, Las Vegas*.

—— (1977b) 'Total hip replacement in cerebral palsy.' *Paper Presented to the Annual Meeting of the American Academy for Cerebral Palsy and Developmental Medicine, Atlanta*.

—— (1982) 'Total hip replacement in young people with neurological disease.' *Developmental Medicine and Child Neurology*, **24**, 186–188. (Annotation.)

—— Brourman, S.N. (1985) 'Combined pelvic osteotomy with open reduction and femoral shortening for dislocated hips.' *Orthopaedic Transactions*, **9**, 942–943.

—— Goss, J.R., Mendes, J. (1986) 'The treatment of the painful hip in cerebral palsy by total hip replacement or hip arthrodesis.' *Journal of Bone and Joint Surgery*, **68A**, 590–598.

—— Laplaza, F.J., Brourman, S.N., Angel, D.H. (1995) 'The severely unstable hip in cerebral palsy. Treatment with open reduction, pelvic osteotomy and femoral osteotomy with shortening.' *Journal of Bone and Joint Surgery*, **77A**, 703–712.

—— Gross, J.R., Mendes, J. (1986) 'The treatment of the painful hip in cerebral palsy by total hip replacement or hip arthrodesis.' *Journal of Bone and Joint Surgery*, **68A**, 590–598.

Rosenthal, D.K., Levine, D.D., McCarver, C.L. (1974) 'The occurrence of scoliosis in cerebral palsy.' *Developmental Medicine and Child Neurology*, **16**, 664–667.

Roye, D.P. Jr, Chorney, G.S., Deutsch, L.E., Mahon, J.H. (1990) 'Femoral varus and acetabular osteotomies in cerebral palsy.' *Orthopedics*, **13**, 1239–1243.

Sage, F.P. (1987) 'Cerebral palsy.' *In* Crenshaw, A.H. (Ed.) *Campbell's Operative Orthopaedics, 7th edn.* St Louis: C.V. Mosby, p. 2894.

Sahlstrand, T., Ortengren, R., Nachemson, A. (1978) 'Postural equilibrium in adolescent scoliosis.' *Acta Orthopaedica Scandinavica*, **49**, 354–365.

—— Lidstrom, J. (1980) 'Equilibrium factors as predictors of the prognosis in adolescent scoliosis.' *Clinical Orthopaedics and Related Research*, **152**, 232–236.

Saito, N., Ebara, S., Ohotsuka, K., Kumeta, H., Takaoka, K. (1998) 'Natural history of scoliosis in cerebral palsy.' *Lancet*, **351**, 1687–1692.

Salter, R.B. (1961) 'Innominate osteotomy in the treatment of congenital dislocation and subluxation of the hip.' *Journal of Bone and Joint Surgery*, **43B**, 518–539.

—— (1966) 'Role of innominate osteotomy in the treatment of congenital dislocation and subluxation of the hip in the older child.' *Journal of Bone and Joint Surgery*, **48A**, 1413–1439.

Salvati, E.A., Wilson, P.D. (1974) 'Treatment of irreducible hip subluxation by Chiari's iliac osteotomy.' *Clinical Orthopaedics and Related Research*, **98**, 151–161.

Samilson, R.L. (1981) 'Orthopedic surgery of the hips and spine in retarded cerebral palsy patients.' *Orthopedic Clinics of North America*, **12**, 83–90.

—— Tsou, P., Aamoth, G., Green, W.M. (1972) 'Dislocation and subluxation of the hip in cerebral palsy.' *Journal of Bone and Joint Surgery*, **54A**, 863–873.

—— Bechard, R. (1973) 'Scoliosis in cerebral palsy.' *In* Ahstrom, J.P. (Ed.) *Current Practice in Orthopaedic Surgery.* St Louis: C.V. Mosby, p. 183.

Sanders, J.O., Herring, J.A., Browne, R.H. (1995) 'Posterior arthrodesis and instrumentation in the immature (Risser-grade-0) spine in idiopathic scoliosis.' *Journal of Bone and Joint Surgery*, **77A**, 39–45.

—— Little, D.G., Richards, B.S. (1997) 'Prediction of the crankshaft phenomenon by peak height velocity.' *Spine*, **22**, 1356–1357.

San Julian, M., Barrios, R.H., Beguiristain, J.L. (1995) 'Lumbosacral instrumentation in patients with scoliosis in cerebral palsy.' *Journal of Pediatric Orthopaedics B*, **4**, 209–212.

Sarwahi, V., Sarwark, J.F., Schafer, M.F., Backer, C., Lee, M., King, E.C., Aminian, A., Grayhack, J. (2001) 'Standards in anterior spine surgery in pediatric patients with neuromuscular scoliosis.' *Journal of Pediatric Orthopaedics*, **21**, 756–760

Schultz, R.S., Chamberlain, S.E., Stevens, P.M. (1984) 'Radiographic comparison of adductor procedures in cerebral palsied hips.' *Journal of Pediatric Orthopedics*, **4**, 741–744.

Scoles, P.V., Boyd, A., Jones, P.K. (1987) 'Roentgenographic parameters of the normal infant hip.' *Journal of Pediatric Orthopaedics*, **7**, 656–663.

Scrutton, D., Baird, G., Smeeton, N. (2001) 'Hip dysplasia in bilateral cerebral palsy: incidence and natural history in children aged 18 months to 5 years.' *Developmental Medicine and Child Neurology*, **43**, 586–600.

Selva, G., Miller, F., Dabney, K.W. (1998) 'Anterior hip dislocation in children with cerebral palsy.' *Journal of Pediatric Orthopaedics*, **18**, 54–61.

Settecerri, J.J., Karol, L.A. (2000) 'Effectiveness of femoral varus osteotomy in patients with cerebral palsy.' *Journal of Pediatric Orthopaedics*, **20**, 776–780.

Sharp, I.K. (1961) 'Acetabular dysplasia: the acetabular angle.' *Journal of Bone and Joint Surgery*, **43B**, 268–272.

Sharrard, W.J.W., Allen, J.M.H., Heaney, S.H., Prendiville, G.R.G. (1975) 'Surgical prophylaxis of subluxation and dislocation of the hip in cerebral palsy.' *Journal of Bone and Joint Surgery*, **57B**, 160–166.

—— Burke, J. (1982) 'Iliopsoas transfer in the management of established dislocation and refractory progressive subluxation of the hip in cerebral palsy.' *International Orthopaedics*, **6**, 149–154.

Shen, J., Qiu, G., Weng, X., Zhao, H., Jin, J., Wang, Y., Ye, Q., Lin, J. (2003) 'Anterior spinal fusion with TSHR instrumentation for scoliosis.' *Chinese Medical Science Journal*, **18**, 41–45.

Shepherd, G.M. (1994) *Neurobiology.* New York and Oxford: Oxford University Press, p. 547.

Sherk, H.H., Pasquariello, P.D., Doherty, J. (1983) 'Hip dislocation in cerebral palsy: selection for treatment.' *Developmental Medicine and Child Neurology*, **25**, 738–746.

Shufflebarger, H.L., Clark, C.E. (1991) 'Prevention of crankshaft phenomenon.' *Spine*, **16**, S409–411.

Sindelarova, R., Poul, J. (2001) 'Prevention of development of hip joint instability in patients with the spastic form of juvenile cerebral palsy.' *Acta Chirurgiae Orthopaedicae et Traumatologiae Cechoslovaca*, **68**, 176–183.

Singhi, P.D., Ray, M., Suri, G. (2002) 'Clinical spectrum of cerebral palsy in north India–an analysis of 1,000 cases.' *Journal of Tropical Pediatrics*, **48**, 162–166.

Sink, E.L., Newton, P.O., Mubarak, S.J., Wenger, D.R. (2003) 'Maintenance of sagittal plane alignment after surgical correction of spinal deformity in patients with cerebral palsy.' *Spine*, **28**, 1396–1403.

Skoff, H.D., Keggi, K. (1986) 'Total hip replacement in the neuromuscularly impaired.' *Orthopaedic Review*, **15**, 154–159.

Smith, R.M., Emans, J.B. (1992) 'Sitting balance in spinal deformity.' *Spine*, **17**, 1103–1109.

Smith, W.S., Ireton, R.J., Coleman, C.R. (1958) 'Sequelae of experimental dislocation of a I weight-bearing ball-and-socket joint in a young growing animal.' *Journal of Bone and Joint Surgery*, **40A**, 1121–1127.

Smucker, J.D., Miller, F. (2001) 'Crankshaft effect after posterior spinal fusion and unit rod instrumentation in children with cerebral palsy.' *Journal of Pediatric Orthopaedics*, **21**, 108–112.

Somerville, E.W. (1959) 'Paralytic dislocation of the hip.' *Journal of Bone and Joint Surgery*, **41B**, 279–288.

Song, H.R., Carroll, N.C. (1998) 'Femoral varus derotation osteotomy with or without acetabuloplasty for unstable hips in cerebral palsy.' *Journal of Pediatric Orthopaedics*, **18**, 62–68.

Sponseller, P.D., McBeath, A.A., Perpich, M. (1984) 'Hip arthrodesis in young patients. A long-term follow-up study.' *Journal of Bone and Joint Surgery*, **66A**, 853–859.

—— Whiffen, J.R., Drummond, D.S. (1986) 'Interspinous process segmental spinal instrumentation for scoliosis in cerebral palsy.' *Journal of Pediatric Orthopedics*, **6**, 559–563.

—— LaPorte, D.M., Hungerford, M.W., Eck, K., Bridwell, K.H., Lenke, L.G. (2000) 'Deep wound infections after neuromuscular scoliosis surgery: a multicenter study of risk factors and treatment outcomes.' *Spine*, **25**, 2461–2466.

Stagnara, P. (1971) 'Traction cranienne par le 'Halo' de Rancho los Amigos.' *Revue de Chirurgie Orthopédique*, **57**, 287–300.

Staheli, L.T. (1981) 'Slotted acetabular augmentation.' *Journal of Pediatric Orthopaedics*, **1**, 321–327.

Stanitski, C.L., Micheli, L.J., Hall, J.E., Rosenthal, R.M. (1982) 'Surgical correction of spinal deformity in cerebral palsy.' *Spine*, **7**, 563–569.

Stasikelis, P.J., Lee, D.D., Sullivan, C.M. (1999) 'Complications of osteotomies in severe cerebral palsy.' *Journal of Pediatric Orthopaedics*, **19**, 207–210.

—— Ridgeway, S.R., Pugh, L.I., Allen B.L. Jr (2001) 'Epiphyseal changes after proximal femoral osteotomy.' *Journal of Pediatric Orthopaedics B*, **10**, 25–29.

Steeger, D., Wunderlich, T. (1982) 'Zur Problematik der Korrekturosteotmie am Hüftgelenk spastisch behinderter Kinder.' *Zeitschrift für Orthopädie*, **120**, 221–225.

Steel, H.H. (1977) 'Triple osteotomy of the innominate bone.' *Clinical Orthopaedics and Related Research*, **122**, 116–127.

Stephenson, C.T., Donavan, M.M. (1971) 'Transfer of hip adductor origins to the ischium in spastic cerebral palsy.' *Developmental Medicine and Child Neurology*, **13**, 247. (Abstract.)

Sussman, M.D., Little, D., Alley, R.M., McCoig, J.A. (1996) 'Posterior instrumentation and fusion of the thoracolumbar spine for treatment of neuromuscular scoliosis.' *Journal of Pediatric Orthopaedics*, **16**, 304–313.

Sutherland, D.H., Greenfield, R. (1977) 'Double innominate osteotomy.' *Journal of Bone and Joint Surgery*, **59A**, 1082–1091.

Suzuki, J., Inoue, S., Tsuji, K., Mitsuhasi, M. (1964) 'Studies on brain changes in scoliosis.' *Journal of the Chiba Medical Society*, **40**, 165.

Szalay, E.A., Roach, J.W. Houkom, J.A., Wenger, D.R., Herring, J.A. (1986a) 'Extension– abduction contracture of the spastic hip.' *Journal of Pediatric Orthopedics*, **6**, 1–6.

—— Carollo, J.J., Roach, J.W. (1986b) 'Sensitivity of spinal cord monitoring to intraoperative events.' *Journal of Pediatric Orthopedics*, **6**, 437–441.

Szoke, G., Lipton, G., Miller, F., Dabney, K. (1998) 'Wound infection after spinal fusion in children with cerebral palsy.' *Journal of Pediatric Orthopaedics*, **18**, 727–733.

Tachdjian, M.O., Minear, W. L. (1956) 'Hip dislocation in cerebral palsy.' *Journal of Bone and Joint Surgery*, **38A**, 1358–1364.

Tahmassebi, J.F., Curzon, M.E. (2003) 'Prevalence of drooling in children with cerebral palsy attending special schools'. *Developmental Medicine and Child Neurology*, **45**, 613–617.

Tanner, J.M. (1962) *Growth at Adolescence, 2nd edn.* Oxford: Blackwell.

Terazawa, K., Nasu, M., Takata, H., Watanabe, T., Hayshi, T. (1980) 'A case of severe scoliosis associated with cerebral palsy showing remarkable improvement following soft tissue release around the hip and axilla and transfer of the m. tensor fasciae latae to the ribs.' *International Orthopaedics*, **4**, 115–120.

Terjesen, T., Hellum, C. (1998) 'Femoral shortening osteotomy for chronic hip dislocation in patients with cerebral palsy.' *Tidsskrift for den Norskelaegeforening*, **118**, 2773–2776. (Norwegian.)

—— Lange, J.E., Steen, H. (2000) 'Treatment of scoliosis with spinal bracing in quadriplegic cerebral palsy.' *Developmental Medicine and Child Neurology*, **42**, 448–454.

Terver, S., Kleinman, R., Bleck, E.E. (1980) 'Growth landmarks and the evolution of scoliosis: a review of pertinent studies on their usefulness.' *Developmental Medicine and Child Neurology*, **22**, 675–684.

Thacker, M., Hui, J.H., Wong, H.K., Chatterjee, A., Lee, E.H. (2002) 'Spinal fusion and instrumentation for paediatric neuromuscular scoliosis: retrospective review.' *Journal of Orthopaedic Surgery (Hong Kong)*, **10**, 144–151.

Thometz, J.G., Simon, S.R. (1988) 'Progression of scoliosis after skeletal maturity in institutionalized adults who have cerebral palsy.' *Journal of Bone and Joint Surgery*, **70A**, 1290–1296.

Thompson, G.H., Wilber, R.G., Shaffer, P.V., Scoles, A., Kalamchi, A., Nash, C.L.F. Jr (1985) 'Segmental spinal instrumentation in neuromuscular spinal deformities.' *Orthopaedic Transactions*, **9**, 485.

Thomson, J.D., Banta, J.V. (2001) 'Scoliosis in cerebral palsy: an overview and recent results.' *Journal of Pediatric Orthopaedics B*, **10**, 6–9.

Tonis, D. (1976) 'Normal values of the hip joint for the evaluation of X-rays in children and adults.' *Clinical Orthopedics and Related Research*, **119**, 39–48.

Trefler, E., Tooms, R.E., Hobson, D.A. (1978) 'Seating for cerebral palsied children.' *Interclinic Information Bulletin*, **17**, 1–8.

Trousdale, R.T., Ekkernkamp, A., Ganz, R., Wallrichs, S.L. (1995) 'Periarticular and intertrochanteric osteotomy for the treatment of osteoarthrosis in dysplastic hips.' *Journal of Bone and Joint Surgery*, **77A**, 73–85.

Tsirikos, A.I., Chang, W.N., Dabney, K.W., Miller, F., Glutting, J. (2003a) 'Life expectancy in pediatric patients with cerebral palsy and neuromuscular scoliosis who underwent spinal fusion.' *Developmental Medicine and Child Neurology*, **45**, 677–682.

—— —— Shah, S.A., Dabney, K.W., Miller, F. (2003b) 'Preserving ambulatory potential in pediatric patients with cerebral palsy who undergo spinal fusion using a unit rod instrumentation.' *Spine*, **28**, 480–483.

—— —— —— —— (2003c) 'Comparison of one-stage versus two-stage anteroposterior spinal fusion in pediatric patients with cerebral palsy and neuromuscular scoliosis.' *Spine*, **28**, 1300–1305.

—— —— —— —— (2004) 'A comparison of parents' and caregivers' satisfaction after spinal fusion in children with cerebral palsy.' *Journal of Pediatric Orthopaedics*, **24**, 54–58.

Turi, M., Kalen, V. (2000) 'The risk of spinal deformity after selective dorsal rhizotomy.' *Journal of Pediatric Orthopaedics*, **20**, 104–107.

Turker, R.J., Lee, R. (2000) 'Adductor tenotomies in children with quadriplegic cerebral palsy: longer term follow-up.' *Journal of Pediatric Orthopaedics*, **20**, 370–374.

Tylkowski, C.M., Rosenthal, R.K., Simon, S.R. (1980) 'Proximal femoral osteotomy in cerebral palsy.' *Clinical Orthopaedics and Related Research*, **151**, 183–192.

Uematsu, A., Bailey, H.C., Winter, W.G., Brouwer, T.D. (1977) 'Results of posterior iliopsoas transfer for hip instability caused by cerebral palsy.' *Clinical Orthopaedics and Related Research*, **126**, 183–189.

Ushmann, H., Bennett, J.T. (1999) 'Spontaneous ankylosis of the contralateral hip after unilateral adductor tenotomy in cerebral palsy.' *Journal of Pediatric Orthopaedics B*, **8**, 42–44.

Vanderbrink, K.D., Beck, K.O., Comfort, T.H. (1984) 'Management of the hip in severe cerebral palsy.' *Orthopaedic Transactions*, **8**, 454.

van der Heide, H.J., Koorevaar, R.T., Schreurs, B.W., van Kampen, A., Lemmens, A. (1999) 'Indomethacin for 3 days is not effective as prophylaxis for heterotopic ossification after primary total hip arthroplasty.' *Journal of Arthroplasty*, **14**, 796–799.

Vauzelle, C., Stagnara, P., Jouvinroux, P. (1973) 'Functional monitoring of spinal cord activity during spinal surgery.' *Journal of Bone and Joint Surgery*, **55A**, 441. (Abstract.)

Vidal, M. (1982) *L'Infirme Moteur Cérébrale Spastique. Troubles Moteurs et Orthopédiques.* Paris: Masson.

Vielpeau, C., Joubert, J.M., Hulet, C. (1999) 'Naproxen in the prevention of heterotopic ossification after total hip replacement.' *Clinical Orthopaedics and Related Research*, **369**, 279–288.

Von Lackum, W.H., Smith, A. de F. (1933) 'Removal of vertebral bodies in the treatment of scoliosis.' *Surgery, Gynecology and Obstetrics*, **57**, 250–256.

Weber, M., Cabanela, M.E. (1999) 'Total hip arthroplasty in patients with cerebral palsy.' *Orthopedics*, **22**, 425–427.

Weinert, C., Ireland, M.L. (1985) 'Abduction osteotomy for the severely contracted hip in spastic quadriplegia—a new technique with rigid fixation using the compression hip screw system.' *Orthopaedic Transactions*, **9**, 101.

Weinstein, S.L., Zavala, D.C., Ponseti, I.V. (1981) 'Idiopathic scoliosis. Long term follow-up and prognosis in untreated patients.' *Journal of Bone and Joint Surgery*, **63A**, 702–711.

Wheeler, J.E., Weinstein, S.L. (1984) 'Adductor tenotomy–obturator neurectomy.' *Journal of Pediatric Orthopedics*, 4, 48–51.

Whitaker, C., Burton, D.C., Asher, M. (2000) 'Treatment of selected neuromuscular patients with posterior instrumentation and arthrodesis ending with lumbar pedicle screw anchorage.' *Spine*, 25, 2312–2318.

Wiberg, G. (1939) 'Studies on dysplastic acetabula and congenital subluxation of the hip joint with special reference to the complication of osteoarthritis.' *Acta Chirurgica Scaninavica*, 83 (Suppl. 58).

Wicart, Ph., Barthas, J., Guillaumat, M. (1999) 'Total joint replacement of the paralytic hip.' *Revue de Chirurgie Orthopédique*, 85, 581–590.

Widmann, R.F., Do, T.T., Doyle, S.M., Burke, S.W., Root, L. (1999) 'Resection arthroplasty of the hip for patients with cerebral palsy: an outcome study.' *Journal of Pediatric Orthopaedics*, 19, 805–810.

Wilber, R.G., Thompson, G.H., Shaffer, J.W., Brown, R.H., Nash, C.L. (1984) 'Postoperative neurological deficits in segmental spinal instrumentation.' *Journal of Bone and Joint Surgery*, 66A, 1178–1187.

Wiles, P. (1951) 'Resection of dorsal vertebrae in congenital scoliosis.' *Journal of Bone and Joint Surgery*, 33A, 151–154.

Wilkins, C., MacEwen, G.D. (1977) 'Cranial nerve injury from halo traction.' *Clinical Orthopaedics and Related Research*, 126, 106–110.

Wilkinson, A.J., Nattrass, G.R., Graham, H.K. (2001) 'Modified technique for varus derotation osteotomy of the proximal femur in children.' *ANZ Journal of Surgery*, 71, 655–658.

Williamson, J.B., Galasko, C.S.B. (1992) 'Spinal cord monitoring during operative correction of neuromuscular scoliosis.' *Journal of Bone and Joint Surgery*, 74B, 870–872,

Winter, R.B. (1986) 'The spine in cerebral palsy.' *Lecture notes from Pediatric Orthopaedic Seminar, Fitzsimmons Army Hospital, Denver.*

Wu, C.T., Huang, S.C., Chang, C.H. (2001) 'Surgical treatment of subluxation and dislocation of the hips in cerebral palsy patients.' *Journal of the Formosa Medical Association*, 100, 250–256.

Yamada, K., Ikata, T., Yamamoto, H., Nakagawra, Y., Tanaka, H., Tesuka, H. (1969) 'Equilibrium function in scoliosis and active corrective plaster jacket for the treatment.' *Yokushima Journal of Experimental Medicine*, 16, 1–7.

Yazici, M., Asher, M.S., Hardacker, J.W. (2000) 'The safety and efficacy of Isola-Galveston instrumentation and arthrodesis in the treatment of neuromuscular spinal deformities.' *Journal of Bone and Joint Surgery*, 82A, 524–543.

Yngve, D.A., Burke, S.W., Price, C.A., Riddick, M.F. (1986) 'Technique. Sublaminar wiring.' *Journal of Pediatric Orthopedics*, 6, 605–608.

Zaoussis, A.L., James, J.I.P. (1958) 'The iliac apophysis and the evolution of curves in scoliosis.' *Journal of Bone and Joint Surgery*, 40B, 442–453.

Zeller, R.D., Ghanem, I., Miladi, L., Dubousset, J. (1994) 'Posterior spinal fusion in neuromuscular scoliosis using a tibial strut graft. Results of a long-term follow-up.' *Spine*, 19, 1628–1631.

Zielke, K. (1982) 'Ventrale Derotationspondylodese. Behandlungsergebnisse bei idiopathischen Lumbalskoliosen.' *Zeitschrift für Orthopädie*, 120, 320–329.

Zimbler, S., Craig, C., Harris, J., Sohn, R., Rosenberg, G. (1985) 'Orthotic management of severe scoliosis in spastic neuromuscular disease—results of treatment.' *Orthopaedic Transactions*, 9, 78.

Zuckerman, J.D., Staheli, L.T., McLaughlin, J.F. (1984) 'Augmentation for progressive hip subluxation in cerebral palsy.' *Journal of Pediatric Orthopedics*, 4, 436–442.

INDEX

Page numbers in *italics* refer to figures and tables.

definition, 3–4
etiology, *6*
dyslexia, 52
dysmetria, definition, 4
Dysport *see* botulinum-A toxin myoneural blocks
dystonia, 104
    clinical findings, 3, 4, *4, 6*
    etiology, *6*
    intrathecal baclofen, treatment responses, 139
    neck muscles, botulinum-A toxin myoneural blocks, 398
    spastic hemiplegia, 214
    stereotactic brain surgery, 126
    total body involved patients, 346, 347, 397–398

Early Motor Pattern Profile, 49
eating utensils, *188,* 188–189
economic factors, 124
education
    conductive, *161,* 161–163
    home-based, 163
        see also Portage Project
    integrated, 120, 160
elbow-flexion deformity
    botulinum-A toxin myoneural blocks, 228
    spastic hemiplegia, surgical procedures, 228
electrical stimulation, 165–166, *166*
    benefits, 165–166
    cerebral, 127
    scoliosis management, 385
    spinal-cord, 127
    types, 165
electrical synaptic transmission, 83
electromyography, 21, 60–62
    biotelemetry systems, 60
    clinical applications, 62
    data presentation, *61, 62*
    hand function evaluation, 218
    H-wave response, 47
    knee-flexion deformity, 303
    lower limb, *60, 61, 62*
    pelvic obliquity, 116
    severity assessment, 8, 47
    spastic diplegia, *263, 270*
electronic communication devices, 181, *181*
electrotherapy *see* electrical stimulation
Elliott and Connolly classification of hand movements, 34
Ely test, 38, *38,* 313
embryonic stem cells, 89
emotional issues, 120
employment, 193, 194–195
encephalomalacia, 105
encephalopathy, 14
endochondral ossification, scoliosis etiology, 383
energetics, 67–69
    data presentation, *68*
energy expenditure analysis *see* energetics
environment
    mobility issues, *124*
    neurobiological effects, 92–93
    see also environmental enrichment
environmental enrichment
    synapse formation and dentritic tree development, 80, 92–93
    use in cerebral palsy, 93, 95
epidemiology, 9–15
episolon aminocaproic acid (Amicar), 395
equilibrium reactions
    analysis, *65,* 65–67, *66, 67*
    assessment, 8, 26–27, *27,* 48

balance training, 158–159
Bobath therapy, 155
deficient, scoliosis etiology, 382
walking prognosis, 102, *102*
equinovarus deformities, 244–245
equinus deformities
    Achilles tendon lengthening, 235, 316
    ankle, 111
    biofeedback devices, 179
    bridle procedure, 245
    forefoot, 42, *43*
    gastrocnemius-soleus lengthening, 316
    in hemidystonia, 238
    kinematics, 315–316
    orthotics, 176
    plaster immobilization, 110, 163–165, 235, 236, 316–317
    spastic diplegia, 266, 314–317
    surgical management, 229–238, 316–317
        postoperative calcaneus deformity, 235, 237–238, 317
        postoperative immobilization, 235, 316–317
esotropia, 32
ethical issues, 16
etiology, *6,* 9–15, *10*
    post-natal acquisition, 14
    prenatal, 9–12, *10*
    preterm birth-related, 12–14
evolution, brain, 94
examination *see* assessment
excess death rate (EDR), 104
exercise, 157–158
exotropia, 32
extensor pollicus longus tendon, rerouting/reinforcement procedure, 223, *223*
extensor thrust, 140
    assessment, 25, *25*
    walking prognosis, 98
external tibial-fibular torsion, 114, *115*
Eye-gaze E-tran Communication Board, *180,* 180–181
eye reflex responses, 32

facial muscles, function assessment, 32
familial cerebral palsy, incidence, 12
family issues, 160, 190–192
Fasano technique, posterior rootlet rhizotomy, 128
fasciotomy, Yount–Ober, 168
feeding devices, *188,* 188–189
feet *see* foot
Feldenkrais method, 166
femoral anteversion, 113, *114*
    excessive in spastic diplegia, *290,* 290–294, *291, 292*
femoral head and neck resection, 375–377, *376, 377*
femoral neck-shaft angles, 114, *114*
femoral osteotomy, 362–365
    complications, 363–364
        heterotopic ossification of hip *see* heterotopic ossification of hip
    derotation *see* derotation femoral osteotomy
    fixation devices, 363
    supracondylar closed wedge extension, 311
    total body involved patients, *362,* 362–364
femoral physeal stapling, knee-flexion deformity, 310–311
Ferguson's angle, 115
fetal alcohol syndrome, 11
fetal electronic monitoring, 12–14, 16
financial issues, 120
fine motor function
    prognosis, 102–103
    skills, *52,* 103

416